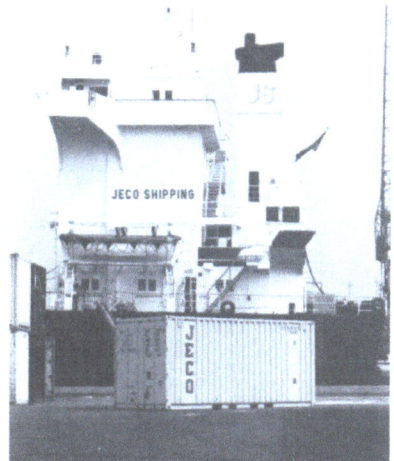
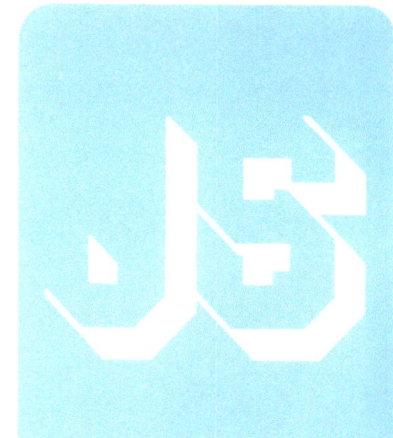
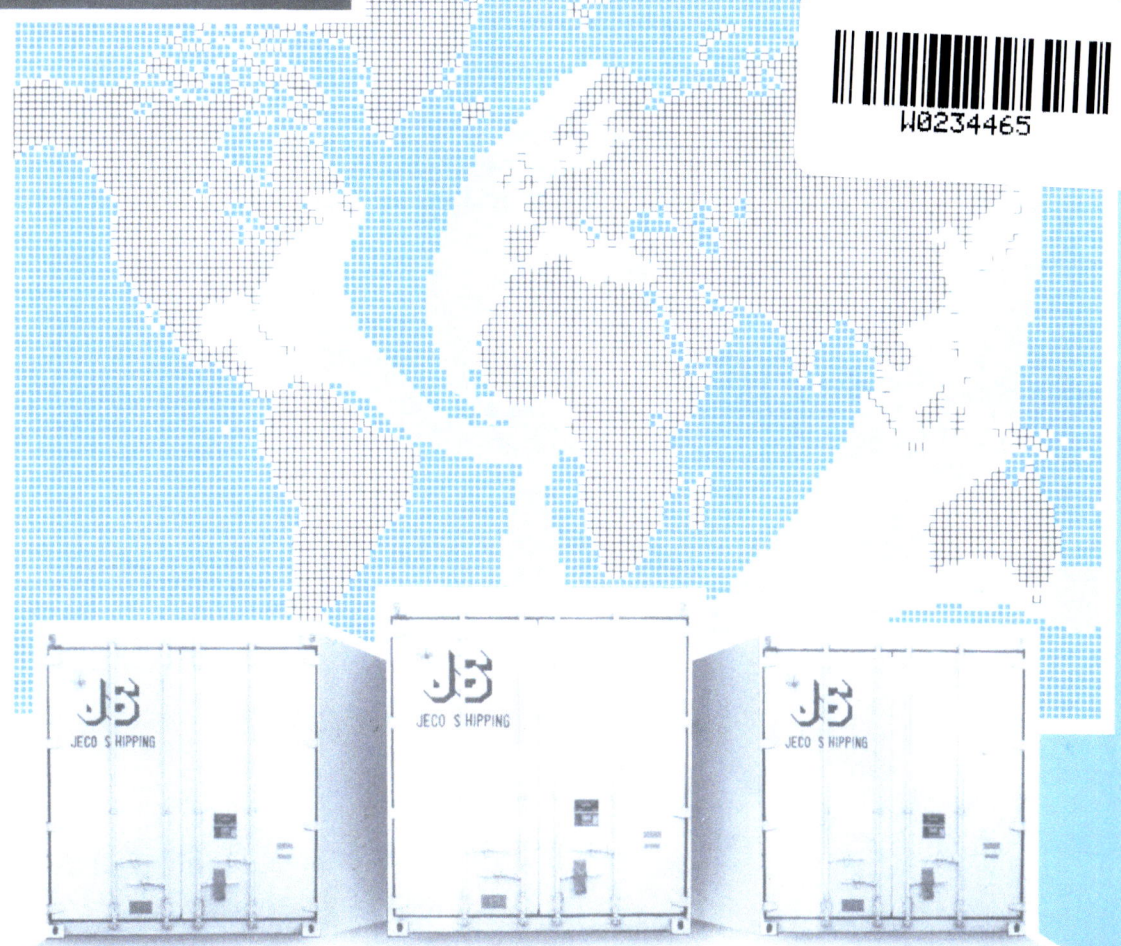

Major Companies
of
Nigeria
1983

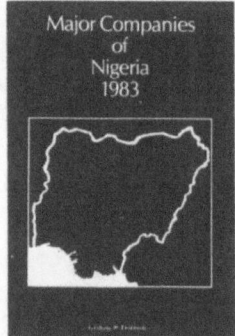
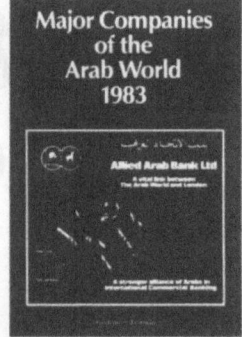
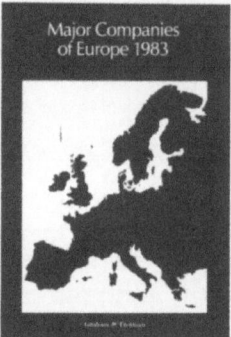
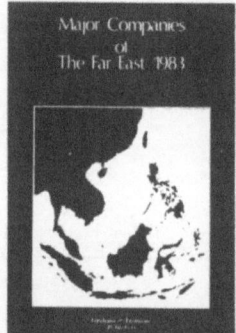
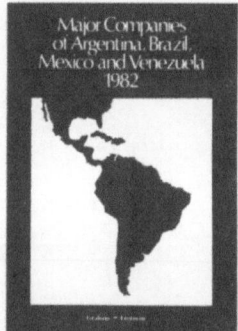

Major Companies
of
Nigeria
1983

Edited by Jennifer Carr

WKAP ARCHIEF

Published by
Graham & Trotman

Sterling House, 66 Wilton Road, London SW1V 1DE
United Kingdom
Telephone: 01-821 1123   Telex: 298878 Gramco G   Cable: Infobooks London

Fourth Edition published in 1983 by
Graham & Trotman Limited
Sterling House, 66 Wilton Road,
London SW1V 1DE, United Kingdom

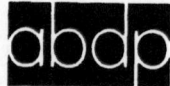

Graham & Trotman Ltd is a member of the
Association of British Directory Publishers

© 1983 Graham & Trotman Limited
Softcover reprint of the hardcover 1st edition 1983

British Library Cataloguing in Publication Data

Major companies of Nigeria — 1983
  1. Corporations — Nigeria — Directories
  338.7' 4' 025669   HD2921

UK ISBN: ISBN-13: 978-94-009-6648-2   e-ISBN-13: 978-94-009-6646-8
       DOI: 10.1007/978-94-009-6646-8

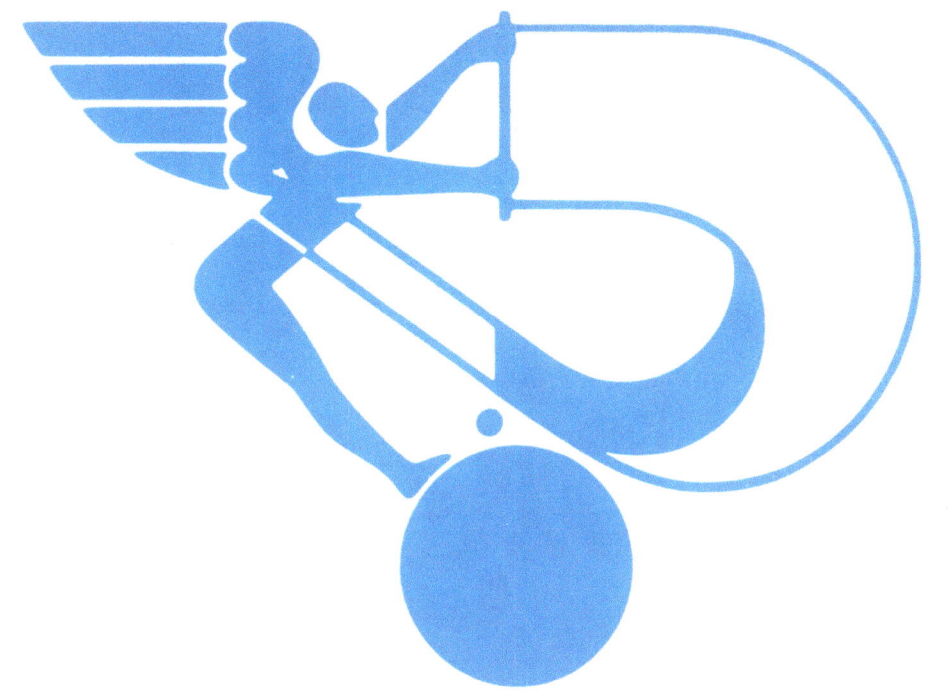

PANALPINA

5 Continents — 1 Forwarder

PANALPINA WORLD TRANSPORT NIGERIA LIMITED

Head Office

APAPA
4, Creek Road,
Tel: 803440-4
    803610-4
Telex: 21347
P. O. Box 69

Postal Address
P. M. B. 12651, Lagos.

Branches

CALABAR
45, Bedwell Street,
P. M. B. 1109,
Tel: 222590

IKEJA-AIRFREIGHT
Tel: 962026, 961690, 932728
P. O. Box 84

KADUNA
18/19, Ahmadu Bello Way
Tel: 212119 P.O. Box 158
Telex: apanika 71109

KANO
59, Tafawa Balewa Road,
Tel: 2572, 5219
P. O. Box 788

PORT-HARCOURT
6, Industry Road,
Tel: (084) 330292
P. O. Box 170
Telex: Panaphng 61106

SAPELE
1, Cemetry Road,
P. O. Box 451

WARRI
Warri/Sapele Road,
Tel: 233818
P. O. Box 135

Telegraphic Address all Branches "PANALPINA"

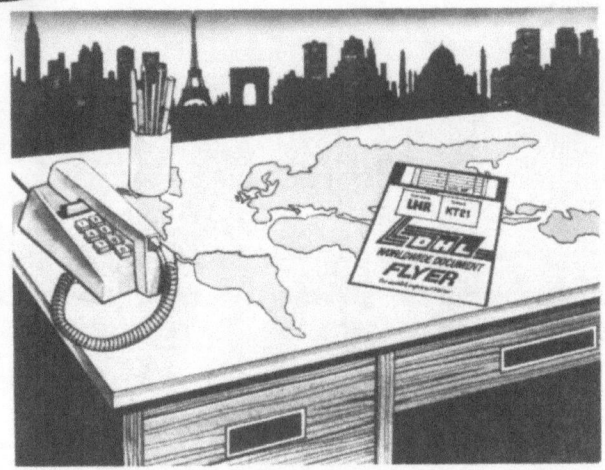
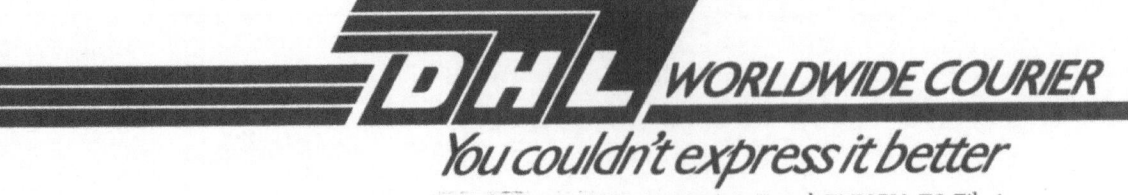

Contents

Introduction   xi

Usage of the index   xii

Advertisers Index   358

MAJOR COMPANIES OF NIGERIA   1

Alphabetical index   326

Index to Business Activities   336

Index Guide to Business Activities

Accountants & lawyers	336	Leisure goods	348
Agents and general trading companies	336	Livestock and animal feeds	348
Agricultural equipment and services	337	Mechanical engineering	348
Agricultural produce	337	Metals, metal processing and	
Air conditioning, heating and		fabrication	348
refrigeration	337	Mining, mineral processing and	
Architecture and town planning	338	quarrying	349
Banks, finance and investment		Motorcycles and bicycles	350
companies	338	Motor vehicles and components	349
Brewing, soft drinks and wine	338	Office equipment/supplies	350
Building materials/cement	338	Oil and gas exploration and production	350
Carpets	339	Oil and gas services and equipment	
Ceramics/sanitary fittings	340	and pipeline contractors	350
Chain stores	340	Oil refining	351
Chemicals	340	Optical and photographic equipment	351
Civil engineering and construction	340	Packaging	351
Commercial and industrial institutes		Paint	351
and associations	342	Paper/paper products	351
Computers	342	Petrochemicals	352
Construction plant	342	Pharmaceutical and medical supplies	
Consultants (business)	342	and services	352
Consultants (engineering)	343	Plant hire	352
Defence and armaments	343	Plastics/plastic products	352
Educational equipment and training		Power equipment	353
services	343	Precision engineering	353
Electrical and electronic equipment	344	Printing	353
Electrical engineering	344	Property or real estate	353
Fertilisers	344	Publishing, broadcasting, films and	
Fishing and fish processing	344	advertising	353
Food and food processing	344	Rubber/rubber goods	354
Freight forwarding and customs agents	345	Safety and security equipment	354
Furniture	345	Scientific instruments	354
Glass and Glass products	346	Shipping, shipbuilding and shipping	
Government bodies	346	services	354
Handicrafts, pottery and jewellery	346	Telecommunications	355
Hardware	346	Textiles and clothing/textile equipment	355
Hotels and catering	346	Timber industries/saw mills	355
Household goods/appliances	346	Tobacco	356
Industrial equipment and heavy machinery	347	Toiletries and cosmetics	356
Insurance/reinsurance	347	Transport	356
Irrigation services/equipment	348	Travel and tourism	356
Leather and shoes	348	Utilities and public services	356

Introduction & Acknowledgements

Over the past two decades rapid development has meant that Nigeria plays an increasingly important role as a major industrial centre among Third World Countries.

Despite the recent economic restraints in Nigeria, the wealth of the country's natural resources and its size guarantee its future as an expanding economy. The publishers remain confident that MAJOR COMPANIES OF NIGERIA contains more information on the major industrial and commercial companies than any other work. The information in the book was submitted mostly by the companies themselves, completely free of any charge.

To all those companies which assisted us in our research operation we express grateful thanks. To all those individuals who also gave us help we are similarly very grateful.

Details of a few very new companies have been included because of their potential significance, although they may not yet be trading actively. Certain companies have been included which, although they may not be very large, are nonetheless important to firms wishing to import and export; shipping agents are an example.

Whilst the publishers have made every effort to ensure that the information in this book was correct at the time of going to press no responsibility or liability can be accepted for any errors or omissions.

About Graham & Trotman Limited

Graham & Trotman Limited, is an independent British publishing company concentrating on the research and publishing of business and technical information for industry and commerce in many parts of the world. The company also runs seminars and conferences for businessmen.

Whilst maintaining and regularly updating a large archive of information on companies, business conditions and markets in Nigeria, the Arab World, South and Central America, the Far East, and Europe, Graham & Trotman also publish books on business management, finance, energy technology, business law, pollution control and several other subjects of international interest.

Graham & Trotman have over 300 publications in print which variously are sold in over 130 countries.

Readers are welcome to write, telephone or telex for a free copy of our complete catalogue of publications.

Usage of the Index

This book has been arranged to allow the reader to locate the company entries easily.

The companies are listed alphabetically allowing any particular company to be located quickly. As for many readers English may be a second or third language the alphabetical ordering used is a strict one and arranged according to international library practice, where each word is considered in turn.

For example:
ADE Engineering appears before
ADE Mechanical Engineering
but after ADE Civil Engineering

At the back of the book there follows an Alphabetical Index and a Business Activity Index. The latter breaks down Nigerian companies into fundamental activities. Under each of these fundamental activities are given the names of the companies practising that activity.

The fundamental business activities under which the companies may be found are as follows:

INDEX CATEGORIES

1   Accountants and lawyers
2   Agents and general trading companies
3   Agricultural equipment and services
4   Agricultural produce
5   Air conditioning, heating and refrigeration
6   Architecture and town planning
7   Banks, finance and investment companies
8   Brewing, soft drinks and wine
9   Building materials/cement
10 Carpets
11 Ceramics/sanitary fittings
12 Chain stores
13 Chemicals
14 Civil engineering and construction
15 Commercial and industrial institutes and associations
16 Computers
17 Construction plant
18 Consultants (business)
19 Consultants (engineering)
20 Defence and armaments
21 Educational equipment and training services
22 Electrical and electronic equipment
23 Electrical engineering
24 Fertilisers
25 Fishing and fish processing
26 Food and food processing
27 Freight forwarding and customs agents
28 Furniture
29 Glass
30 Government bodies
31 Handicrafts, pottery and jewellery
32 Hardware
33 Hotels and catering
34 Household goods/appliances
35 Industrial equipment and heavy machinery
36 Insurance/reinsurance
37 Irrigation services/equipment
38 Leather and shoes
39 Leisure goods
40 Livestock and animal feeds
41 Mechanical engineering
42 Metals, metal processing and fabrication
43 Mining, mineral processing and quarrying
44 Motorcycles and bicycles
45 Motor vehicles and components
46 Office equipment/supplies
47 Oil and gas exploration and production
48 Oil and gas services and equipment and pipeline contractors
49 Oil refining
50 Optical and photographic equipment
51 Packaging
52 Paint
53 Paper/paper products
54 Petrochemicals
55 Pharmaceuticals and medical supplies and services
56 Plant hire
57 Plastics/plastic products
58 Power equipment
59 Precision engineering
60 Printing
61 Property or real estate
62 Publishing, broadcasting, films and advertising
63 Rubber/rubber goods
64 Safety and security equipment
65 Scientific instruments
66 Shipping, shipbuilding and shipping services
67 Telecommunications
68 Textiles and clothing/textile equipment
69 Timber industries/saw mills
70 Tobacco
71 Toiletries and cosmetics
72 Transport
73 Travel and tourism
74 Utilities and public services

INDEX DES GROUPES D'ACTIVITE ECONOMIQUE

1 Conseils financiers et juridiques
2 Représentants, négociants, exportateurs et importateurs
3 Matériel et travaux agricoles
4 Produits agricoles
5 Appareils et matériel de conditionnement d'air, de chauffage et de réfrigeration
6 Architecture et urbanisme
7 Etablissements bancaires et financiers
8 Bières, vins et boissons non-alcoolisées
9 Matériaux de construction
10 Tapis et tapisserie
11 Céramique
12 Grands magasins
13 Produits chimiques
14 Bâtiments, travaux publics et génie civil
15 Etablissements publics et associations commerciales
16 Ordinateurs
17 Equipements et matériel de travaux publics
18 Conseils en affaires du commerce
19 Ingénieurs-conseils
20 Défense et armement
21 Matériel et centres d'éducation
22 Matériel électrique et électronique
23 Constructions électriques
24 Engrais divers
25 Pêche et poissonneries
26 Industrie alimentaire et produits comestibles
27 Fréteurs-expéditeurs et agences en douane
28 Meubles
29 Verrerie
30 Ministères
31 Artisanat, poteries et bijoux
32 Quincaillerie
33 Services hôteliers et restauration
34 Articles ménagers
35 Matériel et équipement industriel
36 Assurances
37 Installation et matériel d'irrigation
38 Maroquinerie
39 Articles et matériel de sport et loisir
40 Bétail et aliments pour animaux
41 Construction mécaniques
42 Métaux, aciers et constructions métalliques
43 Mines et carrières
44 Cycles et motocyclettes
45 Véhicules automobiles et pièces détachées
46 Matériel de bureau
47 Exploration et production du pétrole et du gaz
48 Equipement, services, marketing et transport du pétrole et du gaz
49 Raffinage du pétrole
50 Appareils et matériels photographiques et scientifiques et instruments d'optique
51 Emballage
52 Peintures et vernis
53 Papier
54 Pétrochimie
55 Produits pharmaceutiques et matériel médical
56 Location d'équipements et de matériel
57 Matières plastiques
58 Groupe générateur
59 Instrument de précision
60 Impressions et imprimeurs
61 Biens immeubles et terrains
62 Edition, radiodiffusion et publicité
63 Caoutchouc
64 Matériel et équipement de sécurité
65 Instrument scientifiques
66 Navigation, agences maritimes, constructions et réparations navales
67 Télécommunications
68 Textiles et confection
69 Bois
70 Tabac
71 Produits de toilette et d'entretien
72 Transport
73 Agences de voyage et tourisme
74 Services publics

VERZEICHNIS DER INDUSTRIEGRUPPEN

1 Rechnungsprüfer und Anwälte
2 Vertretungen und allgemeine Handelsgesellschaften
3 Landwirtschaftliche Geräte und Dienste
4 Agrarerzeugnisse
5 Klimaanlagen, Heiz- und Kühlanlagen
6 Architektur und Städteplanung
7 Banken, Finanz- und Investitions- gesellschaften
8 Brauereiwesen, Erfrischungsgetränke, Weine und Nichtalkoholische Getränke
9 Baumaterialen
10 Teppiche
11 Keramik
12 Warenhäuser
13 Chemikalien
14 Bauingenieurwesen und Konstruktion
15 Kommerzielle und Industrielle Institute und Verbände
16 Computer
17 Baumaschinen
18 Beratungsunternehmen (geschäftlich)
19 Beratungsunternehmen (technisch)
20 Verteidigung und Bewaffnung
21 Geräte für das Schulwesen und Ausbildungsdienste
22 Elektro- und elektronische Geräte
23 Elektrotechnik
24 Düngemittel
25 Fischerei und Fischverarbeitung
26 Nahrungsmittel und Nahrungsmittelverarbeitung
27 Güterspedition und Zollagenten
28 Möbel
29 Glas
30 Regierungsbehörden
31 Kunsthandwerk, Töpferei- und Schmuckwaren
32 Eisenwaren
33 Hotelgewerbe und Gastronomie
34 Haushaltswaren
35 Industrieanlagen Ausrüstung
36 Versicherung und Rückversicherung
37 Bewässerungs-Service
38 Leder, Schuhe
39 Freizeitartikel und Sportgeräte
40 Vieh und Futtermittel
41 Maschinenbautechnik
42 Metalle, Metallver- und -bearbeitung
43 Bergbau, Mineralienverarbeitung und -gewinnung
44 Motorräder und Fahrräder
45 Motorfahrzeuge und -komponenten
46 Büroausstattung
47 Öl- und Gas-Exploration und Produktion
48 Öl- und Gas Dienste Auftragnehmer für Anlagen und Pipelines
49 Öl-Raffinerie
50 Geräte für Optik und Fotografie
51 Verpackung
52 Farben
53 Papier
54 Erdölderivate
55 Lieferung und Dienstleistungen betreffs pharmazeutischer Artikel und Arzneimittel
56 Leasing von Anlagen
57 Kunststoffe
58 Energieerzeugungsanlagen
59 Feinmechanik
60 Drückereiwesen
61 Immobilien
62 Verlagswesen, Rundfunkübertragung, Filmproduktion und Werbung
63 Gummi
64 Sicherheits ausrüstung
65 Wissenschaftliche Instrumente
66 Schiffahrt, Schiffsbau und Frachtdienste
67 Femmeldewesen
68 Textilien und Bekleidung
69 Nutzholzindustrie
70 Tabakwaren
71 Toilettenartikel und Kosmetika
72 Transport
73 Reisen und Touristik
74 Versorgungsbetriebe und öffentliche Dienste

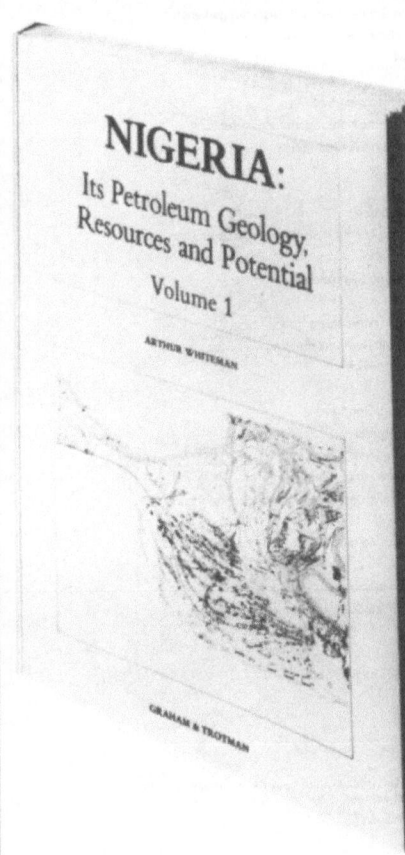

Major Companies
of
Nigeria
1983

158 BARESEL LTD

34 Okesuna St, PO Box 785, Lagos
Tel: 631388

Chairman: O A Braithwaite
Directors: L Spaeth (Vice-Chairman),
  B A Braithwaite,
  Dr G S Braithwaite,
  Mrs L I Imevbore,
  E Fink
Senior Executives: R Weber (Managing Director),
  P O Ajumobi (Personnel Manager),
  L B A Martins (Internal-Auditor),
  K Olorunyomi (Purchasing Manager),
  Tunde Thompson (Public Relations Officer),
  G O Lisboa (Chief Accountant)
PRINCIPAL ACTIVITIES: Civil engineering and construction;
  specialists in infrastructural work
Branch Offices: Savannah Bank of Nigeria Ltd; Standard Bank of
  Nigeria Ltd
Financial Information:
Paid-up capital   ₦ 500,000

Principal Shareholders: O A Braithwaite; Mrs (Dr) G S
  Braithwaite; Mrs L Imevbore; L Spaeth
No of Employees: 473

A A BALOGUN & SONS (NIGERIA) LTD

See BALOGUN, A A, & SONS (NIGERIA) LTD

A B CHAMI & CO LTD

See CHAMI, A B, & CO LTD

A C CHRISTLIEB (NIGERIA) LTD

See CHRISTLIEB, A C, (NIGERIA) LTD

A C E JIMONA LTD

See JIMONA, A C E, LTD

A D GREEN & CO LTD

See GREEN, A D, & CO LTD

A EKERETE LTD

See EKERETE, A, LTD

A G LEVENTIS & COMPANY (NIGERIA) LTD

Iddo House, PO Box 159, Lagos
Tel: 800220/9

Chairman: Alhaji Nuhu Bamalli
Directors: C Leventis, A P Leventis, G E Keralakis, A A David,
  H S A Adedeji, Chief S Ade John, Chief F Edo-Osagie, Alhaji
  Inuwa Usman, Alhaji Isa Abubakar
Senior Executives: J S Robinson (General Manager),
  J E Iriabe (Company Secretary)
PRINCIPAL ACTIVITIES: Co-ordination of operational activities
  of the Leventis Group of Companies and provision of
  business and residential accommodation, management,
  financial and other specialised services. Substantial
  investments in African Insurance Company Ltd; J & P
  (Nigeria) Ltd; Continental Breweries Ltd; Eastern Breweries
  Ltd; Valley Foods (Nigeria) Ltd
Branch Offices: PO Box 41, Ibadan; PO Box 32, Kano; PO Box
  180, Maiduguri; PO Box 210, Kaduna; PO Box 360, Port
  Harcourt
Associated Companies: Leventis Motors Ltd; Leventis Stores
  Ltd; Leventis Technical Ltd; Nigerian Bottling Company Ltd;
  Victoria Beach Hotel Ltd (Mainland Hotel); Continental
  Breweries Ltd; Honda Manufacturing (Nigeria) Ltd; J & P
  (Nigeria) Ltd; Carpet Royal Nigeria Ltd; Valley Foods (Nigeria)
  Ltd; Crown Products Ltd; London Africa & Overseas Ltd;
  Apapa Chemical Industries Ltd; Guinea Construction Co Ltd;
  Iddo Investments Ltd
Principal Bankers: Union Bank of Nigeria Ltd; First Bank of
  Nigeria Ltd; Savannah Bank of Nigeria Ltd

Financial Information:

	₦'000
	1981
Authorised capital	6,000
Paid-up capital	6,000
Turnover	10,166
Profits (after tax)	2,232

Date of Establishment: 24th March 1958

A G S BARMA LTD

See BARMA, A G S, LTD

A H ROBINS INTERNATIONAL COMPANY LTD

See ROBINS, A H, INTERNATIONAL COMPANY LTD

A I CHIAKWELU & BROTHERS

See CHIAKWELU, A I, & BROTHERS

A J MISSRI & CO LTD

See MISSRI, A J, & CO LTD

A J SEWARD (A DIVISION OF UAC OF NIGERIA LTD)

See SEWARD, A J, (A DIVISION OF UAC OF NIGERIA LTD)

A M FALTAS (WEST AFRICA) LTD

See FALTAS, A M, (WEST AFRICA) LTD

A MICHELETTI

See MICHELETTI, A

A O ADESANYA NIGERIA LTD

See ADESANYA, A O, NIGERIA LTD

A O KARUNWI LTD

See KARUNWI, A O, LTD

A O UCHE & SONS (NIGERIA) LTD

See UCHE, A O, & SONS (NIGERIA) LTD

A ONIBUDO & COMPANY LTD

See ONIBUDO, A, & COMPANY LTD

A OTT-ATTAFUA & COMPANY LTD

See OTT-ATTAFUA, A, & COMPANY LTD

A SAVOIA

See SAVOIA, A

A W CROSS LTD

See CROSS, A W, LTD

A W IBE & CO LTD

See IBE, A W, & CO LTD

ABA TEXTILES MILLS LTD

PMB 1125, Aba, Imo State
Tel: 441/2

PRINCIPAL ACTIVITIES: Textile manufacturers

ABAYOMI, OLUFAWO, & PARTNERS

742 Oyo Rd, Opposite Coca Cola Factory, PO Box 2000, Ibadan,
  Oyo State
Tel: 461375 Ibadan, 861222 Lagos
Cable: Olueng
Telex: 31119 Olueng Ng

PRINCIPAL ACTIVITIES: Engineering consultants
Branch Offices: Owo, Ondo State

ABBAS ORGANISATION NIGERIA LTD

26 Itire Rd, Surulere, Near Randle Avenue, Lagos
Tel: 830680, 830705, 848265

PRINCIPAL ACTIVITIES: Estate agents, surveyors, valuers

Date of Establishment: 1975

ABBEY GROUP OF INSURANCE BROKERS, LIFE & PENSIONS CONSULTANTS

4 Igbore St, Onike, Yaba, PO Box 2548, Lagos
Tel: 863823
Cable: Abbeyinsure

Chairman: N A Adeniji
Directors: N A Adeniji, Alex Ojei
Senior Executives: N A Adeniji (Managing Director/Chief
    Consultant),
    Alex Ojei (Executive Director/Senior Consultant),
    E O Omirin (Assistant Senior Manager/Consultant)

PRINCIPAL ACTIVITIES: Insurance consultancy and broking
Branch Offices: 22 Ahmadu Bello Way, Kaduna E9/799 Army
    Barracks, Iwo Rd, Ibadan
Subsidiary/Associated Companies: Abbey Life & Pensions
    Consultants Company; Abbey Nat & Company (Insurance
    Brokers)
Principal Bankers: Union Bank of Nigeria
Financial Information:

	N'000
Authorised capital	100
Paid-up capital	100

Principal Shareholders: Directors as described above
Date of Establishment: 1978
No of Employees: 40

ABBOTT LABORATORIES NIGERIA LTD

Ayefunke House, 3 Olusoji Idowu Street, Ilupeju, PO Box 1427,
Lagos
Tel: 960788, 960789, 960763
Cable: Abbottlab Lagos
Telex: 26135 Abbott NG

Directors: Chief Dr M A Majekodunmi,
    D Dankaro,
    C U Efobi,
    Alhaji M S Kantagora,
    D W Ortlieb,
    A M Ferguson (Alternate),
    R H Morehead,
    D R Lambert (Alternate),
    N Pataky (Managing)

PRINCIPAL ACTIVITIES: Pharmaceuticals and medical supplies

ABDUL AZEEZ ELECTRICAL CENTRE

10/3 Bauchi Rd, PO Box 782, Jos, Plateau State
Tel: 55814, 55920

Chairman: Alhaji Abdul Azeez A Badamasi

PRINCIPAL ACTIVITIES: Wholesalers/retailers of electrical
    fittings and accessories, appliances, radios, televisions, stero
    equipment, refrigerators
Principal Agencies: EMS Nigeria Ltd; Abayomi Stores Ltd; PZ
    Technical Nigeria Ltd; Associated Electronic Products
    (Nigeria) Ltd
Principal Bankers: First Bank of Nigeria Ltd

Date of Establishment: 1967

ABDULLAI GROUP OF COMPANIES NIGERIA LTD

10 Abbey Rd, Off Bode Thomas Street, Igbobi, Lagos
Tel: 962839
Cable: Abdulgroup
Telex: 20202 TDS
Answerback: Box 078

President: Alhaji L O B Abdullai
Directors: R U Depoorter,
    A A Abdullai,
    J O Kanu (Managing),
    G A Van-Sacker
Senior Executives: K Olukoga (Chief Accountant),
    A O Salako (Commercial Manager),
    E O Odubajo (Operations Manager),
    G A Williams (Public Relations Officer)

PRINCIPAL ACTIVITIES: Manufacture of zinc ingots and
    remelted lead. Buyers of non ferrous scrap metal,
    pharmacists; distributors of metals and foundry equipment
Principal Agencies: Afribelgie Foreign Trade Enterprise, Belgium;
    Mac Corporation, USA; Bender Metalle Work, Germany
Branch Offices: Kano; Port Harcourt; Ibadan; Kaduna; Warri;
    Onitsha
Principal Bankers: Societe General de Banque; Wema Bank Ltd;
    National Bank of Nigeria
Financial Information:

	N'000
Authorised capital	1,000
Paid-up capital	600
Turnover	5,000
Profits	302

Date of Establishment: 26th February 1952
No of Employees: 650

ABEBIYI SONAIKE & COMPANY

127/129 Obafemi Awolowo Way, PO Box 3897, Ikeja, Lagos
Tel: 661598, 932313
Cable: Ascoval, Lagos
Telex: 26975

Chairman: Charles Olumide Adebiyi
Directors: Olayinka Adekunle Sonaike
Senior Executives: M Kolawole Diya (Estate Surveyor),
    G Fatimilehin (Estate Surveyor),
    John E Nwadigbo (Estate Surveyor),
    O T Oloniyo (Estate Surveyor)

PRINCIPAL ACTIVITIES: Property management, investment,
    finance and development consultancy, project management,
    valuations, residential and industrial and commercial property
    agency, rating, plant and machinery valuations, land use,
    planning, project analysis
Branch Offices: (City Office) 27/29, Martins Street, PO Box 6879,
    Lagos; 3, Oke Ilewo Street, Ibara, PO Box 1826, Abeokuta;
    55, France Rd, Off Airport Rd, PO Box 5195, Kano
Principal Bankers: United Bank for Africa Ltd; Savannah Bank of
    Nigeria Ltd
Principal Shareholders: Charles Olumide Abebiyi; Olayinka
    Adekunle Sonike
Date of Establishment: 23rd July 1979
No of Employees: 31

ABEREOJE (NIGERIA) LTD

139 Iremo Rd, Ile-Ife, PO Box 229, Oyo State

Chairman: J O Awofisayo
Directors: Mrs Olabisi Bamigbola, Engineer Tunde Awofisayo
Senior Executives: Engineer M A Aboke (Project Engineer),
    Gbenga Akinwale (Accounting/Administrative Manager)

PRINCIPAL ACTIVITIES: Building and civil engineering, mining
    and quarrying, geological consultants, timber contractors and
    sawmill industry
Branch Offices: 70 Idikan St, Ibadan, Oyo State
Associated Companies: Geo-Rock Associates, Nigeria
Principal Bankers: National Bank of Nigeria Ltd
Financial Information:

	N'000
Authorised capital	100
Paid-up capital	100

Date of Establishment: July 1977

ABODERIN & GLAHÉ NIGERIA LTD
208-210 Broad Street, Lagos
Tel: 661432, 661435
Telex: 21817
PRINCIPAL ACTIVITIES: Trade fair consultants

ABUKON NIGERIA LTD
12A Ikorodu Rd, Jibowu, PO Box 217, Ebute-Metta, Lagos State

Tel: 860647
Cable: Abukon Lagos
Telex: 26342 Abukon NG

Chairman: Chief A O Abudu
Directors: Chief O A Akoni,
 E A Awobokun,
 Dr A Adeoba,
 S B Akande,
 M A Abudu (Managing)
Senior Executives: S Bose (Marketing Dev. Manager),
 M A Faniyi (Product Manager),
 L A Adelowo (Production Manager),
 I F Dada (Area Manager)
PRINCIPAL ACTIVITIES: Marketing of food and drinks
Principal Agencies: West Africa Milk Co; Tate & Lyle; West
 African Breweries; F F Scott, UK; Nutrexpa, Spain;
 Ramazzorri, Italy; Brooke Bond; CCF WG Leeuwaden, Holland
Branch Offices: Ibadan, Oyo State; Benin, Bendel State;
 Abeokuta, Ogun State
Principal Bankers: The First Bank of Nigeria Ltd
Financial Information:

	₦'000
Authorised capital	1,000
Paid-up capital	771
Turnover	1,500

Principal Shareholders: Olabopo Investment Co Ltd
Date of Establishment: January 1975
No of Employees: 80

ACADEMY PRESS LTD
Plot D Ilupeju Industrial Estate, Ilupeju, PO Box 3445, Lagos
Tel: 964555, 964556
Cable: Acadpress

Chairman: B A Idris-Animashawun
Directors: O I Akinkugbe, J I Omoniyi, A L Mabogurije, L
 Duval, R Gamble
PRINCIPAL ACTIVITIES: Production of promotional materials,
 calendars, leaflets, publishers of textbooks and magazines
Principal Bankers: Union Bank of Nigeria Ltd

Date of Establishment: 28th July 1964
No of Employees: 500

ACE BUILDERS & BUILDING MATERIAL STOCKISTS (THE)
70 Ayilara Street, Surulere, Lagos
Tel: 835588

PRINCIPAL ACTIVITIES: Builders and builders merchants
Branch Offices: 5 Lakanmi Close, Oritameta, PO Box 1513,
 Ibadan, Tel 411232

ACE METAL CONSTRUCTION (NIGERIA) LTD
Katchia Rd, Kaduna South, PO Box 4009, Kaduna
PRINCIPAL ACTIVITIES: Construction engineers; manufacturers
 of steel
Date of Establishment: 1972

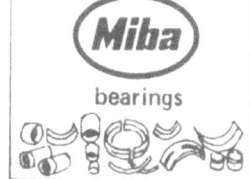
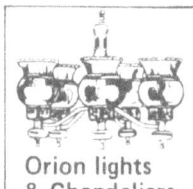
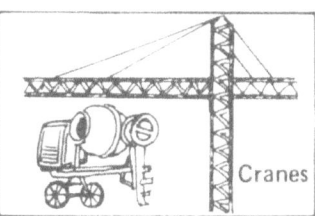
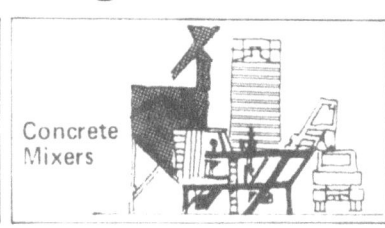
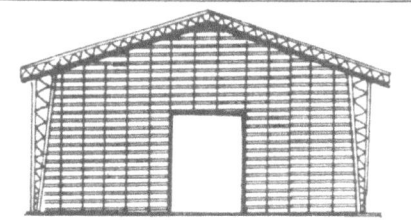
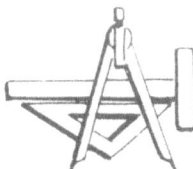

ACIM

17 Commercial Rd, Apapa, Lagos
Tel: 875413, 874985
Cable: Bewac Lagos
Telex: 21244 Lagos

PRINCIPAL ACTIVITIES: Distributors of agricultural and industrial machinery

Principal Shareholders: Division of Bewac

ACM OF NIGERIA LTD

PMB 5077, Port Harcourt, Rivers State
Tel: 21051

PRINCIPAL ACTIVITIES: Oilfield engineering specialists

ACME BUILDERS LTD

Plot 23 Block A, Acme Rd, PO Box 3130, Ikeja, Lagos
Tel: 962701

Chairman: S I Lawal (also Managing Director)
Directors: Mrs E O Lawal
Senior Executives: A B Harvey (General Manager),
  J O Titiloye (Finance Controller),
  B A Groves (Chief Quantity Surveyor/Planning Manager),
  M O Idowu (Administration Manager)

PRINCIPAL ACTIVITIES: Building and civil engineering contractors
Branch Offices: Lagos; Jos; Ibadan; Sapele
Associated Companies: Acme Furniture Ltd; Acme Steel Structures; City Flooring Ind Ltd; Diespeker Ceiling Nig Ltd; Light Machine Ind Ltd; Nippi Ltd
Principal Bankers: Barclays Bank (Nig) Ltd; Societe Generale Bank (Nig) Ltd
Financial Information:

	N'000
Authorised capital	400
Paid-up capital	400
Sales turnover	4,700
Profits	627

Principal Shareholders: S I Lawal; E O Lawal

ACROW LTD

PO Box 4722, Lagos

Directors: E O Emokpae (Director)

PRINCIPAL ACTIVITIES: Suppliers of construction equipment

ADAMU MANAGEMENT INTERNATIONAL

26 Tafawa Balewa Square Complex, PO Box 4195, Ikeja, Lagos
Tel: 681661
Cable: Adadamoko Lagos

Directors: Omokhogie Adamu (Managing)

PRINCIPAL ACTIVITIES: Agricultural equipment and services; agricultural produce; business consultants; office equipment and supplies; travel and tourism
Principal Agencies: Unel International Trading Co Inc
Associated Companies: Adamu Farms Ltd, Bendel State

Date of Establishment: 1981

ADARICE COMPANY LTD

Adani, Uzo Uwani, Anambra State

PRINCIPAL ACTIVITIES: Production of rice

ADDIS ENGINEERING LTD

Plot 9 Block H, Isolo, PO Box 2645, Laogs
Tel: 837953
Telex: 21052 Addis Ng

PRINCIPAL ACTIVITIES: Manufacturers of food processing machines; distribution and after sales service of carrier room air-conditioners and pullen pumps
Principal Agencies: Norman Industries Ltd; Pullen Pumps Ltd, Croydon, UK
Branch Offices: 217-235 Igbosere Rd, Lapal House, Lagos
Principal Bankers: United Bank for Africa Ltd

Date of Establishment: 1963
No of Employees: 100

ADEBOWALE ELECTRICAL INDUSTRIES LTD

5 Shipeolu St, Palm-Grove, Ikorodu Rd, PO Box 1905, Lagos
Tel: 861510, 861576
Cable: Adebstores Lagos
Telex: 21340 Adebo Ng

Chairman: Chief A B Adebowale (also Managing Director)
Directors: M A Kadri (Administrative Manager),
  Adekunle Adebowale,
  Adesoji Adebowale,
  Adewale Adebowale,
  Abiodun Adebowale,
  A S Odutola
Senior Executives: Olutola Oduntan (General Manager),
  Samuel Adebajo (Chief Accountant),
  Zaccheus Oyekunle (Deputy General Manager)

PRINCIPAL ACTIVITIES: Manufacture/importer of electronic/electrical, air conditioning, refrigeration, communication and audio/visual equipment, sets and units; power generating and water pumping engines; pepper and corn grinding engines; cassava grating engines, etc
Principal Agencies: Gibson International Corp, USA; Matsushita Seiko Co Ltd, Japan; Sharp Corporation, Japan; Fernseh and Rund Funk GmbH, West Germany; Industrie A Zanussi SpA, Italy; Delta Enfield Cables Ltd
Branch Offices: 2 Aruosa Sakpoba Rd, PMB 1238 Benin City, Tel 242738; 14 Fagge Takudu Rd, PO Box 905, Kano; SW8/596c Lagos Bye-Pass, Oke Ado, PO Box 53800, Ibadan; 100 Agbani Rd, Enugu, Tel 257585; A8 Junction Rd, Kaduna, Tel 212867, 212163; 61 Idumagbo Ave, Lagos, Tel 657415
Associated Companies: Debo Industries Ltd; Adebowale Stores Ltd
Principal Bankers: Union Bank of Nigeria Ltd; United Bank for Africa Ltd; Savannah Bank of Nigeria Ltd; Chase Merchant Bank Nigeria Ltd
Financial Information:

	N'000
Authorised capital	500
Paid-up capital	500
Sales turnover	27,000
Profits	3,500

Principal Shareholders: Chief Amuzat Beyloku Adebowale
Date of Establishment: 2nd April 1969
No of Employees: 640

ADECENTRO NIGERIA LTD

Samonda, Oyo Rd (Opposite Airport), Bodija, PMB 5549, Ibadan

Tel: 413818, 416729, 416966
Cable: Adecentro Ibadan
Telex: 31170 Univul Ng

Chairman: Chief Amos Olasupo Adegoke
Directors: A D S Odigie (Executive Director),
  J Ade Ojo (Administration Director),
  S Antezza (Purchasing Director),
  N Marfe (Technical Director)
Senior Executives: G A Sobanjo (Chief Accountant),
  J P Minchin (Project Manager),
  A A Olowu (Chief Quantity Surveyor),
  E O Ajibola (Site Manager)

PRINCIPAL ACTIVITIES: Building and civil engineering contractors
Principal Agencies: Government of Oyo State; Government of Ondo State; Institute of Agricultural Research & Training;

University of Ife; The Polytechnic Ibadan
Associated Companies: Universal Valcanizing Co Nig Ltd; Expocentro Nigeria Ltd
Principal Bankers: United Bank for Africa Ltd; Savannah Bank of Nigeria Ltd
Financial Information:

	₦'000
Authorised capital	675
Paid-up capital	675
Turnover	4,000
Profits	200

Principal Shareholders: Chief A O Adegoke (35%); A D S Odigie (5%); Italian shareholders (40%); Other Nigerians (20%)
Date of Establishment: 31st December, 1975
No of Employees: 550

ADEFUSIKA TRADING COMPANY LTD

PO Box 678, Reico House, 71 Apapa Rd, Ebute Metta, Lagos
Tel: 630493, 834215
Cable: Reico Lagos
Telex: 21161 Ng

Chairman: Chief E A Adefusika
Directors: G J P Bouwman, J D Moraal
Senior Executives: M A Alaka (Office Manager),
  G Umohakan (Marketing Manager, Building Materials),
  E Melah (Marketing Manager, Agricultural Div)

PRINCIPAL ACTIVITIES: Agents and general trading; suppliers of building materials, carpets, leisure goods, paint, agricultural equipment, timber
Principal Agencies: Forbo-Krommenie, Netherlands; Gilt Edge Carpets, UK; Briggs & Stratton, USA; Ingersoll Rand, USA; Mather & Platt Ltd, UK
Branch Offices: Aba; Onitsha; Benin; Kano; Kaduna
Associated Companies: Reiss & Co (Nigeria) Ltd; Reiss & Co NV, Netherlands
Principal Bankers: First Bank of Nigeria Ltd

Principal Shareholders: Chief E A Adefusika; Reiss & Co (Nigeria) Ltd
No of Employees: 220

ADEJOBI, ADEOYE, TRADING STORES LTD

SW8/129A, Lagos Bye Pass, PO Box 763, Ibadan, Oyo State
Tel: 413537
Cable: Adejobi
Telex: 31157 Adeoyeng

Chairman: Adeoye O Adejobi
Directors: Flora O Adejobi (Financial Director),
  Adeniyi O Adejobi (Technical Director),
  Adedayo O Adejobi,
  Adesina Adejobi
Senior Executives: Stanley Brown (General Manager/Managing Director),
  Tom Riley (Assistant General Manager/Works Director)

PRINCIPAL ACTIVITIES: Dealers in electrical goods and Electrical Contractors; manufacturers of refrigerators and freezers
Principal Agencies: Eaton Corp; (Samuel Moore Operations), USA; Trimurti Metals, India; Derby A/S, Denmark
Branch Offices: Plot No 1 Osibodu Layout, Olusoji Crescent, Oba Abimbola Rd, Felele Ibadan; 123 Lagos Bye Pass, Oke-Ado, Ibadan; 8 Odo-Ake Street, Ijebu-Igbo
Principal Bankers: National Bank of Nigeria Ltd
Financial Information:

	₦'000
Authorised capital	250
Paid-up capital	250
Turnover	2,900
Profits	87

Principal Shareholders: Adeoye Adejobi; Mrs F O Adejobi; Adeniyi O Adejobi; Adeday Adejobi; Adesina Adejobi
Date of Establishment: May 1976
No of Employees: 125

ADEJORO, S S, & COMPANY LTD

Greenwood Estate, Opebi Village, PMB 21184, Ikeja, Lagos
Tel: 964178, 962843, 963861
Telex: 26879 Sunny Ng

Chairman: S S Adejoro
Directors: Engr T O Ibikunle (Managing),
  G Ola Ramon (Financial Director),
  J A Adejoro (Project Director)
Senior Executives: J S K Atoo (Accounts/Administrative Manager),
  E A Ibikunle (Project Director)

PRINCIPAL ACTIVITIES: Civil engineering and construction
Branch Offices: Kojufoam Industries Ltd, Build Trust Industries Ltd
Principal Bankers: Savannah Bank; Societe Generale Bank (Nigeria) Ltd
Financial Information:

	₦'000
Authorised capital	500
Paid-up capital	400
Turnover	1,500
Profits	0.450

Principal Shareholders: S S Adejoro; T O Ibikunle; G O Ramon; J A Adejoro
Date of Establishment: 16th December 1974
No of Employees: 300

ADEJUMO FAM (NIGERIA) LTD

PO Box 2132, 6 Gab Jinadu St, Off Alhaji Adejumo Ave, Ilupeju Industrial Estate, Ilupeju, Lagos
Tel: 962395/6, 963057
Cable: Adefbros
Telex: 26107 Adefnl Ng

Chairman: Alhaji R A Adejumo (also Managing Director)
Directors: Alhaji T A Aderohunmu (General Manager Operations),
  G E Dotse (Deputy Managing Director),
  L A Adejumo (General Manager Administration),
  Alhaji L R Genty (Marketing),
  Alhaji Ibrahim Iro Kankara
Senior Executives: Alhaji R M Olushesi (Chief Accountant),
  E G D Agbanrin (Senior Accounts Superintendent),
  F O Aluko (Administrative Manager)

PRINCIPAL ACTIVITIES: General merchants: suppliers of industrial chemicals, agro-chemicals, water treatment chemicals, dyestuffs, industrial cleaning machines, pharmaceutical products and general goods
Principal Agencies: ICI; Basf, Hans Mehr, NV Leo de Winter, BV Frado; Dylon International; Bush Boake Allen; Mersey Lime Exporters; Helm; Borax Holdings Ltd; Appleford Ltd; Kermain Ltd; Friese Export-Import GmbH
Branch Offices: 15/17 Daddy Alaja St, Lagos; 3 Matori Rd, Mushin; SW8/945 Liberty Stadium Rd, Ibadan; 6 Airport Rd, Kano; Plots CA 30/31 Matazu Rd & Plot AM8 Abuja Rd, Kaduna
Associated Companies: Adephino Pharmaceutical & Chemicals (Nig) Ltd; Lagos Warehousing & Storage Company Ltd
Principal Bankers: United Bank for Africa Ltd; Nigeria - Arab Bank Ltd; International Bank for West Africa Ltd; Bank of Credit and Commerce Int (Nigeria) Ltd
Financial Information:

	₦'000
Authorised capital	5,000
Paid-up capital	5,000
Turnover	8,800
Profits (1982)	400

Principal Shareholders: Alhaji R A Adejumo; Alhaji T A Aderohumnu; L A Adejumo
Date of Establishment: 1952 (Registered) 1962 (Incorporated)
No of Employees: 250

ADEMOLA, THOMAS, & CO LTD
26 Abibu Oki St, Lagos
Tel: 637687

PRINCIPAL ACTIVITIES: Building and civil engineering
  contractors

ADEOLA BABAFUNKE OVERSEAS TRADING COMPANY
See BABAFUNKE, ADEOLA, OVERSEAS TRADING COMPANY

ADEOME COMPANY LTD
Plot 1108, Victoria Island, PO Box 2534, Lagos
Tel: 611952

PRINCIPAL ACTIVITIES: Suppliers of equipment for the timber
  industry

ADEOYE ADEJOBI TRADING STORES LTD
See ADEJOBI, ADEOYE, TRADING STORES LTD

ADESANYA, A O, NIGERIA LTD
Opposite Cement Factory, Shagamu/Lagos Rd, PO Box 371,
  Shagamu, Ogun State

PRINCIPAL ACTIVITIES: Animal feeds suppliers

ADETONA AWE (NIG) ENTERPRISES
6 Benue St, PO Box 532, Zaria, Kaduna State
Tel: 2368, 3275

Chairman: Sola Awe Akintokun
Directors: Adetona Awe
Senior Executives: Olusesam Awe, Rainu Ogumdipe

PRINCIPAL ACTIVITIES: Agents and general trading, suppliers
  of building materials, electronic equipment, pharmaceuticals
Principal Agencies: Akinlog & Partners
Branch Offices: BJ9 Ikoti St, Ilesha, Oyo State; PO Box 945,
  Ibadan
Principal Bankers: Kaduna Co-operative Bank

ADETUNJI, MADEBAYO, & SONS LTD
N5B/661 Idi-Ape, Iwo Rd, PO Box 3280, Ibadan, Oyo State
Tel: 461696
Cable: Adeplex
Telex: 31210 Main Ng

PRINCIPAL ACTIVITIES: General merchants, importers and
  exporters

ADETUNJI OLOKODANA & CO
Shop 211, Tawalin Bello St, Lagos
Tel: 633032
Telex: 21483 Dokebs Ng

PRINCIPAL ACTIVITIES: General trading

ADEWALE BELLO CONSTRUCTIONS LTD
1 North Station Rd, PO Box 421, Kaduna
Tel: 242540
Telex: 71169 Abccon

Chairman: S Ade-John
Directors: A Bello, Mrs E Bello

PRINCIPAL ACTIVITIES: Civil engineering
Branch Offices: 4 Ogunlowo St, Ikeja, Lagos
Principal Bankers: International Bank for West Africa Ltd
Financial Information:

	N'000
Authorised capital	240
Paid-up capital	240

Principal Shareholders: A Bello; Mrs E Bello; S Ade-John
No of Employees: 500

ADEYEMI COMMERCIAL SYNDICATE SAWMILLS LTD
17 Bola St, PO Box 180, Ebute-Metta, Lagos
Tel: 860610, 861847

Directors: Chief Adeshoja (Director)

PRINCIPAL ACTIVITIES: Distributors of woodworking machine
  tools
Principal Agencies: C D Monniger Ltd, UK

ADMARK (NIGERIA) LTD
15 Warehouse Rd, PO Box 1174, Apapa, Lagos
Tel: 877708, 871650, 875962
Cable: Chadmark, Lagos

Chairman: A S Marinho
Directors: R A M Ozuzu (Managing),
  Mrs E A Robbin,
  A Balogun
Senior Executives: May Nzeribe (Client Service Director),
  Jeff Mistri (Creative Director)

PRINCIPAL ACTIVITIES: Advertising and marketing
Principal Bankers: First Bank of Nigeria Ltd; International Bank
  for West Africa Ltd
Financial Information:

	N'000
Authorised capital	42
Paid-up capital	42

Principal Shareholders: Welan Enterprises Ltd; Akintunde A
  Marinho
Date of Establishment: 1961
No of Employees: 53

ADOBI ORGANISATION
17 Martin St, PO Box 4437, Lagos
Tel: 656366
Telex: 71127

PRINCIPAL ACTIVITIES: Consultants and general contractors

ADOKS ENGINEERING LTD
Block 811, Falomo Shopping Centre, Ikoyi, PO Box 4134, Lagos
  State

PRINCIPAL ACTIVITIES: Suppliers of aluminium and steel
  products; folding doors, security doors, etc

ADVANCE (NIG) LTD
70 Jebba St, Ebute Metta (East), Lagos
Tel: 830200
Cable: Advance Nigeria Ltd

Chairman: Tom C Onyeador
Directors: A Onyeador

PRINCIPAL ACTIVITIES: Suppliers of agricultural equipment,
  chemicals, irrigation equipment, municipal refuse vehicles and
  components, power equipment, toiletries and cosmetics
Branch Offices: 2 Station Ave, Aba
Subsidiary/Associated Companies: Kleen Services (Nig) Ltd,
  Lagos
Principal Bankers: United Bank for Africa Ltd
Financial Information:

	N'000
Authorised capital	100
Paid-up capital	60
Sales turnover	1,000

Principal Shareholders: Tom Onyeador
No of Employees: 150

AERO CONTRACTORS COMPANY OF NIGERIA LTD
PO Box 21090, 8-10 Broad St, Western House, Lagos
Tel: 961551
Cable: Aerocontra Lagos

Chairman: Chief M C Ibru
Directors: P Belgeonne (Managing Director),
  B A M Schreiner,
  N Schreiner,
  F O Ibru,
  A U Ibru,
  E M Ibru
Senior Executives: A Stewart (Technical Manager),
  A Ogunnaike (Head of Administration),
  S Van der Berg (Financial Controller),
  Captain H Koopman (Operations Manager)

PRINCIPAL ACTIVITIES: Aircharter company, oil industry
  aviation services
Branch Offices: Port Harcourt Airport; Warri Airport; PMB 3357,
  16a Dorawa Rd, Kano; Airbase at Murtala Muhammed
  Airport, Ikeja, PMB 1090, Lagos State, Tel 961340, 962570,
  961394
Principal Bankers: United Bank for Africa; International Merchant
  Bank Ltd

Principal Shareholders: Chief M C Ibru; Schreiner Airways BV
Date of Establishment: 1957
No of Employees: 400

AEROMARITIME (NIGERIA) LTD
Kirikiri Wharf, PMB 1193, Apapa, Lagos
Tel: 842152, 873634
Telex: 21556

Chairman: Victor I Odili
Directors: Alhaji Ibrahim Damcida,
  W D Douglass,
  Edugie Idumwonyi,
  W D Everett,
  Alhaji A B Umar,
  E F Pattillo (Managing)

PRINCIPAL ACTIVITIES: Stevedoring, lighterage, and marine
  services
Principal Agencies: Aeromaritime International Management
  Services; Aeromaritime Inc; Lignes Centrafricaines
Branch Offices: PMB 6016, Iwofe Jetty, Port Harcourt, Rivers
  State
Subsidiary Companies: Rhein-Mass - und See-Schiffahrtskontor
  GmbH; Baco Liner GmbH; Pan Atlantic Shipping and
  Transport Agencies Ltd
Financial Information:
Authorised capital   ₦ 1,000,000

Date of Establishment: 19th April 1979
No of Employees: 450

AERONUTRONIC FORD OVERSEAS SYSTEMS
3c Marine Rd, Apapa, Lagos
Tel: 876110

Directors: Chief Ayo Rosini (Director)

PRINCIPAL ACTIVITIES: Telecommunications and power

AFA GATEWAY CONSTRUCTION COMPANY LTD
SW9/6741 Ashanke Close, Challenge, PMB 5242, Ibadan, Oyo
  State

Chairman: A A F Ashanke

PRINCIPAL ACTIVITIES: Construction and civil engineering
Financial Information:
Registered capital   ₦ 200,000

Date of Establishment: July 1977

AFPRINT NIGERIA LTD
Isolo Industrial Estate, Oshodi/Isolo Express Rd, Mushin, PO
  Box 3623, Lagos
Tel: 842445, 843907/9
Cable: Afprint Lagos
Telex: 21394 Afprint Ng

Chairman: D K Chanrai
Directors: G K Chanrai (Managing Director),
  S Maruthi (Director/General Manager),
  M K Chanrai,
  P K Chanrai,
  Chief M N Ugochukwu,
  G O Senbanjo,
  S Nishizawa,
  T S Jones,
  Alhaji I M Damcida,
  Alhaji Sule Katagum,
  I A Tinubu (Personnel)
Senior Executives: S Y Nanal (Mill Manager),
  S A Ashibogun (Company Secretary/Administrative Manager),
  G Okuneye (Chief Accountant),
  P P Mehta (Mill Manager, Iganmu),
  R K Strivastava (Financial Controller)

PRINCIPAL ACTIVITIES: Manufacturers of textile piece goods,
  African prints; furnishings, sheets, etc
Branch Offices: Factory; Iganmu Industrial Estate, Abebe Village
  Rd, Iganmu, Lagos State
Principal Bankers: United Bank for Africa Ltd; Savannah Bank
  Nigeria Ltd; Union Bank of Nigeria Ltd
Financial Information:

	₦'000
Authorised capital	10,000
Paid-up capital	9,450
Turnover	36,564
Profits	1,772

Principal Shareholders: Kewalram Nominees Ltd; Nishizawa
  Nigeria Ltd; Commonwealth Development Corporation,
  Nigeria; Nigerian Industrial Development Bank Ltd
Date of Establishment: 11th December 1964
No of Employees: 3,500

AFRICAN ALLIANCE INSURANCE CO LTD
112 Broad Street, PO Box 2276, Lagos
Tel: 664300, 664373, 664398, 664419

Chairman: Chief S L Edu
Directors: T A Braithwaite,
  Prince Burchard,
  Chief S B Daniyan,
  M O Odele (Managing Director/Chief Executive)
Senior Executives: Ope Oredugba (General Manager),
  E O Olumide (Assistant General Manager),
  Y O Lanlehin (Financial Controller)

PRINCIPAL ACTIVITIES: Life assurance
Branch Offices: Throughout Nigeria
Subsidiary Companies: African Alliance Realty Co Ltd
Principal Bankers: Union Bank; International Bank for West
  Africa; United Bank for Africa; National Bank of Nigeria Ltd
Financial Information:

	₦'000
Authorised capital	500
Paid-up capital	500
Turnover	8,149

Principal Shareholders: Chief S L Edu; T A Braithwaite;
  Munchener Ruckversicherungs Gesselschaft; Prince Burchard;
  Mrs J A Okorodudu
Date of Establishment: 6th May 1960
No of Employees: 282

AFRICAN CONTINENTAL BANK LTD
148 Broad Street, PMB 2466, Lagos
Tel: 662629, 664091, 664163
Cable: Populihead Lagos
Telex: 21282

Chairman: Dr J O J Okezie
Directors: J J Nwobodo, B C Okwo, L D Molokwu, A A
  Uwanamodo, Chief J R Anyaehie, Chief J T S Faafa, J
  Atedoghu
Senior Executives: C N E Olieh (General Manager),
  M S C Nosegbe (Assistant General Manager, Finance),

AEROMARITIME

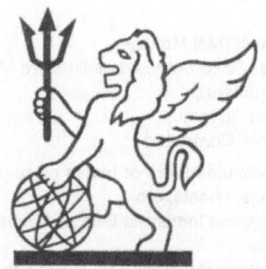

AEROMARITIME (NIGERIA) LIMITED

Aeromaritime has been discharging ocean freight in Lagos and Port Harcourt since 1975. During 1981 Aeromaritime handled 2.4 million tonnes of cargo, including rice, sugar, steel, vehicles, machinery, cement, and 15,000 containers. In 1982 Aeromaritime and LCA began carrying maize in bulk from the United States and bagging it in Lagos through a system which can handle 40,000 tonnes a month. A fleet of 20 tugs and 150 barges of all types makes Aeromaritime the largest lighterage company in Nigeria. Its modern material handling equipment, warehouses, and private security force enable Aeromaritime to deliver cargo rapidly and safely.

AEROMARITIME INVESTMENT COMPANY

Aeromaritime's overseas offices offer a convenient purchasing and delivery service for Nigerian businessmen who are looking for American products. Among the items handled regularly are rice, maize and other grains, communications electronics equipment, prefabricated buildings, agricultural machinery, security systems, helicopters, and specialised vehicles. Other goods can be procured on request. Aeromaritime co-ordinates delivery of such items to West Africa through Lignes Centrafricaines shipping line.

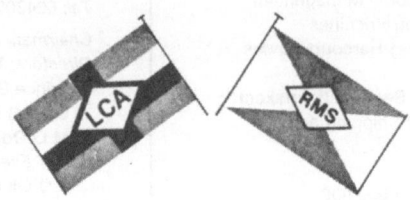

LIGNES CENTRAFRICAINES - RHEIN MAAS UND SEE

LCA and RMS provide liner service and door to door delivery for ocean freight (grain, break bulk, containers, and other heavy lifts) from America, Europe, and the U.K. to the ports of West Africa. They offer many important advantages in addition to very favourable freight rates. LCA and RMS carry most cargoes directly, eliminating the problems and risks of transshipment. As part of a large , fully integrated system, LCA and RMS provide maximum security and minimum loss or damage by keeping cargoes under the control of a single organisation from initial receipt to final delivery.

THE BACO LINERS

These exciting new BArge-COntainer ships eliminate port delay. Each BACO liner carries twelve 800 tonne barges loaded with pre-stowed cargo plus more than 500 containers. This system provides optimum shipping capability and rapid delivery. The use of barges and containers ensures maximum protection of cargo by minimising handling problems. Regular service to Lagos, Warri, and Port Harcourt is provided.

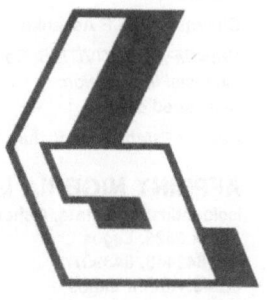

B A Akuazaoku (Assistant General Manager, Planning & Development),
C E Anosike (Assistant General Manager, Operations),
T N George (Assistant General Manager, Personnel)

PRINCIPAL ACTIVITIES: Banking services
Branch Offices: 24-28 Moorgate Rd, London EC2R 6DJ and over a 100 branches throughout Nigeria

Principal Shareholders: Anambra State Government; Imo State Government; Rivers State Government
Date of Establishment: 1948

AFRICAN DESIGNS DEVELOPMENT CENTRE LTD

New Culture Studios, N6A/532A Adeola Crescent, Oremeji, PMB 5162, Ibadan, Oyo State
Tel: 413469
Cable: Newcult Ibadan
Telex: 31117 Edacom Ng

Chairman: Demas Nwoko
Directors: Uche Okeke
Senior Executives: Gbenga Sonuga (Executive Secretary),
E O Chukwuka (Commercial Manager),
P O Nwoko (Technical Manager)

PRINCIPAL ACTIVITIES: Architecture, industrial designs, theatre, films; electronic components distribution
Principal Agencies: Rank Strand Electric of Great Britain
Branch Offices: Project Site: 1 Airport Rd, Benin City, Bendel State
Principal Bankers: United Bank for African Ltd

Principal Shareholders: Demas Nwoko, Uche Okeke

AFRICAN ERA AND COMPANY LTD

13A Obafemi Awolowo Way, Ikeja, PO Box 3849, Lagos
Tel: 961395, 963046
Cable: Aferaco Lagos
Telex: 20117 TDS 260

Chairman: Lt Col C O Adebiyi
Directors: N O Adebiyi (General Manager)
Senior Executives: J O Ogunniyi (Administrative Manager),
Tunde Fasae (Sales Manager),
T Tooley (Production Manager)

PRINCIPAL ACTIVITIES: Manufacturing, assembling and distribution of television, stereo and audio products. Now involved in - cookers fridges, sanitary fittings, and bathroom accessories
Principal Bankers: Nigerian Acceptances Ltd; United Bank for Africa Ltd
Financial Information:

	N'000
Authorised capital	750
Paid-up capital	750
Turnover	3,800

Principal Shareholders: Nigerians
Date of Establishment: February 1976

AFRICAN GLASS COMPANY LTD (FORMERLY CENTRAL GLASS (NIGERIA) LTD)

PO Box 173, Ikeja, Lagos
Tel: 964366

PRINCIPAL ACTIVITIES: Manufacturing of glass containers for the cosmetic and pharmaceutical industries
Branch Offices: Factory Location: Ayodele Diyan Road Industrial Estate, PO Box 1, Ikeja, Lagos

AFRICAN INDUSTRIAL TIMBER CO LTD

PO Box 18, 174 Broad St, Lagos
Tel: 634218

PRINCIPAL ACTIVITIES: Hardwood lumber and log exporters

AFRICAN INSURANCE COMPANY LTD

134 Nnamdi Azikiwe Street, PO Box 274, Lagos
Tel: 661720, 661579, 661877
Cable: Afrinsure

Directors: Chief E O Ashamu, Chief S O Akwiwu, Chief J O Edewor Mazi, C N Obioha, Chief P O Osakwe, A H Sulaiman, B O Ofu, Alhaji Baba Dan Bappa, R A Owusu
Senior Executives: M J C Couch (General Manager),
Y N Mbadiwe (Company Secretary),
T A Okoronkwo (Chief Accountant),
E C M Akamobi (Assistant General Manager)

PRINCIPAL ACTIVITIES: All classes of insurance except life
Branch Offices: Afrinsure House, PO Box 725, Enugu Anambra State; 3 Pound Rd, Aba, Imo State; Eku House, PO Box 109, Warri; PO Box 1331, Ibadan, Oyo State; 19 Kodesho Street, Ikeja, Lagos State; PO Box 2493, 65 Mission Rd, Benin City; 22 Nnamdi Azikiwe Street, PO Box 799, Owerri, Imo State; 85 Ibrahim Taiwo Street, PO Box 11963, Kano; PO Box 1470, Jos; 12 Umuokware Rd, PO Box 665, Orlu; 46 New Market Rd, Onitsha
Principal Bankers: Union Bank of Nigeria Ltd; African Continental Bank Ltd; Savannah Bank of Nigeria Ltd
Financial Information:

	N'000
Authorised capital	600
Paid-up capital	6000
Turnover	3,000

Principal Shareholders: Leventis Group of Companies; Dr K O Mbadiwe
Date of Establishment: 1950
No of Employees: 180

AFRICAN IVORY INSURANCE COMPANY LTD

10 Sanni Adewale St, PO Box 10009, Lagos
Tel: 660514, 660960
Cable: Whitevory

Chairman: Alhaji Mohammed Mustapha
Directors: M A C Chukwudinma (Managing),
Ekong Etuk,
F Agbeyegbe,
Mrs Oriaku Nwosu,
Dr K Abayomi
Senior Executives: L M A Okoye (General Manager)

PRINCIPAL ACTIVITIES: Insurance
Branch Offices: 4 Fagge Takudu, PO Box 2261, Kano; 15 Asu Rd, Aba, Imo State; 31 Ogui Rd, PO Box 250, Enugu, Anambra State
Principal Bankers: African Continental Bank Ltd; Societe Generale Bank (Nigeria) Ltd
Financial Information:

	N'000
Authorised capital	1,000
Paid-up capital	500

Date of Establishment: 31st March 1978

AFRICAN NEWSPAPERS OF NIGERIA LTD

208/212 Broad St, PO Box 2416, Lagos
Tel: 635057, 633699, 632385

PRINCIPAL ACTIVITIES: Publication of newspapers

AFRICAN PAINTS (NIG) LTD

Plot 51, Oregun Industrial Estate, PMB 21538, Ikeja, Lagos State

Cable: Afropaints

Chairman: Alhaji G A Amusan
Directors: Gbenga Akinnawo (Managing),
Dr E O Akinsete,
Eng E Olawoye,
Alhaja A Amusan
Senior Executives: J A Wilkie (Sales Manager),
Kola Osinoiki (Chief Accountant)

PRINCIPAL ACTIVITIES: Manufacturing of paints and allied products

Branch Offices: Opposite 2nd Gate, UI, Oyo Rd, PMB 75 UI Post Office Ibadan, Oyo State; 14B Unity Rd, PO Box 520, Ilorin, Kwara State; 83 1st East Circular Rd, Benin-City, Bendel State; 85 Oyemekun Rd, Akure, Ondo State; NGS 1415, Bosso Rd., Minna, Niger State; 130A Okigwe Rd, PMB 7317, Aba, Anambra State; Onitsha/Owerri Rd, PO Box 4276, Onitsha, Imo State; 53A Muritala Mohammed, PO Box 1617, Jos, Plateau State; 19 Balat Hughes Rd, Kano, Kano State

Principal Bankers: First Bank of Nigeria Ltd

Principal Shareholders: Chairman and Directors as described

Date of Establishment: Incorporated 1974, Commenced Manufacturing, January 1977

No of Employees: 204

AFRICAN PETROLEUM LTD

AP House, 54/56 Broad Street, PO Box 512, Lagos
Tel: 632003/4, 632072, 632144/5
Cable: Ayepee Lagos
Telex: 21242 Ayepee

Chairman: Mohammed Hayatuddini
Directors: O O Shyllon (Managing),
 S M Akpe,
 P C Chigbo,
 J A Cole,
 Ade Ojo
Senior Executives: W N Nwaka (Operations Manager),
 T A Fabyan (Sales Manager),
 S O Odunaike (Manager, Staff Administration),
 E O Olaleye (Finance and Accounts Manager),
 G O Segun (Engineering Manager)

PRINCIPAL ACTIVITIES: Petroleum products marketing

Branch Offices: Club Rd, PO Box 636, Kano; 33 Ali Akilu Rd, Kaduna; PO Box 448, Warri, Bendel State; AP-Shell Rd, PMB 1036, Apapa, Lagos; Ijebu Bye Pass, Oke Ado, PMB 5758,

Oyo State; 11 Moscow Rd, PO Box 266, Port-Harcourt, River State

Principal Bankers: Union Bank of Nigeria Ltd; First Bank of Nigeria Ltd

Financial Information: Year ended 31st December 1981

	₦'000
Authorised capital	11,250
Paid-up capital	11,250
Turnover	217,510
Profits (before tax)	26,590
Profits (after tax)	15,160

Principal Shareholders: Nigerian National Petroleum Corporation

Date of Establishment: 1956 (formerly BP Nigeria Ltd)

No of Employees: 991

AFRICAN PRUDENTIAL INSURANCE COMPANY LTD (THE)

27/29 Martins Street, PO Box 2358, Lagos
Tel: 664435, 663436
Cable: Apico
Telex: 21129 Group Ng

Chairman: Alhaji Mamman Daura
Directors: Chief S Dike Odogwu (Managing),
 Chief M I Agbontaen,
 R T Hart,
 Chief A Ilonzeh,
 Don Abili,
 Arc Oluwole Olumuyiwa,
 Alhaji Ajiya Idris
Senior Executives: J L Spencer (General Manager/Chief Executive),
 O N Ogbonna (Life Manager),
 A H Osuafor (Marine Manager),
 B O Chidozie (Fire/Accident Manager),
 B Ajoku (Accountant)

PRINCIPAL ACTIVITIES: Insurance

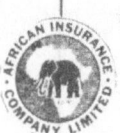

Branch Offices: 77 Azikiwe Rd, Aba; 142 Ikpoba Slope, Benin City; 1A Junction Rd, Kaduna; 35B Bode Thomas St, Surulere, Lagos; 12 Sanni St, Jos
Principal Bankers: United Bank for Africa Ltd; Union Bank of Nigeria Ltd; African Continental Bank Ltd

Date of Establishment: 1964
No of Employees: 42

AFRICAN REINSURANCE CORPORATION

Bookshop House, 50/52 Broad St, PMB 12765, Lagos
Cable: Africare Lagos
Telex: 21505 Accepto Ng; 21239

Senior Executives: Toye Ogunnorin (Public Relations Officer)

PRINCIPAL ACTIVITIES: Reinsurance business; integovernmental, international organisation with full diplomatic status based in Nigeria as the host country

Principal Shareholders: Governments of Independent African States, African Development Bank

AFRICAN TIMBER & PLYWOOD

(A Division of UAC of Nigeria Ltd)

Sapele/Warri Rd, PMB 4001, Sapele, Bendel State
Tel: 41033, 41088
Cable: Unatimply Sapele
Telex: 42275 Sapele

Chairman: E A O Shonekan
Directors: J G A Clegg, Chief S B Daniyan, J C Egri-Okwaji, Alhaji Shehu Idris, H T Mathers, A C I Mbanefo, Chief J O Omidiora, F M O Osifo, J P Rauch, Alhaji Bello Sani, P D Tueart
Senior Executives: L Hodgson (General Manager)

PRINCIPAL ACTIVITIES: Sawmilling, manufacturing of plywood, doors, particle boards, system buildings and various other timber products
Branch Offices: Onibu-Ore House, Block 10, Ikorodu Rd, Maryland, Ikeja, Lagos State
Principal Bankers: First Bank of Nigeria Ltd; Union Bank of Nigeria Ltd

Principal Shareholders: Division of UAC of Nigeria Ltd
Date of Establishment: 1933
No of Employees: 1,500

AFRICAN UNIVERSITIES PRESS

(Pilgrim Books Ltd)

Ibadan Expressway, New Oluyole Estate, PMB 5617, Ibadan, Oyo State
Cable: Pilgrim Ibadan
Telex: 31530

Directors: John E Leigh (Managing Director), Emmanuel A Jaja
Senior Executives: Joseph A Kilanko (General Manager)

PRINCIPAL ACTIVITIES: Publishers of educational and general books
Principal Agencies: Edward Arnold (Publishers) Ltd, UK; John Murray, UK; George Harrap, UK; Ginn Company, UK; Addison Wesley, UK; Elliott Rightway Books, UK
Branch Offices: 74 Oguta Rd, PO Box 21, Onitsha, Anambra State; 17 Ciroma St, Gellesu, Tudun Wada, Zaria, Kaduna State; 21 Ikorodu Rd, Illupeju, PO Box 3560, Lagos
Principal Bankers: First Bank of Nigeria Ltd
Financial Information:

	N'000
Authorised capital	102
Paid-up capital	102

Principal Shareholders: John E Leigh; Daily Times of Nigeria
Date of Establishment: 1st January 1969

AFRO ARAB TECHNI-CHEMICALS LTD

Block H - Plot 2 Isolo Industrial Estate PO Box 1647, Lagos
Tel: 963346
Cable: Arabpharm Lagos

Chairman: Amin Shocair
Directors: Adnan Shocair, Chief Alhaji D S Yaro, Mr Walid, O Sotuminu

PRINCIPAL ACTIVITIES: Pharmaceutical manufacturing
Principal Agencies: Andreu International, Spain; Zambon SPA, Italy; Laboratoires OM, Switzerland
Subsidiary/Associated Companies: Hospitex (Nigeria) Ltd
Principal Bankers: Nigeria Arab Bank Ltd
Financial Information:

	N'000
Authorised capital	1,360
Paid-up capital	1,360
Turnover	1,500

Principal Shareholders: 60% Foreign; 40% Nigerian
Date of Establishment: 17th April 1968
No of Employees: 87

AFRO COMMERCE (WA) LTD

16 Commercial Rd, Apapa, PO Box 1834, Lagos
Tel: 871391
Cable: Afrocom

Chairman: Alhaji Saadu Alanamu
Directors: B V Sokolov (Managing), Alhaji Sani Bakori
Senior Executives: B Ige (Accountant), A Cole (Administrative Manager), G E Ogwu (Sales Manager)

PRINCIPAL ACTIVITIES: Sales and service of machine tools; agricultural equipment etc
Principal Agencies: Balkancarimpex; Agromachinaimpex; Machinoexport; Bearcat
Branch Offices: 1 Kachia Rd, PO Box 592, Kaduna; 32 Ikwere Rd, PMB 5691, Port Harcourt, Rivers State
Principal Bankers: United Bank for Africa Ltd
Financial Information:

	N'000
Authorised capital	500
Paid-up capital	500

Principal Shareholders: Nigerians
Date of Establishment: 1964

AFRO CONTINENTAL NIGERIA LTD

PO Box 2916, Lagos
Tel: 651425
Cable: Acont Lagos
Telex: 21387

Chairman: N D Gaon

PRINCIPAL ACTIVITIES: Importers and exporters; major commodities of importation, grains and cement

Principal Shareholders: Subsidiary of Compagnie Noga d'Importation et d'Exportation SA

AFRO ELEKTRO KONSULT LTD

46 Balogun St, PO Box 3392, Lagos
Tel: 636081, 655891

Directors: John R Richardson (General Manager)

PRINCIPAL ACTIVITIES: Telecommunications and power, consultancy service

AFRO INTERNATIONAL CONSTRUCTION COMPANY

PO Box 4064, Unity House, 37 Marina, Lagos
Tel: 652286
Telex: 21387 Acont Ng

PRINCIPAL ACTIVITIES: Building and civil engineering contractors

AFRO NIGERIAN IMPORT & EXPORT CO LTD
PO Box 80, Sapele, Bendel State
Tel: 42312

PRINCIPAL ACTIVITIES: Manufacturers of crepe rubber;
exporters of rubber

AFROGUARD PUBLICATIONS
4 Falolu Rd, Surulere, Lagos

PRINCIPAL ACTIVITIES: Publishers of banking and insurance
magazines

AFROMEDIA PLASTICS & ENGINEERING LTD
PO Box 2377, Lagos
Tel: 875745, 875664
Cable: Afromedia Lagos
Telex: 21705 Apel Ng

Chairman: Chief J O Nwaburie (also Managing Director)
Directors: T A Owen (General Manager),
Ire Olopade,
S E Olaghere
Senior Executives: W E Evans (Development/Production
Manager),
G C E Glayzer (Mould Design Engineer),
S O Tettey (Accountant)

PRINCIPAL ACTIVITIES: Manufacturers of plastic containers for
oil and kerosine; sundry household items, etc
Branch Offices: Factory: 17b Creek Rd, Apapa, Lagos
Financial Information:

	N'000
Turnover	3,290
Profits	666

Principal Shareholders: Chief J O Nwabunie; Ire Olopade; S E
Olaghere; T A Owen; T M Standfast; E Cappelletti
Date of Establishment: 1975
No of Employees: 129

AFROTEC TECHNICAL SERVICES NIGERIA LTD
Plot 3 Block 'M' Isolo Industrial Estate, PMB 1061, Oshodi,
Lagos State
Tel: 45656, 44706
Cable: Afroman Lagos

Chairman: A O Runsewe
Directors: B G W Harris (Managing Director),
C D J White (Joint Managing Director),
Chief F M Moronu (Deputy Managing Director),
E O Sonubi,
J A Amfani,
E O Banjoko
Senior Executives: A Seivwright (Sales Director),
A Mair (Commercial Manager),
A G Purvis (General Sales Manager),
G O Nwosu (Lagos Sales Manager)

PRINCIPAL ACTIVITIES: Importer and distributor of agricultural
equipment and services; construction plants, power
generation and civil engineering equipment
Principal Agencies: Frederick Parker Ltd, UK; Coronet EM Ltd,
UK; Cement & Steel Ltd, UK; Thwaites Ltd, UK;
Dawson-Keith, UK; Finlay Engineering, UK; Wickham
Engineering, UK; Lef Bishop Ltd, UK; Volvo BM, Sweden;
Dynapac Maskin AB, Sweden; Liebherr-Export AG,
Switzerland
Branch Offices: 705 Hadejia Rd, Kano; 73 Agbani Rd, Enugu; No
2 House, Rumola Junction, Aba Rd, Box 357, Port Harcourt;
16 Mission Rd, Benin City; Off Baga Rd, PMB 1237, Maidugri;
23 Onitsha Rd, Kaduna, Owerri; Oyo Rd, Box 12464, Ibadan;
47 Bedwell St, Calabar; 1A Constitution Hill, Jos
Principal Bankers: First Bank of Nigeria Ltd; International
Merchant Bank; Chase Merchant Bank

Financial Information:

	N'000
Authorised capital	4,000
Paid-up capital	4,000
Turnover	20,000

Date of Establishment: 20th April 1972
No of Employees: 400

AGBARA ESTATES LTD
25 Marine Rd, Apapa, Lagos
Tel: 870225, 873337
Cable: Agbestel

Chairman: Chief A O Lawson
Directors: L A Lawson (Executive Vice Chairman),
B D Tasker (Managing Director),
B E Henshow (Director of Finance),
A A Adetoyo (Legal/Admin. Director),
E Lewis (Technical Diriector)
Senior Executives: A Nmelu (Chief Accountant),
Togonu-Bickerstetly (Senior Architect),
T Longhorn (Contracts Manager)

PRINCIPAL ACTIVITIES: Property and real estate developers
and managers. Major project: Integrated New Town at
Agbara, Ogun State comprising industrial, commercial and
residential sections
Associated Companies: Nationwide Development Company Ltd
Principal Bankers: First Bank of Nigeria Ltd; Union Bank of
Nigeria Ltd; Icon Ltd (Merchant Bankers)
Financial Information:

	N'000
Authorised capital	3,000
Paid-up capital	3,000
Turnover	8,500
Share capital & reserves	12,500

Principal Shareholders: Consolidated Investments Ltd
Date of Establishment: 1974
No of Employees: 150

AGBENOR MINING SYNDICATE
10 Shendam St, PO Box 13, Jos, Plateau State
PRINCIPAL ACTIVITIES: Mining

AGIP (NIGERIA) LTD
Unity House, 37 Marina, PO Box 921, Lagos
Tel: 660255, 662176, 664861
PRINCIPAL ACTIVITIES: Marketing of petroleum products
Principal Bankers: United Bank for Africa Ltd
Financial Information:

	N'000
Authorised capital	6,700
Paid-up capital	6,700

Date of Establishment: 1961

AGRIBUILD NIGERIA LTD
44 Adeoshun St, Ikate, Surulere, Lagos
Tel: 833964
Cable: Agribuild Lagos

PRINCIPAL ACTIVITIES: Suppliers of agricultural machinery and
equipment; construction equipment

AGRICULTURAL DEVELOPMENT CORPORATION (ANAMBRA STATE)
PMB 1024, Enugu, Anambra State
Tel: 253029, 253463, 255251, 255414, 254885
Cable: Agrico Enugu
Telex: 51151 Agrico Ng

Senior Executives: H N Ntephe (General Manager),
G C Okoye (Special Assistant to the General Manager),
Mrs N A Egwuatu (Manager, Secretaries Office)

PRINCIPAL ACTIVITIES: Production of edible palm oil and kernels, fabricated agro-allied equipment and tools, packaged milled rice grain and flour, raw cashew nuts, packaged fried and unfried chashew nuts; liverstock feeds, day-old chickens, turkeys, eggs, broilers, egg-trays and egg cartons, beef and pork etc
Branch Offices: Cold Store: 32 Zik Ave, Enugu, Anambra State; Livestock Feeds: 9th Mile Corner, Enugu, Anambra State
Subsidiary Companies: Adarice Production Nigeria Ltd; Anambra Vegetable Oils Products Nigeria Ltd
Principal Bankers: Union Bank of Nigeria Ltd

Principal Shareholders: Government of Anambra State
Date of Establishment: 3rd February 1976
No of Employees: 600

AGRO INDUSTRIES & DEVELOPMENT SCHEMES CO (NIG) LTD

53 Calcutta Crescent, Apapa, Lagos
Tel: 873201

PRINCIPAL ACTIVITIES: Suppliers of cold drink dispensers and food machines
Principal Agencies: Cretor, Jetspray

AGROLINE (NIGERIA) LTD

3 Adekoyejo Majekodunmi Ave, New GRA Iyaganku, PO Box 11340, Lagos
Tel: 461332, 415303

PRINCIPAL ACTIVITIES: Manufacturers of fungicides, polishes etc
Branch Offices: NW4/371 Ekotedo Iyaolobe, PO Box 1459, Ibadan

Date of Establishment: January 1980

AGROTEC SERVICES LTD

PO Box 377, Mushin, Lagos State
Tel: 861853
Cable: Ashamu Lagos
Telex: 21578 Ng Lagos

Chairman: Chief E O Ashamu
Directors: Mrs P O Ashamu, G F W O Stargardt
Senior Executives: Chief J O Adigun (General Manager),
    J K Fatokun (Sales Manager),
    C Amao (Accountant)

PRINCIPAL ACTIVITIES: Sales and servicing of agricultural equipment, agrichemicals, insecticides, fungicides, herbicides, nematocides, etc; refrigeration equipment; fertilizers; irrigation equipment/installation and maintainance services; livestock feed, especially concentrates
Principal Agencies: IKJ (Agricultural) Ltd, UK; IGB Trading Ltd, Guernsey, Channel Islands; Big Dutchman Ltd, UK; Brodrene Gram A/S, Denmark; Du-Pont De Numours International SA, Switzerland; X Fendt & Co, Germany
Branch Offices: Kaduna, Aba
Principal Bankers: National Bank of Nigeria Ltd; First Bank of Nigeria Ltd; African Continental Bank Ltd; Union Bank of Nigeria Ltd
Financial Information: Member of E O Ashamu Group of Companies

	₦'000
Authorised capital	1,000
Paid-up capital	1,000
Sales turnover	5,411
Profits	265

AIRCOOL METAL INDUSTRIES (NIGERIA) LTD

8-10 Broad St, Western House, Lagos
Tel: 962909

PRINCIPAL ACTIVITIES: Manufacturing of air-conditioners, refrigerators, electric fans
Branch Offices: Plot 2 Isheri Rd, Agidingbi, Ikeja, Lagos, Tel 963988

Principal Shareholders: Adebowale Electrical Industries Ltd

AIREGIN ENTERPRISES & AGENCIES LTD

Airport Rd (Opposite the Airport), PO Box 498, Benin City, Bendel State
Tel: 241027
Cable: Airegin
Telex: 41124 Airgin Ng

Chairman: Mrs Norma Thomas Ojehomon (also Managing Director)
Directors: Mrs A B Asemota, Mrs H R Ogbe, Mrs O Asekun
Senior Executives: P I Ihunde (Manager, Travel Agency)

PRINCIPAL ACTIVITIES: Travel and tourism IATA Agent, retailers of handicrafts, pottery and jewellery
Branch Offices: Benin Exotique, Benin City
Subsidiary Companies: Airegin Travel Agency
Principal Bankers: New Nigeria Bank Ltd; Standard Bank Ltd
Financial Information:

	₦'000
Authorised capital	200
Sales turnover	1,500

Principal Shareholders: Directors as described above

AIROE CONSTRUCTION & CIVIL ENGINEERING CO LTD

PO Box 117, Benin City, Bendel State
Tel: 241241, 241692
Cable: Airoe

Chairman: Anthony Iro Eweka
Directors: Augustine A I Eweka, Sunday I Iro Eweka
Senior Executives: F A Ogedegbe (Administrative/Accounts Manager)

PRINCIPAL ACTIVITIES: Building and civil engineering construction and catering
Branch Offices: 7 Water Resources Rd, Effurun, Warri
Associated Companies: Ikpoba River Motel
Principal Bankers: United Bank for Africa

Principal Shareholders: Anthony Iro Eweka; Augustine A I Eweka
Date of Establishment: 1965

AISA TRADING COMPANY LTD

1A Alhaji Aisa Animashaun Crescent, Off Coker Rd, Ilupeju, PO Box 494, Marina, Lagos

PRINCIPAL ACTIVITIES: Suppliers of ferrous and non ferrous metals

Date of Establishment: March 1974

AJANGA INTERNATIONAL AGENCY

PMB 1273, Enugu, Anambra State

President: John O Uwanaka

PRINCIPAL ACTIVITIES: Agents, general trading company and foreign trade consultant
Principal Bankers: African Continental Bank Ltd

AJAO, J A, BROTHERS

10 Sanusi Olusi Rd, PMB 2278, Lagos
Tel: 632224
Telex: 21519 Ajatex Ng

PRINCIPAL ACTIVITIES: Importers of agricultural machinery and equipment; estate developers

AJAOKUTA STEEL COMPANY LTD
PMB 1123, Okene, Kwara State

Senior Executives: Dr Fidelis Rex Chukwuemeka Ezemenari
(General Manager)

PRINCIPAL ACTIVITIES: Steel production
Financial Information:
Registered capital .... ₦ 500,000

Principal Shareholders: Federal Government of Nigeria
Date of Establishment: November 1979

AJIROTUTU (NIGERIA) LTD
29 Wakeman St, Yaba, Lagos
Tel: 862510

PRINCIPAL ACTIVITIES: Suppliers of electrical machinery
Principal Agencies: Oscar Block Makers
Branch Offices: Kaduna; Kano; Bida

AJOSI OILFIELDS SUPPLY COMPANY LTD
Investment House, Broad St, PO Box 5436, Lagos
Tel: 635240
Cable: Ajosioil Lagos
Telex: 21113 Olopro Ng

Directors: H A Johnson (Director)

PRINCIPAL ACTIVITIES: Equipment supply and services to the
oil and gas industry
Principal Agencies: Sooner Pipe and Supply

AKA AND SONS (NIGERIA) LTD
17 Martins St, PO Box 3371, Lagos
Tel: 633387

PRINCIPAL ACTIVITIES: Importers and distributors of general
merchandise

AKANDE TRADING CO NIGERIA LTD
Plot K3, Ahmadu Bello Way, Kaduna
Tel: 213498

PRINCIPAL ACTIVITIES: Trading company; children's and men's
wear, ladies' fashions, sportswear and general goods

AKANJI COMMERCIAL ENTERPRISES LTD
13 Eyamba St, PO Box 801, Jos, Plateau State
Tel: 2863, 3294

Chairman: D L Akanji
Directors: E O Akanji, N L Ogunlade Akanji

PRINCIPAL ACTIVITIES: Suppliers of building materials,
electronic goods, importers and exporters and general
contractors
Financial Information: Part of Akanji Group of Companies

AKANJI, D L, & CO (NIG) LTD
21 Ahmadu Bello Way, PO Box 801, Jos, Plateau State
Tel: 3294, 2863
Cable: Akangroup

Chairman: D L Akanji
Directors: N L Akanji
Senior Executives: George M Ossai (Accountant)

PRINCIPAL ACTIVITIES: Distributors, suppliers of retail and
wholesale provisions; building materials, consumer electrical
goods, manufacturers' representatives
Principal Agencies: Lever Brothers (Nig) Ltd; Cadbury (Nig) Ltd;
Narakat Biscuits Ltd
Branch Offices: 10 Bola St, Ebute-Metta, Lagos
Principal Bankers: First Bank of Nigeria Ltd
Financial Information: Part of Akanji Group of Companies

	₦'000
Authorised capital	350
Paid-up capital	275
Sales turnover	1,719

AKANJI TRANSPORT
13 Eyamba St, PO Box 801, Jos, Plateau State

PRINCIPAL ACTIVITIES: Transporters and fuel haulage
transporters
Financial Information: Part of Akanji Group of Companies

AKAROLO TECHNICAL COMPANY NIGERIA LTD
Head Office, 13/15 Trans-Amadi Industrial Rd, PO Box 128, Port
Harcourt, Rivers State
Tel: 225740
Telex: 61152 Akatec Ng

PRINCIPAL ACTIVITIES: Estate agents, block moulders and civil
engineering contractors
Branch Offices: Plot 2, Ochonma Layout, Ahoada-Town, Port
Harcourt

AKHIGBE, ODIBO, & CO LTD
4th Floor, 4 Sanni Adewale St, PO Box 4712, Lagos
Tel: 630601, 653886
Cable: Odiboco Lagos
Telex: 21309 Odibo Ng

Chairman: Matthias Odibo Akhigbe
Directors: Boniface U Akhigbe, Patience E Akhigbe
Senior Executives: A S Boyo (Chartered Surveyor),
Mrs C O Akhigbe (Secretary)

PRINCIPAL ACTIVITIES: Property, real estate developers
Branch Offices: 93 Mission Rd, 2nd Floor, PMB 1129, Benin City
Principal Bankers: New Nigeria Bank Ltd; Barclays Bank Nigeria
Ltd
Financial Information:

	₦'000
Authorised capital	200
Paid-up capital	200

Principal Shareholders: M O Akhigbe; B U Akhigbe; P E
Akhigbe; C O Akhigbe

AKIJA HOTEL LTD
43 Murtala Mohammed Way, PO Box 767, Kano
Tel: 3514, 5327/8
Cable: Akijotel

Chairman: Alhaji Ibrahim
Directors: Alhaji Baba Garba (Managing Director)
Senior Executives: Alhaji Yusuf Garba (Manager),
Joseph Olaoye (Accountant),
Ibrahim Jatto (Supervisor)

PRINCIPAL ACTIVITIES: Hotel and catering
Principal Bankers: Bank of the North Ltd
No of Employees: 209

AKIN MARTINS (NIGERIA) LTD
See MARTINS, AKIN, (NIGERIA) LTD

AKINADOD AKINLOYE ABODERIN LTD
208-212 Broad St, 3rd Floor, PO Box 2150, Lagos
Tel: 636853, 634864

PRINCIPAL ACTIVITIES: Suppliers of construction equipment;
manufacturers' representatives
Principal Agencies: Hans Lingl, Anlagenbau und
Verfahrenstechnik GmbH & Co, West Germany

AKIN-GEORGE, J, & COMPANY
40 Balogun St, PO Box 2279, Lagos
Tel: 660570, 661554
Cable: Akinger Lagos

Chairman: Chief J Akin George
Directors: Femi Elugbaju, Miss Abisola George, O A Awoliyi, D Awuah-Darko
Senior Executives: Femi Elugbaju (Executive Director),
  B A Akinsanya (Assistant Director),
  R O Kusanu (Assistant Director),
  M O Akala (Assistant Director)

PRINCIPAL ACTIVITIES: Insurance brokers
Principal Agencies: Lloyds through United African Insurance
Branch Offices: 6A Main St, PO Box 445, Zaria, Kaduna State; 77 Aggrey Rd, PO Box 853, Port Harcourt, Rivers State; 22 Ahmadu Bello Way, PO Box 4131, Kaduna; 51e Ado Bayero Rd, PO Box 4637, Kano
Associated Companies: Sierra Leone Insurance Brokers, Freetown; Marine and General Brokers, Accra; United African Insurance Brokers, London
Principal Bankers: National Bank of Nigeria Ltd
Financial Information:

	₦'000
Authorised capital	20
Paid-up capital	20
Turnover	500
Profits	25

Principal Shareholders: Chief J A George
Date of Establishment: November 1960
No of Employees: 140

AKPENLAMEN CO LTD
9/11 Gbajumo St, PO Box 4891, Lagos
Tel: 664095
Cable: Gregdabs Lagos
Telex: 21276 Godabs Ng

Chairman: Godwin G Daboadzuana
Directors: M Udende, A Dabo
Senior Executives: Christine M Kigundu-Adzuana (Chief Executive, Operations)

PRINCIPAL ACTIVITIES: General merchants, importers and exporters, property development and hotel operators
Branch Offices: Plot 269, Makurdi, Benue State
Subsidiary Companies: ME Ltd; Dabs Nigeria Ltd; ED Publications Ltd; Kenitex Chemicals (Nigeria) Ltd
Principal Bankers: International Bank for West Africa Ltd

AKUTU STRUCTURES LTD
(Formerly Akutu Construction Company Nigeria Ltd)
60 Ziks Avenue, Uwani, PO Box 455, Enugu, Anambra State
Tel: 337036

Chairman: G E Akutu
Directors: Keddy Nwokedi, C Akutu, Mrs P A Akutu
Senior Executives: G O Akutu (Works Manager),
  E C Oranye (Principal Technical Officer)

PRINCIPAL ACTIVITIES: Civil engineering and construction
Principal Agencies: Key power westacre, UK
Branch Offices: 81 Falolu Street, Surulere, Lagos
Subsidiary Companies: Obunike Associates Ltd, Enugu, Anambra State
Principal Bankers: Co-Operative and Commerce Bank Nigeria Ltd

Date of Establishment: 14th December, 1973
No of Employees: 300

AKWIWU MOTORS LTD
20 Ado Avenue, PMB 1145, Apapa, Lagos
Tel: 870542
Cable: Clearhaul
Telex: 21675 Nissco Ng; 22471 Lana Ng

Chairman: Chief Emanuel Akwiwu
Directors: Obi Akwiwu, Joy Akwiwu, Nnamdi Akwiwu
Senior Executives: Obi Akwiwu (Chief Executive),
  Nanmdi Akwiwu (Executive Director),

Law Nduwubah (Operations Manager),
Eugene Ujunwa (Senior Sales Executive)

PRINCIPAL ACTIVITIES: Shipping, transporters, freight
  forwarding, importers of motor vehicles and accessories
Principal Agencies: Sermat SA, France; Fihatra AG (Switzerland);
  Overall Transport, UK; Ellis of Green, UK; Chestergate
  Securities, UK; United Greenfield, UK; Shin-Kobe Elec. Mach.
  Co, Japan; Giant Trading Co, Japan; America-By-Car, UK;
  Gam Purchasing Co, USA; Export Cars, UK; Volvo
  Concessionaires, UK
Branch Offices: 1-2 Umuahia Ave, Gra, Aba
Principal Bankers: Union Bank of Nigeria Ltd
Financial Information:

	N'000
Authorised capital	500
Paid-up capital	500

Principal Shareholders: Directors as described above
Date of Establishment: August 1962
No of Employees: 400

ALADAIRE EXPORT LTD
4/6 Oil Mill St, PO Box 3173, Lagos
Tel: 652416

PRINCIPAL ACTIVITIES: Exporters of hand-printed materials,
  etc

ALADDIN CONSTRUCTION NIGERIA LTD
17 Calcutta Crescent, PO Box 162, Apapa, Lagos
Tel: 875390

Directors: Chuks Anugwom (Executive Director)

PRINCIPAL ACTIVITIES: Construction
Principal Agencies: Ugochukwu & Sons ltd

ALAKIJA & ALAKIJA CONTRACTING SERVICES LTD
6 Ondo Street West, Ebute-Metta, PO Box 7301, Lagos
Tel: 848286

Chairman: Rex I Alakija (also Managing Director)
Directors: Mrs Y Alakija, C Gilmer
Senior Executives: A R Yusuf (Chief Accountant),
  P A Ajakaiye (Chief Buyer),
  Miss Q A Okoh (Secretary)

PRINCIPAL ACTIVITIES: Civil engineering and construction
Branch Offices: 64 Ayilara Street, Surulere, Lagos
Principal Bankers: First Bank of Nigeria Ltd

Principal Shareholders: Rex I Alakija; Mrs Y Alakija; M Alakija; T
  Alakija; B Alakija; A Alakija
Date of Establishment: May 1950
No of Employees: 3,000

ALALADE GROUP OF COMPANIES
9 Ladipo Oluwole Ave, Ikeja, Lagos
Tel: 964897
Telex: 21551 Agroup Ng

PRINCIPAL ACTIVITIES: General merchandise suppliers

ALBAN PHARMACY LTD
128 Broad St, PO Box 461, Lagos
Tel: 630171

PRINCIPAL ACTIVITIES: Importers of pharmaceuticals,
  chemicals photographic equipment and optical goods

ALBISHIR, ALHAJI, & SONS
Shehu Laminu Way, PO Box 233, Maiduguri, Borno State
Tel: 232492, 231164
Cable: Albishir
Telex: 82103 Albish Ng

Chairman: Alhaji Usman Albishir (also Managing Director)
Directors: Alhaji Abubakar Albishir,
  Alhaji Idris Aji (Financial),
  Alhaji Abdusalam Buba (Co-ordinator/Purchasing Manager)

PRINCIPAL ACTIVITIES: Building and Civil engineering
  contractors
Branch Offices: 3 Bompai Rd, Opposite Central Hotel, PO Box
  971, Kano; Bosso Rd, PO Box 256, Minna, Niger State; PO
  Box 785, Yola, Gongola State

ALCAN ALUMINIUM OF NIGERIA LTD
21/22 Marina, Wesley House, PO Box 1071, Lagos
Tel: 636105, 636107
Cable: Alcaniger
Telex: 21947 Alcan Ng

Chairman: Herman W Siemens

PRINCIPAL ACTIVITIES: Manufacturers of aluminium strip, sheet
  and circles
Branch Offices: Trans-Amadi Industrial Estate, PO Box 356, Port
  Harcourt
Associated Companies: Alcan Aluminium Products Ltd
Principal Bankers: Union Bank of Nigeria Ltd; Societe Generale
  Bank Ltd

Principal Shareholders: Alcan Aluminium Ltd, Montreal, Canada
No of Employees: 300

ALCAN ALUMINIUM PRODUCTS LTD
21-22 Marina, Wesley House, PO Box 2160, Lagos
Tel: 636105, 636107
Cable: Flag Lagos
Telex: 21947 Alcan Ng

Chairman: Herman W Siemens

PRINCIPAL ACTIVITIES: Manufacturers of aluminium building
  products
Branch Offices: 85 Aba Rd, PO Box 458, Port Harcourt, Rivers
  State; Ahmed Talib Ave, PO Box 402, Kaduna
Associated Companies: Alcan Aluminium of Nigeria Ltd, Lagos
Principal Bankers: Union Bank of Nigeria Ltd

Principal Shareholders: Alcan Aluminium Ltd, Montreal, Canada
No of Employees: 230

ALEX L M DAVOU FOM & SONS ENTERPRISE LTD
Fom Amegan Fom House, 19 Ahmadu Bello Way, PO Box 701,
  Jos, Plateau State
Tel: 2445
Cable: Alexfom Jos

Chairman: Dr Alexander L M Davou Fom
Directors: Pam Madu (Managing Director),
  Mrs Helen Fom

PRINCIPAL ACTIVITIES: Agents and general trading, building
  materials, suppliers of carpets, ceramics/sanitary fittings;
  civil engineering and construction; hotels and catering;
  medical and surgical equipment; optical and photographic
  equipment
Associated Companies: Speco Ltd, Nigeria
Principal Bankers: Bank of the North; Standard Bank (Nig) Ltd
Financial Information:
Sales turnover (approx)   N 1,000,000

Principal Shareholders: Dr Alex L M Davou Fom; Pam Madu;
  Mrs Helen C Fom

ALEX OGUEJIOFOR COMPANY LTD
See OGUEJIOFOR, ALEX, COMPANY LTD

ALEX TRAVEL AGENCY LTD
39/41 Martins St, PO Box 598, Lagos
Tel: 632480, 651746, 636787, 630160
Cable: Alextravels
Telex: 21592 Alexem Ng

PRINCIPAL ACTIVITIES: Travel and tourist agents (IATA agents),
  car hire
Branch Offices: 7 Aba Rd, Port Harcourt, Tel 21162; Kingsway
  Stores, Ibadan, Tel 21455

ALFA-LAVAL (NIGERIA) LTD
7A Waziri Ibrahim Crescent, PO Box 4068, Kaduna
Tel: 217053
Cable: Alnig

PRINCIPAL ACTIVITIES: Suppliers of plant and equipment services for the agricultural and food industry

Date of Establishment: March 1979

ALGADAMA (HOLDINGS) LTD
Plot 1176 Zaria Rd, PO Box 35, Jos, Plateau State
Tel: 55476, 55525
Cable: Algadama Jos
Telex: 81638 Gadama Ng

Chairman: Alhaji Garba Adama
Directors: Alhaji Ibrahim Maazamu Garba,
    Alhaji Muhammed Nasiru Gurba,
    Alhaji Idirisu Adamu (Purchasing Director)
Senior Executives: Alhaji Mohammed Nasir (Administrative
    Director, Secretary),
    A Musa Karamba (Vice Chairman),
    V V Bhatia (Group Financial Controller),
    R Chibber (Senior Engineer),
    A B Garba (Assistant Director of Admin)

PRINCIPAL ACTIVITIES: Building and civil engineering
    contractors; concrete works and block making industry;
    timber merchandising; cinemas (theatres owners); printers
    and publishers; general merchants
Principal Agencies: Indo Nigeria Films Distributors Ltd, Lagos;
    AMPECA (Nig) Ltd, Lagos; Spillers Ireland Ltd, Dublin;
    Sebelgrove Ltd, London; Adams Worldwide Ltd, Dublin;
    Senerella Enterprises Inc, USA; Omstar Productions,
    Hollywood Calif. USA
Subsidiary Companies: Algadama Cinemas, New Era Cinema
    Masalachi Jumma St, Jos, Plateau State; Algadama
    Construction Ltd, Zaria Rd, Jos, Plateau State; Murna Nigeria
    Ltd, Jos; Algadama (Nigeria) Ltd, Jos; Algadama Nigeria
    Films Distributors Ltd, Lagos; Adams Worldwide Ltd, Jos
Principal Bankers: First Bank of Nigeria Ltd; African Continental
    Bank Ltd; Bank of the North Ltd
Financial Information:

	N'000
Authorised capital	1,000
Paid-up capital	800
Sales turnover	5,700
Profits	500

Principal Shareholders: Alhaji Garba Adama
Date of Establishment: 26th May 1973
No of Employees: 800

ALGADAMA NIGERIA FILM DISTRIBUTORS LTD
34 Balogun Sq, 3rd Floor, PO Box 1902, Lagos
Tel: 632096
Cable: Distinct Lagos

Chairman: Alhaji G Adama

PRINCIPAL ACTIVITIES: Importers, distributors and exhibitors
    of motion pictures; importers and stockists of cinema
    projectors and arc carbons

ALHAJI ALBISHIR & SONS
See ALBISHIR, ALHAJI, & SONS

ALHAJI AUDU BIDA & SONS UNITED COMPANY LTD
See BIDA, ALHAJI AUDU, & SONS UNITED COMPANY LTD

ALHAJI BABA M SALLEH & SONS (NIGERIA) LTD
See SALLEH, ALHAJI BABA M, & SONS (NIGERIA) LTD

ALHAJI M R SHITTU & SONS LTD
See SHITTU, ALHAJI M R, & SONS LTD

ALHAJI MADU MALA SHERIFF GAMBORU
See GAMBORU, ALHAJI MADU MALA SHERIFF

ALHAJI MAI DERIBE & SONS LTD
See DERIBE, ALHAJI MAI, & SONS LTD

ALHAJI MUSTAPHA HARUNA & SONS
See HARUNA, ALHAJI MUSTAPHA, & SONS

ALHAJI NATA'ATA AND SONS
See NATA'ATA, ALHAJI, AND SONS

ALHAJI SANI MASHALL ESTATES
See MASHALL, ALHAJI SANI, ESTATES

ALHAJI SANI MUSA & SONS
See MUSA, ALHAJI SANI, & SONS

ALHAJI USMAN TETENGI & SONS LTD
See TETENGI, ALHAJI USMAN, & SONS LTD

ALHAJI YERIMA HAMMAN WABI & SONS
See YERIMA HAMMAN WABI, ALHAJI, & SONS

ALHAJI ZANNA K MALA & SONS COMPANY
See MALA, ALHAJI ZANNA K, & SONS COMPANY

ALHASSAN DANTATA & SONS LTD
Dantata House, Murtala Mohammed Way, PO Box 84, Kano
Tel: 2011, 4054/5
Cable: Dantatasons Kano
Telex: 77146 Dantco Ng

Chairman: Alhaji Aminu Dantata

PRINCIPAL ACTIVITIES: Building and civil engineering
    contractors; produce marketing and transporting; shipping
Principal Agencies: Mercedes Benz
Subsidiary/Associated Companies: Mamco Nigeria Ltd; Mainline
    Transport Ltd; Dantata Motors Ltd; Sea Dantainer Lines Ltd
    (see separate entry)

ALHERI MINING CO LTD
10 Zaria Rd, PO Box 464, Jos, Plateau State
Tel: 2273

PRINCIPAL ACTIVITIES: Mining

ALINACO (NIGERIA) LTD
10 Bauchi Rd, PO Box 600, Jos, Plateau State
Tel: 53434, 54022

Chairman: Alhaji Baba Inuwa Ali (also Managing Director)
Directors: Alhaji Aminu Ali,
    O U Igwe (Company Secretary/Accountant),
    Alhaji Ali Alhassan (Purchasing Manager)

PRINCIPAL ACTIVITIES: Building and civil engineering
    contractors
Principal Bankers: First Bank of Nigeria Ltd
Financial Information:

	N'000
Authorised capital	500
Paid-up capital	500
Turnover	4,034

Date of Establishment: 29th October 1970
No of Employees: 362

ALL PURPOSE NIGERIA LTD
4 Fasehun Close, Via Nathan St, Lagos
Tel: 874775
Cable: All Purpose Lagos

PRINCIPAL ACTIVITIES: Suppliers of educational equipment and educational toys
Principal Agencies: Gonis Werke Fabrikation Von Neuheiten, West Germany

ALL-AFRICAN WOODWORKING INDUSTRY LTD
51/55 Broad St, PO Box 8453, Lagos
Tel: 635760

PRINCIPAL ACTIVITIES: Sawmillers, timber merchants; manufacturers of furniture and hardboard

ALLEN, J, CO LTD
PO Box 542, 25 Creek Rd, Apapa, Lagos
Tel: 874721, 874812, 874923, 874954, 874565

Directors: J I Holt, W I Pretty, G M Onyluke, B L Saward, G A Johnson, A H Hill

PRINCIPAL ACTIVITIES: Motor vehicle distributors and components, marine equipment distribution and servicing, air conditioning and refrigeration equipment
Principal Agencies: Ford, Volkswagen
Branch Offices: All the principal towns in Nigeria: Startek, 24 Creek Rd, PO Box 217, Apapa, Lagos (refrigeration and air conditioning specialists); Plot 3/4 Adewunmi Estate, PMB 21413, Ikeja, Lagos; 5 Azikiwe Rd, PO Box 8, Port Harcourt; Warri/Sapele Rd, PO Box 490, Warri, Tel 233676; 139 Murtala Mohammed Way, PO Box 1671, Kano, Tel 5745
Principal Bankers: Union Bank of Nigeria Ltd; Mercantile Bank of Nigeria Ltd; First Bank of Nigeria Ltd; United Bank for Africa Ltd

Principal Shareholders: John Holt Ltd
No of Employees: 1,600

ALLGEMEIN BUSINESS ASSOCIATES
129 Apapa Rd, Ebute-Metta, Lagos
Cable: Allgemein Lagos

PRINCIPAL ACTIVITIES: Suppliers of industrial machinery, machine tools, concrete mixers, etc

ALLIED ARCHITECTS
Oluseun House, Opposite ICC Cemetery, Sango, Oyo Rd, Ibadan, Oyo State
Tel: 413842
Cable: Allarch Ibadan

Directors: Chief A O Ojo (Principal Partner),
D O Fadele (Principal Partner),
H O Akinbulumo (Partner),
S A Tijani (Partner)
Senior Executives: F O Omidiora (Associate Partner),
A B Olorunda (Associate Partner)

PRINCIPAL ACTIVITIES: Architects and town planning consultants
Branch Offices: 5th Floor Cooperative Bank Bldg, 30 Marina, PO Box 2658, Lagos, Tel 660548, Cable Allarch Lagos; 68 Marian Rd, PO Box 407, Calabar, Cross River State; 3 Abakpa Rd, PO Box 923, Kaduna; New Nigeria Bank Bldg, Ahmadu Bello Way, Jos, Plateau State; 5 Bunza Rd, PMB 2341, Sokoto; 18 Offa Rd, Ilorin, Kwara State

Date of Establishment: 10th November 1967

ALLIED BANK OF NIGERIA LTD
22 Breadfruit St, PMB 12785, Lagos
Tel: 662976, 664060,664085
Cable: Alliedbank
Telex: 21512 String Ng

Chairman: Chief Obi A Woluchem
Directors: Muthar Bello (Chief Executive)
Senior Executives: S K Banerjee (Executive Director),
D S Udo-Inyang (Executive Director)

PRINCIPAL ACTIVITIES: Commercial banking
Branch Offices: 47/48 Breadfruit St, PO Box 1252, Lagos; 11 Lebanon St, PMB 5417, Ibadan, Oyo State; Plot 11 Block E, Oshodi Ind Estate, PMB 21602 Ilupeju-Lagos; 2 Oguta Rd, PMB 1618, Onitsha, Anambra State; 3A Ahmadu Bello Way, Kaduna; 26 Post Office Rd, Kano; Quary Rd, PMB 2066, Abeokuta; Point Block, Secretariat Complex, Trans Amadi Layout, Port Harcourt - Rivers State
Associated Companies: Bank of India; Chemical Bank; Bankers Trust Co
Principal Bankers: Central Bank of Nigeria
Financial Information:

	₦'000
Authorised capital	10,000
Paid-up capital	6,000
Turnover (gross earning)	17,000
Profits	5,000

Principal Shareholders: Federal Government of Nigeria; Bank of India Bombay; Individual Nigerian Shareholders
Date of Establishment: 10th September 1962 (formerly Bank of India (Nig) Ltd)
No of Employees: 450

ALLIED BENDIX LTD
9 Ibekwe St, PO Box 1797, Onitsha, Anambra State
Tel: 211463

PRINCIPAL ACTIVITIES: Suppliers of steel security doors and safety equipment
Financial Information:
Registered capital ₦ 100,000

Date of Establishment: December 1977

ALLIED BISCUIT COMPANY LTD
Plot 8 Block K, Isolo Express Way, PO Box 5590, Lagos
PRINCIPAL ACTIVITIES: Food manufacturers
Financial Information:
Registered capital ₦ 100,000

Date of Establishment: June 1976

ALLIED ELECTRONICS & TELECOMMUNICATIONS SERVICES LTD
9A, 28 Ogui Rd, PO Box 286, Enugu, Anambra State
Tel: 253673
Telex: 51170 Alecco Ng

PRINCIPAL ACTIVITIES: Suppliers of electronic, electrical and telecommunication equipment; electrical engineering contractors
Branch Offices: 29 Ahmadu Bello Rd, PO Box 967, Jos, Plateau State; Ahmadu Bello Way, PO Box 624, Kaduna, Tel 211409, Telex 71174; Alecco Ng

ALLIED METAL & CHEMICAL WORKS LTD
PO Box 151, Ikeja Industrial Estate, Ikeja, Lagos
Tel: 964449

PRINCIPAL ACTIVITIES: Manufacturing of galvanised buckets, tin bowls, bottle caps, kerosene stoves

ALLIED OILFIELD SERVICES (NIGERIA) LTD (AOS)
39 Norman Williams St, Ikoyl Island, PO Box 5628, Lagos
Tel: 680781, 681243, 682999
Cable: Oiltools Lagos
Telex: 0

Directors: A L Woodworth (Managing Director),
H Fricke (Managing, Port Harcourt)

PRINCIPAL ACTIVITIES: Oil services and equipment suppliers; pipe inspectors
Principal Agencies: Brinadd; Cabot; Hughes Tool; Ingersoll Rand; Joy Petroleum Equipment; AMF Tuboscope; Page Oil Tools etc
Branch Offices: Field Office: PO Box 934, Port Harcourt, River State PMB 1071, Warri, Bendel State

ALLIED TRADING CO LTD
126/130 Nnamdi Azikiwe St, PO Box 655, Lagos
Tel: 663103, 661534
Cable: Alltrades
Telex: 20117 TDS Box 644

Chairman: T H Dalamal
Directors: R H Notaney, Dr Awosika, Mrs M A Agbaje, G Oshuchukwu
Senior Executives: H T Gadhia (General Manager)

PRINCIPAL ACTIVITIES: Importers and wholesalers of general merchandise
Principal Agencies: China National Import & Export Corp
Branch Offices: 69 Balogun St, Lagos; 15 Ereko St, Lagos; 47 Fegge-Takudu, Kano
Subsidiary/Associated Companies: Dalamal Textile Mills Ltd (DALTEX); K R International (Nig) Ltd; K R Textiles & Allied Industries Ltd; Bright Star Industries Ltd
Principal Bankers: Bank of India (Nigeria) Ltd; Union Bank of Nigeria Ltd; United Bank for Africa Ltd; Arab Bank Nigeria Ltd; Allied Bank (Nigeria) Ltd
Financial Information:

	N'000
Authorised capital	240
Paid-up capital	240
Sales turnover	20,000

Principal Shareholders: T H Dalamal; Mrs M A Agbaje
Date of Establishment: 1955

ALLSCOPE COMMUNICATIONS (NIGERIA) LTD
11 Kehinde Akamo Crescent, Ilupeju Estate, Lagos

PRINCIPAL ACTIVITIES: Suppliers, installers, servicers of all ranges of telecommunications equipment

ALLWELL BROWN AND COMPANY
18 Abonnema Wharf Rd, PO Box 242, Port Harcourt
Tel: 335504

Senior Executives: Senibo Allwell-Brown (Partner)

PRINCIPAL ACTIVITIES: Chartered accountants
Branch Offices: 73 Ikwerre Rd, PO Box 242, Port Harcourt
Principal Bankers: Pan African Bank Ltd; International Bank for West Africa Ltd

Date of Establishment: 1974
No of Employees: 30

ALPHA INDUSTRIES (NIGERIA) LTD
PO Box 224, Ikare-Akoko, Ondo State
PRINCIPAL ACTIVITIES: Printing and paper converters
Date of Establishment: 1977

ALRAINE (NIGERIA) LTD
26 Creek Rd, PO Box 2206, Apapa, Lagos
Tel: 803470/4
Cable: Freight Lagos
Telex: 21244 Freight Ng

Chairman: M T Mbu
Directors: Alhaji Shehu Malami, H de Bretteville, Gert J Hjort (Managing Director), R S Martinsen, Rtd Col A Ochefu, Mrs C Mbu
Senior Executives: W Mackenna (Director Shipping and Marine Services Division), D Sigaud (Finance & International Transport Director), H Wichers (Deputy Managing Director), G Hjort (Executive Vice-Chairman/Managing Director)

PRINCIPAL ACTIVITIES: Shipping, marine services, brokerage, chartering, clearing, forwarding, transit, warehousing, container operators, transport, airfreight; deconsolidation terminals
Branch Offices: 26 Yolawa St, PO Box 144, Kano; Plot C Ahmadu Bello Way, PO Box 304, Kaduna; 9 Robert Rd, PO Box 374, Warri; Custom Rd, PO Box 622, Port Harcourt; 65 Marina, PO Box 10, Calabar
Associated Companies: SCAC Paris; Scanafric Copenhagen
Principal Bankers: United Bank of Africa Ltd; First Bank of Nigeria Ltd; International Bank for West Africa Ltd; Chase Merchant Bank
Financial Information:

	N'000
Authorised capital	6,000
Paid-up capital	3,827

Principal Shareholders: Nigerian Capital (60%); Overseas Capital (40%)
Date of Establishment: October 1957
No of Employees: 900

ALUMINIUM MANUFACTURING COMPANY OF NIGERIA LTD
ALUMACO
32 Creek Rd, PO Box 60, Apapa, Lagos
Tel: 803270/2
Telex: 21347 Alumaco

Chairman: Chief S L Edu
Directors: Alhaji Baba Dambappa, F O Ogunlana, Dr E Fot, Dr M Voser, G L Pellow, A Schmidweber
Senior Executives: C Ugboko (Administration Manager), C Ajayi (Company Secretary), J Afolabi (Personnel Manager), Alhaji Kasali (Special Duties/Production Manager), P Orji (Purchasing Manager), Alhaji L Sonubi (Public Relations Manager)

PRINCIPAL ACTIVITIES: Application of aluminium into kitchen utensils, building components, cold rooms, roofing and cladding sheets, vehicle bodies, containers, prefab houses
Principal Agencies: Alusuisse, Zurich
Branch Offices: 26A Zik Ave, Uwani-Enugu; 8 Ahmadu Bello Way, Kaduna; 106 Lagos By Pass, PO Box 1717, Oke-Ado, Ibadan, Oyo State; Plant Location; Off Oshodi/Isolo Expressway, Behind Aswani Textiles, Lagos State, Tel 964907, 960772
Principal Bankers: United Bank for Africa

Principal Shareholders: Swiss Aluminium Ltd
Date of Establishment: 25th January 1960
No of Employees: 1,500

ALUSTEEL CONSTRUCTION LTD
Trans Amadi Layout, PO Box 226, Port Harcourt, Rivers State
Tel: 21115
Cable: Alusteel Port Harcourt

PRINCIPAL ACTIVITIES: Construction in aluminium and steel

AMAGRA INTERNATIONAL MUSIC HOUSE
33 Enugu Rd, PO Box 2538, Kano

PRINCIPAL ACTIVITIES: Wholesalers for records
Branch Offices: 60 Aitken Rd, Sabon Gari, Kano

AMAGROUP ENGINEERS LTD
18 Harbour Rd, Port Harcourt, PO Box 368, Rivers State
PRINCIPAL ACTIVITIES: Structural and civil engineers

AMALGAMATED INDUSTRIES LTD
PO Box 1196, 19a Airport Rd, Kano
Tel: 4430

PRINCIPAL ACTIVITIES: Manufacturing paper bags

AMALGAMATED TIN MINES OF NIGERIA LTD
PMB 2036, Bukuru Headquarters, Jos, Plateau State
Tel: Bukuru 432/4 or Jos 53095
Cable: Amaltinig
Telex: 81367 Atmn Ng

Chairman: D M Dent-Young (also Chief Executive)
Directors: Encik Abdul Rahim Aki, E A Ifaturoti, Alhaji R Lukman, G Gardiner
Senior Executives: C W Bull (Chief Accountant), J A R Wilson (Production Manager), J I Adewale (Company Secretary)

PRINCIPAL ACTIVITIES: Production of tin concentrate from ore and separation of columbite
Subsidiary Companies: A O Nigeria Ltd
Principal Bankers: First Bank of Nigeria Ltd; Union Bank of Nigeria Ltd
Financial Information:

	N'000
Authorised capital	4,000
Paid-up capital	3,000
Turnover	12,163
Profits	260

Principal Shareholders: Nigerian Mining Corporation (58%); Amalgamated Tin Mines of Nigeria (Holdings) Ltd, UK (40%)
Date of Establishment: 1939; deemed to be Nigerian Company in 1968
No of Employees: 1,887

AMALIGHTERAGE & TIMBER EXPORTING CO LTD
18 Harbour Rd, Port Harcourt, Rivers State

PRINCIPAL ACTIVITIES: Lighterage, land transport, ship chandlers and saw mill operations
Branch Offices: Apapa

AMANA CONSTRUCTION CO (NIGERIA) LTD (ACC Ltd)
PO Box 713, Jos, Plateau State
Tel: 2584

Chairman: Ezekiel Washik

PRINCIPAL ACTIVITIES: Building and civil engineering contractors

AMANA CONSULTING ENGINEERS
12 Military Street, CPO Box 4838, Lagos
Tel: 631965, 634630
Cable: Desamamana, Lagos
Telex: 22301 Desam Ng

Directors: Engr Dr E J Amana, Engr A U N Uwe

PRINCIPAL ACTIVITIES: Consulting, civil, structural, water and sewage engineers
Associated Companies: Desam Development Co; International Agroindustries Development Co Ltd
Principal Bankers: First Bank of Nigeria Ltd; Mercantile Bank of Nigeria Ltd; ICON Ltd; United Bank for Africa Ltd

AMARI MINES LTD
Mile 92, Jos-Wamba Rd, PO Box 394, Jos, Plateau State

PRINCIPAL ACTIVITIES: Mining of metal ore
Financial Information: An associate of Selection Trust Ltd, of London

AMARILLO UMBRELLA COMPANY (NIGERIA) LTD

Plot A, Oregun Industrial Estate, PO Box 9361, Lagos
Cable: Umbrella Lagos
Telex: 26234

Chairman: Fred Egbe
Directors: Lachman Hariram, M Aina John, Lachoo Sakhrani, Hadji Bakre Anjorin, Harish Chulani, C Egbe
Senior Executives: Samson Morogbowon (Sales Manager)

PRINCIPAL ACTIVITIES: Manufacture of all type of umbrellas
Principal Bankers: United Bank for Africa Ltd
Financial Information:

	N'000
Authorised capital	400
Paid-up capital	120

Principal Shareholders: Lachman Hariram; M Aina John; Harish Chulani; Hadi Bakre Anjorin; Fred Egbe
Date of Establishment: 1979
No of Employees: 200

AMASS NIGERIA LTD

11 Gbajumo Street, PO Box 4891, Lagos
Tel: 662094
Cable: Amass, Lagos
Telex: 21276 Amass Ng

PRINCIPAL ACTIVITIES: Suppliers of domestic and industrial security products. Insurance investigators, security consultants and general merchants

AMATEMESO SHIPPING AGENCIES LTD

18 Harbour Rd, PO Box 368, Port Harcourt, Rivers State
Tel: 228040
Cable: Amaship
Telex: 21467 Amship Ng

PRINCIPAL ACTIVITIES: Stevedores, shipping agents, ship owners, ship-brokers, clearing and forwarding agents
Principal Agencies: G A Lopez Forwarding & Shipping Co Inc, USA; Adams Transport Co A/S, Denmark; Scandia Liner Agency, Denmark; Scheffler Co, West Germany; Amalighterage & Timber Exporting Co Ltd, Port Harcourt; Amagroup Engineers Ltd, Port Harcourt; Amatemesa Shipping Agencies (UK) Ltd; Amara International Corporation BV, Holland
Branch Offices: Apapa; Warri

AMBROSINI, L, LTD

PO Box 2, 31/32 Niger St, Kano, Kano State
Tel: 2057, 3045

PRINCIPAL ACTIVITIES: Exporters of hides and skins

AMCORD NIGERIA LTD

Mandilas Building, 35 Simpson St, Lagos
President: Harry Akande
PRINCIPAL ACTIVITIES: Construction

AMDUMAC GROUP (NIGERIA) LTD

39 Norman Williams St, PO Box 7403, Lagos
Tel: 681243

PRINCIPAL ACTIVITIES: Oil and gas services
Associated Companies: Porta-Kamp

AMENIGER CONSTRUCTION COMPANY LTD

61 Adelabu St, PO Box 1034, Surulere, Lagos
Cable: Niamerger, Lagos

Chairman: Prince Adeleye Orisagbemi
Directors: Miss Norma Kilway,
James Aluko,
Ademola Adeleye (Director of Administration),
Chief Dapo Daramola (Director for Public Affairs),
Charles Kruse (Projects Director),

Alhaji Kola Animasaun (Associate Projects Director)

PRINCIPAL ACTIVITIES: Architecture; civil engineering and construction; electrical engineering; engineering consultants
Branch Offices: 46 Oyensekun Rd, Akure, Ondo State
Associated Companies: Scandinavian International Consulting Ltd; Kema Nord (Specialty Chemicals Division)
Principal Bankers: Arab Bank (Nigeria) Ltd
Financial Information:

	N'000
Authorised capital	400
Paid-up capital	400
Sales turnover	4,000

Date of Establishment: 500

AMERICAN INTERNATIONAL INSURANCE

200 Broad St, PO Box 2577, Lagos
Tel: 662505, 662573
Cable: Amerlife

Chairman: Alhaji A A Sanusi
Directors: H R Ritter, G A Abonzeid, E C Dobbs, R O U Eronini, D A Marioghae, J I Ahom
Senior Executives: H R Ritter, K O Olufeko, A A Oshodi, P Otojerari, P O'Rourke

PRINCIPAL ACTIVITIES: Insurance and reinsurance
Branch Offices: Aba; Enugu; Benin City; Ibadan; Jos; Kano; Zaria; Ilorin; Lagos
Subsidiary Companies: (ALICO) American Life Insurance Company
Principal Bankers: First Bank Nigeria Ltd; Union Bank of Nigeria; Savannah Bank
Financial Information:

	N'000
Authorised capital	2,000
Paid-up capital	1,200
Turnover	15,860
Profits	820

Principal Shareholders: Nigerian Government, Alico
Date of Establishment: 23rd July 1968
No of Employees: 306

AMERICO LTD

PO Box 1394, 22 Oritshe St, Ikeja, Lagos
Tel: 962808
Cable: Amurulag Lagos

Chairman: Chief Dr G J Amurum (also Managing Director)
Directors: Lucian A Gallinari, P G M Porbeni

PRINCIPAL ACTIVITIES: Manufacturer' representatives, construction management, project consultants, industrial promotions
Principal Agencies: S Marco, SPA, Italy; Brezina Construction Inc, USA; Capp Plastic SPA, Italy
Branch Offices: PO Box 25 Effurun Warri, Bendel State
Subsidiary Companies: Dacota Nigeria Const Ltd
Principal Bankers: Bank of the North Ltd
Financial Information:

Authorised capital	N 100,000

Principal Shareholders: Chief Dr George J Amurun; Dr Lucian A Gallinari
Date of Establishment: 1965

AMEY ROADSTONE COMPANY (NIGERIA) LTD

(ARC (NIG) Ltd)

PO Box 8088, Plot iv, Planning Way, Ilupeju, Ikeja, Lagos
Tel: 962151/2

Chairman: Chief O B Akin-Olugbade
Directors: D V Phillips (Managing),
Chief S O Lambo,
D G S Mardall,
J C Jones

PRINCIPAL ACTIVITIES: Civil engineering and construction
Branch Offices: Badagry Expressway, Lagos; 10 Lamido Crescent, Kano
Principal Bankers: United Bank for Africa Ltd
Date of Establishment: 1974
No of Employees: 1,000

AMICABLE ASSURANCE COMPANY LTD

(Formerly Nigerian Amicable Assurance Company Ltd)

126/130 Nnamdi Azikiwe St, PO Box 4715, Lagos
Tel: 661861, 663511, 66472
Cable: Amicable

Chairman: P A Adeyemo (also Managing Director)
Directors: E Adesioye,
M A Fagbayi,
B A Adeyemo,
M A Awofisayo,
V O Adesakin (General Manager)

PRINCIPAL ACTIVITIES: Insurance
Branch Offices: Ile-Ife; Ibadan; Aba; Onitsha
Financial Information:

	N'000
Authorised capital	500
Paid-up capital	320

AMINCI INTERNATIONAL CO LTD

166 Clifford St, Yaba, Lagos
Tel: 843270

Directors: A D Mohammed (Managing Director)

PRINCIPAL ACTIVITIES: Construction

ANALEX GROUP LTD

5 Railay Commercial Layout, Station Rd, PO Box 1165, Enugu, Anambra State
Tel: 254607
Cable: Analex

Chairman: Engineer Anayo A Nkwonta
Directors: Mrs F O Okoye
Senior Executives: Engineer C Arora (Chief Electrical Engineer), Henry Etche (Assistant Chief Engineer), R N C Nwosu (Transport Manager), Peter Nkwonta (Purchasing Manager)

PRINCIPAL ACTIVITIES: Electrical, mechanical and civil/building engineering contractors
Branch Offices: 372 H Macaulay St, Box 8266, Yaba, Lagos, Tel 960669
Principal Bankers: Co-operative Bank of Eastern Nigeria; African Continental Bank
Financial Information:

	N'000
Authorised capital	1,000
Paid-up capital	1,000
Turnover	4,500
Profits	2,300

Date of Establishment: 1978
No of Employees: 180

ANAMAPHARMACEUTICAL INDUSTRIES LTD

6 Caulcrik, Apapa, Lagos

PRINCIPAL ACTIVITIES: Manufacturing of pharmaceuticals
Financial Information: Associate of Undeco Ltd, Lagos

ANAMBRA MOTOR MANUFACTURING CO LTD

(ANAMMCO)

PO Box 2523, Enugu, Anambra State

Chairman: Sir Joseph Nwankwu
Directors: R Hoh (Managing)

PRINCIPAL ACTIVITIES: Manufacturing of lorries
Branch Offices: Location: Emene Industrial Layout, Emene, Anambra State; 25 Glove Rd, Ikoyi, PMB 12544, Lagos, Tel 681790

Principal Shareholders: Federal, Anambra, Imo, Rivers State Government; Daimler-Benz AG, Germany; Leventis Motors Ltd; Nigerian Public
No of Employees: 1,200

ANAMBRA VEGETABLE OILS PRODUCTS NIGERIA LTD
(AVOP)

Agricultural Development Corporation, PMB 1024, Enugu, Anambra State
Tel: 253029, 253463, 252544
Cable: Agrico Enugu
Telex: 51151 Agrico

PRINCIPAL ACTIVITIES: Production of cooking oil, salad oil, margarine, toilet soap and glycerine

Principal Shareholders: Anambra State Government

ANASORO BUILDERS

3 Amigbo Lane, Uwani, Enugu, Anambra State

PRINCIPAL ACTIVITIES: Building contractors

ANBAR ENTERPRISES LTD

PO Box 445, Apapa, Lagos

PRINCIPAL ACTIVITIES: Building and civil engineering contractors

ANGLO-FRENCH TRADING CO LTD

PO Box 381, 35/37 Martin St, Lagos
Tel: 653546

PRINCIPAL ACTIVITIES: Importers and exporters and distributors of general merchandise

ANGLO-GERMAN COMPANY (INTERCONTINENTAL) LTD

Susannah House, Near Federal Sub Post Office Buildings, PO Box 1700, Warri, Bendel State

Chairman: Chief J A O'Bahor
Directors: HRH Prince J A O'Bahor (Managing Director), W A O'Bahor, Mrs S Bazunu-O'Bahor
Senior Executives: S Orr, R Srinivasan, M Chang

PRINCIPAL ACTIVITIES: Importers and exporters of general merchandise; mechanical engineers; civil engineering and construction; suppliers of computers etc
Principal Agencies: Star Enterprises Investment Corporation; Export Markt Organisation; Isar Rakoll Chemie GmbH; Flosser GmbH & Company; Merkur (Aussenhandel) GmbH & Company; Friedrich Krupp GmbH; Elin-Union AG; Isocommerz GmbH; Voest-Alpine AG; Veba Oel AG; Robotron Export-Import etc
Principal Bankers: Union Bank of Nigeria Ltd
Financial Information:

	N'000
Authorised capital	3,000
Paid-up capital	1,500
Turnover	3,500
Profits	350

Principal Shareholders: Chairman and directors as described
Date of Establishment: 30th October 1978
No of Employees: 150

ANGLO-NORMAN SHIPPING (NIGERIA) LTD
ANSIL

14 Ado Avenue, Apapa, Lagos
Tel: 681482
Cable: Ansiline Lagos
Telex: 21395

PRINCIPAL ACTIVITIES: Shipping

ANOMBEM MOKWUNYE, TWIGG, BROWN & PARTNERS

37 Campbell Street, PO Box 4017, Lagos
Tel: 635149, 633109

Senior Partners: Arc Anombem Mokwunye
Partners: Arc Michael W Twigg, Arc William K Brown

PRINCIPAL ACTIVITIES: Chartered architects and planning consultants
Branch Offices: Imaro House, Murtala Mohammed Way, PMB 1329, Benin City, Bendel State; 4 Rwang Pam Street, PO Box 1240, Jos, Plateau State

ANOPIT LTD

9 Yoruba Rd, PO Box 6263, Kano
Tel: 5503, 5541
Cable: Anopit Kn
Telex: 77150 Anopit Ng

PRINCIPAL ACTIVITIES: Clearing, forwarding, shipping, airfreighting services
Branch Offices: 190 Idewu St, Off Kirikiri-Olodi, PMB 1300, Apapa, Lagos, Cable Anopit Apn Apapa; 8 Jemaa Rd, Off Abubakar Kigo Rd, Kaduna, Cable Anopit Kd Kaduna

APAPA CHEMICAL INDUSTRIES LTD

Malu Rd, PO Box 10, Apapa, Lagos
Tel: 874660, 877169

PRINCIPAL ACTIVITIES: Production of carbon dioxide used in bottling plants
Financial Information: Associate of Nigerian Bottling Co Ltd

APARAKI ENTERPRISES

PO Box 2697, 7th Floor, 9 Nnamdi Azikiwe Street, Lagos
Tel: 660725
Cable: Omoaparaki, Lagos
Telex: 21204 Damex Ng

Chairman: Dayo Megbope
Directors: Mrs Funmi Megbope, Femi Megbope
Senior Executives: Dafe Ebiuwe (Financial Controller), Yomi Odunuga (Sales Executive)

PRINCIPAL ACTIVITIES: Importers and exporters of general merchandise, agricultural equipment and building materials
Principal Agencies: Sidert srl, Italy
Branch Offices: 136 Isolo Rd, Mushin Lagos State
Principal Bankers: Bank of the North, Lagos
Financial Information:

	N'000
Authorised capital	500
Paid-up capital	250
Turnover	4,500

Principal Shareholders: Dayo Megbope; Funmi Megbope
Date of Establishment: 1968
No of Employees: 35

APC INTERNATIONAL NIGERIA LTD

7th Floor, Lapal House, 241 Igbosere Rd, Lagos
Tel: 611539
Cable: Apcin
Telex: 21480

Chairman: Sunday Dankaro
Directors: Chief E A Silva, A Massey, F A Hammond, R Vollenweider
Senior Executives: K J Brett (General Manager), S C Jones (Senior Manager), D B Lamond (Senior Manager)
PRINCIPAL ACTIVITIES: Project management and development consultancy
Branch Offices: Gidan Shehu Ahmed, Bank Rd, Kano, PO Box 422, Tel 2557, Telex 77221
Principal Bankers: United Bank for Africa
Principal Shareholders: Subsidiary of APC International, UK

APEX (EASTERN NIGERIA) LTD

Plot 18, Trans Amadi Industrial Layout, PMB 5073, Port Harcourt, Rivers State
Tel: 227033
Cable: Apex PH
Telex: 61151

PRINCIPAL ACTIVITIES: Stationery manufacturers
Financial Information: Associate of Thomas Wyatt Nigeria Ltd, Ebute-Metta, Lagos

APEX PAINTS LTD

KM 93, Lagos-Abeokuta Rd, PO Box 2073, Abeokuta, Ogun State

Chairman: Chief A O Abudu
Directors: M A Ololade, M A Abudu, R D Chandaria
PRINCIPAL ACTIVITIES: Manufacturers of paint
Branch Offices: 2 Alabi St, PO Box 2410, Ikeja, Lagos; 21 Modube Avenue, PO Box 4090, Onitsha
Principal Bankers: United Bank for Africa Ltd
Financial Information:

	N'000
Authorised capital	1,000
Paid-up capital	370
Turnover	1,500

Date of Establishment: Prodution started May 1981
No of Employees: 60

APROFIM ENGINEERING CONSTRUCTION COMPANY (NIGERIA) LTD

PO Box 2916, Lagos
Tel: 615898, 616762
Cable: Acont Lagos
Telex: 21387 Acont Ng

Chairman: N D Gaon
Directors: Alhaji Yakubu, J O Adalumo
Senior Executives: N G Moore (Managing)

PRINCIPAL ACTIVITIES: Civil engineering and construction
Branch Offices: Location: 23B Idejo St, Plot 976, Victoria Island, Lagos
Associated Companies: Aprofim Agence De Promotion et Financement Immobiliers SA, Geneva, Switzerland
Principal Bankers: International Bank for West Africa Ltd; United Bank for Africa Ltd
Financial Information:

	N'000
Authorised capital	500
Paid-up capital	100

Principal Shareholders: N D Gaon; Alhaji Yakubu; J O Adalumo
Date of Establishment: 11th September 1975

ARATAH, JOSMAN, TRADING COMPANY

26 Odion Rd, Warri, Bendel State

Directors: Joseph O Akpotiwhe (Managing Director)
PRINCIPAL ACTIVITIES: General traders

ARAX AIRLINES LTD

Head Office, 47 Marina, 8th Floor, Lagos Island, PO Box 2310, Lagos
Tel: 653875, 963863
Cable: Araxsi Lagos

Chairman: H O Omenai (also Managing Director)
PRINCIPAL ACTIVITIES: Aviation services to the oil industry

ARBICO LTD

Plot D Block VII Industrial Crescent, Ilupeju, PMB 2040, Lagos
Tel: 962693

Chairman: B C Economides (also Managing Director)
Directors: Chief L O Edet, Chief H O Davies, C S Irune, P Economides, G A David

PRINCIPAL ACTIVITIES: Civil engineering and construction
Branch Offices: Benin City, Bendel State
Subsidiary Companies: Nigeria Button Manufacturing Company Ltd; ECO Furniture Ltd
Principal Bankers: United Bank for Africa Ltd; Union Bank of Nigeria Ltd; First Bank of Nigeria Ltd; New Nigeria Bank Ltd

Date of Establishment: 1958
No of Employees: 3,500

ARBOR SERVICES NIGERIA LTD

23-25 Martins St, PO Box 2778, Lagos
Tel: 651065
Cable: Arboreal Lagos

Chairman: Benjamin Akinboro
Directors: Mrs Esther Ayodele Akinboro
Senior Executives: B A Akinboro (Managing Director), E B Sorinwa (Company Secretary), R A Ogunade (Public Relations Manager), Charles Ogunmodede (Sales Executive)

PRINCIPAL ACTIVITIES: Stationers, booksellers, importers, general merchants and manufacturers' representatives
Principal Agencies: Caffrey Saunders & Co Ltd, UK
Branch Offices: 55B Western Ave, Surulere, Lagos State
Associated Companies: Ben Agency Service, Lagos
Principal Bankers: Union Bank of Nigeria Ltd

Principal Shareholders: B A Akinboro; E A Akinboro

ARCEE TEXTILE INDUSTRIES LTD

PO Box 3982, Lagos
Tel: 843531

PRINCIPAL ACTIVITIES: Textile manufacturers
Branch Offices: Block A Plot 2b Oshodi Industrial Scheme, Mushin, Lagos

ARCHITECHNIQUES

25/27 Raymond St, Yaba, Lagos
Tel: 862904
Cable: Arktekniks Lagos

Directors: Akintunde Olusegun Tejuosos (Partner), Abiodun Oni (Partner)

PRINCIPAL ACTIVITIES: Architectural practice
Principal Bankers: African Continental Bank

Date of Establishment: 1974

ARCHITECTURAL METAL PRODUCTS LTD

Block F Ladipo Street, Oshodi Industrial Estate, PMB 21328, Ikeja, Lagos State
Tel: 964600, 960928
Cable: Mico
Telex: 26232 Manda Ng

Chairman: Chief Adedokun Adeyemi
Directors: R S Cheng (Managing Director),
    S N S Cheng,
    S K MacGregor,
    Chief E O Adeniyi,
    Justice S D Adebiyi,
    Chief O Oyewunmi,
    G O Onabanjo

PRINCIPAL ACTIVITIES: Metal production, aluminium works
Principal Bankers: Savannah Bank of Nigeria Ltd; Icon Ltd
Financial Information:

	N'000
Authorised capital	1,000
Paid-up capital	400
Turnover	3,500
Profits	309

Principal Shareholders: Chiap-Hua Comalco Ltd, Hongkong
Date of Establishment: 1st November 1975
No of Employees: 180

ARC-MODELS COMPANY
Plot 10 Jalupon Estate Extension, Off Bode Thomas Rd,
    Surulere, PO Box 4184, Lagos
Tel: 961821
Cable: Estetiks, Lagos

Chairman: Arc Dr Olawale Odeleye
Senior Executives: Arc O Opoko (Architectural Model
    Maker/Graphic Designer),
    Bayode Edbe (Administrative Manager)

PRINCIPAL ACTIVITIES: Architectural, engineering and town
    planning model markers. Production of finely rendered
    architectural perspective drawings
Associated Companies: Olawale Odeleye Associates (Architects
    & Planners)
Principal Bankers: United Bank for Africa Ltd

Date of Establishment: September 1978

ARCUS CONSULTANT LTD
9B Akarolo Close, PMB 5608, Port Harcourt
Tel: 50279

Chairman: Alhaji A B Umar
Directors: P Keller, A Kessi, Adesupo Odukoya

PRINCIPAL ACTIVITIES: Civil engineers; consultants
Branch Offices: Lagos; Kaduna

AREWA ADVANCEMENT ENTERPRISES LTD
AP2 Gombe Rd, Behind Barclays Bank, PO Box 502, Kaduna
Tel: 243178
Telex: 71154 Araeco Ng

PRINCIPAL ACTIVITIES: Stationers, sales and servicing of office
    and educational equipment
Branch Offices: 3 Crescent Rd, PO Box 382, Zaria, Kaduna
    State, Tel 2588; Kano; Maiduguri; Bauchi; Yola; Minna

AREWA CONSTRUCTION LTD
157/159 Club Rd, PO Box 290, Kano
Tel: 3381, 5173
Cable: Arcol Kano
Telex: 77110 Arcol

Chairman: Alhaji A B Waziri
Directors: P Destefano (Managing Director),
    R Destefano,
    Alhaji Makama Bida,
    Alhaji Abubakar Madi
Senior Executives: J Clough (Financial Controller),
    J Destefano (General Manager)

PRINCIPAL ACTIVITIES: Civil engineering and construction
Branch Offices: Plot H Kaduna South, PO Box 366, Kaduna;
    Kaduna Rd, PO Box 62, Bauchi
Associated Companies: Kano Kiln Ltd
Principal Bankers: United Bank for Africa Ltd
Financial Information:

	N'000
Authorised capital	1,500
Paid-up capital	570
Turnover	12,000
Profits	600

Principal Shareholders: R Destefano; Alhaji A B Waziri; Alhaji M
    Abubakar; Alhaji M Bida; Etsu Nupe; Alhaji S Nogano; Alhaji
    Aminu Dantata; Ahaji Ibrahim El Yanubu
No of Employees: 750

AREWA HOTELS (DEVELOPMENTS) LTD
24 Waff Rd, PMB 2190, Kaduna
Tel: 213076
Cable: Arewotels
Telex: 71124 Arotel Ng

Chairman: Mallam Ahmed Talib
Directors: Mallam Hamza Zayyad, A A Feese, Alhaji T A Sanni,
    Alhaji S U Wunti, Dr H I Adum, Alhaji Halilu Usman Bida,
    Alhaji Tatari Ali, Alhaji Muhammed Suleiman
Senior Executives: Ibrahim Katune (General Manager),
    Isa Yusuf (Financial Controller),
    Ibrahim Dapci (Company Secretary),
    Michael Knight (Operations Manager),
    George Verghese (Senior Development Manager)

PRINCIPAL ACTIVITIES: Hotel investment, development,
    management, consultancy
Branch Offices: Hotels under management: Durbar Hotel, PMB
    2218, Kaduna; Zaria Hotel, PMB 1066, Zaria; Lake Chad
    Hotel, PO Box 368, Maiduguri; Sokoto Hotel, PMB 2199,
    Sokoto; Hamdala Hotel, PO Box 311, Kaduna
Associated Companies: Northern Bakeries Ltd, Kaduna
Principal Bankers: Bank of the North Ltd
Financial Information:

	N'000
Authorised capital	2,500
Paid-up capital	100

Principal Shareholders: New Nigerian Development Company
    Ltd
No of Employees: 1,350

AREWA METAL CONTAINERS LTD (ARMECO)
PO Box 270, Kaduna South, Kaduna State
Tel: 243332, 242443
Cable: Armeco
Telex: 71105 Armeco Ng

Directors: Sig Carlo De Paulis (Director)

PRINCIPAL ACTIVITIES: Metal products manufacturers
Branch Offices: PO Box 4589, Kano, Tel 5030

AREWA STEEL WORKS COMPANY (NIG) LTD
75 Sharada Industrial Area, Phase 2, PO Box 706, Kano
Tel: 3363, 5283, 4751
Cable: Arewa Steel Works, Kano
Telex: 77258 Daye Kh

Chairman: Ali Habib Dayekh
Directors: Hassan A Dayekh,
    Hussein A Dayekh,
    Alhaji Sule Katagun,
    Alhaji K Umor,
    Ibrahim Abdul Aziz (Chief Accountant)

PRINCIPAL ACTIVITIES: Manufacturers of steel structures, water tanks, drying sheds, suppliers of building materials, trailers, grain storage silos, etc
Principal Bankers: Union Bank of Nigeria Ltd; Bank of the North Ltd
Financial Information:

	N'000
Authorised capital	400
Paid-up capital	400
Turnover	2,000

Principal Shareholders: A H Dayekh
Date of Establishment: 1969
No of Employees: 160

AREWA TEXTILES LTD
PO Box 288, Kaduna
Tel: 213495, 211674, 213510
Cable: Arewatex
Telex: 7111 Ng

Chairman: Alhaji Abubakar Tunau
Directors: S Ishii (Managing Director),
  Alhaji Abu Gidado (General Manager),
  K Fukao,
  T Yubisui,
  S Miyoshi,
  E Hori,
  T Ishizaki,
  M M Aliyu,
  Y S Kasimu,
  Alhaji H Abdulkadir

PRINCIPAL ACTIVITIES: Textile manufacturing
Branch Offices: 4th Floor Wesley House, 21/22 Marina, Lagos, Tel 633800, 633802, Telex 21514; 1 Civic Centre, PO Box 4965, Kano Tel 5090
Principal Bankers: Union Bank (Nig) Ltd
Financial Information:

	N'000
Authorised capital	10,000
Paid-up capital	8,107
Turnover	48,000
Profits	4,736

Principal Shareholders: Overseas Spinning Investment Co Ltd, Japan; Northern Nigeria Investment Ltd; International Finance Corporation, USA; Kuwait Investment Co; Barclays Overseas Development Co
Date of Establishment: 1963
No of Employees: 3,600

AREWA TRADEWINDS (NIG) CO LTD
Jingiri Rd, Bukuru Bye Pass, PMB 2089, Jos, Plateau State
Tel: 3589

PRINCIPAL ACTIVITIES: Importers and suppliers of hardware and building materials

AREWA UNITED STORES LTD
18-19 Ahmadu Bello Way, PO Box 454, Kaduna

PRINCIPAL ACTIVITIES: Suppliers of wholesale piece goods and general merchandise

ARIDI INDUSTRIES (NIGERIA) LTD
146 Upper Uselu-Lagos Rd, PO Box 418, Benin City, Bendel State
Tel: 242746
Cable: Aridi Industries, Benin
Telex: 44310 Aini

Chairman: K S Aridi (also Managing Director)
Directors: A S Aridi, E O Adeghe
Senior Executives: B F Magazinovic (General Manager),
  P Umude (Sales Manager),
  P A Mosindi (Chief Accountant)

PRINCIPAL ACTIVITIES: Manufacturers of wooden and steel furniture for schools, offices and home use; steel structures, water tanks, building of motor vehicles and other metal products
Associated Companies: Arigab Construction Company (Nig) Ltd; Maya Building & Construction Co (Nig) Ltd
Principal Bankers: New Nigeria Bank Ltd; Arab Bank Ltd
Financial Information:

	N'000
Authorised capital	400
Paid-up capital	400
Sales turnover	1,500
Profits (approx)	200

Principal Shareholders: K S Aridi; A S Aridi; E O Adeghe
Date of Establishment: 19th December 1969
No of Employees: 130

ARIGAS CONSTRUCTION COMPANY NIGERIA LTD
129 Lagos St, Benin City, Bendel State

PRINCIPAL ACTIVITIES: Civil engineering and construction
Financial Information:
Authorised capital   N 500,000

Date of Establishment: April 1975

ARK STEWART WRIGHTSON
New Africa House, 31 Marina, PO Box 3771, Lagos
Tel: 660346, 662381, 663799
Cable: Insurark Lagos
Telex: 22652

Chairman: F O Awogboro
Directors: J D Rowland,
  A M Soetan,
  G M Whale (Managing Director),
  A I Dasuki,
  L G Stevenson,
  T T Harding,
  M O Adesunloye
Senior Executives: S A Arinoso (Asst. General Manager),
  R B Ajayi (Asst. General Manager - Finance),
  F B Solar (Asst. General Manager - Technical),
  H B E Robson (Training Officer)

PRINCIPAL ACTIVITIES: Insurance brokers
Branch Offices: 41 Allen Avenue, Ikeja Lagos; 33 Murtala Mohammed Way, PO Box 2854, Jos; Murtala Mohammed Way, PO Box 4638, Kano; Plot 268 Trans Amadi Layout, PMB 5525, Port Harcourt
Associated Companies: Stewart Wrightson Group
Principal Bankers: First Bank of Nigeria Ltd; Societe Generale Bank (Nigeria) Ltd

Date of Establishment: January 1976

AROMOLARAN PUBLISHERS NIGERIA LTD
PO Box 1800, Ibadan, Oyo State

Directors: Adekunle Aromolaran (Managing)

PRINCIPAL ACTIVITIES: Publishers of general and educational books

ARONAOUT COMMUNICATIONS LTD
162 Lagos Bye Pass, Oke-Ado, PO Box 3159, Ibadan, Oyo State

Chairman: J O Arowolo (also Managing Director)
Directors: Mohammed Aronaout

PRINCIPAL ACTIVITIES: Telecommunications supply and service
No of Employees: 70

ARROWAYS OF NIGERIA
70/71 Airport Rd, Ikeja, Lagos
Tel: 932780, 961278

Chairman: Jimmy Arogundade

PRINCIPAL ACTIVITIES: Dealers in aquarium and pet products; decorator and glass merchant
Principal Bankers: International Bank for West Africa

ARROWHEAD INSURANCE CO (NIG) LTD

131 Broad St, PO Box 6071, Lagos
Tel: 662183

PRINCIPAL ACTIVITIES: Insurance

ARTHUR ANDERSEN & COMPANY

74B Adetokunbo Ademola St, Victoria Island, PO Box 51204, Falomo, Lagos
Tel: 610774, 610754, 610785
Telex: 21605 Artlag Ng

Directors: R L Kramer (Managing Partner)
Senior Executives: A Bawa, C C Holden, J O Munis

PRINCIPAL ACTIVITIES: Chartered accountants and management consultants

ARTHUR YOUNG OSINDERO & CO

See YOUNG, ARTHUR, OSINDERO & CO

ASABORO, JOSEPH

PO Box 2, Ikare, Ifon via Owo, Ondo State

PRINCIPAL ACTIVITIES: Suppliers of timber, sawmill

ASAGBA, M A, & SONS

18 Odushelu St, Itire, Surulere, Lagos

Chairman: M Asagba

PRINCIPAL ACTIVITIES: Electrical contractors
Branch Offices: 2 Adeola Rd, Sapele, Bendel State
Principal Bankers: United Bank for Africa Ltd

ASANI (NIGERIA) TRADING CO

28 Matanmi St, Via Kayode St, Igbobi, Lagos State

Directors: J A Adesanya (Managing Director)

PRINCIPAL ACTIVITIES: General trading

ASAPE (NIGERIA) COMPANY LTD

PO Box 1880, Apapa, Lagos

PRINCIPAL ACTIVITIES: Suppliers of pumps, electrical motors etc
Principal Agencies: Ercole Marelli Componenti, Italy
Branch Offices: Office location: 2 Alhaji Karimu Akande St, Kirkiri Jetty, Tin Can Island; Zaria Rd, PO Box 2227, Kano; 23 Ekenwa Rd, Benin City; 8 Isoko Rd, Ughelli, Bendel State; 16 Startyong St, Onitsha, Anambra State

ASEMOTA MOTORS (NIGERIA) LTD

Km 6 Alaba, Lagos-Badagry Expressway, PO Box 6135, Lagos
Tel: 830435, 837296

PRINCIPAL ACTIVITIES: Sales and service of motor vehicles

Date of Establishment: March 1977

ASHAKA CEMENT COMPANY LTD

PMB 3276, Kano
Tel: Lagos 630976
Cable: Ashakacem Lagos
Telex: 21299 Wapcem Ng

Chairman: Alhaji A A Waziri
Directors: R N Ezeife,
   S Y Kasimu,
   A D Stirling,
   R J Whale (Managing),
   A Z Gorgoram,
   J K Shepherd,
   Alhaji I Abba,
   Y H Yero,
   Alhaji A Dukku
Senior Executives: M Eccleston (Financial Controller),
   J A Beale (General Works Manager),
   Alhaji S B Gimba (Personnel Manager),
   Ali Gombe (Marketing Manager)

PRINCIPAL ACTIVITIES: Cement manufacturers
Branch Offices: Ashaka Works, Near Gombe, Bauchi State;
   24/26 McCarthy St, PMB 12696, Lagos; 1 Ahmadu Bello Way, Nassarawa, Kano
Principal Bankers: Bank of the North Ltd; Union Bank (Nigeria) Ltd; United Bank for Africa Ltd
Financial Information:

	N'000
Authorised capital	50,000
Paid-up capital	49,000
Turnover (approx)	60,000

Principal Shareholders: Federal Government of Nigeria, Blue Circle Industries (UK); Nigerian Industrial Development Bank Ltd; Nigerian Bank for Commerce and Industry; Northern Nigeria Investments Ltd; Bauchi, Borno and Gongola State Governments
Date of Establishment: August 1974
No of Employees: 1,000

ASHAMU, E O, & SONS (HOLDINGS) LTD

Oke-Afa/Isolo Rd, PO Box 207, Mushin, Lagos
Tel: 831221, 861853, 862456
Cable: Ashamu
Telex: 26340, 21578 Ashamu Ng

Chairman: Chief Emmanuel Oyedele Ashamu
Directors: Mrs Priscilla D Ashamu, Guenter Friedrich Wilhelm Oskar Stargardt
Senior Executives: Dr Oma A Taiga (Executive Director),
   S D Aluma (Group Company Secretary),
   B Adebayo (Group Financial Controller),
   S K Etea (Group Treasurer)

PRINCIPAL ACTIVITIES: General merchandise, agricultural and agro-allied projects, mining, shipping, clearing and forwarding, real estate agents
Principal Agencies: J B Doumeng Group, France
Branch Offices: Ibadan; Jos; Zaria; Kano; Enugu; Benin City; Calabar; Port-Harcourt
Subsidiary Companies: Oke-Afa Farms Ltd; Ikeja Real Estates Ltd; Agrotec Services Ltd; Igbetti Mining Industries Ltd; Oyo Feeds Company Ltd; New Age Shipping Line Ltd; Nigerian Explosives & Plastics Co Ltd; Pioneer Farms Ltd
Principal Bankers: Union Bank of Nigeria; First Bank; International Bank for West Africa; Societe Generale Bank of Nigeria
Financial Information:

	N'000
Authorised capital	20,000
Paid-up capital	20,000
Turnover	30,000

Principal Shareholders: Chief E O Ashamu; Mrs P D Ashamu
Date of Establishment: 1st May 1954
No of Employees: 3,000

ASHLAND OIL (NIGERIA) COMPANY

PO Box 2629, Lagos
Tel: 614277, 611628, 612657, 613334
Cable: Ashland Oil Lagos
Telex: 21103 Ashoil

Directors: Leon R Volterre (General Manager and Managing Director),
W M Varty (Technical Manager)

PRINCIPAL ACTIVITIES: Oil and gas exploration and production, Ashland Oil (Nigeria) Company has a Production Sharing Contract with the Nigerian National Petroleum Corporation

Branch Offices: 53 Trans Amani Industrial Layout, PO Box 802, Port Harcourt

Principal Bankers: Union Bank of Nigeria Ltd

ASIAN AFRICAN CONTAINER (NIGERIA) LTD
Oke-Afa/Isolo Rd, PO Box 377, Mushin, Lagos State

PRINCIPAL ACTIVITIES: Shipping line for trading between the Far East and West Africa

Financial Information: Joint Venture between Orient Overseas Container Line and the Ashamu Group of Companies

ASIATIC INDUSTRIES LTD
Plot B Block 12, Alhaji Adejumo Avenue, Ilupeju Industrial Estate, PMB 21033, Ikeja, Lagos
Tel: 960928, 964600
Telex: 26232

Directors: Chief A A Adeyemi, Mr Stephenhang, Mr Ramonshang

PRINCIPAL ACTIVITIES: Suppliers of steel

No of Employees: 250

ASIATIC INDUSTRIES LTD
Ilupeju Industrial Estate, Alhaji Adejumo Avenue, PMB 21033, Ikeja, Lagos
Tel: 694600, 960928
Cable: Mico
Telex: 26232 Manda Ng

Chairman: Chief Adedokun Adeyemi
Directors: Stephen Cheng (Managing Director),
Raymond Cheng,
Mrs Mary Cheng,
John Siu

PRINCIPAL ACTIVITIES: Steel rods production
Subsidiary Companies: Mandarin Industries Ltd
Principal Bankers: Savannah Bank of Nigeria Ltd; Chase Merchant Bank Nigeria Ltd
Financial Information:

	N'000
Authorised capital	200
Paid-up capital	200
Turnover	6,575
Profits	78

Principal Shareholders: Nigerians 40%; Mandarin Industries Ltd 60%
Date of Establishment: 1978
No of Employees: 170

ASKAR OF NIGERIA LTD
PO Box 581, Eleiyele, Ibadan
Tel: 415480
Cable: Askalin Ibadan

Senior Executives: J O Ajayi (General Manager)

PRINCIPAL ACTIVITIES: Paint manufacturers, putty, glue and varnishes
Branch Offices: 63 Oyemekun Rd, Akure; 93A Ibara Rd, Abeokuta; 147 Ibrahim Taiwo Rd, Ilorin; 94B West Circular Rd, Benin; Std 126C Tunga Minna, Kaduna; BZ 124 Kazaure Rd, Kaduna; Iwo Road Depot, Ibadan
Principal Bankers: National Bank of Nigeria Ltd; Bank of the North

Principal Shareholders: Odu'a Investment Co Ltd
Date of Establishment: 8th September 1961
No of Employees: 87

ASPECT CONSTRUCTION ENGINEERING GROUP (NIG) LTD
PO Box 806, 19 Ojo Giwa St, Lagos
Tel: 635544

PRINCIPAL ACTIVITIES: Building and civil engineering contractors

ASPESI LTD
PO Box 98, Benin City, Bendel State

Directors: A Aspesi

PRINCIPAL ACTIVITIES: Construction

ASPHALT COMPANY OF NIGERIA LTD
Oregun Village Rd, PO Box 2049, Ikeja, Lagos
Tel: 630209, 636353, 636054

PRINCIPAL ACTIVITIES: Road resurfacing

ASRA SEAFOODS (NIGERIA) LTD
Km 10 Badagry Expressway, Lagos
Chairman: Liman Ciroma

PRINCIPAL ACTIVITIES: Fishing and processing
Branch Offices: Port Harcourt

Date of Establishment: November 1978

ASSOCIATED BATTERY MANUFACTURERS (NIGERIA) LTD
PO Box 23, Ikeja Industrial Estate, Ikeja, Lagos
Tel: 933662
Cable: Ablead

PRINCIPAL ACTIVITIES: Manufacturers of automative batteries-lead acid accumulators

ASSOCIATED BREWERIES & COMPANY LTD
PO Box 2246, Lagos
Chairman: Chief A O Lawson
Directors: C Haythorn (Managing Director)

PRINCIPAL ACTIVITIES: Brewing of Lager beer
Branch Offices: Km 31 Lagos-Badagry Expressway, Agbara, Ogun State

Date of Establishment: 500

ASSOCIATED DRUG COMPANY (NIG) LTD
17/19 Old Market Rd, Onitsha, Anambra State
Tel: 212098
Cable: Assodrugs

Chairman: Dr G E Nwokorah
Directors: Anthony O Ibe (Managing Director),
Alhaji Usman Nagado (Public Relations),
L B O Nwajiaku
Senior Executives: E N Onyia (Pharmacist General Manager, Onitsha),
F I Umenduka (Administrative Manager),
Saleh Mohammed Auyo (Pharmacist Manager),
J O Okoli (Secretary)

PRINCIPAL ACTIVITIES: Pharmaceutical importers, manufacturers' representatives and major distributors
Branch Offices: 70 Murtala Muhammed Way, PO Box 6989, Kano, Kano State, Tel 5847
Principal Bankers: United Bank for Africa Ltd; Pan African Bank (Nig) Ltd
Financial Information:

	N'000
Authorised capital	100
Paid-up capital	100
Turnover	1,500
Profits	180

Principal Shareholders: Anthony Okwudili Ibe; Chinweike Erasmus Ikenna; Esther Urobunachi Ibe; Okonkwo Erasmus Chinedu

ASSOCIATED ELECTRONIC PRODUCTS (NIGERIA) LTD

(Formerly Philips (Nig) Ltd)

AEPNL Building, Kilometre 16 Ikorodu Rd, Ojota, PO Box 1921, Lagos

Tel: 900160-9

Cable: Phinig: Lagos

Telex: 21297 Phinig

Chairman: Chief C O Ogunbanjo

Directors: J P Van Dongen Torman (Managing Director),
  S O Oloko (Executive Director),
  H Hoogendijk (Financial Director),
  J T F Iyalla,
  Dr M Tukur,
  O Lijadu,
  Dr G L R Kelder

Senior Executives: R Borgnana (Director of Technical Operations),
  E O P Owelle (General Service Manager),
  J O E Esuturie (Marketing Manager Consumer Products),
  K D Weitz (Products Manager)

PRINCIPAL ACTIVITIES: Manufacturers and importers of electrical and electronic equipment, telecommunication and scientific equipment

Principal Agencies: Philips Groups of Companies

Branch Offices: 41 Ali Akilu Rd, PO Box 335, Kaduna; 50E Ado Bayero Rd, PO Box 2035, Kano; 10B Park Rd, PO Box 475, ABA; 2 Hassan Danlatu Rd, Suleja, Abuja

Subsidiary Companies: N.V. Philips Gloeilampenfabrieken, Holland

Principal Bankers: United Bank for Africa Ltd; Union Bank of Nigeria Ltd; Savannah Bank Nigeria Ltd

Financial Information:

	N'000
Authorised capital	7,500
Paid-up capital	6,834
Turnover	34,000

Principal Shareholders: National Trust Company Ltd of Canada; National Insurance Corporation of Nigeria; Union Securities Ltd

Date of Establishment: 18th October 1955

No of Employees: 1,130

ASSOCIATED EXPORTS (W.A.) LTD

38 Burma Rd, PMB 1157, Apapa, Lagos

Tel: 877848, 870903

Cable: Sweetex

Telex: 20200 Box 074

Answerback: TOS APA Ng

Chairman: Fola Awoboh Pearse

Directors: Richard C Torgerson (Managing)

PRINCIPAL ACTIVITIES: Sales and distribution of strapping and packing systems and equipment

Principal Agencies: Signode Overseas, Inc USA

Branch Offices: FB3 Ibrahim Taiwo Rd, PO Box 1362, Twada, Kaduna

ASSOCIATED LABORATORY SUPPLIES LTD

26 Aba Rd, PO Box 89, Ikot Ekpene, Cross River State

Tel: 39

Cable: Alabscol

Chairman: Dunstan P Inyang

Directors: J U Umana (Financial Controller),
  Nsini Etim Inyang,
  Anselem Umo-Etuk

Senior Executives: J A Hansen (General Manager),
  C U Umoren (General Import Controller),
  Geoffrey D C Echebiri (Area Manager, Aba Branch),
  N I Umo-Ekpo (Senior Sales Executive),
  N W Udoh (General Store Controller),
  Mrs Helen D P Inyang (Warehouse Manager),
  Okon U Umoren (Service Engineer)

PRINCIPAL ACTIVITIES: Importation and distribution of a wide range of scientific equipment, laboratory chemicals, allied medical and diagnostic equipment, apparatus, and reagents

Principal Agencies: Heuer-Leanidas, Switzerland; East Anglia Chemicals Ltd, UK; Glasseport Company Ltd, Czechoslovakia; Shiv Dial India; Laboratory Scientific Export, UK

Branch Offices: 142 Port Harcourt Rd, Aba, Imo State. Representative Offices at Calabar; Kaduna; Maiduguri

Subsidiary Companies: Dunspol Organization Ltd; Associated Manufacturing Company Ltd; Associated Finance Investment Ltd

Principal Bankers: First Bank of Nigeria Ltd

Financial Information:

	N'000
Authorised capital	1,500
Paid-up capital	950
Turnover	3,574 (1980)
Profits	255

Principal Shareholders: Dustan P Inyang; Dunspol Organization Ltd; Associated Manufacturing Company Ltd; Associated Finance Investment Ltd

Date of Establishment: 1969

No of Employees: 99

ASSOCIATED METAL & ALLIED WORKS LTD

PO Box 64, Lagos

PRINCIPAL ACTIVITIES: Manufacturers of household utensils and metalware

Financial Information:

Registered capital	N 400,000

Date of Establishment: May 1975

No of Employees: 130

ASSOCIATED ORES MINING COMPANY LTD

PMB 1021, Okene, Kwara State

Directors: Chief Malomo Barajamu,
  Hajia Hannatu Bature,
  Alhaji Emiola Adeleke,
  Alhaji Yalwaji Azare,
  C N Okezie,
  Engr P U Umunnakwe (General Manager and Chief Executive)

Senior Executives: Engr C Y N Nwaobia (Deputy General Manager),
  Engr L A Adegboye (Deputy General Manager),
  Alhaji Yahaya Mohammed (Company Secretary)

PRINCIPAL ACTIVITIES: Exploration and exploitation of raw materials for the Nigerian steel industry

Branch Offices: 63/71 Broad Street, Lagos

Principal Bankers: National Bank of Nigeria; First Bank of Nigeria Ltd; Bank of the North

Financial Information:

Authorised capital	N 500,000

Principal Shareholders: Federal Government of Nigeria

Date of Establishment: November 1979

No of Employees: 1,051

ASSOCIATED PHARMACEUTICAL PRODUCTS LTD

(Formerly Merck Sharp & Dohme (Nigeria) Ltd)

23 Warehouse Rd, Apapa, PO Box 5571, Lagos

Tel: 874082

Telex: 21214

Directors: Peter H Lange (General Manager)

PRINCIPAL ACTIVITIES: Importation and distribution of pharmaceuticals and cosmetics

31

ASSOCIATED TEXTILE MANUFACTURERS CO LTD

Ilupeju Extension II, Block D Plots 1 and 2, Isolo Express Way, Isolo, PO Box 134, Mushin, Lagos State
Tel: 847825
Cable: Nuzas

Chairman: M A J Zabadne
Directors: Mrs A Zabadne, J Zabadne, Alhaji Ali Fika
Senior Executives: M H Zabadne (General Manager),
   A L O Bakare (Assistant General Manager),
   P E Okpu (Chief Accountant),
   S U Ogbonnaya (Assistant Manager),
   M Idowu (Assistant Manager)

PRINCIPAL ACTIVITIES: Socks manufacturing
Branch Offices: PO Box 673, Jos
Principal Bankers: Nigeria-Arab Bank Ltd
Financial Information:

	₦'000
Authorised capital	1,000
Paid-up capital	600
Turnover	1,000
Profits	200

Principal Shareholders: M A J Zabadne; M R J Zabadne; Mrs A Zabadne
Date of Establishment: 1969
No of Employees: 500

ASSOCIATION OF NIGERIAN CO-OPERATIVE EXPORTERS LTD

New Court Rd, PO Box 477, Ibadan, Oyo State

PRINCIPAL ACTIVITIES: Producers/exporters of cocoa and other cash crops

ASWANI TEXTILE INDUSTRIES LTD

Plot 2d Block A Oshodi Scheme, PO Box 93, Ilupeju, Lagos
Tel: 845543

PRINCIPAL ACTIVITIES: Manufacturing of cotton piece goods, dyeing
Financial Information: Associated company of K Chellaram & Sons (Nigeria) Ltd

ATICON LTD

Kilometer 31, Lagos-Abeokuta Rd, PO Box 1040, Agege, Lagos State
Cable: Consortium Lagos

Chairman: Chief G Akin Taylor
Directors: A Gruvstad, L Sjoborg, R Olsson, M I Kazie
Senior Executives: M I Kazie (Chief Projects Engineer),
   M Odumosu (Finance/Administrative Manager),
   S Somasunderam (Area Manager)

PRINCIPAL ACTIVITIES: Building and civil engineering construction
Branch Offices: 3 Inuwa Wade Rd, PO Box 813, Kaduna
Principal Bankers: United Bank of Africa Ltd; Societe Generale Bank (Nig) Ltd
Financial Information:

	₦'000
Authorised capital	600
Paid-up capital	600
Turnover	5,000

Principal Shareholders: Akin Taylor & Co Ltd; Ab Nils P Lundh; Ab Intong
Date of Establishment: 1974
No of Employees: 350

ATLANTIC MERCANTILE CO LTD

11/13 Warehouse Rd, Apapa, Lagos
Tel: 877231
Telex: 21326 Atmerc Ng

PRINCIPAL ACTIVITIES: Suppliers of general merchandise

ATLANTIC TEXTILE MANUFACTURING CO LTD

Ilupeju Industrial Estate, PO Box 2504, Lagos
Tel: 963191

Chairman: A Jaar
Directors: Alhaji Sule Katagum,
   B De Jaar,
   F L Hinkelmann (Managing Director),
   P A Onokwai (Executive Director)
Senior Executives: P de Waart (Technical Manager),
   S O Ogunmekan (Chief Accountant)

PRINCIPAL ACTIVITIES: Textiles and clothing, textile equipment
Principal Bankers: Union Bank of Nigeria Ltd

Date of Establishment: 1965
No of Employees: 633

ATLAS NIGERIA LTD

Plot 3A Block A, Isolo Industrial Estate, Oshodi Express Rd, Osolo, Mushin West, PO Box 2120, Lagos
Tel: 964072
Cable: Transatlas
Telex: 26237 Atlas Ng

Chairman: Alhaji Ado Ibrahim
Directors: B R T Hill (Managing Director),
   A S Brooker (Executive Director, Technical Manager),
   G K Oladipo (Executive Director, Chief Accountant),
   T A Kafari (Executive Director, Personnel Manager),
   John de T Vischer,
   Mrs R Scott,
   L J Golding,
   Alhaji U E Bello
Senior Executives: R A Yates (Technical Sales Controller),
   G O Ekisola (Controller of Branches),
   I Ogundiran (Data Processing Manager),
   P S Inegbese (Reprographics Sales Manager)

PRINCIPAL ACTIVITIES: Suppliers of office, optical and photographic equipment and scientific instruments
Principal Agencies: Engineering Laboratory Equipment Ltd (UK); Mita Holland BV (Holland); Kern & Co Ltd (Switzerland); GAF (Great Britain) Ltd (UK); Franz Kuhlmann (West Germany)
Branch Offices: PMB 2091, Kaduna; PMB 3092, Kano; PMB 5225, Ibadan; PMB 1133, Benin City; PO Box 656, Ilorin, PO Box 520, Owerri
Principal Bankers: First Bank of Nigeria Ltd
Financial Information:

	₦'000
Authorised capital	3,500
Paid-up capital	2,000
Turnover	12,458
Profits	1,972

Principal Shareholders: Nigerians (60%); British (40%)
Date of Establishment: 1953
No of Employees: 270

ATOKI, FRED, PUBLISHING COMPANY LTD

Plot 25 Kekere-Ekun Street, Orile-Iganmu, PO Box 7313, Lagos
Tel: 880460
Telex: 21619 Nacc Ng

Chairman: F O A Atoki (also Managing Director)

PRINCIPAL ACTIVITIES: Printing and publishing
Associated Companies: Fred Atoki Commercial Services; FAPCO Media

ATSSCO ABBEY OFFICE MACHINE SERVICE STATIONERY (NIG) LTD

40 Niger St, PO Box 918, Kano State
Tel: 4187
Cable: Abbey-Kano

PRINCIPAL ACTIVITIES: Importers, suppliers of general merchandise, manufacturer's representatives
Branch Offices: Lagos State; Borno State
Principal Bankers: Standard Bank (Nig) Ltd

ATTA, M O, & SONS (NIGERIA) LTD
FC3 Ibrahim Taiwo Rd, PO Box 268, Kaduna
Tel: 243363

PRINCIPAL ACTIVITIES: Building and civil engineering contractors; distributors
Principal Agencies: Biscuit Manufacturing Co Nigeria Ltd; Nigerian Breweries Ltd
Branch Offices: Wholesale Office: 005 Jos Rd, Kaduna, Tel 243363, 243500

AUDU LUKAT MOTORS LTD
37E Ado Bayero Rd, PO Box 733, Kano
Tel: 2597, 4336

Chairman: Alhaji M H Koguna
Directors: Alhaji Audu Lukat
Senior Executives: G M Onwuka (Engineer), A C Koyan (Parts Manager)

PRINCIPAL ACTIVITIES: Mechanical engineering; sales and service of motor vehicles
Principal Agencies: Niger Motors; UTC Motors; Vauxhall Motors Ltd; Leventis Motors Ltd
Branch Offices: 17 Murtala Mohammed Way, Kano; Market Roundabout, PO Box 488, Sokoto
Principal Bankers: Bank of the North Ltd
Financial Information:

	N'000
Authorised capital	250
Paid-up capital	200
Sales turnover	211
Profits	135

Principal Shareholders: Alhaji Koguna; Alhaji Audu Lukat

AUGUST REINERS NIGERIA LTD
Unity House, 13th Floor, 37 Marina, PO Box 2288, Lagos
Tel: 636433, 654384

Directors: W H W Schemmel

PRINCIPAL ACTIVITIES: Building and civil engineering contractors

AURORA PRODUCE & SHIPPING CO LTD
15 Wesley St, PO Box 3097, Lagos
Tel: 655075
Telex: 21461 Aurora Ng

PRINCIPAL ACTIVITIES: Shipping and produce marketing
Branch Offices: 3 Joseph St, Lagos, Tel 635197

AUTO COMPONENTS LTD
PO Box 4349, Ikeja, Lagos State
Cable: Pureflow-Lagos

Directors: Segun Abiodun,
  Mr Onwanchu,
  M K Kumar (Production Director),
  C K Rajagopal (Managing Director)

PRINCIPAL ACTIVITIES: Manufacturers of automobile components
Subsidiary Companies: Emir Industries Ltd; Northern Aluminium (Nig) Ltd
Principal Bankers: United Bank for Africa
Financial Information:

	N'000
Authorised capital	300
Paid-up capital	300
Turnover	1,200

Date of Establishment: December 1980
No of Employees: 40

AVERY NIGERIA LTD
Obasa Rd, PO Box 2, Ikeja, Lagos
Tel: 963627, 963657
Cable: Avery Ikeja

PRINCIPAL ACTIVITIES: Suppliers of industrial testing machines
Principal Agencies: Avery Hardoll Petrol and Diesel Pumps
Branch Offices: A1 Block 5 Kakuri, PO Box 942, Kaduna; 88 Tafawa Balewa Rd, PO Box 785, Kano, Tel 24876; 86 West Circular Rd, PMB 1182, Benin City, Bendel State; 280 Trans Amadi Industrial Layout, PMB 5191, Port Harcourt, Rivers State Tel 223635

AVON CROWNCAPS AND CONTAINERS (NIGERIA) LTD
PO Box 2701, Lagos
Tel: 960978, 962716
Cable: Avonind
Telex: 26130 Enpee Ng

Chairman: N P Kirpalani
Directors: S B Akande, Mrs C O Akande, Mrs A O Lasode, S T Lakhani, A S Lakhani
Senior Executives: D Jayaraman (General Manager), D G Kirpalani (Production Manager)

PRINCIPAL ACTIVITIES: Manufacturers of crown corks and metal cans
Branch Offices: Works: Km 38 Lagos-Abeokuta Rd, Otta, Ogun State
Subsidiary Companies: Enpee Industries Ltd
Principal Bankers: United Bank for Africa Ltd
Financial Information:

	N'000
Authorised capital	900
Paid-up capital	900
Turnover	6,000

Principal Shareholders: N P Kirpalani; S B Akande; Mrs C O Akande; Mrs A O Lasode
Date of Establishment: July 1980
No of Employees: 200

AWAYE CONTINENTAL MOTORS CO LTD
15b Wesley St, PO Box 4834, Lagos
Tel: 655916
Telex: 21564 Awacom Ng

PRINCIPAL ACTIVITIES: Suppliers of Motor Vehicles
Branch Offices: 435/437 Herbert Macaulay St, Yaba, Lagos, Tel 861079

AWOSANMI & SONS ENGINEERING WORKS
68/69 Murtala Mohammed Way, PO Box 937, Kano
Tel: 3501

PRINCIPAL ACTIVITIES: Mechanical and electrical engineers; manufacturers' representatives, transporters; distributors of motor vehicles, etc

AYANA MINING SYNDICATE
41 Sarkin Mangu St, PO Box 670, Jos, Plateau State
PRINCIPAL ACTIVITIES: Mining

AYE MARBLE & TERRAZZO INDUSTRIAL WORKS
10 Plymouth Rd, Benin City, Bendel State
Tel: 243164

Directors: Ben U Aye (Managing Director)

PRINCIPAL ACTIVITIES: Suppliers of building materials, marble and terrazzo flooring, marble statuary of all kinds, Benin sculptural art, wood and bronze

AYO, LAWRENCE, & SONS LTD
25 Abonnema Wharf Rd, PO Box 741, Port Harcourt, Rivers
State
Tel: 21272

PRINCIPAL ACTIVITIES: Clearing and forwarding agents
Branch Offices: NW5/197 Adekunle Fajuyi Rd, PO Box 693,
Ibadan

B & C AUTOPANEL ENGINEERING LTD
6 Denton St, Ebute-Metta, PO Box 263, Yaba, Lagos
Tel: 860701
Cable: Autopanel Lagos

PRINCIPAL ACTIVITIES: Manufacturers of vehicle bodies for
buses

B & F NIGERIA LTD
SW8/665 Ijebu Bye-Pass, Oke-Ado, PMB 5359, Ibadan,
Oyo-State
Tel: 411129

Chairman: Jacob Olukayode Falana
Directors: Mrs O Falana
Senior Executives: Olabode Falana (Chief Accountant),
F A Banjo (Chief Mechancial Engineer),
Jide E Omitosin (Sales Controller)

PRINCIPAL ACTIVITIES: Suppliers of general automobile spares,
nuts and bolts, hand tools. Dealers in industrial machinery,
cars and heavy duty vehicles. Servicing
Principal Agencies: Adolf Wurth GmbH & Co Kg, Germany
Branch Offices: 1 Secretariat Rd, Off Ibadan Expressway, Toll
Gate (Oregun), PMB 1126, Oshodi, Lagos
Subsidiary Companies: Machine Tools International Nig Ltd;
Josef Wahler KG (Nig) Ltd
Principal Bankers: United Bank for West Africa Ltd; Union Bank
Ltd
Principal Shareholders: J O Falana; Mrs O Falana
Date of Establishment: 6th December 1977
No of Employees: 43

B B C BROWN BOVERI (NIGERIA) LTD
Industrial Ave, Plot C, Block 1, Ilupeju, PMB 21055, Ikeja, Lagos
Tel: 962187
Cable: Brownbover

Chairman: R L Thomas
Directors: Chief S L Edu,
F Egbe,
K H Eger (Managing Director),
Alhaji S Malami,
Dr W Thommen,
Dr A Wachter

PRINCIPAL ACTIVITIES: Construction; power and electrical
engineering, erection of thermal and gas power stations etc;
power equipment and telecommunication systems

Date of Establishment: Incorporated 24th February, 1977
No of Employees: 800

B C UNIJE & SONS LTD
See UNIJE, B C, & SONS LTD

B K SUTHERLAND & COMPANY LTD
See SUTHERLAND, B K, & COMPANY LTD

B STABILINI & COMPANY LTD
See STABILINI, B, & COMPANY LTD

BABAFUNKE, ADEOLA, OVERSEAS TRADING COMPANY
12 Akanbi St, Onitiri-Layout, Yaba, Lagos
PRINCIPAL ACTIVITIES: Suppliers of general merchandise

BAERTLE, J, & CO (NIG) LTD
1 Gidado Rd, PO Box 68, Kano
Tel: 3357
Telex: 77125

Directors: J Baertle (Managing),
Alhaji Shehu Ahmed,
H D Bollmann

PRINCIPAL ACTIVITIES: Technical advisers and consultants to
industry

BAFCO LTD
46 Ahmadu Bello Way, PO Box 490, Jos, Plateau State
PRINCIPAL ACTIVITIES: Building and civil engineering
contractors

BAGAUDA TEXTILE MILL LTD
17 Ja'afaru Rd, Bompai, PMB 3190, Kano
Tel: 3173 Kano
Cable: Bagauda Kano
Telex: 77229 Baguda Ng

Chairman: Alhaji Isyaku Rabiu
Directors: Alhaji Bala-Rabiu,
Alhaji Mohammed N Rabiu (Managing),
Alhaji Umaru Na Abba,
Alhaji Nababa Badamasi,
M Yusufu Rabiu
Senior Executives: Tuncer Cengiz (General Manager),
Alhaji S M Musa (Commercial Services Manager),
A O Omokaro (Secretary/Accountant),
Alhaji M A Musa (Personnel Manager)

PRINCIPAL ACTIVITIES: Manufacturers of suiting and teteron
materials
Subsidiary/Associated Companies: Isyaku Rabiu & Sons Ltd;
Kano Vehicle & Accessories Ltd; Kano Sugar Co Ltd; Rabiu
Bottling Company
Principal Bankers: First Bank of Nigeria Ltd
Financial Information:

	N'000
Authorised capital	2,000
Paid-up capital	2,000
Turnover	5,000
Profits	500

Principal Shareholders: Kano-Merchant Trading Company;
Chairman and directors as described
Date of Establishment: 27th April 1974
No of Employees: 900

BAKARE, S B, & BROTHERS LTD
18/20 Rhodes Crescent, PO Box 126, Apapa, Lagos
Tel: 873102
Telex: 21401 Essbee Ng

PRINCIPAL ACTIVITIES: Construction, stevedoring; road
haulage, etc

BAKER NIGERIA LTD
PO Box 4011, 8/10 Broad St, Lagos
Tel: 654286
Cable: Bacaso Lagos
Telex: 21543 Bekbek Ng

Directors: Piero G Pieroni (Manager),
C Spannagel (District Manager),
Tom Flick (Production Manager),
N Emmert (Area Manager),
J Jackson (Operations Manager, Warri)

PRINCIPAL ACTIVITIES: Equipment suppliers and services to
the oil and gas industry
Principal Agencies: Gray Tool Company International
Branch Offices: Field Offices: PO Box 385, Warri, Cable
Bacaso-Warri; 8 Emekuku St, PO Box 972, Port Harcourt, Tel
21844, Cable Bacaso-Port Harcourt
Financial Information: As associate of Baker Oil Tools Inc, USA

BAKRIN ENTERPRISES LTD

PMB 1407, Lagos
Tel: 682026

PRINCIPAL ACTIVITIES: General merchants, transporters,
   car-hire and tourist services, manufacturers' representatives
Principal Agencies: Peugeot Ltd
Branch Offices: PMB 2110, Jos, Plateau State, Tel 2437; PMB
   2248, Makurdi, Benue State

BALAKHANY (NIGERIA) LTD

61 Joel Ogunnaike St, PO Box 192, Ikeja, Lagos State
Tel: 964016, 964584
Cable: Balakhany Lagos

Chairman: J O Emanuel
Directors: W H Francis (Managing),
   E A Ola (General Manager),
   A F R Hatfield,
   Alhaji Ali Kotoko
Senior Executives: B Adasonla (Chief Accountant),
   W A Anuku (District Manager)

PRINCIPAL ACTIVITIES: Water drilling, treatment, distribution
   and pump engineers
Principal Agencies: Grundfos A/S Denmark
Branch Offices: 6 Oguta St, PMB 5347, Port Harcourt, Rivers
   State; Warri Rd, PO Box 99, Ughelli, Bendel State;
   Bakin-Kura St, PMB 0049, Bauchi, Bauchi State
Subsidiary/Associated Companies: Balakhany Chad (Nigeria)
   Ltd; Water Surveys (Nigeria) Ltd; Balakhany Ltd, London
Principal Bankers: United Bank for Africa Ltd; Union Bank of
   Nigeria Ltd

Date of Establishment: Over 30 years ago; Longest established
   organisation in the field of ground water supply in Nigeria
No of Employees: 500

BALIN BUILDERS & ALUMINIUM INDUSTRIES LTD

19 Eric Moore Street, Ikeja, PMB 1205, Apapa, Lagos
Tel: 964532

PRINCIPAL ACTIVITIES: Manufacturers of aluminium doors,
   windows etc; civil engineering and construction
Principal Bankers: First Bank of Nigeria Ltd; International Bank
   for West Africa Ltd

BALMORE TRADING COMPANY LTD

PO Box 62, Kano
Tel: 3057, 5770
Cable: Solgodsi
Telex: 77112 Trella Ng

PRINCIPAL ACTIVITIES: Manufacturers of steel engineering
   items; metal doors, etc
Branch Offices: Factory; 181 Club Rd, Kano; Apapa; Lagos;
   Maiduguri; Sokoto
Associated Companies: Northern Steel Works Ltd; Steel
   Construction Ltd

BALOGUN, A A, & SONS (NIGERIA) LTD

13 Labingo St, Alakija, Mushin, Lagos
Tel: 632018, 633062, 833502
Cable: Balinter Lagos

Chairman: Chief A A Balogun
Directors: Waheed A Balogun
Senior Executives: S O Mayungbe (General Manager),
   T Yusuf Ariyo (Personnel Manager),
   F Dada (Accountant),
   S Aghedo (General Foreman)

PRINCIPAL ACTIVITIES: Freighting, general contractors,
   importers and exporters
Principal Agencies: West African Breweries; Cross River State
   Breweries; Mcdermott (Nigeria) Ltd; Tsmpe
Branch Offices: 30 Ginuwa Rd, PO Box 433, Warri, Bendel State,
   Tel 232544, 233534; I50 Marina St, Epe, Lagos State, Tel 10
Associated Companies: Alex Trading Co Ltd; Yorumet (Nigeria)

Ltd
Principal Bankers: First Bank of Nigeria Ltd
Financial Information:

	N '000
Authorised capital	100
Paid-up capital	50
Turnover (approximate)	2,500

No of Employees: 2,000

BALOGUN, J A, WORKS

31 Luther King St, PO Box 652, Lagos
Tel: 630920

PRINCIPAL ACTIVITIES: Building and civil engineering
   contractors

BAMGBOYE ENGINEERING LTD

7/9 Bamgboye St, Ureje, PO Box 218, Ado-Ekiti, Ondo State
Tel: 240616

Chairman: High Chief Obafemi Bamgboye (also Managing
   Director)
Directors: Mrs Adenike Bamgboye, J Oluwafemi Bamgboye

PRINCIPAL ACTIVITIES: Building and civil engineering
   contractors
Financial Information:
Authorised capital   ₦ 250,000

Principal Shareholders: Member of the Bamgboye Group of
   Companies
Date of Establishment: August 1976

BANA CONSULTANTS NIGERIA LTD

J4/5 Ahmadu Bello Way, PO Box 4137, Kaduna

PRINCIPAL ACTIVITIES: Business consultants
Branch Offices: B10 Aminu St, Opposite YMCA, Tudun Wada,
   Kaduna

BANBURY SYSTEMS (NIGERIA) LTD

PO Box 1750, Inuwa Abdul Kadir Rd, Kaduna
Telex: 71160 Topark

Chairman: A H Hayatuddini
Directors: J Neath (Managing),
   A A Ajao,
   V Ndalugi,
   D Kirton

PRINCIPAL ACTIVITIES: Manufacturers of prefabricated
   concrete industrial buildings, bungalows, concrete fencing,
   paving slabs

BANJOKO FIRESAFETY LTD

14 Olabode Close, Ilupeju, PO Box 847, Oshodi, Lagos
Tel: 960614
Cable: Firesafety Lagos

Chairman: J A Banjoko (also Managing Director)
Directors: R O Banjoko, Alhaji A O Badejo

PRINCIPAL ACTIVITIES: Suppliers of fire-fighting equipment and
   fire trucks
Principal Agencies: Foulds clark (London) Ltd, UK; Gebruder
   Bachert, West Germany
Principal Bankers: First Bank of Nigeria Ltd; Wema Bank Ltd
Financial Information:

	₦'000
Authorised capital	200
Paid-up capital	150
Turnover	850

Principal Shareholders: J A Banjoko; R O Banjoko; A O Badejo
Date of Establishment: 1st June, 1979

BANJOKO, L A O, & CO LTD

PO Box 474, Oregun Village, Oyo Rd, Ibadan, Oyo State
Tel: 411641, 411672, 411723

PRINCIPAL ACTIVITIES: Building and civil engineering
   contractors

BANK OF CREDIT & COMMERCE INTERNATIONAL (NIGERIA) LTD

42-44 Warehouse Rd, PMB 1040, Apapa, Lagos
Tel: 870387, 870394
Cable: Crecomnig
Telex: 22377 BCCI AP Ng

Chairman: Alhaji Ibrahim Dasuki
Directors: Chief L O Akindele,
  Chief I A S Adewale,
  Alhaji Ibrahim Katune,
  P F Gutta,
  Sadiq Ali,
  S Qaiser Raza (Managing)
Senior Executives: Mrs W O Ogunmokun (Personnel Manager),
  S A Ojikutu (Marketing Manager),
  B M Gimba (Secretary),
  V A Akinseye (Senior Executive),
  Yinka Onikoyi (Senior Executive)

PRINCIPAL ACTIVITIES: Commercial banking
Branch Offices: 42-44 Warehouse Rd, PMB 1040, Apapa;
  SW8/95A Lagos Bye-Pass, Okebola, PMB 5730, Ibadan; 13C
  Murtala Mohammed Way, PO Box 5488, Kano; 22 Ahmadu
  Bello Way, PMB 2149, Kaduna; 27 Aba Rd, PMB 6193, Port
  Harcourt; Dogondaji House, 5 Birnin Kebbi Rd, PMB 2233,
  Sokoto
Subsidiary/Associated Companies: BCCI Holdings (Luxembourg)
  SA, Luxembourg
Principal Bankers: Central Bank of Nigeria, Lagos; Bank of
  Credit and Commerce International SA, London
Financial Information:

	N'000
Authorised capital	25,000
Paid-up capital	9,000
Profits (net)	7,800
Deposits	297,000
Assets	375,000

Principal Shareholders: Alhaji Ibrahim Dasuki; Chief L O
  Akindele; Chief I A S Adewale; Alhaji Ibrahim Katune; Chief
  Patrick O Bolokor; Alhaji Uba Ibrahim Ringim; BCCI Holdings
  (Luxembourg) SA and others
Date of Establishment: 7 August 1979
No of Employees: 450

BANK OF THE NORTH LTD

5/6 Lagos St, PO Box 211, Kano
Tel: 2895/6, 5175/6
Cable: Northsbank
Telex: 77233 Nortbk Ng

Chairman: A M Mohammed
Directors: Baba Duna,
  E S Yusufu,
  Isa Abubakar,
  Magagji Mu'azu,
  E O Oki,
  J I Ahom,
  Abba Musa Rimi,
  A Bisala,
  Baba Mala Yarema,
  S Muhammed Shanono,
  Mohammed Suleiman Barup Ali Al-Hakim (Managing)

PRINCIPAL ACTIVITIES: Banking
Branch Offices: 118/120 Broad St, Lagos; Kano; Kaduna;
  Maiduguri; Jos; Ibadan; Ilorin; Sokoto; Bauchi; Makurdi;
  Minna; Yola; Zaria etc
Principal Shareholders: The ten Northern State Governments
Date of Establishment: 1959
No of Employees: 2,500

BAO NIGERIA LTD

107 Enu Owa St, PO Box 6349, Lagos
Tel: 663259
Cable: Baolaley

Chairman: Alhaji Iburaimoh Adigun Olaleye
Directors: Hassani Alani Olaleye, Kolawole Akanji Olaleye
Senior Executives: Nurudeen Ali (Sales Manager),
  Abdul Aremu Dawuda (Store Manager)

PRINCIPAL ACTIVITIES: Importers, exporters, general
  merchants and contractors, dealers in motor vehicles and
  components
Principal Agencies: Ashvin Auto Agencies, India; Sys
  Manufacturers, Japan; Luciflex Ind E. Com. Ltda, Brasil
Branch Offices: 116 Enu Owa St, Lagos
Principal Bankers: Savannah Bank of Nigeria Ltd

Principal Shareholders: H A Olaleye; K A Olaleye
Date of Establishment: 13th October, 1972

BARAKA PRESS & PUBLISHERS LTD

5 Ahmadu Bello Way, PO Box 171, Kaduna
Tel: 242625, 216469
Cable: Baraka Kaduna
Telex: 71308 Baraka Ng

Chairman: U J Ekpikhe
Directors: G O Onosode,
  E U Isen,
  W I Adesida (Managing Director)
Senior Executives: J A Bolanta (General Sales Manager),
  P A Ebe (Finance & Administration Manager),
  Z D Baiye (Production Manager),
  U R Umoette (Commercial Manager),
  C C Esonu (Publications Manager)

PRINCIPAL ACTIVITIES: Commercial printing and publishing
Principal Agencies: Western Litho Plate Inc; Sadolin Printing
  Inks Ltd
Branch Offices: 409 Sarkin Yaki, New Airport Rd, Kano
Principal Bankers: Union Bank of Nigeria Ltd; Nal Merchant
  Bank

Principal Shareholders: Christian Witness Team Inc
Date of Establishment: November 1956
No of Employees: 151

BARLOW MINES LTD

Mile 21, Jos-Bauchi Rd, PO Box 123, Bukuru, Plateau State
Directors: Alhaji Dan Mallam (Managing)
PRINCIPAL ACTIVITIES: Mining of Metal ore

BARMA, A G S, LTD

4 Balogun Sq, PO Box 2820, Lagos
Tel: 632168, 633472
PRINCIPAL ACTIVITIES: Construction

BAROID OF NIGERIA LTD

Plot 1192A, Kasumu Ekimode St, Victoria Island, Lagos
Tel: 613622
Cable: Baroid Lagos
Telex: 21093 Baroid Ng

Chairman: W E Parker
Directors: J H Watt, T M House, Chief J A Adeniyi, Chief F H
  Utomi
Senior Executives: J O Onayemi (Chief Accountant),
  C I Nsirim (Administrative Manager),
  G E Hoehn (Operations Manager),
  J David Rogers (General Manager)

PRINCIPAL ACTIVITIES: Oilfield service company and supplier of
  drilling mud chemicals to leading oil prospecting companies;
  work over products; logging services; treating chemicals;
  solids control equipment
Branch Offices: Warri; Port Harcourt; Ebocha
Subsidiary/Associated Companies: Baroid Drilling Chemicals
  and Products Ltd
Principal Bankers: First Bank of Nigeria; Union Bank of Nigeria;
  Nal Merchant Bank

Principal Shareholders: NL Industries Inc; Nigeria National
   Petroleum Corp
Date of Establishment: 1964
No of Employees: 200

BARSHALL, F M, (WEST AFRICA) LTD

PO Box 2068, 122-124 Broad St, Lagos
Tel: 632685, 655995
Telex: 21456 Barges Ng

PRINCIPAL ACTIVITIES: Importers and exporters, general
   trading

BASF (NIGERIA) LTD

Plot C Block 1, Industrial Avenue, Ilupeju, PO Box 2699, Lagos
Tel: 961034, 962259
Cable: Badinig
Telex: 26154 Basf Ng

Chairman: Alhaji M G Lawan
Directors: C Erasmi,
   B Kitzelmann (Managing),
   A O Ogunde,
   Dr O O Ojehomon
Senior Executives: W G Kron (Manager Plastics Department),
   M O E Tiemo (Financial Controller)

PRINCIPAL ACTIVITIES: Suppliers of chemicals, fertilizers,
   pesticides, plastics, dyestuffs, magnetic media
Principal Agencies: Basf Aktiengesellschaft, W Germany and
   group companies
Branch Offices: 11 Lagos St, Kano
Principal Bankers: Union Bank of Nigeria Ltd; Icon Ltd;
   International Bank for West Africa Ltd
Financial Information:
Authorised capital   ₦ 100

Principal Shareholders: Basf Aktiengesellschaft; Alhaji M G
   Lawan; A O Ogunde and other Nigerians
Date of Establishment: December 1965

BATA NIGERIA LTD

Mile 9, Ikorodu Rd, PO Box 548, Lagos
Tel: 900436/9, 964385
Cable: Batashoe Lagostx
Telex: 21278 Lagos

Chairman: J Moore
Directors: L T C Buffin, A Salaun, N Moubayed, Mrs O O
   Olakunri, Alhaji M O Oseni

PRINCIPAL ACTIVITIES: Manufacturing and distribution of
   footwear
Branch Offices: Branches throughout Nigeria
Principal Bankers: First Bank of Nigeria Ltd; United Bank for
   Africa Ltd; Union Bank of Nigeria Ltd
Financial Information:

	₦'000
Authorised capital	4,000
Paid-up capital	4,000
Sales turnover	30,000

Principal Shareholders: Nigerian Citizens and Associations
   (60%); Bata Overseas (40%)
No of Employees: 3,000

BATTERY MANUFACTURING CO (NIG) LTD

PO Box 1096, Adeniyi Jones Ave, Industrial Estate, Ikeja, Lagos
Tel: 963207

PRINCIPAL ACTIVITIES: Manufacturing of dry cell batteries
Financial Information: Subsidiary of West African Household
   Utilities Manufacturing Co Ltd

BAYAJIDA GROUP OF COMPANIES

10 Lebanon Rd, PO Box 778, Kano
Tel: 3523, 3646, 4608
Cable: Batco, Kano
Telex: 77218 Batco Ng

Directors: Alhaji Sani Buhari (Managing Director)

PRINCIPAL ACTIVITIES: Suppliers of textile goods, building
   materials; educational books, stationery and equipment;
   electrical products; manufacturers' representatives;
   construction
Branch Offices: 21 Duala Rd, Apapa, Lagos, Tel 874977; 16
   Industry Rd, Port Harcourt; 4 Marona, Kaduna; 5 Tiga Rd,
   Kano
Subsidiary Companies: Bayajida Amenity Trading Co Ltd;
   Bayajida Construction   Co Ltd; Bayajida Educational Supplies
   Ltd; Bayajida Electrical Stores

BAYER (NIGERIA) LTD

42/44 Warehouse Rd, PO Box 303, Apapa, Lagos
Tel: 876135, 876170
Telex: 21493 Bayap Ng

Directors: J P Hinrichs

PRINCIPAL ACTIVITIES: General trading and representation,
   specialists in technical equipment and services
Principal Agencies: Bayer AG, W Germany
Branch Offices: Principal Branch: Imam House, Ahmadu Bello
   Way, PO Box 411, Kaduna

BAYER PHARMACEUTICALS (NIGERIA) LTD

PO Box 250, 22 Hinderer Rd, Apapa, Lagos
Tel: 876672
Cable: pharmbayer
Telex: 21493 Bayap

Directors: J.-P Hinrichs (Managing)

PRINCIPAL ACTIVITIES: Manufacturing of pharmaceutical
   products

BEC FRERES (NIGERIA) LTD

Western House, 8/10 Broad Street, PO Box 13090, Lagos
Tel: 658426
Telex: 21886

PRINCIPAL ACTIVITIES: Civil engineering and construction

BECCARELLI, P, & CO LTD

Plot 9 Eric Moore Rd, Iganmu Industrial Estate, PO Box 1932,
   Apapa, Lagos
Tel: 873680

Chairman: F P Beccarelli (also Managing Director)
Directors: G Ike (Purchasing Manger),
   F P Beccarell,
   Mrs C Ugwu,
   M Poloni
Senior Executives: J Zannu (Quantity Surveyor),
   A E Nkereuwem (Personnel Manager),
   C E Edet (Accountant)

PRINCIPAL ACTIVITIES: Building and civil engineering
   contractors
Principal Bankers: New Nigeria Bank Ltd; Bank of the North Ltd
Principal Shareholders: G Ike; M Poloni; J A Adeigbo; Professor
   A B Kasunmu; G E Bajomo; F P Beccarelli
Date of Establishment: 1962
No of Employees: 1,000

BECICITI CONSTRUCTION LTD

7 Moleye St, Yaba, PO Box 6374, Lagos
Tel: 860494, 863354
Cable: Fifihouse Lagos

PRINCIPAL ACTIVITIES: Construction

Date of Establishment: 1976

BECKER-VOIGT, H

84 Hawkesworth Rd, Ikoyi, PO Box 1038, Lagos
Tel: 682628

PRINCIPAL ACTIVITIES: Architects and consultants

BEDKANA (NIG) LTD

Trans Amadi Industrial Estate, PO Box 573, Port Harcourt, Rivers State
Tel: 225941
Cable: Bribed
Telex: 61119

Chairman: Bright Emyelike (also Managing Director)
Directors: Tili Sunelay, John Alepor
Senior Executives: Mr Dibia, Gabriel Brown, G O Oleelee, Felix Agibi
PRINCIPAL ACTIVITIES: Importers, suppliers of building materials, concrete block moulding; agriculture
Principal Bankers: Pan African Bank Ltd
Financial Information:

	N'000
Authorised capital	400
Paid-up capital	400

No of Employees: 100

BEECHAM LTD

PMB 1281, Ikeja, Lagos
Tel: 964868, 964869, 900592
Cable: Beechex Ikeja

Chairman: Chief O I Akinkugbe
Directors: G A Soyoye, E N Chesters, V Steel

PRINCIPAL ACTIVITIES: Manufacturers of pharmaceuticals and toiletries
Branch Offices: Aba; Kano; Ibadan; Onitsha; Factory: 20 Industrial Ave, Ilupeju, Lagos
Principal Bankers: United Bank for Africa Ltd

Date of Establishment: 23rd June 1971
No of Employees: 565

BEGGMATIC AUTOMATIONS LTD

303 Herbert Macaulay St, Yaba, Lagos
Tel: 860921

PRINCIPAL ACTIVITIES: Suppliers of Laundry and dry cleaning equipment

BEN AGENCY SERVICE

36 Idumagbo Ave, PO Box 2788, Lagos
Tel: 651065
Cable: Benaser Lagos

Chairman: Benjamin Akinboro
Directors: Christopher Ajetunmobi, Easter Ayodele Akinboro
Senior Executives: Doye Awolola (General Manager), Christopher Ajetunmobi (Shipping Manager)

PRINCIPAL ACTIVITIES: Freight forwarding and customs agents; shipping services; air freight agents
Principal Agencies: P & J Books (Export) Ltd, UK
Branch Offices: 23/25 Martins St, Lagos
Principal Bankers: United Bank for Africa Ltd

BENDEL BREWERY LTD

Benin-Agbor Rd, Benin City, Bendel State
Tel: 242763

Chairman: E K Iseru
Directors: S Bello-Osagie (General Manager),
 J O Aghimien,
 D C Ukah,
 Dr S B Sanni,
 Dr S E Okojie,
 N I I Aihie
Senior Executives: E O Uwagboe (Acting Technical Manager),
 Lt Col S B Nwajei (Transport Manager),
 S A Idahosa (Assistant Chief Accountant),
 C A Ebaghelu (Marketing Manager),
 P Meuller (Chief Engineer),
 B R O Izegbu (Personnel Manager)

PRINCIPAL ACTIVITIES: Brewing of lager beer
Principal Bankers: New Nigeria Bank Ltd; United Bank for Africa Ltd
Financial Information:

	N'000
Authorised capital	1,500
Paid-up capital	1,500
Turnover	15,000

Principal Shareholders: Bendel State Government
Date of Establishment: 1971
No of Employees: 725

BENDEL CHEMICAL INDUSTRIES LTD

188 Sapele Rd, PMB 1130, Benin City, Bendel State
Tel: 242902
Telex: 41109 Michem Ng

PRINCIPAL ACTIVITIES: Production of distilled water, sulphuric acid, industrial flavours, perfumes and chemicals; batteries for all types of vehicles and stand-by generators
Principal Agencies: Du Croco International, Holland
Principal Shareholders: State-owned organisation

BENDEL HOTELS BOARD

GPA, PMB 1054, Benin City, Bendel State
Tel: 241883, 241932
Cable: Benhotel

PRINCIPAL ACTIVITIES: Hoteliers
Branch Offices: Igarra; Auchi; Uromi; Ubiaja; Iguobazuwa; Benin City; Abudu; Agbor; Asaba; Ogwashi-Uku; Sapele; Orerokpe; Kwale; Warri; Ughelli; Oleh; Bomadi

BENDEL INSURANCE COMPANY LTD

129 Ikpoba Slope, PO Box 607, Benin City, Bendel State
Tel: 243184, 243600
Cable: Bendico
Telex: 41135

Chairman: Chief J U E Agbaza
Directors: Dr C A Omozuwa, C K Okoeguale, Chief N A Mene-Afejuku, Chief G I Oviasu, Chief F S Yesufu
Senior Executives: J I Idehen (General Manager),
 E Inoniyegha (Assistant General Manager, Life & Pensions),
 C Onyekuba (Assistant General Manager, Technical),
 O S Iserhierhien (Deputy Chief Accountant),
 Mrs H E Agun (Senior Personnel Manager),
 C Omozokpia (Senior Technical Manager),
 S A Isede (Company Secretary),
 G I Umuerri (Public Relations Manager),
 A Aisien (Senior Manager Sports)

PRINCIPAL ACTIVITIES: Insurance
Subsidiary Companies: Bendel Investment Company Ltd
Principal Bankers: New Nigeria Bank Ltd
Financial Information:

	N'000
Authorised capital	1,000
Paid-up capital	857

Principal Shareholders: Bendel State Government 51; Private Individuals 49%
Date of Establishment: 1969

BENDEL LINE

22 James Watt Rd, PMB 1046, Benin City, Bendel State
Tel: 241199, 241216
Telex: 41155 Midlin Ng

PRINCIPAL ACTIVITIES: Bus services

Principal Shareholders: Bendel State Government
No of Employees: 1,000

BENDEL NEWSPAPERS CORPORATION

18 Airport Rd, PMB 1334, Benin City, Bendel State
Tel: 240050
Cable: Observer
Telex: 41104 Mncben Ng

PRINCIPAL ACTIVITIES: Newspaper publishing

BENDEL PHARMACEUTICALS LTD

188 Sapele Rd, PMB 1130, Benin City, Bendel State
Tel: 242902
Telex: 41109 Michem Ng

PRINCIPAL ACTIVITIES: Manufacturers of surgical cotton wool, bandages, etc; drugs and pharmaceuticals products
Branch Offices: Drug & Chemical Division; 5 Federal Rd, Uselu, PMB 130, Benin City, Tel 240786

Principal Shareholders: State-owned organisation

BENDEL PLASTIC INDUSTRIES LTD

Plot A19 Sapele Rd, PMB 1356, Benin City, Bendel State
Tel: 241433
Cable: Ben Plast

Chairman: J Oni-Ossai
Directors: J O Iluebbey, Chief S S Rone, A Asiwe
Senior Executives: I E Osaghae (General Manager),
E O Adebayo (Secretary/Accountant),
R Uwadia (Sales Executive),
R Osahon (Production Executive)

PRINCIPAL ACTIVITIES: Production of plastics/plastic products
Principal Bankers: First Bank of Nigeria Ltd; New Nigeria Bank of Nigeria Ltd
Financial Information:

	N'000
Authorised capital	500
Paid-up capital	500

Principal Shareholders: Bendel State Government of Nigeria
Date of Establishment: 15th May 1973

BENDEL STEEL STRUCTURES LTD

Enerhen Rd, PO Box 528, Warri, Bendel State
Tel: 231581
Cable: Bensteel, Warri
Telex: 43286

Chairman: E D A Yaduat
Directors: G A U Komori, S E Aganbi, Dr E K Okoh, One representative of Ministry of Trade, Industry and Co-operatives
Senior Executives: Dr A M Nwabuzor (General Manager),
Chief D A Etaluku (Commercial/Administrative Manager),
E T Obodo (Chief Engineer),
Chief S G Odin (Secretary/Accountant)

PRINCIPAL ACTIVITIES: Steel structural engineers
Branch Offices: 235/237 Apapa Rd, Ijora, PMB 12683, Lagos
Principal Bankers: New Nigeria Bank Ltd; First Bank of Nigeria Ltd

Principal Shareholders: Bendel State Government
No of Employees: 400

BENJAMIN NABENA NABENSON PROMOTIONS

See NABENA, BENJAMIN, NABENSON PROMOTIONS

BENNETT-SASORE-DUNN LTD (NIGERIA)

47 Sakpoba Rd, PMB 1158, Benin City, Bendel State
Tel: 241975
Telex: 41125 Betony Ng

Joint Chairmen: John J Dunn (also Managing Director), Joseph E Bennett
Directors: Lander Sasore

PRINCIPAL ACTIVITIES: Civil and building construction
Associated Companies: John J Dunn Construction Co, USA; Joseph E Bennett, Co, USA
Principal Bankers: New Nigerian Bank Ltd

Principal Shareholders: John J Dunn Construction Co; Lander Sasore; Joseph E Bennett Co; Gabby Sasore

BENORA INSTRUMENTS & COMPANY

1-2 Ganiyu Kale St, PO Box 750, PMB 1093, Oshodi, Lagos
Cable: Benotrumen

Directors: B O Anene (Managing Director),
P Essoka,
Disso O Anene,
Alhaji Aliyu Mohammed,
J Ade Balogun
Senior Executives: E Iddaboh (Instrument Engineer),
V C Okoli (Administrative Manager),
E O Anene (Accountant),
A B Salami (Commercial Manager),
Ossy Anene (Works Manager)

PRINCIPAL ACTIVITIES: Sales and service of electrical and electronic equipment, watches, clocks and jewellery, household goods and appliances, optical and photographic equipment. Mechanical engineering, electroplating, engraving, production and reproduction of machine components and spare parts. Sales of paints and petrochemicals, scientific instruments and power equipment
Principal Agencies: Wilh Lambrecht KG, Gottingen Fed Republic of Germany; Meteorology Research Inc California, USA; Telemechanics Ltd, England
Associated Companies: Prime Feathers International Services Ltd, Nigeria
Principal Bankers: Union Bank of Nigeria Ltd; United Bank for Africa Ltd

Date of Establishment: 1974

BENTWORTH FINANCE (NIGERIA) LTD (BFN)

32 Adetokunbo Ademola St, Victoria Island, Lagos
Tel: 611650, 611656, 611730

Chairman: Akintola Williams
Directors: R T Jones (Managing),
A K Gadzama,
J M A Igbon,
F Egbe,
Alhaji A A Idris,
R E Pequignot,
J O Irukwu,
A C Richards
Senior Executives: S A Adesanya (Company Secretary)

PRINCIPAL ACTIVITIES: Provision of hire-purchase and equipment leasing facilities to transport industries etc
Branch Offices: Ibadan, Oyo State
Principal Bankers: Bank for Credit & Commerce International; United Bank for Africa Ltd; Union Bank of Nig Ltd
Financial Information:

	N'000
Authorised capital	3,000
Paid-up capital	3,000
Turnover	30,000

Principal Shareholders: UDT International Ltd, UK
Date of Establishment: 1956
No of Employees: 40

BENUE CEMENT COMPANY LTD

Kilometre 72, Makurdi-Yandev Rd, PMB 063, Gboko, Benue State
Tel: 610766
Cable: Bencem
Telex: 85305 Bencem, 21386 Bencem

Chairman: Alhaji Abdullahi Adamu

Directors: S S Aondona, Alhaji Mamman Idu, G Quirici, Alhaji M Mohammed, Alhaji M Inuwa

Senior Executives: Robert Brenneisen (Manager Director), T M Niagwan (Controller Administration), S P S Gusah (Commercial Controller), W Wildschek (Financial Controller), P Huber (Technical Controller)

PRINCIPAL ACTIVITIES: Manufacturers of cement

Branch Offices: 306 Adeola Odeku St, Victoria Island, PMB 12702, Lagos; Karu Depot, Federal Capital Territory, Abuja

Associated Companies: Benro Packaging Company Ltd

Principal Bankers: Union Bank of Nigeria Ltd; Bank of the North Ltd

Financial Information:

	N'000
Authorised capital	46,200
Paid-up capital	46,200
Turnover	29,000

Principal Shareholders: Federal Ministry of Industries (39%); Benue State Ministry of Trade and Industries (21%); Plateau Investment Company (14%); Bank for Commerce & Industry (7%); New Nigerian Development Company (5%); Nigerian Industrial Development Bank (3%); Cementia Holding Ag (11%)

Date of Establishment: February 1981

No of Employees: 787

BENUE PLATEAU RICE COMPANY LTD

Bukuru Rd, PMB 281, Jos, Plateau State

Tel: 3032, 3343

Cable: Riceco Jos

Telex: 81127 Nascos Ng

PRINCIPAL ACTIVITIES: Parboiling and processing of rice

Financial Information: Associate of Nasreddin Co SAS, Italy

BEPCO (NIG) LTD

113 New Secretariat Rd, PMB 2103, Jos, Plateau State

Tel: 2104, 3005

Telex: 81117 Bepco Ng

PRINCIPAL ACTIVITIES: Building and civil engineering contractors

BEREC NIGERIA LTD

Plot 1 Block J Isolo Industrial Estate, PO Box 2681, Lagos

Tel: 876317, 876413

Cable: Berecbat Lagos

Telex: 21465 Berec Ng

Chairman: Julius Agbaje

Directors: J Ogundeji, Alhaji Hashim, S Deru, M R Sell

PRINCIPAL ACTIVITIES: Manufacturers of batteries

Principal Shareholders: Nigerians; Ever Ready Company (Holdings) Ltd, UK

Date of Establishment: 21st September 1963

BERENSHOT MORET BOSBOOM

25 Boyle St (5th Floor), PO Box 4112, Lagos

PRINCIPAL ACTIVITIES: Engineering consultants

BERG GEOTECHNICAL ENGINEERING (NIGERIA) LTD

4 Kamselem Rd, PO Box 4471, Kaduna

Tel: 210310

Telex: 71118 Kaduna

Chairman: Fernand-Auguste Soeiro (also Managing Director)

Directors: Mrs R A Okezie

Senior Executives: Lucien Nocet (General Manager)

PRINCIPAL ACTIVITIES: Engineering consultants; site investigations, ground water engineering, geological, geotechnical and geophysical surveys, earth and rock dam designers; soil mechanics laboratory

Principal Agencies: PMB 1360, Enugu, Anambra State, Telex 51163; PO Box 5290, Lagos, Telex 21445

Branch Offices: PO Box 5290, Lagos, Telex 21445

Subsidiary Companies: BERG Engineering SA, Paris, Telex 250303

Principal Bankers: Societe Generale Bank (Nigeria) Ltd; International Bank for West Africa Ltd

Date of Establishment: 21st December 1979

BERGER, JULIUS, NIGERIA LTD

Ijora Causeway, Ijora, PO Box 3643, Lagos

Tel: 832810/11, 832901

Cable: Bauberger Lagos

Telex: 21486 Juberg Ng

Chairman: Alhaji Chief A S Adewale

Directors: G Hawranke (Managing), R Wagner, H Wittmann, J Richter (Deputy Managing), M A Braimah, V K Dangin, Alhaji M Fakkai (Executive), Alhaji Chief R I Solomon, M T Usman (Executive)

Senior Executives: O Voise (Commerical Director)

PRINCIPAL ACTIVITIES: Civil engineering and construction

Principal Bankers: Union Bank of Nigeria Ltd

Financial Information:

	N'000
Authorised capital	12,000
Paid-up capital	12,000

Date of Establishment: 18th February 1970
No of Employees: 8,246

BERGER PAINTS (NIGERIA) LTD

Oba Akran Ave, PMB 21052, Ikeja, Lagos
Tel: 900031, 900032, 962312
Cable: Apexior Ikeja

Chairman: Allison Akene Ayida
Directors: Sunday Dankaro, Alex Aofolajuwonio, Akinola Duyile
Senior Executives: Tunji Awobadejo, Akin Adegoke, Parry Owei, J A Ekundayo, Miss F T Carew, Newman Offonry, Tunji Sawyer

PRINCIPAL ACTIVITIES: Manufacturers of all types of paints; automotive finishes, protective coatings, industrial finishes, oil industry coatings, etc
Branch Offices: 70 Trans Amadi Estate, PO Box 681, Port Harcourt, Rivers State
Financial Information: An Associate of the Berger, Jenson & Nicholson Ltd Group of Companies

BERIF INTERNATIONAL COMPANY

PO Box 6855, Lapal House, 7th Floor, Igbosere Rd, Lagos
Tel: 635387
Telex: 21480 Berif

Partners: J I Harry (Principal Partner)
Senior Executives: B Zollinger (Principal Consultant)

PRINCIPAL ACTIVITIES: Commercial and industrial consultants; managing agents
Date of Establishment: 1974

BERIF INTERNATIONAL COMPANY

Commercial and Industrial Consultants

MANAGING AGENTS

MANAGEMENT CONSULTANTS

PROJECT MANAGERS

Feasibility Studies

Techno- and Macro-Economic Surveys

Joint Venture Negotiations

Complete assistance in establishing and incorporating of Companies in Nigeria

Organisation and Re-organisation/Restructuring of Companies/Organisations in Public and Private Sector

Personnel Selection and Supervision

Company Secretarial Services

For advice or assistance, please write to:

Chief Consultant
Berif International Company
PO Box 6855
Lagos

BERLIET NIGERIA LTD

Isolo Expressway, Ilasamaja Industrial Scheme, PO Box 6655, Lagos
Tel: 860645
Cable: Autoberlie Lagos

PRINCIPAL ACTIVITIES: Distribution, servicing, suppliers of spare parts for heavy duty vehicles, agricultural tractors and generating sets
Principal Agencies: Renault, France
Branch Offices: 20 Club Rd, PMB 3114, Kano; Airport Rd, Emene, PO Box 255, Enugu, Anambra State; 43B Upper Siluko Rd, PMB 1430, Benin City, Bendel State
Principal Bankers: Societe Generale Bank Nigeria Ltd; International Bank for West Africa Ltd; United Bank for Africa Ltd
Financial Information:

	N'000
Authorised capital	1,500
Paid-up capital	1,500
Turnover	20,000

Principal Shareholders: Nigerian (60%); French (40%)
Date of Establishment: 30th November 1971
No of Employees: 250

BESTFORM INDUSTRIES CO LTD

54 Ibidun St, Surulere, Lagos

PRINCIPAL ACTIVITIES: Manufacturing of wood and metal furniture, cement blocks

BEWAC AUTOMOTIVE PRODUCTS LTD

PMB 5140, Plot 12 Trans-Amadi Industrial Estate, Port Harcourt, Rivers State
Tel: 333491
Cable: Bap Port Harcourt

Chairman: F I R E Mills
Directors: P A Ogwuma,
M B Phillips,
M O Areh,
G N Mbanefo,
M N A Ukabam (General Manager),
Mrs K I Kemmer,
Dr P N Bassey
Senior Executives: G S Ikemeh (Accountant),
A E Offiong (Sales Manager)

PRINCIPAL ACTIVITIES: Assembly and marketing of landrovers and range rovers, Leyland trucks, Massey-Ferguson Tractors
Principal Agencies: Leyland Nigeria Ltd; Bewac Ltd
Branch Offices: 18 Aba Rd, PMB 5140, Port Harcourt, Rivers State; 5 Okpara Ave, PO Box 372, Enugu, Anambra State; Industry Rd, PMB 7147, Aba, Imo State
Principal Bankers: Union Bank of Nigeria Ltd
Financial Information:

	N'000
Authorised capital	552
Paid-up capital	552
Turnover	2,000

Principal Shareholders: Bewac Ltd; Anambra State Government; Imo State Government; Cross River State Government; Rivers State Government
Date of Establishment: 1964
No of Employees: 250

BEWAC LTD

1 Commercial Rd, PMB 1016, Apapa, Lagos
Tel: 803450/4
Cable: Bewac Lagos
Telex: 21255

Chairman: Chief Alhaji I A S Adewale
Directors: D A Edmonds (Managing),
A A Ayida,
H H Ado Bayero,
A Bello,

Chief (Mrs) D B A Kuforiji,
H G A Lawrence,
D B Otrofanowei,
J W Ritchie,
H A Subair
Senior Executives: S A Gbadebo (Company Secretary),
E O Gbeworo (Marketing Director),
A A Odukoya (Technical Controller),
K O Shaibu (Company Director)

PRINCIPAL ACTIVITIES: Distribution and servicing of motor vehicles, agricultural and industrial machinery, importation and distribution of building and engineering products, hardware, tyres, tubes; importation and installation of irrigation, water and sewage treatment plants, and marine craft. Reprographic, bearing transmission supplies and services. Manufacturers of plastic packaging, air conditioners and generators
Principal Agencies: Leyland; Massey Ferguson; Hanomag; Satec; Wright Rain; Auto diesel; Hitachi; Nashua; Saxon; Crypton; Churchill; Lee Howl-Myers; APE
Branch Offices: PMB 1147, Azikiwe Rd, Aba; PO Box 372, Opara Avenue, Enugu; PO Box 385, Molete, Ibadan; PO Box 504, 23 Queen Elizabeth Way, Jos; PO Box 355, Ahmadu Bello Way, Kaduna; PO Box 153, Maiduguri; 18 Aba Rd, PO Box 5140, Port Harcourt; PO Box 457, Enerhe Rd, Warri
Subsidiary Companies: VYB (Nigeria) Ltd; Bewac Automotive Products Ltd
Principal Bankers: Union Bank of Nigeria Ltd; United Bank for Africa Ltd; First Bank of Nigeria Ltd
Financial Information:

	N'000
Authorised capital	7,500
Paid-up capital	7,500
Turnover	87,300
Profits	(1,900)

Principal Shareholders: Bewac Motor Corporation (40%); State Government (16.7%); Private Individuals (43%)
Date of Establishment: 13th April, 1950
No of Employees: 1,162

BHANDARI & COMPANY (NIGERIA) LTD

66 Eleshin Street, Obalend, PO Box 2232, Lagos
Tel: 963039
Cable: Bhandari Lagos
Telex: 20117 TDS 188

Directors: Chief H Bhandari (Managing),
S A Pitan

PRINCIPAL ACTIVITIES: Manufacturers of sports, scientific and surgical equipment. Importers
Subsidiary/Associated Companies: Metal Industries (Nigeria) Ltd; Raslao & Company Ltd
Principal Bankers: Union Bank of Nigeria Ltd

BHOJSONS & COMPANY (NIGERIA) LTD

49 Marina, PO Box 867, Lagos
Tel: 660990, 660997
Cable: Bhojsons
Telex: 21424

Chairman: B B Chanrai
Directors: M B Chanrai, Chief N O Idowu, Alhaji I M Damcida, G V Melvani, Chief G U Okeke
PRINCIPAL ACTIVITIES: Chain stores, furniture, household goods and appliances; optical and photographic equipment. Textiles and clothing, and textile equipment
Principal Agencies: Bhojsons Industries Ltd; Nigerian Synthetic Fabrics Ltd; Nigerian Embroidery Lace Manufacturing Co Ltd; Nigerian Polyvinly Chloride Products Ltd
Branch Offices: Ebute Metta, Lagos; Ikoyi; Lagos; Ereko St, Lagos; Docemo St, Lagos; Kano; Kaduna; Port Harcourt and Ibadan
Subsidiary Companies: Pantrade & Investment Co Ltd (Gibraltar); Bhojsons (UK) Ltd (UK); Bhojsons & Co (Japan) Ltd (Yokoh ma); Bhojraj Hassomal Private Ltd (Bombay);

Bhojsons & Co (Japan) Ltd (Osaka); Pantrade Dev Co Ltd (Hongkong); Pantrade Dev Co Ltd (Taipei)
Principal Bankers: United Bank for Africa Ltd; Union Bank of Nigeria Ltd; Societe Generale Bank (Nigeria) Ltd; International Bank for West Africa Ltd
Financial Information:
Turnover   Over N 100 Million

Date of Establishment: 1953
No of Employees: 4,000

BHOJSONS INDUSTRIES LTD

PO Box 311, Ikeja, Lagos
Tel: 961223, 961320

PRINCIPAL ACTIVITIES: Textile manufacturers

BIBSON ASSOCIATES LTD

20 Ayinde St, Ojota, PMB 21571, Ikeja, Lagos

PRINCIPAL ACTIVITIES: Importers and distributors of various food products, and building materials. Transporters; motor vehicle distribution and servicing; Plant hire services
Branch Offices: Ibadan; Kano
Subsidiary Companies: Bibson International & Co Ltd; Bibson Land & Coastal Carriers Ltd; Bibson Motors Ltd; Bibson Engineering Co Ltd

BICC CONSTRUCTION (NIGERIA) LTD

50 Warehouse Rd, Apapa, Lagos
Tel: 877171
Telex: 21420 Bictel Ng

PRINCIPAL ACTIVITIES: Construction
Branch Offices: 17 Badagry Rd, Apapa, Lagos, Tel 876744; 38 Warehouse Rd, Apapa, Lagos, Tel 876475, 831290; 5 Ashanti Rd, Apapa, Lagos

BIDA, ALHAJI AUDU, & SONS UNITED COMPANY LTD

Plot A, Ahmadu Bello Way, PO Box 70, Kaduna
Tel: 242897

PRINCIPAL ACTIVITIES: Civil engineering and construction, and general contractors

BIDAT SPORTSWEAR COMPANY LTD

24 Adeyinka St, Ilupeju Industrial Estate, PO Box 5721, Marina, Lagos
Tel: 931363
Cable: Bidatwear
Telex: 11117 Ng

Chairman: Augustine Adesina Buraimoh-Ademuyewo
Directors: William J Rielly, Adelaja Ademuyewo, Brands International Company Ltd
Senior Executives: Donatus Ichentuoye (General Manager), Mrs Yinka Babalola (Deputy General Manager/Financial Controller),
Mrs Bola Bankole (Sales Manager),
Sebastan Nwadike (Production Manager),
Benjamin Okorocha (Sales Manager)

PRINCIPAL ACTIVITIES: Manufacturing of textiles, sports clothing and sports goods
Principal Agencies: Velva Sheen Manufacturing Co Inc (USA); E R Moore Co (USA)
Branch Offices: Factory: PMB 2005, Ijebu-Ode, Ogun State, Tel 434504
Principal Bankers: United Bank for Africa
Financial Information:

	N'000
Authorised capital	500
Paid-up capital	204
Turnover	700

Date of Establishment: 1975
No of Employees: 100

BIDECO (NIGERIA) LTD
PO Box 1311, Ring Rd, Ibadan, Oyo State
Tel: 414686

PRINCIPAL ACTIVITIES: Building and civil engineering
  contractors
Branch Offices: Bideco House, 2A Anthony Rd, Km 12 Ikorodu
  Rd, PMB 21537, Ikeja, Lagos, Tel 960617, 960660

BIMBOTECH (NIGERIA) LTD
53Y Mallam-Kure St, PO Box 1014, Jos, Plateau State
Tel: 55819, 55820
Cable: Bimbotech
Telex: 55820

Chairman: J O Oyegoke
Directors: E A Oyegoke, J O Oyegoke

PRINCIPAL ACTIVITIES: General contracting, civil engineering
  and building construction; transportation; wholesalers
Principal Bankers: Union Bank of Nigeria Ltd
Financial Information:
Authorised capital   ₦ 100,000

Principal Shareholders: E A Oyegoke; J O Oyegoke
Date of Establishment: 20th May 1977

BINATONE ELECTRONICS
7 Oremeji St, Off Medical Rd, PMB 21507, Ikeja, Lagos State
Tel: 960352

PRINCIPAL ACTIVITIES: Suppliers of electrical goods, radios,
  calculators, stereos, etc
Associated Companies: Interworld Enterprises (Nigeria) Ltd

BIOBAKU FABER & PARTNERS
(Formerly Oscar Faber (Nigeria))
Eshugbayi House, 160 Bamgbose Street, PO Box 6685, Lagos
Tel: 635844, 631143
Cable: Fabercon, Lagos
Telex: 22549

Resident Partners: L B Biobaku, I S Ogunbayo, G F Rooke

PRINCIPAL ACTIVITIES: Consulting: civil, structural, electrical
  and mechanical engineering
Associated Companies: Oscar Faber Partnership, UK
Principal Bankers: Union Bank of Nigeria Ltd

BIODE PHARMACEUTICAL INDUSTRIES LTD
PO Box 425, Mile 10, Ikorodu Rd, Ojoto, Lagos
Tel: 900273

PRINCIPAL ACTIVITIES: Manufacturing of pharmaceutical
  products
Branch Offices: 1 Abijoh Close, SW Ikoyi, Lagos, Tel 681864,
  931643

BIOMEDICAL SERVICES COMPANY LTD
10 Ondo Street West, Ebute Metta, PO Box 1228, Surulere,
  Lagos
Tel: 831309
Cable: Bromedical, Lagos
Telex: 376637

Chairman: Dr Umar Farouk Abdulazeez
Directors: Mrs F J Abdulazeez, G G Sonekan, P Y Luguja, G
  Botteron
Senior Executives: Dr A Ibrahim (General Manager),
  M M Salami (Production Manager),
  D O Ogunro (Quality Control Manager),
  M Adeniran (Plant Engineer),
  A Giwah (Company Accountant)

PRINCIPAL ACTIVITIES: Manufacturer and distributor of
  infusions. Distributor of drugs and medicines, hospital,
  surgical and scientific equipment
Principal Agencies: Vifor SA (Switzerland); Sweca (Switzerland);
  Dott Bonapace & Co (Italy)
Branch Offices: 1 Ohimege Rd, PMB 1449, Ilorin, Tel 5295
Principal Bankers: Societe Generale Bank

Financial Information:

	₦'000
Authorised capital	1,000
Paid-up capital	1,000
Turnover	1,650
Profits	382

Principal Shareholders: Dr U F Abdulazeez (51%); NNDC (20%);
  NIDB (11%); Vifor/Andre (10%)
Date of Establishment: 14th April, 1978
No of Employees: 70

BIRMA GENERAL SUPPLIES LTD
13E Bello Rd, PO Box 454, Kano
Tel: 2772, 3823
Cable: Birma Kano
Telex: 77211 Kano

Chairman: Alhaji U S Birma (also Managing Director)
Directors: Alhaji M P Garba,
  Alhaji Usman Kadafur,
  Alhaji U Garba (General Manager)
Senior Executives: Alhaji M Adamu (Accountant),
  Mallam A Birma (Branch Manager),
  Mallam Muhammed (Branch Manager),
  P E Nnaji (Stores Officer)

PRINCIPAL ACTIVITIES: Suppliers of electrical appliances,
  carpets and furniture. Electrical appliances assembly plant to
  be constructed
Principal Agencies: Leventis Group of Companies; Philips Nigeria
  Ltd; Santana Furniture Factory; Nigeria Engineering Works
Branch Offices: PMB 2070, Yola, Gongola State; PO Box 134,
  Zaria, Kaduna State; PO Box 246, Maiduguri, Borno State;
  Bauchi, Bauchi State
Principal Bankers: United Bank for Africa Ltd; Bank of Credit
  and Commerce International (Nigeria) Ltd
Financial Information:

	₦'000
Authorised capital	500
Paid-up capital	500
Sales turnover	6,000
Profits	540

Principal Shareholders: US Birma; Alhaji Usman Kadafur; Alhaji
  G Pindar; Alhaji Usman Garba; Alhaji Dauda Birma
Date of Establishment: 15th April 1970
No of Employees: 135

BIROM MINES LTD
1 Vom Rd, PO Box 75, Bukuru, Plateau State
Tel: 456

PRINCIPAL ACTIVITIES: Mining metal ore

BISCEGLIA BROTHERS & ASSOCIATES
CONSTRUCTION CO (NIGERIA) LTD
27/29 Martins St, PO Box 420, Lagos
PRINCIPAL ACTIVITIES: Construction

BISCUIT MANUFACTURING COMPANY OF NIGERIA LTD
Adinlewa Rd, PMB 1056, Ikeja, Lagos State
Tel: 900152, 900153
Cable: Bisco Lagos
Telex: 21238

Chairman: Chief M N Ugochukwu
Directors: P Best, E J Hamman, Chief G C Ikokwu, Lady D O
  Jibowu, C K N Obih, Chief B O Ofu, Mrs O O Olakunri,
  Alhaji Habib Bello, R I Onyejiaka, D R Simpson, R I
  Ugochukwu
Senior Executives: J N Anozie (General Manager),
  S B McMullen (Deputy General Manager),
  P E Okoronkwo (Financial Controller),
  J A Rockson (Administrative Manager),
  M O Abiola (Accountant),
  F A Bello (Personnel Manager),

V H S Rajawasan (Chief Engineer),
H A Amosu (Factory Manager),
A S Bamgbala (Marketing Manager)
PRINCIPAL ACTIVITIES: Food and food processing, biscuit manufacturers
Principal Bankers: Union Bank of Nigeria Ltd; First Bank of Nigeria Ltd
Principal Shareholders: Ugochukwu & Sons Ltd; John Holt Holdings (Nigeria) Ltd; Nigerian Industrial Development Bank Ltd; Mrs P O Dina
Date of Establishment: 8th November, 1961
No of Employees: 700

BISICHI-JANTAR (NIGERIA) LTD
PO Box 19, Jos, Plateau State
Tel: 229
Cable: Bijanig Jos
PRINCIPAL ACTIVITIES: Tin and columbite mining
Principal Shareholders: Nigerian (60%); Jantar Ltd, London (20%); Bisichi Tin Co, London (20%)

BISIOLU ENTERPRISES LTD
1-3 Warehouse Rd, Apapa, PO Box 3214, Lagos
Tel: 847288
Telex: 21543 Bek Bek
PRINCIPAL ACTIVITIES: Suppliers of sanitary-ware, pipes, floor coverings, adhesives, paints, etc
Principal Agencies: Twyfords Ltd, UK

BISROD FURNITURE COMPANY LTD
PMB 5491, N6A/317 Oyo Rd, Mokola, Ibadan, Oyo State
Chairman: Bisi Rodipe (also Managing Director)
PRINCIPAL ACTIVITIES: Manufacturers of domestic and office furniture. There are plans to expand into sawmilling
Branch Offices: Ijari; Ijebu-Ode; Ogun State
Date of Establishment: 1974

BKI BUILDING & CIVIL ENGINEERING CO LTD
62 Maganda Rd, Kano
Tel: 2769, 2751
PRINCIPAL ACTIVITIES: Building and civil engineering contractors

BLACK & DECKER NIGERIA LTD
PO Box 4199, Ikeja, Lagos
Tel: 610241
Cable: Bladenig
Chairman: F Egbe
Directors: Dr N B Graham Douglas, J B Johnson, R F Leverton, R B N Ditlefsen
Senior Executives: H Mouratides (General Manager),
D J Metcalf (Development Manager),
S A Maduabuchi (Senior Accountant),
E Amromah (Sales Manager),
C O Ladipo (Service/Distribution Manager)
PRINCIPAL ACTIVITIES: Sales and service of domestic and industrial portable electrical tools and accessories, petrol chain saws, radial arm saws, ladders, welders, workbenches
Principal Agencies: Black & Decker Ltd; Dewalt; Tatry-Italy; Star Utensili; Electrici-Italy
Branch Offices: Plot G Ikosi Rd, Dregun, Ikeja, Lagos
Subsidiary Companies: Black & Decker Manufacturing Co, USA
Principal Bankers: First Bank of Nigeria Ltd; Chase Merchant Bank Ltd
Financial Information:

	N'000
Authorised capital	1,000
Paid-up capital	750

Principal Shareholders: 60% Nigerians; 40% Black & Decker Manufacturing, USA
Date of Establishment: August 1970

BLACKWOOD HODGE (NIGERIA) LTD
Asogun Rd, KM 15 Opp Trade Fair Complex, Badagry Express Rd, PO Box 109, Apapa, Lagos
Tel: 875821, 876767, 876839
Cable: Suntract Lagos
Telex: 21393 Suntra Ng, 21870 Suntra Ng
Chairman: Dr Alhaji I B Jose
Directors: M W Davis (Managing Director),
C L Ferguson,
W A Shapland,
F A Afolayan (General Manager/Finance),
S A Salami (General Manager/Operations),
Alhaji Mamman Daura,
Babatunde Edu
Senior Executives: M C Mwabunor (Administrative Controller),
S I Somuyiwa (Parts Controller),
A O Dawodu (Service Controller),
E Osidipe (Financial Controller)
PRINCIPAL ACTIVITIES: Distribution of earth-moving and allied equipment; construction equipment; diesel engines; transmissions and power generators
Principal Agencies: Terex Ltd, Detroit Diesel, Champion Road Machinery Company, P&H Harnischfeger Corporation; Jones Cranes; JCB Sales; ABG; Consolidated Pneumatic Tools Co Ltd; Firestone; Warner Swassey; Eaton International; Grant Galloway & Gear; Fagersta
Branch Offices: 24 Club Rd, Kano; Trans Amadi Industrial Layout, Port-Harcourt, Rivers State; Enerhen Rd, Warri, Bendel State; Baga Rd, Maiduguri, Borno State
Subsidiary Companies: Wholly owned subsidiary; diesel sales and service (Nigeria) Ltd
Principal Bankers: Union Bank of Nigeria Ltd
Financial Information:

	N'000
Authorised capital	5,400
Paid-up capital	5,400
Turnover (1980)	32,653
Profits (Gross)	3,112

Principal Shareholders: John Blackwood Hodge & Company Ltd, UK (40%); Nigerian Nationals (60%)
Date of Establishment: 8th September 1948
No of Employees: 440

BLESSED FURNITURE ENTERPRISES
70 Warri-Sapele Rd, PO Box 546, Warri, Bendel State
PRINCIPAL ACTIVITIES: Manufacturers of all types of furniture

BLUE STRAPS LTD
Owode Industrial Estate, Km 10 Abeokuta Rd, PO Box 2592, Ibadan
Tel: 411277
Cable: Blusco
Telex: 31477 Rosco Ng
PRINCIPAL ACTIVITIES: Manufacturers of steel strappings for packaging and metal seals
Principal Bankers: Allied Bank of Nigeria Ltd
Financial Information:

	N'000
Authorised	650
Paid-up capital	640

Date of Establishment: Came into production July 1980

BODAX INSTRUMENTS & TOOLS LTD
126/130 Nnamdi Azikiwe St, 5th Floor, PO Box 4159, Lagos
Tel: 652199, 636438
PRINCIPAL ACTIVITIES: Suppliers of tools, instruments and spare parts
Branch Offices: Plot 26 Western Ave, Surulere, Lagos

BODE INTERNATIONAL NIG AGENCIES

38 Araromi St, Onike, Yaba, Lagos State
Tel: 862171
Cable: Bodinnag Lagos

Chairman: Chief David Adeleke Olubode
Senior Executives: O A Olubode (Purchasing Manager),
Johnson Opawole (Office Manager)

PRINCIPAL ACTIVITIES: Agents, business consultants; general
procurement of stores and general contract works
Principal Agencies: Federal Government of Nigeria (Consultancy
Services); Engineering Industrial Export Ltd, UK; Thos Storey
Engineers Ltd, UK
Principal Bankers: Union Bank of Nigeria Ltd

Date of Establishment: 1976

BOLADELE BROTHERS & CO LTD

22 Hawley St, PO Box 5878, Lagos
Tel: 634616

PRINCIPAL ACTIVITIES: Colour lithographic printing and rubber
stamps

BOLEX ENTERPRISES

PO Box 3521, 8-10 Broad St, Lagos
Tel: 636821
Telex: 21409 Bolex Ng

PRINCIPAL ACTIVITIES: General merchants

BOLINGO ORGANISATION

74/78 Ziks Avenue, PO Box 161, Onitsha, Anambra State
Tel: 408

PRINCIPAL ACTIVITIES: Companies within the organisation are:
Bolingo Hotels Ltd; Bolingo Electrics Ltd (suppliers of hospital
and scientific equipment, radio transmitters, close circuit
televisions etc); Skyline Construction Co Ltd (building and
civil engineering contractors); Joeson (Suppliers) Ltd
(financiers, export merchants, manufacturers representatives);
Bolingo Fishing Industries Ltd (frozen food stockists); Joeson
Industries Ltd (printing, paper conversion, packaging); Bolingo
(WA) Co Ltd (property investment; general traders); Threads
Industries Co Ltd (textiles)

BOLOKOR MK LTD

Jenta New Layout, PO Box 117, Jos, Plateau State
Tel: 2238

PRINCIPAL ACTIVITIES: Metal ore mining
Branch Offices: Bauchi; Kano; Zaria

BOLORI BROTHERS & CO LTD (BOLBROS)

PO Box 38, Maiduguri, Borno State
Tel: 232932
Cable: Bolbros
Telex: 82152 Bolor Ng

PRINCIPAL ACTIVITIES: Importers and dealers in technical,
electrical and mechanical engineering equipment, and
building materials
Branch Offices: Mubi; Gombe; Yola; 7E Bello Rd, PO Box 6024,
Kano, Tel 5417

BOMA ASSOCIATES (WA) LTD

655 Lagos Rd, PO Box 2675, Ibadan, Oyo State
Tel: 411747
Cable: Boma, Ibadan
Telex: 31531

Principal Consultant: I Olu Ige

PRINCIPAL ACTIVITIES: Industrial business and management
consultants. Manufacturers' representatives. Importers of
office machines, medical disposables, woodmaking machinery
and tools
Principal Bankers: Bank of the North Ltd

BONNY LNG LTD

PO Box 51039, 19 Idejo St, Victoria Island, Lagos
Tel: 614771, 614777, 635442

PRINCIPAL ACTIVITIES: Liquifaction and export of gas, when
the project is completed

Principal Shareholders: NNPC (60%); Shell (10%); AP (10%);
Phillips (7.5%); Agip (7.5%), Elf (5%)

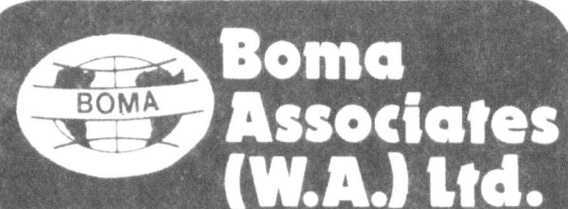

Boma Associates (W.A.) Ltd.

655 LAGOS ROAD, P.O. BOX 2675
IBADAN SW9 NIGERIA
Telephone : (022) 411747,
Telex : 31531 BOMAIG NG,
Cable : 'BOMA' IBADAN NIGERIA

We Are:
Industrial business & Management Consultants.
Industrial Developers.
Market Research and Feasibility Surveyors.
Business Analysts.

Manufacturers' Representatives & Importers of:-
Office Machines & Equipments
Hospital/Medical disposable items
Wood-making Machineries & Tools
Chair base castors, etc.

Office:-
655 Lagos Road, P.O. Box 2675, Ibadan SW9 Nigeria.

BONNY OIL & GAS INDUSTRIES (NIGERIA) LTD
(BOGI)

PO Box 1057, 6 Elsie Femi Pearse St, Victoria Island, Lagos
Tel: 614877, 614586
Cable: Boncon
Telex: 21115

Directors: A F Olaleye (Administrative Manager),
L Berger (General Manager, Port Harcourt),
A P Wright (Engineer),
A Warner (Superintendent Port Harcourt)

PRINCIPAL ACTIVITIES: Oil and gas services; design
engineering, pipeline contractors and construction
Branch Offices: Operations Base; PO Box 649, Port Harcourt,
Rivers State, Tel 285

BONO INTERNATIONAL LTD

138 Warri/Sapele Rd, PO Box 17, Warri, Bendel State
Chairman: Bonus Joel Ogadien (also Managing Director)
PRINCIPAL ACTIVITIES: Suppliers of general merchandise

BONOMI, S G, LTD

162 Mission Rd, PO Box 550, Kano
Tel: 3645

PRINCIPAL ACTIVITIES: Building and civil engineering
contractors and joiners, furniture manufacturers
Branch Offices: 1 Constitution Hill, PO Box 227, Jos; PO Box
245, Kaduna

BOOTS COMPANY (NIGERIA) LTD (THE)

Plots 22/23 Chief T A Doherty Layout, Oregun Industrial Estate,
PMB 21069, Ikeja, Lagos State
Tel: 931701/2/3
Cable: Bootsdrug Lagos
Telex: 26225 Drug Ng

Chairman: C O Lawson
Directors: R A Johnson, J W Dudley, Alhaji I B Jose, Alhaji M
Daura, J W Lewin
Senior Executives: A B Odenusi (Finance Director/Company
Secretary),
Dr M O Abe (Production Director),
A O Ogunsola (Marketing Manager)

PRINCIPAL ACTIVITIES: Manufacturing and selling of
pharmaceutical products, toiletries and cosmetics
Principal Agencies: The Boots Company PLC, UK
Branch Offices: PO Box 468, Kano, Kano State; PO Box 11215,
Ibadan, Oyo State; 51 Aba Owerri Rd, Aba, Imo State
Subsidiary Companies: The Boots Company PLC, UK
Principal Bankers: First Bank of Nigeria Ltd
Financial Information:

	₦'000
Authorised capital	3,000
Paid-up capital	3,000
Turnover	10,000

Principal Shareholders: Nigerians 60%; Boots Nottingham 40%
Date of Establishment: 12th September 1960
No of Employees: 250

BORDPAK PREMIER PACKAGING

5/7 Dockyard Rd, PO Box 369, Apapa, Lagos
Tel: 875644, 875735
Cable: Bordpak Apapa

Chairman: E A O Shonekan
Directors: M G Bloomer, Chief S B Daniyan, Alhaji Shehu Idris,
M C Thompson, H T Mathers, A C I Mbanefo, J O Omidiora,
F M O Osifo, J P Rauch, P D Tueart, Alhaji Bello Sani, J G
A Clegg, J C Egri-Okwaji
Senior Executives: G M Clark (General Manager),
A I Moyo (Commercial Manager),
A Balogun (Marketing Manager),
J L Ojutalayo (General Works Manager),
G Johnson (Resources/Development Manager),
S R Osberghaus (Project Manager),
Dr S N Obidegwu (Technical Services Manager),
M B Ishaku (Personnel Manager)

PRINCIPAL ACTIVITIES: Manufacture of corrugated cases,
packaging cartons, folding boxes, flexibles, labels, wrappers
and systems
Branch Offices: Gidan Goldie Building, 2 Niger Street, PO Box
4149, Kano; 7 Johnson St, PO Box 308, Onitsha
Principal Bankers: First Bank of Nigeria Ltd

Principal Shareholders: Division of UAC of Nigeria Ltd
Date of Establishment: 1964
No of Employees: 1,000

BORINI PRONO & CO LTD

7/9 Burma Rd, PO Box 54, Apapa, Lagos
Tel: 876087, 876058, 831769

Directors: Dr Giuseppe Prono, Dino Camerini, Attilio Del
Mastro, Dr Umberto Camusi

PRINCIPAL ACTIVITIES: Building and civil engineering
contractors
Branch Offices: Kaduna

BORNO ENGINEERING & STEEL MANUFACTURERS LTD

PO Box 6, Maiduguri, Borno State
Tel: 232195
Telex: 82169 Besm Ltd Ng

PRINCIPAL ACTIVITIES: Manufacturers of steel doors and
windows, beds, mattresses, pillows, etc, chairs, desks,
furniture; steel structures

BOSAG BUILDERS

Olakunle Chambers, 1 Ajayi St, Ketu, PO Box 4608, Lagos

Chairman: Bola Abimbola
Directors: Abdul Wazeel Adeleke (Commercial Director),
Sulaiman Abisoye Abimbola (Purchasing Director),
Sikiru Abidemi Abimbola (Project Director)

PRINCIPAL ACTIVITIES: Builders, civil engineers, water
treatment, general contractors
Principal Agencies: Apex Paints Nig Ltd; WTA, Austria;
Aquatechnik, Austria
Branch Offices: 4 Okimogbe St, Egbe, Alimosho, Lagos State
Subsidiary Companies: Kunza Heed (WA) Enterprises
Principal Bankers: National Bank of Nigeria Ltd
Financial Information:

	₦'000
Authorised capital	150
Paid-up capital	100
Turnover	250
Profits	100

Principal Shareholders: Bola Abimbola; Sikiru Abimbola;
Sulaiman Abisoye; T Abim
Date of Establishment: 1979
No of Employees: 100

BOSKALIS NIGERIA LTD

Ibafon Yard, Off Apapa-Ikeja Expressway, Apapa, PO Box 1518,
Lagos
Tel: 834033
Cable: Nidredge Lagos
Telex: 21451

Chairman: Chief Michael C O Ibru
Directors: Dr J A Anaza,
L Verschuren (Managing Director),
P Reydon,
A U Ibru
Senior Executives: N de Jongh (Financial Manager),
J E Larvin (Technical Services Manager)

PRINCIPAL ACTIVITIES: Civil engineering and construction
Principal Agencies: Group member: Royal Boskalis Westminster
Group, (Holland)
Branch Offices: 1 Ihiala Street, Port Harcourt, Rivers State
Principal Bankers: Union Bank of Nigeria; Hollandsche Bank;
Amro Bank Amsterdam Rotterdam Bank NV
Financial Information:

	₦'000
Authorised capital	1,000
Paid-up capital	1,000
Turnover	25,000
Profits	1,120

Principal Shareholders: Oteri Holdings Ltd, Royal Boskalis
Westminster NV
Date of Establishment: 1977
No of Employees: 1,000

BOTAM (NIGERIA) LTD

33 Iga Idungandran St, Lagos
Tel: 632592, 631365
Cable: Botamex
Telex: 22161 Botam Ng

Chairman: Chief A Bisi Badejo
Directors: R A Shafe (Managing),
S A Oladejo (Commercial),
M P B Houdret,

46

F E Okorie (Branch Manager)
PRINCIPAL ACTIVITIES: Importers, industrialists, manufacturers'
    representatives. Distributors, etc
Principal Agencies: Houdret & Co Ltd, UK; Lewis Woolf Griptight
    Ltd, UK; Hesse, Andre & Co, West Germany; Poliscambi
    SRL, Italy; Wirminghams & Funcke, West Germany
Branch Offices: 1 Okwei St, PMB 1563, Onitsha Tel 211861
Principal Bankers: Union Bank of Nigeria Ltd; United Bank for
    Africa Ltd
Financial Information:

	N'000
Authorised capital	500
Paid-up capital	300
Turnover	2,000

Principal Shareholders: Chief A Bisi Badejo; R A Shafe; S A
    Oladejo
Date of Establishment: 1975
No of Employees: 36

BOULOS ENTERPRISES LTD
Oregun Village, Ikeja Industrial Estate, PO Box 879, Ikeja, Lagos

Tel: 934310, 934319
Chairman: F C O Coker
Directors: A G Boulos (Managing),
    G G Boulos,
    Mrs M Tabet,
    J A Ogunbiyi,
    J O Olatunji,
    E I Aleyeideino
PRINCIPAL ACTIVITIES: Motor cycle manufacturers
Principal Bankers: Union Bank of Nigeria Ltd; Savannah Bank of
    Nigeria Ltd
Financial Information:

	N'000
Authorised capital	3,000
Paid-up capital	3,000

No of Employees: 500

BOULOS ENTERPRISES LTD
Plot 10 Block D, Ogba Industrial Scheme, Ikeja, PO Box 241,
    Lagos
Tel: 960948
Cable: Boulos

Chairman: F C O Coker
Directors: A G Boulos (Executive),
    G G Boulos (Managing),
    J A Ogunbiyi,
    E I Aleyideino,
    M Tabet (Mrs),
    J O Olatunji
Senior Executives: C R P Adam (General Manager)

PRINCIPAL ACTIVITIES: Manufacture assembly and distribution
    of motorcycles, power generators, outboard engines and
    spare parts
Principal Agencies: Suzuki, Motor Co Ltd; Nippondenso Spark
    Plugs
Branch Offices: Motorcycle Manufacturing plant plot 10 Block D,
    Ogba, Ikeja
Principal Bankers: Union Bank of Nigeria Ltd; Savannah Bank of
    Nigeria Ltd
Financial Information:

	N'000
Authorised capital	3,000
Paid-up capital	3,000
Turnover	56,000
Profits	6,600

Principal Shareholders: A G Boulds; G G Boulds; A Williams; M
    O Williams; Mrs M Tabet; W Boulos; T Boulos; V Boulos
Date of Establishment: 1963
No of Employees: 750

BOUYGUES (NIGERIA) LTD
200 Awolowo Rd, Ikoyi, PO Box 6513, Lagos

PRINCIPAL ACTIVITIES: Building and civil engineering
    contractors
Financial Information:
Registered capital   N 500,000

Date of Establishment: November 1975

BOZGOMERO OF NIGERIA LTD
9 Harbour Rd, PMB 5199, Port Harcourt, Rivers State
Tel: 330422
Cable: Bozgomero
Telex: 61179 Gomero Ng

Chairman: Gordon Cool Bozimo (also Managing Director)
Directors: Madam Shaka Gomeromo,
    Prince S Y Gomeromo (Executive Director),
    Mrs H I Bozimo
Senior Executives: J C Ibe (Installation Engineer),
    N Gill (Project Engineer),
    P L D Igali ((Accounts/Administrative Manager)

PRINCIPAL ACTIVITIES: Air conditioning and mechancial
    engineering
Principal Agencies: Magic Chef, USA; University Mechanical,
    USA; L & W Equipment Corporation, USA
Branch Offices: Technical Showroom, 20 Liberation Drive, Port
    Harcourt, Rivers State
Principal Bankers: International Bank for West Africa Ltd; Pan
    African Bank Ltd
Financial Information:

	N'000
Authorised capital	100
Paid-up capital	100
Sales turnover	6,000

Principal Shareholders: Gordon C Bozimo; Madam Shaka
    Gomeromo
No of Employees: 150

BRAITHWAITE, T A, (INSURANCE BROKERS) & CO
47 Marina, PO Box 785, Lagos
Tel: 661337, 660598, 661348
Cable: Brokers
Telex: 21921 Injab, Ng

Chairman: T A Braithwaite

PRINCIPAL ACTIVITIES: Insurance brokers
Subsidiary Companies: T A Braithwaite & Associates, UK
Principal Bankers: United Bank for Africa

Date of Establishment: 1958

BRAND CLAY WORKS LTD
15 Edinburgh Rd, Ogui New Layout, PMB 1318, Enugu,
    Anambra State
Tel: 51110 Bracks Ng

PRINCIPAL ACTIVITIES: Manufacturers of bricks
Branch Offices: Factory: Amuro Town, Okigwe Division, Imo
    State; 11 Nottidge St, Onitsha, Anambra State

BRECKWOLDT & CO (NIGERIA) LTD
9 Nnamdi Azikiwe St, PO Box 2114, Lagos
Tel: 634901

Directors: H H Thun

PRINCIPAL ACTIVITIES: General trading and representation
Principal Agencies: Breckwoldt & Co, W Germany

BREMEN NNACHETAM CONSTRUCTION COMPANY (NIGERIA) LTD
10 Ibiam St, Uwani, Enugu, Anambra State
Tel: 254797

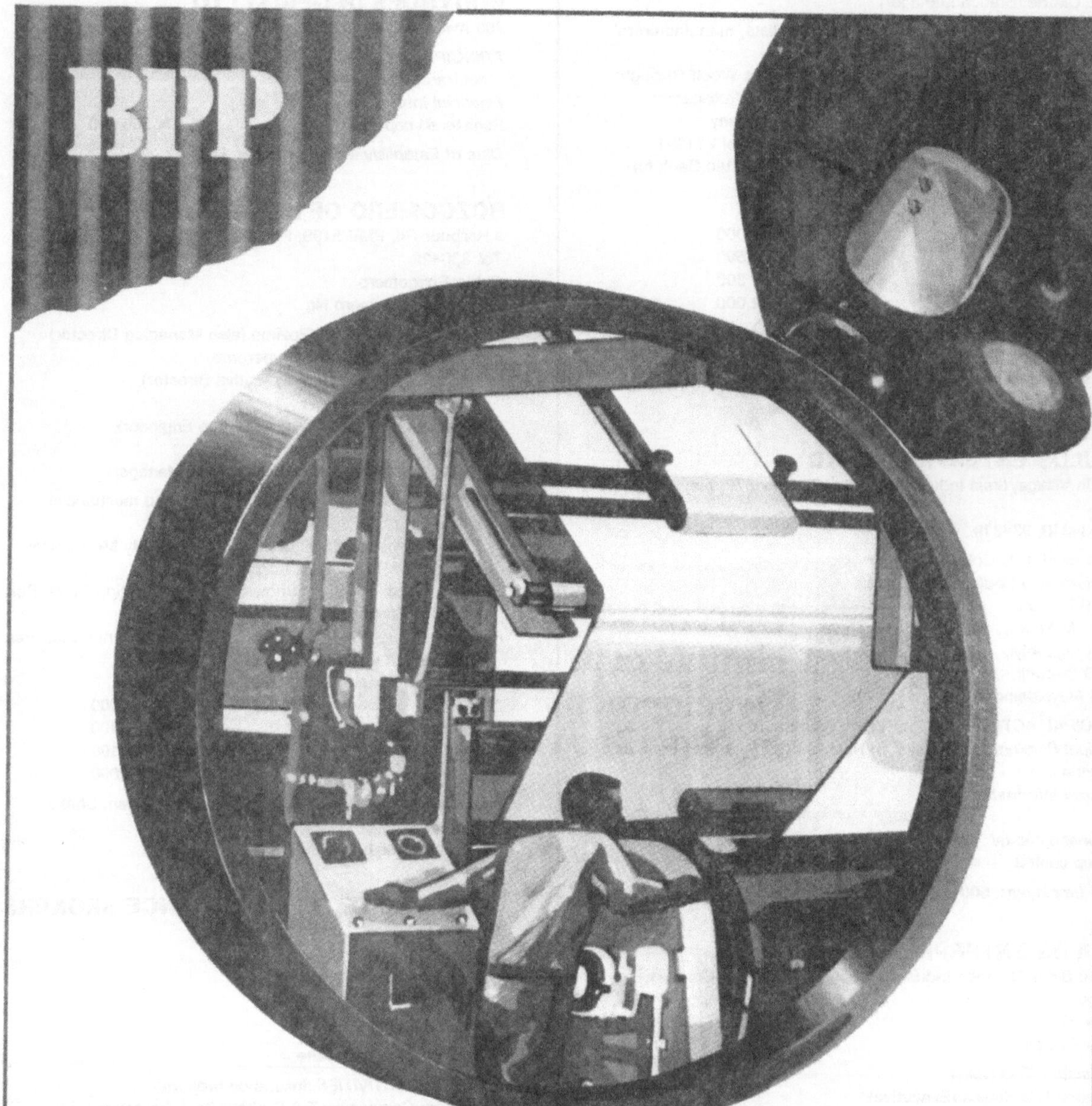

Chairman: Chief C A Nnachetem
Directors: R Viedge (Managing)
Senior Executives: P Diehr (Project Manager),
 K H Sagelsorf (Site Superintendent)
PRINCIPAL ACTIVITIES: Building and civil engineering
 contractors

BRGM (NIGERIA) LTD
69 Awolowo Rd, PO Box 1436, Ikoyi, Lagos
Tel: 681491
Cable: Burgeolog
Telex: 21727 Ng

Chairman: Alhaji Shehu Malami
Senior Executives: J M Vagneron (Managing Director)
PRINCIPAL ACTIVITIES: Geological research; groundwater
 development; mineral prospection and mining
Principal Bankers: International Bank for West Africa Ltd
Financial Information:

	N'000
Authorised capital	200
Paid-up capital	165

Date of Establishment: 1975

BRIAN MUNRO LTD
See MUNRO, BRIAN, LTD

BRIGHT ALUMINIUM PRODUCTS CO LTD
54 Sam Shonibare St, Surulere, Lagos
Tel: 658226, 653336
Cable: Probrital Lagos
Telex: 21511 Ng

PRINCIPAL ACTIVITIES: Suppliers of aluminium products, doors,
 windows, etc

BRIGHT STEEL STRUCTURES CO LTD
4/6 Buli Rd, Industrial Area, PMB 0211 Bauchi, Bauchi State

PRINCIPAL ACTIVITIES: General steel structures and wrought
 iron works, containers and all types of metal work
Branch Offices: PO Box 1457, Kaduna
Financial Information:
Registered capital   N 400,000

Date of Establishment: 1979

BRIGHTSTAR INDUSTRIES LTD
Plot 4 Dada Alah Ogabi Layout, TPA 0829, Apakun, PO Box
 215, Oshodi, Lagos
PRINCIPAL ACTIVITIES: Manufacturers of dry cell batteries

BRISCOE, FRANK
6 Ashenti Rd, Apapa, Lagos
PRINCIPAL ACTIVITIES: Construction

BRISCOE, R T, (NIGERIA) LTD
58 Akanbi Onitiri Close, Off Eric Moore Rd, Iganmu, PO Box
 2104, Apapa, Lagos
Tel: 962075
Cable: Briscoe Lagos
Telex: 21249 Brisco Ng

Chairman: Chief J O Udoji
Directors: F Marcher (Managing Director)

PRINCIPAL ACTIVITIES: Distributors of motor vehicles,
 agricultural equipment, technical equipment, pharmaceuticals,
 telecommunications equipment, printing machinery;
 construction and mining equipment, and other industrial
 machinery
Principal Agencies: Atlas Copco, Sweden
Branch Offices: Ibadan, Telex: 31185 Eastco Ng; Warri; Aba;
 Kano, Telex: 77177 Brisco Ng; Ilorin; Enugu; Jos; Maiduguri

BRISTOL HOTEL
8 Martins St, Lagos
Tel: 630048
PRINCIPAL ACTIVITIES: Hoteliers
Financial Information: Part of Nigeria Hotels Group

BRISTOL MYERS COMPANY
PO Box 261, Lagos
Tel: 876110
Cable: Brimun
Telex: 21756 Sphinx

Senior Executives: E G Payne (Manager)
PRINCIPAL ACTIVITIES: Manufacturers of pharmaceutical
 preparations
Branch Offices: Apapa; Ibadan; Kano; Aba; Benin
Subsidiary Companies: Bristol Laboratories; Mead Johnson

BRISTOW HELICOPTERS (NIGERIA) LTD
Head Office, Murtala Muhammed Airport, PO Box 11, Ikeja,
 Lagos
Tel: 934763, 962885, 931509
Cable: Helicopter Lagos
Telex: 26111 Bristow Ng

Chairman: A O Solaru
Directors: A E Bristow,
 B Collins,
 S A Edu,
 M A Oni,
 K H R Gaston-Parry (Alternate Director)
Senior Executives: K H R Gaston-Parry (General Manager)

PRINCIPAL ACTIVITIES: Aviation service for the oil industry
Branch Offices: Ikeja; Warri; Port Harcourt; Eket; Calabar
Associated Companies: Bristow Helicopters Ltd, UK

Date of Establishment: November 1969
No of Employees: 250

BRITISH INDIA GENERAL INSURANCE CO (NIGERIA) LTD
Inlaks House, 19 Martins St, PO Box 2112, Lagos
PRINCIPAL ACTIVITIES: Insurance

BRITISH-AMERICAN INSURANCE COMPANY (NIGERIA) LTD
35 Simpson St, PO Box 2654, Lagos
Tel: 631861, 631933, 631169, 632840
Cable: Bramlincol Lagos
Telex: 22537

Chairman: Chief Nat A Adibi
Directors: Hilary E Onukogu (Managing),
 G C Davidson,
 Mrs Y Adebonojo,
 Alhaji S Mohammed,
 W Van Zanden
Senior Executives: M N Ononuju (Head of Marketing),
 C E Nwaigwe (Manager, Insurance Operations),
 C C Ndibe (Manager, Data Processing),
 J A Dagbue (Personnel & Public Relations Manager),
 C E Ogali (Financial Controller),
 J Omuederiaye (Superintendent of Agency I),
 Eddy I S Nwosu (Superintendent of Agency II),
 T O Opanuga (Legal Adviser/Company Secretary)

PRINCIPAL ACTIVITIES: Insurance (industrial life), group life
 insurance, mortgage protection insurance
Branch Offices: PO Box 1818, Lagos; PO Box 615, Kaduna; PO
 Box 260, Benin City, Bendel State; PO Box 527, Enugu,
 Anambra State; PMB 1186, Owerri, Imo State
Principal Bankers: Union Bank of Nigeria Ltd

Financial Information:

	N'000
Authorised capital	1,000
Paid-up capital	1,000
Turnover (Premium & Investment)	14,987
Profits	74

Principal Shareholders: Federal Government of Nigeria; British-American Insurance Company Ltd; Nassau, Bahamas
Date of Establishment: 1963
No of Employees: 968

BRONIK MOTORS LTD
400 Herbert Macaulay St, PO Box 511, Yaba, Lagos
Tel: 861553, 861962, 862808
Telex: 21498

PRINCIPAL ACTIVITIES: Distributors of motor vehicles

BROSSETTE (NIGERIA) LTD
PMB 1135, 311 Apapa Rd, Apapa, Lagos
Tel: 846739, 874015, 875312, 860037, 874084, 836739
Cable: Brosetmeto Lagos
Telex: 21316 Broset Ng

PRINCIPAL ACTIVITIES: Manufacturers of scaffolding, glass and aluminium doors and windows; importers of building materials and paints
Branch Offices: PO Box 447, Kachia St, Kaduna, Tel 243413; PO Box 2013, 333 Sultan Rd, Kano, Tel 4611; PMB 5308, 34 Forces Ave, Port Harcourt, Tel 21880

BROWN & ROOT NIGERIA LTD
38 Awolowo Rd, Ikoyi, PO Box 2282, Lagos
Tel: 614168, 683032
Cable: Brownbilt Ng

Directors: Chief Chris Ogunbanjo, Thomas J Feehan, Hugh Gordon, Ben Powell Jr, R O Wilson, Bill Stallworth
Senior Executives: Walter Cowling (Project Manager), O Kalu (Office Manager)
PRINCIPAL ACTIVITIES: Oil and gas services and equipment and pipeline contractors; petrochemicals; paper/paper products; consultants (engineering); metals, metal processing and fabrication
Principal Agencies: Brown & Root Inc, USA; Brown & Root (UK) Ltd, London
Associated Companies: Wimpey-Brown & Root (Nigeria) Ltd; Halliburton Nigeria Ltd; Otis of Nigeria Ltd
Principal Bankers: First Bank of Nigeria Ltd
Principal Shareholders: Brown & Root Inc, Houston, Texas; Union Securities, Lagos

BRUNELLI CONSTRUCTION COMPANY
Km 3 Badagry Expressway, Orile-Iganmu, PO Box 2748, Lagos
Tel: 833115, 870366, 870373
Cable: Brunelli Lagos

Chairman: F Piccolo Brunelli
Directors: E Wilson Ejenobo, D Piccolo Brunelli, Chief J A Ogunfidodo
PRINCIPAL ACTIVITIES: Railways, civil engineering and building contractors; precast and prestressed beams; precast concrete poles and general precastings; piling contractors
Branch Offices: Brunelli Construction Company (Zambia) Ltd, PO Box 32510, Lusaka (Zambia)
Principal Bankers: United Bank for Africa Ltd
Financial Information:
Authorised capital   N 660,000
Date of Establishment: 26th July 1972
No of Employees: 750

BSM LTD
PO Box 1010, 8 Boyle St, Lagos
Tel: 632709

PRINCIPAL ACTIVITIES: Building and civil engineering contractors

BT INTERNATIONAL (NIGERIA) LTD
Stock Exchange House, 17th Floor, 2/4 Customs Street, Lagos
Tel: 66074
Cable: Bantrusrep
Telex: 21748 Btin Ng

Directors: Peter H White (Representative)
Senior Executives: Casimir I Anyanwu (Assistant Representative)
PRINCIPAL ACTIVITIES: Banking (representative office)
Principal Bankers: United Bank for Africa Ltd
Financial Information:
Authorised capital   N 2,000
Principal Shareholders: Bankers Trust Company, New York
Date of Establishment: 1973

BUILDING & CIVIL ENGINEERING CONTRACTORS COMPANY NIGERIA LTD
PO Box 8329, 3 Shagamu Ave, Off Association Ave, Ilupeju, Lagos
Tel: 834084

Directors: S Spyropoulos
PRINCIPAL ACTIVITIES: Building and civil engineering contractors

BULK OIL PLANTS OF NIGERIA LTD
Abonnema Wharf Rd, PO Box 59, Port Harcourt, Rivers State
Tel: 224967, 229675

PRINCIPAL ACTIVITIES: Building materials merchants
Date of Establishment: 1954

BUROMAT DATA SYSTEM LTD
39B Ilupeju Rd, Palmgrove, PO Box 807, Surulere, Lagos
Tel: 960614

PRINCIPAL ACTIVITIES: Data processing
Branch Offices: Block 4 Plot 12, Oluyole Estate, Ring Rd, PO Box 7402, Ibadan, Oyo State

BUSH, W J, & COMPANY (NIGERIA) LTD
168-170 Mission Rd, PO Box 350, Kano
Tel: 4024, 7434, 4495
Cable: Gekatraco

PRINCIPAL ACTIVITIES: Manufacturing of perfumes and cosmetics
Branch Offices: Safara St, Industrial Estate, PO Box 74, Ikeja, Tel 961309; Kano Street, PO Box 350, Onitsha

BUSINESS & INDUSTRIAL CONSULTANTS
PO Box 1029, Lagos

PRINCIPAL ACTIVITIES: Manufacturers' representatives; consultants and suppliers of hand tools, etc
Principal Agencies: Stanley Tools Ltd, UK

BUSINESS EQUIPMENT & MACHINERY LTD (BEAM) (DIVISION OF UAC OF NIGERIA LTD)
58 Marina, PO Box 1081, Lagos
Tel: 662197

Directors: E D Oyinlola (General Manager)
Senior Executives: O S Adebanji (Commercial Manager), R Pairone (Technical Manager), M I Ojo (Personnel/Admin Manager), A O Ogundele (Lagos/West Area Manager), S Coffie-Ukobo (Kalamazoo Factory Manager)

PRINCIPAL ACTIVITIES: Marketing and servicing. Business machines, systems and furniture
Principal Agencies: Chubb, UK; Gestetner, UK; TAV, West Germany; Monroe Business Machines, USA; Canon, Japan; 3M, USA; Kalamazoo, UK; Project, UK
Branch Offices: Branches throughout Nigeria
Principal Bankers: Union Bank of Nigeria Ltd; First Bank of Nigeria Ltd; United Bank for Africa Ltd
Financial Information: Division of UAC of Nigeria Ltd

Date of Establishment: October 1962
No of Employees: 1,100

BUSINESS RESEARCH MANAGEMENT CENTER
(BRMC)
PO Box 2384, Kano
Tel: 5253
Cable: Busresmanter
Telex: 77266

President: Dr A E Ogaba Otokpa, Jr (Founder & President)
Directors: Dr Eileen H Newmark (Executive Vice President)
Senior Executives: Dr Vibart C Stuart (Vice-President Administration),
   Dr G Ramirez (Personnel Director),
   E L Leon (Human Resources Planning & Management),
   Francoise Duranleau (Executive Secretary),
   Andrew E Ehikwe (Manager, Marketing),
   Dr Shraga Serok (Behavioral Scientist/Project Manager)

PRINCIPAL ACTIVITIES: Non profit making sponsored research; provides research services for industry, government agencies and associations
Branch Offices: In 1983 the head office will move to Abuja, Agila Tow and Kano will become the principal branch
Principal Bankers: Savannah Bank Nigeria Ltd; First Bank of Nigeria Ltd; Societe General Bank (Nigeria) Ltd; Bank of Credit and Commerce International

Date of Establishment: 1st September 1976

C C DANIEL MINING INDUSTRY
See DANIEL, C C, MINING INDUSTRY

C C EZEILO
See EZEILO, C C

C FUNCKE & CO (NIGERIA) LTD
See FUNCKE, C, & CO (NIGERIA) LTD

C I F CONSTRUCTION NIGERIA LTD
Km 15 Badagry Rd, PO Box 5276, Lagos
Tel: 873608
Telex: 26754 Onip Ng

Chairman: E O Onipede
Directors: Dr F A Shonubi, Chief J Abimbola Odunlami, M Frot, F Trimouille

PRINCIPAL ACTIVITIES: Construction
Branch Offices: Societe General Bank Ltd; United Bank for Africa Ltd
Financial Information:

	N'000
Authorised capital	400
Paid-up capital	400

C ITOH & CO LTD
See ITOH, C, & CO LTD

C MOORE OBIOHA SONS & COMPANY LTD
See MOORE OBIOHA, C, SONS & COMPANY LTD

C N ONUSELOGU ENTERPRISES LTD
See ONUSELOGU, C N, ENTERPRISES LTD

C NORMANN INTERNATIONAL COMPANY
See NORMANN, C, INTERNATIONAL COMPANY

C O IGUH AND SONS TRADING CO (NIGERIA) LTD
See IGUH, C O, AND SONS TRADING CO (NIGERIA) LTD

C UBA & BROTHERS TRADING COMPANY (WA) LTD
See UBA, C, & BROTHERS TRADING COMPANY (WA) LTD

C WOERMANN (NIGERIA) LTD
See WOERMANN, C, (NIGERIA) LTD

C ZARD & COMPANY LTD
See ZARD, C, & COMPANY LTD

CAASO CONSTRUCTIONAL WORKS LTD
Kilometer 32, Abeokuta Rd, PO Box 611, Lagos

Directors: Dr L O Adegbite, E O Ajala, Engr D A Coker, B A Oni
Senior Executives: Dr S O Olorunfemi (General Manager),
   J O Ogunye (Accountant),
   Engr J O Somoye (Plant Manager)

PRINCIPAL ACTIVITIES: Civil engineering and construction; consultants (engineering); suppliers of construction plant
Principal Bankers: Co-operative Bank Nigeria Ltd
Financial Information:

	N'000
Authorised capital	1,000
Paid-up capital	541
Turnover	3,364
Profits	936

Date of Establishment: 19th August 1968
No of Employees: 400

CADBURY NIGERIA LTD
Isheri Rd, Agidingbi, PO Box 164, Ikeja, Lagos State
Tel: 900395/9, 961545/6, 961504
Cable: CADFRY Lagos
Telex: 26601 Cadbury Ng

Chairman: G O Onosode
Directors: C R Clarke (Managing Director),
   J A Onyesoh (Finance Director),
   B C Dice,
   Dr M Tukur,
   O O Odubogun (Purchasing Director),
   Dr C O Kolade (Administration Director),
   P A Thirkell (Factory Director),
   G W Walsh (Sales/Marketing Director),
   E MacFarlane (Production Director)
Senior Executives: K K Keazor (Company Secretary),
   O O O Sengowawa (Marketing Manager, Services),
   S O Oranyeli (General Sales Manager),
   Dr O A Akinkunle (Personnel Manager),
   M A O Ajiferuke (Marketing Manager, Products),
   B S Majekodunmi (Factory Manager)

PRINCIPAL ACTIVITIES: Manufacturers of food drinks, confectionery, household health and chemical products
Subsidiary Companies: Cadbury Schweppes PLC
Principal Bankers: Union Bank of Nigeria Ltd; First Bank of Nigeria Ltd
Financial Information: As at 31 December 1981

	N'000
Authorised capital	10,000
Paid-up capital	8,307
Turnover	98,849
Profits (After Tax)	5,401

Principal Shareholders: Cadbury Schweppes PLC (40%)
Date of Establishment: 9th January 1965
No of Employees: 2,450

CALABAR CEMENT COMPANY LTD

Old Obutong, PMB 1092, Calabar, Cross River State
Tel: 306/330
Cable: Calcemco
Telex: 65120 Calcem Ng

Chairman: E I Etteh
Directors: Dr A P C Cumming (Managing Director),
  K Onigbanjo,
  B A Olagbegi,
  J A Olugbenie,
  D O Dede,
  Chief J U Udom,
  I E Uboh,
  Magnus O E Williams,
  Alhaji A Ibrahim
Senior Executives: E A Etuk (Company Secretary),
  B O Edet (Financial Controller),
  U J Umo (Administrative Manager),
  A B Siminialayi (Acting Working Manager)

PRINCIPAL ACTIVITIES: Manufacture of cement
Branch Offices: 24/26 Boyle St, Lagos
Principal Bankers: Standard Bank of Nigeria Ltd; Central Bank
  of Nigeria
Financial Information:

	N'000
Authorised capital	20,000
Paid-up capital	15,000
Sales turnover	18,000
Profits	2,200

Principal Shareholders: Cross River State Government, Federal
  Military Government
No of Employees: 600

CALABAR VENEER & PLYWOOD LTD

Esuk Utan, Ikot-Ansa PO Box 333, Calabar, Cross River State
Tel: 222411
Cable: Calvenply

Chairman: H W Akpan
Directors: C E Bassey, A U Ukpong, F A Ugbong, J L Brandler,
  T A B Faleye
Senior Executives: F I Archibong (Company Secretary),
  E O Ayang (General Manager)

PRINCIPAL ACTIVITIES: Timber and plywood production
Principal Bankers: First Bank of Nigeria Ltd
Financial Information:

	N'000
Authorised capital	2,000
Paid-up capital	1,197
Turnover	325

Principal Shareholders: Investment Trust Co Ltd; Nigerian
  Industrial Development Bank Ltd; J L Brandler; Govt. of
  Cross River State
Date of Establishment: 4th May 1965
No of Employees: 312

CALARO OIL PALM ESTATE LTD

Mbarakom, PMB 1114, Calabar, Cross River State

Chairman: E A Opa
Directors: J C F Spiering, P N Ossom, A I Dasuki, Chief Dr B J
  Ikpeme, C Kruegel
Senior Executives: A J Farquharson (General Manager
    Designate),
  S P Udo (Planation Manager),
  I S Hudson (Area Manager),
  W J Henwood (Mill Engineer)

PRINCIPAL ACTIVITIES: Manufacture of palm oil, palm kernals
  and cocoa
Principal Bankers: Union Bank of Nigeria

Principal Shareholders: Nijal/ADC
No of Employees: 4,000

CALEB BOVIS JOHNSON CONSTRUCTION CO LTD

PMB 1264, Plot 23, Adeniyi Jones St, Wemabab Estate, Ikeja,
  Lagos

Directors: A F Odeniyi (Managing Director)
PRINCIPAL ACTIVITIES: Civil engineering and construction

CALEB BRETT & SON (NIGERIA) LTD

29/34 NPA Commercial Block A, Wharf Rd, PO Box 52, Apapa,
  Lagos
Tel: 874706
Telex: 21267

PRINCIPAL ACTIVITIES: Marine, bulk oil surveyors, testing
  laboratories, container cargo inspection and insurance
  valuation, tank calibrators

CAMCO LTD

PO Box 489, Enerhen Rd, Warri, Bendel State
Telex: 775413

Directors: P A Weeks (General Manager),
  Lenwood McWilliams (District Manager, Warri),
  G B Carter (District Manager, Port Harcourt)

PRINCIPAL ACTIVITIES: Oil and gas service and equipment
  suppliers
Branch Offices: Field Office: PO Box 101, Port Harcourt, Tel
  21953

CAMERON IRON WORKS (NIGERIA) LTD

16 Festival Rd, Victoria Island, PO Box 5233, Lagos
Tel: 613477
Cable: Camiron Lagos
Telex: 21787 Cameron Ng

Chairman: J L Harrison (also Managing Director)
Directors: A Olatunji (Finance Director, Company Secretary),
  J O Tomisin,
  Chief S E Idugboe,
  J E Erwin,
  V M Dill
Senior Executives: V E Derval (Base Manager),
  M B Ekpo (Base Manager)

PRINCIPAL ACTIVITIES: Equipment suppliers to the oil and gas
  industry
Principal Agencies: Cameron Iron Works Inc, Houston, USA
Branch Offices: Field Offices: PO Box 995, Trans Amadi Layout,
  Port Harcourt, Rivers State PMB 1066, Oguno Rd, Warri,
  Bendel State;
Principal Bankers: First Bank of Nigeria Ltd

Principal Shareholders: Cameron Iron Works Inc, USA; I T J
  Ordor; S E Idugboe; T O Graham-Douglas; V I Masi; E O
  Abisoye
Date of Establishment: October 1973

CAMPLANT ENGINEERING SALES & SERVICE LTD

223/225 Apapa Rd, Iganmu, PMB 1155, Apapa
Tel: 835142, 834908, 835138, 831444
Cable: Camplant Lagos
Telex: 21324

Chairman: B O W Mafeni
Directors: Dr R W Imishue, Chief A T Amuwo, Dr J A Anaza, J
  U Obere
Senior Executives: A Balogun (General Manager),
  J B Ogunlana (Finance Manager),
  B A Odude (Office Manager),
  S I Clarke (Personnel Manager),
  V D Ojo (Technical Manager),
  R O Ogunleye (Parts Manager)

PRINCIPAL ACTIVITIES: Sales and service of construction and agricultural machines. Generating plants sales, installation and service
Principal Agencies: Komatsu, Tokyo
Branch Offices: Benin; Ilorin; Kano; Lagos
Principal Bankers: Union Bank of Nigeria Ltd; Savannah Bank of Nigeria Ltd; International Bank for West Africa
Financial Information:

	₦'000
Authorised capital	500
Paid-up capital	500
Turnover	10,000

Date of Establishment: January 1978

CANDLES & POLISH WORKS LTD

PO Box 1, Kano
Tel: 2619, 2138
Cable: Candle Works Kano

PRINCIPAL ACTIVITIES: Manufacturers of candles and polish
Branch Offices: Factory: 27 Kundila Rd, Bompai, PO Box 688, Industrial Area, Kano, Tel 5750

CANSULT LTD

5th Floor, New Niger House, PO Box 851, Lagos

PRINCIPAL ACTIVITIES: Engineering consultants

CAPITAL TRUST BROKERS LTD

14th Floor Unity House, 37 Marina, PO Box 2010, Lagos
Tel: 664742, 664729, 664933, 664938

Chairman: Chief Adekunle Ojora
Directors: M O Otutuloro (Managing),
    Mallam Usman Goji,
    E O Ayang,
    G Omoni,
    F A Johnson

PRINCIPAL ACTIVITIES: Stockbrokers
Branch Offices: 2nd Floor, Arm'yau House, 22 Ahmadu Bello Way, PO Box 5054, Kaduna
Principal Bankers: Union Bank of Nigeria Ltd

CAPPA AND D'ALBERTO LTD

72 Campbell St, PO Box 870, Lagos
Tel: 633722, 633794, 633865, 635098
Cable: Capdal Lagos
Telex: 21211 Capdal Ng

Chairman: Chief S B Daniyan
Directors: G Gianotti (Managing),
    Alhaji M S Adewale,
    V Cagna,
    S A Verissimo,
    O Lijadu,
    F Gianotti,
    Chief E O Idowu,
    Chief S A R Anifowoshe,
    G Calvino

PRINCIPAL ACTIVITIES: Building and civil engineering contractors
Branch Offices: PO Box 687, Ibadan, Tel 412777; PO Box 258, Kaduna, Tel 243084
Associated Companies: Clay Industry (Nig) Ltd; Igbobi Development Co Ltd; Stoneroad Prop. Co Ltd
Principal Bankers: United Bank for Africa Ltd; First Bank of Nigeria Ltd; Union Bank of Nigeria Ltd
Financial Information:

	₦'000
Authorised capital	10,000
Paid-up capital	10,000
Turnover	26,972
Profits	2,402

Principal Shareholders: Lagos State (32%); G F D'Alberto (20%); Nicon (10%)
Date of Establishment: 1932
No of Employees: 3,404

CAPPA, G, LTD

8 Taylor Rd, Iddo, PO Box 1673, Lagos
Tel: 800080/1/3, 862110
Cable: Gratocappa
Telex: 26341 Gcappa Ng

Chairman: Charles D Onyeama
Directors: G Cappa (Managing),
    P U Cappa,
    Chief F R A Williams CFR,
    T Poletti,
    Alhaji B U Mandara,
    Ahmadu Yakubu,
    D Valsesia,
    S E da Silva,
    S A Onomakpome,
    G A Williams
Senior Executives: L T Carpenter (General Manager)

PRINCIPAL ACTIVITIES: Building construction and civil engineering
Branch Offices: 35 Ali Akilu Rd, PO Box 105, Kaduna, Tel 212431; Mokola Roundabout, Queen Elizabeth II Rd, PO Box 350, Ibadan, Oyo State, Tel 412666
Subsidiary Companies: Pierugo Ltd, Lagos
Principal Bankers: United Bank for Africa Ltd; First Bank of Nigeria Ltd; Union Bank of Nigeria Ltd
Financial Information: As at 31st March 1981

	₦'000
Authorised capital	5,000
Paid-up capital	5,000
Turnover	38,305
Profits (before tax)	2,011

Principal Shareholders: Nigerian Citizens & Associations (60%); Foundation Gifflenga of Switzerland (40%)
Date of Establishment: 1952
No of Employees: 3,957

CAPRIHANS INDUSTRIES LTD

65 Marina, PO Box 5187, Lagos
Tel: 660298, 660377, 663427, 662079
Cable: Caplas
Telex: 21588 Somoco Ng; 23439 Sonnar Gr

Chairman: S N Jethwani
Directors: P S Pillai (Technical),
    J M Porwal (Financial),
    Chief S O Lambo,
    Dr J A Olubode,
    E O Osindero,
    N Adesiyakan,
    Alhaji K B Okegbenro,
    T O Obafemi,
    Alhaji Sule Katagum

PRINCIPAL ACTIVITIES: Manufacturers of pipes and fittings; industrial mouldings; plastics and plastic products
Branch Offices: Factory: Oregun Industrial Estate, PMB 21593, Ikeja, Lagos
Principal Bankers: International Merchant Bank (Nigeria) Ltd; Icon Ltd (Merchant Bankers); Savannah Bank of Nigeria Ltd
Financial Information:

	₦'000
Authorised capital	2,000
Paid-up capital	2,000

Principal Shareholders: S N Jethwani; Chief S O Lambo; Dr J A Olubode
Date of Establishment: 1st December 1977
No of Employees: 130

CARL-PLOETNER (NIGERIA) LTD
PO Box 587, Ibadan, Oyo State

Directors: R Shipman

PRINCIPAL ACTIVITIES: Public utilities, water supply

CARPET ROYAL (NIGERIA) LTD
PMB 5140, Off Oyo Rd, Moniya Village, Ibadan, Oyo State
Telex: 20311 TDS IBA Ng

Chairman: H R H Prince O A Sijuade
Directors: John Mastoroudes (Managing),
A P Leventis,
Chief A O Ajayi,
G O Philactou,
Alhaji M I Usman,
Sir Desmond Lorimer
Senior Executives: S Van Duren (Production Manager),
Brian Berry (Technical Manager)

PRINCIPAL ACTIVITIES: Carpet manufacturers

Date of Establishment: Incorporated 26th February 1980

CARRARA MARBLE CO LTD
44 Jebba St, Ebute-Metta, PO Box 343, Apapa, Lagos
Tel: 860769

Chairman: A S O Alabi
Directors: Giancarlo Tazzini, Mauro Lagomarsino

PRINCIPAL ACTIVITIES: Suppliers of marble

CASTING NIGERIA LTD
Sango Otto, Ogun State

Senior Executives: D G Kretschmer (Factory Manager)

PRINCIPAL ACTIVITIES: Foundry

Date of Establishment: January 1981
No of Employees: 250

CAVE PLASTICS LTD
PMB 15, Ogidi, Anambra State
Cable: Caveplast Ogidi

Chairman: Mike Ikenze

PRINCIPAL ACTIVITIES: Plastic (polyethylene) extrusion plant for the manufacture of plastic films and shopping bags
Financial Information:
Authorised capital   ₦ 250,000

CAXTON PRESS (WEST AFRICA) LTD
Eleiyele Rd, PMB 5009, Ibadan, Oyo State
Tel: 414491, 461537
Telex: 31103 Caxton Ng

Directors: E U Gbinigie (Managing),
P Medley,
B Popoola,
A Odedina,
Chief Olu I Akinkugbe,
Mrs R M I Odedina
Senior Executives: S O Okeyode (Secretary/Accountant),
V Sibson (Chief Engineer),
J O Ajayi (Factory Manager),
R Oreagba (Litho Manager),
M Williams-Egbah (Commercial Manager),
T Abiodun Ige (Personnel Officer)

PRINCIPAL ACTIVITIES: Printing
Associated Companies: McCorquodale & Company (WA) Ltd
Principal Bankers: First Bank of Nigeria Ltd

Date of Establishment: 1st October 1961
No of Employees: 300

CEC & CO (NIGERIA) LTD
13 Old Cemetry Rd, PO Box 2086, Onitsha, Anambra State

Chairman: Dr C E Chioma
Directors: Mrs Philomena Chioma, Augustine Chioma
Senior Executives: Michael Eseme (Sales Manager),
Geoffrey D C Muruakor (Office Manager),
Cletus Ojinnaka (Printing Manager)

PRINCIPAL ACTIVITIES: Management consultants, economic/project analysts, estate planners and evaluers, printers and publishers
Branch Offices: 10 Umuna Rd, Orlu, Imo State; 47 Douglas Rd, Owerri, Imo State; 29A Nathan St, Surulere, Lagos
Principal Bankers: African Continental Bank Ltd; United Bank for Africa Ltd; Standard Bank of Nigeria Ltd
Financial Information:

	₦'000
Authorised capital	100
Paid-up capital	100
Sales turnover	300
Profits	25

Principal Shareholders: Dr C E Chioma

CECA (NIGERIA) LTD
268 Trans Amadi Industrial Layout, PMB 5241, Port Harcourt, Rivers State
Tel: 222963
Cable: Carbacti

Chairman: Chief G K J Amachree
Directors: J P Soula, C T Cresswell
Senior Executives: J V Rappenne (General Manager),
U J Akpan (Administrative Manager)

PRINCIPAL ACTIVITIES: Supply of drilling mud and chemicals, and oilfield services
Branch Offices: NPA Compound, PO Box 406, Warri
Financial Information:

	₦'000
Authorised capital	175
Paid-up capital	175
Sales turnover	2,300
Profits	250

Principal Shareholders: Ceca SA, Paris; British CA, London; Chief G K J Amachree

CEMENT COMPANY OF NORTHERN NIGERIA LTD
PMB 2166, Kalmbaina Rd, Sokoto
Tel: 2280, 2493
Cable: Sokocem

PRINCIPAL ACTIVITIES: Manufacturers of cement
Branch Offices: Ahmadu Bello Way, PO Box 320, Kaduna, Tel 213499, 210011

CENTRAL BANK OF NIGERIA
Tinubu Square, PMB 12194, Lagos
Tel: 660100-29
Cable: Cebank Ng
Telex: 21350

Governor: Alhaji A Ahmed
Directors: Alhaji A O G Otiti (Deputy Governor)
Senior Executives: Professor G O Nwankwo (Executive Director),
Alhaji A Yelwa (Executive Director)

PRINCIPAL ACTIVITIES: Banking
Branch Offices: Kano; Enugu; Port Harcourt; Ibadan; Benin; Calabar; Jos; Maiduguri; Kaduma; Yola; Minna; Bauchi; Abeokuta; Ilorin; Sokoto; Akure; Owerri; Makurdi; Lagos (Head Office)

Principal Shareholders: Federal Government of Nigeria
Date of Establishment: 1st July 1959

CENTRAL HOTEL
(Nigeria Hotels Ltd)
PMB 3023, Bompai Rd, Kano
Tel: 3051, 5141, 5149
Cable: Bestotel
Telex: 77151 Centel Ng

Directors: S A Alamutu (Managing)
Senior Executives: S O Adesina (Finance Controller),
   A O Akinrinade (Controller of Operations),
   M A Fadipe (Controller of Personnel),
   B Adegbesan (Controller of Corporate Affairs),
   A O Aduyoye (Principal, NHL Training School),
   J A O Eboda (General Manager, Ikoyi Hotel),
   F K Bajomo (General Manager, Central Hotel)

PRINCIPAL ACTIVITIES: Hoteliers
Branch Offices: Ikoyi Hotel, PO Box 895, Club Rd, Lagos
Principal Bankers: Union Bank of Nigeria Ltd
Financial Information:
Paid-up capital   ₦ 2,800,000

Principal Shareholders: Federal Government of Nigeria
Date of Establishment: June 1928
No of Employees: 450

CENTRAL INVESTMENT COMPANY LTD
5 Onitsha Rd, PMB 01212, Enugu, Anambra State
Tel: 253418
Cable: Investco Enugu
Telex: 51223 Invest Ng

Chairman: A A U Odelugwo
Directors: G C Akwaeze, D U Dieke, H O Egbeama, Chief Ike
   Nwokolo, G C Odiari, Dr M O Ude, Dr S C Chukwu
Senior Executives: D O Chuke (General Manager),
   Dr A J C Mogbana (Company Secretary/Controller of
   Administration),
   Mrs C O Edozie (Financial Controller),
   J C Okpukpara (Controller of Operations)

PRINCIPAL ACTIVITIES: Investors, financiers, business and
   management consultants
Subsidiary Companies: Central Building Products Ltd; Afrik
   Enterprises (Nig) Ltd; Aria Chemicals Ltd; Stena Mills Ltd;
   Nigerian Mineral Water Industries Ltd; Ebony Paints (Nigeria)
   Ltd; Central Medical Softwares Ltd; Phina Paint Industries
   Ltd; Life Breweries Co Ltd; Hemason Nigerian Ltd; Madonna
   Bakery Industries Ltd; Francis Builders (Nig) Ltd; Anambra
   Vegetable Oil Products (Nigerian) Ltd
Principal Bankers: First Bank Nigeria Ltd; United Bank for Africa
   Ltd; African Continental Bank Ltd; Union Bank of Nigeria Ltd
Financial Information:

	₦'000
Authorised capital	4,000
Paid-up capital	3,984
Turnover	829
Profits	786

Principal Shareholders: Wholly owned by Government of
   Anambra State
Date of Establishment: 9th February 1974
No of Employees: 50

CENTRAL PACKAGES OF NIGERIA LTD
3 Ayodele Diyan Rd, PO Box 191 or PMB 1311, Ikeja, Lagos
Tel: 964190, 964888
Cable: Cenpack

Senior Executives: C R Thirani (General Manager)

PRINCIPAL ACTIVITIES: Manufacturing cardboard and plastic
   packages and containers
Associated Companies: Nigerian Paper Mills Ltd

CENTRAL WATER TRANSPORTATION
COMPANY LTD
49 New Market Rd, PMB 1784, Onitsha, Anambra State
Tel: 210511, 212436
Cable: Aquaport Onitsha

Chairman: Chief J C Obande
Directors: Young Nwafor (Managing),
   Kaapinen Kwarve,
   Prince B A Afegbua,
   Subaru Sule,
   Alhaji A M M Minna,
   Mrs Ngozi Onyioha,
   O B Etienam,
   Pastor Chief A I Adeyemo,
   Alhaji A B Argungu,
   E A Essiet,
   B O I Anyaoku,
   Alhaji Mani Yangora

PRINCIPAL ACTIVITIES: Transport, shipping; shipbuilding and
   shipping services
Branch Offices: Old NPA Port, PMB 1162, Warri; PMB 12681,
   Lagos
Principal Bankers: New Nigerian Bank Ltd; United Bank for
   Africa Ltd; African Continental Bank Ltd; Investment Bank
   for West Africa Ltd

Principal Shareholders: Federal Government of Nigeria
Date of Establishment: 1st July 1971
No of Employees: 300

CENTURY INSURANCE CO (NIGERIA) LTD
Century Insurance House, Tinubu Sq, PO Box 2837, Lagos
Tel: 634490

PRINCIPAL ACTIVITIES: Insurance

CEP
27 Ikorodu Rd, Igbobi, Lagos
Tel: 848794

PRINCIPAL ACTIVITIES: Suppliers of educational films, all types
   of projectors, communications equipment, scientific and
   laboratory equipment, etc

CEPUZ INTERNATIONAL AGENCIES
68, Igbunabali Rd, PMB 5374, Port Harcourt, Rivers State
Cable: Cepintage

PRINCIPAL ACTIVITIES: Shipping, clearing and forwarding, air
   freight system, warehousing, importers and exporters, general
   contractors, supply services, business consultants and
   confirming agents
Branch Offices: 2 Port Harcourt Rd, Uzuakoli, Umuahia, Imo
   State

CETACONSULT (NIGERIA) LTD
53Y Mallam Kure Street, PO Box 2614, Jos North, Jos, Plateau
State
Tel: 55819, 55820

Chairman: J O Oyegoke (also Managing Director)
Directors: B L Kaul
Senior Executives: K Brenyah (Senior Town Planner)

PRINCIPAL ACTIVITIES: Consultancy services provided in town
   and country planning, civil engineering, architecture and
   project management
Associated Companies: International Planning & Environmental
   Consultants (Nigeria) Ltd; Joe Oyegoke Associates
Principal Bankers: First Bank of Nigeria Ltd
Financial Information:

	₦'000
Authorised capital	100
Paid-up capital	50

Principal Shareholders: J O Oyegoke
Date of Establishment: 2nd December 1977

CFAO (NIGERIA) LTD
Isolo Industrial Estate, PO Box 3034, Lagos
Tel: 632010, 632078, 632150, 632219, 636242
Cable: Senafrica
Telex: 21438 Senafr Ng Lagos; 6118 Faoest Ng Port Harcourt;
77156 Kn Ng Kano

Chairman: G O Onosode
Directors: J Borle (Managing Director),
R Horner (Deputy Managing Director),
M Baudais,
S A Bello,
E D Hindley,
B Danbappa,
A Y Eke,
M O Thomas,
W O Uzoaga
Senior Executives: Chief O A Lampejo (Corporate Secretary)

PRINCIPAL ACTIVITIES: Wholesale suppliers of general goods;
suppliers of motor vehicles, technical equipment, electrical
goods such as air-conditioning equipment and refrigeration,
building materials, agricultural equipment, textiles; export of
non-controlled commodities; supermarket; freight forwarders
Principal Agencies: General Electric Corp; Nigerian Ball-Point
Pens Industries Ltd; Ninetco Ltd; Nigeria Teijin Textiles Ltd;
Galvanizing Industries Ltd; Northern Textiles Manufacturers
Ltd; Hyster Int; etc
Branch Offices: 10/11 Hadejia Rd, PO Box 18, Kano; 8 Azikiwe
Rd, PMB 5130, Port Harcourt; Also at Apapa; Aba; Abeokuta;
Benin City; Enugu; Ibadan; Jos; Kaduna; Maiduguri; Onitsha;
Warri
Subsidiary Companies: Depi Ltd; Nigerian Motors Industries Ltd
(see separate entry); Transcap Ltd (see separate entry)
Principal Bankers: First Bank of Nigeria Ltd; Union Bank of
Nigeria Ltd; United Bank for Africa Ltd; Savannah Bank Ltd;
International Bank for West Africa Ltd; International Merchant
Bank (Nigeria) Ltd
Financial Information:

	₦'000
Authorised capital	15,000
Paid-up capital	12,480
Turnover	253,000
Profits	14,000

Principal Shareholders: CFAO Paris
Date of Establishment: 1892
No of Employees: 4,000

CFC FURNITURE CO (EN) LTD
49 Aba Rd, PO Box 181, Port Harcourt, Rivers State
Tel: 226709
Cable: Cifurco Ph

Directors: Peter Mihedji, Dr Graham-Douglas, F Nyivih, Mrs
Agnes S Mihedji
Senior Executives: Mrs K D Charles (Sales Manageress),
C I Nwachukwu (Factory Manager),
U G Uko (Accountant),
S Mihedji (Purchasing Officer),
C Mihedji (Credit Controller),
A S Nsesay (Secretary)

PRINCIPAL ACTIVITIES: Wooden furniture manufacturers
Principal Bankers: Savannah Bank of Nigeria Ltd; First Bank of
Nigeria Ltd; United Bank for Africa Ltd
Financial Information:

	₦'000
Authorised capital	100
Paid-up capital	100

Principal Shareholders: P Mihedji; Mrs Agnes Mihedji; Stephen D
Mihedji; Cornelius D Mihedji
Date of Establishment: 29th April 1960
No of Employees: 130

CFC FURNITURE CO (WC) LTD
Mile 7, Agege Motor Rd, PO Box 42, Mushin, Lagos
Tel: 841975/6
Cable: Furniture Lagos

PRINCIPAL ACTIVITIES: Manufacturers of wooden furniture and
upholstery
Branch Offices: Ibadan; Kaduna; Warri

CGG NIGERIA LTD
PO Box 6897, Lagos
Cable: Mafric Lagos
Telex: 21226

Directors: B Fajolie (Manager)
PRINCIPAL ACTIVITIES: Geophysical services

CHALLENGE BOOKSHOPS
Agege Motor Rd, Mushin, PMB 12256, Lagos
Tel: 847690
Cable: Challenge Lagos
Telex: 21525 Ecwap Ng

Chairman: Rev S A Ibrahim
Directors: Dr P S Usman (Managing Director),
T T Makanjuola,
Rev D M Olusiyi,
T Arosanyin,
E Oji,
E Mairabo,
I B Majam (Financial Director),
Rev J K Bolarin (Publishing Director),
S N Kolo (Trade Director),
D L Yilwa (Administration Director)
Senior Executives: E M Gara (Import Manager),
A Dogari (Sales Manager),
I Jimba (Personnel Officer),
G Ude (Trade Accountant),
A Suberu (Chief Accountant)

PRINCIPAL ACTIVITIES: Retailers and wholesalers of books and
stationery items; Christian book publishers; media services in
the aspects of audio visuals, filmstrips production cassettes
and records productions; film hire and radio broadcasting
Principal Agencies: Marshall, Morgan & Scott, UK; Collins
Glasgow, UK; Trinitarian Bible Society, UK; Paternoster
Press, UK; George Rowney & Co Ltd, UK; Zondervan
Publishing House, USA; Moody Press, USA; Thomas Wyatt
Nigeria Ltd; Pickering & Inglis, UK; Thomas Nelson Inc, USA;
Rotring-Werke, Germany; Messenger Corportion, USA;
Tyndale House Publishers, USA; Williams Clowes & Sons Ltd,
UK
Branch Offices: 130 Broad Street, PMB 12256, Lagos; Murtala
Mohammed Way, PMB 1346, Ilorin, Kwara State; 45
Akpakpava Rd, PO Box 1286, Benin City, Bendel State;
Challenge Area (Molete), PO Box 298, Ibadan, Oyo State; 38
Zik Avenue Uwani, PMB 1101, Enugu, Anambra State; 106
Nnamdi Azik Rd, PMB 1546, Owerri, Imo State; 2 Oron Rd,
PO Box 8, Uyo, Cross River State; Yakabu Gowon Rd, PO
Box 274, Port Harcourt, River State; 6 Ali Akilu Rd, PO Box
2049, Kaduna; 27A Airport Rd, PO Box 384, Kano; 10 Kano
Rd, PMB 2010, Jos, Plateau State; Hospital Rd, PO Box 13,
Minna, Niger State; 4 Bauchi Trading Layout, Maiduguri Rd,
PO Box 7, Bauchi; Abdulahi Fodio Rd, PO Box 424, Sokoto;
Fed Capital Shop Centre, PO Box 32, Abuja, Fed Capital
Territory. Plus 21 other locations
Principal Bankers: First Bank of Nigeria Ltd; Union Bank of
Nigeria Ltd; Bank of the North Ltd; United Bank for Africa Ltd
Financial Information: A division of Ecwa Publications

	₦'000
Authorised capital	500
Paid-up capital	500
Turnover	6,000

Principal Shareholders: Registered Trustees of Association of
Evangelical Churches of West Africa

Date of Establishment: 1st April 1974, Previously as SIM
  Bookshops, Established 1924
No of Employees: 410

CHAMI, A B, & CO LTD

PO Box 66, Jos, Plateau State
Tel: 2646, 2845
Cable: Barakat Jos
Telex: 81104 Barco

PRINCIPAL ACTIVITIES: General importers, perfumery and
  cosmetics manufacturers
Branch Offices: Kano; Karia; Sokoto; Maiduguri

CHAMPION CONFECTIONERY CO (NIGERIA) LTD

Airport Rd, PO Box 245, Jos, Plateau State
Tel: 54870, 55174
Cable: Platconf
Telex: 81375 Champs

Directors: S Adaji,
  C E J Allanson (Executive),
  C I Ezeh (Alternate),
  J M Bordass,
  S H Gwarlu,
  Dr J S Mamven,
  G Pam
Senior Executives: J M Bordass (General Manager)

PRINCIPAL ACTIVITIES: Boiled sweets and toffee manufacturers
Principal Bankers: First Bank of Nigeria Ltd
Financial Information:

	N'000
Authorised capital	500
Paid-up capital	500
Turnover	3,500
Profits	100

Principal Shareholders: John Holt Ltd; Plateau Investments Co;
  Northern Nigeria Investments Ltd
Date of Establishment: 1970 (Formerly Plateau Confectionery Co
  (Nigeria) Ltd)
No of Employees: 195

CHANRAI, J T, & CO (NIGERIA) LTD

44 Marina, PO Box 362, Lagos
Tel: 636581, 632923

PRINCIPAL ACTIVITIES: Department stores
Subsidiary Companies: H B & Sons Ltd

CHARLIE AND FRANCO LTD

3 Anosike Lane, PO Box 3250, Lagos
Tel: 874353
Cable: Jufrancom

Chairman: Francis Ayeju
Directors: Mrs G Ndiomu, E Egbuson, C Kuye, T O Ogunmoye
Senior Executives: Daniel Ayeju (General Manager),
  Edwin Ayeju (Assistant General Manager),
  Elliott Egbuson (Chief Engineer),
  J Warebi (Operations Manager)

PRINCIPAL ACTIVITIES: Agents and general traders; building
  and civil engineering contractors. Suppliers of building
  materials
Principal Agencies: Frank Komlos and Associates, USA; Favag
  Establishments, Switzerland
Branch Offices: 59 Bonny St, Port Harcourt, Rivers State; A B C
  Orah, 4 Edaiken Primary School Rd, Benin City, Bendel State
Subsidiary Companies: Franco, Brothers and Co; Associated Oil
  Mill; Fena and Atlas Ltd; Fenaju Projects Ltd
Principal Bankers: National Bank of Nigeria Ltd
Financial Information:

Turnover	N over 5,000,000

Principal Shareholders: Chairman and directors as described
Date of Establishment: 20th August 1970

CHARLTON TRADING COMPANY (NIGERIA) LTD

(CTC)

1 Mai Kano Dutse Rd, PO Box 6233, Kano
Tel: 8380

PRINCIPAL ACTIVITIES: Dealers in tools, hardware and building
  materials
Branch Offices: Kano; Sokoto; Yola; Minna

CHASE MERCHANT BANK NIGERIA LTD

23 Awolowo Rd, PMB 12035, Lagos
Tel: 603020/9
Cable: Chase Bank
Telex: 21585 Chas Bk

Chairman: Dr Okoi Arikpo
Directors: Dr John N Abaelu (Managing Director & Chief
    Executive),
  Richard F Cumberland (Deputy Managing Director),
  Alhaji Usman M Goji,
  Alhaji Iguda Inuwa,
  John Charlton,
  Neil J Tedder,
  S S Obaro
Senior Executives: Joshua A Adebayo (General Manager,
    Banking Operations),
  James F Peterson (General Manager, Credit & Marketing),
  . John I Membu (General Manager, Corporate Finance),
  Gbolahan K Olufon (General Manager, Legal Department)

PRINCIPAL ACTIVITIES: Merchant banking
Branch Offices: Dantata House, 66/67 Murtala Muhammed Way,
  PMB 3260, Kano, Tel 4302, Telex 77267; Orosi House, 28
  Forces Avenue, PMB 6178, Port Harcourt, Tel 332474,
  333623, Telex 61138
Subsidiary Companies: Nigerian International Securities Ltd
Principal Bankers: Central Bank of Nigeria; United Bank for
  Africa; Chase Manhattan Bank NA; New York & London
Financial Information: As at 31st December 1981

	N'000
Authorised capital	7,500
Paid-up capital	5,400
Turnover	20,217
Profits (before tax)	6,004
Profits (after tax)	2,965

Principal Shareholders: Federal Ministry of Finance Incorporated
  60%; Chase Manhattan Overseas Banking Corp (USA) 40%
Date of Establishment: 10th April 1975
No of Employees: 260

CHATTALAS BROTHERS LTD

64E Ado Bayero Rd, PO Box 124, Kano
Tel: 2083, 4727, 3065
Telex: 77105

PRINCIPAL ACTIVITIES: Sugar confectionery manufacturers
Branch Offices: Factory: 160 Club Rd, Kano

No of Employees: 400

CHELLARAM, K, & SONS (NIGERIA) LTD

54 Marina, PO Box 117, Lagos
Tel: 801420/24
Cable: Chellaram Lagos
Telex: 26495 Cheram Ng

Chairman: Murli Tahilram Chellaram
Directors: P T Chellaram,
  Alhaji Isa Kaita,
  S P Chugani (Managing),
  Godfrey K Amachree,
  Anofi Guobadia,
  Ram T Chellaram,
  S K Onafowokan (Executive Director),
  Mallam B Shemu
Senior Executives: P C Purohit (Financial Controller),

L K Sharma (General Manager),
S U Manwani (Area Controller - North)

PRINCIPAL ACTIVITIES: Departmental store, supermarket,
wholesale and retail distribution; industrialists

Principal Agencies: K Hattori & Co Ltd; Canon Inc, Japan;
Emerson Electronics, Italy; Nippon Electric Co, Japan; Unisef
Co Ltd, Japan; Noritake Co Ltd, Japan; Rinaser SA, Spain;
Spear & Jackson, UK; SIP (Industrial) Products, UK; Gepic
SA, France; Stanley Tools Ltd, UK; LS Stareet Co Ltd, UK,
Picard, West Germany

Branch Offices: 1-E Liverpool Rd, PO Box 106, Kano; 84
Lebanon Street, PO Box 170, Ibadan, Oyo State; 29/30 Wharf
Rd, Box 165, Zaria; 8 Ahmadu Bello Way, PO Box 33,
Kaduna; 37 Galadima Kyari Drive, PO Box 328, Maiduguri;
Sokoto; Ilorin; Port Harcourt

Subsidiary/Associated Companies: Aswani Textile Industries Ltd;
Dynamic Industries Ltd; Federation Products (Nig) Ltd;
Chellco Industries Ltd

Principal Bankers: Union Bank of Nigeria Ltd; United Bank for
Africa Ltd; Chase Merchant Bank Ltd; International Bank for
West Africa Ltd; Bank of India (Nigeria) Ltd

Financial Information:

	₦'000
Authorised capital	3,000
Paid-up capital	2,400
Turnover	50,000
Profits	2,000

Principal Shareholders: Chellsons (Bermuda) Ltd
Date of Establishment: 1947
No of Employees: 1,200

CHEMDYES NIGERIA LTD

180B Kofo Abayomi St, Victoria Island, PO Box 1746, Lagos
Tel: 613693, 613888
Cable: Chemdyes Lagos
Telex: 21510

Chairman: Godfrey I C Eneli
Directors: S Dankaro, J O B Iroha, Dr Alex C Eneli, Gladys C
Eneli
Senior Executives: Ben C Eneli (Director Shipping and General
Services),
Emman Ochokwu (General Manager)

PRINCIPAL ACTIVITIES: General merchants, manufacturers'
representatives; suppliers of chemicals, educational
equipment, electrical goods, office equipment, scientific
instruments, etc

Principal Agencies: BASF AG, West Germany; Hasbro; Empire
Pencil Co, USA; E J Arnold & Sons, UK; Philip & Tacey, UK

Branch Offices: 28B Ado Bayero Rd, Kano; 22 Kofo Abayomi
St, Apapa; 28 St Michael St, Aba; 7 Ogui Rd, Enugu; 40
Iweka Rd, Onitsha; 42 Akpakpava Rd, Benin City

Associated Companies: Glcen Electronics Ltd; Robertson
Engineering Ltd

Principal Bankers: Barclays Bank Nigeria Ltd; United Bank for
Africa

Financial Information:

	₦'000
Authorised capital	300
Paid-up capital	300
Sales turnover	4,000

Principal Shareholders: Godfrey I C Eneli; Dr Alex C Eneli;
Gladys C Eneli

CHEMEX NIGERIA LTD

29 Forces Avenue, PO Box 808, Port Harcourt, Rivers State
Tel: 332563, 332502
Cable: Chemex Port Harcourt
Telex: 61238

Directors: G U Eleonu (Managing Director),
C B C Uba,
Mrs C Okezie
Senior Executives: A A Chiori (Field Superintendent),
Alex Ori (Field Superintendent),

J N Ijomah (Accountant),
J Tew (Personnel),
S N Boms (Administrative Officer),
A Nwokike (Transport Officer),
E A Alozie (Marketing Representative)

PRINCIPAL ACTIVITIES: Tank cleaning and degassing; tank
sandblasting and coating services, decorative painting,
pollution control, water-proofing of leaking roofs, corrosion
control etc

Branch Offices: Shell Oil Terminal, Bonny, Rivers State; 198
Airport Rd, Effurun-Warri, Bendel State; 28 Pound Rd, Aba,
Imo State

Principal Bankers: Savannah Bank of Nigeria Ltd

Financial Information:

	₦'000
Authorised capital	100
Paid-up capital	95
Turnover	852
Profits	40

Principal Shareholders: G U Eleonu; C B C Uba; Mrs C Okezie
Date of Establishment: 5th June 1973
No of Employees: 113

CHEMICAL & ALLIED PRODUCTS LTD

24 Commercial Rd, PMB 1004, Apapa, Lagos
Tel: 803220/2, 803672/3, 803675/6
Cable: Kemal Lagos
Telex: 21446, 21594, 21096 (Lagos), 26407 (Ikeja)

Chairman: Chief C O Ogunbanjo
Directors: J Potter (Managing Director),
Chief S O Ogunkoya (Deputy Managing Director),
S O Mezu (Secretary/Finance Director),
A O Odusina (Marketing Director),
M I James (Paints Director),
G O Awofusi (Marketing Director),
Mjr-Gen I B M Haruna (Rtd) (Non Executive),
W H Wishart (ICI UK),
P Hamilton (ICI UK)
Senior Executives: Alhaji M A Haroun (Marketing Manager),
B O Elugbaju (Marketing Manger),
D Olatunji (Marketing Manager),
D Adeyemo (Marketing Manager),
K E Kartey (Marketing Manager)

PRINCIPAL ACTIVITIES: Manufacturers of paints,
pharmaceuticals, agrochemicals, industrial chemicals,
explosives, plastics etc

Principal Agencies: Imperial Chemical Industries, UK

Branch Offices: Factories: Paints Division, Adeniyi Jones Avenue,
PMB 21072, Ikeja, Tel 900050-1, Telex 26407;
Pharmaceuticals Division, 14 Burma Rd, PMB 1004, Apapa,
Tel 803220-2, Telex 21446, 21594, 21096; Agrochemicals
Division, Oluyole Industrial Estate, Off Ring Rd, PMB 5016,
Ibadan, Tel 410800; Explosives Division, 104 Ibrahim Taiwo
Rd, Ilorin, Tel 5165; Regional Offices: 9 Industrial Layout, PO
Box 51, Aba, Tel 321; Oluyole Industrial Estate, Off Ring Rd,
PMB 5016, Ibadan, Tel 410800; 107 Maganda Rd, PO Box
829, Kano, Tel 3793, 3036. Depots in Kaduna; Jos; Maiduguri;
Sokoto; Minna; Akure; Benin City; Ilorin; Calabar; Enugu;
Onitsha

Principal Bankers: First Bank of Nigeria Ltd; Union Bank of
Nigeria Ltd; United Bank for Africa Ltd

Financial Information:

	₦'000
Authorised capital	12,500
Paid-up capital	11,666
Turnover	44,382
Profits (before tax)	4,720

Principal Shareholders: Federal Government of Nigeria;
Convenant Industries Ltd (London); Individual Shareholders in
Nigeria
Date of Establishment: May 1955
No of Employees: 782

CHESEBROUGH PONDS INDUSTRIES LTD

35 Creek Rd, PO Box 179, Apapa, Lagos
Tel: 803100/3
Cable: Vasoponds Apapa

Directors: A K A Ogunnuga (Director),
   Bryan J Crowhurst (General Manager),
   David Townsend (Technical Adviser)

PRINCIPAL ACTIVITIES: Manufacturers of pharmaceuticals and cosmetics

CHIAKWELU, A I, & BROTHERS

28 St Michael's Rd, PO Box 485, Aba, Imo State
Tel: 262

PRINCIPAL ACTIVITIES: Importers and distributors of general merchandise

CHIDIEBERE TRANSPORT LTD

PMB 1084, Uzuakoli Rd, Umuahia, Imo State
Tel: 220400, 220039
Cable: Trachidi

Chairman: L C Amazu
Directors: E C Amazu, Mrs A Amazu
Senior Executives: J P Chukwunenye (Financial Controller),
   S O Agomuoh (Administrative Manager),
   J O Nwachukwu (Personnel Manager),
   G N Maduakoh (Business Manager)

PRINCIPAL ACTIVITIES: Transport; motor vehicles and motor-cycles; mechanical and electrical engineering; educational equipment; oil and gas services. A light-scale manufacturing industry is planned
Principal Agencies: Peugeot Automobile Nigeria Ltd; Leventis Motors
Branch Offices: 152 Ogui Rd, Enugu, Tel 252882; 20 Ikorodu Rd, Fadeyi, Lagos, Tel 843838; 130 Cemetery St, Ebute Metta, East Lagos; 110 Akparaya St, Benin City, Tel 240919; 20 Milverton Ave, Aba, Tel 220298; 52 Aba Rd, Port Harcourt, Tel 226336; 15 Constitution Rd, Kaduna; 10 Old Terrace Rd, Opposite Jubilee/Jenta Hotel, Jos; 36A Gold Coast Rd, Kano; Also at Makurdi, Onitsha, Owerri
Associated Companies: Amazu Motors Ltd, Nigeria; L C Automobile, Nigeria
Principal Bankers: Standard Bank (Nig) Ltd
Financial Information:

	N'000
Authorised capital	1,000
Paid-up capital	1,000
Sales turnover	6,000
Profits	50

Principal Shareholders: Chairman and directors as described
No of Employees: 521

CHIYODA CHEMICAL ENGINEERING & CONSTRUCTION CO

Unity House, 15th Floor, 37 Marina, Lagos Island, PO Box 2351, Lagos
Tel: 635005, 635077
Telex: 21218 Lagos

Directors: Mr Yamada

PRINCIPAL ACTIVITIES: Construction and design engineering; construction of refinery and lube oil plant

CHRISLOW ASSOCIATED NIGERIA LTD

9 Olufemi Rd, Surulere, PO Box 1280, Lagos
Tel: 833161
Cable: Chrislow

Chairman: Slowe N Nnochiri (also Managing Director)
Directors: C C Nnochiri, N S Nnochiri Jnr
Senior Executives: B N Nnochiri (Sales Manager),
   S C Okoh (Services Manager)

PRINCIPAL ACTIVITIES: Suppliers of technical equipment, generating sets, etc
Principal Agencies: RTD Swan Ltd, UK; Mars Signal Light Company, USA; Sides, France
Branch Offices: Owerri; Makurdi; Maiduguri; Kano
Principal Bankers: New Nigeria Bank Ltd

Principal Shareholders: Directors as described
Date of Establishment: 1976

CHRISRAY NIGERIA LTD

Development House, 106 Aba-Owerri Rd, PMB 7087, Aba, Imo State
Cable: Chrisray Aba Nigeria
Telex: 63108 Pico Ng; 63115 Onik Ng

Chairman: C N C Ononuji (also Managing Director)
Directors: O O C Ononuju, Mrs C E C Ononuju, A C Ononuju
Senior Executives: Mrs N O Ume (Company Secretary),
   D I Chiabuotu (Secretary),
   J Nduka (Sales Manager),
   J Agomoh (Accountant)

PRINCIPAL ACTIVITIES: Importers and distributors of building materials and general products including Portland cement, roofing, wire nails, galvanised pipes, furniture tubes, angle iron, round iron rods, sanitary-ware, rice, wheat flour, sugar, salt; stockfish and evaporated milk
Branch Offices: 103 Pound Rd, Aba, Imo State
Principal Bankers: African Continental Bank Ltd
Financial Information:

	N'000
Authorised capital	400
Paid-up capital	400
Sales turnover	3,000
Profits	200

Principal Shareholders: Family of Chief Ononuju (100%)
Date of Establishment: April 1973

CHRISTELA CHEMICAL WORKS LTD

102 St Finbarr's College Rd, Akoka, Yaba, Lagos
Tel: 846398
Cable: Chrischem

Directors: Dr P K Idundun, Alhaji Dauda Belel, P U Idundun, Mrs C Idundun
Senior Executives: A O Isaacs (Commercial Executive),
   R Monuaka (Product Executive, Pharmaceutical),
   A E Bassey (Branch Manager),
   B Olabanji (Product Executive, Chemical)

PRINCIPAL ACTIVITIES: Chemicals, pharmaceutical and medical supplies, scientific instruments
Principal Agencies: Knoll AG (West Germany); J T Baker, (USA); Bausch & Lomb, (USA)
Branch Offices: 102B Upper Benin/Sapele Rd, PMB 1495, Benin; PO Box 10395, Kano; PO Box 526, Yola
Principal Bankers: United Bank for Africa
Financial Information:

	N'000
Authorised capital	500
Paid-up capital	500
Turnover	1,900

Principal Shareholders: Dr P K E Idundun
Date of Establishment: 28th January 1974
No of Employees: 61

CHRISTLIEB, A C, (NIGERIA) LTD

35 Creek Rd, PO Box 392, Apapa
Tel: 803100, 803101, 803102
Cable: Christlieb Apapa
Telex: 22378 Accnl Ng

Chairman: A K A Ogunnuga
Directors: A S Marinho (Managing),
   J G Marks,
   W J Taylor,
   Mrs G O Obasa-Porter,

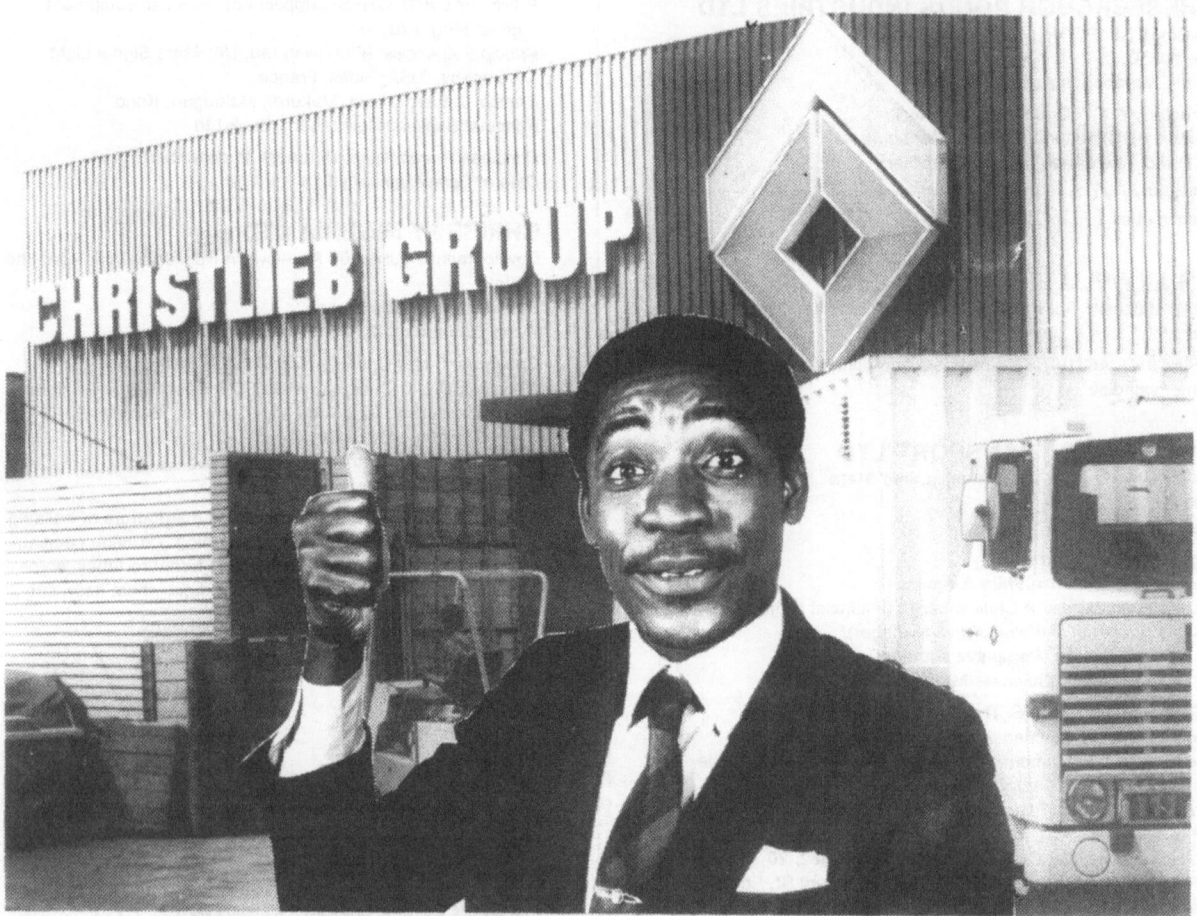

A C Benn,
P F Adepo
Senior Executives: A O Ogundiran (Company Secretary),
F W Baker (Group Technical Adviser),
H A Momoh (Group Financial Controller)

PRINCIPAL ACTIVITIES: General trading; manufacturers'
representatives, manufacturers of plastics, toiletries
pharmaceutical and confectionery products
Principal Agencies: American Kitchen Products Co, USA; Quaker
Oats Ltd, UK
Branch Offices: Plot 82, Sharada Industrial Area, Kano; 2A
Nottidge Street, Onitsha
Subsidiary/Associated Companies: Trebor Nigeria Ltd; Danafco
Nigeria Ltd
Principal Bankers: First Bank of Nigeria Ltd
Financial Information:

	₦'000
Authorised capital	5,000
Paid-up capital	3,000
Turnover	28,000
Profits	2,000

Principal Shareholders: Nigerians 60%; Foreign Interests 40%
Date of Establishment: 1928
No of Employees: 1,500

CHUKWURAH AGRICULTURE INDUSTRIES LTD

Agriculture Rd, Enugwuaja, Ichi, Via Nnewi, Anambra State
Tel: Nnewi 625
Telex: 54333 Ekene Ng

Chairman: S M Chukwurah (also Manging Director)
Directors: C N Chukwurah, E N Chukwurah
Senior Executives: Derek P B Cameron (General Manager),
Dr H Abalos (Technical Sales and Service Manager)

PRINCIPAL ACTIVITIES: Poultry breeding, hatchery, marketing
of poultry and agricultural equipment, animal health products
Principal Agencies: SKA SPA, Italy; Shaver Poultry Breeding
Farms Ltd; Ausculaap BV, Holland; Saeby Jerhstoberi and
Maskinfabrik A/S, Denmark; Laboratorios De Sanidad
Veterinary Hipra SA, Spain
Branch Offices: 128 Owerri Rd, Aba, Imo State; 26 Modebe
Avenue, Onitsha; 28 First East Circular, Benin City, Bendel
State; E9/705E Iwo Rd, Ibadan, Oyo State
Associated Companies: Eziuzo Enterprises Ltd; Ichi Feed
Company
Principal Bankers: African Continental Bank Ltd; United Bank
for Africa Ltd
Financial Information:

	₦'000
Authorised capital	1,000
Paid-up capital	500
Turnover	5,000

Date of Establishment: 9th April 1965
No of Employees: 120

CHUWANG GYANG & SONS LTD

Mile 3 Shen, Near Bukuru, PO Box 8, Bukuru
PRINCIPAL ACTIVITIES: Metal ore mining

CIBA-GEIGY LTD

PO Box 4310, Ikeja, Lagos
PRINCIPAL ACTIVITIES: Drug manufacturers

CIMECO ENTERPRISES (NIGERIA) LTD

41 Edinburgh Rd, Ogui New Layout, PO Box 810, Enugu,
Anambra State
Tel: 257393
Cable: Cimeco Enugu
Telex: 51249 Cimeco Ng

Chairman: Festus Onyekwelu
Directors: Engr C Iloduba (Managing Director),
Mrs Roswitha Iloduba,
Ikechukwu Umeh,
Dr Erich Turba
Senior Executives: Jerry Okoli (Administrative Manager),
Engr John Nwachukwu (Project Engineer),
Ifeanyi Onyekwelu (Senior Technical Officer),
Julian Nwamadi (Secretary),
Clement Nwoye (Chief Accountant)

PRINCIPAL ACTIVITIES: Civil engineering contractors;
proposals for the manufacture of structural ceramic products;
representatives for industrial goods and machineries
Principal Agencies: Agrob Anlagenbau, West Germany;
Rieterwerke GmbH, West Germany; Keller Ofenbau GmbH,
West Germany
Branch Offices: PMB 24, Suleja, Niger State c/o of Federal
Capital Development Authority
Subsidiary Companies: Niteco (Nigeria) Ltd; Blackwood Hodge
(Nigeria) Ltd; Afrotec (Nigeria) Ltd; Scoatrac; UTC (Nigeria)
Ltd; Samphil (Nigeria) Ltd
Principal Bankers: International Bank for West Africa Ltd; First
Bank of Nigeria Ltd
Financial Information:

	₦'000
Authorised capital	400
Paid-up capital	400
Turnover (approx)	2,000

Principal Shareholders: Engineer Chukwuemeka Iloduba; Festus
Onyekwelu
Date of Establishment: Registered 18th July 1977: Actual
bussiness activities started in August 1978
No of Employees: 320

CINSERE SEWING MACHINE INDUSTRIAL COMPANY LTD

5 Badejo Kalesanwo St, Matori, PMB 1005, Mushin, Lagos
Tel: 847860
Cable: Ajenipa Lagos

Chairman: J A Babatayo (also Managing Director)
Directors: T A Oregbemi, B O Babatayo, O O Babatayo, B
Oregbemi
Senior Executives: Isaac Ola Adelowo (Production Supervisor),
Christopher Dele Agboola (Pfaff Sewing Machine Technical
Instructor),
George Adebolu (Sales Supervisor)

PRINCIPAL ACTIVITIES: Assemblers of domestic and industrial
sewing machines
Principal Agencies: Pfaff Industriemaschinen, West Germany;
Sum Cornely, France; Attilio Cornaly, Italy; Sangu Sewing
Machine, Japan
Branch Offices: 26 Obun-Eko St, Lagos; 71 Docemu St, Lagos
Associated Companies: Ajenipa Technical Company
Principal Bankers: United Bank for Africa Ltd; First Bank of
Nigeria Ltd
Financial Information:

	₦'000
Authorised capital	100
Paid-up capital	100
Turnover	450
Profits	150

Principal Shareholders: J A Babatayo; Mrs T A Oregbemi
Date of Establishment: 1950

CISTAR (NIGERIA) LTD

45 Martins St, 3rd Floor, Lagos
Tel: 636882

Directors: J Marchbanks (Managing Director)
PRINCIPAL ACTIVITIES: Construction

CITY GROUP ORGANIZATION

Western House, 8th Floor, 8-10 Broad St, Lagos
Tel: 632293, 632221, 632152
Cable: Citigroup Lagos
Telex: 21179 Cigrup Ng

PRINCIPAL ACTIVITIES: The 15 companies within the
organisation are: City Life & General Assurance Ltd (Life and
Non-Life Underwriting); Land Securities (Land Investment);
City Group Industries Ltd (Joint Venture/Equity Participation
in Companies); City Group Engineering Services Ltd
(Electrical/mechanical, communications, plumbing and water
supply services); City Group Furnishing Company Ltd
(Wholesale and contract furnishing supplies); City Holdings
and Investments Ltd (Investment in town centre commercial
properties); City Group Motors (Nigeria) Ltd (Importation and
distribution of motor vehicles); City Group Finance
Corporation Ltd (Hire purchase/finance and leasing); City
Building Materials Centre Ltd (Importation and distribution of
building materials); City Building Society (Home loans and
savings); City Property Development Ltd (Property
development and residential estates); City Consultants
(Nigeria) Ltd (Consultants in architecture, town planning,
engineering, advertising, management services); City Group
Contruction (Nigeria) Ltd (Building and civil engineering
construction); City Superette Ltd (Wholesale supermarket);
City Distributors Nigeria Ltd (Manufacturers' representatives
and importers of construction plant and machinery,
telecommunications equipment and general engineering
hardware)

CITY SECURITIES LTD

Primrose Tower, 17A Tinubu Street, PO Box 9117, Lagos
Tel: 664503, 660112, 660004
Cable: Ciesel Lagos
Telex: 21925 Ciesel Ng

Chairman: Chief Michael Olasubomi Balogun
Directors: Alhaji Liman Ciroma, Chief Kola Daisi, Ladi Jadesimi,
Mrs Abimbola Adetutu Balogun, Mrs Olaronke Olawunmi
Atere
Senior Executives: Bryan Isaac (General Manager),
Oluwole S Oduyemi (Deputy General Manager),
I Ismail (Deputy Manager),
M A Obunlami (Company Accountant),
Miss O Odunewu (Assistant Manager),
S A A Adedayo (Assistant Manager)

PRINCIPAL ACTIVITIES: Finance and investment services;
capital issues both private and public of equity and
debentures, dealing in securities, finance counselling,
investment management; project finance arrangement and
loan syndication; confirming house services
Principal Agencies: C S L Stockbrokers Ltd
Subsidiary Companies: C S L Stockbrokers Ltd
Principal Bankers: International Bank for West Africa; United
Bank for Africa; Savannah Bank of Nigeria
Financial Information:

	N'000
Authorised capital	1,000
Paid-up capital	902
Turnover	50,000
Profits	157

Principal Shareholders: Primrose Investments Ltd; Blue chip
Holdings Ltd; Chief M O Balogun
Date of Establishment: September 1977
No of Employees: 50

CITYMARK (WEST AFRICA) LTD

Plot 143A-B Gbagada Estate Block E, Expressway, Anthony
Village, PMB 1164, Yaba, Lagos State
Tel: 900730/3
Telex: 26333 Citmak Ng

Chairman: F A O Alade
Directors: Prof M I Jegede,
R O Herbert,

P Huber,
R Kolf,
B Schoepper,
Lucas Da'am Datogoop,
E K Tormerty (Alternate),
James Witte (Alternate),
Alhaji Usman Abdul Kareem (Alternate)
Senior Executives: F A O Alade (Chief Executive),
R O Herbert (Executive Director, Commercial),
Alhaji T.T Jenmi (Manager, International Department),
Henry Ekhator (Chief Administrative Executive)

PRINCIPAL ACTIVITIES: Building, civil, electrical and mechanical
contracting; turn-key projects and commercial activities
Principal Agencies: King Refrigerator Corp, USA; Anti Hyrdo,
USA; Citymark Projektbau, Germany
Branch Offices: Throughout Nigeria
Subsidiary/Associated Companies: Citicon Nigeria Ltd; First
Merchants Ltd; Capital Finance Co Ltd; Citymark Projektbau
GmbH
Financial Information:

	N'000
Authorised capital	1,000
Paid-up capital	750
Turnover	20,000

Principal Shareholders: F A O Alade; Citymark Projektbau
Date of Establishment: 1979
No of Employees: 472

CLARETTA MARITIME SERVICES LTD

126/130 Nnamdi Azikiwe St (5th Floor), PO Box 8590, Lagos
Tel: 630185, 635309
Cable: McJullee Lagos

PRINCIPAL ACTIVITIES: Clearing, forwarding and air freighting
agents

CLARKE, W F, (NIGERIA) LTD

Industrial Estate, Industrial Street, Ilupeju, PMB 21066, Ikeja,
Lagos
Tel: 900350/3
Cable: Tucknip Ikeja

Chairman: Chief M C O Ibru
Directors: Chief S K T Aiyegoro, Alex Ibru, R P A Hornsby
Senior Executives: A R de Paiva Rapozo (General Manager),
D M Aitken (Technical Manager),
W Erewa Meggison (Brand Manager),
Mrs V N Oguocha (Finance Manager)

PRINCIPAL ACTIVITIES: Manufacturers, manufacturers agents
and wholesale distributors
Principal Agencies: Cadbury Schweppes Overseas Ltd; Quaker
Oats; Ovaltine; H J Heinz; Pearse Duff; Thermos; A T Cross;
London Rubber Co; John Harvey & Sons; Cinzano; Royal
Sovereign; Murrey Clarke & Jones
Branch Offices: Kano; Kaduna; Jos; Ilorin; Ibadan; Akure; Benin;
Enugu; Onitsha; Aba; Port Harcourt
Principal Bankers: First Bank of Nigeria Ltd
Financial Information:

	N'000
Authorised capital	1,000
Paid-up capital	1,000
Turnover	27,000

Principal Shareholders: 100% Nigerian owned
Date of Establishment: October 1949
No of Employees: 250

CLARKE, WALTER, & SONS (OVERSEAS) LTD

PO Box 518, Lagos
PRINCIPAL ACTIVITIES: Importers of general merchandise

CLAY INDUSTRY (NIGERIA) LTD

Oregun Industrial Estate, PO Box 319, Ikeja
Tel: 960456, 963529, 963514, 963544
Cable: Nigerclay

Chairman: Chief Adeniyi Coker
Directors: Giulio Gianotti,
  Mrs C Aduke Young,
  Franco Gianotti,
  A R Cordon (General Manager),
  Silvio Bernardi (Production Manager)

PRINCIPAL ACTIVITIES: Manufacturers of structural clay
  products
Principal Bankers: First Bank of Nigeria Ltd; United Bank for
  Africa Ltd
Financial Information:

	₦'000
Authorised capital	2,000
Paid-up capital	2,000

Date of Establishment: Incorporated: 21st July, 1961

CLYDE DIAL CONSTRUCTION (NIGERIA) LTD

4 Balogun Sq, PO Box 2820, Lagos
Tel: 632168, 633472

Directors: Daniel L Carr (Managing Director)

PRINCIPAL ACTIVITIES: Construction

CNEICO (NIGERIA) LTD

12 Keffi Rd, Ikoyi, PO Box 31, Lagos
Tel: 682603, 683062
Cable: Cneico, Lagos
Telex: 21337

Directors: J Vesely (Managing),
  A Oshodi,
  Chief G Eze,
  J B Valenta

PRINCIPAL ACTIVITIES: Importers of machine tools
Principal Agencies: Strojimport, Czechoslovakia
Branch Offices: 5 Decima Rd, PO Box 37, Sapele, Bendel State,
  Tel 41744; 2 Kings Sq, Benin City, Bendel State, Tel 240471;
  54 Ogidi St, Ogui, PO Box 591, Enugu, Anambra State; 74
  Mbaise Rd, Owerri, Imo State; 3 Bompai/Club Rd, PO Box
  176, Kano; Machinery Division and Training Centre; 15
  Commercial Rd, Apapa, PO Box 31, Lagos, Tel 875932,
  873130, 875870
Principal Bankers: First Bank of Nigeria Ltd

CNMD CO
Czechoslovak Nigerian Minerals Development Co Ltd

Tudun Wada, PO Box 424, Jos, Plateau State
Tel: 2522
Cable: Prospect

PRINCIPAL ACTIVITIES: Metal ore mining

COAST TIMBER CO LTD

25 Eric Moore Rd, Ikeja, Lagos
Tel: 21325 Cosco Ng

PRINCIPAL ACTIVITIES: Production of sawn timber
Branch Offices: PO Box 68, Sapele, Bendel State

COASTAL SERVICES (NIGERIA) LTD

42/44 Warehouse Rd, PO Box 97, Apapa, Lagos
Tel: 876290, 876366
Cable: 21226 Cosenil

PRINCIPAL ACTIVITIES: Shipping, warehousing, clearing,
  forwarding, transporters

COATES BROTHERS (WA) LTD

PO Box 395, 7 Henry Carr Rd, Industrial Estate, Ikeja, Lagos
Tel: 961415
Cable: Inkmaker Lagos

PRINCIPAL ACTIVITIES: Manufacturers of printing inks and
  surface coatings for all processes, offset lithography,
  letterpress, etc

COCOA INDUSTRIES LTD

Oba Akran Ave Extension, PMB 1114, Industrial Estate, Ikeja,
  Lagos State
Tel: 900365/7/8
Cable: Cocind
Telex: 21489 Cocind

Chairman: C S O Akande
Directors: O A Iyowu (Managing Director),
  J A Sogo,
  Prof L K Opeke,
  K Fatona,
  Z A Alabi
Senior Executives: S A Osanyingbemi (Administrative Manager
  and Secretary),
  T A Yesufu (Chief Accountant),
  J O Oladoke (Production Manager),
  E E Losa (Chief Engineer),
  S O Olutayo (Chief Chemist)

PRINCIPAL ACTIVITIES: Food and food processing; cocoa
  products
Principal Bankers: United Bank for Africa Ltd; National Bank of
  Nigeria Ltd
Financial Information:

	₦'000
Authorised capital	4,000
Paid-up capital	4,000
Sales turnover	40,000
Profits	4,400

Principal Shareholders: O'Dua Investment Company Ltd
No of Employees: 550

COCOA PRODUCERS ALLIANCE

8/10 Broad St, Lagos
Tel: 635506, 635574, 633995
Telex: 21311 Copal Ng

PRINCIPAL ACTIVITIES: Cocoa production

COGEMAT (NIGERIA) LTD

85 Awolowo Rd, Ikoyi, PO Box 7285, Lagos

PRINCIPAL ACTIVITIES: Suppliers of aluminium products, glass
  products, floor coverings, interior decoration
Principal Agencies: Cogemat, France

COKSEE ENGINEERING WORKS LTD

Amje Bus Stop, Km 35 Agege - Ota Expressway, PO Box 8826,
  Marina, Lagos

PRINCIPAL ACTIVITIES: Structural and steel body building;
  Manufacturers of petrol and water tankers, trailers

COLODENSE NIGERIA LTD

PMB 21505, Ikeja, Lagos
Tel: 960112, 963153

Chairman: Dr I Babatunde Jose
Directors: G Atkinson (Managing Director),
  Alhaji Shehu Ahmed,
  Alhaji Yahya Gusau,
  A O Collinson,
  E B Onifade,
  S O Adesanya,
  N I Ole,
  M Parker
Senior Executives: D E Jordan (Chief Engineer),
  F A Bamwo (Personnel Manager)

PRINCIPAL ACTIVITIES: Converters and suppliers of transparent films; plastics and papers, printed and unprinted for packaging applications throughout Nigeria
Branch Offices: Agbara Industrial Estate, Km 32, Lagos-Badagry Expressway, Ogun State
Associated Companies: British Cellophane Ltd, UK; Colodense Ltd UK
Principal Bankers: First Bank of Nigeria Ltd; Icon Ltd (Merchant Bankers)
Principal Shareholders: British Cellophane Group Ltd; Great Nigeria Insurance Company Ltd; Arewa Associates
Date of Establishment: 1976
No of Employees: 130

COMAZZI, P

PO Box 376, Ibadan, Oyo State
Tel: 411223

Directors: France Fileppi

PRINCIPAL ACTIVITIES: Building and civil engineering contractors

COMBINED MARITIME AGENCIES (NIGERIA) LTD

2 Oroabali Street, PMB 5429, Amadi Flats, Port Harcourt, Rivers State
Tel: 331810, 333736

Directors: Captain Claus Sievers, Monday Ono Imoni
Senior Executives: Captain Harm Palm (General Manager), Conrad Schømer (Financial Controller)

PRINCIPAL ACTIVITIES: Shipping agency, stevedoring, shipping line representation, clearing and forwarding
Principal Agencies: Jeco Shipping Line
Branch Offices: 62 Calcutta Crescent, Apapa, Lagos; Tel 872909, Telex 22407 Cmanig

COMMERCE ASSURANCE LTD

47/48 Breadfruit Street, Lagos
Tel: 661563, 661565

Chairman: Chief K A Adebutu

PRINCIPAL ACTIVITIES: Insurance

Date of Establishment: 1971

COMMERCIAL MEDICINE STORES LTD

23 Nnamdi Azikiwe St, PO Box 89, Lagos
Tel: 633983

PRINCIPAL ACTIVITIES: Pharmacists
Branch Offices: 12 Ojuelegba Rd, Surulere, Lagos, Tel 837121; 93 Kofo Abayomi Crescent, Apap, Lagos, Tel 873839

COMMIND NIGERIA LTD

31 Ikorodu Rd, Fadeyi, Yaba, PO Box 500, Surulere, Lagos
Tel: 862654
Cable: Caropel Ng

Chairman: Chief E O Sonubi (also Chief Executive)
Directors: G O Ogunsanwo (Project Development),
  Mrs O Sonubi,
  Alhaji G A Salami (Vice-Chairman, Finance),
  Alhaji A A Akintunde (Vice-Chairman, Technical)
Senior Executives: A Ojo (Dealership Development Manager),
  A Ajayi (Sales Manager)

PRINCIPAL ACTIVITIES: Suppliers of building materials, chemicals, industrial equipment, construction plant, fertilisers, plastic products, motor vehicles, office equipment, furniture, etc. Telecommunications
Principal Agencies: Acrow; General Motors; Westinghouse
Branch Offices: 40 Ikorodu Rd, Igbobi, Yaba; Badagry Expressway; Shipeolu/Bakare Shomolu
Subsidiary Companies: Keystone Plastics Ltd; ASD Nigeria Ltd; Rock of Ages Investment Co Ltd
Principal Bankers: United Bank for Africa; Wema Bank; National Bank of Nigeria

Financial Information:

	N'000
Authorised capital	1,000
Paid-up capital	1,000
Turnover	10,804

Principal Shareholders: Chairman and directors as described
Date of Establishment: 1975
No of Employees: 350

COMMONWEALTH COMMODITY COMPANY INTERNATIONAL

Susannah House, Near the Federal Sub Post Office Building, PO Box 1700, Warri, Bendel State

Chairman: Chief J A O'Bahor
Directors: HRH Prince J A O'Bahor (Managing),
  W A O'Bahor,
  Mrs S O Bazunu-O'Bahor
Senior Executives: S Orr, S Olympio, R Srinivasan, M Chang

PRINCIPAL ACTIVITIES: Agents and general traders, suppliers of agricultural produce, fish, industrial process plants; electronics engineers
Principal Agencies: Bridgemore Engineering Ltd, GB; Farrel International Inc, GB; Shelsley Engineering Ltd, GB; Powell Duffryn Engineering Company, GB, GP Industries Ltd, India; Australian Meat and Livestock Corporation; New Zealand Meat Exporters Council; Hong Kong Plastic & Metal Products Company; Bee Industrial Corporation Taiwan; Tongkook Trading Company Inc, Korea; W S Craster Ltd, Zimbabwe; Atomic Energy of Canada Ltd etc
Branch Offices: 44 Lower Erejuwa Rd, Warri; 1 Bazunu St, Warri
Principal Bankers: Union Bank of Nigeria Ltd
Financial Information:

	N'000
Authorised capital	3,500
Paid-up capital	3,000
Turnover	7,000
Profits	750

Principal Shareholders: Chairman and directors as described
Date of Establishment: 30th October 1978

COMMUNICATIONS ASSOCIATES OF NIGERIA LTD
COMSAC

Industrial Crescent, Ilupeju Industrial Estate, PMB 21129, Ikeja, Lagos
Tel: 900300/2
Cable: Comdec Ng
Telex: 26363

Chairman: Chief N O Idowu
Directors: Chief Oyebode Oyeleye,
  Y L Akande (Executive Director-Finance),
  J E Lucken,
  D H Smith,
  K Hall (Managing)
Senior Executives: E Forsberg (Technical Manager),
  E S Andrew-Essien (Chief Engineer),
  P M Ikebeli (Administration Manager),
  B M Davies (Marketing Manager),
  E E Etim (Project Manager)

PRINCIPAL ACTIVITIES: Telecommunications
Principal Agencies: Pye Telecommunications, UK; Eddystone Communications Ltd, UK; L M Ericsson, Sweden; Telecomms, Ireland
Branch Offices: PO Box 522, Warri/Sapele Rd, Warri, Tel: 230565; PO Box 517, Aba Rd, Port Harcourt, Tel: 335843; Commercial Avenue, Enugu, PMB 1032, Tel: 255812; Kachia Rd, Kaduna South, Kaduna
Associated Companies: Comden Nigeria Ltd; West African Surveys Ltd; Decca West African Records Ltd
Principal Bankers: First Bank of Nigeria Ltd; Nigerian Acceptances Ltd; International Bank for West Africa

Financial Information:

	N'000
Authorised capital	400
Paid-up capital	400
Turnover	3,600
Profits	271

Principal Shareholders: Nigerians (60%); Decca Ltd, UK (20.40%); Saderete C I Ltd, UK (19.60%)
Date of Establishment: 22nd February 1968
No of Employees: 300

COMMUNICATIONS CONSULTANTS NIGERIA LTD

243 Ijora Causeway, Apapa, Lagos
Tel: 837151, 837154
Telex: 21501 Comcon Ng

PRINCIPAL ACTIVITIES: Communication consultants

COMPAGNIE FRANCAISE DE L'AFRIQUE INTERNATIONALE

Evwreni House, Near UBA/BNP Bank Buildings, PO Box 1700, Warri, Bendel State

Chairman: Chief J A O'Bahor
Directors: HRH Prince J A O'Bahor (Managing),
    W A O'Bahor,
    Mrs S O Bazunu-O'Bahor
Senior Executives: R Amerding, S Olympio

PRINCIPAL ACTIVITIES: Agents and general trading, suppliers of agricultural equipment and produce including fertilisers, livestock and animal feeds
Principal Agencies: Gondard Equipment SA, France; Messrs Dagard SA, France; Messrs Friga-Bohn SA, France; R Tavernier NV, Belgium; Ase Europe NV, Belgium; Atomic Energy of Canada Inc, Canada; Montreal Engineering Company Inc etc
Branch Offices: 44 Lower Erejuwa Rd, Warri, Bendel State; 1 Bazunu St, Warri, Bendel State
Principal Bankers: United Bank for Africa Ltd
Financial Information:

	N'000
Authorised capital	5,000
Paid-up capital	3,000
Turnover	7,000
Profits	750

Principal Shareholders: Chairman and directors as described
Date of Establishment: 30th October 1978
No of Employees: 300

COMPASS TRADING CO LTD

46 Oturkpo Rd, High Level, PMB 2292, Makurdi, Benue State

PRINCIPAL ACTIVITIES: Suppliers of plant and construction equipment, mining equipment, general hardware, automobiles and spares, scientific and graphic equipment
Branch Offices: 53 Western Ave, PMB 3276, Surulere, Lagos; 40B Warri/Sapele Rd, Effurun, PO Box 22, Warri, Bendel State; 31 Zik Ave, PO Box 422, Enugu, Anambra State, Tel 253490; 10B Okigwe Rd, PMB 1253, Owerri, Imo State

COMPLETE HOME ENTERPRISES (NIG) LTD

38 Agege Motor Rd, Alakija, PO Box 97, Mushin, Lagos
Tel: 832615, 844842/3
Cable: Enterhome Lagos
Telex: 21527 Che Ng

Chairman: J C Canaan (also Managing Director)
Directors: E C Cannan
Senior Executives: A Y Madi (General Manager)

PRINCIPAL ACTIVITIES: Suppliers of building materials; furniture; metals; civil engineering and construction
Branch Offices: Building Division: 97 Aba Rd, Port Harcourt; Cement Operation Jetty Offices: Enerhe Rd, Warri
Principal Bankers: Arab Bank (Nigeria) Ltd; Savannah Bank (Nigeria) Ltd; First Bank of Nigeria Ltd

Financial Information:

	N'000
Authorised capital	1,200
Paid-up capital	1,200

Principal Shareholders: J C Canaan; E C Canaan
No of Employees: 1,000

COMPREHENSIVE ENGINEERING CONSULTANTS

13/17 Breadfruit St, PO Box 5382, Lagos
Tel: 636711, 636316

PRINCIPAL ACTIVITIES: Engineering consultants

CONCORDE FURNITURE MANUFACTURING CO LTD

220 Herbert Macaulay St, Yaba, Lagos
Tel: 863221, 861468
Cable: Concordef

Chairman: Dr Adepitan Bamisaiye (also Managing Director)
Directors: Mrs A Bamisaiye, Major General O Olutoye
Senior Executives: M B Fasanya (Factory Manager),
    B Badaru (Accountant),
    J Adelehin (Administrative Manager),
    H J Seyfried (General Manager)

PRINCIPAL ACTIVITIES: Manufacturers of office, hotel, airport and lounge furniture
Branch Offices: Factory Address: Plot 1 Block A, Ilasamaja Industrial Estate, Isolo Dual Carriage Way, Ilasamaja, Lagos
Principal Bankers: First Bank of Nigeria Ltd
Financial Information:

	N'000
Authorised capital	700
Paid-up capital	700
Turnover	1,500-2,000

Principal Shareholders: Dr A Bamisaiye; Major General O Olutoye
Date of Establishment: 29th April 1976
No of Employees: 250

CONCRETE BUILDING CONTRACTORS & GENERAL WORKS LTD

PO Box 70, Sokoto

PRINCIPAL ACTIVITIES: Importers of building materials

CONCRETE POLES INDUSTRIES (NIGERIA) LTD

1 Atekha St, Benin City, Bendel State

Chairman: Jude Irobun Atekha (also Managing Director)
Directors: Emma Atekha,
    Festus Atekha (Financial Director),
    Faith Atekha
Senior Executives: Enrique Paredes (General Manager),
    Emma Onweh (Electrical Engineer),
    Joseph Okunoghae (Plant Manager)

PRINCIPAL ACTIVITIES: Fabrication of all concrete products, mainly electrical distribution poles, concrete blocks, concrete fencing poles; brokerage
Principal Agencies: West African Portland Cement Company; Centricon, West Germany
Branch Offices: Factory: 8 Poles St, Benin City; 9 Ekiomo St, Benin City
Associated Companies: Atekha Brothers & Company Ltd
Principal Bankers: Barclays Bank Nigeria Ltd
Financial Information:

	N'000
Authorised capital	400
Paid-up capital	400
Sales turnover	2,000
Profits	600

Principal Shareholders: Jude Atekha; Emma Atekha; Festus
Atekha
No of Employees: 108

CONCRETE STRUCTURES LTD
Kilometer 8-9 Lagos Rd, PO Box 108, Ibadan, Oyo State
Tel: 410087
Telex: 31209 Morgan Ng

Directors: Rotimi M Morgan (Managing Director),
Omotayo A Morgan (Financial Director)
Senior Executives: B Kamalasena (Chief Design Engineer/Project
Manager)

PRINCIPAL ACTIVITIES: Manufacturers of prestressed/concrete
electric transmission poles; and precast flooring
Principal Agencies: Admac Stressing Ltd, UK
Branch Offices: Branch Liaison Office: 58 Olatilewa St, Surulere,
Lagos
Subsidiary/Associated Companies: Morgan Steel Construction
Co Co Ltd (Subsidiary); Afroware Co Ltd (Associated)
Financial Information:

	N'000
Authorised capital	200
Sales turnover	3,000

Principal Shareholders: R Morgan; A O Morgan
Date of Establishment: 1972
No of Employees: 180

CONSOLIDATED STRUCTURES
10 Ondo St, West Ebute-Metta, PO Box 3903, Lagos

PRINCIPAL ACTIVITIES: Construction

CONSTRUCTION & SUPPORT SERVICES NIGERIA LTD
6B Tafawa Balewa Street, PO Box 375, Jos, Plateau State
Tel: 53297

PRINCIPAL ACTIVITIES: Civil engineering and construction

Date of Establishment: July 1980
No of Employees: 60

CONSTRUCTION MANAGEMENT SERVICES
36 Strachan St, Lagos
Tel: 657197

Directors: Femi Popoola, Michael R Morris

PRINCIPAL ACTIVITIES: Consulting engineers

CONTAINERS (NIGERIA) LTD
PO Box 1, Ikeja, Lagos

PRINCIPAL ACTIVITIES: Packing materials manufacturers

CONTEX NIGERIA LTD
21 Danmole St, Victoria Island, PO Box 1742, Lagos
Tel: 610301
Cable: Structex Lagos

Chairman: L O Akindele
Directors: R L Lawrence (Managing),
R A Gbadamosi,
J Nahman

PRINCIPAL ACTIVITIES: Manufacturers' representatives;
specialists in structural steelworks; suspended ceilings,
partitions; specialist building contractors
Principal Agencies: D Gillespie Associates Ltd, UK; Donn
Products (UK) Ltd
Principal Bankers: United Bank for Africa Ltd
Financial Information:

	N'000
Authorised capital	400
Paid-up capital (to be increased)	200

Date of Establishment: 9th December 1974
No of Employees: 100

CONTINENTAL & GENERAL MERCHANTS LTD
PO Box 6, Warri, Bendel State
Tel: 233944, 232084
Telex: 43284 Kiel Ng

PRINCIPAL ACTIVITIES: Importers and distributors of general
merchandise
Financial Information: Part of Kagho Group of Companies

CONTINENTAL IRON & STEEL CO LTD
Awosika Ave, Industrial Estate, PO Box 161, Ikeja, Lagos
Tel: 961231, 932110, 964367

PRINCIPAL ACTIVITIES: Manufacturing of iron and steel tubes,
bars, rods, flats and wire

CONTINENTAL LINES (AFRICA) LTD
PMB 1073, 24 Wharf Rd, Apapa, Lagos
Tel: 874068, 832582
Cable: Continental Lagos
Telex: 21422 Rbko Ng

PRINCIPAL ACTIVITIES: Shipping, clearing, forwarding,
warehousing, road haulage and air freighting
Branch Offices: 19 Murtala Muhammed Way, PMB 3176, Kano,
Tel 3864, Telex 77213 Taysa Ng; Aba Rd, Opposite Hotel
Presidential, PMB 5254, Port Harcourt, Rivers State; 53
Market Rd, PO Box 565, Warri, Bendel State; 30 Okpe St,
PMB 4067, Sapele, Bendel State; 25 Barracks Rd, PO Box
516, Calabar, Cross River State; Murtala Muhammad Airport,
Ikeja; Apapa Wharf; Owerri

CONTINENTAL MEDICAL COMPLEX LTD
Plot D/106 A Industrial Layout, Oji River, Anambra State
Tel: 255080
Cable: Complex Enugu
Telex: 51180 Lint Nigeria

Chairman: Chief Pius Dim Chikwereuba Okenwa
Directors: Felix O Ihenacho, Samuel Uchenna Chigbo,
Eberhard Seitz, Cyril U Anukam, B A Okafor
Senior Executives: J C Emezie (Company
Secretary/Administrative Manager)

PRINCIPAL ACTIVITIES: Manufacturers of surgical dressings
Principal Bankers: African Continental Bank Ltd; Co-operative
Commerce Bank (Nigeria) Ltd
Financial Information:

	N'000
Authorised capital	3,000
Paid-up capital	1,988
Turnover	640
Profits	10

Principal Shareholders: Markdealers (Nigeria) Ltd; Chief PDC
Okenwa; Anambra State Government; Imo State
Government; Consortex Karl Doelitzsch, West Germany
Date of Establishment: 1973
No of Employees: 300

CONTINENTAL PHARMACEUTICALS LTD
283 Agege Motor Rd, Ilupeju, PO Box 5080, Lagos
Tel: 963753, 963914, 960809, 961042

PRINCIPAL ACTIVITIES: Suppliers of pharmaceutical products

Date of Establishment: December 1974

CONTINUOUS PRINTING INDUSTRY (NIGERIA) LTD
Ewusi Street, Makun Quarters, PMB 2039, Sagamu, Ogun State
Tel: 963099
Cable: Continuous Nigeria

Chairman: O Osimsamya (also Managing Director)
Directors: S O Elebe, Mrs E A Osinsanya, K Adebayo, A Adedoyin
Senior Executives: P Osayamwen (Factory Manager),
    A E Unuoya (Sales Manager),
    F O Adebayo (Accoutant)

PRINCIPAL ACTIVITIES: Printers of computer stationery and preprinted business forms
Branch Offices: Ageso House, 2 Airport Rd, Maryland, PO Box 341, Ikeja
Principal Bankers: National Bank of Nigeria Ltd
Financial Information:

	N'000
Authorised capital	2,000
Paid-up capital	400

Principal Shareholders: Chairman and directors
Date of Establishment: 18th November 1978
No of Employees: 70

CONTROLLED PLASTICS LTD

(Formerly Polyplast Industrial Co Ltd)

Km 8 Hadejia Rd, PO Box 186, Kano
Tel: 7393
Cable: Contro Kano
Telex: 77202 Contro Ng

Directors: V P Sung,
    H A Boukarroum,
    Alhaji A Labaran,
    Alhaji D I Sule,
    Raymond S L Tin (Managing)

PRINCIPAL ACTIVITIES: Manufacturers of plastic houseware, furniture, industrial parts, containers, polythene bags etc
Principal Bankers: Savannah Bank of Nigeria Ltd
Financial Information:

	N'000
Authorised capital	1,000
Paid-up capital	1,000
Turnover	4,000

Principal Shareholders: Directors as described
Date of Establishment: 7th December 1977
No of Employees: 200

CONVEYANCER (NIGERIA) LTD

64 Eric Moore Rd, Iganmu, PMB 1189, Apapa, Lagos
Tel: 837025
Cable: Hydraulics Apapa
Telex: 26991 Conron

Chairman: Alhaji Mogaji Dambatta
Directors: T O Escott (Managing),
    G R Trippas,
    A O Aiyanyo (Executive Director - Personnel),
    C E Dafinone
Senior Executives: A Opeodu (Financial Controller)

PRINCIPAL ACTIVITIES: Agents for mechanical handling, construction and transport equipment
Principal Agencies: Coventry Climax Ltd; Grove Cranes Ltd; Hymac; Ward Power Generators; Polymathic; Watts Tyres; Whale Tankers; Powell Duffryn Eng; Comansa Tower Cranes
Branch Offices: PO Box 815, Warri/Sapele Rd, Benin City, Bendel State; 4 Henry Carr St, Ikeja, Lagos
Associated Companies: Coventry Climax Ltd
Principal Bankers: First Bank of Nigeria Ltd; Chase Merchant Nigeria Ltd; Nigerian-American Merchant Bank Ltd
Financial Information:

	N'000
Authorised capital	2,000
Paid-up capital	2,000
Turnover	10,000
Profits	700

Principal Shareholders: Jediol Corp (40%); Coventry Climax 40%
Date of Establishment: 1964
No of Employees: 120

CO-OPERATIVE AND COMMERCE BANK (NIGERIA) LTD

28 Okpara Avenue, PMB 1321, Enugu
Tel: 253613, 266324
Cable: Encobank Enug
Telex: 51132 Cobank

Chairman: F I Onwadike
Directors: L O Nnaji, M T Ihemadu, M O Wokocha, L M E Ezeofor, Frank Oloto, Dr Agom Eze, Mrs R N Abara, D N Afuecheta, J A Ogbodo, Eddy Obi Okoye
Senior Executives: O T Ajiri (Deputy General Manager),
    G O J Uzoije (Assistant General Manager, Advances),
    P C Okoye (Chief Accountant),
    A Ohabuike (Chief Personnel Officer),
    B Amechi Okoye (Chief Legal Officer),
    B Onyekwelu (Secretary),
    S N Eke (Chief Inspector)

PRINCIPAL ACTIVITIES: Banking
Principal Agencies: 4 Okpara Ave, PMB 1013, Enugu, Anambra State; 84 Azikiwe Rd, PMB 1109, Aba, Imo State; 2 Sokoto Rd, PMB 1779, Onitsha, Anambra State; Okigwe Rd, Owerri, Imo State; Uzuakoli Rd, Umuahia, Imo State; Ogoja Rd, Abakaliki; 17a Nnamdi Azikiwe St, PMB 12738, Lagos; Also at Oguta, Mbawsi, Udi, Awka Afikpo
Principal Bankers: Central Bank of Nigeria
Financial Information:

	N'000
Authorised capital	10,000
Paid-up capital	10,000
Turnover	18,000
Profits	2,000

Principal Shareholders: Government of Anambra State; Government of Imo State; Co-Operative Union of Anambra State; Co-Operative Union of Imo State
Date of Establishment: 1961 (Formerly Co-Operative Bank of Eastern Nigeria Ltd)
No of Employees: 1,700

CO-OPERATIVE BANK LTD

Co-operative Buildings, New Court Rd, PMB 5137, Ibadan, Oyo State
Tel: 23314/6
Cable: Cobank Ibadan
Telex: 31115

President: J B Akinyede
Directors: G O Osoba (General Manager),
    Chief R Obisesan (Vice President)
Senior Executives: T Olajide Olubitan (Chief Accountant)

PRINCIPAL ACTIVITIES: Banking
Branch Offices: Akure; Ife; Lagos; Abeokuta; Ado-Ikiti; Benin; Eruwa; Ibadan; Idanre Ikirun; Lagos etc

Principal Shareholders: Wholly owned subsidiary of Co-operative Investment & Trust Society Ltd
Date of Establishment: 1953

CO-OPERATIVE BANK OF KADUNA STATE

Hospital Rd, PO Box 2121, Kaduna

PRINCIPAL ACTIVITIES: Banking
Financial Information:

	N'000
Capital	1,000
Deposits	20,000

CO-OPERATIVE BANK OF KANO

10E Bello Rd, PO Box 3229, Kano

PRINCIPAL ACTIVITIES: Banking

Financial Information:

	₦'000
Capital	1,000
Deposits	20,000

CO-OPERATIVE INVESTMENT & TRUST SOCIETY

Co-operative Buildings, New Court Rd, PMB 5137, Ibadan, Oyo
   State
Tel: 412294, 412365, 412496, 413795
Cable: Coinvest Ibadan
Telex: 31115

President: J B Akinyede
Directors: G O Osoba (General Manager)

PRINCIPAL ACTIVITIES: Investment, trust society

CO-OPERATIVE SUPPLY ASSOCIATION LTD

349 Herbert Macaulay St, PMB 1046, Yaba, Lagos
Tel: 861587, 861693
Cable: Konsumas Yaba
Telex: 21208 Konsum Ng

PRINCIPAL ACTIVITIES: Importers and distributors of
   agricultural chemicals and equipment, fertilizers, building
   materials, general hardware, groceries and provisions
Branch Offices: Ibadan, Tel 411864; Akure, Tel 2175; Owo, Tel
   65; Benin, Tel 225

COOPERS & LYBRAND ASSOCIATES LTD

Lapal House, PO Box 592, 235 Igbosere Rd, Lagos
Tel: 63220, 632011, 632079, 632151
Cable: Colybrand
Telex: 21551 Coolyb Ng

Directors: C Oyeniyi O Oyediran, Olusola Faleye, Ebenezer F
   Oke, A Oluwole Fadojutimi, Olutola O Sembore, C J Boylan,
   F Afolabi Babalola
PRINCIPAL ACTIVITIES: Business consultants

COOPERS BENLY VENTURES & COMPANY LTD (THE)

See VENTURES, COOPERS BENLY, & COMPANY LTD (THE)

COPE BUILDERS' SUPPLIES LTD

Plot 14 Sapele Rd, Benin City, (Junction Sapele Rd and Murtala
   Mohammed Way), PO Box 686, Bendel State
Tel: 241979, 241559
Telex: 41148 Epoc Ng

PRINCIPAL ACTIVITIES: Suppliers of building materials

COPIERS (NIGERIA) LTD

6 Cow Lane, Lagos
Tel: 634625, 630489

Chairman: A Adebanjo
Directors: Mrs A Adebanjo, B K Adebanjo, Mrs A A Anibaba
Senior Executives: O Akinola (Sales Manager),
   D Agbedare (Accountant),
   Mrs Onu (Sales Supervisor)

PRINCIPAL ACTIVITIES: Suppliers of drawing office, survey,
   graphic and art materials; Hansa plan-printing machines;
   reduction and enlargement of drawings
Principal Agencies: Standardgraph GmbH, West Germany;
   Rotring-Werke Riepe KG, West Germany; J S Staedtler, West
   Germany; Gunther Wagner Pelikan-Werke, West Germany;
   Aaque Systems Ltd, UK; South Wales Chemical Works, UK;
   Royal Sovereign Export, UK
Branch Offices: 83 Igbosere Rd, Lagos
Principal Bankers: First Bank of Nigeria Ltd; National Bank of
   Nigeria Ltd

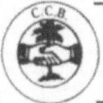
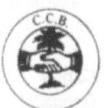

Financial Information:

	N'000
Authorised capital	800
Paid-up capital	800
Turnover	550
Profits	300

Principal Shareholders: A Adebanjo; B K Adebanjo; Mrs A A Anibaba; Mrs O Runsewe
No of Employees: 41

CORNBROUGH PRODUCTS (NIGERIA) LTD

23 Nottidge Street, PO Box 3546, Onitsha, Anambra State
Cable: Assignment, Onitsha

Directors: B O Obi, D C Chukwuma, T C Ifeauyi, B I O Obi

PRINCIPAL ACTIVITIES: Manufacturers, importers, exporters and general merchants

CORNERSTONE ORGANISATION LTD

Plot 4 Block H Isolo Industrial Layout, Isolo, PO Box 12, Apapa, Lagos
Tel: 873318, 877835

PRINCIPAL ACTIVITIES: Transporters of bulk petroleum products

CORPIO CONSTRUCTIONS (NIGERIA) LTD

28 Palace Rd, Olodi, Apapa, PO Box 51565, Falomo, Lagos
Telex: 20117; 11117 International telex

Chairman: Benjamin S C Onwuegbuna
Directors: Chinwe Q Onwuegbuna,
Ojo T Inubile,
Christopher E Ihesiulor,
Benjamin S C Onwuegbuna (Managing),
George C Ndukwe

PRINCIPAL ACTIVITIES: Building and civil engineering; electrical engineering; suppliers of air conditioning equipment
Branch Offices: Plot 343 Sarkin Yaki Rd, Airport Layout, PO Box 4748, Kano PMB 5675, Ibadan
Principal Bankers: United Bank for Africa Ltd

Date of Establishment: 5th October 1977

COSMOS METAL & ELECTRICS LTD

Km 5 Onitsha-Owerri Rd, PMB 1617, Onitsha, Anambra State
Tel: 210465
Cable: Interenam Ikeja
Telex: 54320 Inten

Chairman: Peter Y Y Cheung
Directors: C Udokoro, B Cheung
Senior Executives: T Ho (Assistant Director)

PRINCIPAL ACTIVITIES: Manufacturers of aluminium pots, angle iron and galvanised buckets
Branch Offices: Plot G & H Awosika Ave, Industrial Estate, PO Box 140, Ikeja, Lagos
Associated Companies: International Enamelware Industry Ltd; Cosmos Metal & Electrics Ltd; International Steel Industry Ltd; International Metal Products Ltd; General Steel Mill (Nig) Ltd; Technoflex Co Ltd
Principal Bankers: International Bank for West Africa Ltd

Date of Establishment: 1974
No of Employees: 200

COSTAIN (WEST AFRICA) LTD

PO Box 88, 174 Western Ave, Lagos
Tel: 833474/6, 830271
Cable: Cosdown Lagos
Telex: 21227 Lagos

Chairman: Alhaji Shehu Malami
Directors: R H Carroll (Managing Director),
Chief Dr C M Norman-Williams,
E O Olowo-Okere (Executive Director),
M J Copping (Financial Director),
H D Newell,
A I Ndukwe (Administrative Director)
Senior Executives: S A Aderinlewo (Company Secretary),
J A Idowu (Chief Accountant),
M O Okhiria (Chief Internal Auditor),
O Oladeji (Senior Quantity Surveyors),
O Akande (Personnel Manager),
A A E Inyang (Credit Control Manager)

PRINCIPAL ACTIVITIES: Building and civil engineering contractors, furniture manufacturers
Branch Offices: PO Box 72, Port Harcourt; PO Box 55, Kaduna
Principal Bankers: First Bank of Nigeria Ltd; Union Bank of Nigeria Ltd; United Bank for Africa Ltd

Principal Shareholders: Nigerian Public (60%); Richard Costain (Holdings) Ltd (37.5%); John Holt Investments Ltd (2.5%)
Date of Establishment: Incorporated: 16th July, 1948
No of Employees: 5,000

COTSGAS (NIGERIA) LTD

35 Ikorodu Rd, Yaba, PO Box 2020, Lagos
Tel: 848706, 863014

Directors: C S Adwunmi (Managing)

PRINCIPAL ACTIVITIES: Marketing of liquid petroleum gas and equipment, installations and plumbing
Branch Offices: Throughout Nigeria

COUTINHO, CARO & CO (NIGERIA) LTD

Nasco House, 29 Burma Rd, PO Box 111, Apapa, Lagos
Tel: 877272, 877613, 877626, 873736, 877617, 870834
Cable: Metalcouco
Telex: 21259 Coulag Ng

Chairman: Alhaji Sule Katagum
Directors: Thomas Behrmann (Managing),
Allison A Ayida,
Bukazi L Etete (Executive),
Wolf-Elmar Warning,
Rudi Roesler (Alternate)

PRINCIPAL ACTIVITIES: Engineering consultants and general contractors; planning and construction of industrial plants turn key, high rise buildings, hotels; suppliers and servicers of machinery and spare parts
Principal Bankers: United Bank for Africa Ltd; Societe Generale Bank (Nigeria) Ltd; International Merchant Bank; Union Bank
Financial Information:

	N'000
Authorised capital	800
Paid-up capital	500
Turnover	12,000

Principal Shareholders: A Coutinho; Alhaji Sule Katagum; Allison A Ayida
Date of Establishment: 9th January 1961
No of Employees: 80

CPI-MOORE (NIGERIA) LTD

2 Airport Rd, PO Box 341, Ikeja, Lagos
Tel: 962270, 963099
Telex: 26721 Ageso Ng

Senior Executives: O Osinsanya (Chief Executive),
Mrs E A Osinsanya,
S O Elebe (Technical),
A Adedoyin (Legal),
S K Adebayo (Financial)

PRINCIPAL ACTIVITIES: Suppliers of computer stationery and business forms. Commercial printing
Branch Offices: Factory: Ewusi St, Makun Quarters, PMB 2039, Sagamu

CRITTALL-HOPE NIGERIA LTD

13 Agege Motor Rd, Mushin, PO Box 28, Ikeja, Lagos
Tel: 841409, 845790

Directors: T C F Simpson,
R O Feyisitan,
J Chamberlain (Managing),
S Y Kasimu,
G A Gboyelade,
D R Simpson

PRINCIPAL ACTIVITIES: Manufacturers of metal windows, doors and shutters

Branch Offices: Katchia Rd, Kaduna South, PO Box 231, Kaduna, Tel 242329; 1 Kaduna St, PO Box 398, Port Harcourt, Tel 330005

Principal Bankers: First Bank of Nigeria Ltd

Principal Shareholders: Crittall Windows Ltd; Northern Nigeria Investments Ltd; Odua Investments Ltd; John Holt Investments Ltd

Date of Establishment: 1958
No of Employees: 1,700

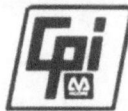
 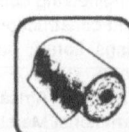 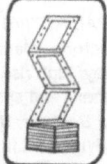
CROCODILE MATCHETS (NIGERIA) LTD

PO Box 4014, Trans Amadi, Plot 29 Trans Amadi Industrial Area, Port Harcourt
Tel: 332514
Cable: Matchets Port Harcourt
Telex: 61145 Cutlas Ng

Chairman: A Spencer
Directors: D Crowley, N Reekie, Alhaji A Onibudo, Chief N Wosu
Senior Executives: J O Ladapo (Works Manager),
N D Agomo (Account Controller),
C Wichay (Production Controller)

PRINCIPAL ACTIVITIES: Manufacturers of matchets
Principal Bankers: United Bank for Africa Ltd; Union Bank of

Nigeria Ltd; Chase Merchant Bank Nigeria Ltd

Financial Information:

	N'000
Authorised capital	500
Paid-up capital	480

Principal Shareholders: G O Ekwelundu; O K Isokariari; C C Onochie; Dr V G Ene; Brig G Kurubo; Florence N Osagie; Ralph Martindale & Co Ltd

Date of Establishment: 4th May 1964
No of Employees: 169

CROSS, A W, LTD

PO Box 337, Ikeja, Lagos

PRINCIPAL ACTIVITIES: Construction

CROSS LINES LTD

140 Calabar Rd, PMB 1073, Calabar, Cross River State
Tel: 222359
Cable: Sescot

Chairman: Major Okon I Essang
Directors: J T Adie,
Chief D D Offong,
Chief D O Enang,
S G Ekere,
A B Assam (General Manager),
S G Ukpanah
Senior Executives: M Anamezie (Company Secretary),
A E Inwang (Workshop Manager),
J A Nami (Assistant General Manager),
N E Ekpe (Senior Accountant)

PRINCIPAL ACTIVITIES: Transportation; Ferry Services; Lighterage, Road Haulage, Passenger Bus Services; clearing and forwarding

Branch Offices: 29 Ikwerre Rd, Port Harcourt

Principal Bankers: Mercantile Bank of Nigeria Ltd; First Bank of Nigeria Ltd

Financial Information:

	N'000
Authorised capital	1,000
Paid-up capital	82
Turnover	1,836

Principal Shareholders: Government of Cross River State
Date of Establishment: 8th January 1970
No of Employees: 400

CROSS RIVER BREWERIES LTD

Industrial Layout, Aka, PMB 1106, Uyo, Cross River State
Tel: 822, 825, 859, 860
Cable: Champbrew Uyo

Senior Executives: Ita D Ekpott (Managing Director),
N Kusi (Assistant General Manager, Finance),
R S Umohette (Assistant General Manager, Marketing),
Karl Liebl (Brewmaster)

PRINCIPAL ACTIVITIES: Brewing and bottling of beer and soft drinks

Principal Bankers: Icon Ltd (Merchant Bankers); African Continental Bank; Mercantile Bank Nigeria Ltd

Principal Shareholders: CRS Investment Trust Company Ltd; CRS Ministry of Finance; Nigerian Industrial Development Bank Ltd; Nigerian Bank for Commerce and Industry; Brauhaase (Technical Partners); Manilla Insurance Company Ltd

Date of Establishment: 31st July 1974
No of Employees: 700

CROSS RIVER ESTATE LTD

PMB 1080, Calabar, Cross River State
Cable: Sesrub

Chairman: Dr F A Egbe
Directors: S O Ekong, Chief G U Otu, E O Ekpenyong, S U Okonedo
Senior Executives: Pastor C O Akpan (General Manager), E B Archibong (Company Secretary/Chief Accountant)

PRINCIPAL ACTIVITIES: Growing and processing of rubber into ribbed smoked rubber sheets, brown crepe and crumb
Principal Agencies: Nigerian Rubber Board; Michelin (Nigeria) Ltd; Dunlop (Nig) Industries Ltd
Principal Bankers: Union Bank of Nigeria Ltd
Financial Information:

	N'000
Authorised capital	5,500
Paid-up capital	4,463

Principal Shareholders: Cross River State Govenment; Nigerian Rubber Board
Date of Establishment: 1956
No of Employees: 1,700

CROSS RIVER STATE AGRICULTURAL DEVELOPMENT CORPORATION

2 Barracks Rd, PMB 1042, Calabar, Cross River State
Tel: 222728
Cable: Crsadc

Chairman: Dr E U Nwa
Directors: U J Udoaka, A E Atta, A T Ukpe
Senior Executives: C N Achima (General Manager), A A Akro (Secretary), D B Ikpeme (Financial Controller)

PRINCIPAL ACTIVITIES: Agricultural development projects
Branch Offices: Calaro Oil Palm Estate, PMB 1114, Calabar, Cross River State; Nko Rubber Estate, PMB 107, Obubra, Cross River State; Ikom Cocoa Estate, PO Box 65, Ikom, Cross River State
Principal Bankers: First Bank of Nigeria Ltd; Union Bank of Nigeria Ltd; Mercantile Bank of Nigeria Ltd

Principal Shareholders: State Government
Date of Establishment: 1969
No of Employees: 5,000

CROSS RIVER STATE NEWSPAPER CORPORATION

Barracks Rd, PMB 1074, Calabar, Cross River State
Tel: 545, 430, 404

PRINCIPAL ACTIVITIES: Newspaper publishing

CROWN AGENTS FOR OVERSEAS GOVERNMENTS AND ADMINISTRATIONS

8-10 Broad St, PO Box 583, Lagos
Tel: 630476, 635889
Cable: Crownagents Lagos
Telex: 21416 Crown Ng

PRINCIPAL ACTIVITIES: Commercial and financial agents for overseas Government and public sector bodies

CROWN CORK AND SEAL COMPANY (NIGERIA) LTD

Henry Carr St, Ikeja Industrial Estate, PO Box 142, Ikeja, Lagos
Tel: 963605
Cable: Crobeal Ikeja

Directors: A A Gill

PRINCIPAL ACTIVITIES: Manufacturing of bottle caps

CRUSADER INSURANCE CO (NIGERIA) LTD

23/25 Martins St, PO Box 2101, Lagos
Tel: 662717, 661507, 662644

Chairman: G O Ogundipe - Alatishe
Directors: E O Efiong (Managing), Alhaji Mala Geidam, Alhaji Isa Ibrahim, M A Adewunmi, G O Onosode, G C Crook, P B Grimshaw

PRINCIPAL ACTIVITIES: Insurance
Branch Offices: 23 Cappa Ave, Palmgrove Estate, Lagos; 41 Ogui Rd, PO Box 149, Enugu, Anambra State; 13A Egunjenmi St, Ekotedo Rd, PMB 5239, Ibadan, Tel 414556; 95 Azikiwe Rd, PO Box 816, Aba, Imo State; Ebu - Oluwa House, 65 Mission Rd, PO Box 547, Benin City, Bendel State; 25 Aba Rd, PO Box 1099, Port Harcourt, Rivers State, Tel 21985

CSS BOOKSHOPS

50/52 Broad St, PO Box 174, Lagos
Tel: 633010, 633081, 633151, 842122

PRINCIPAL ACTIVITIES: Book sellers, stationery, printing and publishing

CSS PRESS (NIGERIA) LTD

PO Box 174, Lagos

PRINCIPAL ACTIVITIES: Commercial printing

CUBITTS (NIGERIA) LTD

2 Mohammed Ladan Rd, Kaduna South, PO Box 227, Kaduna
Tel: 242175

PRINCIPAL ACTIVITIES: Building and civil engineering contractors
Branch Offices: 2 Babani St, Ebute-Metta, PO Box 2033, Lagos, Tel 836776, 833721

CUNIX INDUSTRIAL & COMMERCIAL CO LTD

11 Goldie St, PO Box 134, Calabar, Cross River State
Tel: 2243
Cable: Cunix Calabar

Chairman: C U Nyong
Directors: S A Nyong, J A Nyong, M I Nyong, A J Edoho
Senior Executives: O O Eyo (Accountant/Administrative Manager), M O Achoakawa (Commercial Manager), U A Etukudoh (Engineer)

PRINCIPAL ACTIVITIES: Textile manufacturers; general merchants; distributors of building materials, cement, food items, household goods and appliances, motor cycles, toiletries and cosmetics, beer, soft drinks etc. Building and civil engineering contractors
Principal Agencies: Leventis Motor Ltd; Asbestos Cement Products (Nigeria) Ltd; Turners Building Products (Emene) Ltd etc
Branch Offices: 48/52 Oron Rd, PO Box 145, Uyo, Cross River State, Tel 661; Plot 51 Unity Rd, Ikeja, Lagos; Four Corners, Ikom, Cross River State
Principal Bankers: Mercantile Bank of Nigeria Ltd; First Bank of Nigeria Ltd
Financial Information:

	N'000
Authorised capital	100
Paid-up capital	100

No of Employees: 110

CUTLER-HAMMER NIGERIA LTD

Isolo Expressway (Itire Junction), Ilasamaja Scheme, Isolo, PO Box 1107, Mushin, Lagos
Tel: 847513
Cable: Cutlernig
Telex: 20117 TDS Box 574

Chairman: Chief J A Odeyemi
Directors: N Whiteman (Managing),
  O I Akinnola,
  W Simpson,
  A Hotham,
  V J Meads,
  S D Atayi
Senior Executives: J Starren (Production Manager),
  L Ladipo (Marketing Manager),
  B D Oxborough (Technical Manager)
PRINCIPAL ACTIVITIES: Manufacturers of industrial control
  equipment: motor control centres, starters, automatic
  change-over panels, switch-boards etc
Principal Agencies: Dorman Smith Switchgear Ltd, UK; Watford
  Electric Company Ltd, UK; Klaxon Ltd, UK; Electrical Remote
  Control Co Ltd, UK; Eldon Electrical Ltd, UK; Dorman Smith
  Fuses Ltd, UK
Associated Companies: Cutler-Hammer Milwaukee, USA;
  Cutler-Hammer Europa Bedford, UK; Eaton Corporation, USA
Principal Bankers: Union Bank of Nigeria Ltd
Financial Information:

	N'000
Authorised capital	1,000
Paid-up capital	200 but increasing to 600
Turnover	1,800

Principal Shareholders: Cutler-Hammer Europa Ltd; Mrs V Atayi;
  Chief O I Akinnola; Chief J A Odeyemi; Chief Kola Daisi
Date of Establishment: May 1973
No of Employees: 65

CZECHS (NIGERIA) LTD

Decima Rd, PO Box 37, Sapele, Bendel State

PRINCIPAL ACTIVITIES: Production of rubber

D A JIDEOFO ENTERPRISES LTD

See JIDEOFO, D A, ENTERPRISES LTD

D A NWANDU & SONS ENTERPRISES LTD

See NWANDU, D A, & SONS ENTERPRISES LTD

D B ZANG

See ZANG, D B

D K EJUKORLEM & CO LTD

See EJUKORLEM, D K, & CO LTD

D L AKANJI & CO (NIG) LTD

See AKANJI, D L, & CO (NIG) LTD

D O NKWONTA & SONS ENTERPRISES LTD

See NKWONTA, D O, & SONS ENTERPRISES LTD

D O OLAGBEMIRO & CO (NIGERIA) LTD

See OLAGBEMIRO, D O, & CO (NIGERIA) LTD

DABOUL TRAVEL OFFICE

112 Broad St, PO Box 2110, Lagos
Tel: 680550, 650697

PRINCIPAL ACTIVITIES: Travel and tourist agents
Branch Offices: 94 Frederic McEwen St, Lagos, Tel 633972

DADA-OBE INDUSTRIES (NIGERIA) LTD

Km 4 Badagry Expressway, Coker Bus Stop, 1st Floor, PO Box
  113, Apapa, Lagos

PRINCIPAL ACTIVITIES: Suppliers of vehicle accessories

DADDO INTERNATIONAL (NIGERIA) LTD

95 Awolowo Rd, Ikoyi, PO Box 10303, Lagos
Tel: 683880
Cable: Dadoint
Telex: 21703 Tuks Ng

Chairman: Chief Executive D R Ahuja
Directors: Mrs F Galadima, A Dahiru
Senior Executives: Umesh Chandra (Chief Engineer),
  H K Wadhwani (Commercial Manager),
  P O Ibeh (Sales Organiser)
PRINCIPAL ACTIVITIES: Importers of generators, heavy
  equipment, material handling equipment and tyres;
  manufacturers of candles, steel rolling doors; local agents for
  steel furniture, air-conditioners, refrigerators, household and
  office appliances
Principal Agencies: G Sendker Handels und Transport GmbH,
  Germany; Inver Industrial Leeman Ltd, UK
Branch Offices: 12 Stadium Rd, PO Box 763, Kano Tel 4503;
  22A Creek Rd, PO Box 1055, Apapa Tel 872269; Kakori Rd,
  PO Box 6581, Kaduna Tel 215317; Bank Rd, PO Box 837,
  Jimeta, Yola Tel 24082
Subsidiary Companies: Daddo Candles Divies; Daddo Steel
  Rolling Doors Divison; Daddo Transport Division
Principal Bankers: Union Bank of Nigeria Ltd
Financial Information:

	N'000
Authorised capital	500,000
Paid-up capital	400,000

Principal Shareholders: Mrs R Galadima; A Dahiru
Date of Establishment: September 1979
No of Employees: 50

DAE INTERNATIONAL (NIGERIA) LTD

50 Fagbohun Rd, SW7 Oke-Bola, PO Box 1384, Ibadan, Oyo
  State
Tel: 412128
Telex: 31515 Dae Ng

PRINCIPAL ACTIVITIES: Suppliers and servicers of generating
  plants, electrical appliances and fittings etc
Branch Offices: Workshop: Lagos/Ibadan Rd, Opposite
  Nigerwest, Challenge, Ibadan, Tel 462509; Cooperative St,
  Toro Rd, Ile-Ife

DAFINASI ENTERPRISES LTD

10E Harbour Rd, PO Box 133, Port Harcourt, Rivers State
Tel: 228320
Cable: Dafinasi Port Harcourt

PRINCIPAL ACTIVITIES: Transporters, customs licensed agents
  for clearing, forwarding, shipping, warehousing, general
  importers and exporters

DAGAZAU INTERNATIONAL LTD

Plot 719A Adetokunbo Ademola St, Victoria Island, PMB 1063,
  Apapa, Lagos
Tel: 614205

Directors: Henry J Gauthier (Project Manager)
PRINCIPAL ACTIVITIES: Construction

DAILY NEED CHEMISTS LTD

PO Box 2787, Orogiri St, Lagos
Tel: 632452
Cable: Daychem Lagos

Chairman: M O Jolayemi (also Managing Director)
Senior Executives: S O Olawepo (General Manager)
PRINCIPAL ACTIVITIES: Suppliers of chemicals, food and food
  processing, pharmaceutical and medical supplies and
  services, toiletries and cosmetics
Principal Agencies: Laboratoires Lefrancq, France; Daily Need
  Chemists Works, Hong Kong; Cupal Ltd, UK
Branch Offices: 6 Onikanga Rd, Ilorin, Kwara State
Principal Bankers: First Bank of Nigeria Ltd; Union Bank of

Nigeria Ltd
Financial Information:

	₦'000
Authorised capital	500
Paid-up capital	500
Sales turnover	3,000
Profits	500

Principal Shareholders: Chairman
Date of Establishment: 200

DAILY SOAP LTD
PMB 5317, Km 12 Old Lagos Rd, Ibadan, Oyo State
Tel: 414460

PRINCIPAL ACTIVITIES: Manufacturers of soap

Date of Establishment: February 1974

DAILY TIMES OF NIGERIA
PO Box 139, 3/7 Kakawa St, Lagos
Tel: 661441, 661421, 661431, 661448, 661442, 661453, 661464, 661475, 661291
Telex: 21333

Chairman: Alhaji Aliko Misau Mohammed
Directors: Adagogo Jaja (Managing Director)
Senior Executives: Martin Iroabuchi (Editor)

PRINCIPAL ACTIVITIES: Printing and publishing
Associated Companies: Nigerpak Apapa; Times Press, Apapa
Principal Bankers: First Bank of Nigeria Ltd; Union Bank of Nigeria
Financial Information:

	₦'000
Authorised capital	8,000

Principal Shareholders: Nicom
No of Employees: 650

DALA (NIGERIA) LTD
Plot 12, Aina Layout, Alimoso Rd, Dopema, Ikeja, PO Box 1359, Surulere, Lagos

PRINCIPAL ACTIVITIES: Civil and structural design and construction
Branch Offices: SW8/104 Lagos Bye Pass, PO Box 666, Oke-Ado, Ibadan, Oyo State; 6 Amudipe St, Akure, Ondo State

Date of Establishment: June 1979

DALAMAL TEXTILE MILLS LTD
126/130 Nnamdi Azikiwe St, PO Box 3772, Lagos
Tel: 845740, 847098
Cable: Daltex Lagos
Telex: 21306 Ng

Chairman: G H Dalamal
Directors: T H Dalamal, K Dalamal, D M Dalamal
Senior Executives: B K V Murthy (General Manager)

PRINCIPAL ACTIVITIES: Manufacturers of textile piece goods, shirting, suiting and bedsheets
Subsidiary Companies: First Bank of Nigeria Ltd; United Bank for Africa Ltd; Allied Bank of Nigeria Ltd
Financial Information: 1980 Published Accounts

	₦'000
Authorised capital	3,274
Paid-up capital	3,274
Turnover	11,266
Profits	291

Principal Shareholders: G H Dalamal; T H Dalamal; K Dalamal; D M Dalamal; S Dalama; J D Dalamal; Mrs C Daryanani
Date of Establishment: 1972
No of Employees: 505

D'ALBERTO, E, & GIAMPAOLI LTD
PO Box 8, Kachia Rd, Kaduna
Tel: 212993
Cable: Dalbo
Telex: 71287 Dalbo Ng

Chairman: Alhaji Aliko Mohammed
Directors: E D'Alberto, Mrs D D'Alberto in Motta, Alhaji A Danbaba, Alhaji A B Musa, Mallam M Inuwa Mora
Senior Executives: Allara-Perla Renato (General Manager), Hugh Evans (Quantity Surveyor), T Thurairajah (Chief Accountant), Nino Arcangeli (Branch Manager)

PRINCIPAL ACTIVITIES: Building and civil engineering contractors
Branch Offices: PO Box 41, Maiduguri
Subsidiary Companies: Dalbo Holdings Ltd
Principal Bankers: United Bank for Africa Ltd
Financial Information:

	₦'000
Authorised capital	400
Paid-up capital	400
Turnover	10,000
Profits	250

Principal Shareholders: E D'Alberto; Alh Aliko Mohammed; Mallam Inuwa Mora; Mallam B Kirfi; M T Bature; Alh A B Musa; R Kotey
Date of Establishment: 2nd March 1956
No of Employees: 1,200

D'ALBERTO, L, & CO LTD
SW8/139 Lagos Bye-Pass, PO Box 138, Ibadan
Tel: 411480
Cable: Dalco Ibadan

Chairman: O A Alakija
Directors: Ferruccio Micheletti (Managing), D C Mort, John Adepoju, A C Micheletti, Joseph Ladejo
Senior Executives: J H Stone (General Manager)

PRINCIPAL ACTIVITIES: Building and civil engineering contractors
Branch Offices: PO Box 1231, Ilorin, Kwara State; PO Box 258, Ile-Ife, Oyo State
Principal Bankers: First Bank of Nigeria Ltd

Date of Establishment: May 1954, Incorporated 10th June 1962
No of Employees: 1,500 - 2,000

DALTRADE (NIGERIA) LTD
12 Market St, PO Box 1556, Lagos
Tel: 663160
Cable: Daltrade Lagos
Telex: 21262 Daltd Ng

Directors: W Wyskoczyl (Managing), G Akinsola (Financial)

PRINCIPAL ACTIVITIES: Suppliers of general merchandise
Branch Offices: 38 Ibrahim Taiwo Rd, PO Box 377, Kano; 131 Azikiwe Rd, PO Box 288, Aba, Imo State
Principal Bankers: Union Bank of Nigeria Ltd

Date of Establishment: 1962
No of Employees: 110

DAMBIYOWU NIGERIA LTD
2 Alhaji Tokunbo Alli St/Opebi Village Rd, Off Unity Rd, PO Box 633, Ikeja, Lagos
Tel: 960448

Chairman: M A F Akinde
Directors: Fola Akinde, Dapo Akinde, Kola Akinde
Senior Executives: R A Ajayi (Factory Manager), V Eke (Secretary), Mrs T Abolurin (Sales Manager)

PRINCIPAL ACTIVITIES: Manufacturers of concrete products, blocks, fencing, poles, culverts etc. Distributors of building materials
Branch Offices: Factory: Ijako Village, Abeokuta Motor Rd, Sango-Otta, Ogun State
Principal Bankers: International Bank for West Africa Ltd

Principal Shareholders: M A F Akinde; Fola Akinde; Dapo Akinde; Kola Akinde; N A Deinde; Alhaji W A Akinde

DAMDAVY & COMPANY
100 Isolo Rd, Mushin, Lagos State
Cable: Damco

Chairman: Chief P A N Okafor
Directors: Damien E Obiagwu, David Okafor

PRINCIPAL ACTIVITIES: Agents and general trading
Principal Agencies: Klinor, Italy
Branch Offices: Obiagwu (Nig) Enterprises, 28 Nottidge St, Onitsha, Anambra State
Associated Companies: Mark P Construction Nig Ltd; Shopper Paradise Fashion
Principal Bankers: Co-operative & Commerce Bank (Nigeria) Ltd

Principal Shareholders: Damien Obiagwu; Chief P A N Okafor

DAMEN SHIPYARDS NIGERIA LTD
15 Creek Road, Apapa, Lagos
Tel: 877374, 877379
Telex: 21831 Arelec Ng

Chairman: Chief L O Akindele
Directors: J Phillips,
Mrs Oge Williams,
J A Erchebarne,
K Damen,
E de Rothschild,
Paul L A Veenhuijzen (Managing)

PRINCIPAL ACTIVITIES: Boatbuilding, sales and repairs
Principal Bankers: Societe Generale Bank (Nigeria) Ltd; International Bank for West Africa Ltd
Financial Information:

	N'000
Authorised capital	1,000
Paid-up capital	1,000
Turnover	3,500

Principal Shareholders: Directors as described
Date of Establishment: 6th October 1981
No of Employees: 95

DANIEL, C C, MINING INDUSTRY
Isiagu Afikpo, Anambra State

PRINCIPAL ACTIVITIES: Metal ore mining - lead and zinc

DANIEL MARRYAT (NIGERIA) LTD
See MARRYAT, DANIEL, (NIGERIA) LTD

DANIKSI LTD
1 Shehu Laminu Way, PO Box 201, Maiduguri, Borno State
Tel: 232295
Telex: 82107 Wazco Ng

Chairman: Mohammed Maina Waziri
Directors: M M Waziri, A M Waziri
Senior Executives: Aji Monguno (Administrative Manager), Daniel K O Ladipo (Accountant)

PRINCIPAL ACTIVITIES: General suppliers; business consultants; civil engineering contractors; suppliers of agricultural chemicals, machinery and spare parts, electrical equipment; poultry production
Branch Offices: PO Box 8, Potiskum, Borno State
Subsidiary Companies: Occidental Facilities Ltd, Maiduguri
Principal Bankers: Bank of the North Ltd; International Bank for West Africa Ltd; National Bank of Nigeria Ltd

Financial Information:

	N'000
Authorised capital	250
Paid-up capital	100
Turnover	550
Profits (after tax)	65

Princiap Shareholders: M M Waziri; A M Waziri

DANLON ASSOCIATES
PO Box 6968, 25 Ilupeju Rd, Off Cappa Ave, Palmgrove Estate, Lagos
Tel: 842012
Cable: Danconsult Lagos
Telex: 20117 TDS Bafani 083

Chairman: Daniel L Oni
Senior Executives: Sola Martins (Legal),
S O Ofily (Marketing),
S O Gomenti (Sales),
Olanrewaju Olowofela (Processing)

PRINCIPAL ACTIVITIES: Company formation, etc, business information service and planning and executing of ventures in Nigeria
Branch Offices: 22 Moloney St, (East) Ebute Metta, PO Box 6968, Lagos
Principal Bankers: First Bank of Nigeria Ltd

Principal Shareholders: Daniel Lemose Oni
Date of Establishment: 25th February 1974

DANTATA LAND AND SEA COMPANY LTD
24A Club Rd, PO Box 2291, Kano
Tel: 2511, 4522
Telex: 77152 Tgeltd Ng

Chairman: Alhaji Abdulkadir Sanusi Dantata
Directors: Abusale Dantata, Alhaji Munir Abdulkadir Sanusi Dantata
Senior Executives: Salvatore Spoto (General Manager),
Mohammed El-Zaby (Contracts Manager),
William Anthony Smith (Financial Controller),
Alhaji Abdullahi Danladi (Administrative Manager)

PRINCIPAL ACTIVITIES: Building and civil engineerings. Formerly a haulage business
Associated Companies: Sager & Woerner Construction Company, W Germany; Dantata & Sawoe Construction Company Nigeria Ltd, Kano; Danta Marine Ltd
Principal Bankers: Bank of the North Ltd; First Bank of Nigeria Ltd
Financial Information:

	N'000
Authorised capital	500
Paid-up capital	500
Sales turnover	6,000

Principal Shareholders: Alhaji Abdulkadir Sanusi Dantata; Alhaji Sanusi Dantata
No of Employees: 500

DANWAWU SHIPPING CARGO HANDLING & TRANSPORT CO LTD
Head Office for Airport Operation, 26B Post Office Rd, PO Box 1103, Kano
Tel: 4546
Cable: Nautik
Telex: 77115

Chairman: Alhaji Mohamadu Danwawu
Directors: Alhaji Ibrahim Baba Danwawu
Senior Executives: C O Leonhardt (General Manager),
J F Bolarinwa (Manager),
A A Okwudili (Accountant),
R A Adebowale (Forwarding Manager)

PRINCIPAL ACTIVITIES: Shipping, forwarding, clearing and
transport
Principal Agencies: Northern Textile Manufacturers Ltd, Kano;
Brass & Bed Ornament Ltd, Kano; Kaduna State Distribution
Agency Ltd, Kaduna
Branch Offices: Head Office for Seaport Operations: PO Box
235, 19 Warehouse Rd, Apapa, Lagos
Principal Bankers: United Bank for Africa; First Bank of Nigeria
Ltd

No of Employees: 200

DAPO ALLIED INDUSTRIES (NIGERIA) LTD
32 Niger St, Township, PO Box 194, Kano
Tel: 4074, 4130

PRINCIPAL ACTIVITIES: Manufacturers of metal doors and
windows
Branch Offices: Factory: SW8/685 Lagos Rd, Challenge, PO Box
1606, Ibadan, Oyo State, Tel 461373, 411996; SW6/541
Labaowo St, Ogunpa, Ibadan, Tel 682010; Ahmadu Bello
Way, Near Gwonge Bridge, Maiduguri, Borno State, Tel
232106; Gidan Crankshafts, 005 Jos Rd, Kaduna; SW140 Ibo
Rd, Minna

DAR AL-HANDASAH CONSULTANTS & PARTNERS
PO Box 5018, 60 Awolowo Rd, S W Ikoyi, Lagos
Tel: 680959, 682372
Cable: Darsah
Telex: 22601 Darsah Ng

PRINCIPAL ACTIVITIES: Consultants
Branch Offices: 15/16 Post Office Rd, PO Box 920, Kano; 1
Hotel Close (GRA), PO Box 441, Ilorin, Kwara State, Tel 4654,
Telex 33116 Darsah Ng; 2b Chief Alonge Avenue (GRA), PMB
1305, Benin City, Bendel State, Tel 241152, Cable Darsah; 32
Bukuru Rd, Near Television Centre, PMB 2185, Jos, Plateau
State, Tel 2556, Cable Darsah, Telex 81350 Darjos ng; 173A

Aba Rd, PO Box 535, Port Harcourt, Rivers State, Tel
226097, 227012, Cable Darsah, Telex 61102 Dar Ph Ng Also
at Makurdi, Maiduguri, Sokoto, Yola, Kaduna

DATA PROCESSING MAINTENANCE AND SERVICES LTD
Lapal House, 217-235 Igbosere Rd, Lagos
Tel: 654138
Cable: Compudata lagos

PRINCIPAL ACTIVITIES: Data processing services: suppliers of
data processing equipment and accessories
Principal Agencies: IBM

DATA SCIENCES (NIGERIA) LTD
2 Ola-Ayinde St, Off Airport Rd, Ikeja, PO Box 6352, Lagos

PRINCIPAL ACTIVITIES: Sales and service of computers
Financial Information:
Registered capital ₦ 500,000

Date of Establishment: 1979

DAUPHIN (NIGERIA) LTD
83 Itire Rd, Surulere, PMB 1136, Yaba, Lagos
Tel: 830799
Cable: Daufinders

Chairman: E K Chima
Directors: S I Emenyonu, Mrs J O Nollah
Senior Executives: G S Daniel (General Manager),
E O Emeharole (Accountant/Administrative Manager)

PRINCIPAL ACTIVITIES: Manufacture of leather goods and
shoes; agricultural produce
Principal Agencies: Onfroy, Paris; Chamberlain; UK; Kreuser,
Germany; Phipps-Faire, UK; Resupi AG, Switzerland
Branch Offices: Factory: 51 Park Rd, Aba, Imo State; 43 Bello
Dandogo Rd, Kano
Principal Bankers: International Bank for West Africa Ltd; First

Bank of Nigeria Ltd
Financial Information:

	N'000
Authorised capital	100
Paid-up capital	100
Turnover	1,800

Date of Establishment: 1973
No of Employees: 126

DE FACTO BAKERIES & CATERING LTD

55/59 Oju-Elegba Rd, Surulere, PO Box 31, Yaba, Lagos
Tel: 834522, 834622
Cable: De Facto Lagos

Chairman: Otunba J Ade Toyo
Directors: E O Tuyo (Managing),
  O A Tuyo (General Manager),
  A E Adefeso,
  Alhaji O Omotayo

PRINCIPAL ACTIVITIES: Bakeries and catering
Branch Offices: De Facto Bakery Window & Restaurant, 20
  Olatunde Olabinjo Avenue, Shomobu Lagos; Yaba Bus
  Terminius, Yaba, Lagos
Principal Bankers: Union Bank of Nigeria Ltd
Financial Information:

	N'000
Authorised capital	500
Paid-up capital	150
Turnover	1,094
Profits	96

Principal Shareholders: E O Tuyo; Otunba J Ade Toyo; A E
  Adefeso; Alhaji O Omotayo
Date of Establishment: 15th February 1954
No of Employees: 200

DE PETRACO INDUSTRIES LTD

See PETRACO, DE, INDUSTRIES LTD

DEAZULA TRADING COMPANY (NIGERIA) LTD

95 Ikwerre Rd, PMB 5971, Port Harcourt, Rivers State
Tel: 229091

Chairman: Chief Azunuka Abel (also Managing Director)
Directors: Samuel Abel, John Chinda, Stanley Azunuka
Senior Executives: Lucky E Nwadighoha (Chief Accountant),
  Ebere G Iheanetu (Secretary),
  Michael Akah (Sales Manager)

PRINCIPAL ACTIVITIES: Agents and general trading, suppliers
  of building materials/cement, ceramics/sanitary fittings,
  hardware, property and real estate
Principal Agencies: Crittal-Hope (Nigeria) Ltd
Branch Offices: 33 Ikwerre Rd, PMB 5971, Port Harcourt
Associated Companies: A C Bob-Manuel & Company Ltd; Manila
  Construction Company Ltd
Principal Bankers: International Bank for West Africa Ltd
Principal Shareholders: Chairman and directors as described

DEBS MODERN INDUSTRIES LTD

38E Ado Bayero Rd, PO Box 209, Kano
Tel: 3720

Directors: J K Debs

PRINCIPAL ACTIVITIES: Manufacturers of metal beds and
  furniture

DECCA (WEST AFRICA) LTD

PO Box 412, 4 Faramobi Ajike St, Ikorodu Rd, Lagos
Cable: Deccawa

Directors: Robert Oeges (Managing),
  David G Bennett (Manager),
  Titus I Oloronyomi (Marketing Manager),
  Victor O Nwogwugwo (International Label Executive)
PRINCIPAL ACTIVITIES: Record and tape manufacturers,
  distributors and importers

DEFENCE INDUSTRIES CORPORATION OF NIGERIA

Federal Ordnance Factory, Kaduna South, Kaduna State
Tel: 210511, 243503, 210643
Telex: 71106 Ordfac ng

PRINCIPAL ACTIVITIES: Defence industry

DEJI OYENUGA & PARTNERS

See OYENUGA, DEJI, & PARTNERS

DELCO (NIG) LTD

PO Box 70, Enerhen Rd, Warri, Bendel State

PRINCIPAL ACTIVITIES: Building and civil engineering
  contractors

DELLA GROUP LTD

168 Broad St, PO Box 5680, Lagos
Tel: 637709

PRINCIPAL ACTIVITIES: Suppliers of domestic gas and
  appliances

DELTA BOATYARD LTD

Warri/Sapele Rd, Warri, Bendel State
Tel: 232932

PRINCIPAL ACTIVITIES: Boatbuilding, production of steel
  vessels, wood, fibre-glass river craft
Principal Shareholders: Government-owned Company

DELTA FREEZE LTD

225 Apapa Rd, Iganmu, PMB 1155, Lagos
Tel: 836618
Cable: Deltafreez, Lagos

PRINCIPAL ACTIVITIES: Manufacturers of air-conditioners and
  refrigerators
Financial Information: Subsidiary of the Ibru Organisation

DELTA FURNITURE & FURNISHING IND LTD

5 Ilupeju Bye Pass, PO Box 137, Ilupeju, Lagos
Tel: 961774

Chairman: Chief J K J Amachree
Directors: Segun Abiodun, Sham Chugani, G C Waney

PRINCIPAL ACTIVITIES: Furniture manufacturers

DELTA GLASS COMPANY LTD

PMB 48, Ughelli, Bendel State

Chairman: C B Edo-Osagie
Directors: S Edwards (Managing),
  Chief S Ade John,
  G G O Sonekan,
  Chief A Bubor,
  Justice M A Begho,
  A A David,
  J O Iluebbey,
  H S A Adedeji (Alternate),
  J B Erhuero (Alternate),
  A Socratous (Alternate),
  M O Ogbodu (Alternate)
Senior Executives: M O Ogbodu (Deputy General Manager),
  K Royds (Technical Manager)

PRINCIPAL ACTIVITIES: Manufacturers of beer and mineral bootles and glass tableware
Principal Bankers: Union Bank of Nigeria Ltd; New Nigeria Bank Ltd
Financial Information:

	N'000
Authorised capital	14,625
Paid-up capital	14,625

Principal Shareholders: Nigerian Bottling Company Ltd; Bendel State Government; Nigerian Industrial Development Bank Ltd
Date of Establishment: 26th June 1974
No of Employees: 905

DELTA HOTELS LTD

PMB 5004, Aba Rd, Port Harcourt, Rivers State
Tel: 226704, 226719
Cable: Tourietel

Chairman: Commodore Edwin Kentebe
Directors: Chief Gabriel Gborogbosi, Chief M M Atamata, James Nweke, Chief N T Imo, Bennet Owei, George Mgbor
Senior Executives: I H Wigwe (General Manager),
  G I Agomuo (Financial Controller),
  E F N Hart (Public Relations Manager),
  M O Georgewill (Manager, Hotel Presidential),
  F O Memberrs,
  Miss I D Iyeimo (Personnel Manager),
  I M Sotohn (Internal Auditor),
  S I Tamuno (Purchasing Manager),
  M Khaleel (Principal Engineer)

PRINCIPAL ACTIVITIES: Hoteliers, Hotels within the group are The Hotel Presidential, Port Harcourt and The Olympia Hotel, Port Harcourt. There are also various Catering Rest Houses situated in Port Harcourt, Bori, Degema, Brass and Ahoada
Principal Bankers: Pan African Bank Ltd; International Bank for West Africa Ltd
Financial Information:

	N'000
Authorised capital	1,000
Paid-up capital	1,000
Turnover	7,500
Profits (before tax)	2,500
Profits (after tax)	1,250

Principal Shareholders: Rivers State Government Nigeria
Date of Establishment: 18th January 1974
No of Employees: 963

DELTA OIL NIGERIA LTD

Western House, 8/10 Broad St, PO Box 3606, Lagos
Tel: 635004, 635076
Cable: Jurisconsult
Telex: 21164 Buguma Lagos

Chairman: Chief Godfrey K J Amachree
Directors: Mrs W J Amachree, Chief A S Young-Harry
Senior Executives: Chief Paul R Lanique (Petroleum Consultant), William R Ford (Economic Adviser)

PRINCIPAL ACTIVITIES: Crude oil exploration and production
Subsidiary/Associated Companies: Radiators Nigeria Ltd (Subsidiary); Pan Ocean Nigeria Ltd (Associated)
Principal Bankers: Union Bank of Nigeria Ltd

DELTA PIONEER COMPANY LTD

105 Akpakpava St, PO Box 410, Benin City, Bendel State
Tel: 242373

Chairman: T N Brai (also Managing Director)
Directors: Patrick Inuope (Sales Manager),
  W O Adjekughele,
  A Brai,
  E I Brai,
  J I Brai
Senior Executives: Devidas Gul Ram (Production Manager),
  Isaiah Okoro (Accountant)

PRINCIPAL ACTIVITIES: Suppliers of plastics/plastic signs, rubber goods, neon signs and manufacturers, fabrication of metal and plastic lettering, vehicle and torch light bulbs
Associated Companies: Delta Paper Converters Industries
Principal Bankers: New Nigeria Bank Ltd

Principal Shareholders: T N Brai and Eyewumi; Rone & Associates Ltd

DELTA PROPERTY DEVELOPMENT CO LTD

6B Nzimiro St, Admadi Flats, PMB 5278, Port Harcourt, Rivers State
Tel: 226116
Cable: Ejohnson
Telex: 61116 Nig

PRINCIPAL ACTIVITIES: Real estate investment and development, business consultants

DELTA SCIENTIFIC & TECHNICAL CO LTD

10 Aba Rd, Port Harcourt, Rivers State
Tel: 21925
Telex: 61141 Desben Ng

PRINCIPAL ACTIVITIES: Suppliers of hospital equipment

DELTA STEEL COMPANY LTD

Ovwian-Aladja, PMB 1220, Warri
Tel: 232622, 232064, 232978, 232814, 231900
Telex: 43326, 43327 Desteel Ng

Chairman: Chief Tunji Arosanyin
Directors: Alhaji M A Aziz, Alhaji Yahaya Bawa Jega, Chief T G Ogigbah, Chief Goddy Ezekwe, A Garuba, J E K Oyegun
Senior Executives: Fred A Brume (Chief Executive),
  Tarchia Jooji (Deputy General Manager, Production),
  Stephen N Ojobor (Deputy General Manager, Technical Services),
  Michael O Adiotomre (Deputy General Manager, Co-ordination),
  Lawani A Momoh (Deputy General Manager, Commercial),
  Michael E Ogigirigi (Deputy General Manager, Administration)

PRINCIPAL ACTIVITIES: Production of steel
Principal Agencies: Jos Rolling Mill; Katsina Rolling Mill; Oshogbo Rolling Mill
Branch Offices: Lagos Laison Office, 1 Ozumba Mbadiwe Street, PMB 12786, Lagos, Tel: 617677, 017682; MECON, Ranchi 834002 Bihar India Tel: 20053/21267 Telex: 0625-209 0627-262 Cable: Mecon; European Liaison Office, Graf-Adolf - Strasse 100, Postfach 200442, Fed Rep Germany, Tel: (06) 0211 353757, Telex: 8586274 Elod
Principal Bankers: Central Bank of Nigeria; New Nigeria Bank; Union Bank of Nigeria Ltd; First Bank of Nigeria Ltd; International Bank for West Africa; United Bank for Africa; International Merchant Bank
Financial Information:

	N'000
Authorised capital	220,000
Paid-up capital	220,000

Principal Shareholders: Federal Government of Nigeria
Date of Establishment: 14th November, 1979
No of Employees: 6,729

DELTAPLAST COMPANY (NIGERIA) LTD

Plot 21/22, Sharada Industrial Estate, Phase 2, PO Box 6248, Kano
Tel: 8683
Cable: Deltaplast Kano, Lagos
Telex: 77264 Deltap

Chairman: Alhaji Munir I Shuaibu
Directors: Chief Dogara S Yaro,
  Jacques F Vanmackelberg,
  Ravi K Daryani (Managing)
Senior Executives: Alhaji A Bashir (Administrative Manager),
  S A Adebola (Sales Manager),
  N P Eklahare (Production Manager)

PRINCIPAL ACTIVITIES: Manufacturers of pvc pipes
Branch Offices: 100 Nnamdi Azikiwe St, PO Box 6519, Lagos, Tel 635195
Associated Companies: Shuaib Industries Ltd; Ucodis (Nigeria) Ltd
Principal Bankers: International Bank for West Africa Ltd
Principal Shareholders: Directors as described
Date of Establishment: 26th July 1976
No of Employees: 100

DEMA ENGINEERING LTD

5a Njemanze St, PO Box 476, Port Harcourt, Rivers State
Tel: 22053
Cable: Dema-PH

PRINCIPAL ACTIVITIES: Steel welders, structural and civil engineers

DENCHUKWU GROUP OF COMPANIES

97 Agbani Rd, Uwani, PO Box 717, Enugu, Anambra State
Tel: 2422

PRINCIPAL ACTIVITIES: Distributors of granite chippings, paints, marble, etc

DERIBE, ALHAJI MAI, & SONS LTD

10 Sir Kassim Ibrahim Rd, PO Box 28, Maiduguri, Borno State
Tel: 2465, 2319
Cable: Maideribe, Maiduguri
Telex: 82104 Deribe Ng

Chairman: Alhaji Mai Deribe (also Managing Director)

PRINCIPAL ACTIVITIES: Building/civil engineering contractors, suppliers of all building materials; school stationery suppliers; transporters; produce buying agents
Branch Offices: 7 Ikololu Rd, Surulere, Lagos, Tel 835367; Alhaji Bakari Rd, GRA Jimeta, Yola, Gongola State; 4 Gloucester Sq, London W2, Tel 01-723-3947

DESAM DEVELOPMENT COMPANY LTD

12 Military Street, PO Box 4838, Lagos
Tel: 634630, 630891
Cable: Desamamana
Telex: 22031 Desam Ng

Chairman: Chief (Dr) E J Amana
Directors: Dr O M Amana, Mrs D E Amana, D E Amana
Senior Executives: E O Inyang (General Manager), B A O Akpanim (Operations Manager), L A Ajayi (Financial Controller)

PRINCIPAL ACTIVITIES: Agents and general merchants; food production and processing (flour, bakery and ice cream); importers of building materials, industrial equipment and heavy machinery; shipping agents
Principal Agencies: Incoplan, West Germany; Okpi Dev Co Inc, USA; Structures & Computers, UK; Biedermann International, USA
Branch Offices: 4 Marian Rd, PO Box 349, Calabar, Cross River State, Tel 222679; Plot A11/6 Marian Rd Extension, PO Box 349, Calabar, Cross River State, Tel 22041
Subsidary/Associated Companies: Oil Field Engineering Group Ltd; International Agro-Industries Dev Co Ltd; Amana Consulting Engineers; Desam Industries Ltd; Fortune Insurance Brokers & Consultants
Principal Bankers: Icon Ltd (Merchant Bankers); First Bank of Nigeria Ltd
Financial Information:

	N'000
Authorised capital	1,000
Paid-up capital	1,000
Turnover	3,125
Profits	54

Principal Shareholders: Chief (Dr) E J Amana
Date of Establishment: 1st August 1974
No of Employees: 120

DESIGN GROUP NIGERIA

36 New Court Rd, PMB 5079, Ibadan, Oyo State
Tel: 462320/1
Telex: 31160 Desyn Ng

PRINCIPAL ACTIVITIES: Consultants

DEUTSCHE KAISER GRUPPE (INTERKONTINENTAL)

Evwreni House, (Near UBA Buildings), PO Box 1700, Warri, Bendel State

Chairman: Chief J A O'Bahor
Directors: HRH Prince J A O'Bahor (Managing Director), W A O'Bahor, Mrs S O Bazunu-O'Bahor
Senior Executives: R Amerding, R Srinivasan, M Chang

PRINCIPAL ACTIVITIES: Agency, manufacturers' representatives, import/export trade, wholesale trading, major distributors and suppliers, civil engineering and construction; electronic engineering
Principal Agencies: Nairn International Group of Companies, GB; Francis Shaw & Company, GB; Foster Transformer Ltd, GB; J & T Robinson of Croydon, GB; Kentredder Ltd, GB; Atomic Energy of Canada Ltd, Canada; Borelain International, USA; Australian Meat and Livestock Corp; New Zealand Meat Exporters Council; Pepper Industries, Inc, USA; Cobb International Inc, USA; Westmac International Machinery Company, USA; Japan Machinery Exporters' Association; Tongkook Trading Co Ltd etc
Branch Offices: 1 Bazunu St, Warri, Bendel State; 44 Lower Erejuwa Rd, Warri, Bendel State; 33 Ogida Ave, Ogida Quarters, Benin City, Bendel State
Subsidiary Companies: Anglo-American Company; Anglo-German Company (see separate entry); British-Soviet Company; Compagnie Francaise de l'Afrique (see separate entry); Imperial Japan-American Company; Commonwealth Commodity Company (see separate entry); Eguvbemete Engineering Company; O'Bahor Petroleum Company; J A O'Bahor & Company (see separate entry); Olympio & O'Bahor; J Bazunu & Sons; Bazunu Brothers & Company
Principal Bankers: Union Bank of Nigeria Ltd
Financial Information:

	N'000
Authorised capital	20,000
Paid-up capital	15,000
Turnover	38,000
Profits	3,800

Principal Shareholders: Chief J A O'Bahor, HRH Prince J A O'Bahor, W A O'Bahor, Mrs S O Bazuno-O'Bahor
Date of Establishment: 30th October, 1978
No of Employees: 1,500

DEXSO FURNITURE FACTORY LTD

Plot 135 Trans Amadi Industrial Layout, PO Box 895, Port Harcourt, Rivers State
Tel: 223982

PRINCIPAL ACTIVITIES: Manufacturers of all types of furniture
Branch Offices: 3 Iloro St, Akure, PMB 635, Ondo State, Tel 2088

DHANAMALL & CO (NIGERIA) LTD

49 Martin St, Lagos
Tel: 650226

PRINCIPAL ACTIVITIES: Suppliers of wholesale general merchandise
Branch Offices: 12 Ereko St, Lagos, 650276

DHL INTERNATIONAL NIGERIA LTD

1 Sumbo Jibowu Street, (Corner of Alhaji Ribadu Rd), PO Box 51901, S.W. Ikoyi, Lagos
Tel: 932962, 935299
Telex: 22494 DHLLOS Ng

Chairman: Chief Olajide Oyewole
Directors: Chief R A Komolafe, R A Bowie
Senior Executives: Peter Tribe (General Manager)

PRINCIPAL ACTIVITIES: World-wide international courier service and air cargo service
Branch Offices: Airport Office: 7 Ibadiaran Street, Onigbongbo, Maryland, Ikeja, Tel: 932962, 935299, Telex: 26472 DHL OPS; Development House, 21 Wharf Rd, Apapa; 3 Mission Rd, Benin City; 70 Zik Avenue, Enugu; 1st Floor Investment House, 27 Akilu Rd, Kaduna; 436 Sarkin Yaki Rd, New Airport Layout, Kano; Plot 74 Trans Admadi Industrial Estate, Port Harcourt; 232 Warri/Sapele Rd, Warri
Principal Bankers: First Bank of Nigeria

Principal Shareholders: DHL International (Hong Kong) Ltd

DHV CONSULTANTS NIGERIA LTD

Plot 14 Babatunde Oki St, Ilupeju, PO Box 1391, Ikeja, Lagos

PRINCIPAL ACTIVITIES: Consultants

DIAMOND PLASTICS LTD

13A Burma Rd, PO Box 284, Apapa, Lagos
Tel: 874172, 872654
Cable: Diamond Apapa
Telex: 20200 TDS No 021

Chairman: S M Olakunri
Directors: Mrs O O Olakunri, Simeon M Olakunri
Senior Executives: R G Chandiramani (General Works Manager), B O Osinibi (Accountant)

PRINCIPAL ACTIVITIES: Manufacturers of industrial plastic packaging; plastics/plastic products
Branch Offices: PO Box 48, Koko, Bendel State
Principal Bankers: First Bank of Nigeria Ltd; United Bank for Africa Ltd
Financial Information:
Authorised capital   ₦ 250,000

Principal Shareholders: Simeon M Olakunri; Mrs Olutoyin Olakunri
Date of Establishment: 1969
No of Employees: 200

DIBORSONS BUSINESS ENTERPRISES

75 Jubilee Rd, PO Box 1105, Aba, Imo State
Cable: Diborsons
Telex: 63111 Natbros

Chairman: E O C Dibor (also Managing Director)
Directors: F I O Dibor, K C Dibor, C O Dibor, L C Dibor, C C Dibor

PRINCIPAL ACTIVITIES: Suppliers of general merchandise, ceramics, glass, hardware, paint, plastic products etc
Principal Agencies: Brockhouse Export Ltd, UK; Hyesung Glass Industrial Company Ltd, Korea
Branch Offices: 149 Enugu Rd, PO Box 671, Awka, Anambra State

Principal Shareholders: Chairman and directors as described
Date of Establishment: 21st October 1975

DIESEL GENERATING COMPANY LTD

Km 7, Lagos Rd, PO Box 76, Ibadan, Oyo State
Tel: 412792
Telex: 31164 Servon Ng

Chairman: Sam Oshinowo
Directors: Olatunji Oshinowo, Miss Modupe Oshinowo
Senior Executives: David Shoyemi (Marketing Manager), L A Oshinowo (Administrative Manager)

PRINCIPAL ACTIVITIES: Sales and service of agricultural equipment, diesel generators and electrical materials
Principal Agencies: Merican Curtis Inc, USA
Branch Offices: 46 Oba Akran Ave, Ikeja Industrial Estate, PO Box 7905, Marina, Lagos, Tel 934716, 964626
Associated Companies: Servo Nigerian Enterpises Ltd
Principal Bankers: Co-operative Bank of Nigeria Ltd; Standard

Bank of Nigeria Ltd
Financial Information:

	₦'000
Sales turnover	1,000
Profits (approx)	400

DIESEL SALES AND SERVICE (NIGERIA) LTD

11 Burma Rd, PO Box 109, Apapa, Lagos
Tel: 876767/876839
Cable: Suntract Lagos
Telex: 21393 Suntract

Chairman: Chief Alhaji Shafi Lawal Edu
Directors: Malcolm Walker Davis, William Arthur Shapland, Charles Logan Ferguson, Chief Alhaji Shafi Lawal Edu, Felix Afolabi Afolayan
Senior Executives: J F Coleshill (General Manager)

PRINCIPAL ACTIVITIES: Suppliers of diesel generator sets, industrial and marine diesel engines
Principal Agencies: Detroit Diesel Allison Industrial; Automotive and Marine Engines - Transmissions; Johnson & Towers Inc; Translite
Branch Offices: 24 Club Rd, Kano; Trans Amadi Industrial Layout, Port Harcourt; Enerhe Rd, Warri, Bendel State; Baga Rd, Maiduguri, Borno Stae
Principal Bankers: Union Bank of Nigeria Ltd
Financial Information: A division of Blackwood Hodge (Nigeria) Ltd

Date of Establishment: 29th November, 1957

DIPENTA NIGERIA LTD

Ado Bayero Rd, PO Box 1223, Kano
Tel: 4517

Directors: Michele di Penta, A Di Penta, Z Idris, Usman Goji, M d'Arogona

PRINCIPAL ACTIVITIES: Civil engineering and construction
Branch Offices: PMB 1297, Maiduguri, Borno State

DISSCOL LTD

105 Maganda Rd, PO Box 6409, Kano
Tel: Kano 5503
Telex: 77170

Chairman: A U Ibru
Directors: P Alcan, M C O Ibru, G Broizat, G M Ibru, G Moll
Senior Executives: J G Verlaque (General Manager)

PRINCIPAL ACTIVITIES: Servicing the water industry in supplying drilling rigs and equipment, borehole, consumable products; supplying the agricultural industry with irrigation equipment; pump suppliers for all applications
Principal Agencies: Irrifrance, Pompe Guinard, Foraco
Principal Bankers: Standard Bank of Nigeria

DIXILYN (NIGERIA) LTD

48 Plot 205 Adeleke Adedoyin St, PO Box 1242, Victoria Island, Lagos

Directors: A A Ervin (General Manager),
V Powell (Financial),
L W Christian (Drilling Superintendent)

PRINCIPAL ACTIVITIES: Drilling Contractors

DIZENGOFF WEST AFRICA (NIGERIA) LTD

PO Box 340, 28 Creek Rd, Apapa, Lagos
Tel: 875990, 875549
Cable: Dizeco Lagos
Telex: 21283 Dizeco Ng

Directors: R Yogev, Dr A Sasegbon, Y Menashe, J M Mostard, S O Odugbesan, H E Duke
Senior Executives: Mrs V Duru (Head of Technical Sales and General Goods),
C U Uzoukwu (Personnel/Administrative Manager),
Benson Anorue (Shipping Manager)

PRINCIPAL ACTIVITIES: Suppliers of agricultural equipment and services; telecommunications, building materials, technical equipment, chemicals, etc
Branch Offices: 9 Magazine Rd, Ibadan, Oyo State; 4 Ogui Rd, Enugu, Anambra State; 113 Maganda Rd, Kano; 83A Igun St, Benin City, Bendel State; 1 Ogbunabali St, Orogbun-Diobu, PO Box 637, Port Harcourt, Rivers State; Lagos Rd, PMB 1431, Ilorin, Kwara State; 34 Warri/Sapele Rd, Warri, Bendel State; PO Box 6020, Anglo, Jos, Plateau State; Plot 197 Sokoto Bye Pass, Sokoto
Principal Bankers: Savannah Bank of Nigeria Ltd; Union Bank of Nigeria Ltd; International Bank for West Africa Ltd; Societe Generale Bank Ltd; Chase Merchant Bank Nigeria Ltd; United Bank for Africa Ltd
Financial Information:

	N'000
Authorised capital	2,000
Paid-up capital	1,260
Sales turnover	30,000
Profits	2,000

Principal Shareholders: Balton Handelsonderneming BV, Amersterdam (40%); Nigerian Shareholders (60%)
Date of Establishment: 1959
No of Employees: 450

DLP PHARMACEUTICALS LTD
302 Herbert Macaulay St, PO Box 151, Yaba, Lagos

PRINCIPAL ACTIVITIES: Manufacturers of pharmaceuticals
Branch Offices: Plots 37/39, Iganmu Industrial Estate, Iganmu, Lagos, Tel 833472

DOAL ENTERPRISES LTD
2nd Floor, Western House, 8/10 Broad Street, PO Box 1973, Lagos
Tel: 637676
Cable: Dotoku Lagos
Telex: 21547 Dotoku Ng

Chairman: Chief Dotun Okubanjo
Directors: Mrs A B Okubanjo
Senior Executives: Mrs Funmi Osinowo (Associate Director)

PRINCIPAL ACTIVITIES: Printing, suppliers of paper and paper products. Real Estate. Paper conversion, manufacturers' representatives
Associated Companies: Naija Lion, London
Principal Bankers: Nigeria Merchant Bank Ltd; First Bank of Nigeria Ltd
Financial Information:
Turnover   N 1,000,000

Principal Shareholders: Chief and Mrs Dotun Okubanjo
Date of Establishment: July 1971

DOF CHEMICALS LTD
5 Ikosi Rd, Oregun Village, PMB 21548, Ikeja, Lagos
Telex: 20202 TDS BOX D14

Chairman: D O Onaolapo (also Managing Director)
Senior Executives: E G Harding (General Manager)

PRINCIPAL ACTIVITIES: Distribution of industrial and water treatment chemicals

DOKUNMU, M A, & SONS LTD
PO Box 3252, 4 Balogun Sq, Lagos
Tel: 636271
Cable: Madokstate
Telex: 21557 Madco Ng

PRINCIPAL ACTIVITIES: Estate agents and valuers; importers, exporters of Nigerian produce; manufacturers' representatives; building and civil engineering contractors
Branch Offices: Ikeja, Lagos, Tel 961131, 963963

DOLMECH ENGINEERING (NIG) LTD
44 Hawley St, PO Box 6927, Lagos
Tel: 636633
Cable: Land Motion Lagos

PRINCIPAL ACTIVITIES: Ventilation, air conditioning, metals, metal processing and fabrication
Principal Agencies: Coral Industries, Italy; Expanded Metals; Key Industrial Equipment Ltd, UK; Seedstone Ltd, UK
Branch Offices: PMB 1197, Yaba, Lagos; PO Box 450, Benin, Bendel State
Associated Companies: Nigerian and Overseas Gas Co Ltd; Cotsgas; V Y B Nig Ltd
Principal Bankers: Co-operative Bank Ltd; African Continental Bank Ltd
Financial Information:
Authorised capital   N 400,000

Principal Shareholders: Chairman and directors as described
Date of Establishment: 1976

DOLPHIN DIVE WEST AFRICA
116 Murtala Muhammed Way, PMB 1398, Ikeja, Lagos
Tel: 861850, 963385

PRINCIPAL ACTIVITIES: Suppliers of swimming pools and related equipment; chemicals, agricultural hand tools, etc

DOLPHIN PROPERTIES LTD
PO Box 88, Lagos

PRINCIPAL ACTIVITIES: Building and civil engineering contractors

DOMINO STORES LTD
13 Commercial Avenue, PO Box 431, Yaba, Lagos
Tel: 862558

Directors: M L Murray Bruce (Managing)

PRINCIPAL ACTIVITIES: Retail distribution

Date of Establishment: 1964
No of Employees: 400

DON INTERNATIONAL LTD
4 Adebola St, Off Adeniran Ogunsanya St, PO Box 1253, Surulere, Lagos
Tel: 833831, 835076, 835306
Telex: 26227 Don Ng

PRINCIPAL ACTIVITIES: Suppliers of security items, safes, etc
Branch Offices: 14 Adeniran Ogunsany St, Surulere, Lagos, Tel 832507, 832969; 20 Station Rd, Port Harcourt

DORMAN LONG & AMALGAMATED ENGINEERING LTD
20 Agege Motor Rd, Idi-Oro, PO Box 256, Lagos
Tel: 831886, 831971, 831553
Cable: Amalgam

Chairman: Mallam Turi Muhammadu
Directors: C Wilson (Managing),
   Alhaji M Tafida,
   Alhaji Abdullahi Mahmood,
   A O Onofe-Kohwo (Company Secretary),
   E M Cairney,
   A M Ferguson,
   Isa Yusufu (Deputy Managing)
Senior Executives: K E Bishop (Technical Procurement Manager),
   J M Harrison (Design and Estimating Manager),
   J A O Ogunfuwa (Finance Manager),
   J Diamond (General Manager)

PRINCIPAL ACTIVITIES: Manufacturing and construction of structural steelwork
Principal Bankers: Union Bank of Nigeria Ltd
Financial Information:

	₦'000
Authorised capital	1,250
Paid-up capital	1,046
Turnover	5,500

Principal Shareholders: British Steel Corporation (London); Gongola State; Bauchi State Borno State; New Nigeria Development Company
Date of Establishment: 1949
No of Employees: 650

DORNIER-NIGERIA AERONAUTICAL ENGINEERING

26 Adetokunbo Ademola St, Victoria Island, PO Box 8299, Lagos

Directors: S Genz

PRINCIPAL ACTIVITIES: Aeronautical engineering

DOTUN OKUBANJO & ASSOCIATES LTD

PO Box 1973, 143 Broad St, Lagos
Tel: 637676
Telex: 21547 Dotoku Ng

PRINCIPAL ACTIVITIES: Business consultants; photographers

DOWELL SCHLUMBERGER (NIGERIA) LTD

PMB 12666, 35 Adetokunbo Ademola St, Victoria Island, Lagos
Tel: 615688
Cable: Bigorange Lagos
Telex: 21415 Spelag Ng

Directors: B W Darling (General Manager),
    L Marshall (Manager, Port Harcourt),
    E Wicks (Manager, Warri)

PRINCIPAL ACTIVITIES: Oil and gas services, well cementing
Branch Offices: Field Offices: PO Box 902, Plot 161, Trans-Amadi Layout, Port Harcourt, Tel 330554, Cable Bigorgange Port Harcourt; PO Box 344, Warri, Cable Bigorange Warri

DOYIN INVESTMENTS NIGERIA LTD

Textiles Division, Old Ojo Rd, Off Badagry Expressway, Oluti Amuwo, Lagos

PRINCIPAL ACTIVITIES: Retailers of clothing
Branch Offices: Showroom: 21 Obun Eko St, Lagos, Tel 664134, 663786, 664906

DPMS LTD
(Formerly IBM Nig Ltd)

Lapal House, 217-235 Igbosere Rd, PO Box 1083, Lagos
Tel: 632739, 633969
Cable: Inbusmach
Telex: 21473 DPMSLOS NG

Chairman: B de Luze
Directors: S O Famodimu (Managing),
    Chief Rotimi Williams,
    E O Okeniyi
Senior Executives: Tom Bell (Assistant General Manager),
    Okon Uko (Business Operations Manager),
    A Akerele (Personnel Manager),
    Dapo Ayorinde (Financial Controller)

PRINCIPAL ACTIVITIES: Selling and servicing IBM computers
Principal Bankers: First Bank of Nigeria Ltd; United Bank for Africa Ltd; Wema Bank Ltd
Financial Information:

	₦'000
Authorised capital	1,400
Paid-up capital	1,087
Turnover	3,895
Profits	368

Principal Shareholders: Nigerians 60%; IBM World Trade Corp 40%
Date of Establishment: 1962
No of Employees: 100

DR PEPPER BOTTLING COMPANY OF NIGERIA LTD

8 Second Avenue, Housing Estate, PO Box 9, Calabar, Cross River State
Tel: 221071/2
Cable: Docpepper
Telex: 65166

Chairman: E C D Abia
Directors: A S Abia, S J Umoren, C U Nyong, Dr S N Okpokham
Senior Executives: J Zevenbergen (General Manager),
    F E Okehie (Finance Controller),
    S E Haque (Operations Manager),
    F S Idio (Senior Marketing Manager),
    U J Antigha (Administrative Manager)

PRINCIPAL ACTIVITIES: Manufacturers of soft drinks, plastic crates and carbon dioxide
Principal Agencies: Dr Pepper Company, USA
Branch Offices: Production Centre; 173 Eket Rd, Eket, Cross River State; Branch Office: 10/12 Military Street, B7, Lagos; Depots at: Calabar; Ikom; Uyo; Aba; Onitsha & Enugu
Subsidiary Companies: Kwantala Durables Ltd
Principal Bankers: First Bank of Nigeria Ltd; Merchantile Bank of Nigeria Ltd; Icon Ltd
Financial Information:

	₦'000
Authorised capital	1,800
Paid-up capital	1,800
Turnover	3,793

Principal Shareholders: Nigerians and overseas partners
Date of Establishment: 17th September, 1979
No of Employees: 400

DRAGAGES NIGERIA LTD

9 Alhaji Ribadu Rd, South West Ikoyi, PO Box 60365, Lagos
Tel: 684663
Telex: 21695

PRINCIPAL ACTIVITIES: Design and construction of nuclear power plants, commercial and industrial buildings, dams, tunnels, marine works etc

DRAKE & SCULL (NIGERIA) LTD

90 Lewis St, PO Box 2389, Lagos
Tel: 636549, 631252
Cable: Accumulator Lagos
Telex: 21298 Accumu Ng

Chairman: Alhaji H L Zuru
Directors: L T Bugler (Deputy Chairman),
    A D Scott (General Manager),
    W J J Leslie,
    Alhaji M Inuwa,
    Alhaji M U Ngirna,
    Miss T O Olaniyan
Senior Executives: S A Olusesi (Administrative Manager/Company Secretary),
    E D Edbrook (Commercial Manager),
    M O Solebo (Supply Manager),
    A G Kingston (Contracts Manager),
    O Y Oyelakun (Quantity Surveyor)

PRINCIPAL ACTIVITIES: Mechanical, electrical engineers, plumbing and air-conditioning services; power transmission services
Principal Bankers: Union Bank of Nigeria Ltd

Financial Information:

	N'000
Authorised capital	1,000
Paid-up capital	750
Turnover	15,000

Principal Shareholders: Drake & Scull Engineering Ltd; New Nigerian Development Company Ltd
No of Employees: 1,000

DRESSER NIGERIA LTD

(Dresser Magcobar Minerals Ltd)

Western House, 14th Floor, 8/10 Broad St, Lagos Island, PO Box 912, Lagos
Tel: 653146, 655846
Telex: 21329

Directors: B Barton (Managing Director), A O Sardella (Chief Engineer, Port Harcourt), J R Jordan (Chief Engineer, Warri)

PRINCIPAL ACTIVITIES: Oil services; drilling and equipment suppliers; manufacturers of drilling mud
Branch Offices: PMB 5123, Port Harcourt, Rivers State, Tel 228366; PO Box 435, Warri, Bendel State

DRUG HOUSES NIGERIA LTD

27 Commercial Avenue, PO Box 482, Yaba, Lagos
Tel: 862101, 861814
Cable: Drughouses, Yaba
Telex: 26648 Drugho

Directors: Olayide Theophilus Ososami, Mrs Olujimi Adeola Ososami
Senior Executives: A Ososami (Administrative Manager), Mrs O O Adeniran (Sales Executive)

PRINCIPAL ACTIVITIES: Pharmaceutical, medical supplies and services
Branch Offices: SW9/847C Ring Rd, PMB 5179, Ibadan, Oyo State
Principal Bankers: United Bank for Africa Ltd; Savannah Bank of Nigeria Ltd
Financial Information:

	N'000
Authorised capital	500
Paid-up capital	230
Turnover (March 81)	1,594
Profits	8

Principal Shareholders: O T Ososami; Mrs O A Ososami
Date of Establishment: May 1981
No of Employees: 50

DRUG SPECIALITIES (NIGERIA) LTD

Km 6 Enugu/Onitsha Rd, Nkpor-Agu, Nkpor, PO Box 3546, Onitsha, Anambra State

Directors: B O Obi, J U N I Menakaya, B I O Obi
Senior Executives: Ejike Obadike (Finance), Hope Oneafolu (Marketing), Mike Igweogu (Administration)

PRINCIPAL ACTIVITIES: Suppliers of pharmaceutical and medical products. Hospital and laboratory equipment
Principal Agencies: Laboratories Prodes, Spain
Principal Bankers: First Bank of Nigeria Ltd; Pan African Bank Ltd

DSD NIGERIA LTD

6 Adeola Adeleye St, PO Box 7191, Illupeju, Lagos
Tel: 934915, 932569

Chairman: F A Ayinotu
Directors: Helmut Frommel (Administrative Manager), Wolfgang Schwarz (Technical Manager)

PRINCIPAL ACTIVITIES: Civil engineering and construction, suppliers of construction plant; mechanical engineering
Associated Companies: SHG Saarlandische Handelsgesellschaft mbH; GAV Gesellchaft für Anlagenverwaltung mbH; Verea GmbH; Secometal SA; Socometal SA; DSD Dillinger Service Division for Industry Ltd; Dillinger Ingenieros y Contratistas de Costa Rica SA; CGI Compania General de Industrias CA
Principal Bankers: First Bank of Nigeria Ltd; United Bank for Africa Ltd
Financial Information:
Authorised capital   N 401,000

Principal Shareholders: Torroman International (60%); DSD Dillinger Stahlban, Germany (40%)
Date of Establishment: 21st September 1976
No of Employees: 2,000

DRUG SPECIALITIES (NIGERIA) LIMITED

Name and Address:
DRUG SPECIALITIES NIG. LTD.
KM. 6 Enugu/Onitsha Road, Nkpor-Agu, Nkpor, p.o. Box 3546, Onitsha, Nigeria.

Directors:
B.O. Obi, J.U.N.I. Menakaya LLB, BL, M.P.S., B.I.O. Obi

Senior Executives:
Ejike Obadike (Finance), Hope Oneaflou (Marketing), Mike Igweogu (Administration)

Principal Activities:
Suppliers or Pharmaceutical and Medical Products, Hospitals and Laboratory Equipment.

Principal Agencies:
Laboratores Prodes, Spain

Principal Bankers:
First Bank of Nigeria Ltd, Head Bridge Branch, Onitsha.
Pan African Bank Ltd, Ogidi Branch, Ogidi.

DUBIC BREWERIES LTD

160 Azikiwe Rd, PMB 7394, Aba, Imo State
Tel: 220761, 220206
Cable: Dubic Aba
Telex: 63130 Dike Ng

Chairman: Dike Udensi Ifegwu (also Managing Director)
Directors: C B C Ubah, Manfred Guhl
Senior Executives: Robert J Harbinson (General Manager), Steve-Ben Ikem (Administration/Personnel Manager), R E Mohrbach (Technical Manager)

PRINCIPAL ACTIVITIES: Brewing
Branch Offices: Factory site: Umuode Umuakpara, Obioma Ngwa LGA, Aba, Imo State
Subsidiary Companies: Dubic Industries Ltd; Dubic International Ltd
Principal Bankers: International Bank for West Africa Ltd
Financial Information:

	N'000
Authorised capital	1,500
Paid-up capital	1,500

Principal Shareholders: Directors as described
Date of Establishment: May 1979
No of Employees: 180

DUBIC INDUSTRIES LTD

160 Azikiwe Rd, Box 323, Aba, Imo State
Tel: 220206
Cable: Dubic Aba
Telex: 63130 Dyke Ng

President: Dike Udensi Ifegwu
Directors: Mrs Eunice Dike Udensi
Senior Executives: J G Dhawan (General Manager),
    A Ejindu Agba (Administration/Personnel Manager),
    E Onyekwere (Production Manager)

PRINCIPAL ACTIVITIES: Manufacturers of paper products
Branch Offices: 1/70 Industrial Layout Ogbor Hill, Aba, Imo
    State
Subsidiary Companies: Dubic International Co Ltd; Dubic
    Breweries Ltd
Principal Bankers: International Bank for West Africa Ltd
Financial Information:

	₦'000
Authorised capital	1,500
Paid-up capital	1,500

Principal Shareholders: Directors as described
Date of Establishment: June 1978
No of Employees: 130

DUBIC INTERNATIONAL LTD

160 Azikiwe Rd, Box 323, Aba, Imo State
Tel: 220761
Cable: Dubic Aba
Telex: 63130 Dyke Ng

Chairman: Dike Udensi Ifegwu
Directors: Dike Udensi Dike, O D Udensi, Miss O D Udensi,
    Urum Udensi, Okorie Udensi, Okoji Otisi
Senior Executives: Obewu U Eke (General Manager),
    Eke Agbeze (Administrative Manager),
    Kalu Agwu (Import/Export Manager),
    Agbai Udeagha (Transport Manager),
    Urum Emeri (Building Manager)

PRINCIPAL ACTIVITIES: Import and export agents. Commercial
    distributors
Principal Agencies: Chestershire Ltd, (UK); Faberge International
Subsidiary Companies: Dubic Industries Ltd; Dubic Breweries
    Ltd
Principal Bankers: International Bank for West Africa Ltd
Financial Information:

	₦'000
Authorised capital	1,000
Paid-up capital	1,000

Date of Establishment: April 1976
No of Employees: 75

DUBOSH PLASTICS (NIGERIA) LTD

Matori Estate, Oshodi, Lagos

PRINCIPAL ACTIVITIES: Manufacturers of plastic sheets

DUMEX PHARMACEUTICALS LTD

4B Ijora Cause Way, Ijora, PO Box 7707, Lagos
Tel: 836647, 837158, 833620
Cable: Dumepharm

Chairman: B O Benson
Directors: Chief C Ekwenibe, Alhaji F Uthman, P Chavannaz
Senior Executives: J C Michell (General Manager)

PRINCIPAL ACTIVITIES: Distributors of pharmaceutical
    products, vaccines and milk products
Principal Agencies: A/S Dumex Ltd, Denmark
Branch Offices: Ibadan; Aba; Benin; Kaduna
Associated Companies: A/S Dumex Ltd, Denmark
Principal Bankers: First Bank of Nigeria Ltd; Union Bank of
    Nigeria Ltd; Union Bank for Africa

Financial Information:

	₦'000
Authorised capital	600
Paid-up capital	450
Turnover	6,000
Profits	184

Principal Shareholders: A/S Dumex Ltd, Denmark; CFAO Nigeria
    Ltd
Date of Establishment: 26th September 1960
No of Employees: 100

DUMEZ (NIGERIA) LTD

PO Box 2352, 21 Marina, Lagos
Tel: 636430, 656480
Telex: 21441 Zemud Ng

Chairman: Alhaji B Danbappa
Directors: A Kamel (General Manager/Director)

PRINCIPAL ACTIVITIES: Engineering and construction

DUNLOP NIGERIAN INDUSTRIES LTD

Oba Akran Avenue, Ikeja Industrial Estate, PMB 21079, Ikeja,
    Lagos
Tel: 962506/9, 963421/4, 900410, 900416/9, 962666/8
Cable: Dunlop Ikeja
Telex: 21315 Lagos

Chairman: Malam Mamman Daura
Directors: J E S Hammond (Managing),
    G O Onosode,
    L A Nakpodia (Consumer & Industrial),
    E A Awobokun (Sales, Tyres),
    A Adebowale,
    C A Bushell (Finance),
    C A Griffiths (Works),
    K J Johnson
Senior Executives: M A Gbenro (Finance Controller),
    L A Dairo (General Manager, Dunlopillo),
    Dr S N Anyakora (General Manager, Material Supply Div),
    O O Akinpelu (General Manager, Personnel),
    J C Okporua (General Manager, Flooring),
    G D Isoberenge (General Manager, Marketing Services)

PRINCIPAL ACTIVITIES: Manufactures of tyres, tubes, flooring,
    adhesives and foam products. Marketing of sports
    equipment, general and industrial rubber goods, hoses,
    footwear, power transmissions
Branch Offices: Industrial Products Division, Plot 5C Ijora
    Causeway, PO Box 386, Apapa, Lagos; Ibadan; Benin;
    Kaduna; Kano; Aba; Onitsha
Principal Bankers: First Bank of Nigeria Ltd; Union Bank of
    Nigeria Ltd; United Bank for Africa Ltd; International Bank
    for West Africa Ltd
Financial Information: As at 31st December, 1980

	₦'000
Authorised capital	12,500
Paid-up capital	10,500
Turnover	51,138
Profits (after tax)	1,117

Principal Shareholders: Dunlop International Ltd; Odu'a
    Investment Company Ltd
Date of Establishment: 21st October, 1961
No of Employees: 2,017

DUNON FURNITURE INDUSTRY LTD

156 Zik Ave, Uwani, PO Box 745, Enugu, Anambra State
Tel: 252264
Cable: Dunon Enugu
Telex: 51139 Dunon

Chairman: David Chukwuemeka Egonu
Directors: Ngozi Uchenna Egonu
Senior Executives: Samuel Uchenna Chigbo (Company
    Secretary),
    Jonathan Okpala (Sales Manager),
    Anthony Mgbachi (Accountant)

PRINCIPAL ACTIVITIES: Furniture manufacturers and interior decorators
Branch Offices: 24 Doherty St, PO Box 3588, Lagos; 63 Fosbery Rd, Calabar, Cross River State
Principal Bankers: Union Bank of Nigeria Ltd
Financial Information:

	N'000
Authorised capital	150
Paid-up capital	150
Turnover	1,038
Profits	98

Principal Shareholders: D C Egonu, N U Egonu
Date of Establishment: 8th May 1972
No of Employees: 168

DURO INTERNATIONAL (NIGERIA) LTD
PO Box 3462, Lagos

PRINCIPAL ACTIVITIES: Manufacturers of car parts and accessories, furniture manufacturing; hardware, and accessories

DYNAMIC INDUSTRIES LTD
6 Obasa Rd, Industrial Estate, PO Box 33, Ikeja, Lagos
Tel: 962374
Cable: Dynaplast Ikeja
Telex: 20202 Box 057 NET TDS NG

Chairman: Alhaji I M Damcida
Directors: P T Chellaram,
S P Chugani,
N P Kirpalani,
J K Dina,
R A Vaswani (Managing)
Senior Executives: B A Omotayo (Assistant General Manager),
A A Ibuje (Public Relations Officer),
M D Valecha (Engineer),
J A Deshpande (Engineer),
B N Raha (Engineer),
S Hemachandran (Systems Analyst)

PRINCIPAL ACTIVITIES: Manufacturers of polythene film for all types of packaging applications including shrink film, printed bags, rain sheeting; plastic woven prayer mats and plastic shoes
Subsidiary Companies: Durkosh Industries (Nigeria) Ltd
Principal Bankers: United Bank for Africa Ltd; Nigeria Merchant Bank Ltd
Financial Information:

	N'000
Authorised capital	1,500
Paid-up capital	1,100
Turnover (approx)	3,000

Principal Shareholders: K Chellaram & Sons (Nigeria) Ltd; Anglo Africa Agencies (Nig) Ltd; Nigerian Industrial Development Bank Ltd; Other Nigerians
Date of Establishment: June 1967
No of Employees: 230

DYS TROCCA VALSESIA & COMPANY LTD
2 Babani Street, Ebute Metta, PO Box 317, Lagos
Tel: 833721, 833854
Cable: Italcon Lagos
Telex: 11117 Box 518 NET TDS NG

Chairman: Alhaji M O Oseni
Directors: Mrs D A Alakija,
Chief A O Sanyaolu,
M A Giachetti (Managing),
E Monta (Joint Managing)
Senior Executives: E R Cusworth (Company Secretary),
G Giachetti (Civil Engineering Manager)

PRINCIPAL ACTIVITIES: Building and civil engineering contractors
Branch Offices: PO Box 861, Jos, Plateau State; PO Box 58, Bida, Niger State

Subsidiary Companies: DTV Motors PO Box 2552, Apapa, Lagos
Principal Bankers: First Bank of Nigeria Ltd
Financial Information:

	N'000
Authorised capital	2,400
Paid-up capital	2,400
Turnover	25,000
Profits	1,500

Principal Shareholders: Realestate Financiere SA; Mrs D A Alakija
Date of Establishment: 21st May 1954
No of Employees: 3,000

E OSBORNE NIGERIA LTD
See OSBORNE, E, NIGERIA LTD

E A O CONSTRUCTORS (NIGERIA) LTD
76 Adetokunbo Ademola St, Victoria Island (Faces Eko Hotel), PO Box 2468, Lagos
Tel: 613603

Chairman: Raymond K Okudzeto
Directors: Alhaji Abubakar Jubril, D Yebovi

PRINCIPAL ACTIVITIES: Construction engineers
Principal Bankers: First Bank of Nigeria Ltd
Financial Information: Subsidiary of Promexport International (Nigeria) Ltd
Date of Establishment: 23rd May 1975
No of Employees: 350

E D'ALBERTO & GIAMPAOLI LTD
See D'ALBERTO, E, & GIAMPAOLI LTD

E M MICHELETTI & SON (NIGERIA) LTD
See MICHELETTI, E M, & SON (NIGERIA) LTD

E MOCCI ASSOCIATES
See MOCCI, E, ASSOCIATES

E O ASHAMU & SONS (HOLDINGS) LTD
See ASHAMU, E O, & SONS (HOLDINGS) LTD

EAGLE GROUP LTD
11 Aba Rd, Port Harcourt, Rivers State
Telex: 21178 Air Ng

PRINCIPAL ACTIVITIES: General traders and contractors
Date of Establishment: 1970

EARTH SCIENCES LTD
10 Alakija St, Yaba, PO Box 6352, Lagos
Cable: Earth Yaba

Directors: Don Obot Etiebet (Managing Director)

PRINCIPAL ACTIVITIES: Suppliers of computer equipment, plotters, etc, for the oil and gas industry
Principal Agencies: Digital Equipment Corp; Calcomp; Texas Instruments, Geophysics Divison; SIE, Geophysics Division

EASTERN BULKCEM COMPANY LTD
Site/Office: Rumuolumeni, PMB 5006, Port Harcourt, Rivers State

PRINCIPAL ACTIVITIES: Manufacturers of cement

EASTERN ENAMELWARE FACTORY LTD
PO Box 23, Plot 31, Trans-Amadi Industrial Layout, Port Harcourt, Rivers State
Tel: 21507, 21878

PRINCIPAL ACTIVITIES: Manufacturers of vitreous enamelware and utensils

EASTERN GENERAL CONTRACTORS LTD

4 Okpara Avenue, PO Box 648, Enugu, Anambra State

Directors: E Nwandu (Managing Director)

PRINCIPAL ACTIVITIES: General traders and contractors

Date of Establishment: 1955

EASTERN (OVERSEAS) AGENCIES LTD

27 Kofo Abayomi Ave, PMB 1043, Apapa, Lagos
Tel: 874445, 874018
Cable: Eternoa
Telex: 21291 Eoa Ng; 61114 Eoa Ng

PRINCIPAL ACTIVITIES: Shipping, clearing, forwarding,
  airfreighting, warehousing
Branch Offices: 1 Industry Rd, PO Box 660, Port Harcourt,
  Rivers State, Tel 229774; Telex 61114 Eoa Ng, Cable Eternoa;
  8 Bashiru-Oweh St, PMB 21352, Ikeja, Lagos State, Cable
  Eternoa; 8 Khalil Rd, PMB 1131, Warri; 360B Airport Rd, PMB
  3251, Kano; 67 Marina, Calabar, Tel 222625

EASTERN WROUGHT IRON LTD

Head Office, 47 Trans-Amadi Industrial Layout, PO Box 602,
  Port Harcourt, Rivers State
Tel: 224922, 331194
Cable: Eastwil

Chairman: B A C Okowa
Directors: Apostle N Nkomadu, T A Awoju, C Ogbugo
Senior Executives: I G P Okonny (General Manager),
  H T Inainfe (Secretary/Accountant),
  C E M Owhochukwu (Marketing Manager),
  G Koko (Production Manager)

PRINCIPAL ACTIVITIES: Manufacturers of beds, chairs,
  furniture, hospital beds, mattresses, cushions and pillows
Branch Offices: 23 St Michael Rd, Aba, Imo State
Principal Bankers: First Bank of Nigeria Ltd; Pan African Bank
  Ltd
Financial Information:

	N'000
Authorised capital	160
Paid-up capital	160
Profits	143

Principal Shareholders: Rivers State Government
Date of Establishment: 1960
No of Employees: 200

EBEL BAU NIGERIA LTD

PO Box 5605, Lagos
Tel: 654430, Ext 217

Directors: R E C Harders

PRINCIPAL ACTIVITIES: Engineering consultants

EBUN OLUWA GROUP OF COMPANIES

11 Kosoko St, Lagos
Tel: 635798, 962236
Cable: Felijias Lagos

PRINCIPAL ACTIVITIES: Wholesale and retail traders; property
  and investment
Branch Offices: 33a Ereko St, Lagos

EBURUTU MINING SYNDICATE

13 Kashim Ibrahim St, PO Box 338, Jos, Plateau State

PRINCIPAL ACTIVITIES: Mining

ECWA PRODUCTIONS LTD

Kano Rd, PMB 2010, Jos, Plateau State
Tel: 52230, 53597, 54481
Cable: Challenge Jos
Telex: 81120 Ecwap Ng

Chairman: Rev S A Ibrahim
Directors: T T Makanjuola,
  Rev Dr Nat L Olutimayin,
  E Oji,
  'Tunji Arosanyin,
  U Mallam,
  E G Mairabo,
  Dr P S Usman (Managing Director),
  S N Kolo (Trade Director),
  I B Majam (Financial Director),
  J K Bolarin (Publishing Director),
  Dr D L Yilwa ((Administration Director))
Senior Executives: S K Damah (Personnel Officer),
  G I Ude (Management Accountant),
  A O Suberu (Chief Accountant/Company Secretary),
  J A Babatunde (General Manager, Publications),
  E M Gara (Purchasing Manager),
  S K Diabour (Trade Accountant)

PRINCIPAL ACTIVITIES: Bookselling, stationery supply,
  publishing, Christian broadcasting, film hire service,
  counselling, records and cassettes production, audio visual
  production
Principal Agencies: Zondervan Corporation, (USA); Moody Press,
  (USA), Thomas Nelson, (USA); Marshall Morgan & Scott, (UK);
  Rotring-Werke, (W Germany); George Rowney & Co Ltd,
  (UK); Messenger Corp, (USA); William Clowes & Sons, (UK);
  Pickering & Inglis, (UK); Tyndale House Publishers, (USA);
  Thomas Wyatt (Nigeria) Ltd; Collins Glasgow, (UK); Trinitarian
  Bible Society, (UK); Paternoster Press (UK)
Branch Offices: Challenge Bookshops: Aba Rd, Mile 3 Diobu,
  PO Box 274, Port Harcourt; 130 Broad St, Lagos; 275 Agege
  Motor Rd, Mushin, PMB 12256, Lagos; Kano Rd, PMB 2010,
  Jos; 6 Ali Akilu Rd, PMB 2049, Kaduna; 27A Airport Rd, PO
  Box 384, Kano; 38 Zik Avenue, Uwani, PMB 1101, Enugu;
  Murtala Mohammed Way, PMB 1346, Ilorin; 27 Asa Rd, PO
  Box 1028 Aba, etc
Subsidiary Companies: Challenge Bookshops; Challenge
  Publications; Challenge Enquiry Centre; Elwa Recording
  Studios; Audio Visual Studio
Principal Bankers: Union Bank of Nigeria Ltd; Chase Merchant
  Bank Nigeria Ltd; First Bank of Nigeria Ltd; Bank of the North
  Ltd; United Bank for Africa Ltd
Financial Information:

	N'000
Authorised capital	3,500
Paid-up capital	1,000
Turnover	6,662
Profits	17

Principal Shareholders: Registered Trustees of the Association
  of Evangelical Churches of West Africa (ECWA)
Date of Establishment: 1st April 1974 (Previously as SIM
  Bookshop (1924))
No of Employees: 400

EDDYMAY ENTERPRISES

8 New Market Rd, Onitsha, Anambra State

Directors: Edmund C Ezeani (Managing Director)

PRINCIPAL ACTIVITIES: Importers, exporters, contractors,
  agents and general trading company
Principal Agencies: Broger and Dunner Ltd, Switzerland
Principal Bankers: Union Bank of Nigeria Ltd

EDDY'S ELECTRONICS

5 Breadfruit St, PO Box 7029, Lagos
Tel: 655715

PRINCIPAL ACTIVITIES: Sales and servicing of electronic
  equipment, importers and radios and electrical goods

EDEMSCOT ENGERPRISES NIGERIA LTD

108 Ederly Rd, PO Box 458, Calabar, Cross River State

Directors: Joseph Edemobey (Managing Director)

PRINCIPAL ACTIVITIES: Suppliers of general merchandise

EDEWOR INTERNATIONAL LTD

Eku House, PO Box 257, Warri, Bendel State
Tel: 231511, 233295
Cable: Edewor
Telex: 43295

Chairman: Chief J O Edewor

PRINCIPAL ACTIVITIES: Distributors of trucks
Principal Agencies: Mack Trucks
Branch Offices: J21 Oduduwa Way, GRA Ikeja, PMB 1598, Ikeja,
  Lagos, Tel 961811

EDILIT LTD

219/A Apapa Rd, Iganmu, PO Box 164, Ebute-Metta, Lagos
Tel: 841284, 831755, 833626, 836554

Directors: Piere G Tonella, Umberto Carnazzi

PRINCIPAL ACTIVITIES: Building and civil engineering
  contractors
Branch Offices: Ilorin; Warri; Kaduna

EDISON GROUP & PARNTERS

20 Eric Moore Rd, Iganmu Industrial Estate, PO Box 2975,
  Lagos

PRINCIPAL ACTIVITIES: Engineering consultants

EDMUND & EDMUND (NIGERIA) LTD

PO Box 8150, 10 Ondo St, West, Ebute-Metta, Lagos
Tel: 830264
Cable: Eddylab
Telex: 26613 Edmund

Chairman: E T Lalemi
Directors: E O A Lalemi (Managing Director),
  M Y Lalemi
Senior Executives: A Ogundare (Maintenance Engineer),
  A Awoye (Technical Services Manager),
  S Ogunseun (Field Sales Manager),
  Confort Ogoke (Company Secretary),
  S Ogunsola (Accountant),
  A Jackson (Stock Controller),
  Chucks Okanome (Marketing Manager)

PRINCIPAL ACTIVITIES: Veterinary and medical equipment
  suppliers, air-conditioning, heating and refrigeration,
  chemicals, pharmaceutical and medical supplies and services,
  scientific instrument suppliers. Pest control sprayers
Principal Agencies: Thalheimer Kuehlung, W Germany; Society
  Sterile Catgut, Switzerland; Robinsons & Sons Ltd, UK;
  Vickers Medical, UK; Brillo Magf Company of Great Britain
  Ltd
Principal Bankers: International Bank for West Africa;
  Co-operative Bank Ltd
Financial Information:

	N'000
Authorised capital	100
Paid-up capital	100

Principal Shareholders: Chairman and directors as described
Date of Establishment: 2nd June 1976

EDO TEXTILE MILLS LTD

PO Box 444, Benin City, Bendel State
Tel: 243159

PRINCIPAL ACTIVITIES: Textile manufacturers
Branch Offices: Factory: Eribo Industrial Area, Evbareke, Bendel
  State
Financial Information: Part of Ribway Group of Companies

EDOK-ETER-MANDILAS LTD

Mandilas House, 96-102 Broad Street, PO Box 35, Lagos
Tel: 661967, 662473
Cable: Edeterman
Telex: 21121 Edetma Ng

Chairman: Chief J B Mandilas
Directors: G D Klavidianos, J Alvares, P O Edeoghon, D
  Demetriades, A U Ekwere, Mallam Magaji Inuwa, E C
  Jibuike, G N Sotiriadis
Senior Executives: A Antoniou (Chief Engineer, Design),
  D Jux (Chief Accountant & Financial Controller),
  P Passalaris (Chief Engineer, Mechanical),
  J R Iyasere (Staff Manager)

PRINCIPAL ACTIVITIES: Civil engineering and construction,
  dam, irrigation projects
Branch Offices: 130 Sapele Rd, PO Box 776, Benin City, Bendel
  State; 79 Sir Kashim Ibrahim Rd, PMB 1220, Maiduguri; PO
  Box 109, Bauchi; PMB 1358, Akure
Subsidiary Companies: Mandilas Enterprises Ltd
Principal Bankers: First Bank of Nigeria Ltd; Union Bank of
  Nigeria Ltd; International Bank for West Africa Ltd; United
  Bank for Africa Ltd
Financial Information:

	N'000
Paid-up capital	5,000

Principal Shareholders: Mandilas Trust Company; New Nigeria
  Development Co Ltd; Afrek Ltd; Bendel State Government;
  Edok-Eter
Date of Establishment: 1st June 1974
No of Employees: 3,000

EDOKPOLO, JOHN, & CO LTD

7 Eyaenugie St, PO Box 381, Benin City, Bendel State
Tel: 6212

PRINCIPAL ACTIVITIES: Production of sheet and crepe rubber

EDRITA & COMPANY LTD

20 Bornu Crescent, PO Box 8293, Apapa, Lagos
Tel: 874945, 663668

Chairman: Chief E O Obele
Senior Executives: M I Obele (General Manager)

PRINCIPAL ACTIVITIES: General merchants; haulage;
  distributors of electronic equipment, glass, textiles and
  petroleum products
Principal Agencies: Bendel Glass Co Ltd; African Petroleum Ltd
Branch Offices: 110 Nnamdi Azikiwe St, Lagos; 60 Balogun St,
  Lagos; 21 New Market Rd, Onitsha, Anambra State; 32 New
  Court Rd, Ibadan, Oyo State
Subsidiary Companies: Edrita Containers and Carriers Ltd;
  Obele Industrial Complex Ltd; Green Acres Nigeria Ltd
Principal Bankers: Union Bank of Nigeri Ltd

Date of Establishment: 1972

EDUN COMMERCIAL AGENCY

290 Akaoni St, PO Box 1421, Lagos
Tel: 633411

PRINCIPAL ACTIVITIES: Importers, exporters of clothing;
  jewellery, electrical goods

EFBIKO ENGINEERING LTD

32 Queen St, PO Box 3091, Yaba, Lagos
Tel: 963268

PRINCIPAL ACTIVITIES: Building and civil engineering
  contractors

EGBEMA ENTERPRISES LTD (EEL)

2 Anokwuru St, PMB 5079, Port Harcourt, Rivers State
Tel: 21014, 21758
Cable: Alinso

PRINCIPAL ACTIVITIES: Transport contractors, and importers of
  general merchandise

EGBON MINING SYNDICATE LTD

Dogon Dutse, PO Box 37, Jos, Plateau State
Tel: 2114

PRINCIPAL ACTIVITIES: Metal ore mining

No of Employees: 200

EGBOR AND ASSOCIATES

PO Box 1645, 36/40 Ajani Olujare St, Alaka Estate Surulere,
Lagos
Cable: Planscape Lagos

Chairman: Arc A A Egbor
Directors: Arc O Olusanya
Senior Executives: Arc F R Hickson (Office Manager),
A Salau (Administrative Manager)

PRINCIPAL ACTIVITIES: Architects and planners
Branch Offices: PMB 1322 Benin City, Bendel State; PMB 130
Zaria, Kaduna State
Principal Bankers: First Bank of Nigeria Ltd

Principal Shareholders: Arc A A Egbor; Arc O Olusanya

EJINAKA AND THORNBER LTD

Aba Owerri Rd, PMB 7138, Aba, Imo State
Cable: Ejinaka and Thornber

Directors: Engr G U Meniru,
M O Meniru,
Mrs A I Meniru,
Engr A E Meniru (Managing Director)
Senior Executives: Sunday Esobe (Poultry Manager),
C O Okoro (Feed Mill Manager),
Edward Mayiogu (Broiler Rearing Manager),
J A O Adekale (Lagos Farm Manager),
Josiah Meniru (Hatchery Manager),
S O Ndujiofor (Accountant),
Dr R Brahmakshatriya (Nutritionist)

PRINCIPAL ACTIVITIES: Poultry farming; livestock farming;
livestock feed production and sale, palm plantation for oil
production
Principal Agencies: Dekalb International of Massachusetts, USA
Branch Offices: PMB 1017, Agege, Lagos
Subsidiary/Associated Companies: Subsidiary: Ejinaka Feeds
Ltd; Associated Company: Maince Enterprises Company Ltd
Principal Bankers: Union Bank of Nigeria Ltd; Savannah Bank of
Nigeria Ltd
Financial Information:

	N'000
Authorised capital	100
Paid-up capital	100
Sales turnover	2,500

Principal Shareholders: Directors as described
Date of Establishment: September 1965
No of Employees: 210

EJINKEONYE, L E, BROTHERS TRADING CO LTD

92 Ogui Rd, Asata, Enugu, Anambra State
Tel: 2781

PRINCIPAL ACTIVITIES: Importers of general merchandise

EJIRE HALLELUIH TRADING CO LTD

18 Daminu Rd, PO Box 182, Zaria, Kaduna State
Tel: 2814
Telex: 75247 Ejire Ng

PRINCIPAL ACTIVITIES: Importers and general merchandise

EJUKORLEM, D K, & CO LTD

26 Jingiri Rd, PO Box 250, Jos, Plateau State
Tel: 2830

PRINCIPAL ACTIVITIES: Metal ore mining

No of Employees: 200

EKERETE, A, LTD

Marian Rd Extension, PO Box 555, Calabar, Cross River State
Tel: 2006
Cable: Amekere Calabar

Chairman: Archibong Ekerete
Directors: M Ekerete
Senior Executives: Eric A B Obi (Accountant),
Eno A Ikpe (Sales Manager)

PRINCIPAL ACTIVITIES: Importers/distributors of toys and
educational equipment
Principal Agencies: James Galt Ltd; Combex Ltd; Lew-Ways Ltd
Principal Bankers: First Bank of Nigeria Ltd

Principal Shareholders: A Ekerete; M Ekerete

EKISOLA ELECTRICAL WORKS LTD

PO Box 1878, 123 Lagos Bye Pass, Okeado, Ibadan, Oyo State
Tel: 412144
Telex: 31189 Ekelec Ng

PRINCIPAL ACTIVITIES: Distributors of motor vehicles;
electrical equipment including air-conditioning equipment;
textiles

EKMAN CONSTRUCTION CO LTD

PO Box 554, 12 Ika Ika St, Calabar, Cross River State
Tel: 2101

PRINCIPAL ACTIVITIES: Building and civil engineering
contractors

EKO HOLIDAY INN

PMB 12724, Kuramo Waters, Victoria Island, Lagos
Tel: 615000
Cable: Ekoholiday
Telex: 22650 Eko Hotel Lagos

Chairman: Alhaji Chief Lateef A Dosunmu
Directors: Everett G Thierfelder, Peter C A Thomas, A O Alabi,
C E Okobi, Bode Senbanj, Segun O Samuel
Senior Executives: Samim Akgul (General Manager),
Mrs O Oguneye (Company Secretary),
Carl Prendergast (Financial Controller),
M Eva Maria-Meir (Resident Manager),
Kai Michaelson (Food & Beverage Manager),
Mrs N Atekoja (Executive Housekeeper)

PRINCIPAL ACTIVITIES: Hoteliers
Principal Bankers: Union Bank of Nigeria Ltd

Principal Shareholders: Lagos State Government; Oxy-Holiday of
Africa Ltd
Date of Establishment: 5th March 1967
No of Employees: 1,050

EKO LEATHERWARE FACTORY

61 Enu-Owa St, PO Box 1119, Lagos
Tel: 633985

PRINCIPAL ACTIVITIES: Leather goods

EKSONS (NIG) LTD

Eksons House, 112 Douglas Rd, PO Box 486, Owerri, Imo State
Cable: Eksons-Enugu

Chairman: Chief S O Ekwegh
Directors: Sam Ekwegh, Shed Ekwegh, Alex Ekwegh

PRINCIPAL ACTIVITIES: Designers and engineering contractors
Principal Agencies: AC International, USA; Comfort International,
Italy; Vequip Ltd, UK
Branch Offices: 57 Obioma St, PMB 1286, Enugu, Anambra
State
Associated Companies: Idah Dairy Products Company
Principal Bankers: African Continental Bank; United Bank for
Africa Ltd
Financial Information:
Sales turnover   N 1,000,000

Principal Shareholders: Chairman and directors as described
Date of Establishment: Registered 1970; Incorporated 1974

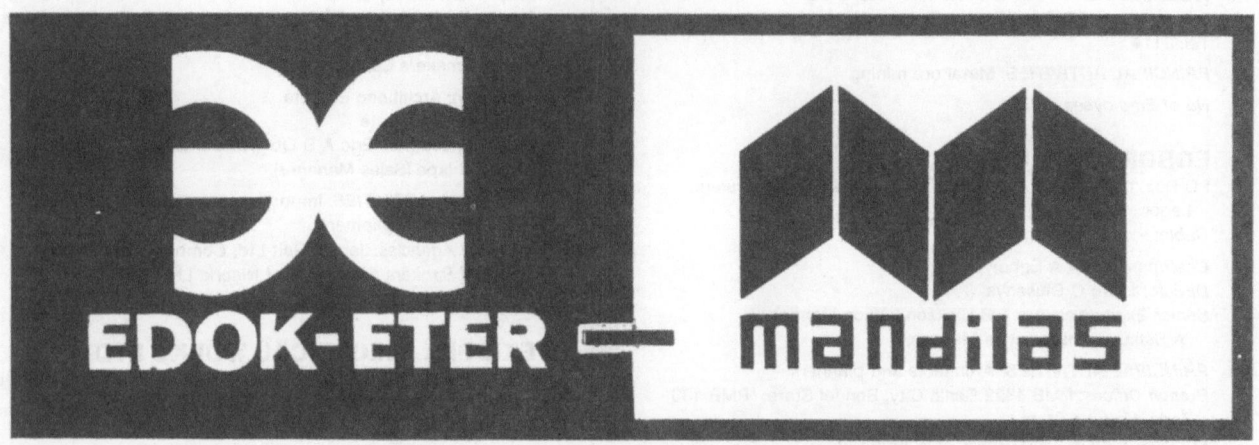

ENGINEERING CONSTRUCTION

LAGOS: REGISTERED OFFICE
96/102 Broad Street
P.O. Box 35
Lagos
Tel: 661967, 662473 Telex: 21121

BENIN: HEAD OFFICE
130, Sapele Road
P.O. Box 776
Benin City
Tel: 243308 Telex: 41127

MAIDUGURI: BRANCH OFFICE
79, Sir Kashim Ibrahim Road
P.M.B. 1220
Maiduguri
Tel: 232995 Telex: 82147

BAUCHI: BRANCH OFFICE
P.O. Box 109 Bauchi
Tel: 42317

EDO86ETL

EKWUEME ASSOCIATES

106 Awolowo Rd, PO Box 5422, Lagos
Tel: 682539
Cable: Atelier Lagos
Telex: 51145 Topark Ng

PRINCIPAL ACTIVITIES: Architects and town planners

ELDER DEMPSTER AGENCIES (NIGERIA) LTD

34 Wharf Rd, PO Box 118, Apapa, Lagos
Tel: 803410
Telex: 21234, 21225 Elder Ng

Chairman: T A Braithwaite
Directors: Chief A O Lawson, I J Ebong, R A Napier, P H D Toosey
Senior Executives: R A Napier (General Manager),
   J B A Olowole (Assistant General Manager, Administration),
   A Barnes (Assistant General Manager, Operations),
   V Usifoh (Apapa Agent)

PRINCIPAL ACTIVITIES: Shipping agents and owners representatives
Principal Agencies: Elder Dempster Lines Ltd, UK
Branch Offices: Custom Rd, PO Box 46, Port Harcourt, Rivers State; Mission Rd, PO Box 42, Bonny, Rivers State
Principal Bankers: First Bank of Nigeria Ltd; Union Bank of Nigeria Ltd

Principal Shareholders: Ocean Linears Ltd, (UK); T A Braithwaite
Date of Establishment: 1970
No of Employees: 350

ELDORADO (NIGERIA) LTD

Henry Carr St, PO Box 237, Ikeja, Lagos
Tel: 962032, 962034, 962036
Cable: Eldonig Ikeja

Chairman: Salem Abu-Hassan
Directors: F S Hassan, S S Hassan, J S Hassan, U Birma
Senior Executives: F A Hassan (General Manager),
   J A Hassan,
   T Petitt (Work Manager)

PRINCIPAL ACTIVITIES: Steel construction, tankers, tippers etc
Principal Agencies: Leventis Motors; Intra Motors
Principal Bankers: First Bank of Nigeria Ltd

Date of Establishment: 1965
No of Employees: 500

ELECTRICAL MATERIAL SUPPLIES (EMS)

Adeola Odutola Estate, Obanikoro, PMB 1110, Mushin, Lagos
Tel: 960736

Senior Executives: I D R Cox (General Manager),
   R W Stainforth (General Sales Manager),
   S Oparah (Commercial Manager),
   R T Chew (Technical)

PRINCIPAL ACTIVITIES: Suppliers of electrical equipment for industrial and domestic installations
Principal Agencies: South Wales Switchgear; MEM; Brooks Motors; AEI Cables; Thorn Lighting; Woods of Colchester; Simplex Fans; Creda Cookers; 3M Jointing Materials; Ottermill Switchgear; I E O Transformers; MK Electric
Branch Offices: Apapa; Ibadan; Kaduna; Kano; Aba; Port Harcourt; Benin
Financial Information: Division of UAC

ELECTRICARE LTD

PO Box 3987, 19 Murtala Muhammed Way, Oyingbo, Ebute Metta, Lagos
Tel: 861243, 862870, 860273, 860016
Cable: Lectricare Lagos
Telex: 26177 Lecare Ng

Chairman: H Ademola Ajayi (also Managing Director)
Directors: C Olatunji Idowu, Adegboyega Oshodi, S I Ajayi, O Osunkeye, Alhayi M O Rotimi, Z O Walter Sannemann
Senior Executives: N E O Ajayi (Operations Manager),
   Mrs T Kuye (Projects Manager)

PRINCIPAL ACTIVITIES: Suppliers of electrical and electronic equipment
Principal Agencies: Kalmar Lighting, Austria; Hume Atkins (Lighting), UK; C M Churchouse/REAL, UK; Maclamp Co Ltd, UK; Julius Sax (Call Systems), UK; Wandsworth Electrical, UK; Access Equipment, UK; Uniline, Denmark; Zerbetto, Italy; Simplex-Ge, UK
Principal Bankers: United Bank for Africa Ltd
Financial Information:

	N'000
Authorised capital	100
Paid-up capital	100

Date of Establishment: 1971

ELECTRO TECHNOLOGIES NIGERIA LTD (ELTEC)

Plot 3F Block 'A' Oshodi Industrial Scheme, Oshodi/Apapa Expressway, PO Box 304, Apapa, Lagos
Tel: 901200
Telex: 26357

Chairman: Sir A Ademola
Directors: Alhaji A I Animashaun,
   G Blaimer,
   Alhaji A Dantata,
   G Goesmann,
   Alhaji I Katune,
   C Ofodile,
   S G Olschewski (Mananging),
   H Troger,
   N Muenz (Deputy Managing Director),
   Prof O Seriki (Executive Director)

PRINCIPAL ACTIVITIES: Suppliers of electrical equipment: electro medical equipment; mainenance and installation of all kinds of electrical and electronic products
Principal Agencies: Siemens AG and affiliated companies
Branch Offices: Kaduna
Associated Companies: Nigerian Cable Manufacturing & Engineering Company, Kano
Principal Bankers: United Bank for Africa Ltd; Societe Generale Bank
Financial Information:

	N'000
Authorised capital	2,000
Paid-up capital	1,572
Turnover	26,000
Profits	1,200

Principal Shareholders: Siemens AG with Nigerian participation
Date of Establishment: 4th September 1970 (Formerly Siemens Nigeria Ltd)
No of Employees: 982

ELECTRODE NIGERIA LTD

137/141 Upper Siluko Rd, PMB 1206, Benin City, Bendel State
Cable: Enimex
Telex: 41145 Enimex

Chairman: H Rau
Directors: T Kiesel, R Fischer, W Erhabor, S I Eweka

PRINCIPAL ACTIVITIES: Manufacturers of mild steel welding electrodes and special welding electrodes such as: surfacing, buffer-layer, tool repairs, cast iron, stainless steel, pipe lines
Financial Information:

	N'000
Authorised capital	1,500
Paid-up capital	400
Sales turnover	1,800

No of Employees: 130

ELECTRONICS INDUSTRIAL COMPANY (NIGERIA) LTD

65 Sapele Rd, PMB 1342, Benin City, Bendel State
Tel: 243436, 243481
Cable: Electrico Benin City
Telex: 1145 Benin City

Chairman: Benson Vincent Aigbadon (also Managing Director)
Directors: Dr Oscar Osche, Letitia Chimela Aigbadon
Senior Executives: P S Amiens (Administrative
 Manager/Accountant),
 P O Ifeta (Sales/Marketing Manager),
 S O P Aganna (Chief Engineer),
 F U Osagie (Administrative Manager)

PRINCIPAL ACTIVITIES: Assemblying and marketing of
 electronic equipment
Principal Agencies: Nordmende, W Germany
Branch Offices: 40 Ezekiel St, Ikeja, Lagos; Q1 Lagos St,
 Kaduna
Principal Bankers: New Nigeria Bank Ltd; United Bank for Africa
 Ltd
Financial Information:

	N'000
Authorised capital	500
Paid-up capital	500
Turnover	2,400

Principal Shareholders: Chairman and directors as described
Date of Establishment: 17th February 1977
No of Employees: 189

ELECTRONICS INSTRUMENTATIONS LTD

N6B/770 Oluseun House, Sango, PO Box 4183 or PMB 5402,
 Ibadan, Oyo State
Tel: 461577
Cable: Theteil
Telex: 20311 TDS IB NG Attn Box 166

Chairman: S A O Odumuye
Directors: E B Osoba, S A Solarin, T O Odufuwa, A M
 Fagbulu, Bayo Majasan

PRINCIPAL ACTIVITIES: Suppliers of electrical and electronic
 equipment, scientific and laboratory instruments,
 telecommunications, agents and general trading
Principal Agencies: Hewlett Packard Inc (USA); Yokogawa
 Electric Works, (Japan); National Air Oil Burner Co Inc, (USA);
 Dinuy SA, (Spain)
Branch Offices: 144 Agege Motor Rd, Atewolara, PO Box 481,
 Mushin, Lagos
Principal Bankers: Cooperative Bank Ltd; Savannah Bank of
 Nigeria Ltd
Financial Information:

	N'000
Authorised capital	100

Principal Shareholders: S A O Odumuye; E B Osoba; S A
 Solarin; T O Odufuwa; A M Fagbulu
Date of Establishment: February 1971

ELEIYELE CASHEW FACTORY

C/o PMB 5085, Eleiyele, Ibadan, Oyo State
Tel: Elecashew

PRINCIPAL ACTIVITIES: Manufacturers of cashew nut shell
 liquid and cashew nuts

ELETTRO ENGINEERING

PO Box 152, 60 Warri/Sapele Rd, Warri, Bendel State
Tel: 233006

Directors: G Maruggi

PRINCIPAL ACTIVITIES: Electrical engineering

ELF NIGERIA LTD

35 Kofo Abayomi Street, Victoria Island, PO Box 927, Lagos
Tel: 614908, 614004, 614075
Cable: Elferap
Telex: 21320 Elf

Chairman: C E Hubault
Directors: P E Godec (Managing Director),
 Chief H O Davies,
 Alj S Iliasu,
 B O Benson,
 E D Hindley,
 J M P Bourgois,
 C Fabre,
 G Gosselin,
 B Polge de Combret
Senior Executives: R Discher (Exploration Manager),
 M Texier (District Manager),
 J C M Mathey (Corporate Affairs Manager),
 C Udenze (Co Secretary/Land & Legal Manager),
 X Daudin (Finance Manager),
 F Van Der Meulen (Project Manager),
 B S Uhuegbulem (Operations Manager),
 S C Iwuchukwu (Administrative Manager),
 A Fanoiki (Gas Affairs Manager)

PRINCIPAL ACTIVITIES: Oil and gas exploration and production
Branch Offices: Plots 3 & 4 Trans Amadi Industrial Layout, PMB
 5160 and PO Box 696, Port Harcourt; Ogunu Base, PO Box
 372, Warri; 1 Tafawa Balewa Rd, Sokoto
Principal Bankers: United Bank for Africa Ltd
Financial Information:

	N'000
Paid-up capital	5,000

EL-KALIL, M, TRANSPORT LTD

251 Apapa Rd, PO Box 1, Apapa, Lagos
Tel: 831686, 331688

PRINCIPAL ACTIVITIES: Haulage contractors

EMANENTO COMPANY AGENCY

44 Tafawa Balewa St, PO Box 878, Jos, Plateau State
Tel: 4418

Chairman: Emmanuel Adoba Entobi (also Managing Director)

PRINCIPAL ACTIVITIES: Agents and general traders, suppliers
 of agricultural equipment, carpets, irrigation equipment,
 motor vehicles, office equipment, scientific instruments etc
Principal Bankers: First Bank of Nigeria Ltd; African Continental
 Bank Ltd

Date of Establishment: 1976

EMBECHEM LTD (FORMERLY MAY & BAKER (NIGERIA) LTD)

Sapara Street, Industrial Estate, PMB 21049, Ikeja, Lagos
Tel: 900201/2, 962832, 962951
Cable: Maybaker, Lagos
Telex: 26258 Mandb Ng Ikj

Chairman: A M Ferguson
Directors: Chief J E A Effah,
 K F Allen (Managing),
 Chief Sir Mobolaji Bank-Anthony,
 I A U Egbuonu (Finance & Co Secretary),
 Prof Deji Femi-Pearse,
 David Dankaro,
 Ronald Bounds
Senior Executives: Dr D J Sheffield (Works Manager),
 M O Famuyide (Admin Manager),
 R M Adams (Pharmaceutical Controller),
 P C Ndukwe (National Sales Manager),
 D O Akinsanmi (Industrial Chemical Manager)

PRINCIPAL ACTIVITIES: Manufacture and distribution of
 pharmaceuticals, chemicals, industrial and agrochemical
 products
Principal Agencies: May & Baker Ltd, (UK); Rhone Poulenc SA,

(France); Whitehall International, (USA); Dr Madhaus &
Company, (West Germany); Lautier Aromatiques, (France)
Branch Offices: 4 Industrial Layout, PO Box 373, Aba, Imo State,
Telex 63125, Tel: 220257; Plot 50 Sharada Industrial Estate,
PO Box 562, Kano, Tel 5519
Subsidiary Companies: May & Baker Ltd, UK; Rhone Poulenc
SA, France
Principal Bankers: First Bank of Nigeria Ltd; Union Bank of
Nigeria Ltd; Societe Generale Bank of Nigeria Ltd;
International Bank for West Africa Ltd; International Merchant
Bank (Nigeria) Ltd
Financial Information:

	₦'000
Authorised capital	2,700
Paid-up capital	2,625
Turnover	15,439
Profits	1,900

Principal Shareholders: May & Baker Ltd (40%)
Date of Establishment: 1943
No of Employees: 450

EMI (NIGERIA) LTD
7 Wharf Rd, PO Box 417, Apapa, Lagos
Tel: 874481, 876036
Cable: Emitron

Chairman: Dr T Abdullahi
Directors: Mallam M I Yahaya,
Alhaji S Makarfi,
M S Wells,
G A Beyering (Managing)
Senior Executives: O A Akinyemi (Chief Executive),
C U Nwaiga (General Manager),
Femi Dairo (Sales Manager),
Bob Okonedo (Creative Manager)

PRINCIPAL ACTIVITIES: Manufacturing and distribution of
gramophone records, cassettes and cartridges; distribution of
musical instruments, etc
Principal Agencies: EMI Worldwide; Labels represented: Arista;
Bell; Cactus; Command; Motown; Mountain; Rare Earth;
Sovereign; MAM; MCA; RAK etc
Principal Bankers: Union Bank of Nigeria Ltd
Date of Establishment: 1962

EMIDSON NIGERIA LTD
18 Obokun St, Ilupeju Estate, Lagos State
Chairman: Duro Oyekanle
PRINCIPAL ACTIVITIES: Manufacturing of household towels and
tissues
Date of Establishment: Started production September 1980

EMIRATE TECHNICAL SERVICES
32 Beirut Rd, PO Box 243, Kano, Kano State
PRINCIPAL ACTIVITIES: Engineering consultants
Financial Information: Subsidiary of Minister Technical Services

EMOS DYNAMICS CO (NIGERIA) LTD
Creek Rd, (Behind Bank of the North), PO Box 1212, Apapa,
Lagos
Tel: 934320
Cable: Emosdyno Lagos

Chairman: Umukoro Ugbede Kesi
Directors: Mrs A Adawa Kesi (Executive Director),
Emonena Kesi
Senior Executives: Ade Oyedele (Financial Controller)

PRINCIPAL ACTIVITIES: General importers and distributors,
business consultants
Subsidiary Companies: Apare Co Ltd

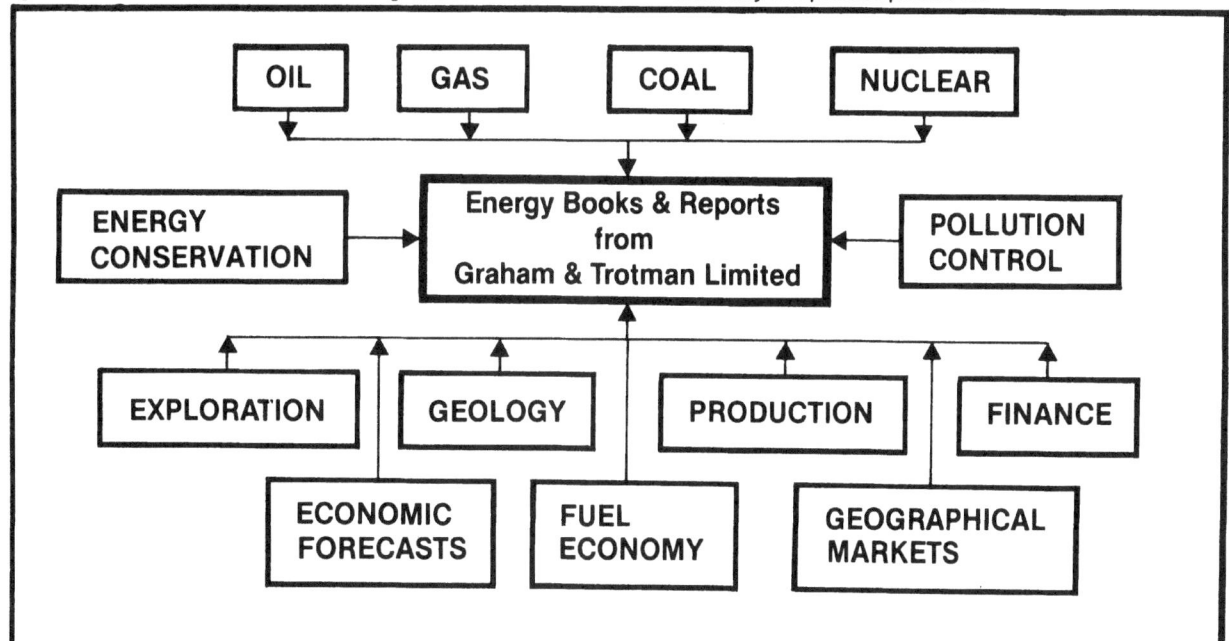

Graham & Trotman Ltd publish a wide range of
titles on energy matters for researchers, scientists,
academics and business executives involved in:
geology, geophysics, geochemistry, soil sciences,
seismology, production engineering, drilling, oil
and gas exploration, energy conservation, pollution
control and many other related fields of study.

For full details of the complete range of energy
titles please write to:
**Marketing Manager (Energy Books and Journals),
Graham & Trotman Ltd, Sterling House,
66 Wilton Road, London SW1V 1DE
Telephone: 01-821 1123
Telex: 298878 GRAMCO G Cables: Infobooks London**

Financial Information:

	N'000
Authorised capital	100
Paid-up capital	50

Principal Shareholders: Emonena Kesi
No of Employees: 166

ENDURANCE LTD
21 New Court Rd, PO Box 1319, Ibadan, Oyo State

Chairman: O I Akinkugbe

PRINCIPAL ACTIVITIES: Suppliers of wholesale and piece goods; building materials

ENGINEERING CONSTRUCTION CO LTD (ECC)
1 Takoradi Rd, Apapa, PO Box 3866, Lagos
Tel: 873469

Directors: H Kunzer

PRINCIPAL ACTIVITIES: Engineering consultants

ENO INDUSTRIES LTD
4a Suzi Gardens, PO Box 516, Jos, Plateau State

PRINCIPAL ACTIVITIES: Mining metal ore

ENOMAH OFFICE EQUIPMENT LTD
102 Murtala Mohammed Way, PO Box 6610, Benin City, Bendel State
Tel: 240606, 241472, 243127, 222472
Telex: 41347 Madona Ng

Chairman: Francis Omo Amadasun
Directors: O T Amadasun, H I Alile
Senior Executives: Godwin Osa Osunde (General Sales Manager),
  Ernest C Odiwanor (Accountant),
  Meshack Duru Godson (Administrative Officer)

PRINCIPAL ACTIVITIES: Office equipment suppliers
Principal Agencies: National Cash Register of Nigeria
Branch Offices: 180 Warri/Sapele Rd, Warri, Bendel State
Subsidiary Companies: Enomah Furniture Factory; Madona Organisation Ltd
Principal Bankers: First Bank of Nigeria Ltd
Financial Information:

	N'000
Authorised capital	50
Paid-up capital	45
Turnover	979
Profits	226

Principal Shareholders: F O Amadasun
Date of Establishment: July 1976
No of Employees: 200

ENPEE INDUSTRIES LTD
Plot K and L, Ilupeju Industrial Estate, PO Box 906, Lagos
Tel: 962200/2
Cable: Enpeeind
Telex: 26130

Chairman: Alhaji I M Damcida
Directors: S V Naik,
  U A Disu,
  N P Kirpalani (Managing)
Senior Executives: M V Vaswani (Production Manager),
  M A K Adekoya (Sales Manager),
  S A Adejobi (Personnel Manager),
  M I Y Oguntibeju (Accountant),
  J O Adeoye (Stores Manager)

PRINCIPAL ACTIVITIES: Manufacturers of suiting, shirting, knitted and printed dress materials, and embroidery lace
Branch Offices: Dalamal House (5th floor), 36 Balogun Sq, Lagos; Factory: Plot 3, Block E, Matori Industrial Scheme, Oshodi, Lagos
Associated Companies: Anglo Africa Agencies (Nigeria) Ltd, Lagos; Globe Commercial Co Ltd, Lagos
Principal Bankers: Union Bank of Nigeria Ltd; United Bank for Africa Ltd
Financial Information:

	N'000
Authorised capital	6,000
Paid-up capital	6,000
Sales turnover	26,000
Profits	3,200

Principal Shareholders: N P Kirpalani and Family; Nigerian Industrial Development Bank Ltd; Anglo Africa Agencies (Nig) Ltd
Date of Establishment: 1969
No of Employees: 2,000

ENVELOPE & FILE CO OF NIGERIA
PO Box 5740, 4 Fasehun Close, Surulere, Lagos
Tel: 835563

PRINCIPAL ACTIVITIES: Suppliers of information storage and retrieval systems, etc
Principal Agencies: Zippel, West Germany

EOM CONSTRUCTION CO LTD
17 Martins St, PO Box 6686, Lagos
Tel: 658486, 830216

PRINCIPAL ACTIVITIES: Civil engineering and construction

EPE PLYWOOD INDUSTRIES LTD
PMB 1009, Epe, Lagos State
Cable: Swinigwood

PRINCIPAL ACTIVITIES: Manufacturers of plywood, veneer, doors, and furniture
Branch Offices: Factory: Erepoto, Epe, Lagos State; Kano

EPPELLION INTERNATIONAL LTD
77/79 Apapa Rd, Ebute-Metta, Lagos

PRINCIPAL ACTIVITIES: Suppliers of computers, calculators, etc
Principal Agencies: International Technical Assistance Corp, USA

EQUATORIAL LINES
3 Ibikunle Akintoye St, PO Box 328, Apapa, Lagos
Tel: 873637
Cable: Torialine Lagos
Telex: 21384 Torial Ng

PRINCIPAL ACTIVITIES: Shipping, shipping agents, clearing and forwarding

EQUITY & GENERAL ACCIDENT INSURANCE COMPANY LTD
Equity House, 29 Zik Ave, PO Box 130, Enugu, Anambra State
Tel: 252485, 253120, 254489
Cable: Equisure

Chairman: Austen Chukwuemeka Nwabude (also Managing Director)
Directors: V K Quist, E O Nwojo, Osita Nwabude, Alhaji U S Ibrahim
Senior Executives: B O Chidozie (Executive Director),
  B C Ezema (Secretary)

PRINCIPAL ACTIVITIES: Insurance
Branch Offices: 51 Idumagbo Ave, PO Box 9677, Lagos; 3 Asa Rd, Aba; 27 Warri/Sapele Rd, Warri; 49B Akpakpava St, Benin City
Associated Companies: Building Materials & Plastic Industries Ltd; Tramet Nigeria Ltd
Principal Bankers: United Bank for Africa Ltd; African Continental Bank Ltd; National Bank Ltd; Co-operative Bank of Eastern Nigeria Ltd
Financial Information:

	₦'000
Authorised capital	500
Paid-up capital	500

Principal Shareholders: A C Nwabude, Osita Nwabude
No of Employees: 250

ERHAHON, R I, & CO LTD

76 Akpakpava St, PO Box 433, Benin City, Bendel State

PRINCIPAL ACTIVITIES: Importers and distributors of general merchandise

ERNESTCO LTD

38 Town Planning Way, Ilupeju, Ikeja, PO Box 4220, Lagos
Tel: 960054, 963613
Cable: Ernestco Ltd

Chairman: Prince Yemi Eweka
Directors: Ernest A Obasuyi (Managing Director), J K Pinheiro
Senior Executives: Ernest Dodoo (Assistant General Manager), Giogio Da Re (Production Manager), Adeleke Adesina (PA to Managing Director), Andrew Ominuta (Personnel Manager), Adesina Banjo (Assistant Production Manager), Godwin Imomoh (Sales/Marketing Manager)

PRINCIPAL ACTIVITIES: Importers/distributors and manufacturing; building materials, furniture, carpets, paints, ceramics/sanitary fittings
Principal Agencies: Linoleum SpA, Italy; Ceramiche le Fiandre, Italy; Amiantite SpA, Italy
Branch Offices: 12 Kachia Rd, PO Box 4009, Kaduna
Subsidiary/Associated Companies: Sellsoman Ltd; Soprog Construction Ltd
Principal Bankers: United Bank for Africa Ltd
Financial Information:

	₦'000
Authorised capital	1,000
Paid-up capital	1,000
Sales turnover	3,500

Principal Shareholders: Prince Yemi Eweka; Ernest A Obasuyi
Date of Establishment: 1974
No of Employees: 225

ERNST & WHINNEY, ONI, LASEBIKAN & COMPANY

PO Box 2442, 25 Boyle St, Lagos
Tel: 636980, 652939, 636053
Cable: Demonstrat
Telex: 21510 Ernst Ng

Directors: A O Lasebikan, J Kirkpatrick, C Cartwright
PRINCIPAL ACTIVITIES: Chartered Accountants

ESLON NIGERIA LTD

8 Inuwa Abdulkadir Rd, PO Box 1427, Kaduna
Tel: 216166

Chairman: Alhaji A S Maiyaki
Directors: S Hosaka (Managing), Mrs E O Daniyan, S Buhari, U Goji, N Badamasi, K Tamaki, Dr N Sagane

Senior Executives: Y A Suleiman (Chief Accountant/Administration Manager), Y Higuchi (Production Manager), M B Girei (Sales Manager), A Horiike (Chief Engineer)

PRINCIPAL ACTIVITIES: Manufacturers of PVC pipes and allied products
Principal Bankers: Union Bank of Nigeria Ltd; ICON Ltd
Financial Information:

	₦'000
Authorised capital	600
Paid-up capital	600
Turnover	2,326

Principal Shareholders: Northern Nigeria Investments Ltd; Sekisui Chemical Company Ltd, Japan; Nichimen Corporation, Japan
Date of Establishment: 1977
No of Employees: 78

ESSDEE FOOD PRODUCTS NIGERIA LTD

Plot 8 Isolo Rd, Mushin, Lagos
Tel: 835868

PRINCIPAL ACTIVITIES: Production of soft drinks

ESTATE ELECTRICAL INDUSTRIES (NIGERIA) LTD

Plot 34 Davies Estate, PO Box 148, Ikeja, Lagos
Tel: 963534
Telex: 26731 Eselin Ng

Directors: M O Adejinmi (Managing)

PRINCIPAL ACTIVITIES: Suppliers of electrical goods, armoured cable, lighting apparatus, etc
Branch Offices: 12 Isheri Rd, Ikeja, Lagos; 52 Olowu Rd, Ikeja, Lagos; 9 Ipodu Rd, Ikeja, Lagos
Associated Companies: Folam International Trading Company
Principal Bankers: United Bank for Africa Ltd

ETCO-ENGINEERING & TECHNICAL COMPANY (NIGERIA) LTD

14 Creek Rd, PO Box 337, Apapa
Tel: 876046, 873627, 876658
Telex: 22481 Etco Ng

Chairman: Chief C O Madarikan
Directors: C Weiss (Managing), A A Balogun, B O Ibru, I Weiss (Acting Managing Director)

PRINCIPAL ACTIVITIES: Electrical, air conditiong, refrigeration and mechanical engineering contractors
Branch Offices: 50B Arigidi Street, Bodija Estate, PO Box 1755, Ibadan, Tel 415426; 3 Saba Close, Rumola Junction, Aba Rd, PMB 5358, Port Harcourt, Tel 330579; 3A Eyo Etta Street, PMB 1111, Calabar, Tel 220497; Also at Warri & Ajaokuta
Principal Bankers: International Bank for West Africa Ltd; First Bank of Nigeria Ltd
Financial Information:

	₦'000
Authorised capital	200
Paid-up capital	100
Turnover	12,000

Principal Shareholders: C Weiss; T O Madarikan; M O Balogun; B O Ibru
Date of Establishment: June 1963
No of Employees: 450

ETERNA ELECTRICAL ENGINEERING WORKS LTD

6 Kachia Rd, PO Box 345, Kaduna
Tel: 213991
Cable: Eterna
Telex: 71138 Etelen Ng

PRINCIPAL ACTIVITIES: Suppliers of metal furniture, air
conditioning and   refrigeration items

ETCO (NIGERIA) LIMITED
Engineering & Technical Company

ELECTRICAL, MECHANICAL AND AIRCONDITIONING ENGINEERING CONTRACTORS

Head office:
14 Creek Road,
PO Box 337,
Apapa NIGERIA.
Tel: 876046, 873627, 876658
Telex: 22481 ETCO NG

Branches:

3A Eyo Etta Street
Housing Estate
PMB 1111
CALABAR
Tel: 087-220497

3 Saba Close
Rumola Junction
Aba Road, PMB 5358
PORT-HARCOURT
Tel: 084-330579

50B Arigidi Street
Bodija Estate
PO Box 1755
IBADAN
Tel: 022-415426

Micheletti compound
Airport Road
PO Box 1595
WARRI
— Also at Ajaokuta

ETERNIT LTD

Sapele-Warri Rd, PO Box 483, Sapele, Bendel State
Tel: 41311
Cable: Eternit
Telex: 42265 Eterok Ng

Chairman: A Piessevaux
Directors: R G Cairns (Managing),
    O Abiola (Finance),
    M Rousseau (Technical),
    J G Rutgers,
    J A Moens,
    S A Onomakpome,
    P Ehizokhale

PRINCIPAL ACTIVITIES: Manufacture of fibre-cement roofing
    and ceiling sheets
Branch Offices: Aba-Owerri Rd, Aba, Imo State; Sakpoba Rd,
    Benin City, Bendel State
Principal Bankers: United Bank for Africa Ltd; Union Bank of
    Nigeria Ltd
Financial Information:

	₦'000
Authorised capital	5,000
Paid-up capital	5,000
Turnover	20,000

Date of Establishment: 1974
No of Employees: 400

ETHIOPE FOOD INDUSTRIES LTD

Jesse, Near Sapele, Bendel State

Directors: Isaac Oghom Onor (Managing Director)

PRINCIPAL ACTIVITIES: Production of glucose and industrial
    starch

ETHIOPE PUBLISHING CORPORATION

PMB 1332, Ring Rd, Benin City, Bendel State
Tel: 243036, 243870
Cable: Ethiope Benin
Telex: 41110 Ethiope Ng

Chairman: Chief G B L Oyakhire
Directors: Chief B E Ugbonwa, C M Aboh, Pius Dongo, Dr Mrs A
    Uduebor
Senior Executives: R U Iredia (Secretary),
    A O Ikuenobe (Acting General Manager)

PRINCIPAL ACTIVITIES: Publishing of books
Principal Bankers: New Nigeria Bank Ltd

Principal Shareholders: Government of Bendel State sponsored
    corporation
Date of Establishment: 1970
No of Employees: 66

ETUK MOTORS TECHNICAL COMPANY LTD

47 Nwaniba Rd, PO Box 346, Uyo, Cross River State
Tel: 729

Chairman: F V Etuk
Directors: A F Etuk,   P F Etuk
Senior Executives: M C Udoh (Engineer),
    Hyacinth P Onwutebe (Secretary)

PRINCIPAL ACTIVITIES: Agents and general traders, mechanical
    engineering and motor vehicles and components specialists
Principal Bankers: African Continental Bank Ltd

Principal Shareholders: P F Etuk; A F Etuk; J V Etuk
Date of Establishment: 28th February 1977

EUROTRADE (NIGERIA) LTD

7A Oduduwa Rd, PO Box 1216, Apapa, Lagos
Tel: 876566/8/9
Cable: Eurotra, Lagos
Telex: 22263 Eurlos Ng

Chairman: Nicolas K Shacolas
Directors: Femi Coker (Deputy Executive Chairman),
    Spyros Phylactis (Vice Chairman),
    Alhaji Kabir Bayero (Executive Director),
    Dimitris Mouskos,
    Abayomi Sogbesan,
    Henry Omo,
    Costas Tsentas,
    J Wariso
Senior Executives: Panikos Papadakis (General Manager),
    Femi Owoyemi (Deputy General Manager),
    Spyros Ioannou (Assistant General Manager),
    Andreas Karkotis (Regional Manager, Port Harcourt),
    Timothy Okelola (Area Manager, Lagos),
    Alex Imoukhuede (Area Manager, Kano)

PRINCIPAL ACTIVITIES: Production of cement, importers of
    maize, concentrates, soyabeanmeal, fishmeal, calcium
    carbonate, building materials, foodstuffs, general
    commodities, machinery and equipment
Principal Agencies: Ruari Europe and World Trade Co Ltd (UK);
    NKS Eurotrade (UK) Ltd, (UK); US Steel International
    Corporation, (USA); Cementa, (Sweden); CBR, (Belgium);
    Heracles General Cement, (Greece); Nestle, (Switzerland)
Branch Offices: 7 Abiriba Street, Port Harcourt, Tel 331267,
    331272, Cables: Eurotra, Port Harcourt; 66 Maganda Rd,
    Kano, Cables, Eurotra, Kano; Akintola Road Extension,
    Sapele Cables: Eurotra, Sapele
Associated Companies: Eurotrade Cement Works (Nigeria) Ltd;
    Gulf Agency and Shipping (Nigeria) Ltd; Gasni Clearing
    International Ltd

Principal Bankers: Savannah Bank of Nigeria Ltd; Societe
  General Bank (Nigeria) Ltd
Financial Information:

	₦'000
Authorised capital	1,000
Paid-up capital	550
Turnover	150,000

Date of Establishment: 18th March 1977
No of Employees: 2,000

EVANS BROTHERS (NIGERIA) LTD

Jericho Rd, PMB 5164, Ibadan, Oyo State
Tel: 417570, 417601, 417626
Cable: Edbooks Ibadan
Telex: 31104

Chairman: Dr S J Cookey
Directors: David da Cunha (Deputy Chairman),
  B O Bolodeoku (Managing Director),
  R A Oyewole (Administrative/Trade Director),
  S A Oke (Sales Director),
  Dr A M Fagbulu,
  F S J Austin,
  E J Lincoln,
  S Pawley
Senior Executives: E A Akinyemi (Chief Accountant/Company
  Secretary)

PRINCIPAL ACTIVITIES: Book publishing and distribution
Principal Agencies: Holt-Saunders Ltd (UK); Scholastics Inc,
  (USA); Financial Training Packs, (UK); Rex Collings, (UK)
Branch Offices: NF12 Maiduguri Rd, PO Box 1511, Kaduna,
  Kaduna State; 120 Orlu Rd, PMB 1541, Owerri, Imo State
Associated Companies: Evans Brothers Ltd, UK
Principal Bankers: United Bank for Africa Ltd; Union Bank of
  Nigeria Ltd; Icon Ltd
Financial Information:

	₦'000
Authorised capital	1,000
Paid-up capital	700

Principal Shareholders: Nigerians: Evans Brothers Ltd, London
Date of Establishment: 6th December 1966
No of Employees: 140

EVANS MEDICAL (NIGERIA) LTD

41 Creek Rd, Apapa, PO Box 2070, Lagos
Tel: 875108, 875430

PRINCIPAL ACTIVITIES: Suppliers of pharmaceuticals

EVERETT TRADING & MANUFACTURING CO LTD
ETAM

Etam House, 19 Alhaji Issa William St, Lagos
Tel: 661902, 662072
Telex: 21858 Etamco

PRINCIPAL ACTIVITIES: Importers and general traders
Branch Offices: 11 Caulcrick Rd, Apapa, Lagos Tel 873089,
  873080; 8 Dele Bakare Rd, Kirikiri, Apapa, Lagos; E9/2607
  New Ife Rd, Opposite Mobile Petrol Station, Ibadan; Plot 116
  Trans-Amadi Industrial Layout, Port Harcourt, Rivers State; 5
  Pategi Rd, Ilorin, Kwara State

EVIAN AFRICA CO LTD

13 Kofo Abayomi Ave, PO Box 6050, Apapa, Lagos
Tel: 875028

PRINCIPAL ACTIVITIES: General importers and exporters

EXCEL PLASTIC INDUSTRIES LTD

PMB 1309, Ikot Ishie, Calabar, Cross River State
Tel: 220240
Cable: Excel
Telex: 65143

PRINCIPAL ACTIVITIES: Manufacturers of plastic pipes
Branch Offices: Kaduna; Jos; Makurdi; Ilorin; Enugu; Benin;
  Lagos

Date of Establishment: November 1976

EXCELSIOR GARMENT FACTORY LTD

Block 2 Units 1 and 2 Industrial Estate, PO Box 1021, Yaba,
  Lagos
Tel: 861322

PRINCIPAL ACTIVITIES: Textiles and clothing manufactures

EXIMPORT & COMPANY NIGERIA LTD

6 Agege Motor Rd, PMB 1399, Ikeja, Lagos
Tel: 834661
Telex: 21563 Ademar Ng; 21173 Cosale Ng

PRINCIPAL ACTIVITIES: Suppliers, importers of domestic
  appliances, scientific equipment, sports and leisure goods

EX-LANDS NIGERIA LTD

PO Barakin Ladi, Via Jos, Plateau State
Tel: 6
Cable: Nigelus

Chairman: T Penhale
Directors: Alhaji M Aliyu, J D Lines, H R Mitchell, I A Olaniyan

PRINCIPAL ACTIVITIES: Mining; production of tin concentrates
Principal Bankers: Barclays Bank Nigeria Ltd
Financial Information:

	₦'000
Authorised capital	700
Paid-up capital	700

Principal Shareholders: Ex-Lands Ltd, London, UK
No of Employees: 900

EXPRESS INSURANCE COMPANY LTD

136 Nnamdi Azikiwe St, Lagos
Tel: 663916, 663840, 662880

PRINCIPAL ACTIVITIES: Insurance
Branch Offices: Ikeja; Apapa; Ibadan; Abeokuta; Ondo; Akure;
  Oshogbo; Benin; Agbor; Warri; Aba; Onitsha; Port Harcourt;
  Calabar; Zaria; Kano; Maiduguri; Sokoto

Date of Establishment: July 1969

EXPRESS INTERNATIONAL MARITIME LTD

78A Old Ojo Rd, Amuwo, Opposite Festac Village, Badagry
  Expressway, PO Box 293, Apapa, Lagos

PRINCIPAL ACTIVITIES: Shipping agents, clearing, forwarding,
  warehousing

EZE, I O, & SONS LTD

1 Aneliaku Close, New Era Layout, PO Box 652, Uwani-Enugu,
  Anambra State
Tel: 254093

Chairman: Chief Innocent O Eze
Directors: R O Eze, Mrs P O Eze, Remy Eze, Ejinkonye Eze
Senior Executives: B I Jidere (Administrative Manager)

PRINCIPAL ACTIVITIES: Building and civil engineering
  contractors; manufacturers of all types of office and
  household furniture
Branch Offices: Wood Working Machines Section: 6 Oba Street,
  Ogui, Enugu
Principal Bankers: First Bank of Nigeria Ltd; African Continental
  Bank Ltd
Financial Information:

	₦'000
Authorised capital	200
Paid-up capital	200
Turnover	213
Profits	17

Principal Shareholders: Directors as described
Date of Establishment: Incorporated as a Limited Liability
  Company in June 1979
No of Employees: 80

EZEILO, C C

26 Oblagu Rd, PMB 1166, Enugu, Anambra State
Tel: 254811
Cable: Cezo

Chairman: Simon Ezeilo
Directors: K Obiajulu,
  Mrs F Ezeilo,
  C Ezeilo (Managing Director)
Senior Executives: C Ochor (Secretary),
  D Obiajulu (Sales Manager)

PRINCIPAL ACTIVITIES: Importing and marketing of furniture;
  chair bases; drawer locks; furniture handles, etc
Principal Agencies: Siso A/S, Denmark
Branch Offices: 13 William St, Onitsha, Anambra State
Principal Bankers: First Bank of Nigeria Ltd; African Continental
  Bank Ltd
Financial Information:

	₦'000
Authorised capital	200
Paid-up capital	120
Sales turnover	700

Principal Shareholders: C Ezeilo; Oliver Ezeilo; Mrs F Ezeilo

EZENNWA, S N, & SONS LTD

5 Railway Layout, Station Rd, PO Box 417, Enugu, Anambra
  State
Tel: 254607

Chairman: Chief S N Ezennwa (also Managing Director)
Directors: E Ezennwa, Mrs H Ezennwa, B O Ezennwa
Senior Executives: E C Udokwu (Manager),
  R Ezenuhe (General Supervisor),
  P Umeis (Inspector of Works),
  A C Ukpabia (Accounting Officer)

PRINCIPAL ACTIVITIES: Civil engineering and construction
Associated Companies: J J Sisca, USA
Principal Bankers: Co-operative Bank of Eastern Nigeria Ltd
Financial Information:

	₦'000
Authorised capital	400
Paid-up capital	400

No of Employees: 400

F G SPIROPOULOS & COMPANY LTD

See SPIROPOULOS, F G, & COMPANY LTD

F M BARSHALL (WEST AFRICA) LTD

See BARSHALL, F M, (WEST AFRICA) LTD

F STEINER & COMPANY LTD

See STEINER, F, & COMPANY LTD

FADO ENGINEERING CO LTD

Phoenix Motors Bldg, 52/54 Murtala Mohammed Way, PO Box
  35, Ebute-Metta, Lagos
Tel: 861160

PRINCIPAL ACTIVITIES: Mechanical engineering

FAGBAMIGBE, OLAIYA, LTD

11 Methodist Church Rd, PO Box 14, Akure, Ondor State
Tel: 2075
Cable: Fagbamigbe Akure

Chairman: Olaiya Fagbamigbe (also Managing Director)
Directors: Mrs Ebun Fagbamigbe, Dr Kole Omotoso, Alex
  Adeniyi Adedipe, Mazi Kalu Okorie, Oluwadare Aguda,
  Bunmi Iyeru, Bode Fagbayibo
Senior Executives: Babatunde Fagbohun (Administrative
    Manager),
  Sunday Ige (Warehouse Manager),
  Jide Solabi (Sales Manager),
  Femi Alabi (Sales Manager, Library Books)

PRINCIPAL ACTIVITIES: Book publishing and distribution;
  publishers' representatives
Principal Agencies: Paddington Press, UK; Harvester Press, UK;
  Wardlock Ltd, UK; Pergammon Press, UK; Mills & Boon Ltd,
  UK; Collins Publishers, UK; Blackie & Sons Ltd, UK; Holmes
  MacDougall Ltd, UK
Branch Offices: Ife Rd, PO Box 1176, Agodi Gate, Ibadan, Oyo
  State
Principal Bankers: Co-operative Bank Ltd; National Bank of
  Nigeria Ltd; Barclays Bank Nigeria Ltd

Principal Shareholders: Olaiya Fagbamigbe; Yetund
  Fagbamigbe; Olugbenga Fagbamigbe; Yemi Fagbamigbe;
  Toyin Fagbamigbe; Dupe Fagbamigbe; Duyi Fagbamigbe

FALCON NIGERIA LTD

Investment House, 21-25 Broad St, PO Box 3820, Lagos
Tel: 632655, 636404
Cable: Falcolin Lagos
Telex: 21523 Falcon Ng

PRINCIPAL ACTIVITIES: Shipping

FALLAD COMMERCIAL ENTERPRISES LTD

2nd Floor, NPA Building, Container Terminal Co, Lily Pond, Ijora,
  Lagos
Tel: 830601

PRINCIPAL ACTIVITIES: Clearing and forwarding agents;
  transportation by sea, land and air; container specialists and
  warehousing

FALTAS, A M, (WEST AFRICA) LTD

PO Box 1915, 62/64 Campbell St, Lagos
Tel: 612174, 613039, 658425

PRINCIPAL ACTIVITIES: Suppliers of graphic art materials and
  equipment, medical and catering equipment

FAN MILK LTD

PO Box 1617, Eleiyele Rd, Ibadan, Oyo State
Tel: 412032
Cable: Niger Fan Ibadan

PRINCIPAL ACTIVITIES: Manufacturers of dairy products
Branch Offices: Apapa

FANZ HOLDINGS LTD

8 Sanni Adewale Street, PO Box 4034, Lagos
Tel: 663158
Cable: Fanze
Telex: 21457 Fanhol Ng

Chairman: Chief Francis Arthur Nzeribe (Executive)
Directors: Chief Frank S Giwa-Osagie,
  Chief (Dr) Vivian G Ene,
  Alhaji M Kabiru Bayero,
  Col Sanni Bello,
  Alhaji Musa T Waziri,
  Chief Olayiwole O Aina
Senior Executives: Chief Olayiwole O Aina (Managing Director,
    Sentinel Assurance Co Ltd),
  J B Nzeribe (Group Financial Director),
  B M A Saldanha (General Manager, Fanz Water Resources),
  V C Oputa (General Manager, Haven Nigeria Computer Co
    Ltd),
  Obi Nzeribe (General Manager, Fanz Scientific & Educational
    Equipment Ltd)

PRINCIPAL ACTIVITIES: Holding company with 14 subsidiaries engaged in: building and civil engineering, discovery and developments of water resources, dams, irrigation schemes, construction, of water works, etc., suppliers of scientific, educational and research equipment; installation and servicing of computer equipment; suppliers of catering and hotel equipment, chemicals for general specialised laboratory work and research; general importers and exporters; manufacturers' representatives; printing, publishing, public relations and contract advertising; insurance; transport contractors, manufacturers of fermented spirits and alcohol; biological microbiological and food manufacturing; suppliers of prefabricated houses, building materials, etc
Principal Agencies: Computer Machinery Company Ltd, UK
Branch Offices: 8 Sanni Adewale Street, Lagos; 4 Presidential Rd, Enugu; 31/33 Martin Street, Lagos; 9a Post Office Rd, Kano; 126 Broad Street, Lagos; 94 Bode Thomas Street, Surulere, Lagos; 65 Grosvenor St, London
Subsidiary Companies: Fanz International Ltd, UK; Fanz Construction Co Ltd; Frank & Frank Construction Ltd; Fanz Water Resources Ltd; Fanz Scientific & Educational Equipment Ltd; Haven Nigeria Computer Co Ltd; Zebra Consultants Ltd; Peninsula Enterprises Ltd; Twilights Public Relations Ltd; Tribita Group (Nigeria) Ltd; Fanz Distillers Ltd; Fanz Transport Ltd; Sentinel Assurance Co Ltd; Fanz Laboratories Ltd; Unifer House (Nigeria) Ltd
Principal Bankers: Savannah Bank (Nigeria) Ltd; Societe Generale Bank Nigeria Ltd; First Bank of Nigeria Ltd; Union Bank of Nigeria Ltd
Financial Information:

	₦'000
Authorised capital	5,200
Paid-up capital	5,200
Turnover (1981)	45,900
Profits	3,400

Principal Shareholders: Chief F A Nzeribe
Date of Establishment: 1962
No of Employees: 4,920

FAR EAST MERCANTILE CO LTD
PO Box 302, 64 Balogun St, Lagos
Tel: 632275

PRINCIPAL ACTIVITIES: Importers and distributors of general merchandise
Branch Offices: Stores: 4b Ijora Causeway, Lagos, Tel 837022

FARAWAMETZ CONSTRUCTION CO LTD
39 Idungaran St, Lagos
Tel: 632883

Directors: G F Moos

PRINCIPAL ACTIVITIES: Construction

FARRELL LINES INTERNATIONAL (NIGERIA) LTD
42/44 Warehouse Rd, PMB 1151, Apapa, Lagos
Tel: 877459, 874118, 874207
Cable: Farship
Telex: 21226 Mafric

Directors: Bronson Hart Fargo, Jnr
Senior Executives: Alhaji G A Shodunke

PRINCIPAL ACTIVITIES: Shipping
Principal Agencies: Farrell Lines Inc, USA

Date of Establishment: 1947

FAS BROTHERS LTD
36 Idumagbo Ave, PO Box 216, Ebute-Metta, Lagos
Tel: 631893, 830878

PRINCIPAL ACTIVITIES: Importers, general merchants, transporters and general contractors

FASHION SHOE COMPANY (NIGERIA) LTD
Alaoji Nwaforunwa, Off Ariaria Market, PMB 7327, Aba, Imo State
Tel: 221676

Chairman: General T Y Danjuma
Directors: J R Anyaehie, T Murai, S Ninagawa

PRINCIPAL ACTIVITIES: Joint venture between Nigeria and Italian industrialists to produce high quality shoes of all types
Branch Offices: Show room: 172 Sam Mbakwe Rd, Aba, Imo State
Principal Bankers: Union Bank of Nigeria Ltd; International Bank for West Africa Ltd
Financial Information:

	₦'000
Authorised capital	400
Paid-up capital	240
Turnover	4,000
Profits	300

Principal Shareholders: TID; SA; Gen T Y Danjuma; J R Anyaehie
Date of Establishment: 24h June 1980
No of Employees: 100

FATMOK ASSOCIATES
PO Box 4274, Ibadan, Oyo State
Tel: 412680

Chairman: J A Adeduntan
Directors: Mrs M O Akintola (Marketing), Kola Akintola (Managing Director)

PRINCIPAL ACTIVITIES: Metal fabrication/manufacturing, agents and general trading, importers and exporters
Principal Agencies: U A C (Textiles); C F A O; Westex Ltd
Principal Bankers: International Bank for West Africa Ltd; National Bank of Nigeria Ltd; Savannah Bank; Cooperative Bank

Date of Establishment: 12th October 1977

FATSPORTS INDUSTRIES LTD
Plot 71 Oyadiran Estate, Sabo, Yaba, Lagos
Tel: 861135
Cable: Fatsports

PRINCIPAL ACTIVITIES: Suppliers of all types of sports equipment

FAWAZ STEELWOOD & CHEMICALS (KANO) LTD
Umaru Babura Rd, Bompai Industrial Area, PO Box 980, Kano
Tel: 4794, 4796
Cable: Fast
Telex: 77141 Fast Ng

Chairman: A K Fawaz
Directors: H K Fawaz (Managing Director),
E H C Ward,
Mallam Ali Baba,
Alhaji Aminu Ibrahim,
Alhaji Farou Mohammed,
Alhaji Kabiru Ahmed,
Mallam Yusufu Abdullah,
Alhaji Ibrahim,
Mallam Kabirumar,
A K Fawaz (Executive Chairman),
Alhaji Mohammed L Mohammed (Director/Administrative)
Senior Executives: T M Halaoui (Production Manager),
William S F Durojaiye (Accountant)

PRINCIPAL ACTIVITIES: Manufacturers of steelwood and wooden furniture, aluminium doors and windows
Associated Companies: Northern Sawmill Ltd; Sokoto Furniture Factory Ltd
Principal Bankers: Bank of the North Ltd

Principal Shareholders: Kano State Investment Co Ltd
No of Employees: 272

FAWEHINMI FURNITURE FACTORY LTD

1 Fawehinmi Furniture Rd, PO Box 408, Onike, Yaba, Lagos
Tel: 860066
Cable: Fagifagi Yaba

Chairman: S I Fawehinmi
Directors: E O A Fawehinmi (Production Manager),
  R A Fawehinmi (Administrative Manager)

PRINCIPAL ACTIVITIES: Office and household furniture
  manufacturing
Principal Bankers: Barclays Bank Nigeria Ltd
Financial Information:

	N'000
Authorised capital	300
Paid-up capital	250
Sales turnover	998
Profits	139

Principal Shareholders: Chairman and directors as described
No of Employees: 300

FEDCO FOAM (NIGERIA) LTD

24 Ja'afaru Rd, PO Box 661, Kano
Tel: 4333
Cable: Fedco Kano
Telex: 77143

PRINCIPAL ACTIVITIES: Manufacturers of polyurethane foam
  articles

FEDERAL MINISTRY OF INDUSTRIES

Federal Secretariat Complex, Phase I, 8th Floor, PMB 12614,
  Ikoyi, Lagos

Chairmen: Alhaji Ibrahim Gusau (Hon Minister of Industries), Dr
  I J Igbani (Hon Minister of State),
Directors: M E P Udebiuwa (Permanent Secretary),
  Alhaji Magaji Muhammed (Director Project Implementation),
  A O Oluwunmi (Director, Industrial Policy and Planning),
  Mrs L B Onafeko (Secretary Administration and Finance),
  D O Ogun (Director, Nigerian Standards Organisation),
  A O Okwura (Director, Industrial Inspectorate),
  Alhaji Lawal Tudunwada (Director-General, Industrial Training
  Fund),
  M W Gadzama (Executive Chairman of Nigerian Enterprises
  Promotion Board)

PRINCIPAL ACTIVITIES: Government body
Branch Offices: Nigerian Standards Organisation, 4 Club Rd,
  Enugu; Industrial Training Fund, 8th Floor, Federal
  Secretariat, PMB 2199, Jos; Industrial Inspectorate Division,
  11 Kofo Abayomi St, Victoria Island, Lagos; Nigerian
  Enterprises Promotion Board, 72 Campbell St, Tafawa Balewa
  Square, Lagos

FEDERAL MORTGAGE BANK OF NIGERIA

11 Breadfruit Street, PO Box 2078, Lagos
Tel: 662860, 662982
Telex: 21840 Fembk

Chairman: O Ukenonu
Directors: Chief S B Falegan (Managing),
  Alhaji M Bature,
  Alhaji M Maude,
  Alhaji M S Agaie,
  F Ola Uddoh,
  Sylvester N B Menegbo,
  Alhaji A Muktar,
  F B O Olokun

PRINCIPAL ACTIVITIES: Provision of finance
Branch Offices: Throughout Nigeria

Principal Shareholders: Federal Ministry of Finance; Central
  Bank of Nigeria Ltd

FEDERAL RADIO CORPORATION OF NIGERIA (FRCN)

Broadcasting House, PMB 12504, Lagos
Tel: 603010/14

Directors: G Bako (Director General)

PRINCIPAL ACTIVITIES: Federal Government owned national
  radio network. This replaced the Nigerian Broadcasting
  Corporation

Date of Establishment: 1978

FEDERATED CORK & SEAL COMPANY LTD

12 Olofin Rd, PMB 1059, Apapa, Lagos
Tel: 876620
Cable: Altransla Lagos

PRINCIPAL ACTIVITIES: Bottle caps manufacturers
Branch Offices: Mile 60 Lagos Rd, Abeokuta, Ogun State

FEDERATED MOTOR INDUSTRIES

17 Creek Rd, PO Box 376, Apapa, Lagos
Tel: 875535, 875539, 875584
Cable: Unavehicle Apapa

Senior Executives: P J Reagan (General Manager)

PRINCIPAL ACTIVITIES: Commercial vehicle assembly plant,
  vehicle body manufacturers

Date of Establishment: 1959

FEDERATION PRODUCTS (NIGERIA) LTD

38 Burma Rd, PO Box 65, Apapa, Lagos
Tel: 875448

PRINCIPAL ACTIVITIES: Leather products manufacturers
Branch Offices: 11 Ashanti Rd, Apapa, Lagos, Tel 874085
Associated Companies: K Chellaram Ltd (see separate entry)

FELICITY ENGINEERING CO LTD

214 Ikorodu Rd, Palm-Grove, PO Box 105, Lagos
Tel: 846385
Cable: Feliceng

Chairman: Felix Abiodun Sodimu
Directors: Biodun Sodimu, Miss Foluso Funmilayo Sodimu
Senior Executives: S O Osiguwa (Contract Manager),
  M A Omokheyeke (Project Engineer),
  M A Yusuf (Administrative Manager),
  M A Sodimu (Purchasing Manager),
  A Adenopo (Accountant)

PRINCIPAL ACTIVITIES: External and internal electrical
  installation contractors
Branch Offices: 25 Eguadase St, PO Box 333, Benin City;
  Reservation Rd, Sagamu Bye Pass, PO Box 268, Sagamu
Principal Bankers: United Bank for Africa Ltd

Principal Shareholders: Felix Abiodun Sodimu Foluso
  Olufunmilayo Sodimu
No of Employees: 200

FELICO INDUSTRIES NIGERIA

PO Box 335, Surulere, Lagos

PRINCIPAL ACTIVITIES: Manufacturers of sodium hypochlorite
  solution
Branch Offices: Office Location: 110 Olatunde Labinjo Ave, Km
  12 Mile 7, Ikorodu Rd, Lagos

FEMCE MARKETING COMPANY

1 Chapel Street, PO Box 2943, Lagos

Chairman: Mike Niyi
Directors: F A Fimihan, Tayo Boje, Prince M F Ade
Senior Executives: Omoniyi Alabi Ade (Import and Business
  Consultant Manager)

PRINCIPAL ACTIVITIES: International importers, purchasing and business consultants
Principal Agencies: Yang & Co, Hongkong; Kawashimaya & Co Ltd, Japan; Thammikary International Corporation USA
Branch Offices: 11 Oladipo Street, Mushin, Lagos
Associated Companies: Michalies Phlemon & Associates
Principal Bankers: Nigeria-Arab Bank Ltd
Financial Information:
Authorised capital   ₦ 400,000

Principal Shareholders: Mike Niyi (40%); F A Fimihan (30%); Wumi Phlemon (30%)
Date of Establishment: March 1974

FEMINA HYGIENICAL PRODUCTS (NIGERIA) LTD

28 Trans Amadi Industrial Layout, PO Box 722, Port Harcourt, Rivers State
Tel: 334018
Cable: Femina
Telex: 61159 Fem Ng

Directors: S L Chellaram,
    L L Chellaram,
    Chief T J Sokoh,
    B Menezes (Managing)

PRINCIPAL ACTIVITIES: Manufacturers of toiletry products; surgical cotton wool etc
Branch Offices: 21 Ibiwe Street, Benin
Principal Bankers: United Bank for Africa Ltd

Date of Establishment: 1973

FEMO (WEST AFRICA) LTD

KM 10 Abeokuta Rd, PO Box 12623, Ibadan, Oyo State

PRINCIPAL ACTIVITIES: Production of fabric leather for furniture, shoes, bags and automotive requirements, vinyl floors, wall papers, tarpaulin etc
Branch Offices: Factory: 2 Orita Rd, PO Box 23, Eruwa, Oyo State

FEMOPE MARKETING COMPANY

83 Palm Avenue, PO Box 1543, Mushin, Lagos State
Tel: 847448, 880965
Cable: Femopemark Lagos

Chairman: I O Moradeyo
Directors: M M Moradeyo
Senior Executives: Mrs E M Oni (Administrative Head of Department),
    S A Balogun (Sales Manager),
    I O Moradeyo (General Manager),
    J Tsakpohore (Stores Manager),
    M M Moradeyo (Accounts Supervisor),
    G Umoh (Workshop Supervisor)

PRINCIPAL ACTIVITIES: Marketing and distributing of specialized surgical instruments, medical disposables and equipment
Principal Agencies: Fra Production, (Italy); Synemed International, (USA); Cooper Medical Devices Corp, (USA); Ipas, (USA); ACM Endoscopy Ltd, (UK); Jhpiego Corp, (USA); Valleylab, (USA)
Branch Offices: 22 Moradeyo Street, Kuje-Amuwo, Lagos-Badagry Expressway; PO Box 1543 Mushin, Lagos State, Tel 880965
Principal Bankers: First Bank of Nigeria Ltd
Financial Information:
Working capital   ₦ 250,000

Principal Shareholders: I O Moradeyo
Date of Establishment: January 1975

FERDINAND ENTERPRISES (NIGERIA) LTD

Plot 16C, Independence Layout, PMB 1263, Enugu, Anambra State
Tel: 254206
Cable: Fenco Enugu
Telex: 51303 Fenco Ng

Chairman: Ferdinand Anyaoha Anaghara
Senior Executives: Fabian N Odudo (General Manager), Joseph U Uga (Financial Controller),
    Clement M Izugbokwe (Marketing Manager),
    H C Ananti (Personnel Manager),
    Mosec C Nwaogu (Foreign Trade Manager)

PRINCIPAL ACTIVITIES: General merchants, contractors, importers, industrialists, estate agents, manufacturers' representatives
Principal Agencies: Anambra Motor Manufacturing Company Ltd; Volkswagen of Nigeria Ltd; Kashima Trading Company Ltd, (Japan); Nishizawa Ltd, (Japan); Leventis Motors Ltd; Kulenkampff & Konitzky, (West Germany)
Branch Offices: 156 Herbert Macaulay Street, Lagos; 25 New Market Road, Onitsha, Anambra State; 141 Aba Rd, Port Harcourt, Rivers State; 100 Okigwe Rd, Owerri, Imo State
Subsidiary Companies: Ferdinand Property Investments Ltd; Ferdinand Industries (Nigeria) Ltd; Fed Motors International Ltd
Principal Bankers: United Bank for Africa Ltd; Union Bank of Nigeria Ltd
Financial Information:

	₦'000
Authorised capital	5,500
Paid-up capital	5,320
Turnover	26,000

Date of Establishment: 1970
No of Employees: 500

FERRERO, A G, & CO LTD

PO Box 125, Kaduna
Tel: 212676

Chairman: Alhaji Baba Duna
Directors: A G Ferrero,
    Giovanni Ferrero,
    Italo Ferrero,
    Alhaji I Kano,
    Maurilio Ferrero,
    Giuseppe Ferrero,
    A Usman-Oyowe (Finance Director)
Senior Executives: A Mather (Chief Quantity Surveyor),
    S Porter (Commercial Manager)

PRINCIPAL ACTIVITIES: Building and civil engineering contractors
Branch Offices: PO Box 435, 56 Yolawa Rd, Kano; PO Box 215, Baga Rd, Maiduguri, Borno State; PO Box 173, 1A River Rd, Zaria, Kaduna State
Associated Companies: Alhaji Ibrahim ltd; IKF Ltd
Principal Bankers: Bank of the North Ltd
Financial Information:

	₦'000
Authorised capital	3,000
Paid-up capital	1,836
Turnover	15,000
Profits	1,000

Principal Shareholders: Alhaji I Kano; A G Ferrero; G Ferrero; I Ferrero; Alhaji Kam Selem
Date of Establishment: 29th July 1959

FESO MIRROR AND GLASS WORKS LTD

8-12 Oyefeso Avenue, Ikorodu Rd, Obanikoro, PO Box 505, Yaba, Lagos State
Tel: 933753, 932617
Cable: Fesoglass Lagos
Telex: 26406 Feglas Ng

FIBREGLASS REINFORCED PLASTICS CO LTD

Chairman: R Olu Oyefeso
Directors: Babatola Oyefeso, Oladipo Oyefeso, Wemimo Oyefeso
Senior Executives: F A Adenodi (Works Manager),
O A Jacob (Works Manager),
C K Pang (Product Manager),
S O Oyefusi (Accountant)
PRINCIPAL ACTIVITIES: Glass merchants and processing, metal processing/fabrication; plastic products
Branch Offices: Bornu St, Ebute Metta, Lagos; Elejina House, Iperu, Ogun State
Subsidiary Companies: Remo Glass Industries Ltd
Principal Bankers: Union Bank of Nigeria Ltd; Allied Bank of Nigeria Ltd; Chase Merchant Bank of Nigeria Ltd
Financial Information:

	N'000
Authorised capital	1,000
Paid-up capital	1,000
Turnover	3,000

Principal Shareholders: R Olu Oyefeso; Babatola Oyefeso; Oladipo Oyefesso; Wemimo Oyefeso
Date of Establishment: 15th August 1958
No of Employees: 105

FIBREGLASS REINFORCED PLASTICS CO LTD

PO Box 206, 144 Ibara Rd, Abeokuta, Ogun State
Tel: 230516, 231007
Cable: Glassplast Abeokuta

Directors: W J Burrows

PRINCIPAL ACTIVITIES: Suppliers of plastics and plastic products; custom moulders in fibreglass/resin

FIDELITY MINING SYNDICATE

79/98 Ahmadu Bello St, PO Box 498, Jos, Plateau State
PRINCIPAL ACTIVITIES: Mining

FIMCON LTD

Ladipo Oluwole Ave, PO Box 98, Ikeja, Lagos
Tel: 963788
Cable: Fimcon Lagos

PRINCIPAL ACTIVITIES: Manufacturers of shoe accessories, immitation jewellery, wiring clips, anodising and plating services

FINANCIAL TRUST COMPANY NIGERIA LTD

Mandilas House, 15th Floor, 96/102 Broad St, PO Box 698, Lagos

Chairman: William Olufemi Olateju Ajayi (also Managing Director)
Directors: Godwin Olusegun Kolawole Ajayi
Senior Executives: Babatunde Pedro (Administrative Manger), Olakunle Osinowa (Investment Executive)

PRINCIPAL ACTIVITIES: Stockbrokers
Branch Offices: Kaduna
Associated Companies: Financial Assurance Co Ltd; Financial Securities Ltd
Principal Bankers: United Bank for Africa Ltd; Central Bank of Nigeria
Financial Information:

	N'000
Authorised capital	100
Paid-up capital	100
Turnover	10,000

Principal Shareholders: G O K Ajayi, W O O Ajayi
Date of Establishment: 11th May 1976

FIRE PROTECTION SERVICES LTD

3rd Floor, Barclays Bank Ltd, PMB 5035, Ibadan, Oyo State
Tel: 410941, 410552, 410624, 414016
Cable: Brokers Ibadan
Telex: 31106

PRINCIPAL ACTIVITIES: Suppliers of fire fighting equipment and alarm systems
Principal Agencies: Chubb Ltd

FIRST BANK OF NIGERIA LTD (FORMERLY STANDARD BANK NIGERIA LTD)

Unity House, 37 Marina, PO Box 5216, Lagos
Tel: 661041, 661043, 661045, 661048, 661057, 660077
Cable: Banking
Telex: 21231

Chairman: Patrick Oguejiofor Nwakoby
Directors: Alhaji Bashiru Hong (Vice Chairman),
Samuel Oyewole Asabia (Managing Director & Chief Executive),
The Rt Hon Lord Barber,
Alhaji Abdullahi Bio Gera,
George Chukwueloka Okonkwo,
Olatunde Olashore,
Simon Momo Onekutu,
Peter William Weller,
Abubakar Ardo Dalil,
Peter Alfred Graham,
John Sneddon Davidson,
Michael Douglas McWilliam,
David Lindsay Millar,
Andrew Ichukwu Obeya

PRINCIPAL ACTIVITIES: Commercial banking
Branch Offices: 170 Offices throughout Nigeria: Including Lagos (22); Ibadan (6); Ikeja (4); Benin City (2); Kaduna (3); Kano (5); Onitsha (5); Port Harcourt (5); Enugu (2); Warri (2); Sapele (2); Jos (3); Maiduguri (2); Zaria (2); Katsina and Apapa
Financial Information: As at 31st December 1981

Liabilities	N'000	Assets	N'000
Share capital (Authorised)	100,000	Cash & Banks	245,293
		Investments loans & other assets	2,334.345
Capital (issued and fully paid)	86,136	Fixed assets	61,909
Reserves (Total)	55,640	Total Assets	2,641,547
Deposits & other liabilities	2,499,771		
Contra a/cs	306,300	Contra a/c	306,300
Total Balance Sheet	2,947,847	Total Balance Sheet	2,947,847

Principal Shareholders: Federal Ministry of Finance (44.8%); The Standard Bank Limited London (38.0%); Nigerian Public (17.2%)

FIRST CHICAGO NIGERIA LTD

18 St Gregory's Rd, Ikoyi, PMB 12028, Lagos
PRINCIPAL ACTIVITIES: Merchant Bank

FIRST CITY INVESTMENT COMPANY LTD

5 Williams St, PO Box 467, Lagos
Tel: 682013
PRINCIPAL ACTIVITIES: Investment and financing

FISAYO HOLDINGS LTD

8 Ojeowere St, Mushin, PO Box 7770, Lagos
Tel: 835790

PRINCIPAL ACTIVITIES: Importers, exporters; motor dealers; manufacturers' representatives; hoteliers, printers

FISCO-CHEMICALS (NIGERIA) LTD

16A Lawani St (Off Isaga Rd), Surulere, Lagos
Tel: 840068

Chairman: D O Ajayi
Senior Executives: U M Ibe (Manager, East),
J O Ajaji (Technical Manager, North),
S O Adegboyegun (Manager, West)

PRINCIPAL ACTIVITIES: Suppliers of laboratory equipment installations, chemicals, hospital equipment; fertilisers
Branch Offices: 85 Oyemekun Rd, Akure, Ondo State
Principal Bankers: Union Bank of Nigeria Ltd

Date of Establishment: 12th January 1974

FISKO CONSTRUCTION ENGINEERING CO LTD

13 Adebambo St, Obanikoro, Ikorodu Rd, Lagos State
Tel: 963934
Cable: Fiskocecon

Chairman: F I Osikoya
Directors: A Osikoya (Administrative Officer),
  O Olajide
Senior Executives: A O Oduyemi (Administrative Manager),
  A Osikoya (Administrative Officer),
  A Rahman (Site Agent)

PRINCIPAL ACTIVITIES: Civil engineering and construction
Branch Offices: PO Box 59, Ijebu-Ode, Ogun State
Subsidiary Companies: Plisson Fisko (Nigeria) Ltd
Principal Bankers: National Bank of Nigeria Ltd
Financial Information:

	₦'000
Authorised capital	500
Paid-up capital	500
Turnover	2,500

Principal Shareholders: F I Osikoya; A Osikoya; O Olajide
Date of Establishment: 1970
No of Employees: 300

FIVE STAR INDUSTRIES LTD

126/128 Nnamdi Azikiwe Street, PO Box 4305, Lagos
Tel: 658055/6
Cable: Fivestar Lagos
Telex: 21522 Ram Ng

Chairman: A H Melwani
Directors: R H Melwani (Managing),
  D J Melwani,
  J F Driver,
  Y A Disu,
  Alhaji Mohammadu Dukku Bello,
  T A Braithwaite
Senior Executives: J F Driver (General Manager),
  A B Ghia (Financial Controller),
  D A Olubi (Personnel Manager)

PRINCIPAL ACTIVITIES: Textiles manufacturers
Branch Offices: Factory: Block E Plot 1, Ilupeju Extension II, Isolo-Expressway, Mushin, Lagos State, Tel 844306, 844526
Associated Companies: Melwanis Company (London) Ltd; Commonwealth Traders Ltd, Hong Kong
Principal Bankers: First Bank of Nigeria; United Bank for Africa; Union Bank of Nigeria; Chase Merchant Bank (Nigeria)
Financial Information:

	₦'000
Authorised capital	5,000
Paid-up capital	3,010
Turnover	30,000

Principal Shareholders: Melwanis Family; Nigerian Industrial Development Bank Ltd; Individual Nigerians
Date of Establishment: 21st July 1969
No of Employees: 1,800

FLAG ALUMINIUM PRODUCTS LTD

Ahmed Talib Ave, PO Box 402, Kaduna
Tel: 243652
Cable: Flag Kaduna
Telex: 71125 Flag Ng

PRINCIPAL ACTIVITIES: Manufacturers of aluminium roofing sheets and building accessories
Branch Offices: 21/22 Marina, PO Box 2160, Lagos, Tel 636105; 85 Aba Rd, PO Box 458, Port Harcourt, Rivers State, Tel

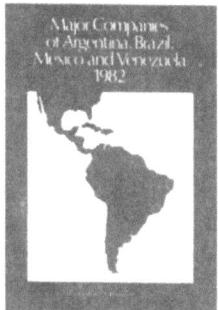 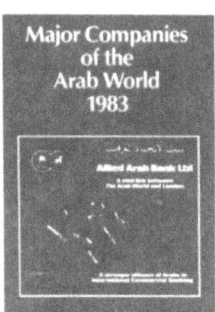 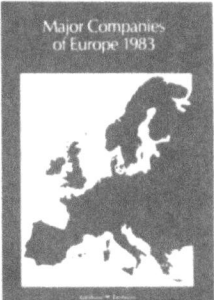 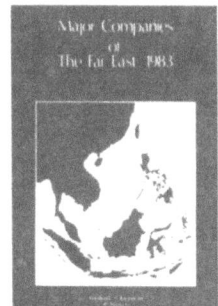 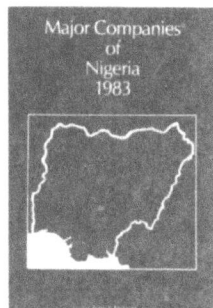

21265; PO Box 1096, Enugu, Anambra State; PO Box 6454,
15 Bello Rd, Kano; PO Box 408, Waziri Rd, Maiduguri, Borno
State; PO Box 914, 200/208 Murtala Mohammed Way,
Calabar, Cross River State

FLOPETROL NIGERIA LTD
Plot 863D Adetokunbo Ademola St, Victoria Island, Lagos
Tel: 614442
Cable: Flotrol Lagos
Telex: 21040 Flolag Ng

Chairman: Chief A Ojora
Directors: E B Sorunke,
 A Yahaya Ahmad,
 P Robinault (Managing),
 H Freyss,
 C Raynaud (Base Manager, Warri),
 J Geneste
Senior Executives: B Goulding (Base Manager, Port Harcourt)

PRINCIPAL ACTIVITIES: Oil and gas services-well testing and
 laboratory analysis services and equipment suppliers,
 snubbing
Branch Offices: 6 Trans-Amadi Layout, PMB 5091, Port
 Harcourt, Rivers State, Tel 225512, Telex 21040; 5 Jeffia
 Crescent, Enerhen Rd, PMB 1092, Warri, Bendel State
Principal Bankers: International Bank for West Africa Ltd

Date of Establishment: August 1970
No of Employees: 200

FLOUR MILLS OF NIGERIA LTD
PO Box 341, 2 Old Dock Rd, Apapa, Lagos
Tel: 803370/3
Cable: Flourmilco Lagos
Telex: 21279 Counman Ng

Chairman: G S Coumantaros
Directors: C Fredericos (Executive Vice-Chairman),
 E Auer (Managing),
 Chief M O Ani,
 J O Fagbemi,
 A M Ferguson,
 M C Ijeh,
 A Joda,
 Alhaji A Kotoko,
 J E Lentakis,
 Chief F C Ozomah,
 J O Sowemimo,
 D L Smith Jnr,
 B M Tukur,
 Chief F R A Williams

PRINCIPAL ACTIVITIES: Manufacturers of flour, pasta, soft
 biscuit flour, whole wheat flour, semovita, self-raising flour.
 Handling and packing of cement
Subsidiary/Associated Companies: Nigerian Bag Manufacturing
 Co Ltd (Subsidiary); Northern Nigerian Flour Mills Ltd
 (Associate)
Principal Bankers: Union Bank of Nigeria Ltd; First Bank of
 Nigeria Ltd; United Bank for Africa Ltd

Date of Establishment: 1960
No of Employees: 2,700

FOLAM INTERNATIONAL TRADING COMPANY
Plot 34, Davies Estate, PO Box 1999, Ikeja, Lagos
Tel: 963534

Chairman: Matthew Oluwole Adejinmi

PRINCIPAL ACTIVITIES: General merchants and contractors,
 importers and exporters; manufacturers' representatives;
 transporters; assembling of agricultural machinery
Branch Offices: 9 Ipodo Rd, Ikeja, Lagos; Factory: 1 Oluwole
 Close, Alagbado Area, Opposite Aticon Ltd, Oko-Oba, Agege
Principal Bankers: United Bank for Africa Ltd

FOOD SPECIALITIES (NIGERIA) LTD
19/21 Industrial Ave, Ilupeju, PMB 21164, Ikeja, Lagos
Tel: 963033, 961597, 961596
Cable: Food Lagos (Ikeja)
Telex: 26280 Food Ng

Chairman: William Mully Murray-Bruce
Directors: Georges Witschi (Managing),
 Olusegun Osunkeye (Executive),
 Ado Ibrahim,
 Jose Daniel,
 Peter Hartwell,
 Innocent Uchendu (Executive)
Senior Executives: D Pomroy (Finance Manager),
 A Schlaepfer (Research & Development Manager),
 R Beachtiger (Factory Manager),
 I A Olayanju (Chief Accountant),
 D Odimgbe (National Sales Manager),
 I Uchendu (Manpower Development Manager),
 Ayo Oginni (Legal Adviser),
 B A T Habib (Company Treasurer)

PRINCIPAL ACTIVITIES: Manufacturers of various canned food
 products
Branch Offices: Kano; Ibadan; Benin; Onitsha; Jos; Port
 Harcourt; Bida; Yola; Maiduguri; Sokoto; Kaduna
Associated Companies: Nestle, Switzerland
Principal Bankers: Union Bank of Nigeria Ltd; First Bank of
 Nigeria Ltd; United Bank for Africa Ltd; International Bank
 for West Africa Ltd; Societe Generale Bank (Nigeria) Ltd

Principal Shareholders: Nestle Holdings Ltd (40%); Nigerians
 (60%)
Date of Establishment: 1969
No of Employees: 1,024

FOODS DIVISION OF UAC OF NIGERIA LTD
PO Box 177, 230 Apapa Rd, Ijora, Lagos
Tel: 831056, 831502, 831594, 831641, 835170
Cable: Unafoods, Lagos

PRINCIPAL ACTIVITIES: Manufacturers of meat products, and
 confectionery
Branch Offices: Ibadan; Enugu; Aba; Port Harcourt; Warri; Kano;
 Benin; Onitsha

FOREMOST DAIRIES (NIGERIA) LTD
1 Ilupeju Rd, PO Box 367, Mushin, Lagos
Tel: 847570, 860316
Cable: Samco, Lagos

Chairman: Sir M Bank-Anthony
Directors: J O Emanuel,
 Mrs E A Vincent,
 D R Moore (Managing)
Senior Executives: N Onwuzulike (Manager, Corporate Affairs),
 G K Odujoko (Manager, Administrative and Accounting),
 M B Lajide (Manager, Plant Operations and Technical),
 J T Alayi (Chief Engineer),
 M O Adekoya (Sales Manager)

PRINCIPAL ACTIVITIES: Food and food processing;
 manufacturers of dairy products
Branch Offices: Ibadan, Oyo State; Shagamu, Ogun State; Lagos
Associated Companies: Foremost McKesson Inc, San Francisco,
 California
Principal Bankers: Savannah Bank of Nigeria Ltd;
 Nigerian-American Merchant Bank Ltd
Financial Information:

	N'000
Authorised capital	1,776
Paid-up capital	1,776
Turnover	5,000

Principal Shareholders: Nigerians (60%); Americans (40%)
Date of Establishment: October 1959
No of Employees: 450

FOREX NEPTUNE OF NIGERIA LTD

88 Norman Williams Street, S W Ikoyi, PO Box 3174, Lagos
Tel: 681181, 681615
Cable: Forexcon
Telex: 21058 Rexcon Ng

Directors: Dr A A Balogun,
   Chief Sambo Adiela,
   A Gould,
   M Jalet (Managing Director),
   P Legręz

Senior Executives: D Brigant (District Manager, Port Harcourt),
   S Tait (District Manager, Warri)

PRINCIPAL ACTIVITIES: Oil drilling contractors, onshore and offshore operations
Principal Agencies: Forex Neptune Group
Branch Offices: 3 Wolu Street, PO Box 5125, Port Harcourt, Rivers State; Tel 335393, 334513; Km 2 Refinery Rd, PO Box 371, Warri, Bendel State, Tel 232711
Principal Bankers: United Bank for Africa Ltd
Financial Information:

	N'000
Authorised capital	400

Principal Shareholders: Nigeria National Petroleum Corporation (NNPC)
Date of Establishment: December 1969
No of Employees: 960

FOSTER WHEELER (NIGERIA) LTD

25 Boyle St, PO Box 4042, Lagos
Tel: 636980, 636053, 652939
Cable: Fosweko Lagos

Directors: Peter Hoskin (General Manager)
Senior Executives: J A Princewill (Sales Engineer)

PRINCIPAL ACTIVITIES: Construction and design engineering

FOUGEROLLE NIGERIA LTD

Plot PC 35, Idowu Taylor St, PO Box 5290, Victoria Island, Lagos
Tel: 617407
Cable: Fougerolle Lagos
Telex: 21445 Enigra

Chairman: Alhaji A A Shasanya
Senior Executives: M Dassonville (General Manager)

PRINCIPAL ACTIVITIES: Civil engineeing and construction
Branch Offices: 3 Colliery Ave, Enugu, Anambra State
Principal Bankers: United Bank for Africa Ltd; Investment Bank for West Africa Ltd
Financial Information:

	N'000
Authorised capital	750
Paid-up capital	750

Principal Shareholders: Nigerians (60%); Fougerolle SA, France (40%)
Date of Establishment: 1974

FOUNDATION CONSTRUCTION LTD

PO Box 2100, 174 Western Ave, Lagos
Tel: 845090, 835393
Cable: Foundations Lagos
Telex: 21100 Fencon Lagos

Chairman: Alhaji Ado Bayero (His Highness the Emir of Kano)
Directors: P Farrington (Managing Director),
   I C Pole,
   M J Gosnell (Financial Director),
   J Muller,
   G A M Hoogeveen,
   L A Ajayi,
   N C Jibunoh,
   E O Adetula
Senior Executives: A J G Bal (Technical Director)

PRINCIPAL ACTIVITIES: Piling and general foundation construction, engineering consultants
Principal Bankers: United Bank for Africa Ltd
Financial Information:

	N'000
Authorised capital	3,000
Paid-up capital	2,800

Principal Shareholders: Richard Costain Holdings Ltd (20%); Nederhorst Grondtechniek BV (20%); Various Nigerian Citizens (60%)
Date of Establishment: 27th September 1960
No of Employees: 500

FOUNDATION ENGINEERING (NIGERIA) LTD

PO Box 2100, 174 Western Ave, Lagos
Tel: 845090, 835393
Cable: Foundations Lagos
Telex: 21100 Fencon Lagos

Chairman: Alhaji Ado Bayero (His Highness the Emir of Kano)
Directors: P Farrington (Managing),
   I C Pole,
   M J Gosnell (Financial),
   J R Boden,
   N C Jibunoh,
   L A Ajayi,
   E O Adetula,
   R H Carroll
Senior Executives: J M Head (Chief Geotechnical Engineer)

PRINCIPAL ACTIVITIES: Soil investigation and ground surveys, laboratory analaysis of rocks and soil samples; reports of bearing capacities of ground conditions; consultancy services
Principal Bankers: United Bank for Africa Ltd; Union Bank of Nigeria Ltd
Financial Information:

	N'000
Authorised capital	1,000
Paid-up capital	900

Principal Shareholders: Richard Costain Holdings Ltd (60%); Various Nigerian Citizens (40%)
Date of Establishment: 21st January 1959
No of Employees: 250

FRANCIS GOODWILL LTD
See GOODWILL, FRANCIS, LTD

FRANCO BUILDERS LTD

12A Station Rd, PO Box 414, Enugu, Anambra State
Tel: 253464
Cable: Franco

PRINCIPAL ACTIVITIES: Building and civil engineering contractors
Branch Offices: 23 Hewett St, Calabar, Cross River State; 22 Wilmer St, Ilupeju, Lagos; PO Box 33, Ikot Ekpene, Cross River State

FRANK BRISCOE
See BRISCOE, FRANK

FRED ATOKI PUBLISHING COMPANY LTD
See ATOKI, FRED, PUBLISHING COMPANY LTD

FRED BALONWU UNIGWE GROUP OF COMPANIES
See UNIGWE, FRED BALONWU, GROUP OF COMPANIES

FREDANO TRADING CO LTD

17/18 Bello Rd, PO Box 5, Kano
Tel: 2038, 2029
Cable: Fredano Kano
Telex: 77138

PRINCIPAL ACTIVITIES: General traders, suppliers to the food, confectionery and construction industries

GOLDEN PENNY PRODUCTS
Health & Energy
Maybe it's just a little grain of wheat — but what a storehouse of nature's nutrients! In fact this golden grain is providing health and energy for the entire nation. Everyday Flour Mills of Nigeria Limited
and its affiliated Companies mill 3,200 tons of wheat to Golden Penny Flour for 4,000 bakers (and their 40,000 assistants) to bake the 5 million loaves we need as our daily bread.
Building a healthy and energetic nation...
GOLDEN PENNY PRODUCTS
Flour Mills of Nigeria Limited
makers of Golden Penny Products

L3P82

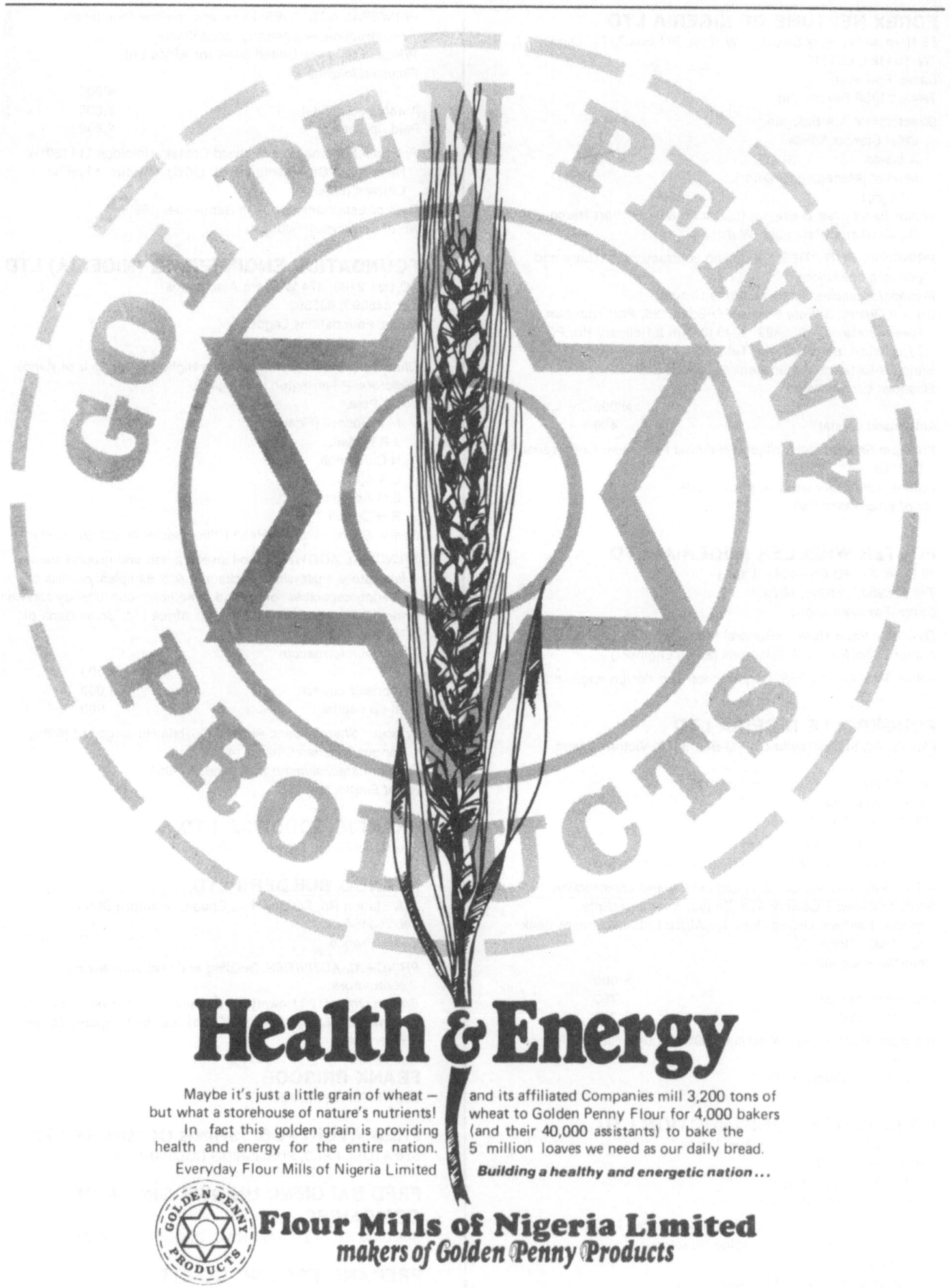

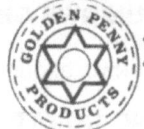

FREEDOM DEVELOPMENT COMPANY LTD

2 Upper Sapele Rd, PMB 1039, Benin City, Bendel State
Tel: 242134, 242190
Cable: Freedom Benin
Telex: 41351 Freeco Ng

President: Vincent E Agenmonmen
Directors: John Agenmonmen, Ehidiamen Agenmonmen
Senior Executives: C D Okoh (Manager),
   P Igene (Manager)

PRINCIPAL ACTIVITIES: Suppliers of various types of doors and
   windows, asbestos products, varieties of wall and floor tiles,
   paints, closets, baths, pipes, plumbing materials and tools,
   water heaters, cement, barbed wire, BRC insulation boards,
   wire nails, keys, mild steel plates etc
Principal Agencies: Nigerian Wire Industries Ltd; Hoesch Pipe
   Mills (Nigeria) Ltd
Branch Offices: Sand Dredging Division: KM 16 Agbor Rd,
   Okhuaihe, Benin City; Stone Quarrying Division: KM 168
   Okene Rd, Okpella, Bendel State
Principal Bankers: African Continental Bank Ltd; Union Bank of
   Nigeria Ltd
Financial Information:

	N'000
Authorised capital	500
Paid-up capital	500

No of Employees: over 100

FREYSSINET NIGERIA LTD

66/68 Eric Moore Rd, Iganmu, PO Box 115, Apapa, Lagos

Senior Executives: A H Bromage (General Manager)

PRINCIPAL ACTIVITIES: Suppliers of pre-stressed material to
   the construction industry

FUASON INDUSTRIES (NIGERIA) LTD

8 Onitsha Rd, PO Box 242, Owerri, Imo State
Tel: 230576, 230938
Cable: Fuason Owerri

Chairmen: HRH Eze Frederick Uwawike Anyanwu, Igwe Odozi
   Obodo I of Mpam
Directors: A U Emeruom (Sales, Marketing),
   H I Anyanwu (Personal Manager),
   Mrs K H Okehi,
   A U Irojiogu,
   F A Duruaku
Senior Executives: M C Anyanwu (Administration Office
   Manager),
   Y Nishino (Factory Manager, Chief Engineer),
   A Bando (Engineer, Chief Technologist),
   C C Anyanwu (Company Secretary/Manager/Planning),
   Cos Anyanwu (Assistant Factory Manager)

PRINCIPAL ACTIVITIES: Manufacturers of galvanised corrugated
   iron sheets
Principal Bankers: Union Bank of Nigeria Ltd
Financial Information:

	N'000
Authorised capital	3,000
Paid-up capital	3,000

Principal Shareholders: HRH Eze F U Anyanwu; Igwe Odozi
   Obodo I of Mpam
Date of Establishment: 24th September 1964
No of Employees: 370

FUBARA ENTERPRISES LTD

14 Idoluwo St, PO Box 4890, Lagos
Cable: Fubenter Lagos

PRINCIPAL ACTIVITIES: General trading

FUNCKE, C, & CO (NIGERIA) LTD

PO Box 5500, 7a Fowler Rd, Ikoyi, Lagos
Tel: 680608
Cable: Funckeco

Chairman: C K H Funcke (also Managing Director)
Directors: G I C Eneli, M N I Ajegbo

PRINCIPAL ACTIVITIES: Management and investment
   consultants
Associated Companies: C Funcke GmbH, West Germany
Principal Bankers: Union Bank of Nigeria Ltd
Financial Information:

	N'000
Authorised capital	30,000
Paid-up capital	30,000

Principal Shareholders: Chairman and directors as described
Date of Establishment: 1974

FUNTUA BRICKWORKS LTD

Funtua, Kaduna State

Chairman: Alhaji Bello Abdulhamid

PRINCIPAL ACTIVITIES: Production of bricks
Financial Information:
Registered capital   N 2,600,000

Principal Shareholders: Kaduna State Government (75%);
   Ceric-Dutreux (25%)
Date of Establishment: 1979

FUNTUA COTTONSEED CRUSHING COMPANY LTD

PO Box 119, Funtua, Kaduna State
Tel: 86
Cable: Cotmill

Chairman: Alhaji Aminu Dantata
Directors: Alhaji Umaro A Mutallab, Alhaji Abdulkadir Abdullahi,
   R V Jones, Alhaji Haruna Danja, Alhaji Mai Deribe, Alhaji
   Nababa Badamasi, Alhaji Idris S Maska, Alhaji Sani Buhari,
   Alhaji Balan Goggo, O Q Hughes, S Max-Okpugo
Senior Executives: Thomas Elliott (General Manager),
   Alhaji Iro Garba (Company Secretary/Financial Controller),
   Ganiyu Adedigba (Deputy Financial Controller/Admin
   Manager),
   M Abdulrahman Mani (Factory Engineer)

PRINCIPAL ACTIVITIES: Processing of vegetable oil seeds,
   livestock and animal feeds
Principal Bankers: Union Bank of Nigeria Ltd
Financial Information:

	N'000
Authorised capital	1,600
Paid-up capital	1,600

Principal Shareholders: Alhaji Aminu Dantata; Kaduna State
   Government; Lewis & Peat Ltd
Date of Establishment: 1971
No of Employees: 140

FURNITURE HOUSE LTD

Railway Ave, PO Box 109, Kaduna South

PRINCIPAL ACTIVITIES: Suppliers of wood and metal furniture;
   upholstery works

FUSI INDUSTRIAL SUPPLIES CO LTD

71 Apapa Rd, Ebute-Metta, PO Box 678, Lagos
Tel: 834215

PRINCIPAL ACTIVITIES: Suppliers of industrial tools
Branch Offices: Kano; Kaduna; Aba; Onitsha; Benin; Warri

G B OLLIVANT & CO (NIGERIA) LTD

See OLLIVANT, G B, & CO (NIGERIA) LTD

G CAPPA LTD

See CAPPA, G, LTD

G I OBASKEKI & SONS LTD

See OBASKEKI, G I, & SONS LTD

G KEWALRAM & SONS (NIGERIA) LTD
See KEWALRAM, G, & SONS (NIGERIA) LTD

G N A HAMZER & CO (NIGERIA) LTD
See HAMZER, G N A, & CO (NIGERIA) LTD

G NDAH & SONS FOUNDATION
See NDAH, G, & SONS FOUNDATION

GABY AND COMPANY (NIGERIA)
72 Ogbunabali Street, PO Box 1175, Port Harcourt, Rivers State

Chairman: Hyacinth Gabriel
Directors: Festus Alozie, Augustine Obilor
Senior Executives: Bright Akudo Gabriel (Secretary), Onyema Alozie (Commercial Manager)

PRINCIPAL ACTIVITIES: Importers, exporters, business consultants, agents and general trading; suppliers of building materials, ceramics/sanitary fittings, electrical/electronic equipment, irrigation services and equipment, office equipment/supplies, paper/paper products; packaging, petrochemicals, oil/gas services and equipment and pipeline contractors; freight forwarding and customs agents, shipping/shipping services, scientific instruments, safety and security equipment; printing; textiles, clothing and textile equipment; timber industries, saw mills; transport services
Principal Agencies: Dr Pepper Bottling Company (Nigeria) Ltd
Branch Offices: 20 Anokwu St, Owerri, Imo State; 111 Hospital Rd, Aba; 29 Oboro St, Umuahia, Imo State
Principal Bankers: African Continental Bank Ltd

Principal Shareholders: Hyacinth Gabriel; Festus Alozie; Augustine Obilor

GALENIKA NIGERIA LTD
27 Commercial Avenue, PO Box 482, Yaba, Lagos
Tel: 861182

Chairman: O T Ososami

PRINCIPAL ACTIVITIES: Manufacturers and distributors of pharmaceuticals
Principal Shareholders: Drug Houses Nigeria Ltd

GALVANIZING INDUSTRIES LTD
Oba Akran Avenue, Industrial Estate, PO Box 96, Ikeja, Lagos
Tel: 960907, 964746, 964756
Cable: Galvanind Ikeja
Telex: 26128 Ng Lggil

Chairman: M Kimura

PRINCIPAL ACTIVITIES: Manufacturers of galvanised roofing sheets
Principal Bankers: First Bank of Nigeria Ltd; United Bank for Africa Ltd; Union Bank of Nigeria Ltd

Date of Establishment: 1962

GAMBORU, ALHAJI MADU MALA SHERIFF
Sir Kashim Ibrahim Ave, PMB 1391, Maiduguri, Borno State
Tel: 232068

PRINCIPAL ACTIVITIES: Building and civil engineering contractors, transporters and suppliers of building materials
Branch Offices: Gombe; Azare; Bauchi

GAS & WELDING (NIGERIA) LTD
Plot 1 Matori Industrial Scheme, Ladipo Street, Mushin, Lagos

Chairman: Alhaji Aliko M Mohammed
Directors: Dr Herm Ch Goldkamp,
Mrs A Ogwuma,
Mr Joerg H Viereck (Managing Director),
Dr Ing Axel Gierhard

PRINCIPAL ACTIVITIES: Production of industrial gases
Branch Offices: Airport Rd, PMB 1225, Warri, Bendel State
Principal Bankers: United Bank for Africa Ltd; Societe Generale Bank (Nigeria) Ltd; Bank of the North
Financial Information:

	N'000
Authorised capital	1,500
Paid-up capital	1,000
Turnover (1981)	4,800
Profits	1,000

Principal Shareholders: Phoenix Maschinentechnik, Switzerland
Date of Establishment: 1976
No of Employees: 120

GAS PRODUCERS LTD
2 Okehi Street, PO Box 502, Port Harcourt, Rivers State
Tel: 331228
Cable: Gases Port Harcourt
Telex: 61109 Gaspor Ng; 81132 Gasjos Ng

Chairman: M Dineur
Directors: V O Allagoa,
J E Andreiessen,
G O Onosode,
R R Riviere (Managing),
E W Somorin (Financial Director),
A Williams
Senior Executives: P Gamberini (General Sales Manager),
N P Amanchukwu (Works Manager),
A K Amogu (Welding Equipment Manager)

PRINCIPAL ACTIVITIES: Producers of industrial and medical gases, oxygen, nitrogen, acetylene and suppliers of welding and medical equipment
Principal Agencies: SAF (Soudure Autogene Francaise) L'Air Liquide; Miller Welding Equipment, Products and Electrodes
Branch Offices: 90B Goldie St, Calabar, Cross River State; Airport Rd, PO Box 41, Jos, Plateau State; 46 Zik Avenue, Uwani Enugu, Anambra State; 334 Iweka Rd Onitsha, Anambra State, Kyari Zorum Rd, Maiduguri, Borno State
Subsidiary Companies: Societe l'Air Liquide
Principal Bankers: United Bank for Africa Ltd; Union Bank of Nigeria Ltd
Financial Information:

	N'000
Authorised capital	1,800
Paid-up capital	1,800
Turnover	4,700
Profits	760

Principal Shareholders: L'Air Liquide (20%); Royal Packaging (20%); Nigerians (60%)
Date of Establishment: 1960
No of Employees: 153

GASKIYA CORPORATION LTD
PMB 1033, Gaskiya Rd, Tadun Wada, Zaria, Kaduna State
Tel: 32203/4
Cable: Gaskiya, Zaria
Telex: 75243

Chairman: Mallam Labo U Yari (also Managing Director)
Directors: Balaraba Abbas Lawal, Saleh Abdu Dutsinwai, Lucas Zamani, Ibrahim Musa Yamadlu, Nuhu Bamalli
Senior Executives: F Fisher (Production Manager),
Manickam Jegatheeswaran (Management Accountant),
M K Bello (Sales Manager),
J D Mohammed (Order Processing Manager),
J J Akpawan (Acccountant),
I Jumare (Administrative Manager)

PRINCIPAL ACTIVITIES: Printing and publishing
Associated Companies: Northern Nigerian Publishing Company Ltd
Principal Bankers: United Bank for Africa Ltd

Financial Information:

	₦'000
Authorised capital	1,400
Paid-up capital	1,050

Principal Shareholders: Kaduna State Government; Jama'atu Nasril Islam; New Nigerian Development Co
Date of Establishment: 1936
No of Employees: 192

GAUFF CONSULTANTS (NIGERIA) LTD

28A Adeola Hopewell St, Victoria Island, PO Lagos 8876, Lagos
Tel: 615188
Cable: Gaufsalta
Telex: 21005 Ibgcn Ng

Chairman: F A Ogbemi
Directors: H Michelmann (Managing),
H P Gauff

PRINCIPAL ACTIVITIES: Civil engineering consultants
Associated Companies: H P Gauff Ingenieure GmbH & Company, Nuremberg, West Germany
Principal Bankers: First Bank of Nigeria Ltd; Union Bank of Nigeria Ltd

Date of Establishment: October 1975

GAZAL INDUSTRIAL ENTERPRISES LTD

27 Kundila Rd, Bompai, PO Box 703, Kano
Tel: 2619, 5750, 2138

PRINCIPAL ACTIVITIES: Manufacturers of candles and polish

GDM TEXTILES MANUFACTURING LTD

26/28 Ereko Street, PO Box 6370, Lagos
Tel: 661662, 901320
Cable: Gdmtextile
Telex: 22140 Gdmtex

Chairman: H G Melwani
Directors: U G Melwani, V G Melwani, Alhaji Jimoh Yusuf
Senior Executives: P E Macchi (Production Manager)

PRINCIPAL ACTIVITIES: Manufacture of textile piece goods of all kinds
Principal Bankers: United Bank for Afica Ltd
Financial Information:

	₦'000
Authorised capital	500
Paid-up capital	500
Turnover	5,000
Profits	200

Date of Establishment: 1972
No of Employees: 400

GEC (TELECOMMUNICATIONS) NIGERIA LTD

26 Creek Rd, PMB 1009, Apapa, Lagos
Tel: 803230/2
Cable: Springjack Lagos
Telex: 21385

Chairman: A E Howson-Wright
Directors: His Highness the Emir of Kano Alhaji Ado Bayero,
J I Ediale,
J M Price,
D B Edwards (Managing)

PRINCIPAL ACTIVITIES: Importation, sales, installation and maintenance of telecommunications equipment
Principal Agencies: General Electric Company Ltd, UK; GEC Telecommunications Ltd of Coventry, UK; Ditchburn Organisation, UK; Marconi Communication Systems Ltd; Marconi Instruments; Gould Advance Instruments; Mitel Telecomms Ltd; Eddystone Radio Ltd; English Electric Valve Co Ltd; Aero Electronics Ltd, UK; Stentofon Communication Systems, Norway
Branch Offices: U7 Katsina Rd, PO Box 363, Kaduna; Central Hotel, PO Box 1200, Kano; 4 Accra Street, PO Box 16, Port

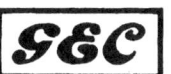

GEC (TELECOMMUNICATIONS) NIGERIA LIMITED

26 Creek Road, PMB 1009, Apapa, Lagos
Tel: 803230/2
Cable: Springjack Lagos
Telex: 21385

PRINCIPAL ACTIVITIES:

Marketing, Installing and Maintaining Private Telephone Systems, Public Telephone Exchanges, Transmission Systems (Radio and Line), Telephones, HF and VHF Communication Systems, Background Music Systems, Telephone Cables and Accessories.

BRANCH OFFICES:

U7 Katsina Road, PO Box 363, Kaduna
Central Hotel, PO Box 1200, Kano
46A Wire Road, PO Box 2275, Benin City
4 Accra Street, PO Box 16, Port Harcourt
Cocoa House, PO Box 1552, Ibadan

Harcourt; Cocoa House, PO Box 1552, Ibadan; 46A Wire Rd, PO Box 2275, Benin City
Subsidiary Companies: Branch Properties Nigeria Ltd; English Electric Nigeria Ltd
Principal Bankers: Union Bank of Nigeria Ltd; Savannah Bank of Nigeria Ltd

GECO ENGINEERING CO (NIGERIA) LTD

27/29 Martins St, 4th Floor, PMB 12608, Lagos
Tel: 660393, 880572

Chairman: Godwin Chukukadibia Ishingene Onah
Directors: Emmanuel Obidi Echetabu, Alhaji Abubakar Wali

PRINCIPAL ACTIVITIES: Geophysicists, drilling, soil sampling and foundation investigation, engineering consultants
Branch Offices: Block E/5 Real Estate, Uwani, PO Box 735, Enugu, Anambra State; PO Box 167, Sokoto
Associated Companies: Kamali Construction Co Ltd; Mintra Contractors Company
Principal Bankers: African Continental Bank Ltd; Union Bank of Nigeria Ltd

Principal Shareholders: Engr G C I Onah; E O Echetabu
Date of Establishment: 28th May 1976

GEM FASTENERS INDUSTRY (NIGERIA) LTD

17 Martins St, PO Box 3325, Lagos
Tel: 636147, 636218
Cable: Gefin Lagos

PRINCIPAL ACTIVITIES: Manufacturers of paper clips, stapplings and office pins
Branch Offices: Factory: Plot 36 Block 56, Ilupeju Industrial Estate, Mushin, Lagos

GENERAL APPLIANCES COMPANY LTD

22 Ikorodu Rd, Jibowu, Yaba, Lagos
Tel: 862778
Telex: 26220

Chairman: Chief M O Akinrele
Directors: Chief J Akin George, C S Adewunmi, Chief O
  Morohundiya, Odu'a Investment Co Ltd
Senior Executives: N O Akinwunmi (Plant Manager),
  L O Olayeye (Public Affairs Manager),
  T Ajibona (Company Secretary Admin. Manager),
  B A Matti (Management Services Manager),
  Y Sulaimon (Engineering Manager),
  G A B Jaiyeoba (Technical Services Manager),
  R F Akintemi (Liaison Manager),
  O C Duyilemi (Sales Manager),
  E O Ayoola (Maintenance Manager),
  M Ajala (Production Controller),
  W Odunlami (Accountant),
  S D Rai (Production Manager)

PRINCIPAL ACTIVITIES: Manufacturers of airconditioners,
  refrigerators, cookers, etc
Principal Agencies: Peugeot Automobile Nigeria Ltd; Startek;
  Kingsway
Branch Offices: Factory: Km 2, Otta Idiroko Rd, Sango Otta,
  Ogun State
Subsidiary/Associated Companies: Gacol Marketing and
  Comfort Centre; Gacol Products Ltd
Principal Bankers: United Bank for Africa Ltd; International
  Merchant Bank Nigeria Ltd; United Bank for Africa Ltd
Financial Information:

	₦'000
Authorised capital	1,000
Paid-up capital	1,000
Turnover	5,816
Profits	321

Principal Shareholders: Mods Holdings Ltd; Odu'a Investment;
  Akin Bayo Investment
Date of Establishment: January 1977
No of Employees: 170

GENERAL CONTRACTORS (NIGERIA) LTD

34 Ogunlana Drive, Surulere, Lagos
Tel: 837607

Directors: E J Halley (Managing Director)

PRINCIPAL ACTIVITIES: General contracting services

GENERAL COSMETICS COMPANY LTD

23B Port Harcourt Rd, Aba, Imo State

Directors: M Ibeh (Managing)

PRINCIPAL ACTIVITIES: Production of soaps and detergents

No of Employees: 200 when in full production

GENERAL ELECTRIC USA OF NIGERIA LTD

Plot 739b Adeola Hopewell St, Victoria Island, PO Box 3912,
  Lagos
Tel: 632965

PRINCIPAL ACTIVITIES: Telecommunications and power
Principal Agencies: General Electric Co, USA

GENERAL METAL PRODUCTS LTD

Plot G2, Apapa Rd, Iganmu, PO Box 442, Apapa, Lagos
Tel: 801400-4
Cable: Gemeprol, Lagos
Telex: 26797 Gmp Ng

Chairman: A K Disu
Directors: R Mueller (Managing),
  W Bachofner,
  Chief S I Fawehinmi
Senior Executives: F Biasi (Deputy Managing Director),
  T O Idagun (Financial Controller)

PRINCIPAL ACTIVITIES: Suppliers of aluminium products,
  building materials
Branch Offices: Textile Rd, Kakuri, PO Box 731, Kaduna;
  Trans-Amadi Ind Layout, PMB 5402, Port Harcourt, Tel
  330821/334434
Principal Bankers: First Bank of Nigeria Ltd; United Bank for
  Africa Ltd
Principal Shareholders: A K Disu; R Mueller; W Bachofner; Chief
  S I Fawehinmi; P G Tonella; A Jordi; R Scherrer; Miss E
  Fischer
Date of Establishment: 1st August 1979
No of Employees: 800

GENERAL METALWARE COMPANY NIGERIA LTD

PO Box 193, Industrial Estate, Ikeja, Lagos
Tel: 90012, 961200, 900111
Cable: Gemetal Lagos

Directors: Y M Cheung (Director)

PRINCIPAL ACTIVITIES: Manufacturing of industrial machinery
  and tools; industrial and domestic plasticware, metal and
  plastic vacuum flasks, sundry metalware products

GENERAL TECHNOLOGY NIGERIA LTD

9 Olufemi Rd, Surulere, Lagos

PRINCIPAL ACTIVITIES: Project co-ordination in the fields of ice
  production plants, cement, plastic etc

Principal Shareholders: General Technology Inc, USA
Date of Establishment: November 1979

GEOCOMSA & CO (NIGERIA) LTD

12 Nnamdi Azikiwe St, PO Box 4702, Lagos
Tel: 636318

Directors: J A Weinmar

PRINCIPAL ACTIVITIES: Engineering consultants

GEODETIC SURVEYS LTD

94 Broad St, Lagos
Tel: 961557
Telex: 21117 TDS167

Chairman: E Keller
Directors: H R Keller (Managing Director),
  E Urhobo,
  G O Heasman (General Manager),
  C T Horsfall (Licensed Surveyor)
Senior Executives: B L Marsh (Contracts Manager),
  A Porter (Admin Manager/Finance Controller),
  H D Smith (Operations Manager),
  R F Horsfall (Personnel Manager),
  I J Bhardwaj (Chief Hydrographer)

PRINCIPAL ACTIVITIES: Surveying: topographical,
  hydrographical, photogrammetrical civil engineering
  consultancy and design; marine geophysics and site
  investigations
Branch Offices: Operations bases: Rumuobiakani, PO Box 901,
  Port Harcourt; Effurun, PO Box 298, Warri; Head Office: 73B
  Tinubu Rd, Palmgrove Estate, Ilupeju, Lagos
Associated Companies: Geodetic & Construction Survey Ltd,
  Switzerland; Geodetic & Construction Survey Pte, Singapore
Principal Bankers: United Bank for Africa Ltd; First Bank of
  Nigeria Ltd

Principal Shareholders: Nigerian (40%); Expatriate (60%)
Date of Establishment: 1966
No of Employees: 100

GEORGE COHEN (NIGERIA) LTD

3 Aerodrome Rd, PO Box 301, Apapa, Lagos
Tel: 876477, 873803
Cable: Coborn Apapa
Telex: 22273 Coborn Ng

Directors: S J Wosko (General Manager/Director)
PRINCIPAL ACTIVITIES: Crane hire and steel stockholders
Date of Establishment: 1960

GEORGE ENGINEERING CO LTD

3 Amaigbo Lane, Uwani, Enugu, Anambra State
PRINCIPAL ACTIVITIES: Electrical and mechanical engineers
Branch Offices: 4 Montgomery Rd, Yaba, Lagos

GEORGE HUNTERS & COMPANY LTD

6 Olaosun Close, (Off 49 Western Ave), PO Box 1381, Surulere,
   Lagos State
Tel: 863727

Chairman: Una Hunters Aigbogun
Directors: G Iyasele, Mrs A E Ajaji, A Ehizuwa
Senior Executives: G I Aletor (General Manager),
   J O Omeike (Financial Controller)
PRINCIPAL ACTIVITIES: Industrial, office and home security
   equipment
Principal Agencies: ACB; UBA; Union Bank; Dormanlong Ltd
Subsidiary Companies: Hunters & Associates
Principal Bankers: Union Bank of Nigeria Ltd
Financial Information:

	₦'000
Authorised capital	500
Paid-up capital	250
Turnover	200
Profits	100

Date of Establishment: 1965
No of Employees: 205

GEORGE KOKU & SONS LTD

See KOKU, GEORGE, & SONS LTD

GEORGE, PATRICK, & SONS LTD

10 Makinde St, Alausa, Ikeja, PO Box 603, Marina, Lagos
Tel: 680496, 931147
Cable: Vicos Lagos

Chairman: Patrick George
Directors: Mrs A Dawodu, M O Osineye, I B Dawodu
Senior Executives: Alhaji K Fasasi (General Manager)
PRINCIPAL ACTIVITIES: Suppliers of air-conditioning
   equipment, building materials, ceramics, civil engineering
   and construction
Principal Agencies: T W Chum Manufacturing Ltd, Taiwan,
   Republic of China
Branch Offices: Factory: 16/18 Okorogbin Rd, Aiyeteju, Isiwo,
   Ijebu-Ode, Ogun State
Principal Bankers: African Continental Bank Ltd

No of Employees: 200

GEORGE WIMPEY & CO (NIGERIA) LTD

See WIMPEY, GEORGE, & CO (NIGERIA) LTD

GEOSERVICES NIGERIA LTD

Office No 8, Federal Place Hotel, Victoria Island, PO Box 7285,
   Lagos
Tel: 610031, Ext 236
Telex: 21432 Palace Lagos

Directors: G Le Rouzic (Managing Director),
   Vincent O Ebuh (General Manager)
Senior Executives: S Ike (Manager, Warri),
   D Chevrotin (Manager, Port Harcourt)
PRINCIPAL ACTIVITIES: Geological and petroleum engineering,
   mudlogging and surveying
Branch Offices: Laboratory: PMB 5027, Port Harcourt, Rivers
   State, Tel 21760; Field Office: Warri, Bendel State

GERMAN-NIGERIAN ENGINEERING COMPANY LTD (GERNIG)

19 Kodesoh St (2nd Floor), PO Box 1979, Ikeja, Lagos

Directors: W Prockl

PRINCIPAL ACTIVITIES: Engineering consultants

GIAMPAOLI CONSTRUCTION (NIGERIA) LTD

PO Box 5077, 7 Agbonyin Ave, Surulere, Lagos
Tel: 11117

Chairman: Ebele Chinye (also Chief Executive)
Directors: Dr Mario Braschi (General Manager),
   Alexis Anielo,
   Alhaji Yahaya Ali,
   Kingsley Ikpe
Senior Executives: Georgio Dallacha (Roads/Drainage),
   Anesimo Dametto (Water System),
   U Awunor (Mechanical Engineer),
   Mr Fagazio (Engineer),
   Mr Mathur (Electrical Engineer),
   Mr Billenci (Engineer)

PRINCIPAL ACTIVITIES: Civil engineering and construction
Branch Offices: Zaria Kano Rd, Basawa, PMB 1136, Zaria,
   Kaduna State
Principal Bankers: Pan African Bank Ltd; Icon Ltd (Merchant
   Bankers); United Bank for Africa Ltd
Financial Information:

	N'000
Authorised capital	2,000
Paid-up capital	2,000

Principal Shareholders: Ebele Chinye; Dr Mario Braschi
Date of Establishment: 14th April, 1976
No of Employees: 700

GICEN TECHNICAL SERVICES LTD

PO Box 1746, 3rd Floor Western House, 8/10 Broad St, Lagos
Tel: 633194
Cable: Gicentech

Chairman: Godfrey I C Eneli
Directors: Dr Alex C Eneli, Ms Chinwe Eneli
Senior Executives: Nnamdi C Oyeka (Group Financial Controller),
   Olu Ologan (Customer Engineering Manager),
   A Mageswaram (Eastern Area Manager),
   H Fernando (Northern Area Manager)

PRINCIPAL ACTIVITIES: Suppliers of office equipment,
   typewriters, dictating equipment etc
Principal Agencies: IBM; Liquid Paper
Branch Offices: Plot 1 Oshodi Layout, Isolo Expressway, Near
   Arab Bank, Lagos State; 39 Awolowo Ave, Bodija Estate,
   Opposite Palm Chemist, Ibadan, Oyo State; 42 Akpakpava St,
   Benin City, Bendel State; 7 Ogui Rd, Enugu, Anambra State
Principal Bankers: Union Bank of Nigeria Ltd; Bank of Credit
   and Commerce International (Nigeria) Ltd
Financial Information:

	N'000
Authorised capital	500
Paid-up capital	200

Principal Shareholders: Chairman and directors as described
No of Employees: 100

GIDA TECHNICAL ENTERPRISES COMPANY

PO Box 2891, Lagos
Tel: 877599
Cable: Academy, Lagos

Senior Executives: Z A Ladipo (Works Manager),
   Lateef Saliu (Equipment Promoter)

PRINCIPAL ACTIVITIES: Suppliers of drilling pipes, pumps and
   control valves; information on location of crude oil, collection
   of data on Nigerian petroleum industry

GILCO NIGERIA LTD

292 Apapa Rd, PO Box 146, Apapa, Lagos
Tel: 873630, 861814, 875084
Telex: 21566; 21286

PRINCIPAL ACTIVITIES: Telecommunications and power; radio
   communication systems specialists
Financial Information: Part of the Gilco group

GINDIRI CONCRETE PRODUCTS LTD

28 Jingiri Rd, Bukuru Bye-Pass, PO Box 713, Jos, Plateau State
Tel: 2584
Telex: 81148 Nig

Chairman: E Washik

PRINCIPAL ACTIVITIES: General contractors, concrete block
   makers, transporters
Associated Companies: Amana Construction Co (Nigeria) Ltd

GION (NIGERIA) LTD

Idaw River Industrial Layout, 96 Agbani Rd, PMB 1122, Enugu,
   Anambra State
Tel: 255597

Directors: Engr G I Onyenso (Managing Director),
   O C Ezeako,
   M O Obiekwe,
   A N Okunna,
   S A Onyenso (Works Manager),
   Mrs F N Udebiuwa
Senior Executives: J U Imeogu (Acting Company Secretary),
   E D Afiakure (Administration Officer),
   U F Azuogu (Project Manager)

PRINCIPAL ACTIVITIES: Wood and metal furniture
   manufacturers; construction of steel structures
Associated Companies: Onys Construction Company Ltd
Principal Bankers: International Bank for West Africa Ltd
Principal Shareholders: Mrs U Offia Nwali; U F Azuogu, P O
   Nwaosuagwu
No of Employees: 150

GLANVILL ENTHOVEN & COMPANY (NIGERIA)

PMB 2273, 14th Floor, Western House, 8/10 Broad St, Lagos
Tel: 651595, 635572, 631951
Cable: Glanniger Lagos
Telex: 21943 Glan Ng

Chairman: P A Adegbemi
Directors: D W Andrew (Deputy Chairman),
   L A C Taylor (Managing),
   B H C Graham,
   M O Longe (Deputy Managing Director),
   Chief C O Fatunmbi,
   Chief J O Ishola,
   Chief S A Olajide,
   A A Oyebadejo
Senior Executives: Alhaji A Adams (Acting General Manager -
   Glanvill Enthoven Life & Pension Consultants),
   E W Zafu (General Manager/Director - Glanvill Enthoven
   Reinsurance Brokers),
   Mrs M B Dawodu (Personnel Manager)

PRINCIPAL ACTIVITIES: Insurance and reinsurance brokers, life
   and pensions consultants
Branch Offices: 18 Boyle St, Lagos; 16th Floor Cocoa House,
   Ibadan; Near Governor's Office, Ibara, Abeokuta; 54A Oba
   Adesida Rd, Akure; 37 Campbell St, Lagos; 47A Trans Amadi
   Layout, Port Harcourt; 12B Post Office Rd, Kano
Associated Companies: Glanvill Enthoven Life and Pensions
   Consultants; Glanvill Enthoven Reinsurance Brokers
Principal Bankers: National Bank of Nigeria
Financial Information:

	N'000
Authorised capital	500
Paid-up capital	500
Turnover	3,500

Principal Shareholders: Odu'a Investment Company Ltd; Jardine Glanvill, UK
Date of Establishment: 1957
No of Employees: 200

GLAXO (NIGERIA) LTD

41 Creek Rd, PMB 1120, Apapa, Lagos
Tel: 803050/1/2
Cable: Glaxo Apapa
Telex: 22256

Chairman: Professor E A Elebute

PRINCIPAL ACTIVITIES: Manufacturers of pharmaceuticals, including antibiotics, etc; foods for infants and invalids
Branch Offices: Aba; Kano; Ibadan; Benin
Financial Information:

	₦'000
Authorised capital	6,000
Paid-up capital	5,880
Turnover (1981)	27,540
Profits (after tax)	4,389

Principal Shareholders: Glaxo Holdings Ltd (40%)
Date of Establishment: 23rd April 1954
No of Employees: 700

GLENDORA ENTERPRISES

Block C Shop 4, Falomo Shopping Centre, Awolowo Rd, SW Ikoyi, Lagos
Tel: 683683

Directors: Mrs Gbemisola Tejuoso (Managing Director)

PRINCIPAL ACTIVITIES: Retail books, stationery, toys, magazines
Branch Offices: Eko Holiday Inn, Victoria Island, Lagos
Principal Bankers: United Bank for Africa

GLOBAL PHARMACEUTICAL AND CHEMICAL AGENCIES LTD

2F Airport Rd, PO Box 1095, Kano
Tel: 2439, 2458
Cable: Global Kano
Telex: 21351 Global Ng

PRINCIPAL ACTIVITIES: Dealers and manufacturers' representatives in chemicals, drugs, dressings, hospital and laboratory equipment, etc
Branch Offices: Maiduguri; Jos; Sokoto; Ilorin; Lagos
Associated Companies: Nigeria & Trading Co

GLOBAL STARS (NIGERIA) LTD

Plot 9 Block A Ogba Scheme, Industrial Estate, PMB 1158, Ikeja, Lagos
Tel: 961486, 961103
Telex: 26462

Chairman: Alhaji A R O Sanusi (also Managing Director)
Directors: A A Sanusi, A Sanusi, G O Sanusi, L O Sanusi, R O Sanusi, F O Sanusi

PRINCIPAL ACTIVITIES: Retailers and distributors of food products
Branch Offices: Throughout Nigeria
Principal Bankers: United Bank for Africa Ltd

No of Employees: 1,000

GLOBE FISHING INDUSTRIES LTD

13a Ijora Causeway, Lagos
Tel: 836794, 836900, 834199

PRINCIPAL ACTIVITIES: Fishing and fish processing

GLOBESTAR ENGINEERING CO (NIGERIA) LTD

68 Hospital Rd, PMB 1167, Aba, Imo State
Tel: 235

PRINCIPAL ACTIVITIES: Building and civil engineering contractors

GLOEDE & HOFF (NIGERIA) LTD

26B Post Office Rd, PO Box 633, Kano
Tel: 2527, 2756

PRINCIPAL ACTIVITIES: General trading and representation
Branch Offices: 21 Wharf Rd, PO Box 979/347, Lagos

GOAS AGENCIES LTD

119 Okumagba Ave, PMB 1165, Warri, Bendel State
Cable: Goas Warri

Chairman: Gabriel Omoko Ande
Directors: Philip Ande, Chief Seritoro Tungbowei, James Otulu, Mrs Agregbalagha Macaulay, S Y T Fiberesima
Senior Executives: S M Obwru (General Manager), Friday O Akeno (Accountant), Stephen Younbai (Transport Manager), Denis Seimokumo (Shipping Manager)

PRINCIPAL ACTIVITIES: Shipping, clearing, forwarding, warehousing, transporters, dealers in building materials, and cement, importers and exporters
Branch Offices: 2A Aggrey Rd, Port Harcourt, Rivers State; 53 Market Rd, Warri, Bendel State; 1 Adjarho St, Essi Layout, Opposite McDermott Yard, Warri, Bendel State
Principal Bankers: First Bank of Nigeria Ltd
Financial Information:

	₦'000
Authorised capital	200
Paid-up capital	100

Date of Establishment: 1970

GOBECCO TRADING COMPANY LTD

9 Awkuzu Street, Uwani, PO Box 346, Enugu, Anambra State
Tel: 335720
Cable: Gobecco
Telex: 51389 Mozulu Ng

Chairman: B C B Eruchalu (also Managing Director)
Directors: B C M Eruchalu, M E B Eruchalu (Secretary)

PRINCIPAL ACTIVITIES: Importers of agricultural machinery, fertilizers, industrial chemicals etc
Principal Agencies: Maria Worner, West Germany; Jordan Electronics, Holland; Etherwest Ltd, UK; Charles Manhardi Machinery Incorp, USA
Subsidiary Companies: Bema Company
Principal Bankers: Union Bank of Nigeria Ltd; African Continental Bank Ltd
Financial Information:

	₦'000
Authorised capital	200
Paid-up capital	150
Turnover	500

Principal Shareholders: B C B Eruchalu; B C M Eruchalu; M E B Eruchalu
Date of Establishment: 1st May 1963
No of Employees: 50

GODBLESS MOTORS NIGERIA LTD

47 Warri/Sapele Rd, Effurun, Warri, Bendel State

Chairman: Alhaji Chief A A Suberu
Directors: P E S Ideh, Alhaji S Adelokun, B A Akanni, J O Ideh

PRINCIPAL ACTIVITIES: Importers of motor vehicles and agricultural machinery
Principal Agencies: General Motors USA (Isuzu)
Branch Offices: Sapele Rd, Benin City, Bendel State
Principal Bankers: New Nigeria Bank Ltd; United Bank for Africa Ltd

Financial Information:

	N'000
Authorised capital	600
Paid-up capital	600
Turnover (approx)	2,000

Principal Shareholders: Chairman and directors as described
Date of Establishment: 29th March 1978

GOLD & BASE METAL MINES OF NIGERIA LTD

Old Airport Rd, PO Box 59, Jos, Plateau State
Tel: 52145
Cable: Basedem

Chairman: I L C Gibb
Directors: H E Croft, A A Kehinde, J D Lines, H R Mitchell
Senior Executives: D H Jones (Chief Engineer),
  M O Nubi-Falowo (Secretary/Chief Accountant)

PRINCIPAL ACTIVITIES: Mining of metal ore, production of tin concentrates
Branch Offices: Jema'a, Kaduna State; Liruie, Kano; Rishi, Bauchi State
Principal Bankers: Union Bank of Nigeria Ltd
Financial Information:

	N'000
Authorised capital	1,400
Paid-up capital	1,400
Turnover	1,763
Profits	551

Principal Shareholders: Nigerian Mining Corporation; Gold & Base Metal Mines Ltd, UK
Date of Establishment: 1934
No of Employees: 1,000

GOLD STAR INDUSTRIES LTD

Km 16 Ikorodu Rd, Ojota, PO Box 704, Lagos

PRINCIPAL ACTIVITIES: Manufacturers and distributors of clothing
Financial Information:
Registered capital   N 400,000

Date of Establishment: 1978

GOLDEN FURNITURE & CONSTRUCTION CO LTD

137 Ikpoba Slope, PO Box 588, Benin City, Bendel State
Tel: 240921

PRINCIPAL ACTIVITIES: Building and civil engineering contractors; manufacturers of furniture

GOLDEN GUINEA BREWERIES LTD

Aba Rd, Afara Industrial Layout, PMB 1031, Umuahia, Imo State

Tel: 220055
Cable: Goldbrew Umuahia

Chairman: Dr Anthony O Okafor
Directors: H E Onukogu, Chief J O Irukwu, Chief T E Nwanosike, B O Uwajumogu, Mrs C O Nkwocha, Owu U Ukoh, O M Wasmuth, Eze G C N Akomas
Senior Executives: A R Williams (General Manager),
  M O Uhiara (Brewery Manager),
  Onyenso Ajiwe (Company Secretary),
  J O Nnaji (Chief Accountant),
  B C Achareke (Chief Engineer),
  P O Okorie (Marketing Manager)

PRINCIPAL ACTIVITIES: Brewing and bottling of lager beer and stout
Branch Offices: 27 Trans-Amadi Industrial Layout, Port Harcourt; Kilometre 7 Aba/Owerri Rd, Osisioma, Aba; 68 Awka Rd, Onitsha; Ehugbo House, Amasiri Rd, Afikpo; 67 Chime Avenue, Enugu; 130 Sam Mbakwe Rd, Owerri
Principal Bankers: First Bank of Nigeria Ltd; Union Bank of Nigeria Ltd

Financial Information:

	N'000
Authorised capital	7,875
Paid-up capital	7,869
Turnover	24,766
Profits (before tax)	6,044
Profit (after tax)	3,569

Principal Shareholders: Imo State Government (51%); Nigerian Investors (39%); Coutinho Caro & Company (10%)
Date of Establishment: 26th September 1962
No of Employees: 750

GOOD-NAME STATIONERY STORES

SW8/676 Adeniji St, Off Oshosami Rd, PO Box 1710, Ibadan, Oyo State
Tel: 410893
Telex: 31109 Zoo Coy Nig

Chairman: Samuel Babajide Senkoya
Directors: O Senkoya, K Babatunde, Dele Olawoyin, O B Boyejo
Senior Executives: L Yinisa (Manager),
  Olu Oduwole,
  Bisi Oresanya,
  Remi Jimoh,
  Daniel Otunbe Atemenu

PRINCIPAL ACTIVITIES: Wholesale suppliers of stationery and office equipment, and general merchants
Principal Agencies: Nigerian Office Stationery Supply Stores, Apapa; Apen Mill Thomas Wyatt Nigeria Ltd; University Press Ltd
Branch Offices: SW9/1151A Challenge Orita Rd, Ibadan, Oyo State
Associated Companies: Igba-Ore-To Commercial (Nigeria) Enterprises Ltd
Principal Bankers: Savannah Bank of Nigeria Ltd

Principal Shareholders: O B Boyejo; Dele Olawoyin; Ola Senkoya; J O Oyetunji
Date of Establishment: 6th March 1970

GOODWILL, FRANCIS, LTD

11 Okesuna Street, PO Box 5032, Lagos
Tel: 636015, 634372
Cable: Franwill
Telex: 22202 Franig Ng

Chairman: Francis Olajide Dairo
Directors: Mrs Emily Adeoti Dairo, Mrs Anthonia Titilayo Carew
Senior Executives: Maclean Francis Hart (Marketing Manager),
  Peter Durojaiye Dairo (Branch Manager),
  Josiah Etteh Anieasaba Mkpah (Accountant),
  Patrick Ofuani (Technical Supervisor)

PRINCIPAL ACTIVITIES: Manufacturers of office furniture; distributors of business machines and security equipment
Principal Agencies: Hobbs Hart & Co Ltd, UK; Carlton Brookes Ltd, UK; Hall-Welter Co Inc, USA; Hermes Precisa International SA, Switzerland
Branch Offices: 16 Awonaike Crescent, Surulere, Lagos; 3 McCullum Street, Ebute Metta, Lagos; Western Liaison Office: A2 Alawode Crescent, Mokola, Ibadan
Principal Bankers: Union Bank of Nigeria Ltd
Financial Information:

	N'000
Authorised capital	100
Paid-up capital	100
Turnover (at 31.3.82)	1,069
Profits (before tax)	194

Principal Shareholders: F O Dairo (75%) and directors as described
Date of Establishment: 10th May 1973
No of Employees: 35

GOODWILL PRESS & BOOKSHOP

PO Box 73, Port Harcourt, Rivers State
Tel: 772

PRINCIPAL ACTIVITIES: Printers

GOODYEAR MIDWEST RUBBER PROCESSING CO (NIGERIA) LTD

Taboga Rd, Ikoba Slope, PMB 1078, Benin City, Bendel State
Tel: 44

Directors: Ian Oneil Roe (Managing Director)
PRINCIPAL ACTIVITIES: Processing of rubber

GOSWIN & CO

Kessington Ikugbade Stores, 163a Warri Sapele Rd, Warri, Bendel State
Tel: 581

PRINCIPAL ACTIVITIES: Suppliers of sanitary fittings

GOTTSCHALCKS BUILDINGS MATERIALS

163/5 Broad St, PO Box 158, Lagos
Tel: 660060, 661139, 664440, 664490, 661142
Cable: Buildsuper

PRINCIPAL ACTIVITIES: Building and civil engineering contractors, importers and distributors of building materials
Principal Agencies: Crittal-Hope; Western Steel; ICI Paints; etc
Branch Offices: 16/17 Ahmadu Bello Way, PO Box 193, Kaduna, Tel 211502; 19 Azikiwe Rd, PO Box 388, Port Harcourt, Tel 229708; 20 Niger St, PO Box 777, Kano, Tel 3767; Murtala Muhammed Way, PO Box 93, Ilorin, Tel 2068; 1 Kano Rd, PO Box 557, Jos, Tel 54014; Sapele Rd, PO Box 340, Warri, Tel 230615; 140 Marina Rd, PO Box 233, Calabar, Tel 222106; 5 Okpara Ave, PO Box 449, Enugu, Tel 255329; Magazine Rd, PO Box 1260, Ibadan, Tel 461475 also at Benin City; Aba; Maiduguri; Onitsha; Sokoto; Obanikoro
Principal Bankers: First Bank of Nigeria Ltd

Principal Shareholders: Division of UAC Nigeria Ltd
Date of Establishment: 26th May 1927

GRACE BAKERIES

68a Jebba St, Ebute-Metta, Lagos
Tel: 861906

PRINCIPAL ACTIVITIES: Bakery
Branch Offices: 2a Party St, Shomolu, Lagos, Tel 843303
No of Employees: 200

GRAND INDUSTRIAL COMPANY LTD

Plot 29 Dantata Rd, Bompai, PO Box 1020, Kano
Tel: 4824, 4825
Cable: Grandinco Kano

Directors: W J Waung
PRINCIPAL ACTIVITIES: Manufacturers of enamelware

GRANDI LAVORI (NIGERIA) LTD

PO Box 2490, Lagos
Tel: 874300

Directors: A Pezzini, A Markus
PRINCIPAL ACTIVITIES: Engineering consultants
Branch Offices: Calabar; Eket

GRÄNGES NIGERIA LTD

45 Saka Tinubu, Victoria Island, Lagos
Tel: 619894
Telex: 22106 Grange Ng

PRINCIPAL ACTIVITIES: Business and engineering consultants
Associated Companies: Gränges Hedlung (Steel builders); Gränges Graver (Tank experts); GIM (Mining and Management); Gränges Metalock (Industrial service and repair); Gränges Engineering (Process Engineering)

GRANT ADVERTISING INTERNATIONAL (NIGERIA) LTD

48 Bode Thomas St, Surulere, PO Box 3930, Lagos
Tel: 833872, 833883

PRINCIPAL ACTIVITIES: Advertising
Date of Establishment: 1970

GREAT BASINS PETROLEUM CO (NIGERIA) LTD

13 Habib House, PO Box 1236, 10 Berkley St, Lagos
Tel: 633921
Cable: Basinoil

PRINCIPAL ACTIVITIES: Exploration

GREAT NIGERIA INSURANCE COMPANY LTD

39/41 Martins Street, PO Box 2314, Lagos
Tel: 662590, 662359, 662288, 664313
Cable: Greatinsur Lagos

Chairman: Olaniwun Ajayi
Directors: D M Faluyi,
Chief Z O Odesola,
M S A Ibitomisin,
Major J S Jolaoso,
Prof D A Olatunbosun,
Dr N A Thomas,
E B Onifade (Managing)
Senior Executives: A B Ajomale (Deputy Managing Director),
O Olaoye (Deputy General Manager, Finance),
D A Adewunmi (Deputy General Manager, Technical),
A O Lucas (Assistant General Manager (Admin)/Company Secretary),
J A Ibitoye (Assistant General Manager, Finance),
A F Kiladejo (Mrs) (Assistant General Manager, Ordinary Life),
S O Asoro (Assistant General Manager (Non-Life)),
B B Banjo (Assistant General Manager, Pensions)

PRINCIPAL ACTIVITIES: All classes of insurance
Branch Offices: 302 Herbert Macaulay Street, Yaba, Lagos; 25 Adeniran Ogunsanya Street, Surulere, Lagos; Plot 13 Afolabi Aina Street, Ikeja, Lagos; 92 Oyemekun Rd, PO Box 15, Akure; 18/19 Ahmadu Bello Street, PO Box 394, Kaduna; 103 Ibrahim Taiwo Rd, PO Box 1227, Kano; Aje House, Lebanon Street, PO Box 1884, Ibadan; 51B Ibadan Rd, PO Box 133, Ijebu-Ode; 49 Akpakpava St, PO Box 404, Benin-City; 4 Rwang Pam Street, PO Box 698, Jos; 4 Ogbagba Street, PO Box 94, Oshogbo; 5 Murtala Mohammed Rd, PO Box 545, Ilorin; 47 Ikwerre Rd, PMB 5481, Port Harcourt; 81D Obafemi Awolowo Avenue, PO Box 1631, Abeokuta; 48 Ajilosun Street, PO Box 784, Ado-Ekiti
Principal Bankers: Union Bank of Nigeria Ltd; Co-operative Bank Ltd; United Bank for Africa Ltd
Financial Information:

	N'000
Authorised capital	1,000
Paid-up capital	800
Turnover	19,297
Profits	967

Principal Shareholders: Odu'a Investment Company Ltd
Date of Establishment: 24th February 1960
No of Employees: 460

GREAT NORTHERN TANNING CO LTD

PO Box 844, 22 Ja'afaru Rd, Kano
Tel: 2148
Cable: Leather Kano
Telex: 77142

PRINCIPAL ACTIVITIES: Tanners, manufacturers of all types of leathers for shoemakers and craftsmen; exporters of tanned Nigerian goatskins and wet blue chrome goatskins
No of Employees: 350

GREEN, A D, & CO LTD
346A Dugbe Market St, Adekunle Fajuyi Rd, PO Box 1329,
  Ibadan, Oyo State
Tel: 413326

PRINCIPAL ACTIVITIES: Electrical contractors

GREEN LIGHT INDUSTRIES LTD
Akoka, Lagos State

Directors: Ola Oteje (Managing Director)

PRINCIPAL ACTIVITIES: Manufacturers of envelopes

GREENHAM PLANT HIRE
PO Box 8, Mushin Industrial Estate, Ikeja, Lagos
Tel: 847428

Senior Executives: G A Cookey-Gam (General Manager)

PRINCIPAL ACTIVITIES: Building and civil engineering
  contractors; plant hire
Financial Information: Division of UAC of Nigeria Ltd

GREENS ENGINEERING LTD
PMB 1031, 36 Rhodes Crescent, Apapa, Lagos
Tel: 873441

PRINCIPAL ACTIVITIES: Building and civil engineering
  contractors

GREGSON TRADING COMPANY LTD
26 Madaki-Ibo, PO Box 1787, Kano

PRINCIPAL ACTIVITIES: Dealers in building materials, electrical
  fittings, plumbing materials, and automobile spare parts

GRENIGAS LTD
Adeyemi Bero Crescent, Ilupeju Industrial Estate, PO Box 3862,
  Lagos
Tel: 961800, 962182
Cable: Grenigas Lagos
Telex: 26655 Vkplas Ng

Chairman: B Akinyemi
Directors: S A Aguele (General Manager),
  T B Oluyide
Senior Executives: C F Akhabue (Sales Manager),
  D A Afemhenkhu (Operations Manager),
  R E Asagba (Accountant)

PRINCIPAL ACTIVITIES: Marketing of domestic and industrial
  gas installations and catering equipment
Principal Bankers: Nigeria Arab Bank Ltd; Bank of Credit &
  Commerce International (Nigeria) Ltd
Financial Information:

	N'000
Authorised capital	400
Paid-up capital	400
Turnover	1,500

Principal Shareholders: As listed above
Date of Establishment: 25th May 1967
No of Employees: 55

GROUP ELEKTRO POWER NIGERIA LTD
9 Abiodun Odeseye St, Off 3rd Lagos Axial Rd,
  Ojota-Oworonsoki Expressway, Ifako Bariga, Lagos
Tel: 860088

Chairman: Oye Elusiyan (also Managing Director)
Directors: Eluyinka Oyewole, Julianah Elusiyan
Senior Executives: A Elusanmi (Administrative Manager),
  D Akande (Assistant Technical Manager),
  P Ansar (Accountant),
  B Koleosho (Commercial Manager),
  Billy Amawampa (Technical Manager)

PRINCIPAL ACTIVITIES: Electrical and mechanical engineering
  contractors, sales and service of electrical and electronic
  equipment; manufacturers representatives
Principal Agencies: Bogard O D'Oscar, France
Branch Offices: 8 Adeleke Adegboyega St, Abule Okuta Bariga,
  Lagos; 29 Bada St, Okeigbo, Ondo State; 79 Jagunmolu St,
  Abule Bariga, Lagos; 1 Okebola St, Akure, Ondo State
Associated Companies: S Oyewole & Brothers (Nigeria) Ltd;
  Elus Electrical & Sons
Principal Bankers: Wema Bank Ltd
Financial Information:

	N'000
Authorised capital	200
Paid-up capital	200

Principal Shareholders: S O Elusiyan
Date of Establishment: 1974
No of Employees: 120

GTE NIGERIA LTD
Adem House, Near Coker Bus Stop, Lagos Badagry Expressway,
  PO Box 5154, Lagos
Tel: 801312, 801310, 801313, 801311, 801314
Telex: 21518 Procon Ng

Chairman: Chief Ade Martins (Executive Chairman)
Directors: D F Molyneux (Managing Director),
  E C Nwankwo (Executive Director - Marketing/Engineering),
  P C Asiodu,
  Liman Ciroma,
  Aminu Wali,
  D D Dudman,
  O M Novick
Senior Executives: N M Powling (Financial Controller & Assistant
  Project Manager),
  A A Oyeman (Operations Manager),
  D J Smith (Project Manager),
  L O Ihejiere (Installation Manager)

PRINCIPAL ACTIVITIES: Comprehensive planning, engineering,
  supply, installation and maintenance support of
  telecommunications systems and telephones, assembly of
  telecommunications products
Principal Agencies: GTE International Corp, USA; AEL Microtel,
  Canada; GTE Atea SA, Belgium; GTE Do Brazil, Brazil; GTE
  Telecommunicazioni Spa, Italy
Branch Offices: 3 Broadcasting Rd, PO Box 3970, Kaduna
Principal Bankers: Union Bank of Nigeria Ltd
Financial Information:

	N'000
Authorised capital	1,000
Paid-up capital	760

Principal Shareholders: GTE International Inc; Chief Ade Martins;
  Alhaji Aminu Wali; P C Asiodu; Oba Otudeko
Date of Establishment: 1970
No of Employees: 140

GUFFANTI (NIGERIA) LTD
1 Kayode St, PO Box 123, Apapa, Lagos
Tel: 964863, 874961, 875513, 875607
Telex: 21323 Gufnig Ng

Directors: Camillo Guffanti, Gabriele Lombardi, G M Uzodike

PRINCIPAL ACTIVITIES: Building and civil engineering
  contractors

GUINEA INSURANCE COMPANY LTD
21/25 Broad St, PO Box 1136, Lagos
Tel: 660630, 660653, 660701
Cable: Golden Lagos
Telex: 21680

Chairman: Chief R A Akinyemi
Directors: Agboola Oke, M D Kinsley, Chief T O
  Shobowale-Benson, K H Williams, Alhaji I Katune, B L
  Roberts, S Y Kasimu, H M J Ramshaw, A A Ukot, Engineer
  E Stow, Oluwole Alaran

Senior Executives: A Oke (Assistant General Manager, Company Secretary),
   F O Aluko (Chief Accountant),
   K K Richards (Northern Area Manager),
   M A Mustapha (Executive Assistant, Technical),
   E O Sonowo (Executive Assistant, Administration),
   H O Dawodu (Executive Assistant, Public Relations),
   B A Afekare (Data Processing Manager),
   A M Adewumi (Assistant General Manager, Finance and Company Secretary),
   O O A Bamigbetan (Production Manager),
   M R Fenton (Assistant General Manager, Technical),
   W R Jones (Manpower Development & Planning Co-ordinator),
   Mrs M M Saseyi (Life Manager)

PRINCIPAL ACTIVITIES: Insurance/reinsurance
Branch Offices: 1st Floor Turaki Ali House, 3 Kanta Rd, PO Box 108, Kaduna, Tel 213031; 5 Beirut Street, PO Box 631, Kano, Tel 3049; 10B Park Rd, PMB 7130, Aba; 77 Sir Kashim Ibrahim Rd, PO Box 479, Maiduguri; 3rd Floor Orosi House, 28 Forces Avenue, PO Box 1131, Port Harcourt, Tel 333995; Gbemisola House, 128 Obafemi Awolowo Way, Ikeja; Tapa House, Imam Dauda Street, Off Eric Moore Rd, Surulere, Tel 834620
Associated Companies: Legal and General International Ltd, UK; Norwich Winterthur Overseas Ltd, UK
Principal Bankers: Union Bank of Nigeria Ltd; Bank of the North Ltd; Savannah Bank of Nigeria Ltd
Financial Information:

	₦'000
Authorised capital	1,000
Paid-up capital	826
Premium Income	13,269
Profits	1,503

Principal Shareholders: Federal Ministry of Finance Incorporated; Northern Nigeria Investments Ltd; Legal and General International Ltd; Norwich Winterthur Overseas Ltd, UK; Ogun State Government; Oyo State Government; Chief T O Shobowale-Benson
Date of Establishment: 3rd December 1958
No of Employees: 158

GUINNESS (NIGERIA) LTD

Industrial Estate, Oba Akran Ave, PMB 21071, Ikeja, Lagos
Tel: 961902, 936348/9
Cable: Guinness Ikeja
Telex: 26254 Guining Ikeja

Chairman: Alhaji S O Gbadamosi
Directors: N E Salmon (Managing Director),
   A K Ubeku,
   S D R Lennox-Boyd,
   Chief V A Ndalugi,
   P T J Banner,
   P M Mbanefo,
   G B Sutton,
   F A Okunola,
   S A Williams
Senior Executives: G R Wilson (General Manager, Ikeja Brewery),
   M F Oteri (General Manager, Benin Brewery),
   C A Ojeikere (Company Secretary)

PRINCIPAL ACTIVITIES: Brewing, stout, lager
Branch Offices: 235 Agbor Rd, Benin City, Bendel State
Principal Bankers: Union Bank of Nigeria Ltd; First Bank of Nigeria Ltd
Financial Information:

	₦'000
Authorised capital	37,500
Paid-up capital	37,500
Turnover	150,000
Profits	12,000

Principal Shareholders: Nigerian Shareholders (60%); Guinness

Overseas Ltd and Atlantaf (40%)
Date of Establishment: 1962
No of Employees: 4,000

GULF OIL COMPANY (NIGERIA) LTD
GOCON

Gocon House, 19 Tinubu Sq, Lagos Island, PMB 2469, Lagos
Tel: 664046, 664081, 614318, 664207
Cable: Gocon
Telex: 21314 Gocon Ng

Directors: L A Turner (Managing Director),
   M J Hill,
   N L DeBay,
   J A Strand,
   D L Garrick,
   H E Hansen
Senior Executives: R L Ambrose (Technical Manager),
   A A Afolabi (Warri Area Manager),
   O Adeyinka (Manager, Human Resources),
   V Ologundudu (Manager, Law),
   P E Howe (Exploration Manager),
   J B Agan (Operations Manager),
   T I Oji (Services Manager),
   J A Williams (Financial Administration Manager),
   I O Ogwuru (Manager, Engineering and Construction)

PRINCIPAL ACTIVITIES: Petroleum exploration and production
Branch Offices: PO Box 1031, Port Harcourt, Rivers State, Tel 226402, 223686; NPA Compound, PO Box 94, Warri, Bendel State, Tel 232103, 230878

GUMO MINING SYNDICATE

Mile 3, Zaria Rd, PO Box 277, Jos, Plateau State
PRINCIPAL ACTIVITIES: Mining

GUOBADIA FURNITURE & CONSTRUCTION COMPANY (NIGERIA) LTD

117 Upper Benin/Sapele Rd, PO Box 414, Benin City, Bendel State
Tel: 241722

PRINCIPAL ACTIVITIES: Construction and furniture manufacturers

GUTHRIE (NIGERIA) LTD

37/39 Iganmu Industrial Estate, PO Box 7585, Lagos
Tel: 833171, 833172
Cable: Guthrie Lagos
Telex: 21355

Chairman: F S K Baron (Rotating with Alhaji M K Bayero)
Directors: Chief S O Lambo, Chief D A Orija, S D H Mosey, Chief J O Oyebanjo, J O Savage
Senior Executives: L O F Odigwe (Financial Controller)

PRINCIPAL ACTIVITIES: Building products, bakery equipment; fire fighting vehicles and equipment; pharmaceuticals; agricultural machinery and services
Principal Agencies: Angus H C B, Angus Fire Armour (fire fighting equipment); Even Products (irrigation equipment); Werner and Pfleiderer; Mono Universal Bakery Machinery; Morton Machinery Co; Globe Bakery Machinery; Woodschow and Company (bakery equipment); Merz, Patentex; Souls; Bieffe; Blendax (pharmaceuticals); Kumpulan Guthrie Sendirian Berhad (rubber processing machinery); Farrow (Irrigation Equipment)
Branch Offices: 16B Post Office Rd, Kano; 3 Katchia Rd, Kaduna; NW4/423 Salvation Army Rd, Ibadan, Oyo State; Uwhe Mansion, PO Box 8, Warri, Bendel State; 62 Aba Rd, Port Harcourt; 49 Port Harcourt Rd, Aba, Imo State; 5 Lugard Rd, Jos, Plateau State
Principal Bankers: First Bank of Nigeria; Union Bank of Nigeria

No of Employees: 375

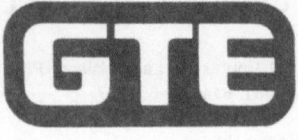

GYARTAGERE EXPLOSIVES & CHEMICALS CO LTD

Km 8 Bukuru Rd, PO Box 403, Jos, Plateau State

Chairman: Paul G Gindiri
Directors: N K Sodan, O A Momoh, H U F Enuha, Christopher Adebayo Alabi, Alhaji Sulei Sale Bimaj
Senior Executives: B Gwong (Accountant), P A Sho-Siver (Sales Manager)

PRINCIPAL ACTIVITIES: Mineral processing and quarrying; chemicals
Principal Agencies: NDCC Ltd, Lagos
Branch Offices: Throughout Nigeria
Principal Bankers: Savannah Bank (Nigeria) Ltd
Financial Information:
Authorised capital ₦ 200,000

Principal Shareholders: Paul G Gindiri; C A Alabi; Alhaji S S Bima

H B & SONS

37/43 Enuowa St, PO Box 3281, Lagos
Tel: 633255, 634292
Telex: 21482 Echbee

PRINCIPAL ACTIVITIES: Importers, general merchants, department stores, supermarkets; wholesalers
Branch Offices: Enugu; Kano; Onitsha; Port Harcourt; Ibadan; Jos; Benin
Financial Information: Subsidiary of J T Chanrai & Co Ltd (see separate entry)
No of Employees: 1,000

H BECKER-VOIGT

See BECKER-VOIGT, H

H CLARKSON EDU & PARTNERS

PO Box 2853, Nasco House, 29 Burma Rd, Apapa, Lagos
Tel: 845871, 873409
Cable: Holdsur Lagos
Telex: 21284 Nidex; 21447 Nerox

Partners: A Edu (Managing Partner), E Edu (Partner), H Clarkson Holdings Ltd, London
Senior Executives: B F Sadler (General Manager), R Godfrey (Marine Manager), A Oyedele (Finance and Administration Manager)

PRINCIPAL ACTIVITIES: Insurance brokers
Branch Offices: 174 Broad St, Lagos; 12B Bello Rd, Kano
Principal Bankers: United Bank for Africa Ltd; Societe Generale Bank (Nigeria) Ltd; International Bank for West Africa Ltd
Financial Information:

	₦'000
Turnover	13,000
Profits	250

Principal Shareholders: Abayomi Edu; Babatunde Edu; H Clarkson Nigerian Holdings
Date of Establishment: 1964

H F SCHROEDER (WA) LTD

See SCHROEDER, H F, (WA) LTD

H H ROBERTSON (NIGERIA) LTD

See ROBERTSON, H H, (NIGERIA) LTD

H W ROMAIN & SON LTD

See ROMAIN, H W, & SON LTD

HABIS TRAVELS LTD

15/16B Post Office Rd, Kano
Tel: 3271, 3272
Cable: Habiskans
Telex: 77174 Kanjet

Chairman: Alhaji Uba Waru
Directors: Alhaji Ado Dandawak
Senior Executives: Nazih Kamal (General Manager)

PRINCIPAL ACTIVITIES: Travel agents
Principal Agencies: All IATA Airlines
Branch Offices: Hamdaua Hotel Complex, Kaduna, Tel 242810
Principal Bankers: International Bank for West Africa Ltd
Financial Information:
Turnover (approx) ₦ 6,000,000

Principal Shareholders: Alhaji Abu Waru; Alhaji Ado Dandawak
Date of Establishment: 1958

HACO LTD

PMB 21061, Ladipo Oluwole Avenue, Ikeja, Lagos
Tel: 900071/2
Cable: Hacol Ikeja

Chairman: Chief Mathias Ugochuku
Directors: C E J Allanson (Managing), R O E Asemota (Executive), D R Simpson (Divisional Chief Executive), G M Onyiuke

PRINCIPAL ACTIVITIES: Manufacturers of toiletries and cosmetics
Principal Agencies: Lentheric; Yardley; Johnson Products, etc
Branch Offices: Principal towns throughout Nigeria
Principal Bankers: First Bank of Nigeria Ltd; United Bank of Africa Ltd

Principal Shareholders: John Holt Ltd
Date of Establishment: 1955
No of Employees: 400

HADEMEC LTD
Formerly Haden (Nigeria) Ltd

PO Box 205, Yaba, Lagos
Tel: 962168
Cable: Coolth Lagos
Telex: 20117 Tds Box 237

Chairman: T B Appta
Directors: Chief S L Edu, Sunday Dankaro, Mrs O O Olakunri, G R Thomas (Managing Director), G Smith, D J Hyam, A A Lasebikah, P J de Vroome
Senior Executives: N A Aro (Chief Accountant/Secretary), G F Miller

PRINCIPAL ACTIVITIES: Building services engineering contractors
Branch Offices: PO Box 206, Zaria, Kaduna State; PMB 116, Agodi Gate, Ibadan, Oyo State; PMB 1195, Maiduguri, Borno State
Principal Bankers: United Bank for Africa

Principal Shareholders: Chief S L Edu; Sunday Dankaro, Mrs O O Olakunri; Haden Carrier Ltd; Haden International Ltd; A A Lasebikah
Date of Establishment: 1951
No of Employees: 350

HAFFAR INDUSTRIAL CO LTD

PO Box 264, 269A Agege Motor Rd, Mushin, Lagos State
Tel: 844536, 835595
Cable: Scissors, Lagos

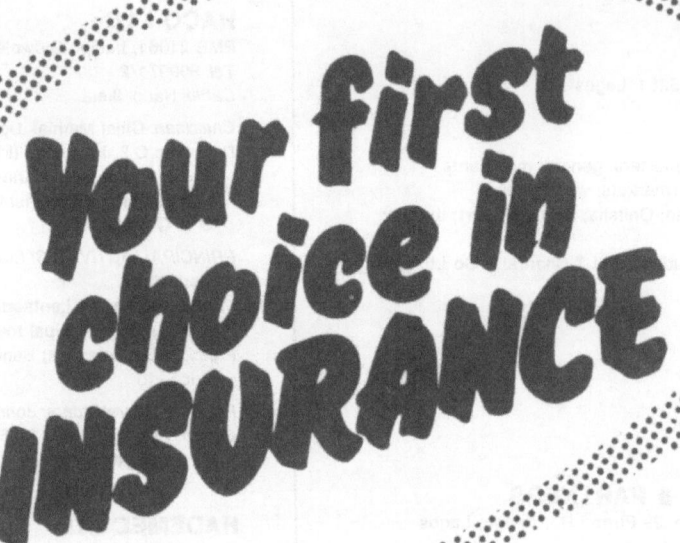
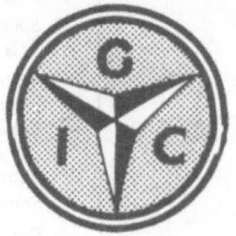

Chairman: M Z Haffar (also Managing Director)
Directors: F F Haffar, E O Salako, Alhaji Yisa Yagboyanju
Senior Executives: S O Adeniran (Personnel Manager),
  Charles Emekobum (Production Manager),
  H T Omotosho (Stores Controller)
PRINCIPAL ACTIVITIES: Textile manufacturers; sewing thread,
  processors of yarn
Principal Bankers: Union Bank of Nigeria Ltd; Arab Bank of
  Nigeria Ltd; First Bank of Nigeria Ltd
Financial Information:

	N'000
Authorised capital	500
Paid-up capital	500
Turnoer	5,000

Principal Shareholders: M Z Haffar; F F Haffar
Date of Establishment: 1968
No of Employees: 300

HAGEMEYER (NIGERIA) LTD

82 Murtala Mohammed Way, Ebuta-Metta, PO Box 179, Lagos
Tel: 800030/2, 860047, 860493

Chairman: Alfred A A Egunjobi
Directors: H P C Butzelaar (Managing),
  Alhaji Babatunde Jose,
  S A Fatiregun

PRINCIPAL ACTIVITIES: Trading company dealing in
  photographic materials, electrical equipment, hardware,
  office equipment, etc
Principal Agencies: Sigma Coatings
Branch Offices: Ibadan; Warri; Kaduna; Kano; Maiduguri; Aba;
  Onitsha; Port Harcourt
Principal Bankers: United Bank for Africa Ltd; First Bank of
  Nigeria Ltd

Principal Shareholders: Nigerians; Hagemeyer and Company;
  Handelmatsahapp NV Naarden
Date of Establishment: May 1960
No of Employees: 400

HALCON ENGINEERING ASSOCIATES LTD

40C Tafawa Balewa Square, PO Box 8028, Lagos
Tel: 632583, 636779

Chairman: Henry C Omo
Directors: J N C Nwangwu, J O Onyeemelukwe

PRINCIPAL ACTIVITIES: Civil engineering and building
  construction
Branch Offices: 5A Aria Rd, PMB 1552, Enugu; Tel 256216; 37
  Constitution Crescent, PO Box 177, Aba; Tel 220262, 221508
Principal Bankers: United Bank for Africa Ltd
Financial Information:

	N'000
Authorised capital	100
Paid-up capital	100

Principal Shareholders: J O Onyemelukwe; Henry C Omo; J N C
  Nwangwu
No of Employees: Over 250

HALLIBURTON NIGERIA LTD

Plot 1153, Gabara Close, Victoria Island, PO Box 3694, Lagos
Tel: 611474, 611478
Cable: Halliburton Lagos
Telex: 21899 Howco Ng

Directors: L F Mermis,
  G J Phillips,
  T A Whitmore (General Manager),
  G A O George,
  F M Adeakin
Senior Executives: G E Pospischil (Operations Manager),
  U K Uzoh (Assistant Company Secretary),
  D D Hale (Field Supervisor, Port Harcourt),
  D J Eelsing (Field Supervisor, Warri)

PRINCIPAL ACTIVITIES: Oil services; wall cementing
Branch Offices: Field Office: Trans-Amadi Layout, PO Box 462,
  Port Harcourt and Enerhen Rd, PO Box 359, Warri
Associated Companies: Brown & Root (Nig) Ltd; Otis Nigeria Ltd
Principal Bankers: First Bank of Nigeria Ltd

HAM DREDGING NIGERIA LTD

Plot 14 Block 5 Oduduwa Crescent, GRA, PO Box 826, Ikeja,
Lagos
Tel: 962772
Telex: 26604 Hamdre Ng

PRINCIPAL ACTIVITIES: Land reclamation, sand supply, channel
  making
Branch Offices: 80 Marian Rd Extension, PMB 1266, Calabar,
  Cross River State; Nigerian Shipbuilders Yard, POB 206, Port
  Harcourt, Rivers State
Subsidiary Companies: Interbeton (Nigeria) Ltd

HAMMOND, MICHAEL, ENGINEERING LTD

228 Apapa Rd, Ijora, PMB 3137, Surulere, Lagos
Tel: 835910
Telex: 21312

PRINCIPAL ACTIVITIES: Electrical engineering; electrical
  equipment suppliers
Principal Agencies: Briamore Manufacturing Ltd, UK; Canadian
  Appliance Manufacturing Company Ltd; Denco Miller & Denco
  Refrigeration
Branch Offices: 40 Aba Rd, Port Harcourt, Rivers State; 70A
  Ibrahim Taiwo Rd, Ilorin, Kwara State

HAMMOND, T A, PROJECTS LTD

Maza Maza Village, Km 7 Badagry Expressway, PO Box 2898,
Lagos
Tel: 880323
Telex: 11117 Net TDS Box 329

Chairman: Col A A Ochefu
Directors: Alhaji Yusuf Katsina,
  Udo Bassey,
  W F Turnbull (Managing),
  Mrs V Lijadu,
  T A Hammond (Chief Executive)

PRINCIPAL ACTIVITIES: Civil engineering and construction
Branch Offices: 15 Ahmadu Bello Way, PO Box 70, Otukpo,
  Benue State
Principal Bankers: First Bank of Nigeria Ltd
Financial Information:

	N'000
Authorised capital	2,000
Paid-up capital	1,500

Principal Shareholders: Nigerians (60%); British (40%)

HAMZER, G N A, & CO (NIGERIA) LTD

19 Kofo Abayomi Ave, PO Box 117, Apapa, Lagos State
Tel: 874957, 876860, 874077
Cable: Galhamzaco Apapa
Telex: 21396 Hamza Lagos; 20117 TDS Box 309 for UK

Chairman: Alhaji Dr Garba Nautan Hamza
Directors: Alhaji Manya Hamza (Manager),
  Alhaji Ysufu Danguru Hamza,
  Mallam M N Hamza

PRINCIPAL ACTIVITIES: Holding company for 19 companies
  engaged in the following activities: property development,
  textiles, furniture, food processing, insurance, consultants,
  travel agency, cargo and shipping services, printing and
  publishing, civil engineering contracting, fishing, agricultural
  machinery suppliers, general trading, importers of agricultural
  produce, building materials, cement exporters of agricultural
  produce including palm kernel and palm oil, cotton, etc

HANEIN & SOLOMONS LTD
PO Box 71, 10 Makoko Rd, Yaba, Lagos
Tel: 862383

PRINCIPAL ACTIVITIES: Building and civil engineering
contractors

HANS MEHR (NIGERIA) LTD
See MEHR, HANS, (NIGERIA) LTD

HANSEN, JOS & SOEHNE (NIGERIA) LTD
31/33 Martins Street, PO Box 141, Lagos
Tel: 664121, 664172, 664212
Cable: Dahanjed
Telex: 21413

Chairman: T A Braithwaite
Directors: K Fritsch, L Omagbemi, Alhaji A Gusau, R Peetz, H
W Oehmchen, Y Amaye

PRINCIPAL ACTIVITIES: Planning, erection and service of
projects for water supply and drainage; expecially large-scale
urban projects; electricity generation; telecommunication and
alarm systems; suppliers of industrial equipment and heavy
machinery
Principal Agencies: Klein, Schanzlin & Becker AG, West
Germany; Paterson Candy International Ltd, UK; Telefonbau
& Normalzeit, West Germany
Branch Offices: 40E Ado Bayero St, PO Box 831, Kano; 49
Akpabio St, Ekulu, PO Box 176, Enugu; Plot 2 Malali Layout,
PO Box 5415, Kaduna
Principal Bankers: First Bank of Nigeria Ltd
Financial Information:

	N'000
Authorised capital	480
Paid-up capital	400

Principal Shareholders: T A Braithwaite; Jos Hansen & Soehne
Aussenhandelsges. mbH Hamburg; Various Nigerian
Shareholders
Date of Establishment: 1955
No of Employees: 170

HAPEL NIGERIA LTD
156 Zik Ave, PO Box 137, Enugu, Anambra State
Tel: 252054, 252515
Cable: Hapel
Telex: 51156 Hapel Ng

Chairman: E N Nwokoro
Directors: Mrs P U Nwokoro
Senior Executives: R G Ewurum (Chief Accountant),
G E Nwokoro (Secretary),
L Ossai (Civil Engineer)

PRINCIPAL ACTIVITIES: Importers of building materials,
electrical goods, gas cookers; suppliers of general
merchandise; transport contractors
Principal Bankers: First Bank of Nigeria Ltd
Financial Information:

	N'000
Authorised capital	100
Paid-up capital	100
Sales turnover	2,500

Principal Shareholders: E N Nwokoro; Mrs P U Nwokoro

HARBONI LTD
PO Box 282, Queen Elizabeth II Rd, Ibadan, Oyo State
Tel: 414011, 414102, 414173
Cable: Harboni Ibadan
Telex: Harboni NG TDS 023

Chairman: Chief E A Ladele
Directors: Felix 'Shokan Oni (Managing),
Engr Thilak Wijesinghe (Technical),
Engr D A Coker,
Alhaji B A Wahabi
Senior Executives: H S de Soysa (Quarry Master),
R Vaithilingam (Mechanical Engineer),

O A Omoniyi (Accountant),
E O Akinwumi (Office Manager),
S I Senathirajah (Senior Accountant)

PRINCIPAL ACTIVITIES: Quarrying
Branch Offices: PMB 1077, Ikeja, Lagos; Sapele Rd, Benin City
Principal Bankers: New Nigeria Bank Ltd
Financial Information:

	N'000
Authorised capital	2,000
Paid-up capital	2,000
Turnover	5,000
Profits	1,000

Date of Establishment: 1946 (Formerly T A Oni & Co Ltd)
No of Employees: 300

HARMONY HOUSE FURNITURE CO LTD
Agege Motor Rd, PO Box 212, Ikeja, Lagos
Tel: 963239, 834136
Cable: Harmofurn

Chairman: I O Ajanaku
Directors: B O Aina
Senior Executives: M Cohen (General Manager)

PRINCIPAL ACTIVITIES: Manufacturing of furniture and allied
products
Branch Offices: Kaduna
Principal Bankers: First Bank of Nigeria Ltd
Financial Information:

Autorised capital	₦ 1,000,000

Principal Shareholders: I O Ajanaku; B O Aina
Date of Establishment: 10th August, 1960
No of Employees: 600

HARMONY INSURANCE CO (NIGERIA) LTD
78 Lagos Bye Pass, Oke-Ado, PO Box 12779, Ibadan, Oyo State

Tel: 412836
Cable: Harmonia

Chairman: Olubunmi Ibitoye (also Managing Director)
Directors: J T F Brown, Mrs P M Ibitoye, D O Akinbote
Senior Executives: S Adeniyi Osho (General Manager),
A A Solanke (Adm Manager),
A G Richards (Claims Manager),
A Ayanwuyi (Accountant),
Ade Atayero (Agency/Underwriting Manager)

PRINCIPAL ACTIVITIES: Insurance
Branch Offices: 37 Ayibara St, Surulere, Lagos; 6 Lagos Bye
Pass, Oke - Bola, Ibadan
Principal Bankers: National Bank of Nigerian Ltd; Arab Bank
(Nigeria) Ltd

Date of Establishment: 1970
No of Employees: 340

HAROLD SODIPO & CO LTD
See SODIPO, HAROLD, & CO LTD

HARRIS INTERNATIONAL TELECOMMUNICATIONS
362 Herbert Macauley St, Yaba, PO Box 7700, Lagos
Tel: 860538, 619399
Cable: Radcom Lagos
Telex: 21550 Domsat Ng

Senior Executives: G W Michael (Managing Director)

PRINCIPAL ACTIVITIES: Telecommunications

HARRISON, PETER, NIGERIA LTD
19 Martins St, PO Box 4889, Lagos
Tel: 660900, 660168
Cable: Petercoms Lagos
Telex: 21515 Pehans Ng; 21945

Chairman: Kayode Ojeseime Ajakaiye (also Managing Director)
Directors: Chief Peter H Ajakaiye
Senior Executives: Francis Akhimie (Sales Officer),
J B Olowojoba (Accountant)

PRINCIPAL ACTIVITIES: General merchants, shippers,
importers, exporters, contractors
Branch Offices: Calabar; Benin City
Subsidiary Companies: Worldwide Traders (Nigeria) Ltd
Principal Bankers: New Nigeria Bank Ltd; African Continental
Bank Ltd
Financial Information:

	₦'000
Authorised capital	100
Paid-up capital	100
Turnover	3,000

Principal Shareholders: K O Ajakaiye; Chief Peter H Ajakaiye
Date of Establishment: 1972

HARRITEDS INTERNATIONAL COMPANY (NIGERIA) LTD

132 Azikiwe Rd, Aba, Imo State

Chairman: Chris Ogbudike
Directors: Chibu Ogbudike, Harrison Ogbudike, Edward
Ogbudike, Egesimba Ogbudike
Senior Executives: C Eze (Secretary),
Caleb Okanume (Manager, Clearing),
Simeon Ogbudike (Manager)

PRINCIPAL ACTIVITIES: Importers, suppliers of general
merchandise
Branch Offices: 1 Okwey St, Onitsha, Anambra State; 158 Ojo
Rd, Lagos
Associated Companies: C Ogbudike and Company
Principal Bankers: Mercantile Bank of Nigeria Ltd
Financial Information:

	₦'000
Authorised capital	1,000
Paid-up capital	500
Turnover	6,000
Profits	600

Principal Shareholders: Chris Ogbudike; Harrison Ogbudike;
Edward Ogbudike
Date of Establishment: 1970

HARUNA, ALHAJI MUSTAPHA, & SONS

PO Box 283, Maiduguri, Borno State
Tel: 2344
Telex: 82108 Haruna Ng

PRINCIPAL ACTIVITIES: Building contractors; general
transporters and produce buyers

HASKONING NIGERIA LTD (FORMERLY NEDECO)

26 Adetokunboh Ademola St, Victoria Island, Lagos
Tel: 617028
Telex: 22511 Hasko Ng

Chairman: R Brouwer
Directors: W Wolters (Managing),
A P A M van Deurzen,
Chuka J Okoli,
Alh Shehu Ahmed,
P L Laboyrie,
M Y L van Berckel,
J O Sonuga,
F C Holthuis,
Y O Beredugo

PRINCIPAL ACTIVITIES: Engineering consultants
Branch Offices: 98 Lamido Crescent, PO Box 973, Kano
Principal Bankers: Savannah Bank of Nigeria Ltd
Financial Information:

	₦'000
Authorised capitakl	100
Paid-up capital	90

Principal Shareholders: Haskoning B V, Holland (60%); Alh
Shehu Ahmed; Y O Beredugo; Chuka J Okoli; J O Sonuga
Date of Establishment: 1978
No of Employees: 40

HASSAN FURNITURE & JOINERY COMPANY LTD

28 Kaga Rd, (Near Shell Depot), PO Box 457, Maiduguri, Borno
State
Tel: 2263, 2372

PRINCIPAL ACTIVITIES: Buildin contractors; manufacturers of
household, school and general purpose furniture
Branch Offices: 2 Ahmadu Bello Way, PO Box 457, Maiduguri,
Borno State

HASSAN TRANSPORT (NIGERIA) LTD

12 Ijora Causeway, PO Box 20, Apapa, Lagos
Tel: 832164, 832215, 837409

PRINCIPAL ACTIVITIES: Fuel-oil haulage specialists and general
haulage
Branch Offices: Port Harcourt
No of Employees: 250

HAVEN NIGERIA COMPUTER CO LTD

Hamburg House, 31-33 Martin St, PO Box 4034, Lagos
Tel: 662383
Telex: 21658 Havcom

PRINCIPAL ACTIVITIES: Computer services
Financial Information:
Authorised capital   ₦ 100,000

Date of Establishment: November 1975

HAY, BARRY, ODUNSI & ASSOCIATES

1st Floor, Lapal House, 235 Igbosere Rd, PO Box 5006, Lagos
Tel: 631480
Cable: Odunhabary Lagos

Chairman: Z A Odunsi
Directors: M S Frost

PRINCIPAL ACTIVITIES: Consulting engineers; structural and
civil engineering design of all types of private commercial
and industrial buildings
Principal Bankers: First Bank of Nigeria Ltd

Principal Shareholders: Z A Odunsi; M S Frost
Date of Establishment: 1971

HEALTH CARE PRODUCTS (NIGERIA) LTD

Formerly Johnson & Johnson (Nigeria) Ltd

25 Industrial Ave, Ilupeju, PO Box 3136, Lagos
Tel: 963210
Cable: Jayandjay

Chairman: A S Guobadia
Directors: G M Brice, K Healey, Chief Dr M Majekodunmi, D L
Garrick
Senior Executives: P Sholola (Chief Accountant),
A Okafor (Marketing Manager)

PRINCIPAL ACTIVITIES: Pharmaceuticals and cosmetics
Principal Agencies: Johnson & Johnson Worldwide; Janssen
Pharmaceuticals; Surgikos
Principal Bankers: Union Bank of Nigeria Ltd; Icon Ltd
(Merchant Bankers); Chase Merchant Bank Nigeria Ltd

Date of Establishment: 1968
No of Employees: 115

HEINEMANN EDUCATIONAL BOOKS (NIGERIA) LTD

PMB 5205, Ighodaro Rd, Jericho, Ibadan, Oyo State
Tel: 462060/1
Telex: 31113 Hebook Ng

Chairman: Alan Hill
Directors: A Higo (Deputy Chairman/Managing Director),
    F S Ehinlaiye (Financial),
    O J Osadolor (Sales),
    Akin Thomas (Publishing)
PRINCIPAL ACTIVITIES: Publishing, educational/general books
Principal Bankers: United Bank for Africa Ltd
Financial Information:

	N'000
Authorised capital	2,000
Paid-up capital	1,292

Date of Establishment: 21st April 1969
No of Employees: 120

HENKEL CHEMICALS NIGERIA LTD
Plot 7 Block K Isolo Expressway, PO Box 4000, Lagos
Tel: 842869, 835360
Cable: Henkelchem Lagos
Telex: 20117 Booth No 226
Chairman: Alhaji Baba Abubakar
Directors: Alhaji H Abdulkadir,
    Alhaji U S Ndayako,
    Peter Saver,
    Karl-Heinz Willemsen (Managing)
Senior Executives: S O Imoru (Financial Controller),
    F A Wodi (Secretary),
    H G Burmann (Marketing Director)
PRINCIPAL ACTIVITIES: Manufacturing of chemicals products
Principal Bankers: Icon Ltd (Merchant Bankers); Societe
    Generale Bank
Financial Information:

	N'000
Authorised capital	2,000
Paid-up capital	1,500
Turnover	16,000

Principal Shareholders: Henkel KG & A, West Germany; Alhaji
    Baba Abubakar
Date of Establishment: 22nd December 1972
No of Employees: 200

HENRY STEPHENS ENGINEERING COMPANY LTD
See STEPHENS, HENRY, ENGINEERING COMPANY LTD

HEPLAC NIGERIA LTD
PO Box 5498, 21 Ikorodu Rd, Lagos
Tel: 960313
Cable: Hepin Lagos
Directors: Eng Olu Awoyinga, Ayo Jegede, Edmund Thompson
Senior Executives: Biodun Ademiji (Group Accountant),
    Eng Roy Blanchette (Technical Manager),
    Eng K Fagbemi (Project Engineer)
PRINCIPAL ACTIVITIES: Electrical mechanical and chemical
    engineering; construction
Branch Offices: Block C, ICC Offices, Agodi, Ibadan, Oyo State;
    127 New Hospital Rd, Akure, Ondo State
Principal Bankers: First Bank of Nigeria Ltd; United Bank for
    Africa; Co-operative Bank Ltd
Financial Information:

	N'000
Authorised capital	250
Paid-up capital	230
Sales turnover	10,000

Principal Shareholders: Directors as described above
Date of Establishment: October 1976
No of Employees: 250

HERBST & NDUSCO CONSTRUCTIONS LTD
Independence Layout, Plot 629, PMB 1469, Enugu, Anambra
    State
PRINCIPAL ACTIVITIES: Construction
Branch Offices: 130 Broad St, Lagos, Tel 20353

HERWA INSURANCE LTD
226 Apapa Rd, Ijora, Apapa, PO Box 9472, Lagos
Tel: 875062
PRINCIPAL ACTIVITIES: Insurance
Branch Offices: Aba; Agbor; Benin; Enugu; Idah; Ibadan; Jos;
    Onitsha; Orlu; Owerri; Kano; Warri

HERWA LTD
Unity House, Marina, PO Box 1681, Lagos
Tel: 636594
Telex: 21358 Herwa Ng
Directors: Carlo Dello Strologo
PRINCIPAL ACTIVITIES: Consultants and general contracting
Branch Offices: 1 Naraguta Ave, PO Box 675, Jos, Plateau State,
    Tel 2871

HIGRADE CONSTRUCTION & ENGINEERING COMPANY LTD
PO Box 732, Lagos
Tel: 863024
Cable: Higrade Lagos
Chairman: E O Uwak (also Managing Director)
Directors: R Becker (Projects),
    Charles Uwak,
    William Uwak,
    Victor Uwak
Senior Executives: Ganiyu Adisa Sarumi (Quantity Surveyor),
    Yinusa Adeyefa Agyifa (Civil Engineer)
PRINCIPAL ACTIVITIES: Civil engineering contractors
Associated Companies: Higrade Poultry Industry Ltd, Lagos
Principal Bankers: Mercantile Bank of Nigeria Ltd; New Nigeria
    Bank
Financial Information:

	N'000
Authorised capital	400
Paid-up capital	250

Principal Shareholders: E O Uwak; Higrade Maritime Services
    Ltd
Date of Establishment: 28th January 1976

HILSON NIGERIA LTD
40 Murtala Mohammed Way, PO Box 999, Jos, Plateau State
Tel: 3589, Ext 4
PRINCIPAL ACTIVITIES: Importers of power equipment,
    electrical goods, scientific instruments, laboratory
    equipment, office machinery, etc
Principal Agencies: Atlas Nigeria Ltd; Philips Nigeria Ltd;
    Adejumo Fam (Nig) Ltd; Black & Decker

HITECH (NIGERIA) LTD
Plot 21 Block 16 Ikorodu Rd, Anthony, PO Box 3914, Ikeja,
    Lagos
PRINCIPAL ACTIVITIES: Fire protection services
Date of Establishment: 1976

HOEGH LINE (NIGERIA) LTD
Nasco House, Plateau/Burma Rd, PO Box 96, Apapa, Lagos
Tel: 877136, 877492
Telex: 21257 Hoegaf Ng
PRINCIPAL ACTIVITIES: Shipping
Branch Offices: 8 Creek Rd, Apapa

HOEK (NIG) LTD

208/212 Broad St, PO Box 2150, Lagos
Telex: 21248 Hoeks Ng

PRINCIPAL ACTIVITIES: Importers of general merchandise

HOESCH PIPE MILLS (NIG) LTD

Henry Carr St, Industrial Estate, PMB 21149, Ikeja, Lagos
Tel: 963643

Directors: H Ruberg

PRINCIPAL ACTIVITIES: Manufacturers and suppliers of pipes

No of Employees: 350

HOGG ROBINSON NIGERIA

11 Jibowu St, Yaba, PO Box 1156, Lagos
Tel: 860491
Cable: Unipen Lagos
Telex: 22626

Chairman: J O Emanuel
Directors: Amos A Adeyeye (Managing)

PRINCIPAL ACTIVITIES: Insurance and reinsurance brokers, specialists in risks related to oil exploration
Branch Offices: 3rd Floor No 1 Obiagu Rd, Enugu; 98/99 Tafawa Balewa Rd, Kano; New Nigeria Development Corporation Building, 18/19 Ahmadu Bello Way, Kaduna; Denden House, Bank Rd, Ibadan, Oyo State; 69 Akpakpava Rd, PMB 1250, Benin City, Bendel State; Edewor Shopping Centre, Warri-Sapele Rd, Warri, Bendel State; 24 Ikwerre Rd, PMB 5725, Port Harcourt, Rivers State
Financial Information:

	N'000
Turnover	2,468
Profits	872

Principal Shareholders: Hogg Robinson Nigeria
Date of Establishment: 1st July 1974
No of Employees: 200

HOLEX TIMBER (NIGERIA) LTD

Mile 3.5 Benin-Lagos Rd, Uselu, PO Box 179, Benin City, Bendel State
Cable: Holex
Telex: 41112

Chairman: Miss Marianne Omoirawua
Directors: M E J Aghagboren (Managing Director),
    O I Afe,
    G B A Egbe
Senior Executives: J Bohlen (General Manager)

PRINCIPAL ACTIVITIES: Saw milling, manufacturing of building materials
Subsidiary Companies: Induscult (Nigeria) Ltd
Principal Bankers: First Bank of Nigeria Ltd; Union Bank of Nigeria Ltd

Principal Shareholders: M Omoirawua (60%); M Aghagboren; O I Afe; G B A Egbe

HOLMAN BROTHERS (NIGERIA) LTD

23 Burma Rd, PO Box 81, Apapa, Lagos
Tel: 877057, 874406, 877128
Cable: Airdrill Lagos
Telex: 21502

Chairman: Sir Mobolaji Bank-Anthony
Senior Executives: M O George (Managing Director)

PRINCIPAL ACTIVITIES: Road construction, civil engineering, suppliers of mining and quarry machinery and construction equipment
Principal Agencies: Compair-Broomwade; Aveling Barford; Hap Cranes; Stothert and Pitt; Mono Pumps; Ruston Bucyrus; Goodwin Barsby
Branch Offices: PO Box 427, Textile Rd, Kaduna South; PO Box

293, Harbour Rd, Port Harcourt
Principal Bankers: First Bank of Nigeria Ltd

No of Employees: 200

HOLT, JOHN, LTD

Ebani House, 149/153 Broad St, PO Box 2508, Lagos
Tel: 661722, 664713, 661756, 664794, 661711
Cable: Holniman Lagos
Telex: 21238

Chairman: Chief M N Ugochukwu
Directors: Alhaji Garba Ja Abdulkadir,
    A A Adio-Moses,
    R H Meadows,
    T R Prentice,
    C V J Allanson (Managing Director),
    P Best (Deputy Chairman),
    J G Storry (Executive Director),
    G M Onyiuke (Executive Director),
    R O E Asemota (Executive Director),
    Dr E Ogbu,
    Alhaji A A Jarma,
    D O Ejiofoh (Managing Director, Holt Engineering)

PRINCIPAL ACTIVITIES: Agents and general trading, distribution of motor vehicles, electrical equipment, agricultural equipment, pharmaceuticals; engineering and shipping services; manufacturers of cosmetics, toiletries and confetionery; assembling of motor cycles
Principal Agencies: Ford Motor Co; Yamaha Electric Motor Corp; Japan; Johnson Products, USA; Proctor & Gamble; Petbow; Clark Equipment; Komatsu
Branch Offices: Over 100 Branches throughout Nigeria; John Holt Ltd, Divisions: Holt Engineering Division, Plot 3 and 4, Adewunmi Estate, Oregun Industrial Estate, PMB 21413, Ikeja, Lagos. (Branches in Kano; Kaduna; Maiduguri; Port Harcourt; Warri; Enugu); Yamaco, Adewunmi Estate, Oregun Industrial Estate, PO Box 542, Ikeja, Lagos (Depots in Port Harcourt; Kaduna); Almarine, Marine Workshop, Ihiala St, Gborokiri, Port Harcourt; Agricon, 25 Creek Rd, Apapa, PO Box 217, Lagos; Trailerways, PO Box 1226, Ibadan, Oyo State; Arewa Bottlers, Plot 25/27, Sharada 2, Industrial Estate, Kano
Subsidiary Companies: J Allen & Co Ltd (see separate entry); West African Drug Co Ltd (see separate entry); Plateau Confectionery Co Ltd (see separate entry); John Holt Shipping Services Ltd (see separate entry); Haco Ltd (see separate entry)
Principal Bankers: First Bank of Nigeria Ltd; Union Bank of Nigeria Ltd; United Bank for Africa; Savannah Bank of Nigeria Ltd; International Bank for West Africa Ltd; New Nigeria Bank Ltd; Pan African Bank Ltd; African Continental Bank Ltd; Mercantile Bank of Nigeria Ltd

Principal Shareholders: John Holt Holdings (Nig) Ltd (40%); Nigerian public (60%)

HOLT'S NIGERIAN TANNERIES LTD

10 Maganda Rd, PO Box 341, Kano

Directors: J G Storry, D P Porter, R H Meadows, P Best, Alhaji A Umar Bamalli, T R Prentice, S Y Kasimu

PRINCIPAL ACTIVITIES: Tanners
Principal Bankers: Union Bank of Nigeria Ltd

Principal Shareholders: Ultimate Holding Co., John Holt Holdings (Nigeria) Ltd

HOME & OVERSEAS TRADING COMPANY LTD

8/10 Broad St, Lagos
Telex: 21430 Hoover Ng

PRINCIPAL ACTIVITIES: General trading and representation

HOME CHARM PAINTS (NIGERIA) LTD
26 St Michael Rd, PMB 1182, Aba, Imo State

Directors: Chief A Mong (Chief Executive),
   A Abosi,
   F Onchua,
   I N Imezurike

PRINCIPAL ACTIVITIES: Production of paint
Branch Offices: Factory: Aba, Imo State
Financial Information:
Registered capital   ₦ 200,000

Principal Shareholders: Silver Paint and Lacquer Company
Date of Establishment: November 1974 Registered

HONDA MOTORS NIGERIA LTD
PMB 1034, Otta, Ogun State
Tel: 960039
Telex: 26286

Chairman: Chief S Ade John
Directors: Koji Mizuguchi (Managing),
   Alhaji Chief Dele Ashiru (Deputy General Manager)

PRINCIPAL ACTIVITIES: Production of motor cycles
Financial Information:
Registered capital   ₦ 4,500,000

Principal Shareholders: Honda Motors Co Ltd, Japan (30%);
   Nigerian Industrial Development Bank Ltd (11%); Nigerian
   Dealers (29%)
Date of Establishment: January 1981 production started
No of Employees: 500

HORST PUKKE & CO (NIGERIA) LTD
See PUKKE, HORST, & CO (NIGERIA) LTD

HOSPITAL EQUIPMENT AND ORTHOPAEDIC SUPPLIES LTD
761 Kofar Mazugai Rd, PO Box 595, Kano
Tel: 5235
Cable: Orthosupply Kano

PRINCIPAL ACTIVITIES: Suppliers and servicers of hospital and
   surgical equipment

HOUSEHOLD PRODUCTS LTD
Bukuru Rd, PMB 2243, Jos, Plateau State
Tel: 52841, 52783
Cable: Detergents
Telex: 81127 Nasco Ng

Chairman: G C Wuyep
Directors: A I Nasreddin, S I Nasreddin, L G Mutbam, P L
   Ramson
Senior Executives: Sanjeev Sarin (General Manager),
   Reda Hamouda (Production Manager),
   R K Mital (Technical Manager),
   H S Chhugani (Quality Control Manager),
   R Mahesh Iyer (Finance Manager),
   I Y Pantuvo (Personnel Manager)

PRINCIPAL ACTIVITIES: Manufacture and sales of detergent
   and allied products
Subsidiary/Associated Companies: Nasreddin Company, SAS
   Italy
Principal Bankers: Bank of the North Ltd; First Bank of Nigeria
   ltd
Financial Information:

	₦'000
Authorised capital	2,000
Paid-up capital	2,000
Turnover	10,000

Principal Shareholders: Plateau State Investment Company Ltd
   (60%); Nasreddin Group of Companies (40%)
Date of Establishment: 12th June 1973
No of Employees: 300

HOWARD CONSTRUCTION CO OF NIGERIA LTD
1 Sunbo Jibowu St, SW-Ikoyi, Lagos
Tel: 681106
Telex: 21539 Howcon Ng

PRINCIPAL ACTIVITIES: Building and civil engineering
   contractors

HULLS SERVICES LTD
PO Box 65, Ebute-Metta, Lagos
Tel: 836394
Cable: Huserv

Chairman: Alhaji K Babs Oke-Gbenro (also Managing Director)
Directors: Kuburatu Oke-Gbenro, Olatunji Kassim, S I Lawal
Senior Executives: Dr M Ola Kassim (Business Consultant),
   Alhaji H H Lawal (General Manager),
   T A Ogundiran (Secretary)

PRINCIPAL ACTIVITIES: Suppliers of electrical equipment,
   air-conditioning, soft drinks, building materials, motor
   vehicles, etc
Principal Agencies: Carr, Day & Martins Ltd, UK; Fleet (Line
   Markers) Ltd, UK
Branch Offices: Location of Head Office: 95 Odutayo St,
   Surulere, Lagos; Branch: 1A Asero Rd, Abeokuta, Ogun State
Associated Companies: Babs Gbenro & Co Ltd; Odunbaku &
   Brothers; Olatunji Kassim & Associate
Principal Bankers: Union Bank of Nigeria Ltd; African
   Continental Bank Ltd
Financial Information:

	₦'000
Authorised capital	250
Paid-up capital	100

Principal Shareholders: Chairman and directors as described

HUNTING SURVEYS (NIGERIA) LTD
Head Office, 1 Francis St, Ikeja, PO Box 4516, Lagos
Cable: Huntopo Lagos

Chairman: D T Sinker
Directors: D A Francis,
   F C Quinn,
   F W Jackson (General Manager),
   J I Ogedegbe,
   K Ogba
Senior Executives: W J Griffiths (Manager, Port Harcourt),
   E O Obazee (Chief Accountant, Company Secretary),
   F O Overare (Projects Supervisor)

PRINCIPAL ACTIVITIES: Geophysical and aerial survey
   contractors; cartography and computer services
Branch Offices: Enerhen Rd, PMB 1045, Warri, Bendel State; 4c
   George's Close, PO Box 708, Port Harcourt, Rivers State
Associated Companies: Survey Services (Nigeria) Ltd
Principal Bankers: United Bank for Africa Ltd; First Bank of
   Nigeria Ltd
Principal Shareholders: J I Ogedegbe; K Ogba; Alhaji I Halilu;
   Hunting Surveys (Nigeria) Employee Trust; Hunting Surveys &
   Consultants Ltd
Date of Establishment: December 1969
No of Employees: 250

HUTTIG-SCHMUCKER CONSTRUCTION (NIG) LTD
9 Alhaji Jimoh Odutola Rd, Ibadan, Oyo State

PRINCIPAL ACTIVITIES: Construction

I I COMMERCIAL SERVICES (IICS)
PO Box 173, Kilometre 3, Bende Rd, Umuahia, Imo State

Chairman: I N U Ibekwe
Senior Executives: O U Ibekwe (Consultant/Services Manager),
   E O Ibekwe (Services Executive),
   F C Ndukwe (Lecturer),
   Miss J U F Onwagba (Lecturer)

PRINCIPAL ACTIVITIES: Advertising, public relations, marketing, business consultancy, education, business research, trade exhibitions, tourism, social research, news coverage, feasibility studies
Subsidiary Companies: I I College of Commerce, PO Box 41, Umuahia, Imo State
Date of Establishment: 16th June 1977 (Formerly Gamp Organisation)

I N ONYENAKAZI & SONS COMPANY
See ONYENAKAZI, I N, & SONS COMPANY

I O EZE & SONS LTD
See EZE, I O, & SONS LTD

I O M NWONYE & SONS COMPANY LTD
See NWONYE, I O M, & SONS COMPANY LTD

IAS CARGO AIRLINES
Old Domestic Terminal, Murtala Muhammed Airport, PMB 1235, Ikeja, Lagos
Tel: 964818, 964972
Telex: 21315 Dunlop Ng

Chairman: Dr F C Okoye
Senior Executives: M O Ogunsanlu (Commercial Manager),
   I K Oladipo (Accountant),
   A J Harvey (Operations Manager)

PRINCIPAL ACTIVITIES: Airfreight Transporters and Courier Services
Principal Agencies: ASA Aeroservices Ltd, UK; UAC International, UK; Redcoat Cargo Airlines; Tradewinds Cargo Airlines; Trans American Airways
Branch Offices: 5 Miller Rd, Bompai, Kano
Associated Companies: IAS Courier Services, Nigeria; IAS Cargo Services, Nigeria
Principal Bankers: Union Bank of Nigeria Ltd; First Bank of Nigeria Ltd

Principal Shareholders: Dr F C Okoye
Date of Establishment: 1974

IBADAN CITY MOTORS (NIGERIA) LTD
Agodi-Ife Rd, PO Box 3328, Mapo Post Office, Ibadan, Oyo State
Tel: 410212
Cable: Citymotors Ibadan
Telex: 31162 Citymo Ng

PRINCIPAL ACTIVITIES: Importers and exporters; manufacturers' representatives; estate agents and general merchants

IBE, A W, & CO LTD
78 Broad St, Lagos
Tel: 634471, 636337
Telex: 21436 Awibe Ng

PRINCIPAL ACTIVITIES: General merchandise suppliers
Branch Offices: 33 Glover St, Ebute-Metta, Lagos; 2 Affa St, Uwani, Enugu, Anambra State

IBEKWE, P A, LTD
30 Silas Works Rd, Fegge, PO Box 394, Onitsha, Anambra State

Tel: 236
Telex: 54334 Pall

Directors: G U Ibekwe

PRINCIPAL ACTIVITIES: Distributors of wholesale general merchandise and building materials

IBILE PROPERTIES LTD
PO Box 907, 8/10 Broad St, Lagos
PRINCIPAL ACTIVITIES: Property developers
Financial Information:
Registered capital   ₦ 500,000
Date of Establishment: 1975

IBRU ORGANISATION (IBRU LTD)
33 Creek Rd, PMB 1155, Apapa, Lagos
Tel: 876533/4, 836618, 836621, 836660
Cable: Ibru Lagos
Telex: 21324

Chairman: Chief Michael Ibru (also Group Chief Executive)
Directors: F O Ibru, G M Ibru, A U Ibru, J Obere, Dr R W Imishue, S O Sekoni, Dr J Anaza

PRINCIPAL ACTIVITIES: Group activities include: industrial refrigeration operating and sales, food and produce importation and distribution, soft drinks manufacture, brewing, sales and distribution, plantations, industrial equipment distribution, plastics, automotive (vehicle distribution), general merchandising, communications
Principal Agencies: Peugeot; Komatsu; Pepsi; Skol; American Motors-Jeep
Branch Offices: 120 Branches throughout Nigeria
Subsidiary Companies: Companies within the Ibru Organisation include: Ibru Sea Foods Ltd (frozen foods); Rutam Ltd (vehicle distribution); W F Clark Ltd (consumer goods distribution); Emsee Shipping Lines Ltd; F Steiner & Co Ltd (scientific equipment and pharmaceuticals, see separate entry); Mitchell Farms (poultry); A J Karouni Ltd (road transport); Aden River Estates Ltd (large-scale industrial farming); together with many other operating subsidiaries
Principal Bankers: United Bank for Africa; National Bank of Nigeria; African Continental Bank
Financial Information:
Sales turnover   ₦ 160,000,000
No of Employees: 8,000

IBRU SEA FOODS LTD
33 Creek Rd, PMB 1155, Apapa, Lagos
Tel: 876533, 876634, 873581
Cable: Ibru Lagos
Telex: 21324

Chairman: Chief M C Ibru
Directors: Mrs E N Ibru, F O Ibru, J U Obere, G O Opara, S O Sekoni, Dr R W Imishue

PRINCIPAL ACTIVITIES: Fishing and fish processing
Branch Offices: Branches all over Nigeria
Principal Bankers: First Bank of Nigeria Ltd; African Continental Bank Ltd; United Bank for Africa
Financial Information:

	₦'000
Authorised capital	1,000
Paid-up capital	800

Principal Shareholders: Oteri Holdings Ltd
No of Employees: 709

IBUKUN TRANSPORT LTD
64 Mba Street, Ajegunle, PO Box 219, Apapa, Lagos
Tel: 834562
Cable: Ibukun Apapa

Chairman: E A A Ososanya (also Managing Director)
Directors: Mrs C O Ososanya, Babs O Ososanya, Miss O A Ososanya, Akinola O Ososanya, Olufunmilayo Ososanya

PRINCIPAL ACTIVITIES: Distribution and road haulage conractors
Principal Agencies: Nigerian Breweries Ltd
Subsidiary Companies: Ore-Ofe Transport Service
Principal Bankers: United Bank for Africa Ltd

Financial Information:

	₦'000
Authorised capital	50
Paid-up capital	50

Date of Establishment: 3rd Spetember 1973
No of Employees: 100

IBUKUN-OLU ENTERPRISES

37/39 Smith St, PO Box 4615, Lagos
Tel: 657386

PRINCIPAL ACTIVITIES: Importers and distributors of heavy
  musical instruments
Branch Offices: 13 Waraola St, Ikate, Surulere, Lagos;
  Showroom: Temple House, Km 22 Thomas Estate, Ikorodu
  Rd, Lagos

ICON LTD (MERCHANT BANKERS)

63/71 Broad Street, PMB 12689, Lagos
Tel: 661812, 660103, 662607, 664174
Cable: Iconbank
Telex: 21437, 21166 Iconbank Ng

Chairman: Alhaji Musa Bello
Directors: Alhaji Abubakar Abdulkadir,
  Dr C E Abebe,
  J Agore,
  N A Adewuyi,
  N H Baring,
  Dr I E Ebong (Managing Director),
  E C Felton,
  Dr Mahmud Tukur
Senior Executives: W H Vogt (General Manager, Banking),
  M Ahmad (General Manager, Administration & Accounts),
  K I Ikpe (Assistant General Manager, Banking Services
  Division),
  C A Udoh (Assistant General Manager, Operations Division),
  G I Fatona (Senior Manager, Accounts)

PRINCIPAL ACTIVITIES: Merchant banking
Branch Offices: NACB Building, Hospital Rd, Kaduna; Desam
  House, Marian Rd, Calabar
Subsidiary Companies: Icon Stockbrokers Ltd
Financial Information:

	₦'000
Authorised capital	5,000
Paid-up capital	5,000
Capital and reserves	12,478
Loans & advances	171,353
Deposits and current accounts	213,252
Profits (before tax)	9,967
Profits (after tax)	4,114

Principal Shareholders: Nigerian Industrial Development Bank
  (45%); Baring Brothers & Company Ltd (15%); Morgan
  Guaranty Trust Company of New York (25%); National
  Insurance Corporation of Nigeria (15%)
Date of Establishment: 22nd February 1975
No of Employees: 225

IDDO PLASTICS LTD

Plot 1 Ijora Causeway, PO Box 2818, Lagos
Tel: 834722, 832581, 831059
Cable: Umbrella Lagos

Chairman: M Aina John
Directors: Harish Chulani,
  Pishu Chulani (Managing),
  Fred Egbe,
  Lachman Hariram,
  Hadj Bakre Anjorin
Senior Executives: Jagdish Mahtani (Administrative Manager),
  Femi Kilo (General Manager)

PRINCIPAL ACTIVITIES: Manufacture of plastic and imitation
  leather shoes
Associated Companies: International Plastics (Nigeria) Ltd;
  Amarilo Umbrella Company Ltd; Nigeria Industrial Auxiliaries

Ltd; Gold Star Industries Ltd; Teevee Industries Ltd; Universal
  Packaging Industries Ltd
Principal Bankers: United Bank for Africa
Financial Information:

	₦'000
Authorised capital	2,000
Paid-up capital	1,400
Turnover	5,000

Principal Shareholders: M Aina John; Fred Egbe; Lachman
  Hariram; Hadj Bakre Anjorin; Harish L Chulani
Date of Establishment: 1962
No of Employees: 400

IDECHEMISTS LTD

5/7 Arochukwu St, PO Box 274, Ogbete, Enugu, Anambra State
Tel: 2309, 2493
Telex: 51133 Idechem Ng

PRINCIPAL ACTIVITIES: Importers of pharmaceutical goods

IDEHEN, J I, & SONS (NIGERIA) LTD

PO Box 42, 137 Upper Igun St, Benin City, Bendel State
Tel: 242283, 241542
Telex: 41107 Idehen Ng

Chairman: George O Ise-Idehen (also Managing)
Directors: F A Idehen (Executive),
  Dr Alex E Idehen,
  Charles I Idehen
Senior Executives: H Omo Idehen (Sawmill Manager),
  Patrick Chuks (Chief Saw Doctor),
  Anthony Odia (Forest Manager)

PRINCIPAL ACTIVITIES: Sawmillers, exporters of lumber and
  round logs and manufacturers of livestock feeds. Poultry
  farmers and general merchants
Branch Offices: Sawmill and Feedmill Factories: Idehen Industrial
  Estate, Oregbeni Branch Sawmill: 126-132 Upper Igun St,
  Benin City, Bendel State
Associated Companies: Idehen Poultry Farms; Idehen Concrete
  Industry
Principal Bankers: First Bank of Nigeria Ltd; New Nigeria Bank
  Ltd
Financial Information:

	₦'000
Authorised capital	200
Paid-up capital	200

Principal Shareholders: Chief J I Idehen; Dr H I Idehen; G O
  Ise-Idehen; F A Idehen; Dr Alex E Idehen; Charles I Idehen
Date of Establishment: 1932 (Established) 1967 (Incorporated)
No of Employees: 120

IDEHEN POULTRY FARM

PO Box 42, 126/132 Upper Igun St, Benin City, Bendel State
Tel: 242283
Telex: 41107

PRINCIPAL ACTIVITIES: Suppliers of poultry

IDEM CONSULTANTS

37 Marina, 14th Floor, Unity House, PO Box 5824, Lagos
Tel: 630512, 631528

PRINCIPAL ACTIVITIES: Business consultants

IFFNA CO LTD

Eastern Nigeria Industrial Estate, PO Box 38, 30 Zik Ave, Enugu,
  Anambra State
Cable: Iffna

Chairman: Dr Nlogha E Okeke (also Managing Director)
Directors: Ifeoma E Okeke (Secretary),
  Emeka A Okeke,
  Ona O Okeke,
  Nnanyelu U Okeke,
  Ifeoma O Okeke

PRINCIPAL ACTIVITIES: Manufacture of paper pins and clips, all types of screws, rivets and wire nails
Branch Offices: Factory: Enugu
Principal Bankers: United Bank for Africa Ltd
Principal Shareholders: Chairman and directors as described

IGBOMINA INVESTMENT CO NIGERIA LTD
151 Ledb Shop, Akanni St, Lagos

Directors: A A Olawepo

PRINCIPAL ACTIVITIES: Manufacturing of leather bags, purses, wallets, suit-cases etc

IGUH, C O, AND SONS TRADING CO (NIGERIA) LTD
7 Bright St, Onitsha, Anambra State

Chairman: C O Iguh
Directors: Benjamin C Iguh (General Manager),
  G Iguh (Deputy Chairman),
  A A Okafor,
  F Igweh,
  Mrs T Iguh

PRINCIPAL ACTIVITIES: General trading and contracting; importers/exporters; manufacturers' representatives
Principal Agencies: Damex Paint Industry (Nigeria) Ltd; Premier Breweries Ltd
Branch Offices: 13b Old Cemetary Rd, Onitsha, Anambra State; Otolo Market, Nnewi, Anambra State
Associated Companies: Ibeh and Sons Enterprises (Nigeria) Ltd; Ibeaniguh Trading Agents (Nigeria) Ltd; Madson Enterprises (Nigeria) Ltd
Principal Bankers: African Continental Bank Ltd
Principal Shareholders: A Aguh; R Madueke; B Uduchukwu; R Ofodum; C Nwoseh
Date of Establishment: 1975

IGWE BROTHERS & CO LTD
12 Udi Rd, Asata, Enugu, Anambra State
Tel: 254276

Directors: C G E Igwe (Managing),
  B Igwe (Works Manager),
  O Okebugwu (Secretary/Administrative Manager),
  C Onwuemedo (Accountant)
Senior Executives: Nnamdi Chukwu (Sites Manager)

PRINCIPAL ACTIVITIES: Civil engineering; electrical engineering works; importers and exporters
Branch Offices: Electrical Stores, 75 Ogui Rd, Asata, Enugu, Anambra State; Workshop, 12 Lagos St, Asata, Anambra State

IJAGBEMI, S A, & SONS (NIGERIA) LTD
1A Murtala Mohammed Way, PO Box 817, Jos, Plateau State
Tel: 2779

Chairman: Chief S A Ijagbemi
Directors: Kola Ijagbemi (General Manager),
  Robert S Ijagbemi (Engineer)
Senior Executives: Lance I Onyeiwu (Sales Manager)

PRINCIPAL ACTIVITIES: General contractors, manufacturers of furniture and metal containers etc
Branch Offices: General Hospital Rd, PO Box 46, Itedo, Isanlu, Kwara State
Principal Bankers: Union Bank of Nigeria Ltd
Financial Information:

	₦'000
Authorised capital	100
Paid-up capital	52
Turnover	138
Profits	28

Date of Establishment: 1968

IJOMAH INTERNATIONAL CO LTD
9-11 Alhaji Karimu Street, Opposite Kiri-Kiri Jetty, Olodi Apapa, GPO Box 8929, Lagos
Cable: Ijomah International

Directors: Edward Ijomah (Managing)

PRINCIPAL ACTIVITIES: Shipping, customs clearing and forwarding; air freighting, inland transportation, warehousing and marine suppliers
Principal Bankers: Societe General Bank

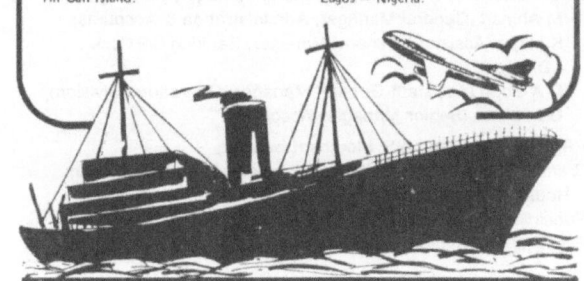
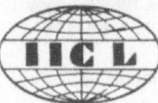
IKEJA RETREADS (NIGERIA) LTD
Oregun Industrial Area, PO Box 220, Ikeja, Lagos
Tel: 964635, 964636

PRINCIPAL ACTIVITIES: Manufacturers of retreaded tyres

IKORODU TRADING COMPANY LTD
39 Iga-Iduganran St, PO Box 395, Lagos
Tel: 630635

PRINCIPAL ACTIVITIES: Textile manufacturers and importers

ILONEX PHARMACEUTICAL COMPANY
PO Box 2852, 1st Floor, 19 William St, Onitsha, Anambra State
Cable: Ilopharm

Chairman: O C Ilongwo (also Managing Director)
Directors: D I Ilongwo,
  F N Udenze (General Manager),
  E C Ilongwo,
  C E Ilongwo

PRINCIPAL ACTIVITIES: Agents and general trading, suppliers of hospital equipment, importers and exporters, manufacturer's representatives
Principal Agencies: Yauns & George Industrial Co Ltd, Taipei, Taiwan; Stayford Export Ltd, London; Finimex Spa, Milano, Italy; Fitch Lovell Exports Ltd, UK; Harng Tai Enterprises Co Ltd, Taiwan; Dott Bonapace & Co, Italy; Bhander Pharmacy,

UK
Branch Offices: Owerri; Enugu; Maiduguri; Jos; Port Harcourt
Subsidiary/Associated Companies: Cydon (Nigeria) Company; Ilonex Drug Company; O C Ilonex Trading Company
Principal Bankers: International Bank for West Africa Ltd; First Bank of Nigeria Ltd; United Bank for Africa Ltd; Union Bank of Nigeria Ltd
Principal Shareholders: Chairman and directors as described
Date of Establishment: 15th March 1979

IMO NEWSPAPERS LTD

PMB 1095, Egbu/Owerri, Imo State
Tel: 230099

Senior Executives: Davey Ozurumba (Editor, Nigerian Stateman)

PRINCIPAL ACTIVITIES: Printers and publishers of Statesman Group of Newspapers

IMPRESIT BAKOLORI (NIGERIA) LTD

12 Creek Rd, Apapa, Lagos
Tel: 875981, 874510
Telex: Impres Ng 22392

Chairman: Alhaji Mohammed Armiya'u
Directors: Enrico Tasso (Managing Director)

PRINCIPAL ACTIVITIES: Civil engineering and construction
Branch Offices: 2 Kontagora Rd, Sokoto; 3/b Tamandu Street, Kano; 16 Sultan Rd, Kaduna; Via P S Mancini 2, Rome, Italy

INACO LTD

117A Agege Motor Rd, Oshodi, PO Box 176, Yaba, Lagos
Tel: 962128

Directors: F Oprandi, A Scandella

PRINCIPAL ACTIVITIES: General contractors

INCAR (NIGERIA) LTD

10 Ijora Causeway, PO Box 2581, Lagos
Tel: 837222, 837274, 837297
Cable: Incar Lagos
Telex: 21382 Ingla Ng

Chairman: Henry Osime Omenai
Directors: Franco Bernardini

PRINCIPAL ACTIVITIES: Distributors of motor vehicles, spare parts, industrial machinery and equipment
Principal Agencies: Fiat; Lancia
Branch Offices: Km 10 Lagos Rd, PO Box 3253, Ibadan, Oyo State; 68 Maganda Rd, PO Box 774, Kano; Hamed Talib Rd, PO Box 3254, Kaduna; Railway Line PMB 1112, Maiduguri, Borno State; Trans Amadi Industrial Layout, PMB 5742, Port Harcourt, Rivers State
Principal Bankers: United Bank for Africa Ltd; Union Bank of Nigeria Ltd; International Bank for West Africa; Bank of the North Ltd; National Bank of Nigeria Ltd

Date of Establishment: 14th March 1963
No of Employees: 1,012

INCO CONSULTANTS (NIGERIA) LTD

72 Awolowo Rd, SW Ikoyi, PO Box 7989, Lagos
Tel: 680849
Cable: Ejinco

Directors: Dr E O Ejike (Managing Director), Dr Silvano Zorzi (Associate Engineer and Director), Dr Lucio Leonardo (Associate Engineer and Director)

PRINCIPAL ACTIVITIES: Structural and civil engineering consultants
Principal Bankers: United Bank for Africa Ltd

Principal Shareholders: Dr E O Ejike; Dr Silvano Zorzi; Dr Lucio Lonardo

INCONTRA NIGERIA LTD

PO Box 9599, Lagos

PRINCIPAL ACTIVITIES: Importers and distributors of automotive spare parts, tools, pharmaceuticals
Branch Offices: 33 Oguntona Crescent, Gbaga Estate, Pedro Bus Stop, Off Apapa-Oworonsoki Expressway, Lagos

Date of Establishment: February 1980

INDIAN BAZAAR (NIGERIA) LTD

69 Balogun St, PO Box 2773, Lagos
Tel: 633789, 635860, 630975

PRINCIPAL ACTIVITIES: Manufacturers of textiles, wholesalers, manufacturers' representatives, general importers and exporters

INDO MINING CO (NIGERIA) LTD

PO Box 6, Bukuru, Via Jos, Plateau State
PRINCIPAL ACTIVITIES: Mining

INDUSTRIAL & SAFETY EQUIPMENT (NIGERIA) LTD

PMB 21531, Ikeja, Lagos
Tel: 963948
Cable: Safequip
Telex: 11117 TDS Box 201; 20117 TDS Box 201 UK only

Chairman: Oluyemi Falade (also Managing Director)
Directors: S O Awe,
 J A Bamgbade,
 Mrs A Falade (Manager, Finance),
 O Abodunde,
 J I Ola Ologbenla
Senior Executives: Ayotunde Falade (Sales Manager),
 Timothy O Sowole (Accountant),
 Richard Ige (Auditor)

PRINCIPAL ACTIVITIES: Importation and marketing of industrial machinery, aluminium scaffolding; security products, fire fighting equipment, navigation warning lights, explosion-proof beam lights, army and police warning lights and general industrial safety
Principal Agencies: Long Products Ltd, UK; Asbestos Rubber Company Ltd, UK; Mistral Glass Ltd, UK; Mini Electronics, Germany; Safety Supply, Canada; Londesborough Oil and Marine Engineering Ltd, UK; Huchinson Mapa, France; Marushichi Metal Industries Ltd, Japan; Joseph Symms & Company Ltd, UK
Branch Offices: Office Location: 12 Faramobi Ajike St, Anthony Village, Lagos
Principal Bankers: Societe Generale; African Continental Bank Ltd
Financial Information:

	N'000
Authorised capital	100
Profits	210

Principal Shareholders: Oluyemi Falade; S O Awe; J A Bamgbade; Mrs Adetole Falade
Date of Establishment: 13th July 1976

INDUSTRIAL CLAYS NIGERIA LTD

Amihe Industrial Complex, Ukpor, Nnewi, Anambra State
Tel: 425
Cable: Amechiclay Ukpor Nnewi

Chairman: F S McEwen
Directors: Mbazulike Amechi (Managing),
 T C M Eneli,
 L Ngozi Anapusim,
 Ben O Amechi,
 Chief M D Okechukwu
Senior Executives: G F Ijoma (Mining Supt),
 Ikem Egbuniwe (Sales Executive)

PRINCIPAL ACTIVITIES: Mining, mineral processing and quarrying, principally quarrying and refining kaolin to various specifications
Associated Companies: Procraft Nigeria Ltd
Principal Bankers: African Continental Bank Ltd
Financial Information:

	₦'000
Authorised capital	200
Paid-up capital	200

No of Employees: 130

INDUSTRIAL GASES LTD
PO Box 53, 224 Apapa Rd, Apapa, Lagos
Tel: 876049, 876294
Cable: Indugas Lagos

Chairman: A B Dijkhoffz
Directors: G O Onosode,
   F O Ogunlana,
   R J Foster,
   M J Moriarty,
   J E Andriessen,
   J Jolles (Managing)
Senior Executives: H J M Molloy (Chief Engineer),
   M G Habgood (Marketing Manager),
   E O O Ogunjobi (Personnel Manager)

PRINCIPAL ACTIVITIES: Manufacturers of industrial gases, oxygen, nitrogen, argon, hydrogen, acetylene, nitrous oxide; distributors of welding equipment, electrodes and a range of medical equipment and gases
Branch Offices: Off McDermott Rd, Warri; 3 Katchia Rd, Kaduna; Sharada Industrial Estate, Kano; 49 Ijebu Bye Pass, Ibadan; State Highway, Oshodi
Associated Companies: Van Leer Containers (Nigeria) Ltd; Royal Packaging Industries Van Leer Bv, Holland; BOC International Ltd, UK
Principal Bankers: United Bank for Africa Ltd
Financial Information:

	₦'000
Authorised capital	3,250
Paid-up capital	3,250
Sales turnover	15,000

Principal Shareholders: Royal Packaging Industries Van Leer BV, Holland; BOC Holdings, UK
Date of Establishment: November 1959
No of Employees: 600

INLAKS LTD
WB 14 Iddo Railway Compound, Behind Lagos Terminus, Lagos
Tel: 800410-3
Cable: Azad

PRINCIPAL ACTIVITIES: Importers, exporters, suppliers of air conditioners and distributors of general merchandise
Branch Offices: Port Harcourt, Tel 334655; Kano, Tel 5873, 2432; Bauchi, Tel 42554; Benin City; Warri; Bauchi

INLAND CONTAINERS (NIGERIA) LTD
Third Floor, 9 Wharf Rd, Apapa, Lagos
Tel: 871563, 872977, 874198
Telex: 21760 Inland Ng

Chairman: O Lijadu
Directors: P H D Toosey, J O Farodoye, N A Adewuyi, I C Ogbue, R A Napier, A P D Bristow, Alhaji Aminu Dantata

PRINCIPAL ACTIVITIES: Transport of customs bonded containers to owned inland container terminal in Kano and Kaduna (bonded inland container service)
Branch Offices: Abdullhai Bayero Rd, Nassarawa, PO Box 7045, Kano, Tel 8409; Kachia Rd, (Off Railway Avenue), Kaduna
Principal Bankers: Society Generale Bank; Icon Ltd; Nigerian-American Merchant Bank

Financial Information:

	₦'000
Authorised capital	3,000
Paid-up capital	1,300
Turnover	2,600
Profits	130

Principal Shareholders: Nicon (50%); Ocean Transport & Trading (40%); Alhaji Aminu Dantata (10%)
Date of Establishment: 6 February 1980
No of Employees: 72

INNOCENT HOPE OVERSEAS COMPANY
PO Box 1613, 71 Hospital Rd, Aba, Imo State
Cable: Innohope

Chairman: Anosikeh N Innocent
Directors: Nnamdi V Anosikeh, Amanze W Anosikeh

PRINCIPAL ACTIVITIES: Importers and suppliers of machinery and equipment for the construction industry
Principal Agencies: Columbia Machine Inc, USA; Edzel Agency Agency Ltd, UK
Branch Offices: 1 Oryema Oji Street, Ariaria Market, Aba, Imo State
Subsidiary Companies: J B Campbell Co, USA
Principal Bankers: Union Bank Ltd

Principal Shareholders: Chairman and directors as described
Date of Establishment: July 1974

INSUMMA (NIGERIA) LTD
20 Little Rd, Yaba, PO Box 6219, Lagos
Tel: 843389

PRINCIPAL ACTIVITIES: Consultants, engineers and architects

INSURANCE BROKERS OF NIGERIA
United House, 37 Marina, PO Box 2010, Lagos
Tel: 662287, 662429, 662838
Cable: Bowinsur
Telex: 21239 Bowsur Ng

Directors: F A Johnson (Managing Director),
   H W Akpan,
   Usman Goji,
   B W Bolton,
   Chief A Ojora,
   P L Eckersley,
   R J Solomon
Senior Executives: M J Egu (Assistant General Manager),
   R A Akerele (Assistant General Manager),
   B K O Kagbare (Assistant General Manager),
   B A Aileru (Assistant General Manager),
   W S Spickett (North Area Manager)

PRINCIPAL ACTIVITIES: Insurance brokers and consultants
Branch Offices: 15C Murtala Mohammed Way, Kano; 1R Barracks Rd, Calabar, Cross River State
Principal Bankers: United Bank for Africa Ltd; Union Bank Ltd; Bank of the North Ltd

Principal Shareholders: Investment Trust Ltd; Marsh & McLennan Inc; Chief Ojora; Alhaji Adamu Ciroma
Date of Establishment: 1955 (Formerly C T Bowring (Nigeria) Ltd)
No of Employees: 80

INTEGRATED CONSULTANTS (NIGERIA) LTD
106 Awolowo Rd, PO Box 5422, Lagos
Tel: 682539
Telex: 51145 Topark Ng

PRINCIPAL ACTIVITIES: Architecture, town planning, civil, structural, electrical and mechanical engineering consultants, quantity surveying

INTER CONTINENTAL FISHING (NIGERIA) LTD

1303A Akin Adesola St, PO Box 50870, Falomo, Victoria Island, Lagos
Tel: 616699, 616752
Cable: Snapper
Telex: 22386

PRINCIPAL ACTIVITIES: Fishing

INTER DESIGNS PARTNERSHIP

83 Falolu Rd, PO Box 168, Surulere, Lagos
Tel: 836011
Cable: Indesigns

Directors: Arc Olusegun Kuti,
    Arc Victor B Attah (Parnter),
    Arc Uduma M Uduma (Partner)

PRINCIPAL ACTIVITIES: Architects, site planners, interior designers
Branch Offices: Main Offices: 3 Alli Akilu Rd, PO Box 742, Kaduna Tel 212618; 26 Carter St, PMB 1933, Enugu, Anambra State Tel 256141 Branch Offices: Airport Rd, PO Box 423, Yola, Gongola State Tel 24570; Plot 268 Trans Amadi Layout, PO Box 417, Port Harcourt, Rivers State; 104 Fosbery Rd, Calabar, Cross River State
Principal Bankers: United Bank for Africa Ltd

Date of Establishment: Apirl 1974

INTERBASIC PRODUCTS CO LTD

19 Shipeolu St, Palm Grove, Ikorodu Rd, PO Box 5199, Lagos

PRINCIPAL ACTIVITIES: Manufacturers of Ceramic tiles
Branch Offices: 119 Agege Motor Rd, Oshodi, Lagos

Date of Establishment: June 1980

INTERBETON NIGERIA LTD

Plot 14 Block 5 Oduduna Crescent, GRA Ikeja, PO Box 826, Lagos

PRINCIPAL ACTIVITIES: Civil engineering contractors

Date of Establishment: 1978

INTERCARE LTD

118 Nnamdi Azikiwe St, PO Box 4901, Lagos
Tel: 636262

PRINCIPAL ACTIVITIES: Freight forwarders, shipping; insurance agents and general merchants

INTERCONTRACTORS (NIGERIA) LTD

Formerly Bartoletti (Nigeria) Ltd

PO Box 439, Apap, Lagos
Tel: 833606, 880142, 880145, 880149, 880170
Cable: Bartoletti Lagos
Telex: 22212 Intcon

Chairman: I Bartoletti
Directors: G Bajlo,
    W Ibrahim,
    Z Mohammad,
    B Olowofoyeku,
    A Parravicini,
    E P Psilogenis,
    G Labigalini (General Manager),
    F Ceruti (Commerical Manager)
Senior Executives: G Galli (Contracts Manager),
    A Guadagni (Assistant General Manager)

PRINCIPAL ACTIVITIES: Civil engineering and construction
Branch Offices: Office location: Km 11 Lagos - Badagry Expressway
Principal Bankers: United Bank for Africa Ltd

Financial Information:

	N'000
Authorised capital	1,150
Paid-up capital	500
Turnover	28,113

Principal Shareholders: I Bartoletti; Herwa Ltd; Chief Olowofoyeku; W Z Mohammad
No of Employees: 3,000

INTERMARK ASSOCIATES LTD

51 Bode Thomas St, Palm Grove, PO Box 4244, Lagos
Tel: 848944

Chairman: Oliver Eniola Johnson (also Managing Director)
Directors: Mrs Margaret A Johnson
Senior Executives: Mrs J Odunewu (Accounts Manager),
    Derek Norman (Creative Manager),
    Adolphus Anyanacho (Office Manager),
    Wale Oyewusi (Client Service/Production Manager)

PRINCIPAL ACTIVITIES: Advertising and public relations
Principal Bankers: United Bank for Africa Ltd; International Bank for West Africa Ltd

Principal Shareholders: Mr and Mrs Johnson
Date of Establishment: November 1970

INTERNATIONAL AGENCIES LTD

PO Box 2288, Unity House, Marina, Lagos

PRINCIPAL ACTIVITIES: Manufacturers' representatives; suppliers of electrical equipment
Principal Agencies: Long & Crawford Ltd, UK

INTERNATIONAL BANK FOR WEST AFRICA LTD

94 Broad St, PMB 12021, Lagos
Tel: 664135, 662301
Telex: 21345 Ibwa Ng

Chairman: Alhaji Aminu Wali
Directors: Antoine G D'Arjuzon (Vice Chairman),
    O Olashore (Managing),
    Marc Blondel,
    Dr Ibrahim A Ayagi,
    Erwin Wehrli,
    Alhaji A Mai Sango,
    Gilbert Nanyiso,
    Benjamin A Wachukwu,
    Angus M Ferguson,
    M Meunier,
    BIAO
Senior Executives: Chief Olayinka O Simoyan, Alhaji A O Arogundade, C Francis, Mr De Montigny

PRINCIPAL ACTIVITIES: Banking
Branch Offices: 42/44 Warehouse Rd, PMB 1108, Apapa, Lagos; 9B Lagos St, PMB 3054, Kano; 27 Aba Rd, PMB 5168, Port Harcourt, Rivers State; 82 Jubilee Rd, PMB 1155, Imo State

Principal Shareholders: Federal Government of Nigeria (60%); BIAO (40%)
Date of Establishment: 1959
No of Employees: Over 1,300

INTERNATIONAL BEER & BEVERAGES INDUSTRIES LTD

Plot 5 Block E Matori Scheme, Oshodi, Lagos

Chairman: Chief Ayo

PRINCIPAL ACTIVITIES: Brewers and bottlers
Financial Information:
Authorised capital   N 500,000
Date of Establishment: April 1978

INTERNATIONAL BISCUITS LTD
1A Barracks Rd, PMB 1117, Calabar, Cross River State

PRINCIPAL ACTIVITIES: Manufacturers of biscuits and allied bakery products (under construction)
Branch Offices: Factory: Ikot Ekpene, Cross River State
Financial Information:
Registered capital ₦ 1,000,000

Principal Shareholders: Investment Trust Company, Nigeria; Nigerian Entrepreneurs
Date of Establishment: Registered January 1980
No of Employees: 200 when in production

INTERNATIONAL BREWERIES LTD
Omi-Asoro, PO Box 104, Ilesha, Oyo State
Tel: 2112
Cable: Interbrews Ilesha

Chairman: Dr Lawrence Omole
Directors: Isaac O Ajanaku,
Adedokun Haastrup,
James Olatunbosun,
E Adegboyega Esan,
Johnson O Fagboyegun,
J Meier Zu Biesen,
Dr Abel O Afolayan,
Alhaji A Adeleke,
Ayanwole A Gbadegesin,
John A Oyalana,
Redford Fiderikumo,
Akinwande A Akinola (Executive/Managing Director),
Adesuyi Folowosele (Executive/Finance Director)
Senior Executives: I O A Farore (Company Secretary),
E Altmann (Brewmaster),
W Karfich (Chief Engineer)

PRINCIPAL ACTIVITIES: Brewing of lager beer and soft drinks
Principal Bankers: First Bank of Nigeria Ltd; International Bank for West Africa Ltd; National Bank of Nigeria Ltd; Union Bank of Nigeria Ltd
Financial Information:

	₦'000
Authorised capital	10,000
Paid-up capital	9,000
Turnover (as at June 30, 1981)	19,097
Profits (as at June 30, 1981;	3,930

Principal Shareholders: Nigerians; Industrial; Finance and Investment Institutions; German Technical Partner
Date of Establishment: 22nd December 1971
No of Employees: 750

INTERNATIONAL COMPUTERS (NIGERIA) LTD
178 Awolowo Rd, SW Ikoyi, PO Box 2134, Lagos
Tel: 684754, 684757, 680421
Cable: Datacomp
Telex: 21132 Comput Ng

Chairman: W W Jackson
Directors: R I Alakija (Vice Chairman),
D J Benson (Managing),
F J Stonehouse,
Alhaji M D Yusufu,
E B Hassan (Executive Financial Director, Company Secretary),
J R Scarlett (Executive Technical Director, Customer Services Manager)
Senior Executives: A J Lavery (Engineering Manager),
W O Edoja (Personnel Manager),
J S MacDonnell (Sales Manager)

PRINCIPAL ACTIVITIES: Computer sales and services
Principal Agencies: International Computers Ltd, UK
Principal Bankers: First Bank Nigeria Ltd; Chase Merchant Bank Nigeria Ltd; International Merchant Bank Nigeria Ltd; Union Bank of Nigeria Ltd

Financial Information:

	₦'000
Authorised capital	833
Paid-up capital	833
Turnover	6,000
Profits	463

Principal Shareholders: International Computers Ltd (UK) 60%; Nigerians 40%
Date of Establishment: Incorporated in October 1969, trading started in 1956
No of Employees: 110

INTERNATIONAL CONTACT CENTRE
4 Wowo St, Olodi, PO Box 44, Apapa, Lagos

Chairman: J O Agbai
Directors: Hyacinth Chukwuneme Uwaoma
Senior Executives: Isaac Ifeagba (General Manager, Marketing Division),
Mrs Josephine Agbai (Secretary/Administrative Manager)

PRINCIPAL ACTIVITIES: Advertising, marketing, sales and servicing of office equipment; suppliers of stationery; importers and exporters; printing
Associated Companies: Joes Tech Centre, Owerri
Principal Bankers: African Continental Bank Ltd; First Bank of Nigeria Ltd; Co-operative Bank of Eastern Nigeria Ltd

INTERNATIONAL CONTRACTORS AGENCY (ICA)
20 Tafawa Balewa Way, PO Box 718, Kaduna

PRINCIPAL ACTIVITIES: Building and civil engineering contractors
Branch Offices: Kano; Sokoto

INTERNATIONAL CONTRACTS & CONSULTANCY SERVICES LTD
Western House (17th Floor), 8/10 Broad St, Lagos
Tel: 653845, 875842
Cable: Danco Lagos
Telex: 21114 Ng

Chairman: Chief J M St Matthew Daniel
Directors: Dr B J St Matthew, Chief Bayo Kehinde

PRINCIPAL ACTIVITIES: Suppliers of air-conditioning and refrigeration, building materials, electrical and electronic equipment; fertilizers, furniture, mechanical engineering plant, petrochemicals, power equipment, oil and gas services and equipment and pipeline contractors; mechanical engineering, electrical engineering
Associated Companies: Marryat Daniel (Nig) Ltd; Danaran (Nig) Ltd
Principal Bankers: United Bank for Africa Ltd

INTERNATIONAL ENAMELWARE INDUSTRY LTD
Km 5 Onitsha-Owerri Rd, PMB 1617, Onitsha, Anambra State
Tel: 210465
Cable: Interenam Ikeja
Telex: 54320 Inten

Chairman: A M Anyoha
Directors: V Umetiti, B Cheung
Senior Executives: T Ho (Assistant Director)

PRINCIPAL ACTIVITIES: Manufacturing of household enamelware
Branch Offices: Plot G & H Awosika Ave, Industrial Estate, PO Box 140, Ikeja, Lagos
Associated Companies: Cosmos Metal & Electrics Ltd; International Steel Industry Ltd; General Steel Mill (Nigeria) Ltd; Mighty Plastic Industry Ltd; International Metal Products Ltd; Technoflex Company Ltd
Principal Bankers: International Bank for West Africa Ltd

Financial Information:

	N'000
Authorised capital	1,500
Paid-up capital	800

Date of Establishment: 1969
No of Employees: 1,100

INTERNATIONAL HOUSING (NIGERIA) LTD

9 Bode Thomas St, PMB 3194, Surulere, Lagos
Tel: 837401

Chairman: A Kanu Oj
Directors: S Heard (Managing Director),
  Agwu A Igbe (Assistant Managing Director)

PRINCIPAL ACTIVITIES: Construction

INTERNATIONAL MARITIME SERVICES

9 Creek Rd, PO Box 319, Apapa, Lagos
Tel: 875887, 875969
Cable: Imarsel Lagos
Telex: 21342 Imas Ng

PRINCIPAL ACTIVITIES: Insurance brokers, buyers agents,
  clearing, forwarding and general warehousing

INTERNATIONAL MERCHANT BANK (NIGERIA) LTD

77 Awolowo Rd, SW Ikoyi, PMB 12028, Lagos
Tel: 684007/9, 684011
Cable: Firstchico
Telex: 21169 FNBCNC Ng

Chairman: Dr D I Saror
Directors: Dr Z H Idilby,
  Dieter F J Juli (Managing),
  Ebitimi E Banigo (Deputy Managing),
  Alhaji U Albishir,
  Alan F Delp,
  Dr Odunayo Olagundoye (Alternate),
  Dr I A Obuzor,
  D B Zang

PRINCIPAL ACTIVITIES: Merchant banking
Branch Offices: 7/8 Lagos St, PMB 3426, Kano

Principal Shareholders: Ministry of Finance Inc (60%); First
  National Bank of Chicago (40%)
Date of Establishment: July 1974 (Formerly First National Bank
  of Chicago (Nigeria) Ltd)

INTERNATIONAL MESSENGERS (NIGERIA) LTD

IMNL

Afrijet House, 17 Laide Tomori St, Off Medical Rd, Ikeja, PO Box
  2780, Lagos
Tel: 963948

Chairman: Chief Rotimi Williams
Directors: Ladi Williams, A R Walters, F R A Williams Jnr
Senior Executives: L Boothright (General Manager),
  George Hillier (Cargo Development Manager)

PRINCIPAL ACTIVITIES: Operators of international air cargo and
  air courier services
Branch Offices: Afrijet House, Sarkin-Yaki Rd, PO Box 1785,
  Kano, Tel 7726, Telex 77150 Anopit Ng; 8 Creek Rd, Apapa,
  Lagos, Tel 876892, 874639, Telex 21332; 87 Wire Rd, PMB
  1504, Benin City, Bendel State, Tel 244508; 1st Floor Block B
  Falomo Shopping Centre, Unit 11, Ikoyi, Lagos, Tel 681275;
  Afrijet House, 22 Ahmadu Bello Way, Kaduna, Tel 213697,
  Telex 71317; Also at Ilorin; Ibadan; Jos; Maiduguri; Port
  Harcourt and Zaria
Associated Companies: IML Air Services Ltd, UK; Holland; Hong
  Kong; UAE; Zambia; USA
Principal Bankers: United Bank for Africa Ltd

Principal Shareholders: United Investment Company; IML Air
  Services (Group) Ltd
Date of Establishment: September 1978

INTERNATIONAL PACKING INDUSTRIES OF NIGERIA LTD

PO Box 113, Industrial Estate, Oba Akran Ave, Ikeja, Lagos
Tel: 961977, 961978

Chairman: Chief S I Nwoke
Directors: Babasola O Thomas (Managing)

PRINCIPAL ACTIVITIES: Packing materials manufacturers; bread
  wrappers, paper bags and other wrapping papers
Branch Offices: Aba

INTERNATIONAL PAINTS (WA) LTD

Oba Akran Avenue, PO Box 67, Ikeja, Lagos
Tel: 963895/6, 961594, 961546
Cable: Corrofoul Ikeja
Telex: 26976

Chairman: Chief Silas B Daniyan
Directors: R F Macmillan (Managing),
  M O Okeke (Administrative Director/Company Secretary),
  C O Williams (Financial Director),
  M A Hamma,
  H M Osha,
  E W Osmond
Senior Executives: C N C Nweke (Works Manager),
  D O Oduah (Marketing Manager),
  J O Esho (Chief Accountant),
  P M Onyemenam (Commercial Manager),
  D L Edwards (Chief Chemist),
  F A Ogbogoh (Special Products Divisional Manager)

PRINCIPAL ACTIVITIES: Manufacturers of international marine
  coatings, industrial finishes, wood finishes, adhesives and
  wide range of subsidiary products: enamel and emulsion
  paints
Branch Offices: Ibadan; Kaduna; Kano; Jos; Benin; Warri; Port
  Harcourt; Akure; Sokoto; Oregun; Owerri; Maiduguri; Ilorin;
  Suleja; Calabar; Enugu
Principal Bankers: Union Bank of Nigeria Ltd; Icon Ltd
  (Merchant Bankers)
Financial Information:

	N'000
Authorised capital	8,000
Paid-up capital	5,200
Turnover (1980)	18,111
Profits (1980)	1,305

Principal Shareholders: International Paints (Holdings) Ltd
  (Subsidiary of of International Paint PLC, UK (40%); Nigerian
  Industrial Development Bank Ltd (20.4%); Nigerian Citizens &
  Associations (39.6%)
Date of Establishment: 23rd January, 1961
No of Employees: 465

INTERNATIONAL PLANNING & ENVIRONMENTAL CONSULTANTS (NIGERIA) LTD

INPLECON

53Y Mallam Kure Street, PO Box 1181, Jos, Plateau State
Tel: 55819, 55820

Directors: J O Oyegoke (Managing Director)

PRINCIPAL ACTIVITIES: Consultancy services provided in town
  and country planning, architecture, estate management,
  surveying and transportation planning
Branch Offices: 29AA Baga Rd, PMB 1008, Maiduguri, Borno
  State
Associated Companies: Cetaconsult (Nigeria) Ltd; Joe Oyegoke
  Associates
Principal Bankers: Bank of the North Ltd; Union Bank of Nigeria
  Ltd

Financial Information:

	N'000
Authorised capital	100
Paid-up capital	100

Principal Shareholders: J O Oyegoke; E A Oyegoke
Date of Establishment: 1st July 1977
No of Employees: 24

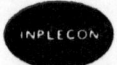

INTERNATIONAL PLANNING & ENVIRONMENTAL CONSULTANTS (NIGERIA) LIMITED
(otherwise known as INPLECON)
53Y Mallam Kure Street
PO Box 1181
Jos
Tel: (073) 55819 & 55820

Principal activities: Consultancy services provided in town and country planning, architecture, estate management, surveying and transportation planning.

Associated Companies: Cetaconsult (Nigeria) Ltd, Joe Oyegoke Associates, Shankland Cox Partnership, UK, Bimbotech (Nigeria) Ltd

INTERNATIONAL PLANNING ASSOCIATES
PO Box 8536, Lagos
Telex: 21432 Palace Ng

Directors: S C Lockwood (General Manager)

PRINCIPAL ACTIVITIES: Consortium consultants to Federal Capital Development Authority

INTERNATIONAL PLASTICS (NIGERIA) LTD
Plot 4C Ijora Causeway, PO Box 2812, Lagos
Tel: 832581, 834722
Cable: Umbrella Lagos
Telex: 26234

Chairman: Hadj Bakre Anjorin
Directors: Harish L Chulani (Managing Director),
    M Aina John,
    Fred Egbe,
    Lachman Hariram,
    Hadj Bakre Anjorin
Senior Executives: Ajit Sadarangani (Quality Control Manager),
    Solomon Oselukwue (Sales Manager),
    Femi Kilo (General Manager)

PRINCIPAL ACTIVITIES: Plastic packaging; polybags, transwrap, shrinkwrap, heavy duty sacks and printed polyethelene packaging. Tarpaulin and PVC sheetings
Principal Bankers: United Bank for Africa Ltd

Financial Information:

	N'000
Authorised capital	500
Paid-up capital	454

Date of Establishment: 1971
No of Employees: 200

INTERNATIONAL STEEL INDUSTRY LTD
Niger Bridge Head, PMB 1610, Onitsha, Anambra State
Tel: 212913
Cable: Interenam Ikeja
Telex: 54320 Inten

Chairman: Peter Y Y Cheung
Directors: Benny Cheung, Alhaji Yau Musa, Y T Cheung, D N Udokoro
Senior Executives: B Cheung (Managing Director),
    T Ho (Assistant Director)

PRINCIPAL ACTIVITIES: Manufacturers of steel pipes and tubes
Branch Offices: Plot G & H, Awosika Ave, Industrial Estate, PO Box 140, Ikeja, Lagos
Associated Companies: International Enamelware Industry Ltd; Mighty Plastic Industry Ltd; Cosmos Metal & Electrics Ltd; International Metal Products Ltd; General Steel Mill (Nig) Ltd; Technoflex Co Ltd
Principal Bankers: First Bank of Nigeria Ltd

Date of Establishment: 1975
No of Employees: 200

INTERNATIONAL TANNERS LTD
PMB 3213, Kano
Tel: 5391, 5392
Telex: 77156

Chairman: Dr Abubakar Imam
Senior Executives: D Hocke (General Manager)

PRINCIPAL ACTIVITIES: Tanning of hides and skins
Subsidiary Companies: CFAO Nigeria Ltd Group
Principal Bankers: Union Bank of Nigeria Ltd
Financial Information:

	N'000
Authorised capital	1,000
Paid-up capital	1,000

Date of Establishment: 1975 (Formerly Intertan Nigeria Ltd)
No of Employees: 280

INTERNATIONAL TRADE (WA) LTD
21/25 Broad St, Lagos
Tel: 654892
Telex: 21379 Intwa Ng

PRINCIPAL ACTIVITIES: General traders

INTERNATIONAL YETTCO (NIGERIA) LTD
PO Box 943, 27 Target Rd, Calabar, Cross River State
Tel: 222193
Cable: Yettco
Telex: 65141 Yettco

Chairman: Moses Akpan Essah
Directors: Uwen Moses Akpan Essah

PRINCIPAL ACTIVITIES: Importers and suppliers of air-conditioning, heating and refrigeration, electrical and electronic equipment
Principal Agencies: United Africa Company (Nig) Ltd; R & A Services
Principal Bankers: Merantile Bank of Nigeria Ltd; African Continental Bank, Calabar

Principal Shareholders: Moses Akpan Essah, Uwem Moses Akpan Essah

INTERSTATE ARCHITECTS

Wesley House, 21/22 Marina, PO Box 1701, Lagos
Tel: 631666, 632725
Cable: Afroarts Lagos

Directors: P A S Gillmore (Senior Partner),
  Arc C R Fisher (Partner),
  Arc A Adeyemi (Partner),
  F A Adesina (Partner),
  K P Smith (Partner)
Senior Executives: H G McCafferty (Manager, Kano Office),
  J C Drummond (Manager, Ibadan Office),
  D O'Connor (Manager, Lagos Office)

PRINCIPAL ACTIVITIES: Architects, specialists in hospitals,
  banks, law courts and industrial commercial buildings
Branch Offices: 4 Noad Rd, PMB 2065, Jos, Tel 54706; 4 Club
  Rd, PMB 3116, Kano, Tel 5794; 6 Stones Rd, Onireke,
  Ibadan, Oyo State, Tel 410011, 410102
Associated Companies: Watkins Gray Woodgate International,
  UK; Zambia; IA/KB Association, Ibadan
Principal Bankers: Union Bank of Nigeria Ltd

INTERWORLD ENTERPRISES NIGERIA LTD

7 Oremeji Street, Off Medical Rd, PO Box 3500, Ikeja, Lagos
Tel: 960852, 964054
Cable: Interworld

Chairman: Chief Ayo Rosiji
Directors: Abimbola Rosiji, Mrs Gbemisola Rosiji, J T Lalvani

PRINCIPAL ACTIVITIES: Manufacturers of domestic appliances
Branch Offices: 12A Festival Stadium Rd, Kano

Date of Establishment: 1975
No of Employees: 87

INTRA MOTORS (NIGERIA) LTD

16 Ijora Causeway, PO Box 712, Lagos
Tel: 837215, 837217, 832171
Cable: Intramobil Lagos
Telex: 21391 Ridala Ng

Chairman: Alhaji Sule Katagum
Directors: H A Agha (Managing),
  O R Lababedi,
  S R Lababedi,
  Alhaji B A O Afariogun (Director of Admin/Company
    Secretary),
  Alhaji I Owodunni,
  B N Unam (Marketing Director),
  J T F Iyalla,
  I A Ikobho
Senior Executives: A O O Olaneye (General Manager),
  A A Adegboye (Chief Accountant)

PRINCIPAL ACTIVITIES: Distributors of motor vehicles, light
  commercial vehicles and spare parts
Principal Agencies: Nissan Motor Company Ltd, Japan
Branch Offices: 16 Umaru Babura Rd, Bompai, PMB 3154, Kano;
  78 Lagos Bye-pass, Oke-Ado, PMB 5243, Ibadan; Diobu, PO
  Box 2371, Port Harcourt
Subsidiary Companies: Rida National Distributors Ltd
Principal Bankers: Savannah Bank (Nig) Ltd; International
  Merchant Bank; Nigeria American Merchant Bank; Icon
  Merchant Bankers; Nigeria-Arab Bank
Financial Information:

As at 31.3.81	₦'000
Authorised capital	7,500
Paid-up capital	7,500
Turnover	87,717
Profits (net)	5,763

Principal Shareholders: S R Lababedi; O R Lababedi; Alhaji I
  Owodunni; Alhaji Sule Katagum; River State Government
Date of Establishment: 3rd December 1960
No of Employees: 700

INTRA TOBACCO MANUFACTURING CO LTD

PO Box 270, Ikeja, Lagos
Tel: 963527
Cable: Cigar
Telex: 21391 Ridala

Directors: A Tayan (General Manager),
  B Ashiru-Balogun (Sales Manager)

PRINCIPAL ACTIVITIES: Tobacco; cigarettes and cigars

INVESTMENT PROMOTIONS LTD

PO Box 1190, Investment House, 21/25 Broad St, Lagos
Tel: 630764
Telex: 21574 Inprom Ng

PRINCIPAL ACTIVITIES: Investment promoters and consultants

IREDE PROPERTIES AND INVESTMENT COMPANY LTD

PO Box 7325, 51 Olonode St, Yaba, Lagos
Tel: 860125

PRINCIPAL ACTIVITIES: Investment and advisory services

IRON PRODUCTS INDUSTRIES LTD

1 Denton St, Ebute Metta, PO Box 342, Lagos

PRINCIPAL ACTIVITIES: Iron casting

Date of Establishment: 1965

ISES LTD

Block 10 Marina Flats, 145 Broad St, PO Box 4587, Lagos

PRINCIPAL ACTIVITIES: Manufacturers of multi-purpose mini
  containers; suppliers of waste disposal equipment and
  through-conduit gate valves etc
Principal Agencies: Adamson & Hatchett Ltd
Financial Information: Part of ACROW Group of Companies

ISIYAKU RABIU & SONS LTD

See RABIU, ISIYAKU, & SONS LTD

ISOKARIARI, O K & SONS (NIGERIA) LTD

8 Ikwerre Rd, PO Box 83, Port Harcourt, Rivers State
Tel: 331045, 331511
Telex: 61218 Oki NG

Directors: O K Isokariari (Managing),
  N K Isokariari,
  G O Isokariari
Senior Executives: E B Ryder (General Manager)

PRINCIPAL ACTIVITIES: Building and civil engineering
  contractors
Branch Offices: Plot 26, Trans-Amadi Industrial Layout, Port
  Harcourt Tel: 331067/330025; Telex: 61108 Klo NG; 126 Bode
  Thomas St, Surulere, Lagos Tel: 837968; Suite 545, Chancery
  House, 53/64 Chancery Lane, London WC2A 1QU, UK, Tel
  831-6925, Telex 21792 Ref. 831
Associated Companies: O K C (Nigeria) Ltd
Principal Bankers: Pan African Bank; Savannah Bank of Nigeria
Financial Information:

	₦'000
Authorised capital	500
Paid-up capital	500
Turnover	10,000

Principal Shareholders: O K Isokariari
Date of Establishment: 4th July 1972
No of Employees: 850

ITAGER (NIGERIA) LTD

57 Jebba St East, PO Box 31, Ebute-Metta, Lagos
Tel: 846205

Directors: E Sola

PRINCIPAL ACTIVITIES: Building and civil engineering
  contractors

ITALAFRO BUILDERS

PO Box 148, Apapa, Lagos
Tel: 634434

Directors: G Scandella

PRINCIPAL ACTIVITIES: Building and civil engineering
contractors

ITIDAL-EPID ENTERPRISES OF NIGERIA

28 Hughes Ave, PO Box 421, Yaba, Lagos

Directors: L O A Dipe (Managing Director)

PRINCIPAL ACTIVITIES: General contractors, suppliers of
general goods, electrical equipment and stationery,
manufacturers' representatives; printers
Principal Bankers: Wema Bank (Nigeria) Ltd; African Continental
Bank Ltd

ITIKU & CO LTD

47 Marina, PO Box 1581, Lagos
Tel: 632985
Telex: 21339 Itiku Ng

PRINCIPAL ACTIVITIES: Financial and industrial development
consultants

ITOH, C, & CO LTD

Unity House, 15th Floor, 37 Marina, PO Box 2351, Lagos
Tel: 635005, 635077
Cable: Citoh Lagos
Telex: 21218 Citoh Ng

PRINCIPAL ACTIVITIES: Construction, contractors

ITT NIGERIA LTD

3A Ikorodu Rd, PO Box 3197, Yaba, Lagos
Tel: 800340 (10 lines)
Cable: Microphone Lagos

Chairman: Alhaji Chief M K O Abiola
Directors: A H Siniawsky (Managing),
   M Okorie (Deputy Managing),
   T O Adeleye,
   R G Wood

PRINCIPAL ACTIVITIES: Telecommunications and power
Branch Offices: Benin City; Port Harcourt; Enugu; Ibadan; Jos;
   Kaduna; Bauchi; Maiduguri; Kano; Sokoto
Principal Bankers: United Bank for Africa Ltd
Financial Information:

	₦'000
Authorised capital	1,400
Paid-up caital	1,300

Principal Shareholders: Alhaji Chief M K O Abiola; David
   Garrick; ISEC; M Okorie; Alhaji F A Oshodi
Date of Establishment: 1957
No of Employees: 3,000

IVORY PRODUCTS LTD

1 Henry Carr St, PMB 1295, Ikeja, Lagos
Tel: 964258, 960365
Cable: Ivorplast Lagos

Chairman: Chief Adekunle Ojora
Directors: S N Okeke,
   E O Evuarherhe,
   Dr C O Williams,
   J A Keji (Managing),
   S B Olupitan,
   R A Gbadamosi,
   S O Adeshina

PRINCIPAL ACTIVITIES: Suppliers of various types of industrial
   and cosmetic plastic wares
Branch Offices: Ibadan; Benin
Principal Bankers: United Bank for Africa Ltd

No of Employees: 165

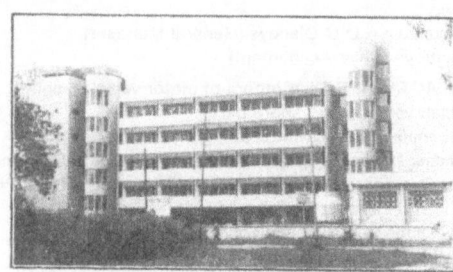

J & H INTERNATIONAL AGENCY

PO Box 1531, Apapa, Lagos
Tel: 877 139

Chairman: J O Agbai
Directors: S I Agbai, J C Agbai, C N Nwachukwu, H C
 Uwaoma
Senior Executives: Mrs Josephine C Agbai (Secretary),
 Daniel Uyimse (Marketing Manager),
 S I Imo (Legal Adviser)

PRINCIPAL ACTIVITIES: Business consultants, suppliers of
 agricultural, electronic and office equipment; printing and
 stationery supplies; importers and exporters; manufacturers
 representatives; advertising and tourism
Principal Agencies: Dainichi, Seiko Co Ltd, Japan; Cep, Italy;
 Brown and Sites Co, USA; Smith Corona; New Canaan; Iecis,
 Italy
Branch Offices: 90 Azikiwe Rd, Aba, Imo State; Douglas Rd,
 Owerri, Imo State; Sabon Gari, Kano
Subsidiary Companies: Joes Tech Centre, Owerri; UOB
 Associates: R & A Services (Division of UAC); NNPC
Principal Bankers: Savannah Bank of Nigeria Ltd; African
 Continental Bank Ltd

Date of Establishment: November 1973
No of Employees: 420

J A AJAO BROTHERS

See AJAO, J A, BROTHERS

J A BALOGUN WORKS

See BALOGUN, J A, WORKS

J A JONES (NIGERIA) LTD

See JONES, J A, (NIGERIA) LTD

J A O'BAHOR & COMPANY LTD

See O'BAHOR, J A, & COMPANY LTD

J A THOMAS RUBBER ESTATES LTD

See THOMAS, J A, RUBBER ESTATES LTD

J AKIN-GEORGE & COMPANY

See AKIN-GEORGE, J, & COMPANY

J ALLEN CO LTD

See ALLEN, J, CO LTD

J BAERTLE & CO (NIG) LTD

See BAERTLE, J, & CO (NIG) LTD

J E NWEKE & SONS LTD

See NWEKE, J E, & SONS LTD

J F OSOSAMI & CO

See OSOSAMI, J F, & CO

J I IDEHEN & SONS (NIGERIA) LTD

See IDEHEN, J I, & SONS (NIGERIA) LTD

J L MORISON SONS & JONES (NIGERIA) LTD

See MORISON, J L, SONS & JONES (NIGERIA) LTD

J MORIN & CO

See MORIN, J, & CO

J NWANKWU & BROS LTD

See NWANKWU, J, & BROS LTD

J O OYEWUMI & CO (NIGERIA) LTD

See OYEWUMI, J O, & CO (NIGERIA) LTD

J T CHANRAI & CO (NIGERIA) LTD

See CHANRAI, J T, & CO (NIGERIA) LTD

JAC-OGHO (NIGERIA) ENTERPRISES

3 Agbarho/Okpara Rd, Agbarho, PO Box 127, Orho-Agbarho,
 Warri, Bendel Stae

Chairman: James Idogho
Directors: Jacob U Omojevbe (General Manager)

PRINCIPAL ACTIVITIES: Building and civil engineering
 contractors; agents and general traders, suppliers of furniture
Branch Offices: 65 Ozolua St, Benin City, Bendel State

JAFCO IMPEX LTD

88 Olatunde Olabinjo Avenue, Ikorodu Rd, PO Box 919, Apapa,
 Lagos
Tel: 962844
Telex: 26937 Jaffal Ng

Chairman: Alhaji Sule Katagum
Directors: John Nassour (General Manager),
 Imad Jaffal

PRINCIPAL ACTIVITIES: Agents and general trading company
Principal Agencies: Kleber Colombes and insecticide
Branch Offices: Ilorin and Kaduna
Subsidiary/Associated Companies: Jafco Industry (Nig) Ltd;
 Jafco Construction (Nig) Ltd
Principal Bankers: International Bank for West Africa Ltd
Financial Information:

	N'000
Authorised capital	400
Paid-up capital	400
Turnover	6,000
Profits	50

JAMES KILPATRICK (NIGERIA) LTD

See KILPATRICK, JAMES, (NIGERIA) LTD

JAMMAL ENGINEERING (NIGERIA) LTD

PO Box 435, 58 Kofo Abayomi Ave, Lagos
Tel: 877315
Cable: Jammal Lagos
Telex: 21392 Jammal Ng

PRINCIPAL ACTIVITIES: Building and civil engineering
 contractors

JARMAKANI INDUSTRIES (NIG) LTD

Ilupeju Industrial Estate, PO Box 118, Ikeja, Lagos
Tel: 963322, 964606
Cable: Jarsprings

Chairman: N E Osundu
Directors: P B Osika, Wilson Yebiboh
Senior Executives: O E Ogbonnayah (General Manager),
 O A Khachmainan (Factory Engineer),
 E B Oni (Works Superintendent)

PRINCIPAL ACTIVITIES: Manufacturers of furniture springs and
 school furniture
Principal Bankers: Pan African Bank Ltd
Financial Information:

	N'000
Authorised capital	500
Paid-up capital	500

Principal Shareholders: Rivers State Government

JAS BUILDERS LTD

173 Zik Ave, PO Box 797, Enugu, Anambra State
Tel: 252800

PRINCIPAL ACTIVITIES: Builders and civil engineers
Branch Offices: Lagos Office: PO Box 7001, Ebute-Metta, Lagos;
 Kwara State; Rivers State; Nsukka and Enugu

JAYBEE INDUSTRIES (NIGERIA) LTD

Ilupeju Industrial Estate, PO Box 2774, Lagos
Tel: 900294/6
Cable: Boolchand

PRINCIPAL ACTIVITIES: Manufacturing of textiles
Financial Information: Associate of Kewalram Jhamatmal, Hong Kong

No of Employees: 500

JBL STAR TRADING COMPANY

54 Hospital Rd, PO Box 639, Aba, Imo State

Chairman: Chief Ben Anyachebelu
Directors: Louis Chidume Nwafor (Managing),
    John Ndukwe Okongwu

PRINCIPAL ACTIVITIES: Importers and traders in building
    materials and general goods
Principal Agencies: African Timber & Plywood Co; Naco Nig Ltd
Branch Offices: 2 Oha Street, Aba, Imo State
Principal Bankers: International Bank for West Africa Ltd

Date of Establishment: 1970

JECIMA MINING SYNDICATE

107 Bauchi Rd, PO Box 667, Jos, Plateau State

PRINCIPAL ACTIVITIES: Mining

JEMINE ENTERPRISES LTD

2 Yesufu Sanusi St, Surulere, Lagos
Tel: 834269

Chairman: N G Ogbemi (also Managing Director)
Directors: Mrs G E Ogbemi,
    Dr Tajudeen Lawal (Technical Director)
Senior Executives: S E Oke (Finance Controller),
    J N Oguh (Project Manager)

PRINCIPAL ACTIVITIES: Agents and general trading; civil
    engineering and construction; hotels and catering;
    transporters
Branch Offices: 69 Okpe Rd, Sapele, Bendel State
Principal Bankers: Union Bank of Nigeria Ltd
Financial Information:
Authorised capital   ₦ 100,000

Principal Shareholders: N G Ogbemi; Mrs G E Ogbemi
Date of Establishment: October 1977

JEPH INTERNATIONAL (NIGERIA) LTD

12B Ugwunabankpa Rd, PO Box 1192, Onitsha, Anambra State
Tel: 212534, 212579
Cable: Jephint Onitsha

PRINCIPAL ACTIVITIES: Building and civil engineering
    contractors
Branch Offices: 23 Raufu Williams Crescent, Surulere, Lagos, Tel
    833132; A05 Junction Rd, Kaduna

Date of Establishment: 1975

JHI LTD

Formerly John Holt Investment Company Ltd

Ebani House, 149/153 Broad St, PO Box 3596, Lagos
Tel: 661711/22
Cable: Holniman Lagos
Telex: 21238

Chairman: Akintola Williams
Directors: P L Cole (Managing),
    Chief S B Daniyan,
    Mrs G Ogbemi,
    E O Bandele,
    L W Dockerill,
    V G Taylor,
    P Best,
    A J Shelley
Senior Executives: A A Adefehinti (General Manager, Finance
    and Investments)

PRINCIPAL ACTIVITIES: Public investment company quoted on
    Lagos Stock Exchange; property investment and equities
Subsidiary Companies: Waterside Properties Ltd
Principal Bankers: Union Bank of Nigeria Ltd

Principal Shareholders: John Holt Group (48%)
Date of Establishment: 1953

JIDEOFO, D A, ENTERPRISES LTD

13 Ogui Rd, PO Box 443, Enugu, Anambra State
Tel: 3411

Directors: D A Jideofo (Managing Director),
    J G Jordan (Project Engineer),
    F I A Jideofo (Company Secretary)

PRINCIPAL ACTIVITIES: Building and civil engineering
    contractors

JIMONA, A C E, LTD

33 Creek Rd, Apapa, Lagos
Tel: 876533, 876634

Chairman: Chief Michael C O Ibru
Directors: J U Obere, G O Sadjere

PRINCIPAL ACTIVITIES: Construction
Branch Offices: Agbara-Otor, Bendel State; Ijora, Lagos
Principal Bankers: African Continental Bank Ltd; First Bank of
    Nigeria Ltd

JIRE ENGINEERING LTD

15 Bello St, Mushin Papa Ajao, PO Box 4831, Lagos

PRINCIPAL ACTIVITIES: Suppliers of surgical instruments;
    furniture, etc

JLGT CONSTRUCTION COMPANY NIGERIA LTD

Plot 1018 Ologun Agbeje St, PO Box 50061, Ikoyi, Victoria
    Island, Lagos
Tel: 618135/6
Telex: 22245 Globes

Chairman: Alhaji Ibrahim Damcida

PRINCIPAL ACTIVITIES: Building and civil engineering
    contractors
Principal Bankers: United Bank for Africa Ltd

Principal Shareholders: Grands Travaux de Marseille

JOART UNITED CONSTRUCTION & ENGINEERING LTD

179 Zik Ave, Uwani, PO Box 553, Enugu, Anambra State

Chairman: A Nwankwo
Directors: Eng Victor U Nwankwo (Managing),
    A Sadiq,
    O Emodi (Director, Co-ordination),
    A Abubakar,
    B E Nwankwo
Senior Executives: C Uduezue (Executive Manager Equipment),
    J Nwokeabia (Quantity Surveyor)

PRINCIPAL ACTIVITIES: Building materials and scientific
    instruments suppliers; civil engineering and construction
Branch Offices: 5 Rimi Rd, PMB 107, Bauchi; 6 Apollo Crescent,
    Jos, Plateau State
Associated Companies: Joart & Co (Nig) Ltd
Principal Bankers: African Continental Bank; First Bank of
    Nigeria Ltd
Financial Information:

	₦'000
Authorised capital	402
Paid-up capital	200

Principal Shareholders: Joart & Co (Nig) Ltd; A Nwankwo; V
    Nwankwo
No of Employees: 700

JOAS ELECTRICAL INDUSTRIES LTD

133/135 Ikorodu Rd, Obanikoro, PO Box 4957, Lagos
Tel: 963262, 963209
Cable: Joas Group
Telex: 26105 NG;

Chairman: Chief J O Amao
Directors: Mrs C A Amao
Senior Executives: J O Famakinwa (General Manager),
   D Idiabana (Group Financial Controller),
   A O Olukotun (Group Admin. Manager),
   O Osinubi (Chief Accountant),
   A Falade (Factory Manager),
   R Awonusi (National Sales Manager)

PRINCIPAL ACTIVITIES: Distributors of household Sound
   Systems, colour televisions, business machines, surveillance
   equipment, language laboratory and audio visual equipment
Principal Agencies: Sony Corporation, Japan; Sony Broadcast,
   UK
Branch Offices: 19 New Court Rd, Ibadan, Oyo State, Tel
   413205; 52 Lagos Rd, Benin City, Bendel State, Tel 240764; 3
   Adua Rd, Kano, Kano State, Tel 7045
Associated Companies: Bode Foam Industries (Nig) Ltd; Atlantic
   Carpets Nigeria Ltd
Principal Bankers: Union Bank of Nigeria Ltd
Financial Information:

	₦'000
Authorised capital	1,000
Paid-up capital	500
Turnover	10,000

Principal Shareholders: Chief J O Amao; Mrs C A Amao
Date of Establishment: January 1972
No of Employees: 300

JOBBA TRADING COMPANY

SW8/166 Ijebu Bye Pass, Oke Ado, PO Box 670, Ibadan, Oyo
   State
Tel: 411100
Telex: 31170 Uniwul Ng

Directors: J B Balogun (Managing)
Senior Executives: G O Aderibigbe (Secretary/Accountant),
   Mrs T O Balogun

PRINCIPAL ACTIVITIES: Manufacturers' representative,
   suppliers of home appliances, electrical and general goods;
   office equipment
Principal Agencies: Siso A/S, Denmark; AEI Ltd, Nigeria
Branch Offices: Behind Unity Hotel, Ofa Rd, PO Box 1580, Ilorin,
   Kwara State
Subsidiary Companies: Balogun Upholstery Furniture Industry;
   Balogun Modern Furniture Company Nigeria Ltd
Principal Bankers: Bank of the North Ltd
Financial Information:
Authorised capital   ₦ 105,000

Date of Establishment: February 1972

JOE ORUCHE TRADING COMPANY LTD

See ORUCHE, JOE, TRADING COMPANY LTD

JOE OYEGOKE ASSOCIATES

PO Box 1014, Jos, Plateau State
Tel: 55819, 55820

Chairman: J O Oyegoke (Principal Partner)
Senior Executives: K Brenyah (Senior Town Planner)

PRINCIPAL ACTIVITIES: Consultancy services provided in town
   and country planning, civil engineering, architecture,
   surveying, estate and project management
Associated Companies: International Planning & Environmental
   Consultants (Nigeria) Ltd; Cetaconsult (Nigeria) Ltd
Principal Bankers: Bank of the North Ltd; Union Bank of Nigeria
   Ltd

Principal Shareholders: J O Oyegoke
Date of Establishment: 1st July 1977

JOELSON & SONS HOLDINGS

3 Agege Motor Rd, Yaba, PO Box 44, Apapa, Lagos

Chairman: J E Nwagbogu
Directors: Prince J H Nwagbogu,
   Miss C I Ndudim (Company/Secretary/Accountant)

PRINCIPAL ACTIVITIES: Importation of general merchandise,
   plans to set up a soft drinks factory are being considered
Principal Bankers: Savannah Bank Nigeria Ltd

Date of Establishment: 1976

JOHN EDOKPOLO & CO LTD

See EDOKPOLO, JOHN, & CO LTD

JOHN HOLT LTD

See HOLT, JOHN, LTD

JOHN HOLT SHIPPING SERVICES

1/3 Burma Rd, PO Box 89, Apapa, Lagos
Tel: 803380/3, 876853, 876864
Telex: 21377

Chairman: Chief M N Ugochukwu
Directors: P Best,
   Alhaji Abdu Abubaker,
   G A Johnson,
   C I Ezeh,
   P L Cole,
   Alhaji G J Abdulkadir,
   A A Adlo-Moses,
   C E J Allanson (Managing),
   R O E Asemota,
   Dr E O Ogbu,
   T R Prentice
Senior Executives: H Onye Osakwe (General Manager)

PRINCIPAL ACTIVITIES: Import/export forwarding, shipping
   agency, travel agency, air freight
Principal Agencies: U.A.C. Nigeria Ltd; Thomas Wyatt; George
   Wimpey and Co Ltd, etc
Branch Offices: Principal towns throughout Nigeria
Principal Bankers: Union Bank of Nigeria Ltd

Principal Shareholders: John Holt Ltd
No of Employees: 500

JOHN OKWESA LTD

See OKWESA, JOHN, LTD

JOHN WEST PUBLICATIONS LTD

See WEST, JOHN, PUBLICATIONS LTD

JOHNSON FOLUSO INTERNATIONAL ENTERPRISES (JOFI)

2 Emiabata St, PO Box 157, Ago-Iwoye, Ogun State

Chairman: Johnson Folorunso Ogunfowokan
Directors: Dayo Ogunfowokan, Miss Toyin Akanni
Senior Executives: Tayo Alli (Manager),
   E A Adenuga (Manager)

PRINCIPAL ACTIVITIES: Importers, exporters, wholesalers and
   retailers, general suppliers of all electrical equipment
Principal Agencies: Adebowa Electrical Ind Ltd; Daddybond Ind
   Ltd
Branch Offices: 48 Emmanuel High St, Ojota, Lagos
Principal Bankers: First Bank of Nigeria Ltd; Wema Bank Nigeria
   Ltd

Date of Establishment: 28th December 1976

JOHNSON PRODUCTS OF NIGERIA LTD

26 Moloney St, Lagos

Chairman: Chief Mrs Opral Benson
Directors: Sunday Dankoro,
  George E Johnson,
  Mrs G Ayo Vaughan Richards,
  M J Cason (Managing)
Senior Executives: S A Lawal (Chief Accountant),
  Adetayo O Ogundehin (Assistant Production Manager)

PRINCIPAL ACTIVITIES: Hair care products manufacturers

Principal Shareholders: Nigerians (60%); Johnson Products
  Company Inc, Chicago
Date of Establishment: 24th October 1980

JOHNSON WAX NIGERIA LTD

PMB 1279, Ikeja, Lagos
Tel: 655995, 632685

Directors: V Awadagin Thomas (Managing Director)

PRINCIPAL ACTIVITIES: Processing and manufacturing of polish
Branch Offices: Factory: Plot 5 Block H Isolo Industrial Estate,
  Lagos

JOHNSON WHITE UNITED LTD

See WHITE, JOHNSON, UNITED LTD

JOINT DESIGN PARTNERSHIP

131 Broad St, PO Box 3402, Lagos
Tel: 634429, 636811

PRINCIPAL ACTIVITIES: Architects and town planning
  consultants

JOKI (NIGERIA) LTD

3 Olofin Rd, Apapa, PMB 3117, Surulere, Lagos
Tel: 873499, 873509
Cable: Joki
Telex: 21259 Apapa; 61233 Port Harcourt

Chairman: J O K Idornigie
Directors: I O Idornigie
Senior Executives: Captain E Massius (Shipping Manager)

PRINCIPAL ACTIVITIES: Shipping, clearing and forwarding
Branch Offices: 12 Eboh Rd, Warri, Bendel State; 14 Industry
  Rd, Port Harcourt; 200/208 Murtala Mohammed Highway,
  Calabar; 24 Mission Rd, Benin City; Shipping Dept; NPA
  Commercial Bldg, 2nd Floor, Tin Can Island Port, Lagos
Associated Companies: Industrial Products (Nigeria) Ltd; Rohlig
  & Co, West Germany
Principal Bankers: United Bank for Africa Ltd; Bank of the North
  Ltd

JOLLITERS CHEMISTS NIGERIA LTD

172 Agege Motor Rd, PO Box 8, Mushin, Lagos
Tel: 834390

PRINCIPAL ACTIVITIES: Wholesalers, retailers, importers and
  dispensers of pharmaceutical products

JONES HOMES INTERNATIONAL NIGERIA LTD

17 Martins St, Lagos

PRINCIPAL ACTIVITIES: Construction

JONES, J A, (NIGERIA) LTD

42 Norman Williams Rd, Ikoyi, Lagos

Chairman: Silas Daniyan
Directors: Forrest Nelson (Managing Director),
  H D McMullin

PRINCIPAL ACTIVITIES: Construction

JOS ALLUVIALS LTD

4a Suzi Gardens, PO Box 516, Jos, Plateau State
Tel: 2054

PRINCIPAL ACTIVITIES: Metal ore mining

JOS INTERNATIONAL BREWERIES LTD

Brewery Rd, PO Box 641, Jos, Plateau State
Tel: 50020

Chairman: Amos A Maren
Directors: Lars Olsen (Managing Director),
  Filibus A Azi,
  Alhaji M S Kurgi,
  Davidson B Gadabuke,
  Alhaji R Yahaya,
  Hajiya L Nimlan,
  Erik Emborg,
  J Dan Jensen

PRINCIPAL ACTIVITIES: Brewing of beer

Date of Establishment: 1975
No of Employees: 600

JOSEF WAHLER (NIG) LTD

See WAHLER, JOSEF, (NIG) LTD

JOSEPH ASABORO

See ASABORO, JOSEPH

JOSIAH PARKES & SONS (NIGERIA) LTD

See PARKES, JOSIAH, & SONS (NIGERIA) LTD

JOSMAN ARATAH TRADING COMPANY

See ARATAH, JOSMAN, TRADING COMPANY

JULI IMPORTERS & EXPORTERS ENTERPRISES

24 Efosa St, PO Box 142, Uzebu Quarters, Off Ekenwan Rd,
  Benin City, Bendel State
Tel: 240510, 241888, 242823
Cable: 41137 Tomdic Ng

PRINCIPAL ACTIVITIES: Importers of stock fish, cement,
  tobacco and general merchandise; exporters of graded crude
  rubber

JULI PHARMACY AND STORES LTD

16 Kodesoh St, Juli House, PMB 21222, Ikeja, Lagos
Tel: 964736
Cable: Handidrugs

Chairman: Julius Adeluyi (also Managing Director)
Directors: Mrs Julia Adeluyi (Executive Director)
Senior Executives: Mrs Idaresit Ekwere (Pharmacist/Branch
    Manager),
  Fola Akinsiku (Pharmacist/Branch Manager),
  Gabriel Farotade (Accountant),
  Miss Dora Omole (Assistant to Managing Director),
  David Akanade (Dispensary Manager),
  Miss Regina Alozie (Senior Sales Supervisor),
  Mrs Funke Agema (Stores)

PRINCIPAL ACTIVITIES: Suppliers of pharmaceuticals goods
Principal Agencies: Roche; Major & Company; Nigerian Hoechst;
  Chemical & Allied; Boots; Glaxo; Pfizer; Sandox etc
Branch Offices: Roundabout Shopping Complex, Ikeja, Lagos;
  Airport Hotel, Ikeja, Lagos; Falomo Shopping Complex, Ikoyi,
  Lagos; Eko Holiday Inn, Victoria Island, Lagos
Associated Companies: Kiddieland (Nigeria) Ltd
Principal Bankers: International Bank for West Africa Ltd
Financial Information:

	N'000
Authorised capital	250
Paid-up capital	250
Turnover	2,000

Principal Shareholders: Julius Adeluyi; Mrs Julia Adeluyi
Date of Establishment: August 1979
No of Employees: 150

JULIUS BERGER NIGERIA LTD
See BERGER, JULIUS, NIGERIA LTD

K CHELLARAM & SONS (NIGERIA) LTD
See CHELLARAM, K, & SONS (NIGERIA) LTD

KABBA CO-OPERATIVE CREDIT & MARKETING UNION LTD
PO Box 25, Kabba, Kwara State

President: Alhaji S O Onundi
Directors: H A Orisafunmi (Manager)

PRINCIPAL ACTIVITIES: Producers of food and cash crops and
dealers in consumer goods

KABELMETAL NIGERIA LTD
28 Henry Carr Street, Industrial Estate, PMB 21253, Ikeja, Lagos

Tel: 900640-2, 961860, 964953
Cable: Kabelmetal
Telex: 26101 KMR NG

Chairman: Chief T Adeola Odutola
Directors: H D Berg (Managing Director),
  Dr J A Sodipo,
  J S P Spaapen,
  M Jeroch,
  G Nwakuche,
  German Development Company (DEG)
Senior Executives: F Benz (General Manager),
  A Anjorin (Assistant General Manager)

PRINCIPAL ACTIVITIES: Manufacturers of electrical wires,
  cables and conductors for power and telecommunication
  transmissions
Principal Bankers: United Bank for Africa Ltd; International
  Merchant Bank Nigeria Ltd
Financial Information:

	₦'000
Authorised capital	6,000
Paid-up capital5	4,000
Turnover (1981/82)	34,000

Principal Shareholders: Kabel Und Metallwerke,
  Gutehoffnungshuette, GmbH, West Germany
No of Employees: 800

KABO BLOCKS LTD
Plot 499/501, Airport Rd, PO Box 1850, Kano
Tel: 5172

PRINCIPAL ACTIVITIES: Manufacturers of building blocks

KADUNA CO-OPERATIVE BANK LTD
Hospital Rd, PO Box 1066, Kaduna
Tel: 213928
Cable: Cobank
Telex: 71156 Cobank Ng

Chairman: Alhaji Ja'afaru Makarfi
Directors: Chief Registrar Co-Operative Societies,
  Ministry of Agriculture & Rural Development,
  Alhaji Shehu Abdullahi (Alternate),
  Permanent Secretary Ministry of Finance,
  Kaduna State,
  Mallam Yusufu M Bamalli (Alternate),
  Permanent Secretary Ministry of Trade,
  Industry & Tourism,
  Kaduna State,
  Mallam Yusufu Abubakar (Alternate),
  Mallam Musa Yarima,
  Dr S E Mosugu,
  Alhaji Nuhu Bayero,
  Mallam Abdurahman Bindawa,

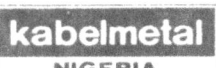
Mallam Zubairu Umar,
Alhaji Abdu Modibbo,
Alhaji Rabe Saidu Dutsin-Ma
Senior Executives: Alhaji M S Kutigi (General Manager),
  Alhaji Aliyu I Kakangi (Acting Chief Accountant),
  M Aliyu Matazu (Senior Inspector),
  M Yakubu Shehu (Research and Development Manager),
  Mallam M T Umar (Acting Advances Manager),
  M Saddik A Mahuta (Senior Legal Officer)

PRINCIPAL ACTIVITIES: Banking
Branch Offices: Katsina, Zaria, Funtua, Saminaka, Birnin-Gwari,
  Kankia, Kachia

Principal Shareholders: Government owned
Date of Establishment: 1974
No of Employees: 200

KADUNA HOTELS CO LTD
Hamdala Hotel, PO Box 311, Kaduna
Tel: 211005
Cable: Hamdala Kaduna
Telex: 71163

Chairman: Alhaji Hamza Zayyad
Directors: Alhaji A M Usman, Alhaji Ladan Zuru, Peter Stone,
  Alhaji Magaji Mohammed, Dr A Y A Aliyu, Alhaji U Dikko,
  Prof A F Ogunsola
Senior Executives: J C Halsall (Hotel Manager)

PRINCIPAL ACTIVITIES: Hotel services
No of Employees: 330

KADUNA INVESTMENTS CO LTD
27 Ali Akilu Rd, PMB 2230, Kaduna
Tel: 211018, 242455, 217094
Telex: 71319 Kaveco NG

Chairman: Muhammad Tukur
Directors: Sani Idris Bagiwa,

M Maikaita Inuwa,
Dr Sa'adu Usman,
M Bature Mashi,
Talat Buhari Balal,
M T Abba Kasim,
M Abubakar Umar,
M Dodo Dabo,
Permanent Secretaries for Ministry of Economic Development
and Ministry of Finance (Kaduna)
Senior Executives: Mallam Samaila Mamman (General Manager),
Mallam S Dalhatu (Investment Manager),
Alhaji D Adamu (Company Secretary),
S J Prathapan (Principal Accountant)

PRINCIPAL ACTIVITIES: Development finance institution
Subsidiary/Associated Companies: Subsidiaries: Katsina Oil
Mills Ltd; Gobarau Bakery Co Ltd; Jema Bakery Co Ltd;
Water & Power Dev Co Ltd; Associates: Peugeot Automobile
(Nig) Ltd; Zaria Industries Ltd; Stirling Civil Engineering Ltd;
Borini Prono & Co Ltd; Tarpaulin Industries (W.A.) Ltd;
Turners Building Products Ltd
Principal Bankers: United Bank for Africa Ltd; Kaduna
Co-operative Bank Ltd
Financial Information:

	₦'000
Authorised capital	6,000
Paid-up capital	6,000
Net profits (December 1980)	919

Principal Shareholders: Kaduna State Government
Date of Establishment: October 1976
No of Employees: 35

KADUNA PROSPECTORS (NIGERIA) LTD

PMB 2045, Jos, Plateau State

Chairman: Alhaji Adamu Garba
Directors: Alhaji A Tambuwal, T D Pwajok, S O Ajetunmobi, A
A Kehinde, E Grayson

Senior Executives: C R Charlton (General Manager)
PRINCIPAL ACTIVITIES: Mining
Financial Information:

	₦'000
Authorised capital	650
Paid-up capital	613

Principal Shareholders: Kaduna Prospectors (UK) Ltd (40%);
Nigerian Mining Corp (55.7%); Individual Nigerians &
Employees (4.3%)

KADUNA TEXTILES LTD

PO Box 68, Kaduna
Tel: 213352
Telex: 71103 Kadtex Ng

PRINCIPAL ACTIVITIES: Spinning and weaving textile mills

No of Employees: 4,500

KAELER (WEST AFRICA) LTD

44 Opebi Rd, PO Box 1417, Ikeja, Lagos State
Tel: 964074
Telex: 20202 TDS 161

Chairman: E A Edouk
Directors: Imeh O Usenekong (Managing Director),
E J Umoh,
Fredy S Reif

PRINCIPAL ACTIVITIES: Sales and service organisation;
suppliers of complete plants and turn-key operations for
complete installations for plastics and packaging
manufacturing machinery. Packaging in-plant operations,
moulds service and spare parts supply
Principal Agencies: Ludwig Engel & Dr Boy (Injection Moulding
Machines); Staehle/Hesta & Moretti (Blow Moulding
Machines); Conair Churchill (Circulating Water Chillers);
Starlinger & Co (Circular Looms and Complete Plant for PP
Woven Bags); Bielloni Castello (Complete Machinery for Film

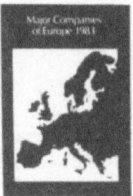
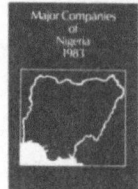
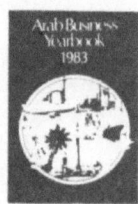
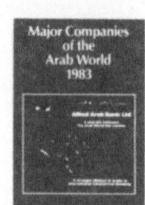
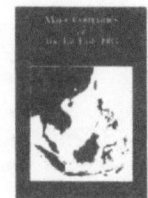
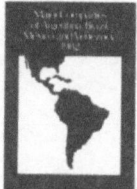

Extrusion Plant); Rapid (Granulators); Coatema GmbH (Complete Coating Plant for Artificial Leather); Moss (Printing equipment); USM International British United (Complete Plant for Shoe Making Industry)
Subsidiary/Associated Companies: Kaeler Holding AG, Switzerland
Principal Bankers: International Bank for West Africa Ltd; First Bank of Nigeria Ltd
Financial Information:

	N'000
Authorised capital	350
Paid-up capital	200

Principal Shareholders: Overseas (40%); Nigerians (60%)
Date of Establishment: 1980

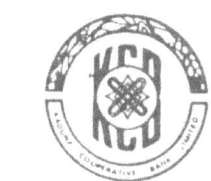

Kaduna Co-operative Bank Ltd.

"THE BANK THAT HELPS YOU TO GROW"
All banking services are provided

Head Office:

Hospital Road, P.O. Box 1066, Kaduna - Nigeria;
Tel: 213928, Telex: 71156 COBANK NG.
Cable: COBANK

Branches:

Kaduna	— Hospital Road (Main Branch) P.M.B. 2121, Kaduna
Kaduna	— Central Market
Kaduna North	— N.D.A.
Katsina	— Kofar-Kaura, Kano Road
Zaria	— 2/4 Liverpool Avenue, P.M.B. 1071. Tel: 32936
Funtua	— 51 Katsina Road
Saminaka	— Jos Road
Birnin-Gwari	— c/o Local Government Secretariat
Kankia	— Dutsin-ma Road
Kachia	— Kafanchan Road

CORRESPONDENTS THROUGHOUT ALL MAJOR FINANCIAL CENTRES OF THE WORLD

KAGHO INDUSTRIAL ENTERPRISES LTD
84A Warri/Sapele Rd, PO Box 6, Warri, Bendel State
Tel: 230938

PRINCIPAL ACTIVITIES: Importer and distributor of paper products
Branch Offices: 10 Lower Erejuwa Rd, Warri, Bendel State, Tel 233336

KAILASH INDUSTRIES (NIGERIA) LTD
17 McEwan St, Yaba, Lagos
Tel: 862488
Cable: Kailash

PRINCIPAL ACTIVITIES: Manufacturing of cosmetics, paints, surface coatings, polishing preparations

KAILASH WEAVING & GARMENT MANUFACTURING CO (NIGERIA) LTD
30/32 Murtala Mohammed Way, Ebute-Metta, Lagos
Tel: 846254, 862225, 862302

PRINCIPAL ACTIVITIES: Textile Manufacturing

KANDARA PALACE HOTEL LTD
2 Unity Rd, PO Box 2016, Kano
Tel: 3612, 3680
Cable: Kandotel
Telex: 77136 Kassim Ng

PRINCIPAL ACTIVITIES: Hoteliers

KANO CITIZENS TRADING COMPANY LTD
Masaka Mills, Gwamaja, PMB 3024, Kano
Tel: 2413
Cable: Masaka Kano

PRINCIPAL ACTIVITIES: Manufacturers of cotton drills, cords, towels, cellular, panama baft and shirting

KANO CONFECTIONERY LTD
127 Club Rd, PO Box 1192, Kano
Tel: 4318, 5734
Cable: Amka Kano
Telex: 77148 Elhoss Ng

Directors: S C El-Hoss

PRINCIPAL ACTIVITIES: Manufacturers of sweets and confectionery

KANO COOPERATIVE BANK LTD
11c Murtala Muhammed Way, PO Box 4636, Kano
Tel: 7181/8
Cable: Bankop
Telex: 77279

Chairman: Mallam Ahmed Sani
Directors: Haruna Aliya, Hajiya Dina Hassan, Gwadabe Wudilawa, Sharu Gambo Salihu, Shazali Ali, Ibrahim D Mudi
Senior Executives: Farouk Ahmed (General Manager), Yusufu Abubakar (Deputy General Manager), Mikailu Abdullahi (Secretary/Legal Adviser), Isaal O Anikwue (Asst. General Manager Admin), Wilcox B Alalibo (Asst. General Manager, Finance)

PRINCIPAL ACTIVITIES: Commercial banking
Branch Offices: 10E Bello Rd, PMB 3229, Hadejia, Kano State; Birnin Kudu; Wudil; Dawakin Kudu; Danbatta; Kafin Hausa; Karaye; Tsakuna Dala Hotel Agency, Kano State
Financial Information:

	N'000
Authorised capital	10,000
Paid-up capital	3,889
Turnover	41,862
Profits	171

Principal Shareholders: Kano State Government; Kano Cooperative Societies
Date of Establishment: April 1976
No of Employees: 300

KANO DYEING AND PRINTING CO LTD
9 Independence Rd, PO Box 422, Kano

PRINCIPAL ACTIVITIES: Manufacturing of piece goods
No of Employees: 600

KANO MERCHANTS TRADING CO LTD
73 Ibrahim Taiwo Rd, PO Box 896, Kano
Tel: 4489

Directors: A I Rabiu

PRINCIPAL ACTIVITIES: Suppliers of general merchandise, wholesalers

KANO OIL MILLERS LTD
123-131 Maganda Rd, Kano
Tel: 2384, 3068
Telex: 77116 Komkan Ng

PRINCIPAL ACTIVITIES: Oil millers
Branch Offices: Oil Mill: 93 Tafawa Balewa Rd, Kano, Tel 2300

KANO RESIDENTIAL HOTEL
24 Murtala Mohammed Way, PO Box 2147, Kano
Tel: 3168

Directors: Alhaji Sani Mashall (Managing Director)

PRINCIPAL ACTIVITIES: Hoteliers

KANO STATE HOTELS MANAGEMENT BOARD
150 Murtala Muhammed Way, PMB 3339, Kano
Tel: 5311, 5314
Telex: 77241

Chairman: Alhaji Muhammadu Gayyama (Madakin Hadejia)
Directors: Alhaji Isa Abubakar, Hajia Sa'adatu Baffa Usman,
Alhaji Mohammed Olo Kote, Alhaji Mohammed Sabo Nanono,
Alhaji Sule Dandauda, Alhaji Miyitaba Dankani,
Commissioner of Home Affairs and Information, Hajia Delu
Garba, Alhaji Babaji Gwaram
Senior Executives: Alhaji Umar Abdulwahab (General Manager),
Aminu Muhtar (Assistant General Manager),
Mahmoud Sani Bello (Secretary),
Usman Haruna (Group Accountant),
Tafida Mohammed Bello (Group Personnel Manager),
Yusuf Othman (Hotel Manager),
Shuaibu Isa Dale (Hotel Manager),
Shehu Buddaraini (Hotel Manager)

PRINCIPAL ACTIVITIES: Hoteliers; hotels include the Daula
Hotel; the Bagauda Lake Hotel; the Rock Castle; Magwan
Water Restaurant and Catering Rest Houses
Principal Bankers: Bank of the North Ltd; Kano Co-Operative
Bank Ltd; International Bank for West Africa Ltd; Bank of
Credit and Commerce International Ltd
Principal Shareholders: Wholly owned by the Kano State
Government
Date of Establishment: October 1976
No of Employees: 1,000

KANO STATE INVESTMENT & PROPERTIES LTD
4th Floor Gidan Murtala, PMB 3119, Kano
Tel: 5331
Cable: Investco
Telex: 77281

Chairman: Alhaji Saleh Jibril
Directors: M S Nanono (Managing Director),
Alhaji Sani Gule,
Alhaji Dogara,
Alhaji Garba,
Alhaji Dali Danbatta,
J A Koguna,
Alhaji Shehu Ibrahim,
Hayiya T Abdulsalam,
Alhaji Sani A Daura,
Alhaji Abdussamadu Iliyasu
Senior Executives: Alhaji Masa'abu Mohammed (Investment
Manager),
Alhaji Rufa'i Shehu (Estate Controller),
P K Gosh (Financial Controller),
I L Modi (Senior Investment Executive),
Alhaji U F Abdullani (Deputy Company Secretary)

PRINCIPAL ACTIVITIES: Investment in industrial, commercial
and agricultural projects; management of housing estates
Principal Bankers: Bank of the North Ltd

Principal Shareholders: Wholly owned by Kano State
Government
Date of Establishment: 20th October 1971 Incorporated
No of Employees: 108

KANO SUGAR INDUSTRY NIGERIA LTD
13 Ibrahim Taiwo Rd, PO Box 582, Kano
Tel: 5011, 4489
Telex: 77229 Baguda

PRINCIPAL ACTIVITIES: Sugar manufacturers
Branch Offices: Throughout Nigeria

Date of Establishment: 1978
No of Employees: 170

KANO SUIT AND PACKING CASES FACTORY LTD
PO Box 896, Kano
Tel: 4489

Directors: Alhaji Mustapha Danlami

PRINCIPAL ACTIVITIES: Manufacturing of suitcases and packing
cases
Branch Offices: Factory: 4 Sule Gaya Rd, Bompai, Kano

KANO WELDING & STEEL CONSTRUCTION CO LTD
PO Box 1422, 45 Murtala Mohammed Way, Kano

Directors: A I Hassan (Managing Director)

PRINCIPAL ACTIVITIES: Steel construction

KANOTEX LTD
329 Kundila Rd, Bompai, PO Box 1132, Kano
Tel: 4077
Cable: Kanotex
Telex: 77184 Kantex Ng

Directors: Suhail Akar (Managing Director),
Aminu Dantata
Senior Executives: Nazih Kamal (General Manager),
T Akar (Technical/Production Manager)

PRINCIPAL ACTIVITIES: Manufacturers of textiles
Principal Bankers: Union Bank of Nigeria Ltd

Date of Establishment: 1970

KAPITAL INSURANCE COMPANY LTD
Gidan Dan Baskore, 15c Murtala Muhammed Way, PO Box
2044, Kano
Tel: 5666
Cable: Kaninsure Kano
Telex: 71108 Newdev Ng

Chairman: H B Mohammad
Directors: M S Nanono,
M S Kutigi,
K A Kere,
L W Hammick,
C O Rowe,
T Ibrahim,
M S Umar (Executive),
A Soppet (Managing)
Senior Executives: A O Aderemi (Accountant),
A R Bello (Senior Underwriter)

PRINCIPAL ACTIVITIES: Insurance and reinsurance
Branch Offices: Kaduna; Minna; Bauchi
Principal Bankers: Bank of the North Ltd; Bank of Credit and
Commerce (Nigeria) Ltd
Financial Information: As at 31st December 1980

	₦'000
Authorised capital	337
Paid-up capital	337
Turnover	2,700
Profits	171

Principal Shareholders: New Nigeria Development Corporation
Ltd; Kano State Investment and Properties Ltd; Bauchi State
Investment and Property Development Ltd; Niger
Development Co Ltd; Commercial Union Assurance Co Ltd
Date of Establishment: 18th April 1974
No of Employees: 50

KAROPHARM LABORATORIES LTD
150A Mission Rd, PO Box 648, Benin City, Bendel State
Tel: 242598
Cable: Karopharm

Chairman: Gabriel I Oviasu
Directors: I K Omorede Oviasu
Senior Executives: Joseph A Ehidiamhen (Secretary/Accountant)

PRINCIPAL ACTIVITIES: Drug manufacturing
Principal Bankers: Union Bank of Nigeria Ltd; New Nigeria Bank
    Ltd
Financial Information:

	N'000
Authorised capital	60
Paid-up capital	60
Turnover (1981)	173

Principal Shareholders: G I Oviasu; Mrs P O Oviash; I O Oviasu
Date of Establishment: 1972

KARUNWI, A O, LTD
PO Box 54, 6 Lancaster Rd, Yaba, Lagos
Tel: 842643

PRINCIPAL ACTIVITIES: Building and civil engineering
    contractors

KASSA MINES LTD
Q34 Adetutu St, PO Box 612, Jos, Plateau State

PRINCIPAL ACTIVITIES: Mining

KAURA BISCUIT AND MACARONI FACTORY LTD
12 and 15 Club Rd, PO Box 2147, Kano
Tel: 4292

Directors: Alhaji Sani Mashall (Managing Director)

PRINCIPAL ACTIVITIES: Manufacturers of biscuits

No of Employees: 400

KAY INDUSTRIES NIGERIA LTD
Henry Carr St, Industrial Estate, Ikeja, Lagos
Tel: 963839, 964055, 962102
Cable: Wondertex

Directors: D G Uttamchandani

PRINCIPAL ACTIVITIES: Manufacturing of lace and embroidered
    textiles

No of Employees: 200

KAYCEE (NIGERIA) LTD
45 Marina, PO Box 4619, Lagos
Tel: 663258, 662302, 664733
Cable: Kaycee
Telex: 21559 Kaycee Ng

Chairman: L L Chellaram
Directors: S L Chellaram,
    G H Dayal (Managing Director),
    Alhaji Isa Kaita,
    Chief T J Sokoh,
    Chief F R A Williams,
    A Otulana
Senior Executives: K T Tulsiani (Merchandise Manager),
    M K Khatri (Financial Controller),
    P J O Arifalo (Administrative Manager)

PRINCIPAL ACTIVITIES: Department stores: suppliers of
    wholesale goods including building materials, hardware,
    textiles and electrical goods; manufacturers' representatives;
    importers and exporters of general merchandise
Principal Agencies: JVC Nivico, Japan; Rising, Japan (Electrical
    Products); Coleman, USA (Jugs and Coolers); Thomas A
    Edison, USA (Airconditioners); Norton Bicycles, India;
    Crompton and Greaves, India; Hawkins Pressure Cookers,
    India; Fides Products, Italy; Citizen Co, Japan (Calculators
    and Typewriters); Mikasa and National Generators, Japan

Branch Offices: 28 Wharf Rd, Apapa, Lagos; 5/6 Lagos St,
    Kano; 25 Ahmadu Bello Way, Jos; Nelly Thomas Hausa Rd,
    Warri, Bendel State; 2 Ibiwe St, Benin City, Bendel State;
    Market Rd, Sapele; 4 Anokwuru St, Port Harcourt; 4 Bright
    St, Onitsha, Anambra State; 17 Okpara Ave, Enugu, Anambra
    State
Principal Bankers: Union Bank of Nigeria Ltd; United Bank for
    Africa Ltd; First Bank of Nigeria Ltd; Societe Generale Bank
    (Nigeria) Ltd; International Bank for West Africa Ltd; Chase
    Merchant Bank Nigeria Ltd
Financial Information:

	N'000
Authorised capital	4,000
Paid-up capital	2,550
Turnover	45,000
Profits	2,000

Principal Shareholders: Kaycee (Bermuda) Ltd (40%); Nigerian
    Shareholders (60%)
Date of Establishment: 1972
No of Employees: 500

KAYSON COMPANY LTD
12 Ajigbeda St, Off Agege Motor Rd, Mosalasi Bus Stop, PO
    Box 4449, Surulere, Lagos
Tel: 831492

President: Emmanuel Kayode Okeowo
Directors: Tunde Oyefodunrin, Femi Songonuga
Senior Executives: Kamar Jimoh (Credit Controller),
    S M Ayoola (Underwriting/Claims Manager),
    S O Ofori (Accountant/Office Manager)

PRINCIPAL ACTIVITIES: Insurance and reinsurance
Principal Agencies: Royal Exchange Assurance Nig Ltd; Great
    Nigeria Insurance Co Ltd; Crusader Insurance Co (Nig) Ltd;
    United Nigeria Insurance Co Ltd; Unity Life and Fire
    Insurance Co Ltd; Mercury Assurance Co (Nig) Ltd; National
    Insurance Corporation of Nigeria; Niger Ins Co Ltd; Sentinel
    Ass Co Ltd
Branch Offices: 1B New Ikang Rd, PO Box 885, Calabar, Cross
    River State
Principal Bankers: African Continental Bank Ltd

Principal Shareholders: E K Okeowo; O A Songonuga
Date of Establishment: 7th June 1972

KCA DRILLING (NIGERIA) LTD
156-157 Trans-Amadi Estate, PO Box 711, Port Harcourt, Rivers
    State

PRINCIPAL ACTIVITIES: Drilling contractors

KEDAM HOLDINGS (NIGERIA) LTD
48 Upper Drive, Palm Grove Estate, Ikorodu Rd, Ilupeju, PO Box
    888, Ikeja, Lagos

PRINCIPAL ACTIVITIES: Management and financial investment
    group, involved in the manufacture and distribution of
    aluminium, timber and metal products, the manufacture and
    canning of Nigerian food products, civil engineering and
    building contracting, real estate and property development
Branch Offices: 4 Oremeji St, Off Medical Rd, PO Box 888, Ikeja,
    Lagos
Subsidiary Companies: K-Indal (Nigeria) Ltd; K-Total
    Construction (Nigeria) Ltd; K-Timber Metal (Nigeria) Ltd;
    K-Foods Products (Nigeria) Ltd; K-Realestate (Nigeria) Ltd

KENNEDY TRANSPORT (NIGERIA) LTD
10 Aba Rd, PO Box 810, Port Harcourt, Rivers State
Tel: 333335, 335328
Cable: Kentrans
Telex: 61111 Rozzy Ng

Chairman: Chief Dr E S Amadi (also Managing Director)
Directors: A E Nyong, Dr M T Akobo, Dr Obi Wali, O O Ngei,
    M O Harrison
Senior Executives: O B Martins (Shipping Manager),
    E R Antezzia (General Manager, Operations)

145

PRINCIPAL ACTIVITIES: Transportation (haulage), shipping, clearing/forwarding, air freight, travel agents, catering, real estate agents, import/export, business consultants, manufacturers' representatives

Principal Agencies: Amway Corporation of Michigan City, USA; Danish Turnkey Dairies Ltd, Denmark; Wusin Enterprises Inc, Taiwan; Owen's Commercial Syndicate, UK; Ippec Equipment/Commercials, UK; Fairies Industrial Co Ltd, Republic of China; H W Port/Korner GmbH, Germany; Century Shipping Corporation, Korea; Brabant (International) Ltd; BGN International SA, Spain; Container-Lloyd (USA) Inc

Branch Offices: 12 Nnamdi Azikiwe St (1st Floor), PO Box 3439, Lagos, Tel 632460

Associated Companies: Kennedy Dairies (Nigeria) Ltd; Equipment Gesellschaft, West Germany

Principal Bankers: Pan African Bank Ltd; African Continental Bank Ltd; Union Bank of Nigeria Ltd; National Bank of Nigeria Ltd

Principal Shareholders: Chief Dr E S Amadi; A E Nyong; Dr Obi Wali

Date of Establishment: 11th June 1971

No of Employees: 176

KENT ENGINEERING NIGERIA LTD

PO Box 7955, Lagos
Tel: 833257
Cable: Kenteng

Chairman: Alhaji Y A Alashe
Directors: R O Bennett (Contract Director),
Alhaja I A Alashe
Senior Executives: S O Ola (Plumbing Manager),
Felix Aniakor (Supervisor),
B Nkwoji (Office Manager)

PRINCIPAL ACTIVITIES: Plumbing, mechanical, electrical engineering, air-conditioning equipment suppliers; sewage contractors

Branch Offices: PO Box 743, Port Harcourt
Principal Bankers: African Continental Bank Ltd
Financial Information:
Sales turnover   N 2,000,000

Principal Shareholders: Alhaji Y A Alashe; Alhaja A Alashe
No of Employees: 300

KENTING AFRICA RESOURCE SERVICES LTD

53 Lawson St, PO Box 1658, Lagos
Tel: 636239, 636555
Cable: Kentingaf Lagos
Telex: 21308 Kentaf Ng

Chairman: Chief R O Coker
Directors: A V Vanden Brink,
J A Thomas,
D G Mackay,
Chief A O Morgan,
J Srath (Managing)
Senior Executives: F A Adepetun (Financial/Administrative Manager),
A A Kobiti (Accountant),
Mrs J U Okolie (Personnel Assistant)

PRINCIPAL ACTIVITIES: Geophysical services; mapping and aerial photography and resource surveys

Principal Agencies: Federal Government Ministeries; State Ministries

Branch Offices: 10A Bompai Rd, PO Box 589, Kano; 2A Zaria Rd, PO Box 994, Jos, Plateau State

Subsidiary Companies: Kenting Ltd, Canada; Kenting Earth Sciences, Canada

Principal Bankers: First Bank of Nigeria Ltd; Savannah Bank of Nigeria ltd

Date of Establishment: 21st March 1973
No of Employees: 150

KEPPLER HAUSBAU (NIGERIA) LTD

8/10 Broad St, 9th Floor, PO Box 1258, Lagos

Directors: J Janssens

PRINCIPAL ACTIVITIES: Engineering consultants

KESINGTON INDUSTRIES LTD

2nd Floor, Face-to-Face Bldg, 112 Western Ave, Surulere, PO Box 2041, Lagos
Tel: 831973, 834463
Cable: Kessco Lagos

Directors: Chief Kesington A Adebutu (Managing Director)
Senior Executives: Miss Abimbola Onayemi (General Manager)

PRINCIPAL ACTIVITIES: Manufacturing all types of paints, protective coatings, adhesives, metal containers and plastic containers

Branch Offices: Factories: Km 70/72, Lagos-Ibadan Rd, PO Box 58, Iperu, Remo, Ogun State

Associated Companies: Kesington & Company Ltd, Nigeria
Principal Bankers: United Bank for Africa Ltd; Allied Bank of Nigeria Ltd

Principal Shareholders: Chief Kesington A Adebutu

KEWALRAM, G, & SONS (NIGERIA) LTD

48 Marina, PO Box 320, Lagos
Tel: 630357, 630428
Telex: 21421 Geekay Ng

PRINCIPAL ACTIVITIES: Department stores and wholesalers

KEYDRIL NIGERIA LTD

10 Waziri Ibrahim St, Victoria Island, PO Box 50229, Falomo, Ikoyi, Lagos
Tel: 611214

Directors: C Durham (Managing Director)

PRINCIPAL ACTIVITIES: Drilling contractors

KHALIL & DIBBO TRANSPORT LTD

PO Box 323, Ibadan, Oyo State
Tel: 413645
Telex: 31124 Khadib Ng

PRINCIPAL ACTIVITIES: Transport contractors

KIKACHUKWU AGRICULTURAL ENTERPRISES LTD

19 Martin St, 4th Floor, PO Box 50463, Falomo, Ikoyi, Lagos
Tel: 663574

PRINCIPAL ACTIVITIES: Suppliers of agricultural equipment
Branch Offices: 175B Aba Rd, Port Harcourt, Rivers State, Tel 332912; 64 Warri/Sapele Rd, PO Box 210, Warri, Bendel State; 12 Edo Crescent, PMB 1346, Benin City, Bendel State, Tel 244345, Telex 41124 Ng; Hatchery Site, Mile 2, Ogwashi-Uku/Isha Rd, PO Box 27, Ogwashi-Uku, Bendel State

Financial Information:
Registered capital   N 100,000

Date of Establishment: May 1977

KILPATRICK, JAMES, (NIGERIA) LTD

Plot 10 Block B, Isolo Expressway, Itire Junction, Ilasamaja, PO Box 2646, Lagos
Tel: 876475, 877171
Cable: Jelectrick Lagos
Telex: 21420 Jelectrick Ng TDS Box 379

Chairman: Chief J Akin George
Directors: John B Dennis (Managing Director),
  John A Odeyemi (Deputy Managing Director),
  Chief G E Mabiaku,
  Mahmoud Gashash,
  B Haywood,
  D Watt Kilpatrick,
  H N Jeffery (Alternate),
  J Stevenson (Alternate)
Senior Executives: M J Bovingdon (Commercial Manager),
  T A Adekanmbi (Personnel Manager),
  B O Eroju (Senior Contracts Manager),
  I L Archibald (Chief Quantity Surveyor),
  S U Egbuche (Technical Manager),
  J A Idowu (Secretary/Administrative Manager),
  S R Foster (General Manager, Civil Division),
  M F Onitilo (Chief Accountant),
  J J Hodder (Divisional Manager, Electrical)

PRINCIPAL ACTIVITIES: Electrical, mechanical and civil
  engineering services and contractors
Principal Agencies: Balfour Kilpatrick International; Balfour
  Beatty Contruction, BICC Group
Branch Offices: Plot C Ahmadu Bello Way, Kaduna, Tel 243328,
  Telex 71127 Jelectric Ng (Kaduna); 1B Ewah Rd, Benin City,
  Bendel State; 19B Sultan Rd, PO Box 5436, Kano
Principal Bankers: First Bank of Nigeria Ltd; Union Bank of
  Nigeria Ltd

Principal Shareholders: Nigerians
Date of Establishment: 1962 (Established) 1969 (Incorporated)
No of Employees: 2,000

KING CARPET MANUFACTURING CO LTD

PO Box 500, Mushin, Lagos State
Tel: 901180
Cable: Kingcarpet
Telex: 26688 Carpet Ng

Chairman: Sunder Dalamal
Directors: O Oyewole,
  H Pujara,
  Alhaji U S Birma,
  N W Dalamal,
  H Pujara (Managing)

PRINCIPAL ACTIVITIES: Manufacturers of carpets, rugs and
  allied products
Principal Bankers: First Bank of Nigeria Ltd
Financial Information:

	N'000
Authorised capital	1,500
Paid-up capital	1,250

Date of Establishment: 1978

KINGSTON LTD

12 Aliyu Street, Iju Ishaga, PO Box 2501, Agege, Lagos
Cable: Kingspub Lagos
Telex: 20202-123

Chairman: R Shola Taiwo
Directors: S Ojurongbe, Alhaja B Taiwo
Senior Executives: S A Olaitan (Sales Manager),
  Alhaji A Kokiyan (Administrative Manager),
  T Atanda Taiwo (Production Manager)

PRINCIPAL ACTIVITIES: Printing
Principal Agencies: Volkswagen of Nigeria Ltd; Jolliters
  Chemists (Nig) Ltd; Ademuyiwa Lighting & Electronics Co Ltd;
  Ogun State Housing Corporation; Agro Services Corporation
  Ogun State
Branch Offices: 102 Shokenu Street, PO Box 638, Abeokuta,
  Ogun State
Subsidiary Companies: Kingston International
Principal Bankers: United Bank for Africa Ltd

Financial Information:

	N'000
Authorised capital	100
Turnover	150
Profits	20

Date of Establishment: 10th August 1978

KINGSWAY CHEMISTS LTD

Billingsway, Oregun Industrial Estate, PO Box 1063, Ikeja, Lagos

Tel: 901030/9

Senior Executives: P R Batchelor (General Manager)

PRINCIPAL ACTIVITIES: Importers and distributors of
  pharmaceuticals, photographic and surgical
  equipment/hospital supplies
Branch Offices: Aba; Benin; Enugu; Ibadan; Jos; Kaduna; Kano;
  Lagos; Maiduguri; Onitsha; Sokoto and Zaria
Financial Information: Division of UAC of Nigeria Ltd

KINGSWAY STORES OF NIGERIA LTD

49/51 Marina, PO Box 562, Lagos
Tel: 662544
Cable: Unakinway
Telex: 21233

Chairman: E A O Shonekan
Directors: Chief S O Adebo, C A Ince, Alhaji J P Rauch, M G
  Bloomer, Isa Kaita, Chief S B Daniyan, F M O Osifo, H T
  Mathers, P D Tueart, A P Graham, A C I Mbanefo, J O
  Omidiora
Senior Executives: M C Thompson (General Manager),
  I O Adeworan (Personnel Manager),
  J O Allen (Commercial Manager),
  A L Brown (Merchandise Manager, Nigeria)

PRINCIPAL ACTIVITIES: Department stores, supermarkets
Principal Agencies: Lever Brothers Nigeria Ltd; Nigeria
  Breweries Ltd; Food Specialities Nigeria Ltd
Branch Offices: Liberation Drive, Port Harcourt; Airport Rd,
  Kano; Akpakpava Rd, Benin City, Bendel State; Okpara Ave,
  Enugu, Anambra State
Principal Bankers: First Bank of Nigeria Ltd; Union Bank of
  Nigeria Ltd
Financial Information: Division of UAC of Nigeria Ltd

Principal Shareholders: Nigerian Public (60%)
Date of Establishment: 1948
No of Employees: 1,600

KLF LTD

12 Adenuga Taiwo Street, Obanikoro, PO Box 1172, Ikeja,
  Lagos
Tel: 963470
Telex: 26441 Klf Ng

Chairman: Adedehin Ebunolu Adefeso (also Managing Director)
Directors: D O Uhimwem, G Yaroson
Senior Executives: S E A Uwakwe (Project Engineer),
  C O N Egwu (Company Secretary),
  S O Ogba (Accountant)

PRINCIPAL ACTIVITIES: Consultants in kitchen and laundry
  operations; planning, delivery and installation. After sales
  maintenance services
Principal Agencies: Stott Benham (UK) Ltd; Hobart
  Manufacturing Company, USA; Moorwood Vulcan (UK) Ltd
Associated Companies: Dou Associates; Yaroson & Partners
Principal Bankers: Bank of Credit & Commerce International;
  United Bank for Africa Ltd
Financial Information:

	N'000
Authorised capital	50
Paid-up capital	50
Turnover	1,200
Profits	(5% of turnover)

Principal Shareholders: A E Adefeso; D O Uhimwem; G Yaroson
Date of Establishment: 4th April 1977

KLIFCO (NIGERIA) LTD

NTA/Choba Rd, PO Box 2511, Port Harcourt, Rivers State
Tel: 333141
Telex: 61255 Klifco Ng

Chairman: Clifford C Nwuche
Directors: G A Graham-Douglas,
  Festus Ngochindo,
  Chibudo Nwuche,
  Orabule Adele,
  S Mukherjee (Managing)
Senior Executives: I Zakai (General Manager),
  S Hinkis (Engineer),
  B H Kim (Financial Controller),
  O T Akpan (Engineer),
  C O Ogbonda (Business Administrator)

PRINCIPAL ACTIVITIES: Building and civil engineering
  contractors; trading and commodity distributors; drilling of
  water boreholes, treatment and supply
Principal Agencies: Haitai International Inc, South Korea; Sanofi
  Pharma International, France
Branch Offices: 731 Apollo Crescent, Jos, Plateau State; 64A
  Okosi Rd, Onitsha, Anambra State; 67 Okupe Estate,
  Maryland, Ikeja, Lagos
Subsidiary Companies: Afro Aqua, NTA/Choba Rd, PO Box
  2511, Port Harcourt
Principal Bankers: International Bank for West Africa Ltd;
  Societe General Bank (Nig) Ltd; Chase Merchant Bank Ltd
Financial Information:

	₦'000
Authorised capital	40
Paid-up capital	25
Turnover	500

Principal Shareholders: C C Nwuche; Festus Ngochindo
Date of Establishment: 23rd July 1973
No of Employees: 250

KLOECKNER INA NIGERIA LTD

Plot 713A Adetokunbo Ademola St, Victoria Island, PO Box
  5473, Lagos

Directors: F A Claassen,
  Hans H Garbe (Managing)

PRINCIPAL ACTIVITIES: General trading and representation.
  Joint venture project to build the largest flat glass factory in
  Nigeria at Okitipupa in Ondo State is underway Production is
  planned to start 1983

KNIGHT, FRANK & RUTLEY (NIGERIA)

47 Marina, PO Box 221, Lagos
Tel: 664221, 664226
Cable: Knitefrank, Lagos
Telex: 21428

Chairman: A J Shelley
Partners: J I Ojo-Osagie, S N Okeke, S Udo-Akagha, P C
  Nwankwo, O J A Idudu, M O Jawando, S A Otegbola, M A
  Ogunbodede
Senior Executives: W O Olowonyo (Partnership Secretary)

PRINCIPAL ACTIVITIES: Chartered surveyors
Branch Offices: 58A Tafawa Balewa Rd, Kano; NACB Building,
  Hospital Rd, Kaduna; Orosi House, Port Harcourt; 68 Marian
  Rd, Calabar, Cross River State; 19 Ogun Rd, Enugu;
  Kingsway Building, Benin-City; Standard Building, 5 Zaria Rd,
  Jos
Subsidiary Companies: Knight Frank & Rutley, London
Principal Bankers: Union Bank of Nigeria Ltd; United Bank for
  Africa Ltd; Societe Generale Bank Nigeria Ltd

Principal Shareholders: Partners as described

KOJUSOLA FOAM INDUSTRIES LTD

PMB 4398, Oshogbo, Oyo State
Tel: 34178, 32912

Chairman: S S Adejoro
Directors: Engr T Ola Ibikunle,
  J Ade Ibikunle (Managing Director)
Senior Executives: G Ogunremi (Accountant),
  O Omoloye (Sales Manager)

PRINCIPAL ACTIVITIES: Manufacturing of foam mattresses,
  cushions and pillows
Associated Companies: S S Adejoro & Co Ltd; Buildtrust
  Investment Co Ltd
Principal Bankers: Wema Bank Ltd
Financial Information:

	₦'000
Authorised capital	200
Paid-up capital	200
Sales turnover	1,500

Principal Shareholders: Chairman and directors as described
No of Employees: 120

KOKU, GEORGE, & SONS LTD

17th Floor, Western House, 8-10 Broad St, PO Box 3116, Lagos
Tel: 614066, 636865
Cable: Yodel Lagos
Telex: 21475 Debora Ng

PRINCIPAL ACTIVITIES: Suppliers of building materials and
  building equipment; supermarkets

KOLE-JAMES & CO LTD

12 Abibu-Oki St, Lagos
Tel: 633990

PRINCIPAL ACTIVITIES: General merchants, hoteliers

KOLINAH INDUSTRIES NIGERIA LTD

Dayo Williams Estate, Suberu-Oje, Km 32 Abeokuta Express
  Way, PO Box 1906, Agege, Lagos State
Tel: 963534
Cable: Kolinah, Lagos
Telex: 26731 Eselin

Directors: Olusoga Ayo Ogunjale,
  Bisi Kofoworola,
  Funwulayo Bandele,
  S Kola Ogunjale (Managing)
Senior Executives: Kunle Oke (Marketing Manager),
  F Lindsay (General Manager),
  Olu Ogunjale (Executive Director)

PRINCIPAL ACTIVITIES: Suppliers of agricultural equipment and
  produce; building materials, ceramics, construction plant,
  household goods, livestock and animal feeds, timber etc.
  Supermarkets
Branch Offices: Abuja; Ibadan; Enugu; Ondo; Benin; Kano;
  Kaduna; Abeokuta; Port Harcourt
Subsidiary/Associated Companies: Mono Kosters & Co; Kolinah
  Supermarkets; Kolinah Farms Ltd
Principal Bankers: United Bank for Africa Ltd

Principal Shareholders: Directors as described
Date of Establishment: 1980
No of Employees: 400 (including casuals)

KOLINTON TECHNICAL INDUSTRIES LTD

Block M Plot 2 Isolo Industrial Estate, Isolo, PMB 1060, Ebute
  Metta, Lagos

PRINCIPAL ACTIVITIES: Suppliers of domestic electrical
  equipment
Branch Offices: Showrooms: 62 Simpson St, Ebute Metta,
  Lagos; 87 Agege Motor Rd, Oshodi, Lagos

Date of Establishment: 1972

KOLOKO IMPORTS & EXPORTS CO LTD

PMB 3014, 105 Ojuelegba Rd, Surulere, Lagos
Tel: 833585, 833866
Telex: 21590 Koloko Ng

PRINCIPAL ACTIVITIES: Exporters and importers of general merchandise

KOLYNSON CO LTD

57 Western Ave, Surulere, PO Box 1191, Lagos
Tel: 830641

PRINCIPAL ACTIVITIES: Suppliers of stationery and office equipment
Branch Offices: 68 Enu-Owa St, Lagos, Tel 635740

KOSM (WEST AFRICA) LTD

179 Zik Avenue, PO Box 2460, Enugu, Anambra State
Tel: 332902
Telex: 51319 FDPUBS

Chairman: Chief Arthur A Nwankwo
Directors: Engr V U Nwankwo (Managing),
 D M Unonu (Projects Administration),
 E R Nwankwo
Senior Executives: B C Ndigwe (Project Engineer),
 L C Onyewuchi (Admin Secretary),
 O Obeagha (Site Agent)

PRINCIPAL ACTIVITIES: Civil engineering and construction, engineering and business consultants
Principal Bankers: International Bank for West Africa Ltd
Financial Information:

	N'000
Authorised capital	402
Paid-up capital	200

Principal Shareholders: Joart & Co (Nig) Ltd; A Nwankwo; E Nwankwo
Date of Establishment: 1976
No of Employees: 1,500

KPOHRAROR & SONS GROUP OF COMPANIES

Kagho Omomadia Crescent, Enerhen Rd, PO Box 530, Effurun, Warrri, Bendel State
Tel: 233575, 233448

PRINCIPAL ACTIVITIES: Building and civil engineering contractors; transporters

KRABO NIGERIA LTD

25B Folaiwyo Bankole Street, End of Alhaji Masha Rd, Surulere,
 PO Box 5685, Lagos
Tel: 833256
Cable: Krabo-Lagos

Directors: Ben O Omanukwue (Managing),
 Emman A Nwobodo (Executive),
 Alfred C Okongwu

PRINCIPAL ACTIVITIES: Dealers in office equipment; machines, safes, stationery and printing materials, signs specialists
Principal Agencies: Tipp-Ex Vertrieb & Co GmbH, West Germany; Citraco Development Internaional NV, Belgium
Principal Bankers: African Continental Bank Ltd; Union Bank of Nigeria Ltd
Financial Information:

	N'000
Authorised capital	100
Paid-up capital	50

Principal Shareholders: Ben O Omanukwue; Emman A Nwobodo
Date of Establishment: Incorporated in 1977

KRAGHA & ASSOCIATES

Head Office, 1 Oyekan Rd, Apapa, PO Box 4216, Lagos
Tel: 830216
Cable: Kagrasoc Lagos

Directors: Moses O Kragha (Managing Director)

PRINCIPAL ACTIVITIES: Mining and petroleum consultants

KRAMER-ITALO LTD

13 Shonola Street, Ebute Metta, PO Box 3578, Lagos
Tel: 846290/5
Cable: Italo Build Lagos
Telex: 21889 Gudwal Ng

Chairman: Chief R A Fani-Kayode
Directors: W Bleiker (Deputy Chairman),
 B W O Bailey (Managing Director),
 Kayode Osun-Benjamin,
 Mrs A A Fani-Kayode,
 Alhaji Sani Zangon Daura
Senior Executives: C Potts (General Manager),
 A R Parker (Construction Manager)

PRINCIPAL ACTIVITIES: Building and civil engineering contractors
Principal Agencies: International Housing Ltd; Con-Tech Forming System
Branch Offices: Minna; Bauchi
Associated Companies: Kramer International Ltd (UK); Kramer Ltd (Switzerland); Kramico SAE (Egypt); SAC (Swiss Arabian Contracting) Ltd (Saudi Arabia); Kramer/Walser Consortium (Iraq); Kramer Alamnor Construction SDN BHD (Malaysia); Wong Yock Liet (Singapore)
Principal Bankers: United Bank for Africa Ltd
Financial Information:

	N'000
Authorised capital	500
Paid-up capital	500

Principal Shareholders: Chief R A Fani-Kayode; W Bleiker
Date of Establishment: December 1959
No of Employees: 1,500

KUCENA-DAMIAN (NIGERIA) LTD

12 Adeniyi Adefioye Street, Ikate, PO Box 581, Surulere, Lagos
Tel: 830236
Cable: Kucena Lagos

Chairman: Damian Orogbu
Directors: M A I Orogbu, Peter Damian
Senior Executives: S O Okafor (Production Manager),
 M O Obi (Administration),
 C Chukwurah (Sales Executive),
 E K Emetu (Accounts)

PRINCIPAL ACTIVITIES: Printing, publishing and manufacture of business forms/stationery and audio visual display systems
Principal Agencies: H H Drent Machinefabriek; Magiboards Ltd UK
Branch Offices: 89A Enugu Rd, Awka, Amambra State
Associated Companies: Ekkodelta (Nigeria) Ltd
Principal Bankers: Union Bank of Nigeria Ltd
Financial Information:

	N'000
Authorised capital	50
Paid-up capital	50
Turnover	300
Profits	22

Principal Shareholders: Chairman and directors as described
Date of Establishment: 27th November 1977

KUEPPERS (NIGERIA) LTD

10 Ilaka St, Ilupeju Estate, PO Box 1522, Ikeja, Lagos
Tel: 963850

Chairman: Alhaji Yahaya Gusau
Directors: I Isa,
  J O Sonuga,
  Dr T Kueppers,
  B Kueppers,
  N Stein,
  U Birnbaum,
  S Winkel (Managing Director),
  W W Schueler (Alternate Director),
  J Richter (Alternate Director),

PRINCIPAL ACTIVITIES: Civil engineering and construction
Branch Offices: 7 Dan Amar Rd, PO Box 1408, Kaduna; New
  Central Market, PO Box 186, Sokoto
Principal Bankers: Bank of the North Ltd; United Bank for Africa
  Ltd
Financial Information:

	N'000
Authorised capital	750
Paid-up capital	500
Turnover	11,800

Date of Establishment: 31st October 1975
No of Employees: 1,140

KUFENA TRADING CO LTD

1 Old Motor Park, Main St, PO Box 369, Zaria, Kaduna State
Tel: 2327

Chairman: Horst Schwandt
Directors: Alhaji M Bello (Managing),
  Alhaji M T Bello (Planning/Control),
  Alhaji Baba Zaria (Contracts Director),
  Dr Horst J Bloch (Marketing/Planning Director),
  Mal Samaila Mohmed (Marketing Director),
  Mal Othman Mohmed (Marketing Director)

PRINCIPAL ACTIVITIES: General contractors; suppliers of
  scientific, educational and office equipment etc; prospecting
  for minerals
Principal Agencies: Geoexplor & Geochem, West Germany;
  Herrn Apotheker Horst Schwandt; Geoexplor & Kufena (Int)
  Ltd; Alsalmans (Nigeria) Ltd; Zaria Nasara Enterprises Co Ltd
Principal Bankers: Bank of the North Ltd; United Bank for Africa
  Ltd

Date of Establishment: 4th August 1969
No of Employees: 500

KUNZA HEED (W.A.) ENTERPRISES

Olakunle Chambers, PO Box 8291, Lagos
Cable: Kunza Lagos

Chairman: Hadji Minkaila Bola Abimbola
Directors: Abdul Wazeel Adeleke,
  Olabisi Tolanikawo,
  J Pedro (Technical Director),
  Zaheed Olakunle (Commercial Director)
Senior Executives: Olabisi Abimbola (Public Relations Officer)

PRINCIPAL ACTIVITIES: Transport and haulage services;
  clearing, forwarding agents; industrial representatives;
  imports, exports; general contractors
Principal Agencies: DAF (Products), Holland; Switchgear,
  London; International Paints; ICI Products; African Paints
Branch Offices: 1 Ajayi Street, Ketu, Lagos; 22C Ikorodu Rd,
  Ketu, Lagos
Subsidiary Companies: Balume Engineering Services and Supply
  Co; WTA Salzburg Austria
Principal Bankers: National Bank Nigeria Ltd; Savannah Bank
  Nigeria Ltd
Financial Information:

	N'000
Authorised capital	150
Paid-up capital	100
Turnover	250
Profits	50

Principal Shareholders: J Pedro; E O Fadamitan
Date of Establishment: 1974
No of Employees: 50

KURU LTD

Jos, Plateau State

Directors: J Thomson (Managing Director)
PRINCIPAL ACTIVITIES: Mining of metal ore
Principal Shareholders: Bisichi-Jantar (Nigeria) Ltd

KUSBA SHIPPING AGENCIES LTD

13 Commercial Rd, Apapa, Lagos
Tel: 874027
Telex: 21589 Kusba Ng

PRINCIPAL ACTIVITIES: Shipping services
Branch Offices: 1 Banji Adewole Lane, Akoka, Lagos, Tel 42677

KWA FALLS OIL PALM ESTATE LTD

Aninge, PMB 1050, Calabar, Cross River State
PRINCIPAL ACTIVITIES: Manufacturing of palm oil and kernel
No of Employees: 1,000

L A O BANJOKO & CO LTD

See BANJOKO, L A O, & CO LTD

L AMBROSINI LTD

See AMBROSINI, L, LTD

L D'ALBERTO & CO LTD

See D'ALBERTO, L, & CO LTD

L E EJINKEONYE BROTHERS TRADING CO LTD

See EJINKEONYE, L E, BROTHERS TRADING CO LTD

L R NABENA & SONS LTD

See NABENA, L R, & SONS LTD

LAAS LTD

25 Abonnema Wharf Rd, PO Box 741, Port Harcourt, Rivers
  State
Tel: 228422

PRINCIPAL ACTIVITIES: Shipping, clearing, forwarding
Branch Offices: NW5/197 Adekunle Fajuyi Rd, PO Box 693,
  Ibadan, Oyo State; 30 Bowen Ave, Behind Catholic School 1,
  Warri, Bendel State; 1 Basiru Owe St, Ikeja, Lagos

LABSTOCK (NIGERIA) LTD

284C Murtala Mohammed Way, PMB 1106, Yaba, Lagos
Tel: 863882
Cable: Labap Yaba
Telex: 21681 Jerima Ng

Chairman: Dr N I C Nwachuku
Directors: Dr J O Odugbose,
  Dr N I C Nwachuku,
  C A Nwachuku (Administrative Director),
  D O Odugbose,
  Alhaji Ahamdu Mohammed
Senior Executives: O A Kalejaiye (General Marketing Manager),
  K E Oyeka (Eastern Area Sales Manager),
  Mrs N C Oyeka (Personnel Assistant to Managing Director),
  J O Njoku (Assistant Commercial Manager),
  V O E Ajayi (Assistant Sales/Service Engineer),
  Mrs A M Fosu (Northern Area Sales Manager)

PRINCIPAL ACTIVITIES: Importation and distribution of
scientific, medical and laboratory instruments and chemicals
Principal Agencies: MSE Scientific Instruments Ltd, UK; Grant
Instruments Ltd, UK; Technicon Instruments Company, UK;
Sartorius-Werke GmbH, Germany; Griffin & George Ltd, UK;
Difco Laboratories, UK; Fluka AG, Switzerland; BDH
Chemicals Ltd, UK
Branch Offices: 67 New Lagos Rd, Benin City, Bendel State; 167
Oyo Rd (Nr Airport), Ibadan, Oyo State; 7 Funtua Rd, PMB
13, Samaru, Zaria, Kaduna State; 3 Emir Yahaya Rd, PO Box
647, Sokoto; 28 Onitsha Rd, PMB 1498, Owerri, Imo State
Associated Companies: Transtron Ltd, Lagos
Principal Bankers: Union Bank of Nigeria Ltd; Bank of Credit
and Commerce International (Nigeria) Ltd
Financial Information:
Authorised capital ₦ 100,000

Principal Shareholders: Dr N I C Nwachuku; C A Nwachuku; Dr J
O Odugbose; D O Odugbose; Alhaji Ahmadu Mohammed
Date of Establishment: 12th February 1971

LACON NIGERIA LTD
Baiyeku Rd, Igbogbo, PO Box 238, Ikorodu, Lagos State

Chairman: Chief S A Agoro
Directors: Prince Alhaji F A Alagbe, J A Adegboye, N A
Bakare, A O Ogunkoya, G K Ajayi, J Kruttke
Senior Executives: John T Page (Factory Manager and Chief
Executive),
S Afolabi Noah (Sales and Marketing Manager)

PRINCIPAL ACTIVITIES: Manufacture of clay bricks, blocks and
course floor tiles

Principal Shareholders: Lagos State Government; Nigerian
Industrial Development Bank; Battenfeld Encon
Anlagentechnik, Hamburg
Date of Establishment: Commissioned 27th April 1979
No of Employees: 100

LADEJOBI PRODUCTS NIGERIA LTD
Development House, 21 Wharf Rd, PO Box 399, Apapa, Lagos
State
Tel: 872730
Cable: Ladepharm
Telex: 22259 Ogadem Ng

Chairman: Bode Ladejobi
Directors: Foluso Ladejobi, Bendele Ladejobi
Senior Executives: Alex Ladipo (Manager Water Division),
M Y Annan (Chief Accountant),
Bode Ladejobi (Chief Executive)

PRINCIPAL ACTIVITIES: Brewing; chemicals; defence and
armaments; food and food processing; pharmaceuticals and
medical supplies
Principal Agencies: Stella Meta Filters; Portacel Ltd; Newton
Chambers Engineering Ltd; Aeronautical and General
Instruments Ltd (AGI); Bedford Wine, USA
Subsidiary Companies: Nigerian Pharmaceutical and Medical
Company
Principal Bankers: Union Bank of Nigeria Ltd
Financial Information:

	₦'000
Authorised capital	200
Paid-up capital	200

Principal Shareholders: Bode Ladejobi; Foluso Ladejobi; Bandele
Ladejobi
Date of Establishment: January 1980
No of Employees: 32

LADGROUP LTD
Plot 1 Block H, Isolo Industrial Estate, PO Box 3795, Lagos

Directors: B A Onafowokan (Managing),
V A Onafowokan,
A A Adesina,
V O Kwechime,
O A Onafowokan

PRINCIPAL ACTIVITIES: Manufacturing and marketing of food
products
Branch Offices: 56 Akenzua Rd, PO Box 2088, Benin City,
Bendel State
Principal Bankers: Societe Generate Bank; First Bank of Nigeria
Ltd; NAL Merchant Bank

Date of Establishment: June 1972
No of Employees: 76

LAFA SOAP & COSMETIC INDUSTRY
Omu, Ijebu-Ode, Ogun State

PRINCIPAL ACTIVITIES: Manufacturers of bath and laundry
soaps, detergents and cosmetics

LAFIA CANNING FACTORY
Cocoa House, PMB 5085, Ibadan, Oyo State
Tel: 462661
Cable: Lafican Ibadan

PRINCIPAL ACTIVITIES: Manufacturers of tinned fruit
Branch Offices: Factory; PMB 5068, Moor Plantation, Ibadan

LAGO (NIGERIA) LTD
Mile 7.5 Ikorodu Rd, PO Box 418, Yaba, Lagos
Tel: 961159, 961582

Directors: F Lombardo, R Muzzicato, G Cacciani

PRINCIPAL ACTIVITIES: Building and civil engineering
contractors

LAGOS & NIGER SHIPPING AGENCIES LTD
PO Box 192, 4 Creek Rd, Apapa, Lagos
Tel: 875692, 875739
Cable: Lansal Lagos
Telex: 21317 Lansal Ng

PRINCIPAL ACTIVITIES: Shipping agents, clearing and
fowarding
Branch Offices: PO Box 361, Port Harcourt; PO Box 1132, Warri,
Bendel State; 131 Goldie St, Calabar, Cross River State

LAGOS AIRPORT HOTEL LTD
Obafemi Awolowo Way, PMB 21041, Ikeja, Lagos
Tel: 901001/5
Cable: Airpotel Lagos
Telex: 21303 Airotl Ng

Chairman: Surv J O Daramola
Directors: Chief A K Jowosimi, H A Jabaru, Chief A B Kolawole
Senior Executives: M O Ogundana (General Manager),
J O Awoyinfa (Chief Accountant/Company Secretary)

PRINCIPAL ACTIVITIES: Hotel and catering industry
Principal Bankers: National Bank of Nigeria Ltd; Savannah Bank
of Nigeria Ltd; Nigeria-Arab Bank Ltd
Financial Information:

	₦'000
Authorised capital	2,400
Paid-up capital	2,400
Turnover	5,902
Profits	963

Principal Shareholders: Odu'a Investment Company Ltd
Date of Establishment: 9th May 1966
No of Employees: 532

LAGOS PLANT HIRE SERVICES (NIGERIA) LTD
4 Commercial Rd, Apapa, Lagos
Tel: 873579, 876542

PRINCIPAL ACTIVITIES: Plant hire
Branch Offices: Plot 109 Calabar St, Surulere, Lagos, Tel 841918

LAGOS STATE DEVELOPMENT & PROPERTY CORPORATION

Ilupeju Industrial Estate, Ikorodu Rd, PMB 21050, Ikeja, Lagos

Directors: G B Jinadu (General Manager)

PRINCIPAL ACTIVITIES: Planning and development of Lagos

LAGOS STATE TRANSPORT CORPORATION

State Highway, Isolo Express Rd, Ilupeju, PO Box 2137, Lagos
Tel: 963455, 900770/2
Telex: 21577

Chairman: Olatunde Soetan
Directors: S O Joseph, L Oyenuga, A A Somide, Alhaji R O Sadiq, B A Ogunlewe, Mrs C A Awodeinde, Mrs S O Bayagbona, Alhaji S T Hallid, Alhaji R A Aguntasholo
Senior Executives: Alhaji A A Awelenje (Acting General Manager),
    Gboyega Isikalu (Secretary to the Corporation)

PRINCIPAL ACTIVITIES: Public transportation
Principal Bankers: First Bank of Nigeria Ltd

Principal Shareholders: Lagos State Government
Date of Establishment: 1977
No of Employees: 1,424

LAING CONSTRUCTION LTD

142A Adekunle Fajuyi Way, GRA, Ikeja, PMB 12715, Lagos
Tel: 960314
Cable: Laingcon
Telex: 21641 Laing Ng

Chairman: Alhaji Umaru Sanda Birma
Directors: M Spence (Managing Director),
    F Awumolo,
    Alhaji Sani Zangon Daura,
    J F Meddins,
    R Pawsey
Senior Executives: B A Adegoke (Company Secretary),
    I J Rogers (Chief Quantity Surveyor)

PRINCIPAL ACTIVITIES: Building and civil engineering contractors
Branch Offices: Kano Rd, Auno, PMB 1440, Maiduguri, Borno State; 2 Arakan Rd, Kano
Principal Bankers: United Bank for Africa Ltd
Financial Information:
Turnover   ₦ 20,000,000

No of Employees: 2,500

LAKATI CONSTRUCTION & COMPANY

13 Eyamba St, PO Box 801, Jos, Plateau State

PRINCIPAL ACTIVITIES: Builders and general construction work
Financial Information: Part of Akanji Group of Companies

LAKE CONCRETE INDUSTRIES LTD

22 Mbanugo St, Ogbete, PO Box 62, Enugu, Anambra State
Tel: 254303
Cable: Lacrete Enugu
Telex: 51164 Lake Ng

Chairman: Gogo Nwakuche
Directors: Uzoma Nwakuche

PRINCIPAL ACTIVITIES: Manufacturers of prestressed concrete poles, slabs, beams, blocks, road kerbs, sewage pipes, etc
Branch Offices: Port Harcourt Rd, Aba, Imo State
Principal Bankers: International Bank for West Africa Ltd

LANDMARK INDUSTRIAL SUPPLIES LTD

39, 50 Ibadan St, Ebute Metta (West), PO Box 1552, Lagos
Cable: Darltaba Lagos

Chairman: Darlington T Baiyewu (also Managing Director)
Directors: Elliot O Yemitan, Mosunmola Apinke, Oluwaseyi Baiyewo
Senior Executives: Michael 'Dola Baiyewu (Administrative Manager),
    Augustine Nwabuisi (Technical Sales Manager)

PRINCIPAL ACTIVITIES: Importers and distributors of general goods and handtools, power, air and pneumatic tools; welding equipment and accessories; electrical and general contractors suppliers; garage equipment; abrasive products; hardware, etc
Principal Agencies: Aga Welding Ltd; Abrasive Specialities Ltd, UK; Consolidated Pneumatic Tool Company Ltd, UK; Tandarc Woodbridge Meadows, UK; James Stead & Co Ltd, UK
Branch Offices: NW5/67 Salvation Army Rd, Ibadan, Oyo State; 4 Baiyewu Close, Ijaiye Agege, Lagos State; 23 Oke Ejigbo St, Abeokuta, Ogun State
Associated Companies: Witt and Bush Ltd; Black and Decker Nigeria Ltd
Principal Bankers: First Bank of Nigeria Ltd; New Nigeria Bank Ltd

Date of Establishment: 3rd November 1976

LANLEK (NIGERIA) ASSOCIATES

Ajibike Chambers, E7/263 Ode Aje Oloolu, PO Box 2110, Ibadan, Oyo State

PRINCIPAL ACTIVITIES: Agents and general trading, educational equipment and training services, office equipment supplies, paper/paper products; publishing and advertising, business consultants
Branch Offices: Oyekale House, Erunmu Postal Agency, Erunmu, Ibadan, Oyo State; S4/672 Aperin Oniyere, Adesola Rd, Ibadan, Oyo State
Associated Companies: Lanlek Transport Services; Lanlek Typing and Secretarial Services
Principal Bankers: Co-operative Bank Nigeria Ltd

Principal Shareholders: Chairman and directors as described
Date of Establishment: April 1977

LANRAY & SONS

PO Box 123, Ebute Metta, Lagos

PRINCIPAL ACTIVITIES: General merchandise importers

LANRE BHADMUS INDUSTRIES LTD

26 Calcutta Crescent, PO Box 516, Apapa, Lagos
Tel: 870639, 875216
Cable: Carcare Lagos
Telex: 22476 Cacare Ng

Chairman: Lanre Bhadmus (also Managing Director)
Directors: Mrs E D Bhadmus
Senior Executives: Emmanuel E O Umejiaku (Sales Manager),
    Young Ogwuegbu (Administration Manager),
    Biola Kudaisi (Accountant)

PRINCIPAL ACTIVITIES: Suppliers of car-care products, accessories and spare parts; rubber goods, toiletries and generating sets; manufacturers representative
Principal Agencies: Holt Lloyd Export Ltd, UK; Cannon Rubber Ltd, UK; ASM (Accessories) Ltd, UK; Herbert Richter, West Germany; Kex International, USA; Auto-Plas, UK; Otto Golze & Sohnes, West Germany
Branch Offices: Ikeja Roundabout Shopping Arcade, PO Box 274, Ikeja, Tel 962973; 42 Balogun Street, Lagos
Principal Bankers: United Bank for Africa Ltd
Financial Information:

	₦'000
Authorised capital	1,000
Paid-up capital	450

Principal Shareholders: Lanre Bhadmus; Mrs E D Bhadmus
Date of Establishment: Incorporated 1974
No of Employees: 100

LAS & CO LTD

81 Olateju St, Challenge, Mushin, PO Box 312, Yaba, Lagos
Tel: 844160, 862646, 862862
Cable: Lascolim Lagos
Telex: 21368 Chacom Ng

Chairman: Chief L A Shoyombo
Directors: E A Adeboye,
   A I Shoyombo (Marketing),
   A A Shoyombo

PRINCIPAL ACTIVITIES: Manufacturers' representatives; real
   estate agents, civil engineering contractors; importers and
   exporters, suppliers of beer, soft drinks and foods
Branch Offices: SW8/538 Shoyombo St, Oke Ado, Ibadan, Oyo
   State
Associated Companies: L A Shoyombo and Sons Ltd
Principal Bankers: First Bank of Nigeria Ltd; Savannah Bank of
   Nigeria Ltd
Financial Information:
Turnover (approx)   ₦ 1,500,000

Principal Shareholders: Chief L A Shoyombo
Date of Establishment: 11th April, 1968

LASTRA CONSTRUCTION (NIGERIA) LTD

76 Adetokunbo Ademola St, Victoria Island, PO Box 2468,
   Lagos

Chairman: R K Okudzeto

PRINCIPAL ACTIVITIES: Construction
Financial Information: Subsidiary of Promexport International
   (Nigeria) Ltd

LATADEK CONSTRUCTION COMPANY LTD

87 Agege Motor Rd, Oshodi, Lagos

PRINCIPAL ACTIVITIES: Building and civil engineering
   contractors
Branch Offices: Works Yard: Edun Alaran Estate, Ojokoro
   Abeokuta Express Rd, Agege, Lagos; 7 Kole Balogun
   Crescent, Ikirun Rd, Oshogbo, Oyo State

Date of Establishment: June 1980

LATDERMA ENTERPRISES

PO Box 50049, Ikoyi, Lagos State
Tel: 636721
Cable: Latma

Chairman: Lateef Adekunle Martins
Directors: Mrs A A Martins, Tunde Martins, Adelola Martins
Senior Executives: Gbolaham Loakman (General Manager)

PRINCIPAL ACTIVITIES: Importers and exporters,
   manufacturers' representatives; suppliers of toys, textile
   materials, footwear, electrical equipment
Branch Offices: Ibadan; Kaduna; Enugu; Kano
Principal Bankers: Bank of the North
Financial Information:

	₦'000
Authorised capital	2,000
Paid-up capital	500
Sales turnover	1,500
Profits	350

Principal Shareholders: Chairman and directors as described
No of Employees: 150

LAVALIN NIGERIA LTD

PO Box 1214, Maiduguri, Borno State
Tel: 2665
Telex: 82106

PRINCIPAL ACTIVITIES: Engineering consultants

LAW UNION AND ROCK INSURANCE CO OF NIGERIA LTD

PO Box 944, 88-92 Broad St, Lagos
Tel: 663356, 663526, 662245, 663214
Cable: Lawrok

Chairman: Col Sani Bello (Rtd)
Directors: V H Twyford (Managing)

PRINCIPAL ACTIVITIES: Insurance
Principal Agencies: Enugu; Ibadan; Kano; Makurdi
Financial Information: Associate of Royal Insurance Co Ltd, UK

LAWAL ARAROMI COMMERCIAL STORES

3 Alagbede Court, Oshodi St, PO Box 6883, Lagos

PRINCIPAL ACTIVITIES: Importers, exporters, general
   merchants, manufacturers' representatives and commission
   agents
Principal Bankers: Mercantile Bank Nigeria Ltd

LAWAN SCHUTTE & CO (NIGERIA) LTD

Nigerian Food Company Bldg, Iddo Railway Terminus, PO Box
   1190, Lagos

Directors: L Miller

PRINCIPAL ACTIVITIES: General trading and representation

LAWRENCE AYO & SONS LTD

See AYO, LAWRENCE, & SONS LTD

LAWRENCE OMOLE & SONS LTD

See OMOLE, LAWRENCE, & SONS LTD

LEADWAY ASSURANCE COMPANY LTD

Leadway House, NN28/29 Constitution Rd, PO Box 458, Kaduna

Tel: 211145, 211146, 210026
Cable: Leadassure

Chairman: Alhaji Hassan Hadejia

PRINCIPAL ACTIVITIES: Insurance
Branch Offices: Throughout Nigeria

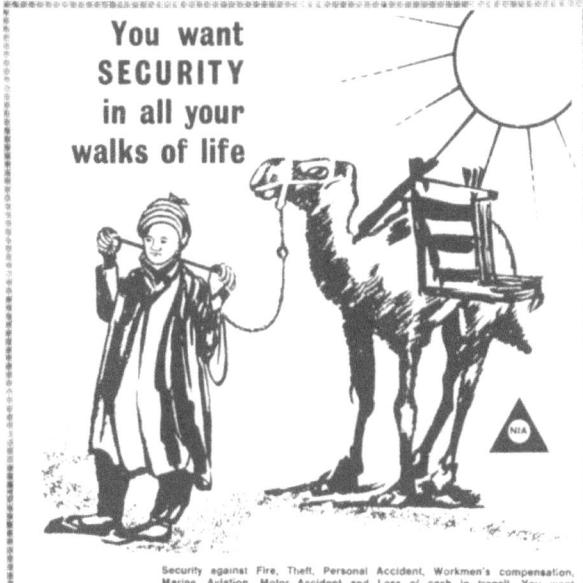

LEATHER TANNING INDUSTRY NIGERIA LTD

PO Box 28, Owerri, Imo State

Chairman: G N Nwankwere

Directors: Dr A E Okorafor, S E Aluge, B U Ekanem, M U Onyewuenyi

Senior Executives: J N Onyeforo (Acting General Manager),
A Fadare (Secretary/Accountant),
F E Wali (Personnel and Staff Manager),
V O Anyanwu (Accountant),
A Nwankwere (Leather Technologist)

PRINCIPAL ACTIVITIES: Tanning
Principal Bankers: Standard Bank of Nigeria Ltd
Financial Information:

	₦'000
Authorised capital	200
Paid-up capital	162

Principal Shareholders: G N Nwankwere; Imo State Government; A C Nlemadim; M U Onyewuenyi; O Nnaji; J Nwaneri; V O Anyanwu

LECCO ENGINEERING CONSTRUCTION CO LTD

11 Chief Nduka St, PO Box 254, Port Harcourt, Rivers State
Tel: 21764

Directors: Dr G Leton

PRINCIPAL ACTIVITIES: Manufacturers of furniture, wire nails; body building for vehicles

LEMAN INDUSTRIES (KADUNA) LTD

Nassarawa Rd, Industrial Estate, Kaduna South, PMB 2194, Kaduna
Tel: 210393
Telex: 71341 Leman Ng

Chairman: Alhaji Lema Jibrilu

Directors: Mr P Brito, Alhaji Sani Jibrilu, Alhaji S Hamisu Kano, Nigerian Bank for Commerce & Industry

Senior Executives: Duarte O Ofonso (General Manager),
Danladi Nyam (Co-Ordinator of Services and Head of Administration),
John de Courcy (Commercial & Technical Manager),
Manuel Abrantes (Production Manager),
Antonio de Jesus (Financial Manager)

PRINCIPAL ACTIVITIES: Manufacturers of metric precision finished bolts, screws and nuts, nails, roofing accessories; motor vehicles components

Branch Offices: (Warehouse) Plot 15, Block B Ilasamaja Scheme, Oshodi/Isolo Express Way, PMB 1903, Apapa, Lagos

Principal Bankers: Union Bank of Nigeria Ltd; United Bank of Nigeria Ltd; First Bank of Nigeria Ltd; International Bank of Nigeria Ltd

Financial Information:

	₦'000
Authorised capital	1,000
Paid-up capital	1,000

Principal Shareholders: Alhaji L Jibrilu; Nigerian Bank for Commerce & Industry; Mr P Brito
Date of Establishment: November 1976
No of Employees: 230

LENNARDS NIGERIA LTD

Km 16 Ikorodu Rd, PO Box 143, Ikeja, Lagos
Tel: 960170, 962982

Chairman: Otunba J Ade Tuyo

Directors: S O Lawal (General Manager),
Chief N A Mene-Afejuku,
Chief H N Ugwunze,
K Land (Managing),
A Ferguson,
J Durbin,
Alhaji A B Fashola (Vice-Chairman),
Alhaji F Adesina (Company Secretary),

A A Degun

PRINCIPAL ACTIVITIES: Retailers and wholesalers of footwear
Principal Bankers: United Bank for Africa Ltd; First Bank of Nigeria Ltd

Principal Shareholders: Nigerians: Greenless Lennards Ltd, UK
No of Employees: 350

LEO-JIMBUS MERCANTILE AGENCIES (NIGERIA)

1st Floor, 41 Moore St, PO Box 3550, Onitsha, Anambra State

PRINCIPAL ACTIVITIES: Manufacturers of wallpaper

LEO'S GROUP OF COMPANIES LTD

91 Payne Crescent, Apapa, PO Box 4664, Lagos
Tel: 874585, 874309, 877850
Cable: Leosgroup Apapa/Lagos

Chairman: Toye Leoshe

Directors: Mrs Olayemi Laoshe, Fadeke Majekodunmi, Dr G B Onipinla

Senior Executives: Mrs M F Akinyanju (Chief Executive)

PRINCIPAL ACTIVITIES: Engineering equipment, sales and services of air-conditioners, refrigerators, sewage treatment plants, mortuary plants, hospital and laboratory equipment, importers of machinery

Principal Agencies: Westinghouse Electric International Company, USA; Control Systems Ltd, UK; Clow Corporation, USA; Tappan International, USA; Sybron Corporation, USA

Branch Offices: Leo's Construction Ltd, PO Box 4664, Lagos
Principal Bankers: National Bank of Nigeria Ltd

No of Employees: 172

LEVER BROTHERS NIGERIA LTD

15 Dockyard Rd, PO Box 15, Apapa, Lagos
Tel: 874291, 874362, 874443, 874064
Cable: Neptune Apapa
Telex: 21520 Levers Ng

Chairman: Dr Michael Olawole Omolayole (also Managing Director)

Directors: J H Kempster (Vice-Chairman and Deputy Managing Director),
A A Abidogun,
S O Alatise,
A A Ayida,
C O Enuke,
J Derwig,
M L Duns,
S C Ikenze,
S O R Vannerus,
R F Giwa

PRINCIPAL ACTIVITIES: Manufacturing and marketing of detergents, soaps, edible products, toilet preparations and fruit squashes

Branch Offices: Factory Rd, Aba, Imo State, Telex 63101 Levers Ng

Principal Bankers: United Bank for Africa Ltd; Union Bank of Nigeria Ltd; First Bank of Nigeria Ltd

Financial Information:

	₦'000
Authorised capital	31,875
Paid-up capital	31,875
Sales turnover (1980)	166,517
Profits (after tax 1980)	7,081

Principal Shareholders: Unilever (Commonwealth Holdings) Ltd
Date of Establishment: April 1923
No of Employees: 3,500

LEVITT INDUSTRIES

C/O Gulab Group of Companies, 126/130 Nnamdi Azikwe St, Lagos

PRINCIPAL ACTIVITIES: Construction

LEWIS & PEAT (NRI) LTD

PMB 4059, Sapele, Bendel State
Tel: 60003, 60029, 60030
Telex: 42262 Lepen Ng

Chairman: Nelson Ogowewo
Directors: A S Guobadia, Mrs C N Eke, R V Jones, T A Smith
Senior Executives: S C D Ugorji (Acting General Manager),
  P C Okongwu (Assistant General Manager),
  B G Willington (Chief Engineer),
  C Kaduru (Shipping Manager),
  R Akpotoma (Accountant)

PRINCIPAL ACTIVITIES: Processing of rubber and manufacturing of rubber products, shipping
Principal Agencies: North Delta Lines Ltd, UK
Subsidiary Companies: Guinness Peat International Ltd, UK; Northern Expellers Ltd, Nigeria
Principal Bankers: Union Bank of Nigeria Ltd
Financial Information:

	N'000
Authorised capital	2,000
Paid-up capital	1,872
Turnover	4,000

Principal Shareholders: Nigerian Rubber Board; Guinness Peat International Ltd
Date of Establishment: 1961
No of Employees: 241

LEYLAND NIGERIA LTD

PMB 29, University of Ibadan Post Office, Ibadan, Oyo State
Tel: 413311, 413362
Telex: 31414; 31211

Chairman: Prince Isaac Adebayo
Directors: Peter V Quick (Managing Director),
  Alhaji Shuaibu Bello,
  M A Oyero,
  Alhaji Abubakar Abdulkadir,
  Alhaji Magaji Mohammed,
  R J Hancock,
  A M Cameron (Company Secretary),
  M J Sheehan,
  R J Dunn,
  O A Smith

PRINCIPAL ACTIVITIES: Manufacturing and distribution of commercial vehicles
Principal Bankers: Union Bank of Nigeria Ltd; First Bank of Nigeria Ltd; National Bank of Nigeria Ltd; United Bank of Africa Ltd
Financial Information:

	N'000
Authorised capital	15,000
Paid-up capital	15,000

Principal Shareholders: Federal Government; State Goverments; Development Banks; Nigerian Private Investors (60%); Leyland International (40%)
Date of Establishment: 12th August 1976
No of Employees: 1,300

LIFE FLOUR MILL LTD

PO Box 547, Sapele, Bendel State
Tel: 834467, 832572, 832576 (Lagos); 42590, 42628, 42195 (Sapele)
Telex: 42270 Lifeco, 26816 Lfour, 42268 Wasl

Chairman: Chief Alfred Ogbeyiwa Rewane
Directors: H Harry Bresky,
  R G Myers,
  A Enahoro,
  S Asemota,
  E Akpata,
  J Dediare,
  S Babajide,
  A Ede,
  M Tutun,

J E Rodrigues (Managing)
Senior Executives: Ted B Wiest (Operations Manager),
  William Shreve (Financial Controller),
  Ken Cole (Chief Miller),
  Tunde Babajide (Director of Shipping),
  Alex Ede (Director of General Administration)

PRINCIPAL ACTIVITIES: Production of wheat flour, millfeed and bagging of maize
Branch Offices: 11 Idita St, Surulere, PO Box 7008, Lagos
Associated Companies: West African Shrimps Ltd; Top Feeds Ltd; Deltapac Ltd
Principal Bankers: United Bank for Africa Ltd; International Merchant Bank Ltd
Financial Information:

	N'000
Paid-up capital	400
Turnover	60,000

Principal Shareholders: Seaboard Overseas Ltd; Wheat and Mills (Nig) Ltd; West African Holdings Ltd
Date of Establishment: 25th March 1971
No of Employees: 450

LIGHT INDUSTRIES (NIGERIA) LTD

7B Onike Rd, Yaba, GPO Box 1451, Lagos
Tel: 860291, 862308
Cable: Lightind
Telex: 22190 Plstik Ng

Chairman: P E Okoronkwo
Directors: M A R Farri,
  Raju Mahtani (Managing),
  A O Ndubuisi,
  M N Sadhwani

PRINCIPAL ACTIVITIES: Manufacturers of plastics and plastic products. Printing
Principal Bankers: United Bank for Africa Ltd
Financial Information:

	N'000
Authorised capital	250
Paid-up capital	250

Date of Establishment: 1969
No of Employees: 150

LILLESHALL (NIGERIA) LTD

48 Burma Rd, PO Box 1293, Apapa, Lagos
Tel: 877584
Cable: Linbuild
Telex: 21324

Chairman: Chief M C O Ibru
Directors: Goodie M Ibru, A K Shogbamimu, J A Balogun
Senior Executives: J A Adeniji (Acting General Manager),
  Hadji M A Olanipekun III (Administrative Manager),
  Paul O Lee Jnr (Technical Manager),
  J N Emegha (Company Accountant),
  J U Ogoke (Lagos Sales Manager)

PRINCIPAL ACTIVITIES: Agents and general trading company, building materials, civil engineering and construction
Principal Agencies: GKN, UK; Modular Technology Corp, USA
Branch Offices: 67 Ibrahim Taiwo Rd, PMB 3423, Kano; PO Box 721, Jos, Plateau State; E101 Babanlayi Rd, Maiduguri, Borno State; 34 Warri/Sapele Rd, Warri, Bendel State; AN7 Kazaure Rd, Behind Radar Cinema, PO Box 797, Kaduna; 12B Victory St, Benin, Bendel State
Principal Bankers: First Bank of Nigeria Ltd
Financial Information:

	N'000
Authorised capital	300
Paid-up capital	300
Turnover	1,929
Profits	14

Principal Shareholders: Subsidiary of Ibru Organisation
Date of Establishment: 1962

LIMSON & CO LTD
24 Breadfruit St, PO Box 1112, Lagos
Tel: 962301
Cable: Limson Lagos

PRINCIPAL ACTIVITIES: Leather and shoe manufacturers

LINBOLSEN MULTI-LINGUAL SERVICES LTD
1st Floor, Mainland Hotel, PO Box 2808, Ebute-Metta, Lagos
Tel: 860171, Ext 217

Directors: Linda Arokodare, Morin Agboola, Lawrence
Arokodare, Ette Etteh
Senior Executives: Yewande de Silva (Administrative Manager)

PRINCIPAL ACTIVITIES: Business consultants; conference
interpreting
Branch Offices: 146 Awolowo Rd, Ikoyi, Lagos; Airport Hotel,
Ikeja
Principal Bankers: United Bank for Africa Ltd

LINK GROUP INTERNATIONAL LTD
19 Ogui Rd, PO Box 42, Enugu, Anambra State
Tel: 253204
Cable: Links Enugu
Telex: 51138

Chairman: Jim I Nwobodo
Directors: Alhaji M D Galadima, Dr Correa Lima, J N I
Nwobodo
Senior Executives: P N Onwumechili (Secretary/Accountant)

PRINCIPAL ACTIVITIES: Pharmaceuticals and medical supplies;
scientific instruments; suppliers and servicers of scientific,
medical and technical equipment for education, research and
health-care
Principal Agencies: Sorvall Division of Dupont; AEI Scientific
Apparatus Ltd
Branch Offices: 18 Biaduo St, SW Ikoyi, PO Box 5274, Lagos;
116A Akpoba Slope, PMB 1318, Benin City; 32 Beirut Rd,
PMB 3313, Kano; 41 Aba-Owerri Rd, Umungasi, Aba
Associated Companies: Jimson International Cargo Agencies
Principal Bankers: African Continental Bank Ltd

LION OF AFRICA INSURANCE CO LTD
149/153 Broad Street, Lagos
Tel: 664730
Cable: Zaki Lagos
Telex: 22141

Chairman: Alhaji Ahmed Talib
Directors: Chief G K J Amachree,
Alhaji H A Ahmadu,
J D Brennan,
Alhaji Aliko M Mohammed,
A V Caddick,
Chief J K Agbaje,
M J S Bedi (Managing Director),
Alhaji Baba Jimeta
Senior Executives: R S Gambhir (Underwriting Controller),
J G Hill (Controller, Technical),
N S Brooks (Controller, Technical),
E D Okafor (Controller Administration/Development),
B N Ugwu (Senior Fire Manager),
E S Ajayi (Senior Claims Manager),
O K Oji (Assistant Controller, Audit),
C I Membu (Senior Accident Manager)

PRINCIPAL ACTIVITIES: All classes of insurance business
Principal Agencies: 208 Apapa Rd, Ijora, Lagos; 6 Lagos
Bye-Pass Rd, POB 1482, Ibadan; Sir Kashim Ibrahim Rd,
PMB 1194, Maiduguri; Edewor Shopping Centre, Effurum,
POB 484, Warri; Numan Rd, POB 366, Yola; Bello Rd, PO
Box 574, Kano; Plot C Ahmadu Bello Way, POB 149, Kadura;
22 Okpara Ave, POB 35, Enugu; 35 Ahmadu Bello Way, POB
697, Jos; 20 New Market Rd, PMB 2235, Onitsha
Subsidiary Companies: Guardian Royal Exchange Assurance
Group
Principal Bankers: First Bank of Nigeria Ltd; United Bank for

Africa; Bank of the North
Financial Information:

	N'000
Authorised capital	1,000
Paid-up capital	800

Principal Shareholders: Governments of Borno; Gongola and
Bauchi State; Guardian Royal Exchange Assurance Ltd
Date of Establishment: 1952
No of Employees: 250

LIPTON OF NIGERIA LTD
10/12 Burma Rd, PO Box 165, Apapa, Lagos
Tel: 803360/3
Cable: Lipton, Apapa

Chairman: A A Abidogun (also Managing Director)
Directors: Alhaji S A Sanusi (Commercial Director),
J O Odunsi (Sales Director),
F O Osibo (Technical Director),
J Pick (New Inv-Development Director),
J P Lusty

PRINCIPAL ACTIVITIES: Manufacturing and marketing of tea
and coffee and other beverages
Branch Offices: 8 Factory Rd, PO Box 108, Aba, Imo State; 48
Murtala Mohammed/Tafawa Balewa Rd, PO Box 1110, Kano;
SW9/2298 Ago-Taylor, Abeokuta Rd, Ibadan, Oyo State
Associated Companies: Lever Brothers of Nigeria Ltd; Lagos;
UAC of Nigeria Ltd, Lagos
Principal Bankers: First Bank of Nigeria Ltd; Union Bank of
Nigeria Ltd
Principal Shareholders: Lipton Tea Company Ltd; Walton on
Thames, UK
Date of Establishment: 1959
No of Employees: 637

LISABI MILLS (NIGERIA) LTD
Km 14, Ikorodu Rd, Maryland, PO Box 404, Yaba, Lagos
Tel: 861576, 960102

Chairman: Mrs V I Ladipo
Directors: Chief O A Adeosun,
Dr J Kehinde Ladipo (Managing),
Ms J Kayode Ladipo (Personnel & Administration)
Senior Executives: J T Ogun (Accoutant),
D A Mabo (Sales Manager)

PRINCIPAL ACTIVITIES: Food processing; marketing of
agricultural equipment
Branch Offices: 39 Commercial Avenue, Yaba, Lagos
Principal Bankers: International Merchant Bank (Nigeria) Ltd;
Union Bank of Nigeria Ltd
Financial Information:

	N'000
Authorised capital	100
Paid-up capital	100
Turnover (March 1981)	1,270

Date of Establishment: 1938
No of Employees: 109

LISABI MINING ASSOCIATION LTD
7 Ahmadu Bello St, PO Box 498, Jos, Plateau State

PRINCIPAL ACTIVITIES: Metal ore mining

No of Employees: 500

LISTER MOTORS (NIGERIA) LTD
Plot 7 1CC Layout, Ring Rd, PMB 5546, Ibadan, Oyo State
Tel: 413231
Telex: 31142 Al Ng

Chairman: Chief Alhaji A A Alao
Directors: Chief Alausa
Senior Executives: J Tidy (General Manager)

PRINCIPAL ACTIVITIES: Distributors of motor vehicles and spare parts
Principal Agencies: Datsun/Nissan Products
Branch Offices: Aba; Sokoto; Lagos; Kano
Principal Bankers: Bank of the North; Icon Bank

Date of Establishment: 1974
No of Employees: 250

LITIGO ENTERPRISES (NIGERIA) LTD
9/11 Gbajumo St, PO Box 4628, Lagos
Tel: 630867

PRINCIPAL ACTIVITIES: General merchants; importers and exporters

LITTLEWAYS INTERNATIONAL LTD
Isola Olateju Estate, 25 Abeokuta Rd, PMB 0003, Aiyetoro, Egbado North, Ogun State
Tel: 846445, 683546
Cable: Littleways Lagos

Chairman: Chief Isola Olateju (Engineer)
Directors: Ola Aremu Sanni, Akinbambo Olateju
Senior Executives: S A Adeyemi (Production Engineer), G A Fadipe (Field Supervisor)

PRINCIPAL ACTIVITIES: Manufacturers of electrical parts and wall brackets; electrical and telecommunication contractors and distributors
Principal Agencies: Molecz and Sohn, Austria; Fraba Ag, West Germany; Futurit Werk Kg, Austria
Subsidiary Companies: 'Olateju Ota-Okunkun Ltd; Ayetoro Fashions Ltd
Principal Bankers: Union Bank of Nigeria Ltd
Financial Information:

	₦'000
Authorised capital	100
Paid-up capital	100

Principal Shareholders: Chief Olateju; Mrs Olateju and 5 others
Date of Establishment: 8th December 1972

LIVESTOCK FEEDS LTD
1 Henry Carr St, PMB 1097, Ikeja, Lagos
Tel: 900375/77, 964020
Cable: Feeds Ikeja

Directors: R E Cawthorn, R J Dron (Managing Director), A N A Modebe, G O Olukoya, H K Aderibigbe (General Manager, Executive Director), R A Salami
Senior Executives: G O Olukoya (Director Finance and Administration), J K O Osinaike (Finance Manager), A O Bello (National Production Manager), J U Onwunali (Sales Manager)

PRINCIPAL ACTIVITIES: Production and marketing of animal feeds, concentrates and premixes
Branch Offices: Waziri Ibrahim Crescent, Abakpa Rd, PMB 2115, Kaduna; PMB 1203, Sapele Rd, Benin City, Bendel State; PMB 7119, Aba, Imo State
Principal Bankers: Union Bank of Nigeria Ltd
Financial Information:

	₦'000
Authorised capital	2,000
Paid-up capital	1,467
Sales turnover	12,925
Profits (after tax)	1,511

Principal Shareholders: Pfizer Corporation, New York; A N A Modebe
No of Employees: 250

LODIGIANI (NIGERIA) LTD
1/7 Abulenla Rd, PO Box 133, Ebute Metta, Lagos
Tel: 831854

PRINCIPAL ACTIVITIES: Building contractors

LOMBARD INSURANCE CO LTD
1/3-7 Nnamdi Azikiwe St, PO Box 9155, Lagos
Tel: 664371, 662020
Cable: Lombardy

Chairman: Chief A Koleoso
Directors: R A Williams (Managing), Prince Yemi Eweka, Alhaji R A Adejumo
Senior Executives: J Ganesan (General Manager), M A Bakare (Assistant General Manager)

PRINCIPAL ACTIVITIES: All classes of insurance except life
Branch Offices: PO Box 2184, Kano; PO Box 463, Enugu; 37 St Michael Rd, Aba; 6 William Street, Onitsha
Principal Bankers: National Bank of Nigeria Ltd
Financial Information:

	₦'000
Authorised capital	300
Paid-up capital	300
Turnover (net)	1,500
Profits (1980)	26

Date of Establishment: 23rd October 1970
No of Employees: 50 (approx)

LONDON & KANO TRADING CO LTD
56 Marina St, Lagos
Tel: 650995

PRINCIPAL ACTIVITIES: Leaf tobacco importers, etc

LONDON AFRICA & OVERSEAS LTD
Iddo House, Iddo Island, PO Box 556, Lagos
Tel: 832192, 876799

PRINCIPAL ACTIVITIES: Importers of spare parts for motor vehicles

LONGMAN NIGERIA LTD
PMB 21036, 52 Oba Akran Ave, Industrial Estate, Ikeja, Lagos
Tel: 964370, 963176, 963007
Cable: Longman Ikeja

Directors: F A Iwerebon (Managing Director), Chief J F Odunjo, T J Rix, C J Rea, J D Williamson
Senior Executives: J A Olowoniyi (Chief Accountant), O Bankole (Marketing Manager), O Agboole (Publisher)

PRINCIPAL ACTIVITIES: Book publishing
Principal Agencies: Longman Group Ltd, UK
Branch Offices: PO Box 442, Zaria; PO Box 425, Enugu; PMB 1122, Owerri; PMB 1236, Maiduguri; PO Box 224, Ilorin; PO Box 1192, Ibadan; PMB 1104, Benin
Principal Bankers: First Bank of Nigeria Ltd
No of Employees: 150

LONOGU ENTERPRISES LTD
PO Box 4397, Lagos

Chairman: W Chukwuru
Directors: P Adekunle, S Abijun
Senior Executives: G Cartland (Project Manager), P Floyd (Sales Manager), D Murphy (Design Engineer), Ade Adeyeyo (Accountant)

PRINCIPAL ACTIVITIES: General traders and multi-service engineering contractors
Branch Offices: Kaduna

LOUIS BERGER INC NIGERIA

14B Ilupeju Bye Pass, Ilupeju, PMB 21376, Ikeja, Lagos
Tel: 964517
Cable: Bergereng Lagos

Chairman: F J Farhi
Directors: G O Obembe,
  Dr J O Jackson,
  F S Berger (Managing),
  D M Wolff

PRINCIPAL ACTIVITIES: Engineering consultants, road design, realignment; railroad design; town planning; waste disposal; drilling and subsurface soil investigation; pedological surveys, construction project management; agro-industrial and irrigation services
Branch Offices: Kaduna; Port Harcourt; Abuja; Jos
Associated Companies: Nigeria Foundation Services and Soil Research Co Ltd
Principal Bankers: Union Bank of Nigeria Ltd

Principal Shareholders: Louis Berger International Inc
Date of Establishment: 1961
No of Employees: 275

LOVELL STEWART NIGERIA LTD

Plot 16 Akinola Cole Crescent, PMB 1452, Ikeja, Lagos
Tel: 960156
Cable: Lovestew Lagos

Chairman: Dr Adetunji Adeoba
Directors: E G Vassar (Managing),
  C O Lawson,
  A Adeyemi,
  N E Wakefield,
  R M I Stewart,
  H A V Omooba (General Manager, Administration),
  B J Howard (General Manager)
Senior Executives: Mrs M O Ogun (Chief Accountant),
  A B Alabi (Company Secretary)

PRINCIPAL ACTIVITIES: Building and civil engineering contractors
Associated Companies: Acceptance Concrete Products Ltd
Principal Bankers: First Bank of Nigeria Ltd; International Bank for West Africa Ltd
Financial Information:

	₦'000
Authorised capital	445
Paid-up capital	445
Turnover	5,900

Date of Establishment: 20th April, 1976
No of Employees: 250

LOWU INTERNATIONAL (NIGERIA) LTD

18 Upper Offin Lane, Balogun Sq, Quatar Ariyo, Lagos
Chairman: Alhaji M O Olorunoje (also Managing Director)
PRINCIPAL ACTIVITIES: General trading and contracting

LUNCHEON VOUCHERS NIGERIA LTD

25/25A Montgomery Rd, Yaba, PO Box 7438, Lagos
Tel: 862289

Chairman: Chief E A Osindero
Directors: L O A Fadipe, Chief C S Sankey, Chief Joseph Kagho-Omommadia, Dr J M Garba, Alhaji M I Hadejia, B E Ogbuagu, Dr C B Fadipe, M F Adewunmi, Ibrahim Abba Ganna

PRINCIPAL ACTIVITIES: Provision of luncheon voucher services
Branch Offices: 9 Nnamdi Azikiwe Street, Lagos; Abdulai House, Abdulai Rd, Ago-Taylor, PO Box 1811, Ibadan; 36 Ibrahim Taiwo Rd, Kano; 125 Bello Rd, PO Box 6959, Bompal, Kano; 1A Ahmadu Bello Way, PO Box 4512, Kaduna; 144 Sirk Kashim Ibrahim Rd, PO Box 400, Maiduguri; 10 Egbede Street, Off New Lagos Rd, Benin City; 65B Ogbunabali Street, Port Harcourt; 36 Zik Avenue, (Afrinsure House), Uwani, Enugu; 121A Oba Adesida Rd, Akure; 115 Ibrahim Taiwo Rd,

Ilorin
Subsidiary Companies: Luncheon Vouchers Investments Ltd
Principal Bankers: First Bank of Nigeria Ltd; Union Bank of Nigeria Ltd
Financial Information:

Authorised capital	₦1,000,000

Date of Establishment: 3rd June 1976
No of Employees: 200

M A ASAGBA & SONS
See ASAGBA, M A, & SONS

M A DOKUNMU & SONS LTD
See DOKUNMU, M A, & SONS LTD

M A ONIGBINDE & SONS LTD
See ONIGBINDE, M A, & SONS LTD

M EL-KALIL TRANSPORT LTD
See EL-KALIL, M, TRANSPORT LTD

M O ATTA & SONS (NIGERIA) LTD
See ATTA, M O, & SONS (NIGERIA) LTD

MAACHI-VALLE AND ASSOCIATES

PMB 1135, Enugu, Anambra State
Cable: Vallenugu

Directors: P Mercurelli

PRINCIPAL ACTIVITIES: Engineering consultants

MAAS (NIGERIA) LTD

PO Box 197, Ebute-Metta, Lagos
Tel: 630243

PRINCIPAL ACTIVITIES: General merchants

MAASARANT INDUSTRIES LTD

PO Box 269, 47 Maganda Rd, Kano
Tel: 2433
Cable: Maasarani, Kano
Telex: 77234 Maasra Ng

Chairman: Fawzi Maasarani
Directors: Umaru Baba, Abdel Aziz Maasarani, Jouseph Lukie
Senior Executives: Festus Adegbulugbe (Company Secretary), Issam Ghader (Engineer)

PRINCIPAL ACTIVITIES: Manufacturers of plastic products
Principal Agencies: Northern Plastics Industries Ltd, Kano
Principal Bankers: Union Bank of Nigeria Ltd
Financial Information:

	₦'000
Authorised capital	2,000
Paid-up capital	2,000
Turnover	5,399
Profits	276

Principal Shareholders: Fawzi Maasarani; Umaru Baba
Date of Establishment: 1970
No of Employees: 350

MCDERMOTT (NIGERIA) LTD

PO Box 2841, Plot 293 Akin Olugabade St, Victoria Island, Lagos
Tel: 613800, 613722
Cable: Jaramac
Telex: 21321

Directors: W D Howell (Managing Director),
  L Bennett

PRINCIPAL ACTIVITIES: Oil services, all types of offshore construction
Branch Offices: McDermott Rd, PO Box 94, Warri, Bendel State, Tel 233433

No of Employees: 1,900

MACGREGOR & OJUTALAYO
19 Military St, Onikan, PO Box 3114, Lagos
Tel: 654865
Cable: Ojumacco
Telex: 21409 Bolex

Directors: Kole Ojutalayo, Yomi Macgregor
Senior Executives: G I Adara,
   Ademakinwa Ademiluyi,
   Olabiyi Silva (Senior Administrative Officer)

PRINCIPAL ACTIVITIES: Chartered surveyors, real estate
   consultancy, project managers
Branch Offices: 5th Floor, Finance Corporation Building, Ibadan,
   Oyo State
Principal Bankers: United Bank for Africa; International Bank for
   West Africa

Principal Shareholders: Directors as described
Date of Establishment: May 1973

MACLISLE COMPLEX LTD
133 Agbani Rd, Uwani, PMB 1153, Enugu, Anambra State
Tel: 252887
Cable: Mactraco Enugu

PRINCIPAL ACTIVITIES: Importers and servicers of machinery,
   suppliers of agricultural machinery and accessories; electrical
   appliances; mining equipment; wood working machinery and
   building materials etc
Branch Offices: 3 Tetlow St, Owerri, Imo State; General Goods
   Department, 129 Zik Ave, Enugu, Anambra State, Cable
   Intermako Enugu

MACMILLAN NIGERIA PUBLISHERS LTD
Oluyole Industrial Estate, Scheme 2, PO Box 1463, Ibadan, Oyo
   State
Tel: 413917
Cable: Macbooks Ibadan
Telex: 31141 Mabook Ng

Directors: Olu Anulopo (Managing Director)
Senior Executives: J O Dada (Financial Controller),
   A O Amori (Publishing Manager),
   E C Ohuka (Marketing Manager Zone A),
   S L Asere (Marketing Manager Zone B),
   I Ademokun (Marketing Manager Zone C)

PRINCIPAL ACTIVITIES: Book publishing
Principal Agencies: Macmillan Education Ltd; Macmillan Press
   Ltd

Date of Establishment: 1965

MACPON ENGINEERING AND CONSTRUCTION COMPANY LTD
46 New Market Rd, PMB 1554, Onitsha, Anambra State
Tel: 374 Onitsha
Cable: Macpon Onitsha

Chairman: Chief D C Nwosu
Directors: Igwe P C Ezenwa (Eze-Okpoko I of Oba),
   C D C Ufondu,
   F A Ojukwu,
   O Osolu,
   M Chukwulozie,
   I C Onwuarolu,
   A O Orakwusi
Senior Executives: Chief P C Ezenwa (Managing Director),
   C U Anyaeche (Accountant/Administrative Manager),
   M O Udeaja (Manager, Furniture Division),
   G C Okoli (Engineer),
   M A Jideofor (Purchasing Officer)

PRINCIPAL ACTIVITIES: Civil engineering and construction and
   excise licence furniture manufacturers
Branch Offices: Furniture Showrooms: 71 Old Market Rd,
   Onitsha; Factory Building Oba, Idemili Local Government
   Area, Mile 7 Onitsha Nnewi Rd, Oba; Factory: 39 Campbell
   St, Lagos

Principal Bankers: United Bank for Africa Ltd; African
   Continental Bank Ltd; Co-operative Bank of Eastern Nigeria
   Ltd
Financial Information:

	N'000
Authorised capital	200
Paid-up capital	150

Principal Shareholders: Chairman and directors as described
No of Employees: 100

MADEBAYO ADETUNJI & SONS LTD
See ADETUNJI, MADEBAYO, & SONS LTD

MADONA ORGANISATION LTD
55 Akpakpava St, PO Box 782, Benin City, Bendel State
Tel: 243127
Telex: 41347 Madona Ng

PRINCIPAL ACTIVITIES: Importers, exporters, manufacturers'
   representatives, suppliers of building materials
Principal Agencies: Midland Galvanising Products Ltd; Bendel
   Cement Factory Ltd; Turners Building Products Ltd
Principal Bankers: First Bank of Nigeria Ltd

No of Employees: 50

MADRAS MANUFACTURING CO LTD
PO Box 530, Plot 8 Isolo Rd, Ilupeju, Lagos
Tel: 845868

PRINCIPAL ACTIVITIES: Manufacturers of textile equipment
Branch Offices: 1 Adegunwa St, Yaba, Lagos, Tel 45869

MADUKA, U, ENTERPRISES (NIGERIA) LTD
Block 82 Achara Layout, Agbani Rd, PO Box 567, Enugu,
   Anambra State
Tel: 3422

PRINCIPAL ACTIVITIES: General merchants and contractors

MAG FURNITURE AND INTERIOR DESIGNS LTD
Olusosun Oregun Industrial Estate, PMB 1287, Ikeja, Lagos
   State

Chairman: Major General R A Adebayo
Directors: Mrs M Adebayo, Mrs M O Aderem, Miss A A
   Adebayo
Senior Executives: David Child (General Manager),
   J Kehinde (Accountant)

PRINCIPAL ACTIVITIES: Manufacturers and wholesalers,
   contract and retail sale of furniture
Principal Agencies: Harrison Jones (UK) Ltd
Principal Bankers: United Bank for Africa Ltd
Financial Information:

	N'000
Authorised capital	750
Sales turnover	3,000
Profits	300

Principal Shareholders: Chairman and directors as described
No of Employees: 200

MAIDEN ELECTRONICS WORKS LTD
PO Box 158, Ikeja, Lagos State
Tel: 934368/9, 931773
Cable: Maiden Lagos
Telex: 21371 Maiden Ng

Chairman: Anofi S Guobadia
Directors: D L Garrick, Mrs G A Guobadia
Senior Executives: Raymond Hart (General Manager),
   Michael Uzamere (Marketing Manager)

PRINCIPAL ACTIVITIES: Assembling electrical and electronic equipment, telecommunication equipment
Principal Agencies: Racal Communications Ltd; Dymar Electronics Ltd; PYE/TMC Ltd; Decca Communications Ltd
Branch Offices: F13 Kaduna Rd, Kaduna; 95 Asa Rd, Aba, Imo State; 22A Mission Rd, Benin, Bendel State
Principal Bankers: Arab Bank (Nigeria) Ltd; United Bank for Africa Ltd; First Bank of Nigeria Ltd
Financial Information:

	N'000
Authorised capital	500
Paid-up capital	300

Principal Shareholders: A S Guobadia; Mrs G A Guobadia; D L Garrick
No of Employees: 200

MAIDEN MARITIME (NIGERIA) LTD
37 Calcutta Crescent, PMB 1062, Apapa, Lagos
Tel: 877240
Cable: Maidco

PRINCIPAL ACTIVITIES: Shipping, shipping services, clearing and forwarding, warehousing, freight, general agents

MAI-NASARA & SONS LTD
Head Office, 13A Club Rd, PO Box 1115, Kano
Tel: 4141, 4734

PRINCIPAL ACTIVITIES: General block makers, printers and auctioneers, general merchants

MAINLAND BROS LTD
20 Payne Crescent, Apapa, Lagos
Tel: 876756
Telex: 21584 Osena Ng

PRINCIPAL ACTIVITIES: General trading and contracting

MAINLAND HOTEL
PO Box 2158, Lagos
Tel: 860121, 860010
Telex: 21595 Mainla Ng

PRINCIPAL ACTIVITIES: Hoteliers

MAINTENANCE BUILDING CONTRACTORS LTD
MBC
4 Ikorodu Rd, PMB 1011, Yaba, Lagos
Tel: 877489

Directors: Giovanni Visinoni

PRINCIPAL ACTIVITIES: Building contractors

MAIS TYRES SERVICE (CITY RETREADING SERVICE)
64 Freeman St, PO Box 557, Lagos
Tel: 650296
Cable: Citread Lagos

Chairman: Chairman of Lagos Mainland and Island Local Governments
Directors: Lagos Mainland and Island Local Government Committee Council
Senior Executives: 'Tayo Sam Elegbe (General Manager)
PRINCIPAL ACTIVITIES: Retreading tyres and suppliers of new tyres
Principal Agencies: Dunlop & Michelin
Principal Bankers: First Bank of Nigeria Ltd

Principal Shareholders: Lagos Mainland & Island Local Governments
Date of Establishment: 1968
No of Employees: 200

MAJAND & COMPANY
22 Alhaji Olubuade Street, Near Gaskiya College Cardoso, PO Box 659, Apapa, Lagos

PRINCIPAL ACTIVITIES: Office equipment sales and services
Principal Bankers: First Bank of Nigeria Ltd

MAJEK SOETAN INDUSTRIES ENTERPRISES
8/10 Broad St, Lagos
Telex: 21295 Antoma Ng

PRINCIPAL ACTIVITIES: General contractors, supplies of general merchandise

MAJEM TRADING COMPANY
22 Alhaji Olubuade Street, Near Gaskiya College Cardoso, PO Box 659, Apapa, Lagos

PRINCIPAL ACTIVITIES: Importers, exporters, manufacturers representives, general merchants, clearing and forwarding, general goods suppliers and contractors
Principal Bankers: Savannah Bank Ltd

MAJOR & COMPANY (NIGERIA) LTD
44 Burma Rd, PO Box 351, Apapa, Lagos
Tel: 803321/2/3
Cable: Majorcom Lagos
Telex: 21378 Majcom Ng

Chairman: Alhaji Shehu Othman Malami
Directors: Douglas James Fielding,
  Detlef Bernhard Hoernecke (Managing),
  Francis Yerima Imhagwe,
  Alhaji Raimi Akande Adejumo,
  Francis Xavier Monahan,
  Alternate David George Oakenfold,
  Isaac Pius Obi,
  Isreal Akanbi Sholola,
  Godwin Andrew Ukekwe
Senior Executives: I A Sholola (Financial Controller),
  D G Oakenfold (Technical Manager),
  G A Ukekwe (Area Manager),
  A O Erebor (Area Manager),
  M A Okogie (Personnel Manager)

PRINCIPAL ACTIVITIES: Importation and wholesale distribution of hospital diagnostics and laboratory technology apparatus, immunobiological preparations, oxygen therapy and anaesthetic apparatus; surgical instruments and equipment (including the provision of complete modular operating theatres), veterinary pharmaceuticals and agricultural chemicals, etc
Principal Agencies: Ames; Ameda; Ashe; Bayer; Beecham; Beiersdorf; BCLO; Berk; Ethicon; Fisons Howmedica; ICC Institut; Pasteur; Kirby; Lepetit; Lloyds; Medic; Nordmark; Penlon; Reckitt & Colman; Schering (USA); Smith & Nephew; Travenol (Baxter); Whitehall; Wyeth; Porges
Branch Offices: 4 Lagos Bye-Pass, PO Box 1431 Ibadan, Oyo State; PO Box 750, 100/4 Murtala Muhammed Way, Kano; PO Box 96, 1 Dogon Dutse, Jos, Plateau State; PO Box 850, 10 Industrial Layout, Aba, Imo State; PMB 1375, Plot 17A Sapele Rd, Benin, Bendel State
Associated Companies: Major & Company (Ghana) Ltd; Major & Company (Sierra Leone) Ltd; Nigerian Chemical Services Ltd, Lagos
Principal Bankers: Union Bank of Nigeria Ltd; First Bank of Nigeria Ltd

Principal Shareholders: Nigerians 60%; Others 40%
Date of Establishment: 1952
No of Employees: 700

MAKE LTD
13 Commercial Rd, PMB 1279, Apapa, Lagos
Tel: 870006, 870008
Telex: 22108

Directors: Chief S N Ebinum,
   Alhaji R A O Majekodunmi,
   C Agbo (Managing),
   M O A Majekodunmi

PRINCIPAL ACTIVITIES: Importation and distribution of iron and steel products
Principal Agencies: Krupp Handel GmbH, West Germany
Branch Offices: Trans-Amadi Estate, Port Harcourt; Oluyole Estate, Ibadan; Enerhen-Effurun Rd, Warri
Principal Bankers: Societe Generale Bank (Nig) Ltd; United Bank for Africa Ltd
Financial Information:

	₦'000
Authorised capital	750
Paid-up capital	750
Turnover	10,000
Profits	250

Principal Shareholders: Directors as described
Date of Establishment: 21st February 1978
No of Employees: 138

MAKELLA & PARTNERS

45 Campbell St, Lagos
Tel: 653336, 841482
Cable: Kellapat Lagos
Telex: 21511 Elapat Ng

PRINCIPAL ACTIVITIES: General contractors

MAKERI SMELTING COMPANY LTD

PO Box 653, Jos, Plateau State
Tel: 2841
Cable: Makeri Jos
Telex: 81114

Chairman: M M Murray
Directors: R J Tolley (Managing Director),
   Alhaji H R Zayyad,
   P J Keenan,
   A R Williams,
   M F Garner
Senior Executives: A S C Paton (Chief Accountant),
   J G Rwang (Works Manager)

PRINCIPAL ACTIVITIES: Smelting and refining of tin, lead and white metal alloys
Subsidiary Companies: Plateau Development Co Ltd (wholly owned)
Principal Bankers: First Bank of Nigeria Ltd

Principal Shareholders: Amalgamated Metal Corporation; Nigerian Mining Corporation; New Nigerian Development Corporation
No of Employees: 105

MAKIN LTD

20 Obokun St, Ilupeju, Industrial Estate, PO Box 4354, Lagos
Tel: 961727
Cable: Maxiken, Lagos

Chairman: Engr Chief A A Bodede
Directors: Joseph Bodede (Director of Operations)

PRINCIPAL ACTIVITIES: Manufacturers' representatives, suppliers of food products, pharmaceuticals, etc
Principal Agencies: Casburt Pharmaceutical Equipment; Apotex Pharmaceuticals Inc., Toronto, Canada; Novo Pharmaceuticals, Toronto, Canada
Principal Bankers: First Bank of Nigeria Ltd; Savannah Bank of Nigeria

Date of Establishment: September 1976

MAKIRA KWARIN MABUGA METAL WOOD MANUFACTURING COMPANY LTD

177 Independence Rd, PO Box 2568, Kano
Tel: 3076

Chairman: Alhaji Abdullah Ibrahim

PRINCIPAL ACTIVITIES: Manufacturers of furniture

MALA, ALHAJI ZANNA K, & SONS COMPANY

14 Sir Kashim Ibrahim Rd, PO Box 202, Maiduguri, Borno State
Tel: 232820

Directors: Alhaji Zama U Malal

PRINCIPAL ACTIVITIES: General contractors, licensed buying agents, and transporters

MANAGEMENT ENTERPRISES LTD

5A Aerodrome Rd, PO Box 1269, Lagos
Tel: 874726
Cable: Promoters Lagos
Telex: Promote 21556

Chairman: A F Bouri
Directors: D M Nicholson (Shipping),
   Chief O B Akin-Olugbade,
   V N Khouri (Managing),
   G F Bouri,
   A S Guobadia,
   B G Popo (Admin),
   S C Beresford-Cole (Sales),
   Alhaji K Ojomu,
   Alh I R Fagbemi

PRINCIPAL ACTIVITIES: Importers and suppliers of cement and other building materials; edible products; hospital equipment; motor accessories; day old chicks; agricultural equipment and ceramics
Branch Offices: 3 Industry Rd, Port Harcourt; Chief Odibo Estate, Warri
Associated Companies: Industrial Cartons Ltd
Principal Bankers: Nigerian Arab Bank Ltd; Bank of Credit and Commerce International Ltd; Societe Generale Bank (Nig) Ltd
Financial Information:

	₦'000
Authorised capital	5,000
Paid-up capital	500
Turnover	85,000

Principal Shareholders: Bouri Investment Corporation; OBA Transport Ltd; A S Guobadia
Date of Establishment: 11th February 1963
No of Employees: 1,000

MANATEC COMPANY LTD

28 Kaduna St, PO Box 1121, Port Harcourt, Rivers State
Tel: 222912

PRINCIPAL ACTIVITIES: Hoteliers; industrial caterers; building, structural and civil engineers, general contractors

MANDARIN INDUSTRIES COMPANY LTD

Block 'F' Ladipo Street, Oshodi Industrial Estate, PMB 21033, Ikeja, Lagos State
Tel: 964600, 960928
Cable: Mico
Telex: 26232 Manda Ng

Chairman: Chief Adedokun Adeyemi
Directors: Stephen Cheng (Managing),
   Raymond Cheng,
   Mrs Mary Cheng,
   John H Siu
Senior Executives: C Y Fong (Factory Manager)

PRINCIPAL ACTIVITIES: Foundry work, steel rods production
Principal Bankers: Savannah Bank of Nigeria Ltd; Chase
  Merchant Bank Nigeria Ltd
Financial Information:

	N'000
Authorised capital	500
Paid-up capital	400
Turnover	1,117
Profits	355

Principal Shareholders: Nigerians (40%); Chiap-Hua Overseas
  Development of Hongkong (60%)
Date of Establishment: 1966
No of Employees: 150

MANDILAS LTD
Mandilas House, 96/102 Broad St, PO Box 35, Lagos
Tel: 661967, 662473
Cable: Mandilas
Telex: 21121 Mandla Ng

PRINCIPAL ACTIVITIES: Distribution of motor vehicles,
  air-conditioning equipment, technical and electronic
  equipment; car hire and travel agents; engineering and
  planning consultants; building and civil engineering
  contractors
Principal Agencies: RCA Corporation; AEG Telfunken; Sulzer
  Bros Ltd; Doxiadis Associated International; Stone-Platt
  Crawley Ltd; Henry Sykes Ltd; AG Petzetakis SA, etc
Branch Offices: 130 Sapele Rd, PO Box 776, Benin City, Tel
  243308, Telex 41127; 79 Sir Kashim Ibrahim Rd, PMB 1220,
  Maiduguri, Tel 232995, Telex 82147; PO Box 109, Bauchi, Tel
  42317
Associated Companies: Norman Industries Ltd

MANDRIDES, P S, & CO LTD
64 Murtala Muhammed Way, PO Box 42, Kano
Tel: 2477, 2181, 4636, 2479
Cable: Mandrides Kano
Telex: 77147 Ng

Chairman: Alhaji Shehu Ahmed
Directors: Thomas Joannou Frederick (Managing Director),
  Alhaji Baba Danbappa,
  Alhaji Inuwa Umoru,
  Peter Best,
  Alhaji Dodo Mustapha,
  Mallam Danjuma Hassan Abdu,
  Dr Sulemanu Kumo
PRINCIPAL ACTIVITIES: Manufacturers of vegetable oils and
  animal feeds, importers and exporters
Branch Offices: 7-9 Auno St, Maiduguri, Borno State; 1 Old
  Wharf Rd, Apapa, Lagos State; 40 Harbour Rd, Port
  Harcourt, Rivers State
Subsidiary/Associated Companies: Nigerian Bulk Oil Company
  Ltd (Associated); Maiduguri Oil Mills Ltd (wholly owned
  subsidiary)
Principal Bankers: United Bank for Africa Ltd; Chase Merchant
  Bank Nigeria Ltd; Savannah Bank of Nigeria Ltd
Financial Information:

	N'000
Authorised capital	2,000
Paid-up capital	2,000

Principal Shareholders: Nigerian (60%) and foreign investment
  (40%)
Date of Establishment: 1949
No of Employees: 500

MANILA CONSTRUCTION CO (NIGERIA) LTD
25 Ikot Ekpene St, PO Box 1132, Port Harcourt, Rivers State
Tel: 222938
Telex: 61143 Maclit Ng

Chairman: Prince S O Amadi
Directors: Chief O Wonodi, E C Amadi
Senior Executives: A Sankaralingam (Chief Engineer),
  Chief C C S Amadi (Site Manager),

  E O Amadi (Purchasing Officer),
  L N Eguzoro (Supervisor)

PRINCIPAL ACTIVITIES: Construction and transportation
Associated Companies: Deazula Trading Co (Nigeria) Ltd

MANILLA INSURANCE COMPANY LTD
1 Barracks Rd, PMB 1085, Calabar, Cross River State
Tel: 222188
Cable: Manilla
Telex: 65105

Chairman: Julius Abang
Directors: O E U Ekong, Chief E R Akpan, B J Ukpong, E B
  James, O N Udo, H W Akpan, Chief J S Inyang, Chief E B
  Ntekim
Senior Executives: E U Uko (General Manager),
  A A Akpabio (Head of Underwriting Assistant General
    Manager),
  B A Oworen (Head of Administration),
  A J Udoubo (Company Secretary/Head of Claims),
  P A Etim (Head of Finance),
  E T N Edoho (Head of Life)

PRINCIPAL ACTIVITIES: All types of insurance
Branch Offices: 4 Sanni Adewale St, PO Box 6601, Lagos, Tel
  658194; 7/13 Aka Rd, PMB 1040, Uyo; 49 Ikwere Rd, PO Box
  1010, Port Harcourt; Also at Ikom; Ogoja; Oron; Aba; Eket;
  Ikot Ekpene; Abak; Ikot Abasi; Etinan; Ugep; Ukanafun
Principal Bankers: Mercantile Bank (Nig) Ltd
Financial Information:

	N'000
Authorised capital	800
Paid-up capital	800
Turnover	4,000
Profits	818

Principal Shareholders: Government of Cross River State
Date of Establishment: 11th July 1970
No of Employees: 295

MANSA CONSTRUCTION CO LTD
PO Box 561, 706 Hadeija Rd, Kano
Tel: 4421
Telex: 77127 Mansco Ng

PRINCIPAL ACTIVITIES: Building and civil engineering
  contractors, water supply engineers, mining
Branch Offices: 13 Commercial Rd, PO Box 296, Apapa, Lagos;
  35 Harbour Rd, Port Harcourt, Rivers State; Maiduguri Rd,
  PO Box 42, Bauchi
Principal Bankers: African Continental Bank Ltd; Bank of the
  North Ltd

MANUFACTURERS AGENCIES
19 Martins St, PO Box 1574, Lagos

PRINCIPAL ACTIVITIES: Tobacco products importers

MANUFACTURING & MARKETING CO (NIG) LTD
15 Commercial Avenue, Yaba, PO Box 3579, Lagos
Tel: 863350, 863839
Cable: Mamcom Lagos
Telex: 22180 Mamco Ng

PRINCIPAL ACTIVITIES: Distributors of prefabricated buildings;
  manufacturers representatives
Principal Agencies: Portakabin Ltd; Glasdon Ltd; Portasilo Ltd
Branch Offices: Agbara Industrial Estate, KM 31 Badagry
  Expressway, Lagos
Principal Bankers: First Bank of Nigeria Ltd

Date of Establishment: December 1966
No of Employees: 60

MAPCOTEC (NIGERIA) LTD

5 Badagry Street, Off Adeniyi Jones Ave, PO Box 750, Ikeja,
  Lagos State
Tel: 964491
Cable: Mapcotec Lagos
Telex: 31181 Ng

Chairman: Alhaji R A Kadiri
Directors: Segun Osifeso (Head Air Survey Section),
  Mr Majiyagbe,
  Moshe Orem (Managing),
  M Aharoni

PRINCIPAL ACTIVITIES: Land surveying, photo flights,
  photogrammetry, mapping and hydrography
Branch Offices: SW1/261 Maya Street, Gege Olopa, Ibadan, Oyo
  State; Federal Capital, Abuja
Subsidiary/Associated Companies: Pantomap
Principal Bankers: Co-operative Bank Ltd; International Bank for
  West Africa Ltd
Financial Information:

	N'000
Authorised capital	100
Paid-up capital	100
Turnover	850
Profits	75

Principal Shareholders: Chairman and directors as described
Date of Establishment: January 1978
No of Employees: 100

MARBS FURNITURE INDUSTRY LTD

9 Harbour Rd, PO Box 141, Port Harcourt, Rivers State
Tel: 8019

PRINCIPAL ACTIVITIES: Manufacturers of furniture of all kinds,
  interior decoration

MAREEN INDUSTRIES LTD

99 Agbani Rd, PO Box 2031, Enugu, Anambra State
Tel: 253377, 253072
Cable: Mareen Egugu
Telex: 51124 Enugu Nigeria

Chairman: E E Ndubuisi (also Managing Director)
Directors: Mrs M N Ndubuisi, L E Ndubuisi
Senior Executives: E Okoli (Technical Assistant),
  E Attah (Manager, Concrete Works),
  Mrs R N Anidobi (Medical Sales Representative)

PRINCIPAL ACTIVITIES: Supplies/distribution of
  hospital/scientific equipment; products for water analysis;
  audio-visual educational material
Principal Agencies: Hach Chemical Company, USA; Seiwa
  Optical Company Ltd, Japan; Chemicals & Products Co,
  USA; Schuco International Nachf (Karl Riewesell GmbH),
  West Germany; Meiji-Labax Co Ltd, Japan; Aesculap Werke
  AG; Activated Chemical Co, USA
Branch Offices: Makurdi; Lagos; Onitsha
Associated Companies: Mareen Concrete Works
Principal Bankers: International Bank for West Africa Ltd;
  African Continental Bank Ltd; Co-operative Bank of Eastern
  Nigeria Ltd

Principal Shareholders: E E Ndubuisi and family
Date of Establishment: January 1975

MARGHI ENTERPRISES LTD

15 Ahmadu Bello Way, PMB 1073, Maiduguri, Borno State
Tel: 232236
Cable: Marghi

Chairman: Alhaji Bukar Petrol Marghi (also Managing Director)
Directors: Alhaji Madu Gambomi, Alhaji Bukar Umara, Alhaji
  Antar Mohammad
Senior Executives: Bukar Kotokori (Contracts Manager),
  L Nafiu (Commercial Manager),
  Malam Mastafa Madu (Accounts/Administration),

MANILLA INSURANCE COMPANY LIMITED

Incorporated in Nigeria

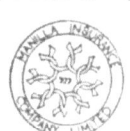

1 Barracks Road, PMB 1085, Calabar,
Cross River State
Tel: 222188
Cable: Manilla
Telex: 65105

Chairman: Julius Abang
Directors: O E U Ekong, B J Ukpong
O N Udo, Chief E R Akpan,
E B James, H W Akpan, Chief J S Inyang
Chief E B Ntekim
Senior Executives:
E U Uko (General Manager)
A A Akpabio (Asst. General Manager/
  Head of Underwriting)
B A Oworen (Head of Administration)
A J Udoubo (Company Secretary/Head
  of Claims)
P A Etim (Head of Finance)
E T N Edoho (Head of Life)

PRINCIPAL ACTIVITIES: All types of insurance

Branch Offices:
4 Sanni Adewale Street, PO Box 6601, Lagos. Tel: 658194
49 Oron Road, PMB 1040, Uyo
49 Ikwere Road, PO Box 1010, Port Harcourt
Also at: Ikom, Ogoja, Aba, Eket, Ikot Ekpene, Ikot Abasi,
Abak, Ugep, Etinan, Ukanafun

Principal Bankers: Mercantile Bank of Nigeria Limited

Financial Information:

	N '000
Authorised Capital	800
Paid-up capital	800
Turnover	4,000
Profits	818

Principal Shareholders: Government of Cross River State

Number of Employees: 295

Jeremiah Umokoro (Works Supervisor),
N Adze (Sales)

PRINCIPAL ACTIVITIES: General merchants, distributors, transporters, civil engineering contractors and agents
Principal Agencies: Vitaform Nigeria Ltd; Raccaform Nigeria Ltd; Leventis Motors Ltd; J Allen Motors Ltd; John Holt Ltd; PZ Ltd; UTC Ltd; CFAO Ltd; R T Briscoe Ltd; Yamaco
Branch Offices: Gombe; Potiskum; Mubi; Gamboru; Yola; Damaturu; Damagum; Biu; Bauchi; Jos; Kano; Lagos
Associated Companies: Marghi Line Transport Service
Principal Bankers: Union Bank of Nigeria Ltd; Nigeria Bank of Nigeria Ltd
Financial Information:

	N'000
Authorised capital	1,000
Paid-up capital	500
Sales turnover	5,800

Date of Establishment: 20th July, 1971
No of Employees: 180

MARINE AND GENERAL ASSURANCE COMPANY LTD

194 Broad Street, Lagos
Tel: 663849, 661912, 661907
Cable: Magopol

Chairman: F S McEwen
Directors: Chief J Akin-George (Deputy Chairman),
Chief Michael Ibru,
T B Oluyide,
Chief A O Lawson,
Alhaji U S Birma,
Chief O B Akin-Olugbade,
Professor O Akinla,
S O Ogunniyi (Deputy Managing Director)
Senior Executives: V A Onabanjo (Acting Deputy General Manager),
A O Peters (Acting Deputy General Manager),
A A Puddicombe (Chief Accountant)

PRINCIPAL ACTIVITIES: Insurance
Branch Offices: PO Box 416, Kano; PO Box 303, Maiduguri; PMB 5202, Ibadan; PO Box 524, Jos and also at Benin; Auchi; Sokoto; Aba; Onitsha; Makurdi; Ondo; Isolo; Warri; Calabar
Principal Bankers: Union Bank of Nigeria Ltd; First Bank of Nigeria Ltd; National Bank of Nigeria Ltd
Financial Information:

	N'000
Authorised capital	1,000
Paid-up capital	800
Turnover	4,566
Profits	507

Principal Shareholders: H Stephens & Sons Ltd; T B Oluyide; M C O Ibru; J Akin-George & Co; A O Lawson; Professor O Akinla; F S McEwen; Alhaji US Birma; Ago Ebga Stores; Chief C O Ogunbanjo; Nigerian Maritime Services
Date of Establishment: March 1969
No of Employees: 194

MARINI GROUP

Victoria Island, Lagos

PRINCIPAL ACTIVITIES: Suppliers of civil engineering equipment
Principal Agencies: Officina Meccanica Marini, Italy

MARITIME ASSOCIATES (INTERNATIONAL) LTD

PO Box 2288, 37 Marina, Apapa, Lagos
Tel: 636433, 654385
Telex: 21380 Marita Ng

PRINCIPAL ACTIVITIES: Genral merchants and contractors
Branch Offices: 43/47 Balogun St, Lagos

MARITIME STORES LTD

12 Gbaja St, Surulere, PO Box 224, Yaba, Lagos
Tel: 837793

PRINCIPAL ACTIVITIES: Importers, exporters, general merchants, manufacturers' representatives

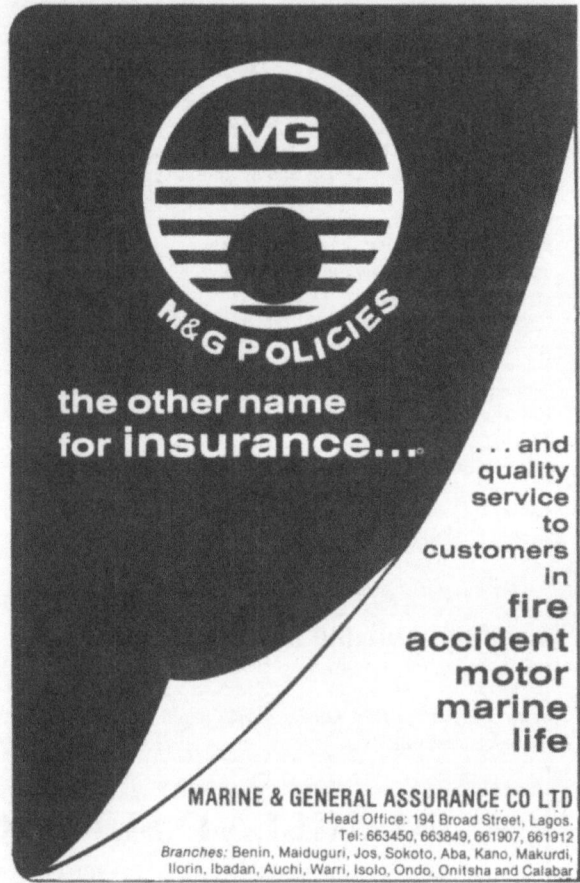

MARKDEALERS (NIGERIA) LTD

Continental Medical Complex Building, Plot D/106 A Industrial Layout, Oji River, PO Box 436 or PO Box 11, Enugu, Anambra State
Tel: 255080
Cable: Markdeals Enugu
Telex: 51180 Lint

Chairman: Chief P D C Okenwa (also Managing Director)
Directors: F O Ihenacho,
S U Chigbo,
D D Okpara (Director of Finance & Investment)
Senior Executives: J C Emezie (Group Company Secretary)

PRINCIPAL ACTIVITIES: Trade distributors; industrial promotion and investments development
Principal Agencies: Continental Medical Complex Ltd, Anambra State
Branch Offices: Markdealers (UK) Ltd, 103 Loampit Vale, London, SE13 7TG, UK
Subsidiary Companies: Continental Medical Complex Ltd
Principal Bankers: African Continental Bank Ltds; Cooperative & Commerce Bank Ltd; Union Bank Ltd
Financial Information:

	N'000
Authorised capital	1,000
Paid-up capital	712
Turnover	1,800

Principal Shareholders: Chief P D C Okenwa
Date of Establishment: 9th April 1970
No of Employees: 37

MARKETING AND SHIPPING ENTERPRISES LTD

26 Kodesoh Street, PO Box 1990, Ikeja, Lagos
Tel: 961305, 961817
Cable: Mascodist Lagos

Chairman: Chief Ayo Rosiji
Directors: Edward G Hanna (Managing),
  S A Adesope,
  Mrs R R Ogun

PRINCIPAL ACTIVITIES: Supermarket/wholesale food importers
Principal Agencies: B V Vleeswarenfabriek; Th Van Huystee BV Holland
Principal Bankers: United Bank for Africa Ltd; First Bank of Nigeria
Financial Information:

	N'000
Authorised capital	40
Paid-up capital	40
Turnover	3,500

Principal Shareholders: Chief Ayo Rosiji; Starco Ltd, Switzerland; Edward G Hanna
Date of Establishment: August 1964
No of Employees: 85

MARRYAT, DANIEL, (NIGERIA) LTD

PO Box 453, 17th Floor, Western House, 8/10 Broad St, Lagos
Tel: 653845
Telex: 21114 Danco Ng

Chairman: Chief J Mobolaji St Matthew Daniel
Directors: H E Maber (Managing Director),
  E Aleyideino,
  G Morgan,
  D Reynolds,
  B St Matthew Daniel
Senior Executives: E Idiong (Administrative Manager),
  Z A Aina (Chief Accountant)

PRINCIPAL ACTIVITIES: Electrical and mechanical services contractors
Associated Companies: Marryat Jackson Norris, UK (Joint Venture)
Principal Bankers: First Bank of Nigeria Ltd
Financial Information:

	N'000
Authorised capital	500
Paid-up capital	400

Principal Shareholders: Chief J M St Matthew Daniel; Marryat Jackson Norris Ltd, UK
Date of Establishment: 26th September 1976
No of Employees: 400

MARTIN MUKORO CONSTRUCTION COMPANY

See MUKORO, MARTIN, CONSTRUCTION COMPANY

MARTINS, AKIN, (NIGERIA) LTD

PO Box 4032, Lagos
Cable: Keencall Lagos

Chairman: Akin Martins (also Managing Director)
Directors: Yomi Martins

PRINCIPAL ACTIVITIES: Trade and industrial consultants, commercial information and marketing enquiries, claims collection, etc
Branch Offices: 22 Osoro Street, Behind Wema Bank Staff Training School, Papa Ajao, Lagos
Principal Bankers: First Bank of Nigeria Ltd
Financial Information:

Turnover	N 30,000

Principal Shareholders: Akin Martins; Yomi Martins
Date of Establishment: Established: 1955, Incorporated: 23rd April 1965

MARUBENI ENGINEERING (WA) LTD

3/5 Gbajumo St, PO Box 917, Lagos
Tel: 662417, 663401
Cable: Marubeni Lagos
Telex: 21410 Mareni Ng

Chairman: Y Ochi
Directors: M Ogihara (Managing),
  V A Haffner,
  H Watanabe,
  T K Sagoe

PRINCIPAL ACTIVITIES: Engineering contractors, town planners
Principal Agencies: Marubeni Corporation, Japan
Branch Offices: Hope Lodge Close, PMB 0018, Ibadan, Oyo State
Subsidiary Companies: Sumitomo Electric Industries Ltd; Nippon Electric Company
Principal Bankers: United Bank for Africa Ltd; Union Bank of Nigeria Ltd
Financial Information:

	N'000
Authorised capital	500
Paid-up capital	125

Principal Shareholders: Marubeni Corporation, Japan
Date of Establishment: 3rd April 1978

MAS-CHRISCO AND ASSOCIATES

70A Kekereowo St, Igbein, Ilasamaja, PMB 1130, Oshodi, Lagos State
Cable: Mca Lagos

Chairman: Amos Olagoke Ogunjimi (also Managing Director)
Senior Executives: O John (Project Manager)

PRINCIPAL ACTIVITIES: Building and civil engineering contractors general merchants, importers, exporters, manufacturers' representatives
Principal Bankers: First Bank of Nigeria Ltd

No of Employees: 1,000

MASCOT I ABALI & BROTHERS LTD

2 Awolowo St, PO Box 109, Enugu, Anambra State
Tel: 253279
Cable: Mascot

PRINCIPAL ACTIVITIES: Civil engineering and electrical contractors; importers of mining equipment and building materials
Principal Agencies: Dowty Mining Equipment Ltd
Branch Offices: Umuahia; Lagos; Port Harcourt

MASHALL, ALHAJI SANI, ESTATES

12 Club Rd, PO Box 2147, Kano
Tel: 4292

Directors: Alhaji Sani Mashall (Managing Director)

PRINCIPAL ACTIVITIES: Building contractors, transporters

MASS STATIONERY STORES CO (NIGERIA)

11 Bishop Street, Lagos

Chairman: M A Shoyombo
Directors: Miss Oluwakemi Shoyombo, Alhaji Ladode

PRINCIPAL ACTIVITIES: Suppliers of office equipment and general contractors
Principal Agencies: Apex Mill of Nigeria
Branch Offices: 32 Lawanson St, Surulere, Lagos; 19 Odunsi St, Lagos
Principal Bankers: Savannah Bank of Nigeria Ltd

MATCO AGENCIES

PO Box 1761, Lagos

PRINCIPAL ACTIVITIES: Importers of general merchandise

MATEF LTD

103 Ibadan St, PO Box 31, Ebute-Metta, Lagos
Tel: 860022

Directors: Helmut Panella

PRINCIPAL ACTIVITIES: General consultants

MATSON & COMPANY (NIGERIA) LTD

PO Box 2384, 21 Obun Eko St, Lagos

PRINCIPAL ACTIVITIES: Fire fighting and security equipment

Date of Establishment: 1975

MATSONS (NIGERIA) ENTERPRISES

27 John St, PO Box 6107, Lagos
Cable: Matsdiary Lagos

PRINCIPAL ACTIVITIES: Agents and general traders
Principal Bankers: First Bank of Nigeria Ltd

MATTEM (NIGERIA) ENTERPRISES

181 Tapesu St, PO Box 765, Apapa, Lagos
Tel: 873059, 871472

Directors: M Emuh (Managing Director)

PRINCIPAL ACTIVITIES: Telecommunications equipment
suppliers

MATUWO ELECTRONICS CO

PO Box 7934, Lagos
Tel: 657886
Cable: Matuwo Lagos

PRINCIPAL ACTIVITIES: Suppliers of electrical equipment

MATZEN & TIMM (NIGERIA) LTD

50 Burma Rd, PO Box 333, Apapa, Lagos
Tel: 877180, 877101
Cable: Omatimo Lagos
Telex: 21119 Mati Ng

Directors: Dr O E Awani,
P F Wiechers (Managing),
H Leiser

PRINCIPAL ACTIVITIES: Semi-trailer plant suppliers; dealing and
consulting in industrial and construction equipment, such as
flooring, shelving, ceilings, panels, etc; diesel generators
Branch Offices: PMB 5806, Trans Amadi Industrial Layout, Port
Harcourt, Telex 61174
Principal Bankers: First Bank of Nigeria Ltd; United Bank for
Africa Ltd; Union Bank of Nigeria Ltd
Principal Shareholders: M & T Associates Leiser KG,
Zug/Switzerland; Dr O E Awani, Lagos
No of Employees: 150

MAURICE PROJECT CENTRE LTD

6 Olaosun St, Off 49 Western Ave, PO Box 1445, Surulere,
Lagos
Tel: 831642

Chairman: Alexis Anielo
Directors: Ebele Chinye, Mrs Lilia Aneni, Henry Hackney
Senior Executives: Mr Mensah-Woode (Senior Consultant, Head
of Projects Division),
Vijay Khetarpal (Consultant, Head of Business Division),
Christopher Amadi (Administrative Consultant),
Ravi Bhavnani (Consultant, Industrial Engineer),
S Okoro (Marketing Consultant),
Anthony Ebube (Accounting Consultant),
Anthony Emechi (Control Consultant)

PRINCIPAL ACTIVITIES: Consultants, business management and
engineering; travel services
Principal Agencies: Management Consultants to Giampaoli
Organisation, Lagos; Mid-Enterprises (Nig) Ltd, Lagos;
Abrasive Industries (Nigeria) Ltd; Anochie Foundation Nigeria
Ltd
Branch Offices: 1 Eziama Rd, PO Box 3160, Aba, Imo State;
Kano Rd, PMB 1136, Zaria, Kaduna State; Onu Isii Industrial
Estate, Eke/Enugu, Anambra State
Associated Companies: Maurice Industries Ltd; Maurice Travel
Ltd; Maurice Farms Ltd; Mr Maurice Fresh Drinks Ltd; Anco
Nigeria Ltd
Principal Bankers: Union Bank of Nigeria Ltd; United Bank for
Africa Ltd; Pan African Bank Ltd; Mercantile Bank of Nigeria
Ltd
Financial Information:

	₦'000
Authorised capital	500
Paid-up capital	500

Principal Shareholders: Alexis I Anielo; Ebele Chinye; Mrs Lilia
Aneni
Date of Establishment: 6th May 1974
No of Employees: 100

MAX O URBAHN INTERNATIONAL LTD

See URBAHN, MAX O, INTERNATIONAL LTD

MBANEJO BROTHERS LTD

18 Church St, PO Box 563, Jos, Plateau State

PRINCIPAL ACTIVITIES: Metal mining

MBATA, SAM, & COMPANY LTD

Calvary House, 24 Ikwerre Rd, PO Box 674, Port Harcourt,
Rivers State
Tel: 229659

Directors: S A Mbata, Mrs A A Mbata
Senior Executives: Onyema Mbata (Sales Manager),
B O Amabibi (Accountant),
Miss Boma Hart (Secretary)

PRINCIPAL ACTIVITIES: Building material merchants and
contractors; agents and general traders
Branch Offices: 27 Hospital Rd, PO Box 674, Port Harcourt

MBK NIGERIA LTD

Formerly Mitsui & Co (Nigeria) Ltd

5th Floor, 138/146 Broad St, Lagos
Tel: 664412, 664292, 664220
Cable: Mitsui Lagos
Telex: 21549 Mitsui Lg

Chairman: M Nakano (also Managing Director)
Directors: S Kishi (Director, Group Co-ordinator),
S O R Uwhubetine (Executive Director)
Senior Executives: M Shiozawa (Group Technical Manager),
T Aida (Investment Adviser)

PRINCIPAL ACTIVITIES: Trading company; importing, exporting,
joint investments, engineering and technical service, shipping
and delivery
Principal Agencies: Mitsui Group
Principal Bankers: United Bank for Africa; Savannah Bank
Nigeria Ltd
Financial Information:

	₦'000
Authorised capital	500
Paid-up capital	250

Principal Shareholders: Mitsui & Co Ltd (Tokyo)
Date of Establishment: 14th May 1969

MEDAC (NIGERIA) LTD
26 Commercial Ave, Yaba, PO Box 973, Lagos
Tel: 861578
Cable: Medac Lagos

Directors: K Steinhauser, S A Oduneye
Senior Executives: Matthew Oyovwevotu (Science Manager),
  A O Smith

PRINCIPAL ACTIVITIES: General trading and representation
Principal Agencies: Tafesa, West Germany; Asta Werke AG,
  West Germany; E Merck AG, West Germany; Biotest Serum
  Institute, West Germany, W Weimer, West Germany
Branch Offices: Zaria; Agbor
Principal Bankers: Savannah Bank of Nigeria Ltd
Financial Information:
Turnover   ₦ 800,000

Principal Shareholders: K Steinhauser; Chief L S Akintola; S A
  Oduneye
Date of Establishment: 1968

MEDAL BROTHERS CO LTD
2 Railway Ave (off Makera Rd), PO Box 83, Kaduna South,
Kaduna State
Tel: 213573
Telex: 71171 Abenco

PRINCIPAL ACTIVITIES: General merchants and distributors of
  building materials

MEHR, HANS, (NIGERIA) LTD
10 Awori Crescent, Ilupeju, PO Box 979, Lagos
Tel: 960634, 960638
Telex: 21270 Merolg Ng

Directors: C Vink, E Friese

PRINCIPAL ACTIVITIES: Consulting engineers and
  representation, importers of machinery
Branch Offices: 26B Post Office Rd, PO Box 633, Kano
Associated Companies: Gloede & Hoff (Nigeria) Ltd

MEMCO STEEL CO LTD
Km 8-9 Old Lagos Rd, PO Box 42, Ibadan, Oyo State
Tel: 461382
Cable: Lubarico
Telex: 31159

Directors: S O Daodu, William Bouari
Senior Executives: Mario Messi (General Manager),
  E I Akinwunmi (Financial Controller),
  Robin Alakija (Managing Director)

PRINCIPAL ACTIVITIES: Manufacturers of trailers, low-loaders
  and all steel structures
Principal Bankers: Bank of the North Ltd
Financial Information:

	₦'000
Authorised capital	420
Paid-up capital	420
Turnover	6,500

No of Employees: 400

MEMUDU AROWOLO & BROTHERS
PO Box 51026, Falomo, Lagos

PRINCIPAL ACTIVITIES: Importers, exporters and general
  merchants

MENTHOLATUM (NIGERIA) LTD
Plot 50 Sharada Industrial Estate, PO Box 348, Kano
Tel: 4875
Cable: Mentholatum

Chairman: Alhaji Aminu Dantata
Directors: Chief J A O Olopade, Dr D Edo Awani, Dr K M
  Henderson, H Oglesby
Senior Executives: R G Scarr (General Manager)

PRINCIPAL ACTIVITIES: Pharmaceutical manufacturers and
  suppliers
Branch Offices: 100 Ekot Epene Rd, Aba, Imo State
Principal Bankers: Union Bank of Nigeria Ltd; Societe Generale
  Bank Nigeria Ltd; Savannah Bank of Nigeria Ltd
Financial Information:

	₦'000
Authorised capital	615
Paid-up capital	615
Turnover	6,000

Principal Shareholders: Alhaji Aminu Dantata; Chief J A
  Olopade; Mentholatum Co Ltd, UK
Date of Establishment: 1969
No of Employees: 160

MERCANTILE BANK OF NIGERIA LTD
1 Barracks Rd, PMB 1084, Calabar, Cross River State
Tel: 222603, 222605
Cable: Mercbank
Telex: 65118 Ng

Chairman: Okon Akpan Una
Directors: O J Okpoyo, Chief Bassey Asuquo Okokon, Dr
  Simon Nje Okpokam, Timothy Udondek, T F Ntuen, E A
  Okpo, I J Johnson, J F A Ekum, E M Ekong
Senior Executives: I Okokon (Chief Inspector),
  O U Nsek (Controller of Personnel),
  F Ekpo (Chief Accountant, Chairman of Management
    Committee),
  Chief J L E Duke (Controller of Operations),
  I W Inyang (Company Secretary)

PRINCIPAL ACTIVITIES: Banking
Branch Offices: Ikot Ekpene Rd, Uyo; 65 Ikwere Rd, Port
  Harcourt; 69 Hospital Rd, Aba; 34 Nnamdi Azikiwe St, PMB
  12687, Lagos; Ikom; Ogoja; Oron; Ikot Ekpene; Obudu; Abak;
  Ukanafun
Financial Information:

	₦'000
Authorised capital	12,000
Paid-up capital	6,100

Principal Shareholders: Government, private companies and
  individuals
Date of Establishment: 28th July 1970
No of Employees: 764

MERCHANT BANKING CORPORATION NIGERIA LTD (MBC)
16 Keffi Street, SW Ikoyi, Lagos

Chairman: Chief Dr M A Mejekodunmi
Directors: C de Mailly-Nesle (Managing),
  Alhaji Aminu Sanusi,
  Sunday Dankaro,
  Dr Duro Ogunbiyi,
  Chief Sobo Sowemimo,
  H de Saint Amand,
  O Michon,
  P Deveaud,
  Prof T Belo Osagie

PRINCIPAL ACTIVITIES: Merchant banking

MERCURY ASSURANCE CO LTD
17 Martins St, PO Box 2003, Lagos
Tel: 651816, 658346

Chairman: A Ekineh
Directors: Chief D O Ogugua, Alhaji Ahmadu Habibu, Dr F
  Ukoha, Alhaji B Dange

PRINCIPAL ACTIVITIES: Insurance
Branch Offices: Throughout Nigeria
Principal Bankers: African Continental Bank Ltd; National Bank
  of Nigeria Ltd

Principal Shareholders: Federal Ministry of Finance Inc; Alhaji
  Ahmadu Habibu
Date of Establishment: 1966
No of Employees: 500

MEREOLEH BROTHERS CO (NIGERIA) LTD
26 Lafia Rd, Northbank, GPO Box 797, Makurdi
Cable: Merekaduru

Chairman: Romanus Enyeribe Kaduru
Directors: Patric O Kaduru,
  Nicholas Mereoleh Kaduru (Managing),
  Mrs Leti Kaduru,
  Mrs Marthina Kaduru

PRINCIPAL ACTIVITIES: Importers, exporters, agents;
  agro-animal husbandry
Principal Agencies: Olehson's Agro-Animal Kingdom
Branch Offices: 24 Nekede Rd, Owerri, Imo State; B37
  Northbank Market, Makurdi
Associated Companies: Anaesoro-Onye-AGro-Animal Farm
Principal Bankers: Union Bank of Nigeria Ltd

Principal Shareholders: Patric O Kaduru; Mrs Leti Kaduru; Mrs
  Philomena N kaduru; Anthony Adikwu
Date of Establishment: 6th June 1973
No of Employees: 50

MESACOM ELECTRONICS INSTRUMENTATIONS LTD
Plot 6, Block G Oshodi Industrial Scheme, Isolo, PO Box 5707,
  Lagos
Tel: 614360, 961680, 843325
Cable: Mesacom Lagos

Chairman: Eng E Okusanya (also Managing Director)
Directors: S A Ogunade,
  Mrs F O Okusanya,
  Mrs Ibi Olubajo,
  J B O Okusanya (Public Relations Director),
  G O Okusanya (Director, Business Development)
Senior Executives: Clarkson E Obasi (Office Manager)

PRINCIPAL ACTIVITIES: Suppliers of computers, educational
  equipment and training services, electrical and electronic
  equipment, office equipment/supplies: telecommunication and
  power equipment
Principal Agencies: Feedback Instruments Ltd, UK; Gould
  Advance Ltd; Electronics Associates Inc; Swan Electronics;
  Eccles Technical Services Ltd
Branch Offices: Mesacom (UK) Ltd, PO Box 27, East Grinstead,
  Sussex, UK
Principal Bankers: National Bank of Nigeria Ltd
Financial Information:
Sales turnover   ₦ 2,500,000

Principal Shareholders: Eng E O Okusanya; Mrs F O Okusanya

MESTEROM (NIGERIA) LTD
PMB 1216, 1 Atewologun St, Maryland, Ikeja, Lagos
Tel: 963313

PRINCIPAL ACTIVITIES: Building and civil engineering
  contractors

METAL & WOOD FURNITURE CONSTRUCTION COMPANY LTD
142 Aba Rd, PMB 5066, Port Harcourt, Rivers State
Tel: 229315
Cable: Mewood

Directors: P N Ehoro (Managing),
  G A Hardy (Executive Director)
Senior Executives: C A Ihunwo (Administrative Manager),
  C J O Ikwuagwu (Company Accountant),
  L F Solbrich (Factory Manager)

PRINCIPAL ACTIVITIES: Manufacturers of household, office and
  school furniture
Branch Offices: 61 Mbaise Rd, Owerri, Imo State
Associated Companies: Meewood (Africa) Ltd, UK
Principal Bankers: Pan African Bank Ltd; International Bank for
  West Africa Ltd
Financial Information:

	₦'000
Sales turnover	1,681
Profits (gross)	418

No of Employees: 263

METAL BOX NIGERIA LTD
31 Creek Rd, PMB 1179, Apapa, Lagos
Tel: 876656, 874791
Cable: Metalboxes Apapa
Telex: 21549 LG

Chairman: Chief S B Daniyan
Directors: K Puri (Managing Director),
  El Lawale (Financial Director),
  F A B Longe (Regional Coordinator),
  A C I Mbanefo,
  G O Obatoyiubo,
  Arthur Roberts,
  P K Nanda
Senior Executives: A Fowokan (Company Secretary),
  G O Okiu (Chief Accountant),
  V Ugbade (Personnel Manager),
  J Shotonwa (Purchasing Manager),
  B Bankole (Commercial Manager),
  A Makuu (Production Manager)

PRINCIPAL ACTIVITIES: Manufacturers of processed food cans
  and other cans for the chemicals, paint, oil, agro-allied and
  costmetic industries, beer, beverage and aerosol cans
Branch Offices: 3-5 Metal Box Rd, Ogba, Ikeja, Lagos State
Associated Companies: Metal Box plc, UK
Principal Bankers: First Bank of Nigeria Ltd, Chase Merchant
  Bank
Financial Information:

	₦'000
Authorised capital	7,000
Paid-up capital	6,480
Turnover	36,000
Profits	6,000

Principal Shareholders: Metal Box Overseas Ltd (40%); Nigerians
  (60%)
Date of Establishment: 22nd January 1960
No of Employees: 1,386

METAL BOX TOYO GLASS NIGERIA LTD
MBTG
138/146 Broad St, PO Box 2515, Lagos
Tel: 633362, 633220, 633292
Cable: Metaltoyo Lagos

Chairman: Chief Christopher Oladipo Ogunbanjo
Directors: S A Fox (Managing Director),
  J G Gilbertson,
  Chief A O Lawson,
  F A B Longe (Regional Co-ordinator),
  T Matsumura,
  A O Ogunshola,
  H M Osha,
  Dr K Saeki,
  I R M Willis

PRINCIPAL ACTIVITIES: Manufacturing of glass bottles including
  beer and soft drink bottles; cosmetic jars
Branch Offices: Factory: Km 32, Lagos/Badagry Express Rd,
  Agbara Estate, Ogun State
Principal Bankers: First Bank of Nigeria Ltd

Financial Information:

	N'000
Authorised capital	8,500
Paid-up capital	8,500
Turnover	18,667
Profits	1,200

Principal Shareholders: Metal Box Ltd (Overseas Division) UK; Toyo Glass Co Ltd, Tokyo, Japan
Date of Establishment: 24th July 1974
No of Employees: 1,250

METAL CONSTRUCTION (WA) LTD

13 Burma Rd, PO Box 141, Apapa, Lagos
Tel: 803010, 803011, 803012
Cable: Metanks Lagos
Telex: TDS 036 Apapa

Chairman: T Okeowo (also Managing Director)
Directors: G A Okeowo

PRINCIPAL ACTIVITIES: Structural steel designers and fabricators of steel structures, barges, house-boats, pontoons, pressure vessels, silos, underground and aboveground tanks, tankers, trailers, motor bodies, bridge beams, spiral weld casings, railway wagons and civil engineering contractors
Branch Offices: Trans-Amadi Industrial Layout, Port Harcourt; Rainbow Town, PO Box 578, Port Harcourt, Tel 2191; 4 Club Rd, Kano, Tel 5794; Lagos Main Works, Klm. 36 Lagos/Abeokuta Rd, Near Otta

METAL FABRICATOR (NIGERIA) LTD

Km 16 Ikorodu Rd, PO Box 3819, Ikeja, Lagos

PRINCIPAL ACTIVITIES: Manufacturers of metal furniture

METAL FURNITURE (NIGERIA) LTD

Airport Rd, PO Box 106, Ikeja, Lagos
Tel: 964674/5

PRINCIPAL ACTIVITIES: Suppliers of metal furniture

METALLOPLASTICA (NIGERIA) LTD

9/11 Queens Barracks Rd, PO Box 309, Apapa, Lagos State
Tel: 803090/2
Cable: Eloplastic
Telex: 22296 Metallo

Chairman: B B A Ndiomu
Directors: M M Azar (Deputy Chairman),
    Michael Azar (Managing Director),
    Chief S S Ogboka,
    J O Edema
Senior Executives: Nabil Faddoul (Acting Managing Director),
    Pastor M Olu Aoko (Chief Accountant),
    Alhaji A A Akeredolu (Public Relations/Labour Officer),
    A Wilso (Technical Adviser),
    Ahmad Minkara (Chief Executive)

PRINCIPAL ACTIVITIES: Manufacturers of plastic products
Branch Offices: 102/105 Trans-Amadi Industrial Layout, PMB 5171, Port Harcourt, Rivers State
Principal Bankers: Union Bank of Nigeria Ltd
Financial Information:

	N'000
Authorised capital	1,000
Paid-up capital	1,000
Turnover	8,761
Profits	559

Principal Shareholders: Rivers State Government; Port Harcourt
Date of Establishment: 1961
No of Employees: 500

METALS & MINERALS (NIGERIA) LTD

A198 Isokun Street, PO Box 222, Ilesa, Oyo State
Tel: 2207, 2161
Cable: Diatomite Ilesa

Chairman: A O Apapa
Directors: D M O Akinbiyi, Mrs A T Ifaturoti, Mrs M O Oyawoye
Senior Executives: E A Ifaturoti (Principal Mining Consultant), P B Ilori (Mining Engineer)

PRINCIPAL ACTIVITIES: Mining, petroleum, geological and geotechnical consultants; groundwater exploration and development; quarry management; borehole equipment suppliers
Branch Offices: 59 Ajakaiye Street, Onipetesi, Ikeja
Associated Companies: Allied Quarries Ltd, Ilesa
Principal Bankers: First Bank of Nigeria Ltd

Principal Shareholders: Mrs A T Ifaturoti; E A Ifaturoti; Mrs M O Oyawoye; A O Apara; D M O Akinbiyi
Date of Establishment: 14th November 1968

METALUM LTD

PMB 21471, Ikeja, Lagos State
Cable: Alcomet
Telex: 11117 TDS 108 Lagos

Chairman: T A Braithwaite
Directors: Mrs R A Braithwaite, A T Ogedengbe, R Fijabi, W Stauffacher
Senior Executives: K E Davies (General Manager)

PRINCIPAL ACTIVITIES: Metals, metal processing and fabrication
Principal Bankers: First Bank of Nigeria Ltd
Financial Information:

	N'000
Authorised capital	1,000
Paid-up capital	1,000
Turnover	12,000

Principal Shareholders: Investment Holdings Ltd; T A Braithwaite
Date of Establishment: June 1976
No of Employees: 400

METOXIDE (NIGERIA) LTD

Kilometre 8 Lagos Rd, PO Box 1821, Abeokuta, Ogun State
Cable: Metoxide Abeokuta
Telex: 26408 Tower Ng

Chairman: Chief A O Abudu
Directors: D K Chandaria,
    Alhaji A Dantata,
    S Adedoyin,
    S R Das (Managing)
Senior Executives: M L Bhatia (Manager)

PRINCIPAL ACTIVITIES: Manufacturers of zinc oxide used in the manufacture of tyres, rubber products, paints, pharmaceuticals, ceramics, agriculture, insecticides and other industrial products
Principal Bankers: United Bank for Africa Ltd

Principal Shareholders: Olabopo Industrial Investments Nigeria Ltd; S Adedoyin; Dantata Investment and Securities Co Ltd; Metoxide International Ltd
Date of Establishment: 1979

METRA NIGERIA

132 Broad St, PO Box 4397, Lagos

PRINCIPAL ACTIVITIES: Business consultants
Financial Information: Joint venture between Walter Solomon & Associates Ltd of Nigeria and Metra Consulting Group Ltd of UK

METRISCOPE NIGERIA LTD

23 Calcutta Crescent, Apapa, Lagos
Tel: 75242 Cotpro Ng

Chairman: Goodie M Ibru
Directors: B A Olaogun,
    G V Austin (Technical Manager),
    P W Brassington

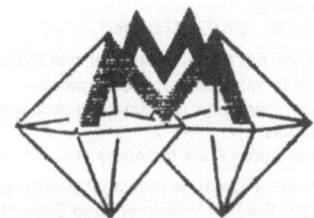
PRINCIPAL ACTIVITIES: Design and installation of laboratories and furniture suppliers
Principal Agencies: Sintacel Ltd, UK
Branch Offices: Sales Address: PO Box 347, Western Way, Zaria Kauna State
Principal Bankers: United Bank for Africa Ltd
Financial Information:
Authorised capital ₦ 100,000

METROCOM INTERNATIONAL LTD
11 Olatunde Ayoola Ave, Obanikoro, PO Box 1550, Ikeja, Lagos
Tel: 963146

Senior Executives: I Stocco (Group General Manager), M J Davies (General Manager, Unimer), D Cassels (General Manager, Metro-Technical)

PRINCIPAL ACTIVITIES: Sales and service of industrial equipment; building materials, ceramics etc
Branch Offices: Parts/Service Depot: Km 33, Lagos Badagry Expressway, Agbara, PO Box 2919, Lagos State
Subsidiary Companies: Unimer; Metro-Technical
Date of Establishment: 4th July 1969
No of Employees: 150

METROPOL MANAGEMENT CONSULTING SERVICES LTD
MMCS Ltd
PO Box 476, Murtala Muhammed International Airport, Ikeja, Lagos

Directors: A O Adeniji (Senior Consultant Electrical Engineering), J I Adeniji (Managing Director and Principal Consultant)

PRINCIPAL ACTIVITIES: Management consultants and agents
Principal Agencies: Plastak Service, Italy; Sifa, France; Euro Business Publications (UK)
Branch Offices: Location: Plot 122, 53 Afariogun St, Expressway, Via Charity Hotel, Oshodi, Lagos
Subsidiary Companies: Scientific Advertising Services: Oliver Clearing Associates
Principal Bankers: African Continental Bank Ltd; International Bank for West Africa Ltd

Principal Shareholders: J I Adeniji; A O Adeniji
Date of Establishment: 1967; 1975 as a limited liability company

METROPOLITAN DISTRIBUTORS LTD
18 Burma Rd, Apapa, PO Box 1550, Lagos
Tel: 875103

PRINCIPAL ACTIVITIES: Distributors of ceramic tiles and floor coverings

METROPOLITAN INDUSTRIES (NIG) LTD
16 Industrial Avenue, Ilupeju, PO Box 1239, Lagos
Tel: 961884, 961885, 961528
Cable: Hindustan Lagos

Chairman: C G Bhakta
Directors: Olajide Oyewole, Alhaji Ali Lawan, Chhaganbhai Gopalji Bhakta, Mrs Nike Akande, Naranbhai Copalji Patel

PRINCIPAL ACTIVITIES: Manufacturers of PVC and leather footwear, polythene products, etc
Branch Offices: Operations in Port Harcourt
Subsidiary Companies: Nigeria Model Industries Ltd; Wab Terry (Nig) Ltd

MICCOM ENGINEERING WORKS LTD
4 Odebunmi St, Off Akowonjo Rd, Agege, PO Box 3375, Ikeja, Lagos

Chairman: Engr Tunde Ponnle
Directors: Mrs Olufunke Ponnle, T Eng Mite (Technical Director)
Senior Executives: Lasun Tela (Administration Manager), Jai Ram (Production Engineer), Krishore Sachdev (Maintenance Engineer), Emmanuel Nwabueze (Accounts Manager)

PRINCIPAL ACTIVITIES: Manufacturers of electrical cables
Principal Bankers: First Bank of Nigeria Ltd
Financial Information:

	₦'000
Authorised capital	400
Paid-up capital	400

Principal Shareholders: Chairman and directors as described
Date of Establishment: 1974
No of Employees: 155

MICHAEL HAMMOND ENGINEERING LTD
See HAMMOND, MICHAEL, ENGINEERING LTD

MICHELETTI, A
1 Nsukka St, PO Box 262, Port Harcourt, Rivers State
Tel: 21078, 22216
Cable: Miclet
Telex: 61122 Miclet Ng

Directors: Arrigo Micheletti

PRINCIPAL ACTIVITIES: Building and civil engineering
contractors
Branch Offices: Warri; Benin City

MICHELETTI, E M, & SON (NIGERIA) LTD
8 Okpara Avenue, PO Box 388, Enugu, Anambra State
Tel: 338846, 254860
Telex: 51171 Etmami

Chairman: I Micheletti
Directors: C N Achugbu, B Mora, B O Achugbu, Alhaji A
Gusau
Senior Executives: A Deiro, I Squara, F Polla, S N Onuoha, E
O Aguene

PRINCIPAL ACTIVITIES: Building and civil engineering
contractors
Branch Offices: 3 Kalapazin Avenue, PO Box 569, Kaduna; 17
Wharf Rd, Box 64, Zaria, Kaduna Stae
Principal Bankers: Union Bank of Nigeria Ltd
Financial Information:

	₦'000
Authorised capital	500
Paid-up capital	500

Principal Shareholders: I Micheletti; C N Achugbu; B Mora
Date of Establishment: September 1955
No of Employees: 1,000

MICHELIN (NIGERIA) LTD
Plot 129/132 Trans-Amadi Industrial Estate, PO Box 527, Port
Harcourt, Rivers State
Tel: 334981
Cable: Pneumiclin
Telex: 61104

Chairman: J W Porter
Directors: M de Demo,
H Ossmann,
Chief J O Udoji,
R Abah,
S Amukele,
G Rouzier (Managing Director)
Senior Executives: J Grepin (Factory Manager),
M B Williams (Company Secretary/Financial Director)

PRINCIPAL ACTIVITIES: Manufacturers of pneumatic products
Principal Bankers: United Bank for Africa; Union Bank of Nigeria
Ltd; International Bank for West Africa Ltd
Financial Information:

	₦'000
Authorised capital	2,667
Paid-up capital	2,667
Turnover	50,000

Principal Shareholders: Michelin Tyre Co, UK; Rivers State
Government
Date of Establishment: 5th January 1962
No of Employees: 1,750

MICHELJOHNSON LTD
SW9/533B Ago Taylor Rd, PO Box 4015, Ibadan, Oyo State
Telex: 31232 Mepic Ng

PRINCIPAL ACTIVITIES: Suppliers of laboratory, medical,
surveying equipment, floor tiles, etc

MIDDLETON RIVER BROTHERS (NIGERIA) LTD
16 Ndoki St, New Layout, PMB 5589, Port Harcourt, Rivers
State

PRINCIPAL ACTIVITIES: Rivers and land haulage, civil
engineering and construction, dredging engineers,
warehousing, clearing and forwarding, lighterage etc

MID-LAND BOTTLING COMPANY LTD
Ondo State Investment Corporation, Acquinas College Rd,
Akure, Ondo State

PRINCIPAL ACTIVITIES: Soft drinks production
Financial Information:
Registered capital ₦ 1,500,000
Date of Establishment: 1978 registered
No of Employees: 120

MIDLAND GALVANIZING PRODUCTS LTD
PMB 2153, Abeokuta, Ogun State
Cable: Midgal
Telex: 24660 Midgal

Chairman: Chief A O Abudu
Directors: Chief O Akoni,
A M Ferguson,
R D Chandaria,
S M Chandaria,
Chief D R Borkar (Managing)

PRINCIPAL ACTIVITIES: Manufacturing of flat galvanized and
corrugated roofing sheets
Branch Offices: Oregun; Ikeja; Lagos State
Associated Companies: Metoxide (Nig) Ltd; Apex Paints Ltd;
Architectural Products Ltd
Principal Bankers: United Bank for Africa Ltd
Financial Information:

	₦'000
Authorised capital	4,000
Paid-up capital	2,100
Turnover	14,000
Profits	1,200

Principal Shareholders: Charnley Dev Co Ltd, Bermuda; Olabopo
Industrial Inv Ltd
Date of Establishment: January 1979
No of Employees: 376

MIDLAND SUPPLIES LTD
PO Box 1438, Ilorin, Kwara State
Tel: 4449
Telex: 33109 Midlan Ng

PRINCIPAL ACTIVITIES: State Government bulk purchasing
organisation

MID-MOTORS NIGERIAN COMPANY LTD
Urubi St, Benin-Lagos Rd, PMB 1140, Benin City, Bendel State
Tel: 242609, 240903
Cable: Midmotors Benin
Telex: 41131 Midmot Ng

Chairman: Chief G O Igbinedion, The Esama of Benin (also
Managing Director)
Directors: P O Igbinedion, O Igbinedion, M L Igbinedion
Senior Executives: J Luchetti (General Manager)

PRINCIPAL ACTIVITIES: An indigenous automative company, importation, assembly, distribution and servicing of motor vehicles; spare parts
Principal Agencies: Chrysler; Hino, Japan; TCM; etc
Branch Offices: PO Box 2212, Lagos, Telex 21528 Midmot Ng; Ibadan; Ilorin; Enugu; Aba; Jos; Benin
Subsidiary Companies: Okada Dry (Nigeria) Ltd; Gabdion Motors Ltd
Principal Bankers: Savannah Bank of Nigeria Ltd

Date of Establishment: 6th June 1968
No of Employees: 450

MIDWEST TEXTILE MILLS LTD

PO Box 102, Asaba, Bendel State
Tel: 19

Directors: W Y Annkpe

PRINCIPAL ACTIVITIES: Manufacturing of cotton piece goods
Branch Offices: 27/29 Martins St, Lagos, Tel 656474

No of Employees: 300

MIDWESTERN TIMBER MANUFACTURERS SYNDICATE

PO Box 63, Sapele, Bendel State
Cable: Afrikander

Directors: R I Omuamuanor

PRINCIPAL ACTIVITIES: Timber exporters
Principal Bankers: New Nigeria Bank Ltd

MIFI (NIGERIA) LTD

2 Galadima Rd, PO Box 328, Kano
Tel: 5063, 5525, 4426, 5137
Cable: Mifi Kano
Telex: 77188 Mifi Ng

PRINCIPAL ACTIVITIES: Manufacturers of furniture for schools, homes etc; suppliers of building materials, cosmetics, electrical equipment etc
Branch Offices: Kano; Zaria

MIKE MERCHANDISE CO LTD

10A Asa Rd, PMB 1157, Aba, Imo State
Tel: 205

PRINCIPAL ACTIVITIES: Importers of building materials, electrical and electronic equipment

MILLET NIGERIA LTD

PO Box 44, Sapara Rd, Ikeja Industrial Estate, Lagos
Tel: 961666, 961312
Cable: Millet Lagos
Telex: 26759

Chairman: E S Millet
Directors: F S Millet, H T Minakiri, Chief T D Rapu, Mrs S E Millet
Senior Executives: Horsfall Tasiere Minakiri (General Manager), William Esealuke (Accountant), George Garba (Personnel Manager), Obi Anachuna (Dyehouse Manager)

PRINCIPAL ACTIVITIES: Manufacturing of towels, etc
Principal Bankers: First Bank of Nigeria Ltd

Principal Shareholders: Foreign (60%); Nigerians (40%)
Date of Establishment: 1963
No of Employees: 500

MINARFOL TRANSPORT CO LTD

4 Kofo Abayomi Ave, Apapa, Lagos
Tel: 875525
Telex: 21593 Minfol Ng

PRINCIPAL ACTIVITIES: Transporters

MINGI MINING CO LTD

Dogon Dutse, PO Box 489, Jos, Plateau State
PRINCIPAL ACTIVITIES: Mining metal ore
No of Employees: 1,000

MINISTER TECHNICAL SERVICES

32 Rhodes Crescent, PO Box 541, Apapa, Lagos

PRINCIPAL ACTIVITIES: Engineering consultants
Branch Offices: 1 Dutse Close, Kano, Tele 3875, 5532, Telex 77129 Mintek Ng
Subsidiary Companies: Emirate Technical Services (see separate entry)

MINNESOTA NIGERIA LTD

Isolo Expressway, PO Box 3062, Lagos
Tel: 801600, 801610, 801602
Cable: Triminco Lagos
Telex: 26404

Chairman: Chief C O Ogunbanjo
Directors: B J Purdy (Managing Director), R S Priebe, Alhaji M Mai-Sango, Chief M N Ugochukwu
Senior Executives: Dr B A Masha (Production Manager/Chief Engineer), A B Kuku (Financial Manager), E N Iroha (Distribution Manager)

PRINCIPAL ACTIVITIES: Manufacturers of industrial and commercial pressure sensitive tapes, and scouring pads; distribution of electrical products; industrial and commercial chemicals; fire fighting agents; medical and dental products; graphic products
Principal Agencies: 3M Company, USA
Branch Offices: 71 Agbani Rd, Enugu
Principal Bankers: Savannah Bank of Nigeria Ltd; First Bank of Nigeria Ltd

Date of Establishment: 13th May 1975
No of Employees: 144

MISR (NIGERIA) LTD

15 Martins St, PO Box 997, Lagos
Tel: 662230, 662370, 664455
Cable: Misr or Shintam Lagos
Telex: 21273 Misr Ng

Chairman: Kamal Hilali
Directors: Alhaja Morohunranti Dosunmu, A I Mansour (Managing)
Senior Executives: A H I Fouad (Financial Controller), H N M Nafadi (Import/Sales Manager), M B Bisada (Import/Sales Manager)

PRINCIPAL ACTIVITIES: Importers and exporters of general goods, manufacturers' representatives
Principal Agencies: Sole representative for all Arab Republic of Egypt products in Nigeria
Associated Companies: Egyptian General Trade Organisation; Ministry of Economy & Foreign Trade, Egypt
Principal Bankers: Allied Bank (Nigeria) Ltd; Arab Bank Ltd; Bank of Credit and Commerce International

Principal Shareholders: El Nasr Export & Import Co, Cairo; A I Mansour; Alhaja Morohunranti Dosunmu
Date of Establishment: 28th October 1961

MISSRI, A J, & CO LTD

117 Nnamdi Azikiwe St, PO Box 417, Lagos
Tel: 658096

PRINCIPAL ACTIVITIES: Suppliers of wholesale general merchandise

MISTING EVERHOT
PO Box 7059, Lagos
Cable: Mistinghot Lagos

Chairman: S O Olayeye (also Managing Director)
Directors: A O Jonathan (Import Manager)

PRINCIPAL ACTIVITIES: Manufacturers' representatives, and general trading
Principal Bankers: Savannah Bank of Nigeria Ltd

No of Employees: 450

MISR (NIGERIA) LTD

INCORPORATED IN NIGERIA
IMPORTERS EXPORTERS & EGYPT TRADE
REPRESENTATIVE
CABLES & TELEGRAMS: MISR OR SHINTAM
TELEX 21273

LAGOS OFFICE:
15, MARTINS ST.
P.O. BOX 997
TEL: 662230
664455
662370

WE ARE NOTABLE IMPORTERS AND EXPORTERS OF BASIC NECESSITIES AND THE ONLY EGYPT TRADE REPRESENTATIVE IN NIGERIA. WHY NOT CONTACT US FOR ALL YOUR IMPORTATION AND EXPORTATION PROBLEMS.

MITSUBISHI SHOJI KAISHA (NIGERIA) LTD
11th Floor, Unity House, 37 Marina, PO Box 7384, Lagos
Tel: 636906
Cable: Mitsubishi Lagos
Telex: 21569 Mskigs Ng

Directors: A Tanaka (Managing Director)

PRINCIPAL ACTIVITIES: Steel contractors
Principal Agencies: Mitsubishi Corp, Japan

MITTON REFRIGERATION SERVICE
19 Onasanya St, Via Ishaga Rd, Surulere, PO Box 5593, Lagos
Tel: 832297, 832083

Directors: S I Adigwe (Managing Director)

PRINCIPAL ACTIVITIES: Suppliers and servicers of air conditioners, refrigerators and all electrical appliances
Branch Offices: 14A Ishekpe St, Ogwashi-Uku, Bendel State

MOBIL OIL NIGERIA LTD
Bookshop House, 8-14th Floors, 50 Broad Street, PMB 12054, Lagos
Tel: 635171, 635176
Cable: Mobiloil Lagos
Telex: 21228 Mobil Ng

Chairman: Richard M Leonard Jr (also Managing Director)
Directors: Godwin T S Adokpaye (Executive),
Ibrahim B M Haruna,
H R H Alphonsus O O Okagbue I Obi of Onitsha,
Eugene A Renna,
Stanley C Rosenstein,
Robert D Wales
Senior Executives: S A Adeyoyin (Manager, Sales),
P A Awolaja (Manager, Accounting & Finance),
C F Cronheim (Manager, Systems/Credit Servicers),
S U U Eka (Manager, Employee Relations),
E A Leigh (Manager, Planning/Supply),
A C Osokolo (Manager, Operations)

PRINCIPAL ACTIVITIES: Marketing and distribution of petroleum and petroleum products
Principal Agencies: Mobil Oil Corporation, USA
Branch Offices: Western Branch Office, PO Box 8, Apapa; Eastern Branch Office, PMB 1029, Benin; Northern Branch Office, PMB 3008, Kano
Principal Bankers: Union Bank of Nigeria Ltd; United Bank for Africa Ltd; Societe Generale Bank (Nigeria) Ltd; Savannah Bank of Nigeria Ltd; Chase Merchant Bank Nigeria Ltd; International Bank for West Africa Ltd; First Bank of Nigeria Ltd; International Merchant Bank (Nigeria) Ltd
Financial Information:

	N'000
Authorised capital	34,800
Paid-up capital	34,800
Turnover	261,361
Profits	27,541

Principal Shareholders: American (60%); Nigerian (40%)
Date of Establishment: 31 December 1951
No of Employees: 474

MOBIL PRODUCING NIGERIA (MPN)
Bookshop House 8-14th Floors, 50 Broad St, PMB 12054, Lagos

Tel: 653517, 653527, 653567
Cable: Mobiloil Lagos
Telex: 21228 Mobil Ng

Chairman: Carl J Burnett Jr (also Managing Director)
Directors: Alfred K Koch (General Manager),
A A Olukoya (Finance Director)

PRINCIPAL ACTIVITIES: Exploration and production of crude oil

Principal Shareholders: Nigerian National Petroleum Corp; Mobil Oil Corporation
Date of Establishment: 1962
No of Employees: 800

MOCCI, E, ASSOCIATES
283/8 Akin Olugbade St, Victoria Island, PO Box 2063, Lagos
Tel: 610849

Directors: E Mocci, V Bruno

PRINCIPAL ACTIVITIES: General contractors
Branch Offices: Calabar

MODEARO (NIGERIA) LTD
6 Azikiwe Rd, 1st Floor Leventis Stores Building, PO Box 817, Port Harcourt, Rivers State
Tel: 330448
Cable: Modearo Port Harcourt
Telex: 61123 Leveco Attention Modearo

Chairman: Sulaimon A Hameen
Directors: Waidi A Kareem (Managing),
Dapo Akinde
Senior Executives: Moshood A Bola (Director of Operations, East),
Dapo Akinde (Director of Operations, West)

PRINCIPAL ACTIVITIES: Shipping, clearing and forwarding, transporting, warehousing, air freighting, marine and lighterage, international trade
Principal Agencies: Nigerian Bottling Company Ltd; Dr Pepper

Bottling Company Ltd, Danit; A/S Dansk Haardmetal, Denmark; Livestock Feeds Ltd; Cocoa Industry Nigeria Ltd; Oyo State Water Corporation

Branch Offices: Shipping, clearing & Forwarding Division, PO Box 965, Calabar, Cross River State, Cable Monetrens Calabar; Poultry and Farming Division, Jagun Alaro Lane, Ede, Oyo State; 14 Alhaji Kareem St, Opposite Kirikiri Jetty, Tin Can Island, Port Area, PO Box 1575, Apapa, Lagos, Tel 872419, 872421, Telex 20200 NET TDS Ng

Principal Bankers: Union Bank of Nigeria Ltd; National Bank of Nigeria Ltd; Savannah Bank of Nigeria Ltd; Societe Generale Bank of Nigeria Ltd

Financial Information:

	₦'000
Authorised capital	100
Paid-up capital	60
Turnover	2,300

Principal Shareholders: S A Hameen; W A Kareem; M A Bola
Date of Establishment: 1973 (Incorporated 1978)
No of Employees: 115

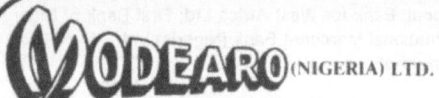

DIVISIONS:
* SHIPPING
* CLEARING AND FORWARDING
* AIR FREIGHTING
* BUILDING MATERIALS
* AGRICULTURAL MACHINERY
* LIGHTERAGE OPERATORS
* POULTRY AND FARMING
* INTERNATIONAL TRADE

Head Office:
6 Azikiwe Road
(1st Floor, Leventis Stores Building)
PO Box 817
PORT HARCOURT
NIGERIA
Cable: "MODEARO PHARCOURT"
TELEX: 61123 LEVECO
Telephone: 330448

Branch Offices:
(1) Lagos:
14 Alhaji Kareem Akande Street
(Opposite Kirikiri Jetty, Tincan Island Port Area)
PO Box 1575
APAPA
Cable: "MODEARO LAGOS"
Telephone: (01) 872419 & 872421
TELEX: 20200 NET TDS NG.

(2) Calabar:
PO Box 965
Calabar
NIGERIA
Cable: "MODEARO CALABAR"

MODELOR DESIGN AIDS LTD

295 Ikorodu Rd, PO Box 573, Lagos
Tel: 964939
Cable: Dimensions
Telex: 21926 Modulor Ng

Chairman: Chief O O Balogun
Directors: Mrs F Balogun, Miss Bolanle Balogun
Senior Executives: Kunle Balogun (Project Manager),
Biodun Adekoya (Senior Engineer),
Dr J O M Jibowu (Computer Engineer),
Musud Malak (Computer Superintendent)

PRINCIPAL ACTIVITIES: Computer analysts, programmers, scale modelmakers, offset printers, bureau service in respect of engineering, architecture and surveying hardware; software; comprehensive structural engineering services, architecture,

surveying
Principal Bankers: United Bank for Africa Ltd

Principal Shareholders: Modulor Group
Date of Establishment: 1979

MODERN CERAMICS INDUSTRIES LTD

Aba Rd, PMB 1040, Umuahia, Imo State
Tel: 220222, 220892, 220019
Cable: Moceram

Chairman: Eng D N Ugwudi
Directors: N P D Ngbaraonye, L E Nwachukwu, V Chukwu, Mrs S E Abiakam, F O S Ozurumba
Senior Executives: J C Nwabugwu (General Manager),
Bona B Uhegbu (Company Secretary),
C C Okpara (Marketing Manager),
J A Ekwuribe (Deputy Chief Accountant)

PRINCIPAL ACTIVITIES: Manufacturers of ceramics wares
Associated Companies: Eurotecnica Italy
Principal Bankers: First Bank of Nigeria Ltd; African Continental Bank Ltd; Union Bank Nigeria Ltd
Financial Information:

	₦'000
Authorised capital	3,500
Paid-up capital	3,500
Turnover	1,000

Principal Shareholders: Government of Imo State
Date of Establishment: 1964
No of Employees: 350

MODERN DOMUS LTD

15 Gbajumo St, PO Box 6266, Lagos
Tel: 635923, 633275, 836382, 832944

PRINCIPAL ACTIVITIES: Suppliers of furniture and furnishings

MODERN FOUNDRY PRODUCTS LTD

243 Ijora Causeway, Ijora, PO Box 28, Apapa, Lagos State
Tel: 832411, 832188
Cable: Jarmakani, Apapa
Telex: 21030 Nassar, 26788 Blues

Directors: Alhaji Jalo Waziri, H N Jarmakani, S N Jarmakani

PRINCIPAL ACTIVITIES: Casting of brass, aluminium and iron
Branch Offices: Factory: Blue 5 Way, off Billings Way, Oregun Industrial Estate, Lagos State
Principal Bankers: First Bank of Nigeria Ltd
Financial Information:

	₦'000
Authorised capital	500
Paid-up capital	400

Principal Shareholders: Directors as described
Date of Establishment: 1969
No of Employees: 100

MODERN INDUSTRIES LTD

17 Dantata Rd, Bompai, PO Box 417, Kano
Tel: 2227/4
Telex: 77186 Nornit Ng

PRINCIPAL ACTIVITIES: Suppliers of sanitary-ware and ancillary equipment

MODERN SHOE INDUSTRY LTD

PO Box 49, Owerri, Imo State

PRINCIPAL ACTIVITIES: Manufacturing of footwear

MODULOR GROUP

295 Ikorodu Road, PO Box 573, Lagos
Tel: 964939, 901310/2
Cable: Dimensions
Telex: 21926 Modulo NG; 26345 Modelo NG

Chairman: Chief O O Balogun
Senior Executives: A A Ajibola (General Manager),
  Mrs S O Ajomo (Group Administrative Manager),
  A A Adeyemi (Personnel Manager),
  Kunle Balogun (Project Manager),
  Mrs R H Sodipo (Company Secretary/Legal Adviser),
  U Shrestha (Chief Architect - Housing),
  R E Long (Principal Project Coordinator)

PRINCIPAL ACTIVITIES: Architects, planning consultants, project development
Branch Offices: 2nd Floor, Bank Chambers, 27/29 Martins Street, Lagos, Lagos State; 83 Francis Okediji Street, Off Adeyi Avenue, Bodija Estate, Ibadan, Oyo State; C/O Physical Planning Unit, University of Ilorin, PMB 1515, Ilorin, Kwara State; C/O Project Office, Metallurgical Training Centre, Ajaokuta, Kwara State; Ist Avenue, Miango Rd, PO Box 6575, Anglo, Jos, Plateau State
Associated Companies: Promana Associates; Modelor Design Aids Ltd
Principal Bankers: United Bank for Africa Ltd; Union Bank of Nigeria Ltd

Date of Establishment: 1967
No of Employees: 192

MOFAT ENGINEERING COMPANY LTD
8 Agege Motor Rd, Shogunle, PO Box 6369, Lagos
Tel: 960744
Cable: Mofateng Lagos
Telex: 20202 Ikeja Tds B.131

Chairman: Mrs Irene Fatimilehin
Directors: Bola Ige, Seyi Fatimilehin
Senior Executives: Dayo Esuruoso (Technical Manager),
  Oluseyi Fatimilehin (Managing)

PRINCIPAL ACTIVITIES: Sales, installation and servicing of electrical and electronic equipment
Principal Agencies: Fluke International Corporation; B&K Precision Instruments
Branch Offices: SW8/131 Ijebu Bye-Pass, PO Box 3464, Ibadan, Oyo State
Principal Bankers: Union Bank of Nigeria Ltd
Financial Information:

	₦'000
Authorised capital	50
Paid-up capital	27

Principal Shareholders: Chairman and directors as described
Date of Establishment: 17th November 1972

MOGAJI OSONA ENTERPRISES LTD
28 Rotimi St, Surulere, PO Box 5160, Lagos
Cable: Entegloria Lagos

Chairman: G A Onasanya (also Managing Director)
Directors: Mrs M A Onasanya,
  S A Adeleye (Marketing Director)

PRINCIPAL ACTIVITIES: General merchants and manufacturers' representatives; large-scale importers of food items such as wheat flour, rice, milk, sugar, poultry products, sea foods, etc
Branch Offices: Branch offices will be opened very soon
Principal Bankers: Union Bank of Nigeria Ltd

Principal Shareholders: G A Onasanya; M A Onasanya; S A Adeleye

MONEME & SONS BOOKSHOPS
PO Bos 779, 78 Hospital Rd, Aba, Imo State

PRINCIPAL ACTIVITIES: Booksellers and stationers; suppliers of sports goods and artists materials

MONIER CONSTRUCTION COMPANY (NIG) LTD
PO Box 8919, Lagos
Tel: 617666, 610750
Telex: 61230 Monier Ng

Chairman: Chief Mike Nkwoji
Directors: G Haass (Managing),
  Engr W Siegel,
  Engr Josiah O Akinseye,
  Alhaji Aliko Mohammed

PRINCIPAL ACTIVITIES: Engineering design, construction, building and civil engineering contractors
Branch Offices: 18/19 Abonnema Wharf Rd, PO Box 304, Port Harcourt, Tel 333100, 333482; Uratta Rd, PMB 1163, Owerri; Emene Rd, PMB 1576, Enugu

Date of Establishment: Incorporated 24th May 1958

MONOTYPE NIGERIA LTD
3 Ilupeju Bye Pass, Ilupeju, PO Box 8824, Lagos
Tel: 963815
Cable: Monotype
Telex: 26692 Mono Ng

Chairman: Dr Babatunde Jose
Directors: Dr B A Masha (Managing),
  Chief O A Adeosun,
  Alhaji Mamman Daura,
  R C Day,
  J W Mawle,
  D H J Schenck

PRINCIPAL ACTIVITIES: Distribution and service of printing machines equipment and printing consumables
Principal Agencies: Monotype Corporation Ltd; Salfords, UK; Pictorial Machinery, UK; AM Varityper, USA; Hans Herold, West Germany; Challenge, USA; Como Maskin, West Germany; Horsell Graphics, UK; NuArc, USA; Solna Offset, Sweden; T C Thompson, UK; Vandersons, USA; Worsley Brehmer, UK; Derncliff Engineering Pattern, UK
Branch Offices: 22 Okigwe Rd, Aba, Imo State; S7/372A Oba Abimbola Rd, Felele Layout, Challenge, Ibadan, Oyo State; Z1 Jos/Abeokuta Rd, Kaduna, Kaduna State
Principal Bankers: Union Bank of Nigeria Ltd
Financial Information:

	₦'000
Authorised capital	300
Paid-up capital	300
Turnover	3,000
Profits	500

Principal Shareholders: Monotype Corporation Ltd, Salfords UK (40%); Monotype Nigeria Ltd, (60%)
Date of Establishment: 3rd January 1970
No of Employees: 50

MONTUBI
4 Thorburn Ave, PO Box 8960, Yaba, Lagos State
Tel: 860694
Telex: 22626

Senior Executives: A Paoli (Project Manager),
  G L Ferretti (Area Representative)

PRINCIPAL ACTIVITIES: Construction of petroleum pipelines

MOON CONFECTIONERY LTD
PO Box 556, Kano
Tel: 4696, 3191
Cable: Moonco Kano

PRINCIPAL ACTIVITIES: Manufacturers of confectionery, sweets
Branch Offices: Factory: 583 Umaru Babura Rd, Bompai, Kano

MOONE CONSTRUCTION CO LTD
Head Office, 173 Zik Ave, PMB 1148, Enugu, Anambra State
Tel: 252800

PRINCIPAL ACTIVITIES: Civil engineering, specialists in road construction and construction of military barracks

MOORE OBIOHA, C, SONS & COMPANY LTD

125/127 Aba/Owerri Rd, Abayi Umuocham, PO Box 165, Aba, Imo State
Tel: 506
Cable: Moscol

Chairman: Chief C Moore Obioha
Directors: N E Obioha, G Nnamdi Obioha
Senior Executives: Z I Igwe (General Manager),
E C Obiedelu (Transport Manager)

PRINCIPAL ACTIVITIES: Suppliers of electrical and electronic equipment, motor-cycles, motor vehicles and components; transporters
Principal Agencies: Leventis Motors Ltd, Nigeria; Saba-Werke GmbH, West Germany
Branch Offices: 65a Ojuelegba Rd, Surulere, Lagos; 174a Aba Rd, Port Harcourt; 103 Upper New Market Rd, Onitsha; 41a Aba/Owerri Rd, Aba; 36c St Michael's Rd, Aba; 29 Ogoja Rd, Abakaliki
Subsidiary Companies: Moscol Transport Company Ltd
Principal Bankers: International Bank for West Africa Ltd; First Bank of Nigeria Ltd

No of Employees: 350

MORIN INTERNATIONAL GROUP LTD

Plot 74/78, Segun Industrial Estate, PMB 1233, Apapa, Lagos
Tel: 850866
Telex: 46812 Cdlegroup

Directors: T H Samuel

PRINCIPAL ACTIVITIES: General traders and contractors

MORIN, J, & CO

61 Enu-Owa St, PO Box 1119, Lagos
Tel: 633985

Directors: J O Ogunsanya

PRINCIPAL ACTIVITIES: General trading and representation
Branch Offices: Principal Branch: 15 Affar St, PMB 1623, Onitsha, Anambra State

MORISON, J L, SONS & JONES (NIGERIA) LTD

10 Lancaster/Onike Rd, Yaba, PMB 2084, Lagos
Tel: 860301
Cable: Conflict Lagos

Chairman: A K Onwude
Directors: P A Hoare, L J Walters, C W Freyer, A V Omenka, Chief A A Daniel, R Walli

PRINCIPAL ACTIVITIES: Importers, distributors and manufacturers of pharmaceuticals, agro-veterinary, medical supplies, writing instruments and giftware, wines and spirits, cosmetics and toiletries, domestic appliances
Branch Offices: SW8/350 Lagos Rd, Molete, PO Box 566, Ibadan, Oyo State; 11 Jingiri Rd, PMB 2246, Jos, Plateau State; Warama House, 17D Civic Centre, PO Box 804, Kano; 39A Siluko Rd, PMB 1139, Benin City, Bendel State; 30 Haruna St, PMB 1573, Onitsha, Anambra State; 66 Jubilee Rd, PMB 7133, Aba, Imo State
Principal Bankers: Union Bank of Nigeria Ltd

MORPOL INDUSTRIAL CORPORATION LTD

PO Box 187, 4 Warehouse Rd, Apapa, Lagos
Tel: 873201, 876372
Cable: Morcor Lagos
Telex: 21517 Morcor Ng

Chairman: Albert D Paulus
Directors: Malam Ibrahim Abdurrahman Okene (Personnel), Samir D Paulus (Managing), Alhaji M B Nasidi, L T Ogidan, Farouk D Paulus
Senior Executives: Sunday Sanusi (Accounts Manager), Peter Otulu (Stocks Controller),

Samuel Osanyintade (Service Engineer)
PRINCIPAL ACTIVITIES: Building and civil engineering contractors; suppliers of construction equipment filtration equipment and automotive spare parts
Principal Agencies: Braham Millar Group Ltd, UK; Ransomes & Rapier Ltd, UK; Fram Europe Ltd, UK; Inprodex Establishment, Switzerland; Muller S/A Industria e Comm, Brazil; Dresser Industries, Brazil; Kato Machine Company, Japan; Yammar do Brasil S/A, Brazil
Branch Offices: 12 Kodesoh St, Ikeja, Lagos, Tel 962007
Principal Bankers: United Bank for Africa Ltd; Savannah Bank of Nigeria Ltd; National Bank of Nigeria Ltd
Financial Information:

	N'000
Authorised capital	400
Paid-up capital	270
Turnover	3,000

Principal Shareholders: Ibrahim Abdurrahman; Albert D Paulus; L T Ogidan; F D Paulus; Alhaji N B Nasidi
Date of Establishment: 1968
No of Employees: 100

MORRIS, PHILIP, NIGERIA LTD

International Cigarette Company Ltd

PO Box 524, Commercial House, 1/11 Commercial Ave, Yaba, Lagos
Tel: 800250/2
Cable: Philmorris Lagos
Telex: 21123 Lagos; 33128 Ilorin

Chairman: Chief G K J Amachree
Directors: G H Courtier (Vice-Chairman and Managing Director), A Ayida, Mallam M I Yahaya, R W Murray, H H Schedel, O O Ajayi (Leaf Controller), E G Charnaud (Marketing Manager)
Senior Executives: H Tabel (Manufacturing Manager), S B O Rhodes (Head of Corporate Affairs), J A Ibidapo (Company Secretary), A Akinyemi (Personnel Controller)

PRINCIPAL ACTIVITIES: Manufacturing of cigarettes
Branch Offices: Ibadan; Enugu; Kano; Port Harcourt; Kaduna; Jos; Benin; Maiduguri; Factory: Industrial Area, Offa Rd, PO Box 106, Ilorin, Kwara State, Tel 2294, Telex 33128 Morris Ng; Leaf Office: PO Box 107, Zaria, Tel 2478, 2611
Principal Bankers: Union Bank of Nigeria Ltd
Financial Information:

	N'000
Authorised capital	7,750
Paid-up capital	7,734
Turnover (approx)	15,000
Profits (approx)	500

Principal Shareholders: Philip Morris Inc, New York; Northern Nigeria Investments Ltd
Date of Establishment: 1969
No of Employees: 900

MOSHESHE GROUP OF COMPANIES

A22 Warri/Sapele Rd, Effurun, PO Box 552, Warri, Bendel State
Tel: 232553
Telex: 43297 Mogeme Ng

PRINCIPAL ACTIVITIES: Importers of general goods and cement, cold storage and distribution of fish and meat; shipping services, property development, light metal construction; bakeries; motel
Branch Offices: 143 Apapa Rd, PO Box 281, Ebute-Metta, Lagos, Tel 831470; 3 Mosheshe Industrial Ave, Kirikiri Creek, Apapa, Lagos
Associated Companies: Mosheshe (General) Merchants Ltd;

Mosheshe Fisheries Ltd; Mosheshe Motel; Sino Bakery Ltd; Haouchar Bakery Ltd; Casson (Nigeria) Ltd; Mosheshe Shipping Lines Ltd; Mosheshe Property Development Co

MOTHERCAT OVERSEAS (NIGERIA) LTD

PO Box 1244, 13/17 Breadfruit St, Lagos
Tel: 636556
Cable: Mothercat Lagos
Telex: 21019 Cat Ng

Chairman: Dr E O Urhobo
Directors: Z Shammas (Managing Director),
 J Ifidon-Ola,
 T Campbell,
 S Sarkis (Agents),
 E N Nwokoro
Senior Executives: T Threapleton (Area Plant Manager),
 G Bitar (Resident Engineer, Lagos),
 S Sayegh (Resident Engineer, Port Harcourt)

PRINCIPAL ACTIVITIES: Mechanical engineering and contracting
Branch Offices: PO Box 402, Enerhen Rd, Warri, Bendel State; PMB 1214, 42 Ihama St, Benin City, Bendel State; PO Box 617, Trans-Amadi Industrial Layout, Port Harcourt, Rivers State
Associated Companies: Niger Construction Ltd
Principal Bankers: Union Bank of Nigeria Ltd

Principal Shareholders: Mothercat (Overseas) Ltd (40%); Nigeria Economic Welfare Services Ltd (41%); Ministry of Finance Inc, Imo State (17%); Company's Employees (2%)

MOTOR AND GENERAL INSURANCE COMPANY

19 Martins St, Lagos
Tel: 633433
Telex: 21400 Bim Ng

PRINCIPAL ACTIVITIES: Insurance
Branch Offices: 69 Awolowo Rd, Ikoyi, Lagos, Tel 681491

MOTOR PARTS INDUSTRY LTD

233 Apapa Rd, PO Box 198, Apapa, Lagos
Tel: 836131, 831280

Directors: G Cava, C Vegezzi

PRINCIPAL ACTIVITIES: Distributors of spare parts for motor vehicles

MOTOROLA

Communications Division, 28 Creek Rd, PO Box 340, Apapa, Lagos
Tel: 875990, 875549

Directors: Zeev Halperin (Managing Director)
Senior Executives: H Guterman (Communications Engineer)

PRINCIPAL ACTIVITIES: Telecommunications and power
Branch Offices: PO Box 637, Port Harcourt, Tel 21470

MOTORWAYS NIGERIA LTD

SW8/665 Ijebu Bye-Pass, Oke-Ado, PMB 5359, Ibadan, Oyo State
Tel: 411129
Cable: Motorways Ibadan
Telex: 31145 Motorba Ng

PRINCIPAL ACTIVITIES: Distributors and services of commercial and municipal vehicles and spare parts; dealers in industrial and precision machinery, agricultural equipment and hand tools
Branch Offices: PO Box 6, Yaba, Lagos, Tel 844803; 102 Ikorodu Rd, Igbobi; Ikosi Rd, Oregun Industrial Estate, Oregun

MOUKARIM INDUSTRIES LTD

Industrial Area, Keffi Rd, PO Box 54, Kaduna South
Tel: 210743
Cable: Moukind
Telex: 71150 Mokind Ng

PRINCIPAL ACTIVITIES: Furniture manufacturers, steel containers and structures, subsidiary companies that deal with bedding, air-conditioning, wholesale supplies of large and small electrical appliances
Principal Bankers: Barclays Bank Nigeria Ltd

MOUKARIM METALWOOD FACTORY LTD

51 Sharada Industrial Estate, PO Box 602, Kano
Tel: 4051, 5106, 4845, 3204, 2493
Cable: Moukarim Kano
Telex: 77140 Mouka Ng

Directors: A F Moukarim

PRINCIPAL ACTIVITIES: Engineering; manufacturers of steel structures, windows, doors, etc; metal and wood furniture, etc
Branch Offices: PO Box 160, Ikeja, Lagos State, Tel 962480; PO Box 160, Oregun, Tel 934789; PO Box 33, Katsina; PO Box 482, Jos
Associated Companies: Borneo Engineering & Steel Manufacturers Ltd

MOULDEX LTD

PMB 21622, Ikeja, 22 D Ogundipe Rd, Maryland Village, Lagos State
Tel: 960426
Telex: 26875 Mouldex Ng

Chairman: A A Akintola

PRINCIPAL ACTIVITIES: Production, installation and service of diesel electric generating sets, production and marketing of diesel welders and diesel waterpumps, marketing of welding transformers and industrial hoses
Principal Agencies: Birnbaum Export GmbH, West Germany; Kleber, France; Petzetakin, Greece
Principal Bankers: Nigeria Arab Bank; Nigeria-American Merchant Bank
Financial Information:

	N'000
Authorised capital	400
Paid-up capital	100
Turnover	2,000

Date of Establishment: 1971
No of Employees: 50

MRT CONSULTING ENGINEERS (NIGERIA) LTD

2nd Floor, 20 Johnson Street, Off Coker Rd, Ilupeju, PO Box 3188, Lagos
Tel: 631014
Cable: Meritcon Lagos
Telex: 21383 Edetma

Chairman: Ahmed Joda
Directors: G F Albany Ward (Managing),
 Dr J O Sonuga,
 G Courtney,
 T S Kowobari,
 E M T Powell,
 A J Price,
 Dr F I Soribe (Deputy Managing Director),
 M I Ufoeze

PRINCIPAL ACTIVITIES: Engineering consultants
Branch Offices: 13B Ahmadu Bello Way, PO Box 1620, Kano; PMB 2251, Sokoto; PMB 1089, Maiduguri; PMB 104, Gombe
Associated Companies: Sir M Macdonald & Partners Ltd; Mott, Hay & Anderson International Ltd; Enplan Group; John Taylor & Sons; Rendel, Palmer & Tritton

Principal Bankers: Union Bank Nigeria Ltd

Date of Establishment: 1972

No of Employees: 540

MUKORO, MARTIN, CONSTRUCTION COMPANY

138 Oladipo St, Mushin-West, Lagos

Tel: 844680

Chairman: Chief Martin M Emretiyoma

Directors: S O Babatunde, S K Emretiyoma, A M Egoh, Miss Patricia E Emretiyoma

Senior Executives: J W Ovien (Administrative Manager/Public Relations Office),
George Teichert (Chief Engineer),
S Ndugbaghwa (Accountant),
Y Emretiyoma (Supervisor)

PRINCIPAL ACTIVITIES: Civil engineering and construction

Branch Offices: Km 28 Badagry Expressway, Lagos

Associated Companies: Mamco Services Ltd

Principal Bankers: United Bank for Africa; African Continental Bank Ltd; New Nigeria Bank Ltd

Financial Information:

	N'000
Authorised capital	200
Paid-up capital	86
Turnover	2,500

Principal Shareholders: M M Emretiyoma; S K Emretiyoma; P Emretiyoma

Date of Establishment: 2nd July 1971

No of Employees: 500

MULTI ALUMINIUM MANUFACTURING COMPANY LTD
MULMACO

PO Box 47, Mushin, Lagos

Tel: 935512, 935733

PRINCIPAL ACTIVITIES: Manufacturers of aluminium sheets for roofing and cladding; earthenware household utensils

Branch Offices: Factory: 6 Coker St, Orile, Agege, Lagos State

MULTIMALT LTD

Berti, Tin Can Island Port, Apapa, Lagos

Tel: 610915

Telex: 21833 Tincan

Chairman: Chief J Akin-George

Directors: Chief A O Rewane,
R J Haythornethwaite,
D W Ringrose,
Alhaji A Dahiru,
E Enwerem,
J A Odeyemi (alternate),
T Dediare (alternate)

Senior Executives: C D Earley (General Manager)

PRINCIPAL ACTIVITIES: Importation, storage and distribution of malt in bulk to the brewery and allied trades

Principal Bankers: First Bank of Nigeria Ltd

Date of Establishment: Incorpoated February 1977, Date of Operation October 1982

MUNRO, BRIAN, LTD

PO Box 261, 22b Creek Rd, Apapa, Lagos

Tel: 876110, 876157

Cable: Brimun

Chairman: Chief Ayo Rosiji

Directors: S K G Powell (Managing Director),
N J Rapp,
E Kanu,
S Oni

PRINCIPAL ACTIVITIES: Distribution of all foodstuffs

Principal Agencies: Colgate Palmolive, UK; John Walker & Sons Ltd; UK; Unigate, UK; Reckitt & Coleman, UK; General Foods, USA; Bovril, UK; Spillers; Smedley HP Foods; Cross Paperware

Branch Offices: Ghana; Sierra Leone

Principal Bankers: Savannah Bank Ltd; United Bank for Africa Ltd

MUSA, ALHAJI SANI, & SONS

25 Adakawa St, PO Box 345, Kano

Tel: 3811

PRINCIPAL ACTIVITIES: General contractors and transporters; concrete block manufacturers

N VIKTORS INTERNATIONAL AGENCIES

See VIKTORS, N, INTERNATIONAL AGENCIES

NAAFCO (SCIENTIFIC SUPPLIES) LTD

Plot 56, Akanbi Onitiri Close, PO Box 2734, Lagos

Tel: 835975, 832340

Cable: Naafco Lagos

Chairman: F O Ogunlana

Directors: M A Aboderin,
J B F Haller,
J E Jackson (General Manager),
J C Z Martin,
C R Schaefer,
A B Umar,
O O Bello (Sales),
Professer M O Kayode

Senior Executives: S O Okubote (Chief Accountant),
E C Ekpo (Purchasing/Distribution Manager),
P O Bojeghre (Technical Service Manager)

PRINCIPAL ACTIVITIES: Suppliers of scientific instruments for education, research, and industry

Principal Agencies: Naafco, USA; Corning Ltd, UK; A Gallenkamp, UK; Philip Harris Ltd, UK; Edwards High Vacuum, UK; BDH Chemicals Ltd, UK; G H Zeal Ltd, UK; Griffin & George Ltd, UK; Manesty Machines Ltd, UK etc

Branch Offices: 47 Port Harcourt Rd, PO Box 321, Aba; SW8/101 Ijebu Bye Pass, Ibadan; 40 Niger St, PO Box 1785, Kano

Associated Companies: A Gallenkamp, UK; Philip Harris, UK

Principal Bankers: United Bank for Africa Ltd

Financial Information:

	N'000
Authorised capital	2,000
Paid-up capital	2,000
Sales turnover	6,000

Principal Shareholders: Rockabrand Corporation, USA; A Gallenkamp & Co Ltd, UK; Philip Harris Holdings Ltd, UK; Frederich Holdings Ltd, Nigeria; Rafco International Ltd, Nigeria; Universal Holdings Ltd, Nigeria; Cool Penny (Nig) Ltd

Date of Establishment: 1962

No of Employees: 140

NABENA, BENJAMIN, NABENSON PROMOTIONS

90 Kirikiri Rd, Olodi-Apapa, Lagos State

Tel: 333857

Chairman: Benjamin K Nabena

Directors: Ebisiro R Nabena, Miss Ebilayifa M Nabena, Ndukagpo Y Nabena, Harcourt L Nabena

Senior Executives: Peter Ngere (Secretary),
Samuel Akaluwa (Electrical Engineer),
George Efeludu (Civil Engineer),
Edward Wemigha (Public Relations Officer),
A Nabena (Sales Manager)

PRINCIPAL ACTIVITIES: Agents and general trading; suppliers of building materials/cement; Civil engineering and construction; educational equipment; electrical equipment and electronics; office equipment/supplies; real estate; consultants; mechanical engineering
Branch Offices: 19 Harbour Rd, Port Harcourt, River-State; 26/28 Mbonu St, D/Line, Port Harcourt, Rivers-State; Tel 333857
Principal Bankers: Bank of the North

Principal Shareholders: Chairman and directors as described
Date of Establishment: 5th October 1968

NABENA, L R, & SONS LTD
90 Kirikiri Rd, Olodi-Apapa, Lagos State
Tel: 333857

Chairman: Benjamin K Nabena
Directors: George K Nabena, Patricia M Nabena
Senior Executives: W A Nabena (Accountant),
    B Opukeme (Administrative Manager),
    N Isu (Architect),
    F I Eguaoje (Civil Engineer)

PRINCIPAL ACTIVITIES: Civil engineering and construction; transporters; suppliers of building materials, hardware; industrial equipment; timber; real estate agency; engineering consultants
Branch Offices: 19 Harbour Rd, Port Harcourt, Rivers State; 26 Mbonu St, D/Line, Port Harcourt, Rivers State, Tel 333857
Principal Bankers: Bank of the North; Pan African Bank; United Bank for Africa Ltd

Principal Shareholders: Chairman and directors as described
Date of Establishment: 18th May 1972
No of Employees: 150

NACO NIGERIA LTD
Behind Leventis Motors, PO Box 108, Apapa, Lagos
Tel: 876564, 876950
Cable: Apapanac

Chairman: D O Dafinone
Directors: M C M Thorpe (Managing),
    Mrs D B A Kuforiji,
    A Ainsworth,
    D E Davey,
    G D Harding
Senior Executives: S A Fadare (General Manager),
    M O Makanjuola (Field Sales Manager, Nigeria),
    A Dixon (Technical Manager),
    J O Afisunlu (Accountant)

PRINCIPAL ACTIVITIES: Metal fabrication in steel and aluminium, aluminium and steel windows and doors
Branch Offices: PMB 1181, Benin City, Bendel State; PO Box 302, Jos, Plateau State; PMB 1274, Maiduguri, Borno State; PO Box 233, Calabar, Cross River State; PO Box 1323, Aba, Imo State; PO Box 2165, Kano; PO Box 93, Ilorin, Kwara State; Also Ibadan; Akure; Kaduna
Principal Bankers: First Bank of Nigeria Ltd

Principal Shareholders: VYB (Nigeria) Ltd; Pillar Industries Pty Ltd
No of Employees: 245

NAGARTA DRUG COMPANY LTD
BZ172 Junction Rd, PO Box 678, Kaduna
Tel: 210809
Cable: Nagadrug Kaduna

Directors: K Sambo (Managing Director)

PRINCIPAL ACTIVITIES: Distributors of pharmaceutical and veterinary products, surgical and hospital equipment
Branch Offices: 5-A Suzi Gardens, PO Box 742, Jos

NAILS & GENERAL STEEL MANUFACTURING INDUSTRY LTD
Onwuka Interbiz House, 27 Ikorodu Rd, Yaba, Lagos
Tel: 861014
Telex: 26685

PRINCIPAL ACTIVITIES: Manufacturers of nails, wire etc

NAL MERCHANT BANK LTD
Bookshop House, 50/52 Broad Street, PO Box 2432, Lagos
Tel: 600222, 633294, 635843, 600420/9
Cable: Acceptor, Lagos
Telex: 21505 Accepto Ng

Chairman: Alhaji M O Atta
Directors: W L Gunlicks (Vice Chairman),
    Chief O A Adeosun (Managing Director & Chief Executive),
    K S Tenny (Deputy Managing Director),
    D Anyanechi,
    C E Ekpiken,
    Chief G A Esan,
    O Lijadu,
    H B Mohammed,
    I C Ogbue,
    D R Simpson
Senior Executives: O K Belo (General Manager - Capital Issues, Trustees and Investment Department),
    Brian Kurtz (General Manager, Credit II),
    J A Oyetan (General Manager, Credit I),
    J O Fatinikun (Company Secretary/Deputy General Manager, Staff)

PRINCIPAL ACTIVITIES: Merchant banking: including banking services; corporate finance; bonds; loan stock and issue of equities; investment advisory service and portfolio management
Branch Offices: Imam House, Ahmadu Bello Way, PMB 2172, Kaduna, Tel 213667, 242476; 19 Onitsha Rd, Owerri, Tel 230363
Subsidiary/Associated Companies: Nigerian Stock Brokers Ltd, Lagos; Continental Illinois National Bank & Trust Company of Chicago
Principal Bankers: Central Bank of Nigeria Ltd; Union Bank of Nigeria Ltd
Financial Information: As at 31st March 1982

	₦'000
Authorised capital	7,500
Paid-up capital	4,900
Profits (unaudited)	6,425

Principal Shareholders: Federal Ministry of Finance Incorporated; National Insurance Corporation of Nigeria; New Nigeria Development Corporation; Continental Bank of Chicago; Credit Lyonais; John Holt Investment Ltd; John Holt Holdings Nigeria Ltd
Date of Establishment: 25th November 1960 (Formerly Nigerian Acceptances Ltd)
No of Employees: 188

NAMCO NIGERIA LTD
66/7 Fagge ta Gabas, Hadejia Rd, Dantata House, PO Box 84, Kano
Tel: 4054/5
Telex: 77146

PRINCIPAL ACTIVITIES: Suppliers of electronic equipment, generating sets, etc
Principal Agencies: Thomas W Ward Ltd, UK

NAPAK SERVICES (NIGERIA) LTD
63 Akogun St, PMB 1213, Apapa, Lagos
Tel: 961659, 963427
Cable: Napservis, Lagos

Chairman: S O Adebakin
Directors: Chief E O Adebaki
Senior Executives: A O Odubayo (Senior Accountant),
    M O Yesufu (Administrative Manager)

PRINCIPAL ACTIVITIES: Internaional shipping, air freighting, forwarding and clearing agents; general traders
Branch Offices: 16 Ladipo St, PMB 1213, Apapa, Lagos; Murtala Mohammed International Airport, PO Box 232, Ikeja, Lagos; 360B Airport Rd, PMB 3226, Kano; 14 Industrial Rd, PO Box 736, Port Harcourt; NPA Yard, PMB 1097, Warri
Principal Bankers: United Bank for Africa Ltd
Financial Information:

	₦'000
Authorised capital	500
Paid-up capital	500
Turnover	1,300

Principal Shareholders: S O Adebakin
Date of Establishment: 18th October, 1971
No of Employees: 200

NARUMAL & SONS (NIGERIA) LTD

65 Marina, PO Box 1300, Lagos
Tel: 653427, 658947
Cable: Khizmat
Telex: 21453 Sonnar Ng; 21588 Somoco Ng

Chairman: S N Jethwani
Directors: I M Bharwani, T K Surendran, J A Cole, Alhaji Sule Katagum, G K Ola
Senior Executives: Jagdish Chandra Sethi (General Manager),
V I Bhandari (Production Manager),
C S Srinivasan (Data Processing Manager),
A K Sen (Deputy Data Processing Manager),
K Sadhuram (Wholesale Manager),
E Larmie (Programmer/Analyst),
J I K Edu (Senior Internal Auditor),
B D Pai (Financial Controller)

PRINCIPAL ACTIVITIES: Data processing and tabulating services, manufacturing of textiles; storage, warehousing, cold storage
Branch Offices: Factory: Oregun Industrial Estate, PO Box 1149, Ikeja, Lagos, Tel 932740, 933559
Principal Bankers: International Merchant Bank Nigeria Ltd; New Nigeria Bank ltd
Financial Information:

	₦'000
Authorised capital	1,000
Paid-up capital	1,000

Principal Shareholders: Sonnar (Jersey) Inc, Jersey; Channel Islands (60%); J A Cole; Dr J A Sodipo; Alhaji Sule Katagum (40%)
Date of Establishment: 4th April 1962
No of Employees: 250

NASCO BISCUITS (NIGERIA) LTD

Formerly Benue Plateau Biscuits Co Ltd

Bukuru Rd, PO Box 576, Jos, Plateau State
Tel: 52551/2
Cable: Biscuits Jos
Telex: 81127

Chairman: Ahmed Nasreddin
Directors: Abdulrahim I Nasreddin, Saleh I Nasreddin, Plateau Investment Company Ltd, Attia A Nasreddin
Senior Executives: Kamal Kamel (General Manager),
Nath Madueke (Commercial Manager),
Stephen Yepwi (Personnel Manager),
Fazal Mahmood (Finance Manager),
Y M E Anwar (Production Manager),
A H Tawfik (Technical Manager)

PRINCIPAL ACTIVITIES: Food and food processing; manufacturers of assorted types of biscuits
Subsidiary Companies: Household Products (Nig) Ltd; Nasco Pack (Nigeria) Ltd; Northern Nigeria Fibre Products Ltd
Principal Bankers: First Bank of Nigeria Ltd

Principal Shareholders: Nasreddin Group International & Plateau

Investment Co Ltd, Jos
Date of Establishment: April 1974
No of Employees: 600

NASCO ESTATE COMPANY (NIGERIA) LTD

PO Box 261, Apapa, Lagos
Tel: 874238
Telex: 21513

PRINCIPAL ACTIVITIES: Estate development and management

Principal Shareholders: Part of the Nasreddin Group International Ltd

NASCO PACK LTD

Formerly Benue Plateau Packages Ltd

Bukuru Rd, PO Box 6286, Jos, Plateau State
Tel: 55707, 54093
Cable: Naspack Jos
Telex: 81127 Nascos Ng

PRINCIPAL ACTIVITIES: Manufacturers of packaging

Principal Shareholders: Part of the Nasreddin Group International Ltd

NASREDDIN GROUP INTERNATIONAL (NIGERIA) LTD

PMB 2722, Old Airport Junction, Yakubu Gowon Way, Jos, Plateau State
Tel: 50030
Cable: Nasredd Jos
Telex: 81127 Nascos Ng

Chairman: Ahmed Idris Nasreddin
Directors: Abdurrahim Idris Nasreddin, Saleh Idris Nasreddin

PRINCIPAL ACTIVITIES: To provide central administration for the companies under the Group
Branch Offices: 21 Wharf Rd, PO Box 261, Apapa, Tel 870945, 870934, 874238, Telex 21513
Subsidiary Companies: Household Products Ltd (see separate entry); Nasco Biscuits (Nigeria) Ltd (see separate entry); Northern Nigeria Fibre Products Ltd; Nascon (Nig) Ltd (Construction); Fimsa (Nig) Ltd; Nasbro Trading Company Ltd; Nasco Pack Ltd (see separate entry); Nasco Estate Company (Nigeria) Ltd (see separate entry)
Principal Bankers: First Bank of Nigeria Ltd; Union Bank of Nigeria Ltd
Financial Information:

	₦'000
Authorised capital	6,850
Paid-up capital	6,850
Sales turnover	30,000
Profits	2,500

Principal Shareholders: Nasreddin Company SAS, Milan; New Nigeria Development Company Ltd, Kaduna; Government of Plateau State, Jos
No of Employees: 4,000

NASSAR, S, & SONS (NIGERIA) LTD

20 Abibu Oki St, PO Box 541, Lagos
Tel: 637117, 657195

PRINCIPAL ACTIVITIES: Investment company

NATA'ATA, ALHAJI, AND SONS

B340, Wunti St, Bauchi
PRINCIPAL ACTIVITIES: Tin mining

NATIONAL BANK OF NIGERIA LTD

82/86 Broad St, PMB 12123, Lagos
Tel: 662438, 662840
Cable: Nationbank (Branches in Nigeria), Natbaniger (London)
Telex: 21348 Nabank; 884462 Natbaniger London

Chairman: Chief Michael Adedapo Omisade
Directors: Samson Olatunde Banjo (Managing Director),
 Joseph Akinwumi Ogunbiyi,
 Reuben Olorunfemi Adewusi (Deputy Managing),
 M A Adeniran,
 G L Oyawala,
 Chief Femi Oyebanjo,
 Tunde Oyefodunrin,
 J O Tuki
Senior Executives: Olufunmiso Babafemi Ewedemi (Staff Director
 of Finance),
 C T A Milton-Job (Staff Director, Operations),
 Leye Ajayi (Staff Director, Administration and Service)

PRINCIPAL ACTIVITIES: General commercial banking
Branch Offices: 32 Balogun St, PMB 12123, Lagos, Tel 664299,
 661341; Cocoa House, 16th Floor, PO Box 5086, Ibadan; 86
 Broad St, PMB 800, Akure; 2B Akpakpava Rd, PMB 1031,
 Benin City; 1B Niger Rd, PO Box 100, Kano; 2 Devonshire
 Square, London EC2M 4TA
Associated Companies: Glanvil Enthoven and Company Nigeria
 Ltd
Financial Information:

	N'000
Authorised capital	15,000
Paid-up capital	10,000
Profits	8,000

Principal Shareholders: Governments of Oyo (44%); Ondo (31%)
 and Ogun States (25%); Minority founder shareholders
Date of Establishment: 11th February 1933
No of Employees: 3,700

NATIONAL CASH REGISTER (WA) LTD
NCR

6 Broad St, PO Box 509, Lagos
Tel: 634217, 634287, 634358
Cable: Nacareco Lagos
Telex: 21108 NCR Ng

Chairman: A S Gillan
Directors: George E Ellis (Managing),
 O O Adebule,
 M R Chukwuedo,
 P C Akujobi,
 W S Anderson,
 J E Rambo,
 P Kilmartin

PRINCIPAL ACTIVITIES: Suppliers of office equipment, and
 complete computer systems; cash registering systems and
 equipment; printers. There are plans to build a paper roll
 manufacturing plant and a rotary press for the production of
 computer stationery
Principal Agencies: NCR Corp, USA
Principal Bankers: First Bank of Nigeria Ltd; United Bank for
 Africa Ltd; International Bank for West Africa Ltd

Date of Establishment: 9th December 1949
No of Employees: 368

NATIONAL ELECTRIC POWER AUTHORITY
(NEPA)

24-25 Marina, PMB 12030, Lagos
Tel: 651370, 650563

Directors: Alhaji Mohammed Tata Askira (General Manager),
 M M Kafaru (Assistant General Manager)

PRINCIPAL ACTIVITIES: Generation, transmission and
 distribution of electric power
Financial Information: Government body

NATIONAL FREIGHT COMPANY

21 Inuwa Abdulkadir Rd, Industrial Layout, PMB 2175, Kaduna
 South, Kaduna
Tel: 216992
Telex: 71128 Nafco

Chairman: Alhaji Bello Alkamawa
Directors: Alhaji Saidu Isa Balarabe,
 E O Ologunde,
 Chief James Spiff,
 D F Babalola,
 M O Onoja,
 Alhaji Abubakar Ladan (General Manager)
Senior Executives: Olukayode Bawa-Allah (Assistant General
 Manager, Operations),
 J I Audu (Assistant General Manager, Technical Service)

PRINCIPAL ACTIVITIES: Transporters; freight forwarders
Principal Bankers: Societe Generale Bank; Bank of the North
 Ltd; United Bank for Africa Ltd
Financial Information:

	N'000
Authorised capital	2,500
Paid-up capital	2,500
Turnover	6,400

Principal Shareholders: Wholly owned by the Federal
 Government
Date of Establishment: 1976
No of Employees: 874

NATIONAL GRAINS PRODUCTION COMPANY
LTD

Grains House, Ali Akilu Rd, PMB 2182, Kaduna
Tel: 243407
Cable: Grains Kaduna
Telex: 71305 Nagren Ng

Chairman: V G Sanda
Directors: Alhaji Kasimu Aliyu, Alhaji Abu Dagawa, Alhaji Waziri
 Duci Kura, U G Otu, E C Unachukwu
Senior Executives: Alhaji M Alkali (General Manager),
 D E Oyakhilome (Assistant General Manager),
 H M Fernando (Chief Accountant & Financial/Company
 Secretarial Adviser),
 B F Iyiola (Chief Storage Manager),
 Alhaji M M Dambala (Company Secretary)

PRINCIPAL ACTIVITIES: Production, storage, processing and
 marketing of grains such as cereal grain (maize, sorghum,
 rice) and grain vegetables (cowpeas, soyabeans, etc) grain
 flour and breakfast cereal; animal feeds processing and
 raising of stock
Branch Offices: Integrated large scale mechanised farm project
 at Mokwa in Niger State; maize and rice project at Kazuntu in
 Kaduna State; rice project at Jesse in Bendel State; grain
 processing mill at Kaduna in Kaduna State
Subsidiary Companies: Jema'a Mechanised Farms Ltd; Ilero
 Mechanised Farms Ltd; Bansara Rice Farms Ltd; Imo Grain
 Farms Ltd; Gaya Mech Farms Ltd; Ondo Mech Farms Ltd;
 Ogun Farms Ltd; Maiwa Mechanised Farms Ltd
Principal Bankers: First Bank of Nigeria Ltd; United Bank for
 Africa Ltd; Union Bank of Nigeria Ltd; Societe Generale Bank
 (Nig) Ltd
Financial Information:

	N'000
Authorised capital	10,000
Paid-up capital	1,959

Principal Shareholders: Federal Government of Nigeria
Date of Establishment: 1975
No of Employees: 174

NATIONAL INSURANCE CORPORATION OF
NIGERIA
NICON

96/102 Broad St, PO Box 1100, Lagos
Tel: 662708
Cable: Nicon Lagos
Telex: 22651

Chairman: Barrister Y Shantali
Directors: O Adejuwon,
 Dr Sa'ad Abubakar,

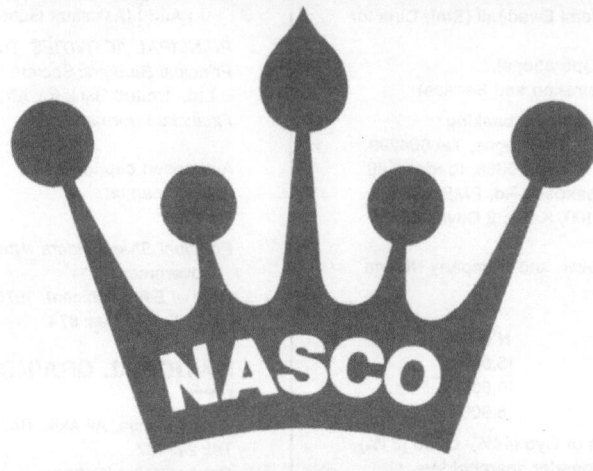

Chief C Imegwu,
O Lijadu (Managing),
Chief S A Ajayi,
J U Edozie,
Hajiya Binta Maisango
Senior Executives: N A Adewuyi (General Manager, Technical),
J O Farodoye (General Manager, Finance and Administration),
I C Ogbue (General Manager Staff Development and
Training),
B A Lawson (Deputy General Manager, Production)

PRINCIPAL ACTIVITIES: Insurance
Branch Offices: PMB 2036, Kaduna, Tel 212880, 211935; PO
Box 340, Enugu, Tel 255632; PMB 5452, Ibadan, Tel 410046;
13B Post Office Rd, Kano, Tel 5356; PMB 2085, Jos, Plateau
State; PMB 1255, Maiduguri, Borno State; Kingsway House,
PMB 1343, Benin City, Bendel State, Tel 240521; 45 Bedwell
St, PO Box 972, Calabar, Cross River State, Tel 222241;
Ahmadu Bello Way, Opposite Gusau Garage, PO Box 815,
Sokoto; 38 Murtala Mohammed Rd, Ilorin, Kwara State; 24
Ikwerre Rd, Port Harcourt, Rivers State, Tel 331419; PMB
7100, Aba, Imo State; 43 Okigwe Rd, Owerri, Imo State; PO
Box 1214, Akure, Ondo State; PO Box 2397, Abeokuta, Ogun
State; PO Box 1277, Makurdi, Benue State; PO Box 1210,
Yola, Gongola State; PO Box 1079, Minna, Niger State
Subsidiary Companies: Niger Insurance Co Ltd; National
Properties Ltd
Principal Bankers: United Bank for Africa Ltd; National Bank of
Nigeria Ltd; Central Bank of Nigeria; Societe Generale Bank
(Nigeria) Ltd; Bank of the North Ltd
Financial Information:

	₦'000
Authorised capital	10,000
Paid-up capital	10,000
Gross premium	56,200
Profits	8,600

Principal Shareholders: Federal Government of Nigeria
Date of Establishment: 1st July 1969
No of Employees: 827

NATIONAL MOTORS (NIGERIA) LTD
PO Box 12011, Ebute-Metta, Lagos

PRINCIPAL ACTIVITIES: Suppliers of automobiles, trucks, spare
parts, etc

NATIONAL OIL AND CHEMICAL MARKETING COMPANY LTD
38/39 Marina, Eagle House, PMB 2052, Lagos
Tel: 662313, 660070, 663290
Cable: Nolchem Lagos
Telex: 21235 Nolchem Lagos

Chairman: M A Gbegbaje
Directors: I J D Durlong, S M Akpe, K S Atkinson, J
Cordingley
Senior Executives: M O Akanbi (General Manager/Chief
Executive),
E I Okoye (Sales Manager),
I B Ekarika (Chemicals Manager),
A O Onafuwa (Administrative Manager),
S A Makinwa (Finance Manager),
S I C Okoli (Operations Manager)

PRINCIPAL ACTIVITIES: Marketing of petroleum and refined
petroleum products, agricultural, industrial and domestic
chemicals; plastics
Branch Offices: PO Box 45, Apapa, Tel 873453 (Installation
Manager); Installation Yard, Apapa, Tel 873510, 873601,
873672, 873936, 873628, 873723, 873794, 873865, 873537;
(Bitumen Plant), Apapa, Tel 875867; Chief Engineer, Apapa,
Tel 873537; Purchasing & Stores Section, Apapa, Tel 873137;
PO Box 360, Benin City, Tel 249451; PO Box 189, Calabar,
Tel 222268; Upper Ogui Rd, PO Box 681, Enugu, Tel
253338/9; National Oil Depot, Gusau, Tel 4233; PO Box 401,
Ibadan, Tel 462790/1/2; Murtala Muhammed Airport, Ikeja
(Domestic) Tel 961746; Murtala Muhammed Airport, Ikeja

(International) Tel 901082, 901351, 834201, 861394, 834206;
PO Box 36, Jebba, Tel 9; Jingiri Rd, PMB 30, Jos, Tel 2326,
2897, 2822; Kakuri Rd, PMB 2053, Kaduna, Tel 210911,
210932, 211404; PMB 3012, Airport Rd, Kano, Tel 4316,
4662, 4317; Northern Aviation Field Manager, Kano Airport,
Tel 2575; PO Box 164, Maiduguri, Tel 2516; PO Box 28,
Reclamation Rd, Port Harcourt, Tel 225151, 225181; PMB
1023, Warri, Tel 233465; 17 Industrial Ave, Illupeju Estate,
Lagos, Tel 962226; PMB 66, Gombe
Principal Bankers: Union Bank of Nigeria Ltd; First Bank of
Nigeria Ltd; United Bank for Africa Ltd; International
Merchant Bank Ltd; Icon Ltd

Principal Shareholders: Nigerian National Petroleum
Corporation; Shell International Petroleum Company; Asiatic
Petroleum Company
Date of Establishment: 30th June 1970
No of Employees: 1,500

NATIONAL ROAD CONSTRUCTION COMPANY OF NIGERIA LTD
PMB 1048, 11A Hinderer Rd, Apapa, Lagos

PRINCIPAL ACTIVITIES: Building and civil engineering
contractors

NATIONAL ROOT CROPS PRODUCTION COMPANY LTD
R/8 Independence Layout, PMB 01347, Enugu, Anambra State
Tel: 253134
Cable: 'Roots'
Telex: 51162 Cesmak Ng

Chairman: Chief Dr O A Fagbenro Beyioku
Directors: V E Nwode, A M Tiohn, M A Okoji, Alhaji M B Rijau
Senior Executives: Nelson A Nwosu (General Manager),
John C Obi (Assistant General Manager, Production),
Matthew U Echeozo (Assistant General Manager, Marketing),
Donatus S O Eneh (Financial Controller),
B J Umeh (Company Secretary)

PRINCIPAL ACTIVITIES: Production, purchase, processing,
storage and marketing of root and tuber crops. Mechanised
gari processing at Ugwuoba (Anambra), Mgbirichi (Imo),
Agbor/Alidinma (Bendel) and Ikot Usop (Cross River)
Branch Offices: Area Office, 72 Campbell Street, Lagos; 69
Jebba Street (East), Ebute Metta, Lagos; PMB 2186, Makurdi;
1 Imam Street, Kaduna; PMB 2064, Agbor; PMB 1304,
Owerri; PMB 1207, Ogoja; PMB 1003, Ankpa; PMB 048, Ikot
Abasi, Cross River State
Principal Bankers: First Bank of Nigeria Ltd; African Continental
Bank Ltd; International Bank for West Africa
Financial Information:

	₦'000
Authorised capital	2,000
Paid-up capital	1,200
Turnover (1980 - 9 months)	219
Profits (Net loss 1980)	(1,307)

Principal Shareholders: Ministry of Finance Incorporated
Date of Establishment: Incorporated September 1975, Started
Field Operations April 1976
No of Employees: 331

NATIONAL SALT COMPANY OF NIGERIA LTD
PO Box 5212, Lagos

Senior Executives: R Spallasso (General Manager),
P O Akinyele (Public Relations Manager),
G Savio (Technical Manager)

PRINCIPAL ACTIVITIES: Refining and packing of table salt,
industrial edible salt and agricultural salt
Branch Offices: Location: PO Box 39, Salt City, Ijoko, Near
Sango Otta, Ogun State, Cables Saltcity Lagos, Telex 26257

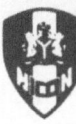
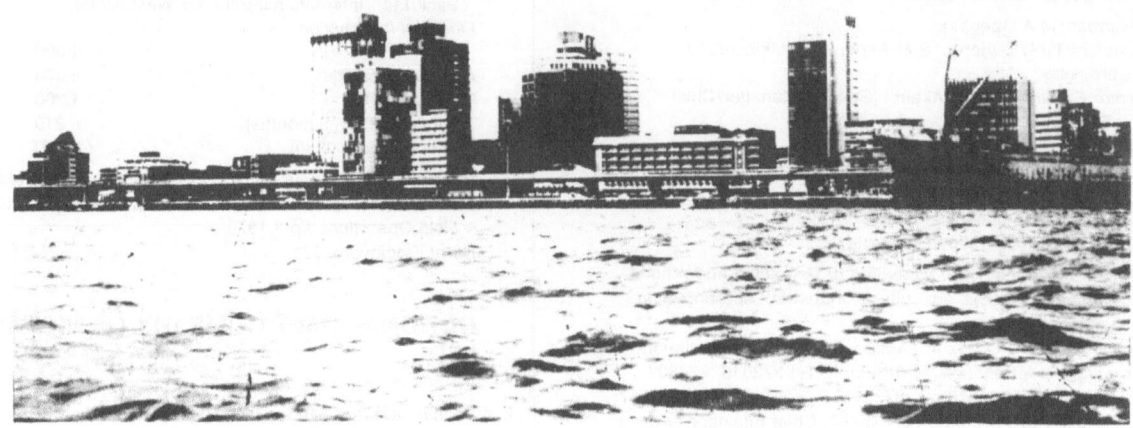

Principal Bankers: First Bank of Nigeria Ltd

Date of Establishment: 1976

No of Employees: 200

NATIONAL TRUCKS MANUFACTURERS LTD

Km 8 Kano-Zaria Rd, Kano

PRINCIPAL ACTIVITIES: When in full production the factory will produce trucks and farm tractors

Principal Shareholders: Federal Government (35%); Kano State (10%); Sokoto State (2.5%); NNDC (2.5%); Private Nigerian Investors and Dealers (10%); Fiat-Iveco (40%)

Date of Establishment: 1975 (Incorporated), June 1980 (Started Production)

No of Employees: 1,800 when in full production

NATIONAL VETERINARY RESEARCH INSTITUTE

PO Vom, Plateau State

Tel: Vom 1

Governing Board: Alhaji Aliyu Zungun

Directors: Dr A G Lamorde

Senior Executives: Dr B Y Owolodun (Assistant Director),
Dr I Umo (Chief Vet Research Officer),
D O Onoviran (Chief Vet Research Officer),
Dr E N Okeke (Chief Vet Research Officer),
Dr M C Njike (Chief Res Officer),
Dr J P Fabiyi (Chief Research Officer),
Dr D R Nawathe (Chief Vet Research Officer),
S D Lot (Admin Secretary)

PRINCIPAL ACTIVITIES: Research and diagnostic services; production of vaccines and sera; training

Date of Establishment: 1924 (Formerly Federal Department of Veterinary Research)

No of Employees: 1,000

NAVARRO INTERNATIONAL (NIGERIA) LTD

48 Isheri Rd, PO Box 182, Ikeja, Lagos

PRINCIPAL ACTIVITIES: Construction

NCIE LTD

Plot 4 Block B, Gbagada Industrial Estate, PO Box 837, Lagos

Tel: 900380

Chairman: J C Emeka

Directors: Alhaji Y Kaltungo, Chief N N Onugu, M Ade, H Hirsch, M O Soremi, D Berger, M Lengfeld, T Dortschy

PRINCIPAL ACTIVITIES: Steel importers

Branch Offices: Throughout Nigeria

Date of Establishment: 1960

No of Employees: 950

NCO MERCHANTS BROTHERS COMPANY

AB2 Ibrahim Taiwo Rd, Kaduna

Chairman: N C Etu

Directors: R O O Odide, A O Egwuronu

Senior Executives: O O Ogbuagu (Financial Controller),
E Otaka (Import Manager),
O C Etu (Distribution Manager)

PRINCIPAL ACTIVITIES: Suppliers of hardware, paper/paper products, plastic/plastic products, textiles and clothing/textile equipment

Branch Offices: 108 Azikiwe Rd, Aba, Imo State; 258 Ehi Rd, Aba, Imo State

Associated Companies: S Omazi and Brothers; O O Ogbuagu and Brothers

Principal Bankers: First Bank of Nigeria Ltd

NDAH, G, & SONS FOUNDATION

1 Aba Rd, PO Box 721, Port Harcourt, Rivers State

Tel: 21816

PRINCIPAL ACTIVITIES: Real estate management; furniture manufacturers; wholesale merchants

NEDLLOYD LINES

42/44 Warehouse Rd, Apapa, PO Box 20, Lagos

Tel: 877582

Cable: Nedship Lagos

Telex: 21261 Nedlld Ng

Senior Executives: Th A R Strauss (Resident Representative)

PRINCIPAL ACTIVITIES: Shipping

Date of Establishment: 1920

NEITAL NIGERIA LTD

PO Box 90, Maiduguri, Borno State

Tel: 232448

Telex: 82105 Ng

Chairman: Alhaji Moh Bello Damaturu

Directors: Dr Saidu Mohammed, Thagama B Kirawa, Alhaji Moh Allamin, Alhaji Hayatu Deen, Bata Mshelia, T O Maduemezia

Senior Executives: K O Ja'Afar (Managing Director),
G Sala (Production Manager)

PRINCIPAL ACTIVITIES: Manufacturers of shoes and leather

Principal Bankers: United Bank for Africa Ltd

Financial Information:

	₦'000
Authorised capital	1,000
Paid-up capital	910
Turnover	2,000

Principal Shareholders: Borno State Government; Effe SPG, Italy

Date of Establishment: 1974

No of Employees: 107

NELSON, THOMAS (NIGERIA) LTD

8 Ilupeju Bye Pass, PMB 21303, Ikeja, Lagos State

Tel: 961452

Cable: Thonelson Ikeja

Chairman: Professor C O Taiwo

Directors: John G Jermine (Deputy Chairman),
Samuel O Daramola (Managing),
Ezekiel B Iyekolo (Marketing),
Seyi Mabogunje (Publishing),
Chief G A Alawode,
Dr F C Ogbalu,
Nicolas Thompson,
Christopher Nott

Senior Executives: William K Tella (Warehouse Manager),
Stephen Oyedemi (Finance Manager)

PRINCIPAL ACTIVITIES: Textbook publishing and warehousing

Principal Agencies: Pitman Publishing Ltd; W H Allen Ltd; Thomas Nelson & Sons Ltd; Van Nostrand Reinhold Co Ltd; Harcourt Brace Jovanovich; Panaf Books Ltd

Branch Offices: 1 Main St, Zaria, Kaduna State; 18A Aba-Owerri Rd, Aba, Imo State

Associated Companies: Thomas Nelson & Sons Ltd, UK

Principal Bankers: Union Bank of Nigeria Ltd

Financial Information:

	₦'000
Authorised capital	501
Paid-up capital	500

Date of Establishment: 1968

NEM INSURANCE COMPANY (NIGERIA) LTD

12/14 Broad St, Lagos

Tel: 600040/5

Cable: Emplomutua Lagos

Telex: 20117 MET TDS FOR BOX 366

Chairman: Alhaji Halliru Abdullahi
Directors: B A Lawson (Managing),
  T R Usher,
  Ibo Wu Sofola
Senior Executives: E K Gasper, N M Onianwah, O A Adebiyi, J U Akaraiu

PRINCIPAL ACTIVITIES: Insurance
Branch Offices: 12/14 Broad Street, PO Box 654, Lagos, Lagos State, Tel: 600040/1-5; 127/129 Obafemi Awolowo Way, PO Box 3280, Ikeja, Lagos State; 6th Floor, Aje House, Lebanon Street, PMB 5328, Ibadan, Oyo State, Tel: 411899, 411992; 1st Floor, African Continental Bank Building, 3 Ogui Rd, PO Box 187, Enugu, Anambra State, Tel: 255556, 252694; 24 Ikwerre Rd, PO Box 1947, Port Harcourt, Rivers State, Tel: 333513; 2/4 Liverpool Avenue, PO Box 415, Zaria, Kaduna State, Tel: 2044; 3rd Floor, 65 Ibrahim Taiwo Rd, PO Box 1185, Kano, Kano State, Tel: 5027; 143 Ikpoba Slope, PMB 1230, Benin-City, Bendel State, Tel: 244905; 2nd Floor, 38 Murtala Muhammed Rd, Ilorin, Kwara State, Tel: 5251; 3rd Floor, 27 Michael's Rd, PO Box 2839, Aba Imo State; 10 Rwang Pam Rd, PO Box 1261, Jos, Plateau State, Tel: 54882
Principal Bankers: United Bank for Africa Ltd
Financial Information:

	N'000
Authorised capital	800
Paid-up capital	800

Date of Establishment: June 1965
No of Employees: 230

NEPTUNE CONSTRUCTIONS LTD

Behind J Berger (Nig) Ltd, Apapa Ikeja Expressway, Kirikiri, Apapa, PO Box 2254, Lagos
Tel: 872932, 872934
Cable: Nepstruct

Chairman: Bola Adeleke
Directors: Alhaji Isa Tahir

Senior Executives: H Mukoro (Accountant),
  R Akinrolabu (Structural Engineer),
  B Shita-Bey (Production Manager),
  A Zara (Contracts Manager)

PRINCIPAL ACTIVITIES: Manufacturers of steel truck bodies; fabrication of steel framed structures; building construction
Principal Agencies: GRS International, UK
Principal Bankers: Savannah Bank (Nig) Ltd
Financial Information:

	N'000
Authorised capital	1,000
Paid-up capital	800
Turnover	3,500
Profits	140

Principal Shareholders: Bola Adelere; Mrs J Bona
Date of Establishment: January 1968
No of Employees: 350

NEPTUNE TRANSPORT SERVICES LTD

21 Wharf Rd, 6th Floor, Development House, PMB 1056, Apapa, Lagos
Tel: 848293
Cable: Neptranser, Lagos

PRINCIPAL ACTIVITIES: Shipping, clearing, forwarding; insurance agents

NETARCOMMS NIGERIA LTD

30 Palace Road, Olodi, Apapa, Lagos State
Tel: 870517, 870507
Telex: 22484, 20117 UK Only

Chairman: Stephen Chiejile (also Chief Executive)

PRINCIPAL ACTIVITIES: Suppliers of electrical goods and communication equipment
Principal Bankers: Savannah Bank of Nigeria Ltd; Societe General Bank Ltd

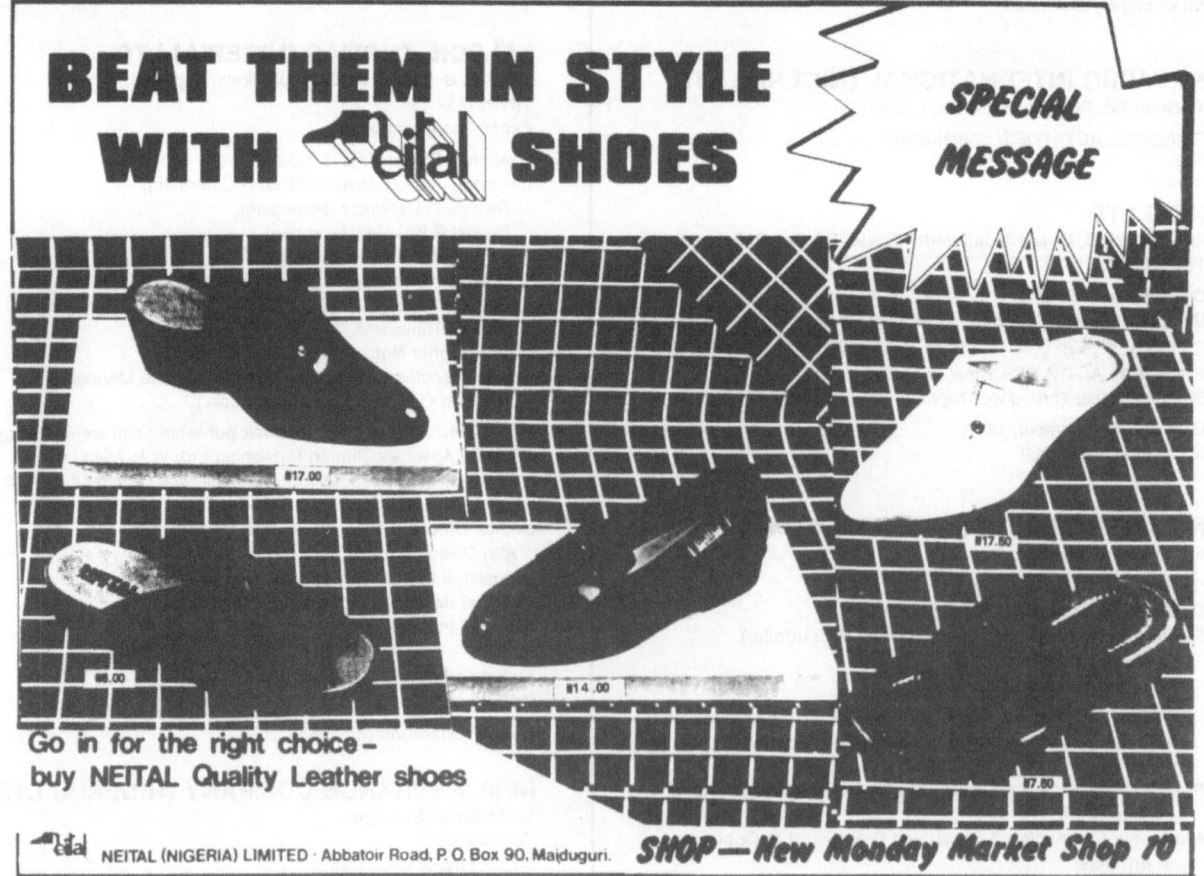

NETHERLANDS HARBOURWORKS (NIGERIA) LTD

Plot 1, Chief Okupe Estate, Maryland, PMB 21086, Ikeja
Tel: 962970
Cable: Builders Ikeja
Telex: 26391 Nehab Ng

Chairman: Chuka J Okoli
Directors: A A Fowora, A V Leeuwen
Senior Executives: M E Versluis (General Manager),
 A C Goeting (Financial Manager),
 H Kos (Technical Logistic Manager)

PRINCIPAL ACTIVITIES: Civil engineers, consultants and
 building contractors
Branch Offices: Ikom Highway, PMB 1232, Calabar, Cross River
 State
Associated Companies: Foundation Engineering (Nigeria) Ltd,
 Ham Dredging (Nigeria) Ltd; Interbeton (Nigeria) Ltd
Principal Bankers: First Bank of Nigeria Ltd
Financial Information:

	N'000
Authorised capital	800
Paid-up capital	800
Turnover	55,000

Principal Shareholders: Hollandsebeton Groep (HBG) (40%);
 Nigerian Shareholders (60%)
Date of Establishment: 1975
No of Employees: 1,250

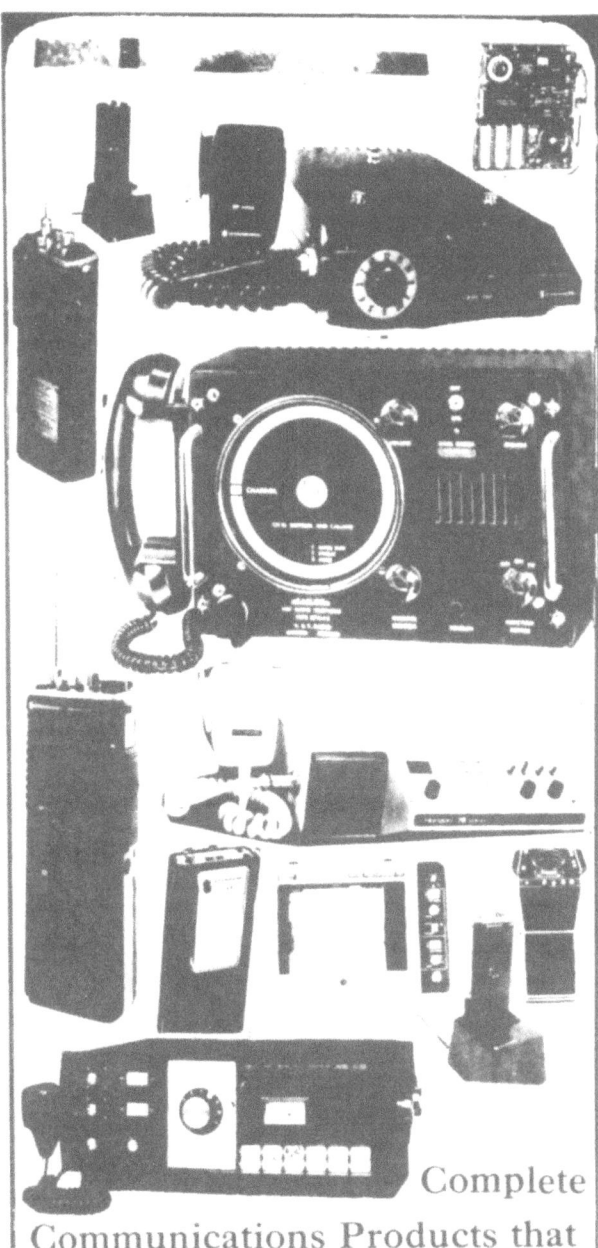

Complete
Communications Products that
work for business and Industry
Sold and Serviced by:-
NETARCOMMS NIG LTD
No 30 Palace Road, Olodi Araromi Apapa,
off Tin Can Island Port Express Way,
PMB 1257 Apapa Post Office,
Telex: 22484 (20117 UK only)
Telephone: 870517 & 870507
We Deal on :-
x Hf SSB Radio telephone for BASE, Mobile & Aircraft.
x VHf / UHf fM.
x Micro Computer for Learning Languages by yourself.
x HRO for purifying salt water to fresh clear drinking water.
x PAGERS.
x Radar for Merchant Vessels.
x Echo Sounder for Fishing & Surveying
x Gyro Compass
Please Contact us for further details and free demonstration.

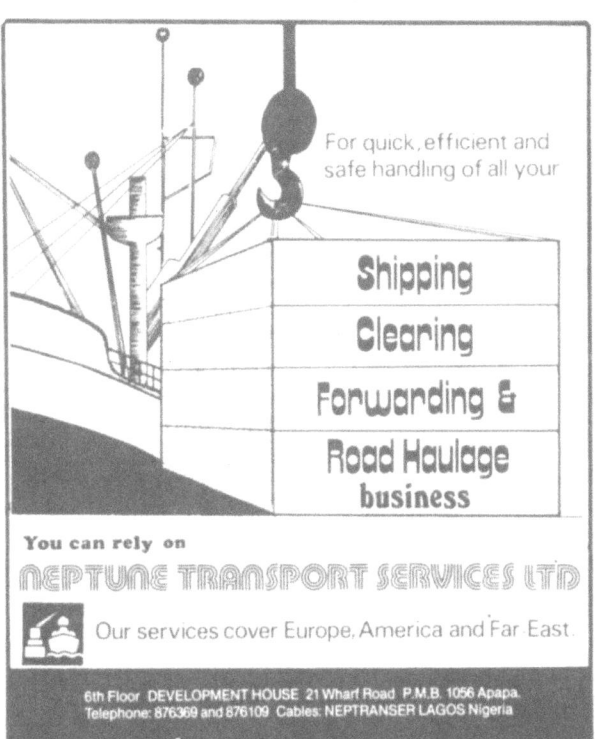

NEVLON PHARMACEUTICAL (REVLON) LTD

Warma Development House, 21 Wharf Rd, Apapa, Lagos
Tel: 876176

Directors: Chief Remi Fami-Kayode

PRINCIPAL ACTIVITIES: Pharmaceuticals and cosmetics

NEW AFRICA DEVELOPMENT COMPANY LTD

37 Marina, Unity House, 12th Floor, PO Box 4256, Lagos
Tel: 662365, 660118
Cable: Monafdec
Telex: 21408 Artin Ng

Chairman: Chief M A Omisade
Directors: Engr L A Okunola, Mrs M F Orafidiya
Senior Executives: Engr L A Okunola (Executive Director),
Patrick Jeribe (Technical Sales Manager),
T A Aboderin (Technical Sales Manager),
M A Alowdoja (Development Manager)
PRINCIPAL ACTIVITIES: Sales representatives; distributors of
electrical materials
Principal Agencies: General Electric Trading Company, USA;
Honeywell Controls Inc, USA; Sierra Research Corporation,
USA
Branch Offices: 15 Agoro Odiyan St, Victoria Island, Lagos, Tel
615728; SW8/105, Okeado, Ibadan, Tel 410550
Principal Bankers: Union Bank of Nigeria Ltd; Icon (Merchant
Bankers) Ltd
Financial Information:

	₦'000
Authorised capital	1,000
Paid-up capital	1,000
Turnover	500,000

Principal Shareholders: M A Omisade
Date of Establishment: 1976
No of Employees: 30

NEW AFRICAN INDUSTRIES LTD

33 Ogedegbe St, Warri, Bendel State
PRINCIPAL ACTIVITIES: Production of crepe rubber

NEW AGENCY OF NIGERIA

National Theatre, Iganmu, PMB 12756, Lagos
Tel: 801290/3
Cable: Nannan Lagos
Telex: 22648

Chairman: Professor Alfred E Opubor
Directors: M O Odebode,
G Bako,
V I Maduka,
Mamman Daura,
I S Moemeke,
Tom Borha,
Hamra Imam,
E O Amona,
J O Nzekwu (General Manager)
Senior Executives: V O Adefela (Editor in Chief),
I O A Adeleye (Chief Engineer),
C I Fadare (Secretary/Head of Administration),
Akin Rotibi (Commercial Manager)
PRINCIPAL ACTIVITIES: News gathering and distribution
Principal Agencies: The Associated Press, USA; Agence France
Presse; Reuters
Principal Bankers: African Continental Bank Ltd; Union Bank of
Nigeria Ltd
Principal Shareholders: Federal Government of Nigeria
Date of Establishment: 1978

NEW BREED ORGANISATION LTD

35 Ogunlana Drive, Surulere, PO Box 5414, Lagos
Tel: 831506

Directors: Chief C Okolie, Chief A Ibru, Mrs M Okoli, P Alfuwa
PRINCIPAL ACTIVITIES: Publishing
Principal Bankers: United Bank for Africa Ltd; Union Bank of
Nigeria Ltd

NEW INDEPENDENT RUBBER COMPANY LTD

Amukpe Village, Sapele/Warri Rd, PO Box 150, Sapele, Bendel
State
Tel: 42258
PRINCIPAL ACTIVITIES: Production of crepe rubber

NEW INDIA ASSURANCE COMPANY (NIGERIA) LTD

34 Balogun Sq, PO Box 650, Lagos
Tel: 664995, 661213, 664110
Cable: Niassurance

Chairman: Chief T A B Olatunji
Directors: H B Dandiwala (Managing Director),
Chief N Idowu,
Tijani A Baba,
Alhaji S M A Damagum,
K C Ponnappa,
V K Mody
Senior Executives: A Ogunubi (Assistant General Manager)
PRINCIPAL ACTIVITIES: Insurance
Branch Offices: 68E Bello Rd, PO Box 809, Kano
Associated Companies: The New India Assurance Company Ltd,
Bombay, India
Principal Bankers: Allied Bank of Nigeria Ltd; Bank of the North
Ltd
Financial Information:

	₦'000
Authorised capital	500
Paid-up capital	300
Turnover	5,480
Profits	700

Principal Shareholders: Federal Ministry of Finance Inc (49%);
Nigerian Government
Date of Establishment: 1970

NEW INSURANCE COMPANY (NIGERIA) LTD

12/14 Broad St, PO Box 944, Lagos
PRINCIPAL ACTIVITIES: Insurance

NEW NIGERIA BANK LTD

Mission Rd, PMB 1193, Benin City, Bendel State
Tel: 200200, 200201/3
Cable: Nigerbank, Head Office Benin
Telex: 41103 Nebank

Chairman: Chief G E Mabiaku
Directors: Chief F A Agbaje, Chief M I Agbontaen, Chief S
Obukowho, Chief A O Okolocha, Chief O Ezekiel, Professor
O Nwanwene, Dr S T Aiokwe, Dr M O Odaro, F S Uwahe,
Ministry of Finance Incorporated
Senior Executives: Dr M O Odaro (General Manager),
G O Okoubo (Deputy General Manager),
C O Okpiabhele (Assistant General Manager, Legal),
Chief A J Sule (Assistant General Manager, Inspection and
Management),
S O Ikeneku (Assistant General Manager, Administration),
E N Aganmwonyi (Assistant General Manager, Operations),
L E Ugbo (Assistant General Manager, Finance),
J U E Agbaza (Assistant General Manager, Manpower
Development)
PRINCIPAL ACTIVITIES: Banking services
Branch Offices: Ring Rd Branch, Benin City; Mission Rd Branch,
Benin City; Murtala Muhammed Way Branch, Benin City; 4
Sanni Adewale St, Lagos; PMB 1048, Warri, Bendel State; 7C
Muritala Mohammed Way, Kano; PMB 2132, Jos; 1 College
Hill, London, EC4R 2RA, UK
Financial Information:

	₦'000
Authorised capital	11,600
Paid-up capital	5,600
Turnover	22,860
Profits	2,780

Principal Shareholders: Bendel State Government of Nigeria
Date of Establishment: 2nd October 1970
No of Employees: 1,590

NEW NIGERIA CONSTRUCTION COMPANY LTD

3 Kanta Rd, Turaki Ali House, PMB 2173, Kaduna
Tel: 210386
Cable: Satom Kaduna
Telex: 871102 Satom Ng

Chairman: Alhaji Magaji Inuwa
Directors: Alhaji Hassan Mu'Azu,
   Adewale Bello,
   Rene Vitry,
   Charles Calier,
   Engr Abdullah Nuhu (Managing),
   Mrs Folake Ndalugi
Senior Executives: Ademola Amos Elufowope (Company
   Secretary/Financial Controller),
   James McKenna (Technical Manager)
PRINCIPAL ACTIVITIES: Building and civil engineering
   contractors
Principal Bankers: International Bank for West Africa Ltd;
   United Bank for Africa Ltd
Financial Information:

	N'000
Authorised capital	500
Paid-up capital	500

Principal Shareholders: New Nigeria Development Company Ltd;
   Satom of France; Other Businessmen/Employees
Date of Establishment: May 1973
No of Employees: 980

NEW NIGERIA DEVELOPMENT COMPANY LTD

Ahmed Talib House, 18/19 Ahmadu Bello Way, PMB 2120,
   Kaduna
Tel: 216833, 210909, 210082, 210153
Telex: 71108

Chairman: Dr Ibrahim Tahir
Directors: A Abdurrahim (Group Managing Director & Chief
   Executive),
   B W Juta,
   M Oyeyipo,
   R Dantoro,
   S Y Hamma,
   Dr Aliyu Mohammed,
   Yerima A A Sani,
   I Aliyu,
   D Tebu,
   S S Gofwen,
   S Mustafa,
   B Takaya
Senior Executives: Alh. H B Mohammed (Director, Manufacturing
   Division),
   Mal. Magaji Inuwa (Director, Textiles Division),
   Mal. Moh. Hayatudeen (Director, Construction Division),
   Alh. S D Umar (Director, Finance, Institution & Commerce),
   Dr Tunji Olagunju (Director, Agriculture),
   C G Danjuma (Director, Hotels, Food & Beverage),
   ALH M M Maishanu (Drector, Administration)

PRINCIPAL ACTIVITIES: Planning, identification, preparation and
   implementation of projects; Provision of long-term loans;
   Equity participation, consultancy services foreign capital
   investment through joint ventures. Hotel management and
   promotion of the textile industry
Subsidiary Companies: There are 12 Subsidiaries and 133
   Associate Companies within the NNDC Group
Principal Bankers: Union Bank of Nigeria Ltd; Bank of the North
   Ltd; United Bank for Africa Ltd; First Bank of Nigeria Ltd

Financial Information:

	N'000
Authorised capital	50,000
Paid-up capital	50,000
Turnover	6,000
Profits	2,700

Principal Shareholders: Government of Bauchi; Benue; Borno;
   Gongola; Kaduna; Kano; Kwara; Plateau; Niger; Sokoto
   States
Date of Establishment: 1956
No of Employees: 330

NEW NIGERIA INSURANCE COMPANY LTD

118/120 Broad St, PO Box 3698, Lagos
Tel: 636151, 636222

PRINCIPAL ACTIVITIES: Insurance

NEW NIGERIA MERCHANTS LTD

PO Box 3380, Plot 83/84 Odusote St, Anthony Mile 8, Ikorodu
   Rd, Lagos
Tel: 964123
Cable: Nenigmerc Lagos

Chairman: F K Odusote
Directors: R O Odusote
Senior Executives: A A Nehemiah (Transport Manager),
   Z A Adebanjo (Accountant),
   S Olashore (Workshop Engineer),
   D D Meme (Administrative Manager),
   B A Sofenwa (Wharf Manager)

PRINCIPAL ACTIVITIES: Clearing, forwarding, shipping, haulage,
   warehousing and freight services; customs agents
Principal Agencies: West Africa Milk Company Ltd; Sodick
   ASEA; Adebowale Electrical Industries; Best Stores Ltd;
   Food Specialities etc
Principal Bankers: Co-operative Bank Ltd; Union Bank of Nigeria
   Ltd
Financial Information:

	N'000
Authorised capital	200
Paid-up capital	200

Principal Shareholders: F K Odusote; R O Odusote
Date of Establishment: 1971
No of Employees: 200

NEW NIGERIA PRESS

PO Box 263, Ebuta-Metta, Lagos

Directors: E A Atilade (Managing Director)
PRINCIPAL ACTIVITIES: Publishing

NEW NIGERIA SALT COMPANY LTD

PMB 4071, Oghareki, Sapele, Bendel State

Directors: B U N Igwe
PRINCIPAL ACTIVITIES: Production of edible and industrial salt

NEW NIGERIAN NEWSPAPERS LTD

Newspaper House, Ahmadu Bello Way, PO Box 254, Kaduna
Tel: 243386/8
Cable: Nornews Kaduna
Telex: 71120 Newnig Ng

Chairman: Chief I I Morphy
Directors: Bukar Petrol,
   Gab Idigo,
   Isa Ozi Salami,
   Ma'Azu Maiyaki,
   Abubakar A Gwandu,
   Goke Ajiboye,
   Tukur Othman (Managing),
   Laminu Baba Gana (Company Secretary)
Senior Executives: Abbat Ahmed (Chief Accountant),
   Dan Agbese (Editor)

PRINCIPAL ACTIVITIES: Printing and publishing
Branch Offices: 220A Apapa Rd, Ijora, Lagos; Also offices all
over the country
Associated Companies: New Nigerian Packaging Company
Principal Bankers: First Bank of Nigeria Ltd; Bank of the North
Ltd
Financial Information:

	N'000
Authorised capital	600
Paid-up capital	600
Turnover	4,000

Principal Shareholders: Federal Government
Date of Establishment: January 1966
No of Employees: 1,000 (approx)

NEW-GATE INSURANCE CO LTD
Star Suite, Ebani House Complex, 149/153 Broad St, PO Box
9186, Lagos
Tel: 630504, 630644

PRINCIPAL ACTIVITIES: Insurance
Branch Offices: Plots 9, 10 & 11, Awodi-Ora Estate, Via Mile 2
Isolo-Apapa Express Rd, Kirikiri, Apapa, PO Box 4088, Lagos

NEWMARK ELECTRIC CO LTD
40 Oyekan Rd, PO Box 4543, Surulere, Lagos
Cable: Nectecnec Lagos

Chairman: P A Idaewor (also Managing Director)
Directors: Ben Idaewor, R Idaewor, A Idaewor
Senior Executives: M Saliu (Administrative Manager),
I B Julius (Chief Accountant)

PRINCIPAL ACTIVITIES: Suppliers of power, audio-visual,
electronics and telecommunication systems
Branch Offices: SW7B/700 Orita Challenge, Ibadan, Oyo State
Associated Companies: Peter Block & Partners, Lagos
Principal Bankers: Union Bank of Nigeria Ltd

Principal Shareholders: Chairman and directors as described
Date of Establishment: 25th July 1978

NEWMARK ELECTRIC COMPANY LTD
65 Ilesanmi St, Surulere, Lagos
Tel: 836033

Directors: Benjamin Idaewor,
Rosemary Idaewor,
Agnes Idaewor,
Pat A Idaewor (Managing and Engineering)
Senior Executives: A Mohammed (Administration, Personnel and
Industrial Relations),
E Okonjo (Senior Accountant),
P Idaewor (Sales Manager),
E Amechi (Operations Manager)

PRINCIPAL ACTIVITIES: Distribution, installation and
maintenance of electrical, electronic, audio-visual and
telecommunication equipment, including air-conditioning and
refrigeration
Principal Agencies: Barkway Electronics Ltd; UK (Duplex
Intercom Systems); Rank Pullin Controls, UK (VHF/UHF Radio
Telephones); Communication Associate Inc, USA (HF/SSB
Transceiver); Redifusion Industrial Services Ltd, UK (Audio
Visual Systems); Italtel, Italy (PABX Telephone Systems)
Branch Offices: Branches to be established at Kano, Enugu, Port
Harcourt and Benin City
Associated Companies: Peter Black & Partners, Lagos; Industrial
Consultants Ltd, Lagos
Principal Bankers: African Continental Bank Ltd

NFS (FOOD AND COLD STORAGE) LTD
1 Harbour Rd, PO Box 128, Apapa, Lagos
Tel: 877337
Cable: Eldorado, Lagos
Telex: 22243 Nfs Ng

Chairman: Wm M Murray-Bruce
Directors: W R Murray-Bruce

PRINCIPAL ACTIVITIES: Wholesale fresh and frozen provisions;
agents and general traders
Branch Offices: 17 Ohiamini Street, PO Box 635, Port-Harcourt,
Rivers State
Principal Bankers: First Bank of Nigeria Ltd

Principal Shareholders: Domino Stores Ltd; The Union
International Company Ltd, UK
Date of Establishment: December 1956

NICHEDOS AND COMPANY LTD
23 Ondo St (West), Ebute-Metta, Lagos
Tel: 833470
Cable: Nichedos Lagos

Chairman: N A O Edomwande
Senior Executives: D Iroakazi (Sales Manager),
E A Adegile (Marketing Executive),
S Erobame (Administrative Manager)

PRINCIPAL ACTIVITIES: Agents and general trading company
Principal Agencies: Toyo Radio Co Ltd, Japan; General Cold
Corporation, New York, USA; Nairn Floors International, UK
Branch Offices: 26 Latunde Ave, Onipanu Bus Stop, Ikorodu Rd,
Lagos
Associated Companies: Bendel Electronics Co, Lagos; Prestige
Furniture Co, Lagos
Principal Bankers: United Bank for Africa Ltd
Financial Information:

	N'000
Authorised capital	100
Paid-up capital	100

NICHEMTEX INDUSTRIES LTD
808 Investment House, 21/25 Broad St, PO Box 4815, Lagos
Tel: 650545, 636010, 636080
Cable: Nichemtex Lagos
Telex: 21296

Chairman: Cha Chi Ming
Directors: L A Salako,
Payson Cha,
Y A Disu,
G O Senbanjo,
Richard Young,
Jan A Dekker (Controller),
Camille Zillikens,
Frans de Maat,
Thomas T L Tung (Joint Managing Director),
Mrs A A Ajao
Senior Executives: J Van Veldhoven (Plant Manager),
S C Wo (Plant Manager),
L A Aiyenigba (Administration Manager),
E A Fabiyi (Sales Manager),
W A Akerele (Chief Accountant)

PRINCIPAL ACTIVITIES: Production of textile cloth, polyester
staple fibre, dyed textile cloth, polyester filament
Branch Offices: (Factory) Ibeshe Rd, Ikorodu, Lagos State
Principal Bankers: Union Bank of Nigeria Ltd; First Bank of
Nigeria Ltd; United Bank for Africa; National Bank of Nigeria
Ltd

Principal Shareholders: Cha Chi Ming Ltd (29.3%); Akzo NV
(29.3%); Lagos State Government (13.3%); Federal
Government (10%); Nigerian Industrial Development Bank
(10%), other (8.1%)
No of Employees: 2,500

NICHIMEN COMPANY (NIGERIA) LTD
35 Kingsway Rd, Ikoyi, PMB 2761, Lagos
Tel: 682778, 683442
Cable: Nichimen Lagos
Telex: 21207

Chairman: Alhaji Umaru Mutallab
Directors: T Fujino (Managing Director),
H Kawahara,
Alhaji Abdu Alhassan,

P S Achimugu

PRINCIPAL ACTIVITIES: Business information, technical surveys and research on projects and investment opportunities

NICHOLAS LABORATORIES NIGERIA LTD

PMB 21118, Ikeja, Lagos
Tel: 962001
Cable: Nichlabs Lagos

PRINCIPAL ACTIVITIES: Manufacturers of toiletries and pharmaceuticals
Branch Offices: Onitsha; Zaria; Factory: 6 Industrial St, Ilupeju, Lagos

NIDANCONSULT

16B Shonibare Estate, Maryland, Ikeja, PO Box 2223, Lagos
Tel: 963630
Cable: Cowiconsult Lagos
Telex: 77206 Nidan Ng

Senior Executives: N Thorsboll (General Manager)

PRINCIPAL ACTIVITIES: Consulting engineers and planners; projects completed for ministries of works in most Nigerian States, as well as for the Federal Government

Date of Establishment: 1960
No of Employees: 100

NIDOCO LTD

7 Onike Rd, PMB 1070, Yaba, Lagos
Tel: 862294
Cable: Snacfoods

Chairman: Alhaji N K Gbajabiamila
Directors: Mrs A A Gbajabiamila, Mrs E O Ebie
Senior Executives: P O Bamgbose (Acting General Manager),
F O Ogunjumelo (Chief Accountant),
C A Oghuma (Production Manager),
A A Oshundiya (Administrative Manager)

PRINCIPAL ACTIVITIES: Food manufacturing; importers of cereals
Principal Agencies: Gist Brocades; National Oats
Branch Offices: M23 Kuban Rd, Tudan Wada, Kaduna
Associated Companies: African Research Development Company (Nigeria) Ltd
Principal Bankers: Union Bank of Nigeria Ltd; NAL
Financial Information:

	₦'000
Authorised capital	180
Paid-up capital	180

Principal Shareholders: Chairman and directors as described
Date of Establishment: 31st August 1961
No of Employees: 222

NIDOGAS COMPANY LTD

23 Creek Rd, PO Box 443, Apapa, Lagos
Tel: 803330, 803331, 803332
Cable: Nidogas
Telex: 22117

Chairman: Dr D E Awani
Directors: A A Ayida, Chief J O Akinpelu, Dr M Gorla, M Quattrini, Mrs B N Wachukwu, Aliyu Bello
Senior Executives: S Y Laryea (AG General Manager)

PRINCIPAL ACTIVITIES: Importation, assembly, and marketing of gas appliances; processing and distribution of LPG
Branch Offices: 27B Post Office Rd, Kano; 167 Aba Rd, PM Box 5789, Port Harcourt; 9 Alhaji Jimoh Odutola Rd, Gbagi Commercial Area, PO Box 587, Ibadan; 11 New Lagos Rd, PM Box 1575, Benin City; 26 Wharf Rd, PO Box 516, Zaria; 2 Ahmadu Bello Way, PM Box 538, Maiduguri
Principal Bankers: United Bank for Africa Ltd

Financial Information:

	₦'000
Authorised capital	2,417
Paid-up capital	2,417
Turnover	4,000

Principal Shareholders: Liquigas SpA, Italy; Odua Investment Co Ltd, Ibadan; NNDC, Kaduna; Dr D E Awani
Date of Establishment: 1955
No of Employees: 121

NIFEIPIRI POULTRIES LTD

Poultry Farm Chokocho, PMB 5461, Port Harcourt
Tel: 331993

Chairman: Rev Godknows M Nifeipiri
Directors: Inye Nifeipiri, S M O Amachree
Senior Executives: Mioye Nifeipiri

PRINCIPAL ACTIVITIES: Rearing of chickens, processing and marketing
Branch Offices: Nifeipiri Farm; Obamafor, Buguma City; Secretariat Complex Block C, Room 626, PMB 5461, Port Harcourt, Tel 331993
Subsidiary Companies: National Council of Nigerian Farmers
Principal Bankers: Union Bank of Nigeria Ltd
Financial Information:

	₦'000
Authorised capital	100
Paid-up capital	50
Turnover	115
Profits	30

Principal Shareholders: Directors as described
Date of Establishment: June 1976

NIGER AGENCIES INTERNATIONAL (NIGERIA) LTD

PO Box 553, 42 Sakpoba Rd, Benin City, Bendel State
Tel: 243100

PRINCIPAL ACTIVITIES: State Government bulk purchasing organisation

NIGER BISCUITS COMPANY LTD

35 Creek Rd, Apapa, PO Box 1568, Apapa, Lagos
Tel: 876821, 876827/6
Cable: Nibisco Lagos
Telex: 21134

PRINCIPAL ACTIVITIES: Manufacturing of biscuits, confectionery

NIGER CONSTRUCTION LTD

PO Box 1244, 13/17 Breadfruit St, Lagos
Tel: 662906
Cable: Mothercat Lagos
Telex: 21019 Cat Ng

Chairman: L A Ilegbodu
Directors: Z Shammas (Managing Director),
S Sarkis (General Manager),
S B I Ikoh-Ogbetta,
J A Ibe
Senior Executives: G Bitar (Engineer),
S Sayegh (Engineer)

PRINCIPAL ACTIVITIES: Civil engineering and construction, electrical engineering, mechanical engineering, oil and gas services and equipment and pipeline contractors
Branch Offices: PO Box 402, Enerhen Rd, Warri, Bendel State; PMB 1214, Ihama St, Benin City, Bendel State; PO Box 617, Trans Amadi Industrial Layout, Port Harcourt, Rivers State, Cable Mothercat Port Harcourt
Associated Companies: Mothercat Overseas (Nigeria) Ltd
Principal Bankers: New Nigeria Bank Ltd; Union Bank of Nigeria Ltd

Financial Information:

	N'000
Authorised capital	5,000
Paid-up capital	5,000
Sales turnover	63,000

Principal Shareholders: Mothercat (Overseas) Ltd (40%); Nigerian Economic Welfare Services Ltd (41%); Ministry of Finance Inc, Imo State (17%); Company's Employees (2%)
Date of Establishment: 1961
No of Employees: 4,500

NIGER CONSULTANTS LTD

PO Box 671, Kaduna

PRINCIPAL ACTIVITIES: Engineering consultants architects

NIGER DELTA SHIPPING AGENCIES LTD

41 Yoruba Rd, Sapele, Bendel State
Tel: 42710

Chairman: Prince Kenekueyero B Omotseye (also Managing Director)

PRINCIPAL ACTIVITIES: Shipping agency

NIGER INSURANCE COMPANY LTD (THE)

PO Box 2718, 47 Marina, Lagos
Tel: 664452, 662191, 662186
Cable: Gerins

Chairman: Dr Sa'ad Abubakar
Directors: O Lijadu, Alhaji Umaru A Yelwa, Alhaji Ado Dandawaki, Chief A Akomolafe, Chief Bayo Oluwole, Vin Adikibe
Senior Executives: Ajibola O Ogunshola (General Manager), A K Oniwinde (Deputy General Manager), Bola Oyesanmi (Assistant General Manager, Finance), C Ehirim (Senior Manager, Life & Pensions Department), A O Owokalade (Administration Manager), O Adeyemi-Wilson (Company Secretary/Legal Adviser), E O Osikoya (Chief Accountant), G E Ibe (Manager, Fire & Accident Department), B O Lewis (Manager, Marine & Aviation Department), I F Unuakhalu (Agency Manager)

PRINCIPAL ACTIVITIES: Insurance
Branch Offices: SW8/101 Ijebu-Bye Pass, Opposite St Theresa's College, Oke Ado, Ibadan; 24 Ikwerre Rd, PMB 5428, Port Harcourt; 69 Akpakpava Street, PMB 1517, Benin City; 27 Asa Rd, PO Box 3281, Aba; 47 Muritala Mohammed Way, PO Box 2712, Ilorin; SW32 Bosso Rd, PO Box 1517, Minna; 1136 Ahmadu Bellow Way, Sokoto; Warama House, 17D Civic Centre, PO Box 4639, Kano
Principal Bankers: Union Bank of Nigeria Ltd; United Bank for Africa Ltd
Financial Information:

	N'000
Authorised capital	800
Paid-up capital	800
Turnover	10,684
Gross Profit	1,504

Principal Shareholders: National Insurance Corp of Nigeria

NIGER MATCH COMPANY LTD

Eleiyele Industrial Layout, Ibadan, PO Box 1499, Ibadan, Oyo State
Tel: 412248, 411042
Cable: Nigermatch Ibadan
Telex: 31107 Nigmat

Directors: V Allam (Managing Director)

PRINCIPAL ACTIVITIES: Manufacturers of safety matches
Branch Offices: PO Box 315, 125, Trans-Amadi Industrial Layout, Port Harcourt, Rivers State

NIGER MOTORS LTD

17 Creek Rd, PO Box 350, Apapa, Lagos
Tel: 876695, 874803, 873704

PRINCIPAL ACTIVITIES: Commercial vehicle distributors

NIGER OIL RESOURCES LTD (NORCO)

Crusader House, 23/25 Martins St, PO Box 8088, Lagos
Tel: 635116
Cable: Norcoil Lagos
Telex: 21168 Norco Ng

Chairman: Chief O B Akin-Olugbade
Senior Executives: J B Jones (Office Manager)

PRINCIPAL ACTIVITIES: Oil and gas services, holding company

NIGER PETROLEUM CO LTD

5 Williams St, 2nd Floor, Lagos Island, PO Box 467, Lagos
Tel: 636590
Cable: Nigpetro Lagos

Chairman: Chief S L Sdu

PRINCIPAL ACTIVITIES: Oil and gas services, holding company

NIGER RAW MATERIALS LTD

PO Box 1167, 112 Broad St, Lagos
Tel: 631275, 650225
Telex: 21447 Nerox Ng; 21284

PRINCIPAL ACTIVITIES: Management consultants, project development; commodity exporters

NIGER RIVER TRANSPORT LTD

PO Box 1, Burutu, Bendel State
PRINCIPAL ACTIVITIES: Shipbuilding

NIGER SANITARY INDUSTRY LTD

1 Damson Street, Industrial Scheme Ogba, PO Box 4072, Ikeja, Lagos
Tel: 836374
Cable: Sanidos Lagos

Chairman: Alhaji Adamson Olatunji Bamisedun
Directors: Alhaji Mokiram Rotimi Bamidedun, Alhaji Serifat Modupe Bamisedun

PRINCIPAL ACTIVITIES: Manufacturers of surgical dressings; toiletries and paper products
Principal Bankers: Union Bank of Nigeria Ltd
Financial Information:

	N'000
Authorised capital	1,000
Paid-up capital	750
Turnover	8,101
Profits	324

Principal Shareholders: Alhaji Adamson Olatunji Bamisedun
Date of Establishment: 1962
No of Employees: 500

NIGER SEA FOODS LTD

Plot 181, Trans-Amadi Industrial Estate, PO Box 1044, Port Harcourt, Rivers State
Tel: 333921, 333936, 335645
Cable: Fisherman Pharcourt
Telex: 61158 Fisher

Chairman: Chief Tamunobere Oforiokuma (also Managing Director)
Directors: A D Eremie, M Agbamuche, Mrs I Oforiokuma, S Allweli-Brown
Senior Executives: I T Temmeh (Financial Controller), L A Wilkey (Company Secretary/Legal Adviser)

PRINCIPAL ACTIVITIES: Sea foods, fishery
Branch Offices: Liaison Office: 37 Awolowo Rd, South West
Ikoyi, PO Box 51490, Falomo, Lagos, Cables Fishermen
Lagos, Telex 21720 Fisher Ng; Sub-Main Depot; Ibuot Obot,
Calabar, Cross River State, Tel 683026, 684361
Associated Companies: Taminy Agencies (Nigeria) Ltd
Principal Bankers: Pan African Bank Ltd; African Continental
Bank Ltd
Financial Information:

	N'000
Authorised capital	500
Paid-up capital	500

Principal Shareholders: Chief Tamunobere Oforiokuma; Mrs
Inyang Oforiokuma
Date of Establishment: 22nd January 1975
No of Employees: 156

NIGERCARE INTERNATIONAL COMPANY (NIGERIA) LTD
PO Box 7653, 9 Ajao Rd, Surulere, Lagos
Tel: 837377

Chairman: Dr Isaac O Ayodeji
Directors: Chief S A Oladapo
Senior Executives: Taposh K Shome,
J Niyogi,
Sam B Carter (Director of Operations, Sokoto),
Dr Dalim Majumdar (Consulting),
Engr R O Akintoye (Director of Engineering)

PRINCIPAL ACTIVITIES: Building and civil engineering, soils
and foundation, irrigation, sewage and sanitary engineering,
hotel management, and investment studies; land development
Branch Offices: 121 Odosida St, Ondo; SW8/448 College
Crescent, Ibadan, Oyo State; 15B Lodge Rd, Sokoto, Sokoto
State
Associated Companies: Safe Associates of Nigeria; Safe
International Inc, USA
Principal Bankers: Co-operative Bank Ltd; United Bank for
Africa
Financial Information:

	N'000
Authorised capital	400
Paid-up capital	100

Principal Shareholders: Dr I O Ayodeji; Chief S A Oladapo
Date of Establishment: 1976

NIGERCHIN ELECTRICAL DEVELOPMENT COMPANY LTD
1 Ayodele Diyan Rd, PM Box 21096, Ikeja, Lagos
Tel: 964578, 964579
Cable: Nedevco

Chairman: Chief J O Udoji
Directors: N O George-Taylor, Alhaji Usman Goji, D Chuang, J
Huang, L D Trillwood, A Fenn
Senior Executives: L A Hill (General Manager)

PRINCIPAL ACTIVITIES: Manufacturers of electrical wires and
cables, wiring and mains cables of copper and aluminium
Associated Companies: Canada Wire & Cable (International)
Principal Bankers: International Bank for West Africa Ltd;
International Merchant Bank (Nig) Ltd; Icon Ltd (Merchant
Bankers)
Financial Information:

	N'000
Authorised capital	2,000
Paid-up capital	1,584
Turnover	22,040

Date of Establishment: March 1970
No of Employees: 300

NIGERGAS LTD
PO Box 441, Enugu, Anambra State
Tel: 252695
Cable: Nigergas Enugu
Telex: 51159 Enugu

Chairman: Justic G C M Onyiuke
Directors: Mrs M C Obanye, Aka Ogbobe, I Micheletti
Senior Executives: A E O Ugwumba (General Manager),
G N Ani (Company Secretary/Administration Manager),
B C Ikejiaku (Chief Accountant),
A A Chikwendu (Chief Engineer/Production Manager),
C Okwu (Marketing Officer),
L M C Igwemezie (Engineer Grade 1)

PRINCIPAL ACTIVITIES: Gas production
Branch Offices: 171 Warri/Sapele Rd, Warri, Bendel State; 7B
Oguta Rd, Onitsha, Anambra State; PMB 7072, Aba, Imo
State
Principal Bankers: Co-operative Bank of Eastern Nigeria Ltd;
United Bank for Africa Ltd; African Continental Bank Ltd
Financial Information:

	N'000
Authorised capital	1,500
Paid-up capital	1,500

Principal Shareholders: Government of Anambra State,
Micheletti & Sons
No of Employees: 150

NIGERGROB CERAMICS LTD
PO Box 658, Abeokuta, Ogun State

Chairman: Dr S O Biobaku
Directors: E Rudlaff, Dr K Schieferdecker, Dr E Turba, A A
Alikah, R Kuppers, A Puschmann, R Goettin, Dr Lo Dare,
G O Badmus, A Adenekan
Senior Executives: E Rudlaff (Managing Director)

PRINCIPAL ACTIVITIES: Manufacturer of wall and floor tiles and
sanitary-ware
Principal Agencies: Agrob Aktiengesellschaft, Germany
Principal Bankers: United Bank for Africa Ltd; National Bank of
Nigeria Ltd
Financial Information:

	N'000
Authorised capital	2,350
Paid-up capital	2,350

Principal Shareholders: Agrob Anlagenbau, West Germany;
Odu'a Investment Co; NIDB; Edico; DEG, West Germany;
UTC, Switzerland; Sifida, Switzerland; Private Nigerians
No of Employees: 380

NIGERGUARDS LTD
PO Box 760, Jos, Plateau State

Chairman: W K R Hallam
Directors: Mrs M I Hallam, W O R Hallam

PRINCIPAL ACTIVITIES: Security services
Branch Offices: Abuja Federal Capital: Bauchi; Benue; Borno;
Gongola; Kaduna; Kano; Kwara; Niger; Plateau; Sokoto

NIGERIA AIRWAYS LTD
Airways House, PO Box 136, Murtala Muhammed Airport, Ikeja,
Lagos
Tel: 900476
Cable: Westafair
Telex: 21509 Wtlos Ng

Chairman: Alhaji M A Sanusi
Directors: Alhaji Mai Deribe, Chief D O Onu, Prince A Lamuye,
Alhaji S Adesada, Mrs A White, Alhaji M Yerima Balla, G O
Mogaji

PRINCIPAL ACTIVITIES: National airline

NIGERIA CANDLE STICK MANUFACTURING COMPANY LTD

PMB 3324, 27 Ibrahim Taiwo Rd, Kano
Tel: 2822

PRINCIPAL ACTIVITIES: Manufacturers of candles

NIGERIA COACH CONSTRUCTION LTD

Faleye Industrial Site, Yebu, Lagos Rd, PMB 5288, Ibadan, Oyo
   State

Directors: G Zamlera (Managing Director)

PRINCIPAL ACTIVITIES: Bus assemblers

NIGERIA COLD STORES LTD

PO Box 358, 21 Dockyard Rd, Apapa, Lagos
Tel: 837631, 873161
Cable: Nigercold, Lagos
Telex: 21358 Herwa Ng

Chairman: F S McEwen
Directors: Jidda Ibrahim, Chief S A Iredia
Senior Executives: W Sonta (Group General Manager)

PRINCIPAL ACTIVITIES: Suppliers of wholesale food products;
   frozen fish
Branch Offices: 2 Igbokwe St, D Line, PO Box 951, Port
   Harcourt, Tel 221693, Cable Nigercold PH
Associated Companies: Mesurado Fishing Company (Nigeria)
   Ltd; Herwa Ltd
Principal Bankers: First Bank of Nigeria Ltd
Financial Information:

	₦'000
Authorised capital	200
Paid-up capital	200

Date of Establishment: 4th November 1961
No of Employees: 150

NIGERIA CONSTRUCTION AND FURNITURE COMPANY LTD (NCFC)

NCFC House, 5 Onitsha Rd, PO Box 345, Enugu, Anambra State

Tel: 255452
Cable: Enigsol
Telex: 51131 Enisol NG

Chairman: T C M Eneli
Directors: I N Ani, F O Umunna, U N Anya, Dr N Ike
Senior Executives: E C Madubike (Acting General Manager),
   B K Kundu (Financial Controller),
   Agodi Ibegi (Chief Engineer),
   F B I Egolum (Company Secretary)

PRINCIPAL ACTIVITIES: Civil engineering and construction
Branch Offices: Iva Valley, Enugu; Niger Bridge Industrial Layout,
   Onitsha, Anambra State; 94A Abark St, Aba, Imo State
Associated Companies: Vanguard Industries Ltd
Financial Information:

	₦'000
Authorised capital	200
Paid-up capital	200
Turnover	5,000

Principal Shareholders: Anambra State Government
Date of Establishment: 1960
No of Employees: 2,000

NIGERIA DISTILLERIES LTD

Km 40 Abeokuta Expressway, Sango Otta, Ogun State
Tel: 960507
Cable: ALCOHOL, Ikeja
Telex: 26890 NDL Ng

PRINCIPAL ACTIVITIES: Blending and bottling of wines and
   spirits
Branch Offices: Mailing address: PO Box 2077, Ikeja, Lagos
Principal Bankers: Societe General Bank Ltd; United Bank for
   Africa Ltd

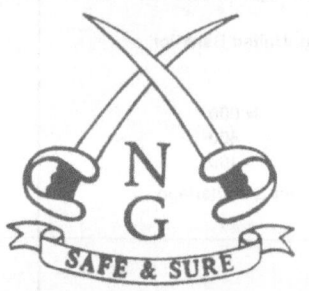

Financial Information:
Registered capital   ₦ 100,000

Date of Establishment: 1961
No of Employees: 250

NIGERIA DRILLING COMPANY LTD
PO Box 1242, Apt 1, 239D Kofo Abayomi Rd, Victoria Island,
    Lagos
Tel: 613558
Cable: Nidco-Lagos

Senior Executives: J W Brinlee (Division Manager),
    Alex Ofurum (Warehouseman)

PRINCIPAL ACTIVITIES: Offshore drilling contractors
Subsidiary Companies: Associate Co; Loffland Brothers Co

NIGERIA ENGINEERING WORKS LTD
49 Trans Amadi Industrial Layout, PO Box 519, Port Harcourt,
    Rivers State
Tel: 331180, 334090
Cable: Nigeng
Telex: 61142 Nigeng

Chairman: G P Birla
Directors: Mrs N D Birla,
    J A Olugbenle,
    Ine A D Ikhobo,
    M L Pachisia (Managing),
    A Kalio,
    Mrs E Akuta
Senior Executives: R M Aron (Chief Engineer),
    K P Bhutada (Works Manager, Maiduguri Factory)

PRINCIPAL ACTIVITIES: Manufacturing of air-conditioners, fans,
    water-coolers, steel furniture, school furniture, office
    equipment, shelving racks, library shelving and designing,
    fabrication and erection of steel structures, bulk storage
    tanks
Branch Offices: PMB 1414, Maiduguri, Telex 82126; PO Box
    3682, 134 Awolowo Rd, Lagos, Tel 680578, Telex 21289; PO
    Box 2081, 69 Ibrahim Taiwo Rd, Kano, Tel 5285
Associated Companies: The Birla Group, India
Principal Bankers: United Bank for Africa Ltd; Chase Merchant
    Bank Nigeria Ltd
Financial Information:

	₦'000
Authorised capital	2,000
Paid-up capital	1,920
Turnover (approx)	27,000
Profits (approx)	2,500

Principal Shareholders: Birla Brothers & Associates;
    Government of Rivers State of Nigeria; Nigerian Industrial
    Development Bank Ltd
Date of Establishment: 4th June 1964
No of Employees: 1,025

NIGERIA FIBRE INDUSTRY COMPANY LTD (NIFINCO)
PO Box 1644, Ibadan, Oyo State
Tel: 410402

PRINCIPAL ACTIVITIES: Textiles
Branch Offices: Badagry

NIGERIA GENERAL MOTORS LTD
65 Marina, PO Box 4694, Lagos
Tel: 661059, 663477
Cable: Somoco Lagos
Telex: 21588 Somoco Ng

Chairman: S N Jethwani (also Managing Director)
Directors: Chief A F Odulana, T O Obafemi, B E Dalvie, Alhaji
    Sule Katagum
Senior Executives: A A Akinbowale (Assistant General Manager,
    Administration),
    E K Ubah (Assistant General Manager, Imports),
    O Odegbami (Company Accountant),

J O Eyayo (Chief Accountant),
    L J Jashnani (Production Manager)

PRINCIPAL ACTIVITIES: Manufacturing of miscellaneous
    fabricated metal products, welding electrodes and allied
    equipment, assembly and progressive manufacture of diesel
    engines, gasoline/diesel generating sets, pump sets, grinding
    mills, sugar cane crushers, rice hullers and allied agricultural
    machinery/equipment
Principal Agencies: Daihatsu Motor Co Ltd, Japan; Homelite
    Textron Inc, USA; Batliboi & Co Ltd, India; Steelage
    Industries Ltd, India; Ishihara Kikai Kogyo Co Ltd, Japan;
    Greaves International Ltd, India; Larsen & Toubro Ltd, India;
    Ford of Europe, UK; Hobart Brothers International AG; USA
    and Europe; Mahindra & Mahindra Ltd, India
Branch Offices: 42/44 Burma Rd, PMB 1068, Apapa, Lagos; 152
    Uselu Benin-Lagos Rd, PO Box 728, Benin City; 119/120
    Ibrahim Taiwo Rd, PMB 3111, Kano; SW8/172 Ring Rd, PO
    Box 1798, Ibadan; Factory: Old Ojo Rd, Off Km 11, Badagry
    Expressway, Lagos
Principal Bankers: International Merchant Bank (Nigeria) Ltd;
    Societe Generale Bank (Nigeria) Ltd
Financial Information:

	₦'000
Authorised capital	1,000
Paid-up capital	1,000

Principal Shareholders: Sonnar (Jersey) Ltd (60%); Nigerians
    (40%)
Date of Establishment: 20th October 1969
No of Employees: 190

NIGERIA GREEN LINES LTD
Unity House, 37 Marina, 13th Floor, PO Box 2288, Lagos
Tel: 636433, 654385
Telex: 21380 Marita NG

Chairman: Alhaji Chief W L Folawiyo

PRINCIPAL ACTIVITIES: Ship owners

NIGERIA GROUP FOUR CONSTRUCTION COMPANY LTD
10 Taslim Elias Close, Victoria Island, Lagos
Tel: 611365

Directors: Gilbert George Odiase

PRINCIPAL ACTIVITIES: Construction

NIGERIA HOTELS LTD
18 Club Rd, Ikoyi, PO Box 895, Lagos
Tel: 682295, 684349
Cable: Bestotel
Telex: Bestel Ng

Chairman: Chief Livinus Ogbonna
Directors: Chief S A Alamutu (Managing Director),
    S O Adeshina (Director-Finance),
    Mrs K N Agundu,
    Dr G A Adeosun
Senior Executives: O A Akinrinade (Controller of Operations),
    M A Fadipe (Controller of Personnel),
    Otunba A A Adegbesan (Controller of Corporate Affairs),
    T Oke (Chief Accountant),
    'Seni Oduyoye (Hotel Inspectorate Executive),
    C A Abisuga (Chief Internal Auditor)

PRINCIPAL ACTIVITIES: Hotels and catering
Branch Offices: Ikoyi Hotel, Kingsway Rd, Ikoyi, Lagos; Central
    Hotel, Bompai Rd, Kano
Subsidiary Companies: Bristol Hotel, 8 Martin Street, Lagos;
    Trade Fair Hotel, Lagos/Badagry Expressway, Lagos; Hill
    Station Hotel, Tudun Wada Rd, Jos; Metropolitan Hotel,
    Murtala Muhammed Way, Calabar
Principal Bankers: Union Bank of Nigeria Ltd

NIGERIA INDUSTRIAL GROUP LTD

Financial Information:

	N'000
Authorised capital	15,000
Paid-up capital	2,840
Turnover	10,500
Profits	373

Principal Shareholders: Federal Government; Kano State Government; Nigeria Railway Corporation; National Insurance Corporation of Nigeria; Nigerian Industrial Development Bank; New Nigeria Development Company; Northern Nigeria Investment Ltd
Date of Establishment: June 1928
No of Employees: over 2,000

NIGERIA INDUSTRIAL GROUP LTD

1A Independence Rd, Bompai, PO Box 1041, Kano
Tel: 3888
Cable: Nigroup

Chairman: Alhaji Usman S Dantata
Directors: Y A Adisa (Managing Director),
Chief S O Lambo,
Y Wakita,
D C L Nichols,
Alhaji A G Getso,
G Haltead

PRINCIPAL ACTIVITIES: Manufacturer of wire nails, chain link fencing, barbed wire and welded wire mesh
Principal Agencies: Nigerian Wire Industries Ltd
Branch Offices: Plot No 5, Inuwa Abdul Kadir Rd, PO Box 6647, Kakuri, Kaduna
Associated Companies: Nigerian Wire Industries Ltd, Ikeja
Principal Bankers: First Bank of Nigeria Ltd

Principal Shareholders: Alhaji Usman S Dantata; Chief S O Lambo; Bridon Mitsui
Date of Establishment: 1971
No of Employees: 100

NIGERIA KRAFT BAGS LTD

Oregun Industrial Estate, Ikeja, PO Box 20, Ikeja, Lagos
Tel: 963726, 964637
Cable: Nigerkraft Ikeja

Chairman: Chief Bola Adefemi
Directors: P Bolarinwa (Managing),
Raymond W Baker,
Alhaji Jalo Waziri,
O Adewumi (Executive),
A O Falope,
Chief J O Ogunyemi,
Raymond Innes,
J O Oladapo
Senior Executives: David Danby (Factory Manager),
Cornelius Sunday Elegbe (Deputy Factory Manager),
Kristian I Ukah (Company Secretary/Accountant)

PRINCIPAL ACTIVITIES: Manufacturers of industrial and consumer packaging, mainly for cement products, animal feeds and other consumer paper packages
Principal Bankers: First Bank of Nigeria Ltd; International Merchant Bank (Nigeria) Ltd, NAL Merchant Bank Ltd
Financial Information:

	N'000
Authorised capital	500
Paid-up capital	498

Principal Shareholders: Nigerian Diversified Investments Ltd; Lagos; Odu'a Investment Co Ltd; Ibadan, Oyo State; West African Portland Cement Company Ltd, Lagos
Date of Establishment: 1966
No of Employees: 400

NIGERIA MARINE & TRADING COMPANY LTD

2 Warehouse Rd, PO Box 19, Apapa, Lagos
Tel: 877557
Cable: Sacwal

Chairman: Chief M C O Ibru
Directors: G M Ibru, S O Alabi, F O Porbeni, J Simon, T G Townshend, J A Balogun
Senior Executives: G O Oriowo (General Manager),
J R Fakar (Accountant),
S N Adolor (Branch Manager, Lagos),
G A Ado-Imoisili (Branch Manager, Warri),
S A Echemunor (Branch Manager, Port Harcourt)

PRINCIPAL ACTIVITIES: Marine contractors to oil industry and importers of marine and industrial equipment, rubber and PVC hoses, marine fittings and marine paints, etc
Principal Agencies: Kleber-Colombes, France; Societe Industrie De Transmissions, France; Zodiac, France; Newton Collier Ltd, UK; Griflex Products Ltd, UK
Branch Offices: 27 Mcdermott Rd, Warri, PMB 1083 Bendel State; 3 Njemanze St, PO Box 624, Port Harcourt, Tel 225671/2
Principal Bankers: International Bank for West Africa Ltd
Financial Information:

	N'000
Authorised capital	200
Sales turnover (approx)	2,000

Principal Shareholders: Oteri Holdings Ltd, Apapa
No of Employees: 400

NIGERIA MERCHANT BANK LTD

25 Nnamdi Azikwe Street, PO Box 2413, Lagos
Tel: 664307, 664377, 664417
Cable: Cowrie Lagos
Telex: 21475

Chairman: Alhaji Dabo Sambo
Directors: Alhaji U A Mutallab (Vice-Chairman),
Chief S O Falae (Managing),
I Usman (Deputy Managing),
S S Baffa,
Madam O Omoniyi,
A A Coker,
Chief K B Omatseye
Senior Executives: H A Omisore (Controller of Corporate Finance),
J O Ekundayo (Controller of Operations)

PRINCIPAL ACTIVITIES: Merchant banking
Branch Offices: 3 Azikiwe Rd, Port Harcourt

Principal Shareholders: Ministry of Finance Inc, United Bank for Africa Ltd
Date of Establishment: 1960; became a Merchant Bank in 1973

NIGERIA NATIONAL FISH COMPANY LTD

31A Airport Rd, PMB 1427, Benin City, Bendel State
Tel: 242191
Telex: 41375

Chairman: Chief D N Oronsaye
Directors: A Dale (Managing),
J O Ajibola,
F B Giwa,
Chief Eneh,
Price Ogei,
P Larinde,
Mr Olagbeji,
Mr Hirsch

PRINCIPAL ACTIVITIES: Fishing and fish processing

Date of Establishment: 1975
No of Employees: 600

NIGERIA NATIONAL SUPPLY COMPANY LTD

Nasco House, 5th Floor, 29 Burma Rd, Apapa, PMB 12662, Lagos
Tel: 876606
Cable: Procurers
Telex: 21560

Chairman: Chief G C Okuia
Directors: S A Fagbemi, Alhaji S Ringim, A G K Onikoye, M B Dogon-Yaro, Alhaji S Idris, S O Isiadinso
Senior Executives: Alhaji A D Mohammed (General Manager),
  C P N Okafor (Procurement Manager),
  C S Audu (Marketing Manager),
  J O Babayemi (Acting Finance Manager),
  Y M Wanka (Branch Manager, London Office),
  Administration Manager/Secretary

PRINCIPAL ACTIVITIES: Federal Government agency for the procurement and distribution of essential commodities and stores requirements of ministries, corporations, companies, and government institutions. Retail shops to be opened
Branch Offices: 5 Kennedy Ave, Trans-Amadi Industrial Layout, PMB 5179, Port Harcourt; C/O Co-operative Movement Office, Gombe-Biu Rd, PMB 9, Gombe; Eku House, PMB 1142, Warri; C/O Co-operative & Credit Marketing Union Office, Kano Rd, PMB 6031, Funtua; 59 Calabar Rd, PO Box 869, Calabar; 2 Maimalari Rd, Bompai, PO Box 3030, Kano; PMB 1459, Nguru Rd, Maiduguri; Minna Rd, PO Box 71, Bida, Niger State; Amakohia, Okigwe, C/O Min of Trade, Industry & Co-operative, Owerri, Imo State; C/O Min of Trade, Industry & Co-operative, Oyo State, Ibadan; 7 Onitsha Rd, PMB 1534, Enugu; Shipping & Forwarding Div, 46, Burma Rd, Apapa; Warehouses and Lagos Distribution Centre, Plot 5 Block K Isolo; Industrial Layout, Isolo Express Way, Isolo; Purchasing Office, 61 Broad St, Lagos; Imperial House, 15/19 Kingsway, London WC2; Quantity Control Division, 42 Burma Rd, Apapa, Lagos
Principal Bankers: United Bank of Africa Ltd
Financial Information:

	₦'000
Authorised capital	25,000
Paid-up capital	25,000

Date of Establishment: 24th January 1972

NIGERIA PUBLISHERS SERVICES LTD

PO Box 62, Ibadan, Oyo State
Tel: 462726
Telex: 31478

Chairman: Chief G Osiname
Directors: T D Otesanya (Managing),
  O Oloko,
  R Fowles,
  O Odusote,
  Chief S O Sotanwa
Senior Executives: A A Falore (Warehouse Manager),
  S D Idowu-Kuola (Marketing Manager),
  Dare Arokoyo (Area Manager)

PRINCIPAL ACTIVITIES: Warehousing and books distribution
Principal Agencies: Cambridge University Press, UK; George Allen & Unwin Ltd, UK; Hodder & Stoughton Ltd, UK; Hutchinson Publishing Group, UK; Routledge & Kegan Paul Ltd, UK; Collins Publishers, UK; Lea & Febiger, USA; Little, Brown & Company, US; Medical Examinations Publishing Company, USA; Rand McNally & Company, US
Branch Offices: PO Box 722, Zaria, Kaduna State, Tel: 3470; PO Box 4073, Onitsha, Anambra State
Principal Bankers: Union Bank of Nigeria, Icon Merchant Bankers
Financial Information:

	₦'000
Authorised capital	100
Paid-up capital	50
Turnover	2,500

Principal Shareholders: Hodder & Stoughton Ltd
Date of Establishment: 1st April 1978
No of Employees: 66

NIGERIA REINSURANCE CORPORATION

50/52 Broad St, PMB 12766, Lagos
Tel: 634141, 631200
Cable: Nigeriare
Telex: 21092

Chairman: Chief Toye Coker
Directors: J O Irukwu (Managing Director),
  Chief A J Uka,
  Alhaja M Y Amu,
  Chief A J Ukpanah,
  Alhaji M Galadanci,
  Alhaji Bala Hassan,
  Alhaji Sidi Aliyu,
  K B Orubebe,
  J A Amaichigh
Senior Executives: O Osoka (Manager, Life, Marketing Department),
  G Adesina (Manager, General Accident Department),
  C Oyolu (Manager, Marine/Aviation Departments),
  O Alao (Deputy Chief Accountant),
  E Zango (Deputy Secretary to the Corporation)

PRINCIPAL ACTIVITIES: National and international professional reinsurer; channel through which reinsurance business is ceded to African reinsurance corporations and reinsurers all over the world
Branch Offices: Plot G5 Ahmadu Bello Way, PMB 225, Kaduna, Tel 212485; Cocoa House, 12th Floor, Ibadan, Oyo State, Tel 461163, 461160; Valid House, Colliery Avenue, Enugu, Anambra State, Tel 256828
Principal Bankers: African Continental Bank; Bank of the North; United Bank for Africa; Union Bank of Nigeria
Financial Information:

	₦'000
Authorised capital	10,000
Paid-up capital	6,000
Turnover (approx)	50,000

Principal Shareholders: Public corporation, owned by the Federal Government of Nigeria
Date of Establishment: 1st July 1976
No of Employees: 380

NIGERIA RELIANCE FURNITURE COMPANY

3 Neki Commercial Layout, PO Box 625, Gangere, Jos, Plateau State
Tel: 2313

Chairman: Peter James Onah
Senior Executives: John Ona Ajeibi (Manager),
  Stephen Ujah (Foreman),
  Bashiru Gbadamosi (Foreman)

PRINCIPAL ACTIVITIES: Furniture manufacturing for schools, offices, hospitals and hotels

NIGERIA STEEL PRODUCTS LTD

PMB 5288, Ibadan, Oyo State

Directors: Guido Zamblera

PRINCIPAL ACTIVITIES: Manufacturers of road tankers, trailers, steel bodies, storage tanks, structural steel buildings, barges
Branch Offices: Enerhen Rd, Warri, Bendel State Tel: 616, 390

NIGERIA TEIJIN TEXTILES LTD

Israel Adebajo Rd, Industrial Estate, PO Box 1128, Ikeja, Lagos
Tel: 900573, 900572, 961054
Cable: Teijin, Ikeja
Telex: 21503 Latjn Ng

Directors: F Ola Ijiti (Assistant General Manager)

197

PRINCIPAL ACTIVITIES: Manufacturing of polyester and viscose rayon blended fabrics; Teijin Tetoron suitings

No of Employees: 1,200

NIGERIA REINSURANCE CORPORATION

Head Office:
Bookshop House,
50/52 Broad Street,
Lagos.

Tel: 636394, 631200
Cable: Nigeriare
Telex: 21092 Nigrin ng

Chairman: H O Mohammed MBE
Directors:
Mr J O Irukwu *(Managing Director)*
Chief Toye Coker Chairman, Alhaja MY AMU
Chief A J Ukpanah, Alhaji M Galadanci
Alhaji Bala Hassan, Alhaji Sidi Aliyu
Mr K B Orubebe and Mr J A Amaichigh
Senior Executives:
Mr O Osoka *(Senior Manager, Life/Marketing Department)*
Mr G O Adesina *(Senior Manager, Accident/Fire Department)*
Mr C O Oyolu *(Senior Manager, Marine/Aviation Department)*
Mr D B Hart *(Secretary to the Corporation)*

Principal Activities: National and international professional reinsurer; channel through which reinsurance business is ceded to African reinsurance corporation and reinsurers all over the world.
Principal Bankers:
African Continental Bank
Bank of the North
United Bank for Africa
Union Bank of Nigeria

Financial Information:	N,000
Authorised Capital	10,000
Paid-up Capital	6,000
Turnover (approx)	50,000

Principal Shareholders: Public corporation, owned by the Federal Government of Nigeria
Number of Employees: 220

NIGERIA-ARAB BANK LTD

Mandilas House, 96/102 Broad St, Lagos
Tel: 662398, 661955, 662098, 662320
Cable: Bankarabi (all branches)
Telex: 21973 NARABH

Chairman: Alhaji Ibrahim El Yakubu
Directors: Alhaji S A Sule (Managing),
M Fahoum (Vice Chairman),
Alhaji U Nagogo (Executive),
A S T Obeidat (Executive),
M Beydoun,
I A Ademiluyi,
M Gaiya,
Mrs B Onyeador,
H A Darwish
Senior Executives: A M Okkeh (Manager, Isolo Branch),
A S T Obeidat (Manager, Apapa Branch),
M A Majeed (Manager, Kano Branch),
M H El-Mongy (Manager, Ibadan Branch)

PRINCIPAL ACTIVITIES: Commercial banking
Branch Offices: 36 Balogun Square, Lagos, Telex 21488; 4E Bello Rd, PO Box 318, Kano; 300 Apapa Rd, PO Box 537, Apapa, Lagos; Plot No 1 Block F, Ilupeju Industrial Ext 11, PMB 1083, Mushin, Lagos; Intra Motors Building, 78 Lagos By-Pass, PMB 5518, Ibadan, Oyo State; Gwarzo and Kazaure, Kano State; Owode Egbe, Ogun State; Bichi, Ado-Odo, Odeda, Oregun, Kaduna, Tudun-Wada, Minna, Fiditi, Kafin Maiyaki, Odeomu Oyo State

Financial Information: As at 31st December 1980

Liabilities	N'000	Assets	N'000
Share capital	5,000	Cash & banks	993
Reserves (total)	5,142	Investments, loans	
Deposits, taxation,		& other assets	
Dividends & other		(less tax & dividends	
Liabilities	99,520	etc)	106,701
		Fixed assets	1,968
		(Total assets	109,662)
Contra a/cs	35,633	Contra a/cs	35,633
		Total Balance Sheet	145,295

Principal Shareholders: Federal Ministry of Finance Incorporated Lagos; Arab Bank Ltd, Amman, Jordan
Date of Establishment: 12th November, 1969
No of Employees: 400

NIGERIAN & OVERSEAS PRODUCTS LTD

Head Office, 2 Dala Junction, PO Box 701, Kano
Tel: 4086, 3852
Cable: Noped

Chairman: Alhaji Salihi Lliasu
Directors: A Lliasu
Senior Executives: B G Oladodu (Accountant),
A O Martins (Lagos, Manager),
Alhaji R Modiu (Transport Manager)

PRINCIPAL ACTIVITIES: General transportation of goods including heavy machines, containers; sale of windscreens, generators, batteries, etc
Principal Agencies: Expo Visual Ltd, UK
Branch Offices: 4 Creek Rd, PO Box 130, Apapa, Lagos, Tel 873216; 36 Ruwam-Godiya Close, off Dawaki Rd, Kaduna
Principal Bankers: International Bank for West Africa Ltd; Bank of the North Ltd; United Bank for Africa Ltd

Date of Establishment: 3rd December 1968

NIGERIAN AGIP OIL COMPANY LTD

9/11 Macarthy St, PO Box 1268, Lagos
Tel: 651590/1, 630709, 630833
Cable: Agipoil Lagos
Telex: 21268

Chairman: P Carotenuto
Directors: P Maioli (Vice-Chairman),
S Iazzolino (Managing),
O Bassani (Deputy Managing),
J Iyalla,
L Lamberti,
Alhaji A Mutallab
Senior Executives: A Celenza (Finance Manager),
A Pirocchi (District Manager),
M E Arinze (Materials Manager),
J A Olatunji (Administration Manager),
P O Amaechi (Organisation & Dev. Manager),
S N Uwechie (Engineering Manager)

PRINCIPAL ACTIVITIES: Oil and gas exploration and production
Branch Offices: District Office, Mile 4 Port Harcourt/Ikwere Rd, PO Box 923, Port Harcourt, Tel: 21691/2, 21325/6, Cable: Agipoil Port Harcourt; Warri Base, Enehren Rd, PO Box 334, Warri
Subsidiary Companies: AGIP S.p.A and associated companies
Principal Bankers: United Bank for Africa Ltd
Financial Information:

	N'000
Authorised capital	1,800
Paid-up capital	1,800
Turnover	266,000

Principal Shareholders: AGIP SpA and associated companies
Date of Establishment: 1962
No of Employees: 1,366

NIGERIAN AGRICULTURAL AND COOPERATIVE BANK LTD

PMB 2155, Hospital Rd, Kaduna
Tel: 242203, 210111, Ext 290, 242204 (Projects)
Telex: 71115 Nabank Ng

PRINCIPAL ACTIVITIES: Financing of agricultural projects
Financial Information:
Capital   ₦ 24,000,000

Date of Establishment: 1973

NIGERIAN AGRICULTURAL PROMOTIONS COMPANY LTD

18/19 Ahmadu Bello Way, PO Box 1595, Kaduna
Cable: Agrico
Telex: 71108 Newdev Ng

Chairman: Alhaji Usman Nagogo
Directors: Mallam Abdu Abdurrahim, S B Oloruntoba, Alhaji M Zakari, Alhaji M Nimlan, Alhaji Ali Ndimi, Mallam A Idris, Dr Tunji Olagunju, Alhaji S D Umar
Senior Executives: Dr N O O Ejiga (General Manager), Dr C A M Lakpini (Livestock Specialist), Mallam Y Shehu (Agronomist)

PRINCIPAL ACTIVITIES: Agricultural consultants; agricultural and agro-allied project management and agricultural investment promotion
Principal Bankers: Bank of the North
Financial Information:

	₦'000
Authorised capital	1,000
Paid-up capital	400

Principal Shareholders: New Nigeria Development Company Ltd
Date of Establishment: 1973

NIGERIAN ALLUVIALS LTD

Dogon Dutse, PO Box 52, Jos, Plateau State
Tel: 2052

PRINCIPAL ACTIVITIES: Mining of metal ore

NIGERIAN ALUMINIUM DEVELOPMENT CO LTD (NADECO)

5 Williams St, PO Box 467, Lagos
Tel: 636590, 637065

PRINCIPAL ACTIVITIES: Distributors of aluminium sheets and ladders etc; consultants
Principal Agencies: Alusuisse Swiss Aluminium Ltd
Branch Offices: 32A Creek Rd, PO Box 360, Apapa, Lagos, Tel 874034, 874186

NIGERIAN ALUMINIUM ENGINEERING COMPANY LTD (NAECO)

5 Adeyemo Close, Off New International Airport Rd, Mafoluku, Oshodi, Lagos State
Tel: 934472, 934481

Chairman: Alhaji M Taiwo Odunuga
Directors: J O Bankole, B O Odunuga
Senior Executives: Tunde Obayemi (Personal Assistant to Managing Director), C A Oyelakin (Accountant)

PRINCIPAL ACTIVITIES: Manufacturers of building materials
Principal Bankers: United Bank for Africa Ltd; Nigeria-Arab Bank Ltd
Financial Information:

	₦'000
Authorised capital	500
Paid-up capital	200
Turnover	750
Profits	25

Principal Shareholders: Chairman and directors as described
Date of Establishment: March 1978
No of Employees: 61

NIGERIAN ALUMINIUM EXTRUSIONS LTD (NIGALEX)

PMB 21275, Plot No 5 Block H, Expressway, Oshodi Industrial Scheme, Ikeja, Lagos
Tel: 961426, 901160/4
Cable: Nigalex Ikeja
Telex: 26152

Chairman: Dr A Wachter
Directors: R Goettin, Dr M Voser, O Lijadu, A A Alikah, A Schmidweber, H Zayyad, E B Onifade, Sifida Investment Company SA (Luxembourg)
Senior Executives: H R Schaffner (General Manager), Bruno Klaus (Works Manager), Norman Skene (Chief Works Engineer), Joe I G Nzeka (Public and Industrial Relations Officer), Max Siegrist (Product Development Manager)

PRINCIPAL ACTIVITIES: Extrusion and anodising of aluminium sections, clear or in colour
Associated Companies: Swiss Aluminium Ltd (Alusuisse); UTC International Ltd
Principal Bankers: United Bank for Africa
Financial Information:

	₦'000
Authorised capital	1,200
Paid-up capital	1,200

Principal Shareholders: Alusuisse; UTC Basle; Great Nigeria Insurance Company; National Insurance Corporation of Nigeria; Nigerian Industrial Development Bank; International Finance Corp, Washington; Sifida Investment Company SA; New Nigeria Development Co, Ltd; Bendel Insurance Co Ltd; Odu'a Investment Co Ltd
No of Employees: 200

NIGERIAN AMERICAN MERCHANT BANK LTD

25 Boyle Street, Onikan, Lagos
Tel: 630935, 631707, 632363

Chairman: Chief Dr Ngbo Bekinbo Grahem-Douglash
Directors: P J Robb (Managing), Alhaji Ibrahim M Damcida, Rex I Alkija, G B Yurchyshyn

PRINCIPAL ACTIVITIES: Merchant banking

Date of Establishment: 1979
No of Employees: 75

NIGERIAN ASBESTOS INDUSTRIES LTD

Industrial Estate, PO Box 51, Bauchi
Cable: Babestos, Bauchi
Telex: 21003 Panaf Ng

PRINCIPAL ACTIVITIES: Manufacturers of building materials and cement
Branch Offices: 22 Idowu Taylor Street, PO Box 6776, Lagos
Principal Bankers: Union Bank of Nigeria Ltd
Financial Information:

	₦'000
Authorised capital	3,000
Paid-up capital	3,000
Turnover	2,000
Profits	235

Principal Shareholders: Bauchi State Government; M/S Hyderabad Asbestos Cement Product; Nigerian Industrial Dev Bank Ltd; Northern Nigerian Investment Ltd; Nigerians
Date of Establishment: 1st July 1974
No of Employees: 200

NIGERIAN AVIATION HANDLING COMPANY LTD

Murtala Mohammed Airport, Ikeja, Lagos

PRINCIPAL ACTIVITIES: Cargo and freight forwarders
Financial Information:
Registered capital   ₦ 1,000,000

Date of Establishment: 1979

NIGERIAN BAG MANUFACTURING COMPANY LTD

Eric Moore Rd, Iganmu, PO Box 589, Apapa
Tel: 832625
Cable: Bagco Lagos
Telex: 26153 Bagco Ng

Chairman: G S Coumantaros
Directors: D B Bentley (Managing),
  S A Oluwo,
  J O Fagbemi,
  A Plytas,
  J O Sowemimo
Senior Executives: R Mason (Technical Co-ordinator),
  R I Stoney (Production Co-Ordinator),
  A Oshogwemoh (Production Manager Plant 1),
  D A Ikujenyo (Production Manager Plant 2),
  D Ogunfowokan (Production Services Manager),
  P Barraclough (Technical Manager),
  O S Bello (Development Manager),
  S S Oyedele (Chief Accountant),
  J O Famoye (Personnel Manager),
  C O Dasilva (Training Manager)

PRINCIPAL ACTIVITIES: Manufacturers of woven polypropylene sacks
Principal Bankers: First Bank of Nigeria Ltd

Principal Shareholders: Flour Mills of Nigeria Ltd
Date of Establishment: 1972
No of Employees: 1,600

NIGERIAN BALL-POINT BEN INDUSTRIES LTD

PMB 1424, Israel Adebajo Close, Ikeja, Lagos
Tel: 964218

PRINCIPAL ACTIVITIES: Manufacturers of ball point pens

NIGERIAN BANK FOR COMMERCE AND INDUSTRY (NBCI)

1/9 Berkley St, PO Box 4424, Lagos
Tel: 632675/7, 632687, 632670
Cable: Nibacind
Telex: 125276

Chairman: Alhaji Sule Katagum
Directors: C Okobi (Managing Director),
  Alhaji Mahmud Gashash,
  E A Taiwo,
  D D Achakpa,
  Mallam M Ngileruma,
  Col Hilary Njoku,
  Dr S D Olaoye,
  Lt Col B B Awodeyi,
  Dr S A David-West,
  C F I Olaniyan,
  Dr J E Okundaye,
  Rev B Ikobi,
  Alhaji Dawuda Kutigi
Senior Executives: G C Akwaeze (Investment Appraisal),
  E E Okpiabhele (Administration/Secretary),
  M O Shodunke (Accounts),
  Alhaji Dangana (Investment Supervision),
  G Omoni (Legal Adviser),
  B a Olateru-Olagbeji (Merchant Banking)

PRINCIPAL ACTIVITIES: Provides equity capital and medium and long-term loans
Branch Offices: 1 Akpakpava St, PMB 1134, Benin City; 4 Lagos St, PMB 3252, Kano; 22 Station Rd, PMB 5849, Port Harcourt; 3 Kirikasama Rd, PMB 1547, Maiduguri; PO Box 2772, Jos; PMB 1160, Ikot-Ekpene, Cross River State
Financial Information:

	₦'000
Authorised capital	50,000
Paid-up capital	50,000

Principal Shareholders: Federal Government of Nigeria (60%); Central Bank of Nigeria (40%)
Date of Establishment: 1973
No of Employees: 280

NIGERIAN BOOK SUPPLIERS LTD

28 Akinremi St, PO Box 4440, Ikeja, Lagos
Tel: 631742
Cable: Nigerbook
Telex: 20202 Tds Box 052

Chairman: Mrs I Fatayi-Williams
Directors: Babatunde Fatayi-Williams (Managing Director),
  Oladele Fatayi-Williams
Senior Executives: Mrs Olatunde Williams (General Manager),
  R John (Marketing Manager),
  Mrs J C Coker (Orders Manager, Library Supplies),
  Mrs V P Oseni (Orders Manager, Bookshop Supplies),
  A C Ofoegbu (Legal Publications Manager),
  Olaniyi O Erinle (Accountant),
  Hakeem A Sanni (Credit Controller)

PRINCIPAL ACTIVITIES: Booksellers and library suppliers: suppliers of audio-visual materials, management and training films
Principal Agencies: Butterworths (UK); Open University; Harper and Row; Elsevier/North Holland; Nisbet; Associated Book Publishers (Sweet & Maxwell); Institute of Building; Brierley Price Prior
Associated Companies: Universal Distributors Ltd; Nigerian Cards Ltd

NIGERIAN BOTTLING COMPANY LTD

Head Office: Obafemi Awolowo Way, Ikeja, Lagos
Tel: 800220/9, 900901/9
Cable: Bottling Lagos

Chairman: H S A Adedeji
Directors: G E Keralakis, C Leventis, A A David, Chief S Ade John, Alhaji I El Yakubu, J T F Iyalla
Senior Executives: J E Iriabe (Company Secretary),
  A A Adesanya (General Manager)

PRINCIPAL ACTIVITIES: Manufacturers of soft drinks; bottlers of carbonated beverages
Principal Agencies: Holds franchise from the Coca-cola Company, USA
Branch Offices: Registered Office: Iddo House, Iddo, PO Box 159, Lagos; Benin City; Enugu; Ibadan; Ikeja; Ilorin; Jos; Kaduna; Kano (2); Owerri; Port Harcourt (2); Warri
Subsidiary Companies: Apapa Chemical Industries Ltd; Crown Products Ltd
Principal Bankers: Union Bank of Nigeria Ltd; Chase Merchant Bank Nigeria Ltd
Financial Information:

	₦'000
Authorised capital	25,000
Paid-up capital	24,511
Turnover (1981)	124,665
Profits (1981)	20,336

A member of the A G Leventis Group

Principal Shareholders: Nigerians (60%); Foreign (40%)
Date of Establishment: 22nd November 1951
No of Employees: 5,400

NIGERIAN BREWERIES LTD

PO Box 545, Abebe Village Rd, Iganmu, Lagos
Tel: 834651/6, 834003
Cable: Nibruserv Nibrusuper
Telex: 26370

Chairman: C E Abebe
Directors: C Allport (Managing, Technical),
  A O Adeaga,
  T J Davies (Deputy Chairman and Managing Director),
  Mrs M C Eneli,
  J Hunt,
  M A Makinde,
  F O A Ohiwerei,
  Chief E A Silva,
  J W den Hond,
  P van Eerde (Alternate Director),
  G A Oke (Alternate Director)
Senior Executives: W Kool (Aba Brewery Manager),
  H Timmer (Kaduna Brewery Manager),
  A De Voogd (Lagos Brewery Manager),
  W Kool (Nigeria Technological Controller),
  P O Onono (Public Relations Adviser),
  O A Yusuf (General Sales Manager),
  G Balogun (Chief Accountant),
  O A Peters (Company Secretary)
PRINCIPAL ACTIVITIES: Brewing and soft drinks
Branch Offices: PO Box 86, Apapa, Lagos State; PO Box 496, Aba, Imo State; PMB 2116, Kaduna
Associated Companies: Progress Trust Ltd
Principal Bankers: United Bank for Africa Ltd; First Bank of Nigeria Ltd; Union Bank of Nigeria Ltd
Financial Information:

	₦'000
Authorised capital	36,600
Paid-up capital	36,600

Principal Shareholders: CWA Holdings Ltd, UAC International Ltd, Heineken Brouwrijan BV, 43,000 Nigerians
Date of Establishment: 16th November 1946
No of Employees: 3,088

NIGERIAN BRICKS & CLAY PRODUCTS LTD

PMB 2154, Jos, Plateau State

PRINCIPAL ACTIVITIES: Production of clay bricks

NIGERIAN CARDS LTD

28 Akinremi St, PO Box 4440, Ikeja, Lagos

Chairman: Mrs Irene Fatayi-Williams
Directors: B A R Fatayi-Williams (Managing Director),
  Dr A A Fatayi-Williams,
  O A Fatayi-Williams
Senior Executives: Mrs O Williams (General Manaer),
  T O Oduyebo (Marketing Manager)

PRINCIPAL ACTIVITIES: Producers and distributors of greeting cards and allied products with a nationwide chain of card boutiques
Principal Agencies: Hallmark Cards Incorporated, UK
Associated Companies: Nigerian Book Suppliers Ltd; Universal Distributors Ltd
Principal Bankers: First Bank of Nigeria Ltd

NIGERIAN CARPET MANUFACTURING CO LTD

SW8/89 Lagos Bye Pass, Oke-Ado, Ibadan, Oyo State

PRINCIPAL ACTIVITIES: Manufacture of carpets
Financial Information: Part of Ribway Group of companies (see separate entry)

NIGERIAN CARTON & PACKAGING MANUFACTURING COMPANY LTD

23 Industrial Avenue, Ilupeju, PO Box 296, Ikeja, Lagos State
Tel: 961505, 964145
Cable: Nicapaco
Telex: 26129, 26121 Multip Ng, Nicapa Ng

Chairman: Jameson Shu
Directors: Anthony H O Shu (Managing Director),
  Chief C M Smith,
  Chief D S Yaro

PRINCIPAL ACTIVITIES: Manufacturers of packaging, corrugated cartons, paper/paper products, plastics, printing
Branch Offices: 1 Sapara Street, Ikeja Industrial Estate, Lagos
Principal Bankers: United Bank for Africa
Financial Information:

	₦'000
Authorised capital	500
Paid-up capital	500

No of Employees: 350

NIGERIAN CATERERS & SUPERMARKETS LTD

PO Box 3646, 132 Awolowo Rd, Sw Ikoyi, Lagos
Tel: 680831, 682910
Cable: Alabela Lagos

Chairman: Edwin G P Abela
Senior Executives: Fouad Chamma (Manager),
  Jamil Bitar (Superintendent, Warri),
  Ibrahim Jeha (Superintendent, Port Harcourt)

PRINCIPAL ACTIVITIES: Industrial catering for the oil industry; food suppliers, traders and contractors
Branch Offices: PO Box 352, Chief Obido Estate; Warri, Bendel State; Tel: 233749/231951; PO Box 448, 45 Trans-Amadi Industrial Layout, Port Harcourt, Rivers State, Tel: 334118/333420
Principal Bankers: First Bank of Nigeria Ltd

Principal Shareholders: Albert Abela, Lebanon and UK

NIGERIAN CEMENT COMPANY LTD (NIGERCEM)

Nkalagu, PO Box 331, Enugu, Anambra State
Tel: 259001/4
Cable: Nigercemco Enugu

Chairman: G I Onyenso
Directors: S O Ilodibia, M E Ibekwe, L U Ukwu, A Okoro, M B Yesufu, C C Amobi, E O Onwuka, M Yesufu, E O Ezigbo
PRINCIPAL ACTIVITIES: Manufacturers of cement and paper bags
Branch Offices: Aba

Principal Shareholders: Federal Government (10%); Commonwealth Development Corporation (10%); Private Investors (25%); Imo and Anambra State Government (55%)

NIGERIAN CEMENTATION & DRILLING CO LTD

37 Marina, Unity House, 11th Floor, Lagos
Tel: 636792

Chairman: E A Adewusi
Directors: L Ponzan,
  G Dugnani,
  L Ginetti (Managing)

PRINCIPAL ACTIVITIES: Civil engineering
Principal Bankers: United Bank for Africa Ltd

Principal Shareholders: Chairman & directors as described
Date of Establishment: 1975
No of Employees: 150

NIGERIAN CEREALS PROCESSING COMPANY LTD

Umaru Babura Rd, PO Box 523, Kano
Tel: 3170, 2333

Directors: M A Fadlallah (Director)

PRINCIPAL ACTIVITIES: Manufacturers of macaroni, rice and
animal feeds

NIGERIAN CHEMICAL SERVICES LTD (NCS)

PO Box 83, 26 Henry Carr St, Ikeja, Lagos
Tel: 931187, 961012, 962324
Cable: Chemserve Ikeja
Telex: 21378 Majcom Ng

Chairman: D J Fielding
Directors: C B Ruffell (Managing Director)

PRINCIPAL ACTIVITIES: Manufacturers of cosmetics,
insecticides, expanded polyestyrene, industrial chemicals
Branch Offices: Aba; Kano

NIGERIAN COAL CORPORATION

29 Okpara Ave, PMB 01053, Enugu, Anambra State
Tel: 255314, 255325
Cable: Coals Enugu
Telex: 51115

Directors: Alhaji Ibrahim Omar, Alhaji L O Omotosho, Alhaji Isa
Haruna, R N Mba, E Ashieaka, C N Okezie
Senior Executives: A O Udemah (Administrator/Acting General
Manager, Finance),
F N Ugwu (Acting General Manager, Production),
E E Mbanugo (Acting General Manager, Administration),
U O Okpara (Principal Commercial Officer),
I M Chukwu-Ike (Chief Planning Officer),
N Ukaejiofor (Senior Med Officer),
D A Sowade (Secretary)

PRINCIPAL ACTIVITIES: Mining and marketing of Nigerian coal
Branch Offices: Ijora Coal Office, Lagos
Principal Bankers: International Bank for West Africa; African
Continental Bank

Principal Shareholders: Federal Government of Nigeria
Date of Establishment: 12th October 1950
No of Employees: 3,072

NIGERIAN COCOA BOARD

Cocoa House, PMB 5032, Ibadan, Oyo State
Tel: 462840/3
Cable: Nicob Ibadan
Telex: 31230 Nicob; 31442 Nicob

Chairman: Dr Abiola Ojo
Directors: His Highness Emmanuel o Efeizomir (The Obi of Owa),
Y Oyeleke,
Mallam H B Mohammad,
Chief C A Oluwasina,
Raymond Kotey,
M N Agbor,
Alhaji A Dangana,
The Permanent Secretary (Federal Ministry of Agriculture and
Water Resources),
The Permanent Secretary (Ministry of Trade),
A O Udo (Central Bank of Nigeria),
Chief M O Akinode,
J A Akinsipe (General Manager)
Senior Executives: A A Coker (Assistant General Manager,
Shipping),
J A Afuwape (Assistant General Manager, Administration),
M O Mafe (Assistant General Manager, Finance),
A Akinlose (Assistant General Manager, Sales)

PRINCIPAL ACTIVITIES: Marketing of cocoa, coffee and tea on
a national and international basis
Branch Offices: Ikeja; Apapa; Akure; Ikare; Ado-Ekiti; Calabar;
Abeokuta; Ondo; Port Harcourt; Ile-Ife; Umuahia; Osogbo;
Sapele; Owo; Benin; Ikom; Kabba

Principal Bankers: Central Bank of Nigeria; Cooperative Bank of
Nigeria Ltd; United Bank for Africa Ltd; African Continental
Bank Ltd
Financial Information:
Turnover   ₦ 242,194,762
Principal Shareholders: Federal Government of Nigeria
Date of Establishment: 1st April 1977
No of Employees: 1,592

NIGERIAN COMMERCIAL & INDUSTRIAL ENTERPRISES LTD

State Highway, Ilupeju Industrial Estate, Mushin, PO Box 837,
Lagos
Tel: 900385, 900386/7
Cable: Yabco Lagos

Chairman: John C Emeka
Directors: D Berger,
T Dortschy,
H Hirsch,
M Lengfeld,
A Rotzler (Managing Director),
M O Soremi
Senior Executives: K H Lindemann (Financial Controller),
B R Theuss (General Manager)

PRINCIPAL ACTIVITIES: Suppliers of building materials, steel
sections and plates, metals, metal processing and fabrication,
paper/paper products
Principal Agencies: Hoesch Handel AG, West Germany;
Salzgitter Stahl GmbH, West Germany
Branch Offices: PO Box 133, Kaduna; PO Box 354, Warri;
Zaramaganpa Bukuru Rd, Jos; 54 New Lagos Rd, Benin City;
PO Box 3424, Ibadan; PO Box 644, Port Harcourt; Oyo Bye
Pass, Ilorin; PMB 1272, Maiduguri; PMB 1189, Calabar; 4
Okpara Ave, Enugu; PO Box 527, Sokoto; PO Box 647, Kano
Principal Bankers: United Bank for Africa Ltd
Financial Information:

	₦'000
Authorised capital	5,000
Paid-up capital	2,400
Sales turnover	30,000

Principal Shareholders: Salzgitter Stahl GmbH, Germany;
Hoesch Handel AG, Germany; J C Emeka
No of Employees: 1,000

NIGERIAN COMMERCIAL FACTORY LTD

PO Box 5780, Plot A Block IV Area Planning Authority Rd,
Ilupeju Industrial Estate, Lagos
Tel: 964102
Cable: Plastishoe

Chairman: Bashir Lababedi
Senior Executives: Khaldoun Adi (Managing Director)

PRINCIPAL ACTIVITIES: Plastic footwear manufacturers
Principal Bankers: Arab Bank (Nigeria) Ltd
Financial Information:

	₦'000
Authorised capital	300
Paid-up capital	300

No of Employees: 200

NIGERIAN COMMERCIAL PRESS

41 Commercial Ave, Yaba, PO Box 1266, Lagos
Tel: 860786

PRINCIPAL ACTIVITIES: Printers and stationers
Branch Offices: Depot: 7 Oyebajo St, Igbobi, Lagos

NIGERIAN COMPANY FOR ENERGY ENGINEERING LTD (NICOGEN)

Lapal House, 215/235 Igbosere Rd, Lagos
Tel: 630139, 632560, 632540, 632561
Telex: 21656

Directors: J I C Igbe, J Ways, Dr G U Damachi, Chief J U Odey, G Wayas
PRINCIPAL ACTIVITIES: Civil engineering, construction, mechanical and electrical contractors
Branch Offices: 73B Marine Rd, PO Box 2002, Apapa, Lagos
Principal Bankers: United Bank for Africa Ltd; Mercantile Bank of Nigeria Ltd; Union Bank Ltd
Financial Information:

	₦'000
Authorised capital	500
Paid-up capital	500

Date of Establishment: 1976
No of Employees: 600

NIGERIAN CONCRETE INDUSTRIES LTD
191 Agege Motor Rd, PO Box 20, Mushin, Lagos
Tel: 836756, 831382

Chairman: Otunba J Ade Tuyo
Directors: L O Hertel

PRINCIPAL ACTIVITIES: Production of concrete and other building materials, spun pipes, blocks, etc
Branch Offices: Ring Rd, PMB 5198, Ibadan, Oyo State; College Rd, PO Box 122, Akure, Ondo State

NIGERIAN CONSOLIDATED FOOD PRODUCERS LTD
Western House, 12th Floor, PO Box 10171, 8/10 Broad St, Lagos

PRINCIPAL ACTIVITIES: Poultry production
Branch Offices: Imeke Village, Ilado Imeke Rd, Badagry Division, Lagos State
Financial Information:
Registered capital ₦ 400,000

Date of Establishment: October 1977

NIGERIAN CONSTRUCTION & HOLDING CO LTD
11 Alhaji Ribadu Rd, SW Ikoyi, PO Box 183, Apapa, Lagos
Tel: 680070, 681340
Cable: Conhold Lagos

Chairman: Chief S B Bakare
Directors: B H Beany, Chief Dr Norman Williams, Barbar Beany, Chief Bola Adedipe
Senior Executives: Khalil M Khouri (General Manager), Derek A White (Purchasing Manager), B Ali (Financial Controller)

PRINCIPAL ACTIVITIES: Construction of industrialised system buildings and conventional buildings
Branch Offices: PO Box 56, Auchi, Bendel State
Principal Bankers: Societe Generale Bank Nigeria Ltd
Financial Information:

	₦'000
Authorised capital	500
Paid-up capital	500
Sales turnover	15,000

Principal Shareholders: Chairman and directors as described
No of Employees: 2,000

NIGERIAN CONSTRUCTION AND WATER RESOURCES DEVELOPMENT LTD
Oyo Rd, Opposite University of Ibadan, PO Box 1420, Ibadan, Oyo State
Tel: 416410, 416431, 416464
Cable: Waterdev Ibadan
Telex: 31129 NWRD Ng

Chairman: Layi Ogunsola
Directors: E Porat, M Shawkan, Y Melman (Managing), Chief A K Alimikhena, Chief S F Onabanjo,

Chief F T Okpomu
Senior Executives: E Serlin (Branch Manager - Oyo State), M Feldman (Branch Manager - Bendel State), R A Gordon (Branch Manager - Cross River State), G Ben-Abraham (Branch Manager - Anambra State), R Adivi (Branch Manager - Ondo State), S Ofek (Operation Manager of Works), N Shay (Financial Controller), C F K Amavi (Secretary/Chief Accountant), S E Usiholo (Personnel Manager), S O Olagoke (Chief Supplies Officer), J O Ladele (Project Manager)

PRINCIPAL ACTIVITIES: Building and civil engineering contractors
Branch Offices: Sapele Rd, PO Box 409, Benin City, Bendel State; 4P Atimbr St, Off Airport Rd, PO Box 1346, Calabar, Cross River State; 62 Park Avenue, GRA PO Box 8149, Enugu, Anambra State; Ijero Rd, PO Box 179, Ido-Ekiti, Ondo State
Principal Bankers: First Bank of Nigeria Ltd
Financial Information:

	₦'000
Authorised capital	2,431
Paid-up capital	2,431

Principal Shareholders: Odu'a Investment Company Ltd; Bendel State Government; Water Resources Development (International) Ltd, Israel
Date of Establishment: 1959
No of Employees: 3,000

NIGERIAN COTTON BOARD
Tarkwa House, PMB 6035, Funtua, Kaduna State
Tel: Funtua 176
Cable: Cotboard Ng

Chairman: Alhaji Lema Jibrilu
Directors: Alhaji Mohammed Jabbi, Alhaji Usman Tahir, Alhaji Mohammed A Kollere, Alhaji Abubakar Kwakuru, Alhaji Usman A Bichi, Alhaji Sani Sigona Kotangora, Dr J S Odama, O Ajetunmobi, Ex-Officio Members, Representatives of Federal Ministries of Agriculture, Trade, Economic Planning, Central Bank of Nigeria, General Manager of Nigerian Cotton Board
Senior Executives: Alhaji Bello Adamu (General Manager/Chief Executive), J C Udokwu (Assistant General Manager, Sales), Alhaji Baba Mairami (Assistant General Manager, Finance), Alhaji A Tunau (Assistant General Manager, Operations), Adekunle Adeyemo (Chief Marketing Research Officer), Mallam A M Koki (Board Secretary/Legal Adviser), Alhaji Inua Muhammed (Personnel Manager), Alhaji Maikudi Kankia (Purchasing Manager, Tobacco), Alhaji A A Adebesin (Assistant Chief Accountant)

PRINCIPAL ACTIVITIES: Cotton and kenaf marketing
Principal Agencies: Cotton and Agricultural Processors (Nig) Ltd, Zaria; Nigerian Tobacco Company Ltd; Philip Morris (Nig) Ltd; Northern Nigeria Fibre Ltd, Jos; Jamaa Fibre Scheme, Jos
Branch Offices: Biu; Challawa; Funtua; Gombe; Gusau; Kontagora; Keffi; Kumo; Kuru; Lamurde; Lokoja; Mai Inchi; Mallumfashi Misau; Osogbo; Zaria
Associated Companies: Cotton & Agricultural Processors (Nigeria) Ltd
Principal Bankers: Bank of the North

Principal Shareholders: Nigerian Federal Government
Date of Establishment: 1st April 1977
No of Employees: 600

NIGERIAN CUTLERY LTD
PO Box 135, Ikeja, Lagos

PRINCIPAL ACTIVITIES: Manufacturing of cutlery, scissors, and agricultural implements

NIGERIAN DIVERSIFIED INVESTMENTS LTD

Investment House, Room 911, 21/25 Broad Street, Lagos
Tel: 664778, 663651
Cable: Overecho

Chairman: Raymond W Baker
Directors: Chief C O Ogunbanjo,
  Alhaji Jalo Waziri,
  B W Isaac,
  Philip C Broughton,
  Chief G O Osuchukwu (Executive Director/Company
    Secretary)
Senior Executives: P Bolarinwa (Executive Director),
  E U Konyeshi (Executive Director)

PRINCIPAL ACTIVITIES: Investment holding company
Associated Companies: Continental Office Products Ltd; Nigeria
  Kraft Bags Ltd; Jim Corporation Ltd
Principal Bankers: First Bank of Nigeria Ltd
Financial Information:

	N'000
Authorised capital	400
Paid-up capital	400

Principal Shareholders: Overecho Inc New York; Chief C O
  Ogunbanjo
Date of Establishment: 21st August 1969
No of Employees: 500

NIGERIAN DIVING SERVICE LTD

Savannah Bank Chamber, 6th Floor, 138/146 Broad St, PO Box
  2151, Lagos Island
Tel: 664759, 663277
Cable: Dodco Lagos
Telex: 21037 Dodco Lagos

Chairman: D O Dafinone
Directors: C E Dafinone,
  T Lindsay (Managing)
Senior Executives: T Salami (Chief Accountant),
  E A Luggard (Diving Superintendent)

PRINCIPAL ACTIVITIES: Diving services for the oil and
  construction industries
Branch Offices: 9 Kofo Abayomi Ave, Apapa, Lagos, Tel:
  870496, 870498 Cable: Dodco Lagos
Principal Bankers: Union Bank of Nigeria Ltd

Principal Shareholders: D O Dafinone; C E Dafinone
Date of Establishment: January 1972

NIGERIAN DOOR FABRICATION COMPANY LTD

Plot 2 Block L Industrial Estate, Isolo, PO Box 325, Surulere,
  Lagos State
Tel: 847569
Cable: Sikco

Chairman: S A Kasali (also Managing Director)
Senior Executives: P Eitel (Factory Manager)

PRINCIPAL ACTIVITIES: Manufacturers of flush doors, window
  frames and door frames
Principal Agencies: Compagnie Forestiere du Gabon
Associated Companies: S Kasali & Company Ltd
Principal Bankers: First Bank of Nigeria Ltd
Financial Information:

	N'000
Paid-up capital	1,000
Sales turnover (approx)	4,000

No of Employees: 100

NIGERIAN DREDGING AND MARINE LTD

1 Adeola Hopewell Street, Victoria Island, Lagos
Tel: 615129, 615130
Telex: 21362 Habwok Ng

Chairman: Alhaji Nuhu Bamali
Directors: R C W Brouwer (Managing),
  O Akinwumiju (Financial),
  I S Usman,
  Alhaji Balarabe Ismaila,
  A J Hoekstra,
  T A Anenih
Senior Executives: J van Mameren (Dredging Manager),
  A D van der Veen (Pipeline Manager),
  R W Boogaard (Civil Manager),
  S O Smith (Financial Controller)

PRINCIPAL ACTIVITIES: Dredging and land reclamation, pipeline
  construction, civil engineering and housing
Principal Agencies: Royal Volker Stevin, Holland
Branch Offices: Merogun Waterside, PO Box 361, Warri;
  Abuloma, PO Box 290, Port Harcourt
Associated Companies: Roads Nigeria Ltd; Adriaan Volker Civil
  Engineering (Nigeria)
Principal Bankers: First Bank of Nigeria; Union Bank of Nigeria

Principal Shareholders: Nigerian Citizens (60%); Van Hattum en
  Blankevoort (Royal Volker Stevin) (40%)
Date of Establishment: 14th April 1960
No of Employees: 3,000

NIGERIAN ELECTRIC FITTING LTD

150 Club Rd, PO Box 195, Kano
Tel: 2513
Cable: Voltelec

PRINCIPAL ACTIVITIES: Manufacturers of electric fittings

NIGERIAN ELECTRICITY SUPPLY CORPORATION (NIGERIA) LTD

PO Box 15, Bukuru, Plateau State
Tel: Bukuru 171
Cable: Nigercorp

Chairman: C R de Kretser (also Managing Director)
Directors: Hon Trevor Trefgarne, S J Cockburn, S Miner, S O
  Ajose, B A Lawson, R K Adewale, Plateau Investments Co
  Ltd

PRINCIPAL ACTIVITIES: Electricity generation and supply
Principal Bankers: First Bank of Nigeria Ltd
Financial Information:

	N'000
Authorised capital	5,000
Paid-up capital	5,000
Turnover	2,500

Principal Shareholders: Plateau State Government; Benue State
  Government; National Insurance Corporation of Nigeria;
  Nigerian Mining Corporation; Nesco Investments Ltd, London
No of Employees: 340

NIGERIAN ELECTRONICS COMPANY LTD

34/36 Ojuelegba Rd, PMB 3073, Surulere, Lagos
Tel: 833261/2, 831803

PRINCIPAL ACTIVITIES: Importation and assembly of electrical
  products, refrigerators, air-conditioners, cookers, etc
Branch Offices: 71 Ibara Rd, Abeokuta, Ogun State; 8 Agbado
  St, Benin City, Bendel State; SW8/880 Liberty Stadium Rd,
  Ibadan, Oyo State

NIGERIAN EMBEL TIN SMELTING COMPANY

Jos, Plateau State

PRINCIPAL ACTIVITIES: Tin smelting

NIGERIAN ENAMELWARE COMPANY LTD (NEWCO)

1 Adinlewa Rd, PO Box 3, Ikeja Industrial Estate, Ikeja, Lagos
Tel: 963075
Telex: 26659 Newco Ng

Chairman: Alhaji Inuwa Wada
Directors: Alhaji Inuwa Wada,
   Eric N Y Chu (Managing Director),
   S K Ying (Deputy Chief Executive),
   John Turf,
   P Best,
   O A Adeosun,
   A A Adio-Moses,
   R J Whitfield,
   D R Simpson,
   Alhaji O Omodeni (Chief Accountant)

PRINCIPAL ACTIVITIES: Manufacturers of enamelware
Financial Information:

	N'000
Authorised capital	2,400
Paid-up capital	2,400
Turnover (1981)	24,146
Profits (1981)	366

Principal Shareholders: John Holt Holdings (Nigeria) Ltd; I Feng Co Ltd
Date of Establishment: 1961
No of Employees: 1,335

NIGERIAN ENGINEERING AND CONSTRUCTION COMPANY LTD (NECCO)

Km 14 Lagos Badagry Expressway, PMB 12684, Lagos
Tel: 861458
Cable: Neccolim Lagos
Telex: 11181 Yu Energo; 11862

Chairman: Malam Aminu Wali
Directors: Mallam A B Wali, Alhaji Maina Waziri, Dr T Onoge, T Anineh, A C Asadu, M Novakovic, M Boskovic, D Stojanovic, D Radulovic
Senior Executives: P O Ilugbo (Chief Accountant),
   R O Fajemisin (Deputy Commercial Manager),
   T A Babalola (Senior Administration Officer Personnel, Acting Secretary),
   B Bogetic (Technical Manager, Acting),
   V Krunic (Managing),
   Kabiru Rabiu (Company Secretary),
   M Popnovakovic (Commercial Manager)

PRINCIPAL ACTIVITIES: Civil engineering, construction and consulting services; furniture making
Branch Offices: PO Box 5105, Kano (Irrigation Project); PMB 26, Yola, Gongola State (Kiri Dam Project)
Principal Bankers: United Bank for Africa; Union Bank of Nigeria Ltd
Financial Information:

	N'000
Authorised capital	2,000
Paid-up capital	1,244
Sales turnover	35,000

Principal Shareholders: Federal Government of Nigeria (60%); Energoprojekt of Belgrade (40%)
Date of Establishment: April 1974
No of Employees: 3,844

NIGERIAN ENTERPRISES PROMOTION BOARD (NEPB)

Constanza House, 72 Campbell St, PMB 12553, Race Course, Lagos
Tel: 680975

PRINCIPAL ACTIVITIES: Government body set up to carry out the indigenisation programme in Nigeria
Branch Offices: Inspectorate Division; 15/19 Keffi St, SW Ikoyi, PMB 12553, Lagos

NIGERIAN EXPLOSIVES & PLASTICS CO LTD

PO Box 149, Oke-Afa, Isolo, Mushin, Lagos State
Tel: 862456, 831221, 831226
Cable: Neplasco Lagos
Telex: 21578 Ashamu Ng

Chairman: Chief E O Ashamu
Directors: O O Fashola
Senior Executives: C A Alabi (General Manager),
   S A Okunade (Marketing Manager),
   K A Ipadeola (Chief Accountant),
   Y O Obe (Store Controller),
   V I Anyafulu (Office Manager),
   Miss O A Awoyemi (Market Research Officer)

PRINCIPAL ACTIVITIES: Distributors of industrial explosives, personal firearms, industrial chemical products, goodrich tyres, paints and typar
Principal Agencies: E I Dupont De-Nemours, USA; South Western Pipe, USA; Goodrich Co, USA; Remington Arms Inc, USA; Gevelot, France; British Steel Co, UK
Branch Offices: 18 Park Rd, Zaria; Mile 5 Bukuru Rd, Jos; 167 Ikwere Rd, Diobu, Port Harcourt; Merogun Waterside, Ifugbe, Warri; Okpanam Rd (just after Nnebisi College), Asaba; N6A/405 Adekemi Chamber, Ibadan, Oyo State; 106 Ibrahim Taiwo, Kano
Associated Companies: IkJ (Agricultural) Ltd, UK; AWATCO, USA
Principal Bankers: United Bank for Africa Ltd; National Bank of Nigeria Ltd; ICON Ltd
Financial Information:

	N'000
Authorised capital	1,000
Paid-up capital	1,000

No of Employees: 155

NIGERIAN EXTERNAL TELECOMMUNICATIONS LTD

15 Marina, PO Box 173 and PMB 12742, Lagos
Tel: 659666
Cable: Necom Lagos
Telex: 11001 Netad Ng

Chairman: J E K Oyegun
Directors: I O A Lasode, Malam Muhammed Mahe, Chief Bassey E Bassey
Senior Executives: Y A Raji (Director of Engineering),
   F H O Akindele (General Manager),
   M Ogunmoyero (Director of Finance),
   K Fields (Head of Company Services Department),
   R Adu Agbede (Chief Personnel Officer),
   F K Olowu (Company Secretary),
   J A Soetan (Chief Traffic Officer)

PRINCIPAL ACTIVITIES: Provision of telecommunication services
Principal Bankers: United Bank for Africa

Principal Shareholders: Federal Ministry of Finance Incorporated holding shares on behalf of the Federal Government of Nigeria
Date of Establishment: 31st December 1962
No of Employees: 3,042

NIGERIAN FAR EAST COMPANY LTD (NIFECO)

Development House (5th Floor), 21 Wharf Rd, PO Box 645, Apapa, Lagos
Tel: 874074, 873485
Cable: Nifechouse Lagos
Telex: 21201 Nifeco Ng

Chairman: Dr P C Onianwa

PRINCIPAL ACTIVITIES: Construction, systems engineering and

telecommunications engineering
Principal Agencies: United Technologies Corp, USA; Western
Electric Int, USA

NIGERIAN FIBRE INDUSTRIES COMPANY LTD

Floor 23, Cocoa House, PO Box 1644, Ibadan, Oyo State
PRINCIPAL ACTIVITIES: Fibre manufacturers

NIGERIAN FOOD COMPANY LTD

Iddo Railway Terminus, PO Box 3115, Lagos
Tel: 862580, 832827, 861726
Cable: Nigerfoods
Telex: 21516 Bobeef

Chairman: A I Obeya (also Permanent Secretary, Federal
Ministry of Agriculture and Rural Development)
Directors: G A Bukar-Kolo (Managing Director),
H Kano,
M Deribe,
Dr I M Khalil,
Aji K Alkali
Senior Executives: Hamma Damaturu (General Manager),
W A Nzewi (Chief Accountant, Secretary)

PRINCIPAL ACTIVITIES: Food and food processing
Branch Offices: Kaduna, Maiduguri
Principal Bankers: Bank of the North Ltd; International Bank for
West Africa Ltd
Financial Information:

	N'000
Authorised capital	800
Paid-up capital	480
Sales turnover	4,000
Profits	27

Principal Shareholders: Nigerian Livestock & Meat Authority;
Borno Local Government
No of Employees: 100

NIGERIAN FOUNDRIES LTD

Ilupeju Industrial Estate, PO Box 3574, Lagos
Tel: 963266, 963267, 962387, 964602
Cable: Foundries Lagos
Telex: 26276 NF Ltd Ng

Chairman: R V Barberopoulos
Directors: J V Barberopoulos
Senior Executives: S L Vacanas (General Manager)

PRINCIPAL ACTIVITIES: Manufacturers of cast iron fittings for
civil engineering and construction works/irrigation
Principal Bankers: United Bank for Africa Ltd
Financial Information:

	N'000
Authorised capital	1,500
Paid-up capital	1,200
Sales turnover	6,500

Principal Shareholders: R V Barberopoulos; J V Barberopoulos;
S I Nwazue
Date of Establishment: 26th June 1969
No of Employees: 150

NIGERIAN GAS INDUSTRIES

41 Jebba St (East), PO Box 72, Ebute-Metta, Lagos
Tel: 860393
Cable: Oxygases

PRINCIPAL ACTIVITIES: Importation and distribution of welding
equipment and gas welding material
Principal Agencies: Arcum Arc Welding Products

NIGERIAN GENERAL INSURANCE COMPANY LTD (THE)

1 Nnamdi Azikiwe Street, Tinubu Square, PO Box 2210, Lagos
Tel: 664507, 664578, 664698, 664686
Cable: Nigesure Lagos

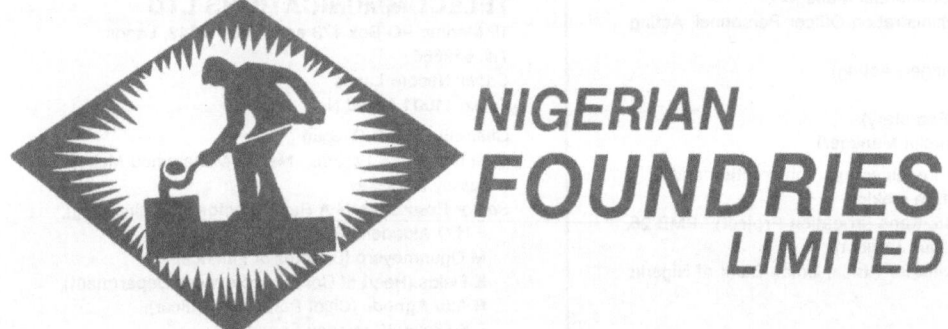

Chairman: J S Olawoyin
Directors: Alhaji S O Gbadamosi,
 Alhaji Agbo Alausa,
 Chief E O Adebimpe,
 Chief M A Adegborioye,
 Chia Surman,
 D O Babalola,
 Ariyo Adebayo,
 H T Durojaiye (Managing)
Senior Executives: A O Awopetu (Assistant Managing Director),
 A A Ogunmade (Financial Controller),
 I L Agboola (Company Secretary),
 A B Akanni (Controller of District, Ibadan),
 Alhaji A Ogunsanya (Controller of District, Lagos)

PRINCIPAL ACTIVITIES: All types of insurance
Branch Offices: PO Box 1538, Abeokuta; 15 Kodesoh Street,
 Ikeja; Cocoa House, PO Box 1285, Ibadan; PO Box 1210,
 Kano; PO Box 131, Akure
Subsidiary Companies: Great Nigeria Insurance Company Ltd;
 Glanvill, Enthoven & Co
Principal Bankers: National Bank of Nigeria Ltd; Wema Bank
 Ltd
Financial Information:

	N'000
Authorised capital	1,000
Paid-up capital	800
Turnover	10,000
Profits	800

Principal Shareholders: Odu'a Investment Company Ltd
Date of Establishment: 21st April 1951
No of Employees: 400

NIGERIAN GENERAL SECURITY & SAFETY COMPANY LTD

125 Lewis Street, PO Box 4811, Lagos
Tel: 653269, 653876

Chairman: G Y Adebanjo (also Managing Director)
Directors: S O Ismaji, K B Adebanjo

PRINCIPAL ACTIVITIES: Safety and security services

Date of Establishment: 1971
No of Employees: 400

NIGERIAN GENERAL SUPERINTENDENCE CO LTD

3/5 Sapele Rd, PO Box 315, Apapa, Lagos
Tel: 875558, 875639, 875470
Telex: 21347

Directors: B M Whiteman (Managing Director)

PRINCIPAL ACTIVITIES: Cargo superintendents
Branch Offices: Kano; Port Harcourt; Warri

NIGERIAN GLASS CONTAINERS & METAL MANUFACTURERS LTD

PO Box 1, Ikeja, Lagos
Tel: 963610, 962116

PRINCIPAL ACTIVITIES: Manufacturing of glass containers and
 packaging materials

NIGERIAN GROUNDNUT BOARD

1 Bida Rd, Civic Centre, PMB 3067, Kano
Tel: 4169, 2886, 3562
Cable: Grabod, Kano
Telex: 77240 Ng

Chairman: Alhaji Na Funtua
Directors: Alhaji Muhammadu Ningi,
 Shehu Mamman,
 Alhaji Rabiu Dan Sista,
 Mr Idachaba,
 S A Sammuel,
 Rowland Nwosu,
 Alhaji Mamman Kaura,

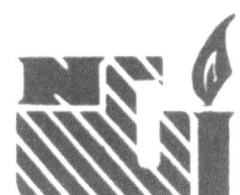

Alhaji Geraima Geidam,
Alhaji Baba Mayobalwa (Representative of Federal Ministry of
 Agriculture),
Representative of Central Bank of Nigeria,
Representative of Federal Ministry of Commerce
Senior Executives: Alhaji U B Danfulani (General Manager),
 S O Ajayi (Assistant General Manager, Finance),
 S A Moito (Assistant General Manager, Sales),
 E A I Agum (Board Secretary)

PRINCIPAL ACTIVITIES: Sole exporters of groundnuts,
 sheanuts, soya beans, benniseed and ginger
Branch Offices: Offices at Gusau; Zaria; Bauchi; Jos; Lagos; Sub
 Zonal Offices: Bida; Kontagora; Funtua; Kafanchan; Katsina;
 Ilorin; Maiduguri; Makurdi; Port Harcourt; Kama Namoda;
 Yola
Principal Bankers: Bank of the North Ltd; United Bank for Africa
Principal Shareholders: Federal Government of Nigeria
Date of Establishment: 1st April 1977
No of Employees: 500

NIGERIAN HARDWARE INDUSTRIES LTD
Block M Plot 7, Oshodi Industrial Scheme, Isolo, PMB 1051,
 Mushin, Lagos
Cable: Nighar Apapa

PRINCIPAL ACTIVITIES: Manufacturers of aluminium building
 products, doors, windows, etc
Branch Offices: Office: 139 Broad St, Lagos; Ibadan; Aba;
 Enugu; Kaduna; Benin City; Kano
Principal Bankers: United Bank for Africa Ltd
Financial Information: Associate of Union Trading Company

NIGERIAN HARDWOOD COMPANY LTD
Idiale-Urhonigbe, Abraka Via Sapele, PO Box 44, Sapele, Bendel
 State
Tel: 93
Cable: Nigerhard Abraka
Telex: 21324 Lagos

Chairman: Chief M C O Ibru
Directors: F O Ibru,
 G H Robertson,
 H A Blackburne (Managing Director),
 Chief J J Adjarho,
 Chief A O Eguavoen (Administrative/Personnel Manager)
Senior Executives: Chief S E Ogefere (Chief Accountant)

PRINCIPAL ACTIVITIES: Production of sawn timber
Principal Bankers: First Bank of Nigeria Ltd; New Nigeria Bank
 Ltd; Icon Ltd (Merchant Bankers)
Financial Information:

	N'000
Authorised capital	100
Paid-up capital	100

Principal Shareholders: Oteri Holdings Ltd; Chief M C O Ibru
Date of Establishment: 1919
No of Employees: 568

NIGERIAN HOECHST LTD
Plot 144 Oba Akran Ave, PO Box 261, Ikeja Industrial Estate,
 Lagos
Tel: 961184, 964082, 900131
Cable: Hoprod Lagos
Telex: 21381 Hoprod Ng

Chairman: Chief E O Ashamu
Directors: Dr J-U Mohr (Managing),
 Dr N O Olambiwonnu,
 Alhaji A Mohammadu,
 Engineer S I Omotoso,
 D Cord,
 B S Oloruntoba,
 J M Schoeler,
 Dieter Cron
Senior Executives: R A Ayanwale (Personnel Manager),
 Z O Odusoga (Company Secretary),

C I Onyemenam (Sales Manager),
H W Borger (Administrative Manager),
A Woerpel (Pharmaceutical Manager),
F Bergmann (Projects Manager),
A Ogbonna (Depot Manager)
PRINCIPAL ACTIVITIES: Manufacturers of polyvinlacetate for
 paint adhesive and textile industry; suppliers of
 pharmaceutical products
Branch Offices: 5 Industry Rd, PO Box 585, Aba; Plot 1A
 Ahmadu Bello Way, PO Box 464, Kaduna; 63 Murtala
 Muhammed Way, PO Box 1760, Sabon Gari, Kano; 70
 Trans-Amadi Layout, PMB 5229, Port Harcourt; UI Post
 Office, PMB 55, Ibadan
Principal Bankers: United Bank for Africa Ltd; First Bank of
 Nigeria Ltd; Nigerian Acceptances Ltd; Icon Ltd (Merchant
 Bankers)
Financial Information:

	N'000
Authorised capital	3,000
Paid-up capital	3,000
Turnover	33,468

Principal Shareholders: Hoechst Ag, West Germany; E O
 Ashamu & Sons (Holdings) Ltd; Nigerian Citizens
Date of Establishment: 1964
No of Employees: 530

NIGERIAN HOLLOWBLOCK INDUSTRIES LTD
Mile 4, Sapele Rd, PO Box 349, Benin City, Bendel State
Tel: 240227, 243991
Cable: Hollowblocks

PRINCIPAL ACTIVITIES: Concrete products manufacturers

NIGERIAN INDUSTRIAL AUXILIARIES LTD
Kilometre 16, Ikorodu Rd, PO Box 2818, Lagos
Tel: 832581, 834722
Cable: Umbrella Lagos
Telex: 26234

Chairman: Fred Egbe
Directors: Hadj Bakre Anjorin,
 J A Cole,
 M Aina John,
 Lachman Hariram,
 Harish Chulani,
 Lachoo Sakhrani (Managing Director)
Senior Executives: Femi Kilo (General Manager)

PRINCIPAL ACTIVITIES: Production of beach sandals and other
 rubber and plastic products
Principal Bankers: United Bank for Africa Ltd
Financial Information:

	N'000
Authorised capital	600
Paid-up capital	400

Principal Shareholders: Fred Egbe; Hadj Bakre Anjorin; J A
 Cole; M Aina John; Lachman Hariram; Harish Chulani
Date of Establishment: 1974
No of Employees: 100

NIGERIAN INDUSTRIAL COMPLEX AMALGAMATION LTD
4 Auno Street, PO Box 4210, Maiduguri, Borno State
Tel: 2044
Cable: Nicamaiduguri

Chairman: Alhaji A Aliyu Mahmud
Directors: Alhaji Hasson Adamu (Managing Director),
 Alhaji S F Abubakar,
 Alhaji Musa Tafida,
 S K Somany,
 A C Onochie
Senior Executives: Alhaji Musa Abba (Sales/Administrative
 Director),
 R S Somani (General Manager)

PRINCIPAL ACTIVITIES: Manufacturers of steel doors and windows
Branch Offices: 25B Niger St, PO Box 56, Kano
Associated Companies: MCC Blocks Ltd; UP (Nigeria) Ltd
Principal Bankers: United Bank for Africa Ltd; International Bank for West Africa Ltd
Financial Information:

	N'000
Authorised capital	400
Paid-up capital	400

Principal Shareholders: Alhaji Aliyu Mahmud; Alhaji Hassan Adamu; Alhaji S K Abubakar; Alhaji Mahmud Waziri; NBCI
No of Employees: 100

NIGERIAN INDUSTRIAL DEVELOPMENT BANK LTD

NIDB House, 63/71 Broad Street, PO Box 2357, Lagos
Tel: 663470, 663495
Cable: Nidbank Lagos
Telex: 21701, 21708

Chairman: Chief Gbadegesin Ajeigbe
Directors: Alhaji Abubakar Abdulkadir (Managing Director & Chief Executive),
L K Omosebi,
P E Okit,
Alhaji I W Masaka,
Chief S M Amoye,
Alhaji A Y Saleh,
Alhaji Isa Mohammed,
O Durojaiye,
M S Udom,
Chief J O Okoroafor
Senior Executives: J A Olugbenle (Deputy General Manager), G O Senbanjo (Deputy General Manager)

PRINCIPAL ACTIVITIES: Financial development company
Branch Offices: 27 Ali Akilu Rd, PMB 2141, Kaduna; 58 Aba/Owerri Rd, PMB 7086, Aba, Imo State; 3 Dass Rd, GRA PMB 0245, Bauchi, Bauchi State; 15A Oba Adesida Rd, PMB 804, Akure, Ondo State
Subsidiaries Companies: Icon Stockbrokers Ltd; Commonwealth Development Company (Nigeria) Ltd
Principal Bankers: Central Bank of Nigeria; International Bank for West Africa Ltd
Financial Information: As at 31st December 1980

	N'000
Authorised capital	100,000
Paid-up capital	99,352
Turnover	19,507
Profits (before tax)	6,911

Principal Shareholders: Federal Government of Nigeria (Through Ministry of Finance Inc) 59%; Central Bank of Nigeria 40%; Private Nigerian Individuals 1%
Date of Establishment: 22nd January 1964
No of Employees: 667

NIGERIAN INSTITUTE OF MANAGEMENT

PO Box 2557, 58 Adelabu St, Surulere, Lagos
Tel: 830565
Cable: Nimrod

Chairman: G O Onosode
Directors: Chief O I A Akinyemi (Director-General),
M A Oworen (Deputy Director-General),
Kayode Ajasin (Director of Administration),
F N Ikpong (Director of Institute Services)
Senior Executives: G Oviogbodu (Editor and Manager Publications),
I O O Olonge (Business Manager, Publications),
C Oloruntuyi (Administrative Manager),
A O Lawrence (Accountant),
R O Nwatulegwu (Lecturer Consultant),
P O A Emefiele (Membership Manager),
B O Awosika (Lecturer, Consultant)

PRINCIPAL ACTIVITIES: Business consultants; publishing of business journals; executive training services, advisory body
Branch Offices: 7 Alhaji Muritala Animashaun Close, Surulere, Lagos; Port Harcourt; Ibadan; Kano; Benin City; Kaduna; Jos; Enugu; Zaria; Aba; Calabar; Owerri; Abeokuta; Akure
Principal Bankers: First Bank of Nigeria Ltd
Financial Information:
Sales turnover (approx) N 1,000,000
Date of Establishment: 1961
No of Employees: 150

NIGERIAN INTERNATIONAL CONSTRUCTION COMPANY LTD

PMB 1354, 95B Wetheral Rd, Owerri, Imo State
PRINCIPAL ACTIVITIES: Construction

NIGERIAN INTERNATIONAL EXCHANGE LTD

9 Nnamdi Azikiwe St, Lagos
PRINCIPAL ACTIVITIES: Manufacturing of textile piece goods

NIGERIAN INVESTIGATION AND SAFETY COMPANY LTD

43 Massey St, PO Box 2636, Lagos
Tel: 633822
PRINCIPAL ACTIVITIES: Security guards and services
Date of Establishment: 1965

NIGERIAN IRON & WOOD FACTORY LTD

15 Bello Rd, PO Box 651, Kano
Tel: 2690, 3332
Cable: Niwfact Kano
Telex: 77167 Niwfact Ng

PRINCIPAL ACTIVITIES: Manufacturers of iron and wood furniture
Branch Offices: Factory: Plot 46/47, Sharada Industrial Estate Phase II, Kano; 7 Umar Ali Rd, Maiduguri, Borno State

NIGERIAN JOINT AGENCIES LTD

PMB 2130, 52 Warehouse Rd, Apapa, Lagos
Tel: 875181 875185
Telex: 21256 Nijal Ng

PRINCIPAL ACTIVITIES: Business consultants

NIGERIAN LEATHER WORKS COMPANY LTD

2-5 Independence Rd, PO Box 998, Kano
Tel: 2415
Cable: Leatherworks Kano

Chairman: Alhaji H R Zayyad
Directors: Alhaji Shehu Ahmed, Alhaji Sanusi Dantata, Ibrahim El-Tayeb El Rayah, Alhaji Ibrahim Ilatune, Suleimmy Baffa
Senior Executives: Alhaji T A Sanni (Chief Executive),
P R Sawyer (Operations Manager),
R N Okwoli (Accountant),
Olu Omirin (Administrative Officer)

PRINCIPAL ACTIVITIES: Manufacturing of leather footwear
Principal Bankers: Union Bank of Nigeria Ltd
Financial Information:

	N'000
Authorised capital	400
Paid-up capital	281

Principal Shareholders: New Nigeria Development Company Ltd
Date of Establishment: 1960
No of Employees: 122

NIGERIAN LIFE & PENSIONS CONSULTANTS

9 Jibowu Street, Yaba, PO Box 1156, Lagos
Tel: 860383, 863228
Cable: Unipen Lagos
Telex: 26486 Hoggs Ng

Chairman: Justin Olabode Emanuel
Directors: S A Alao (Managing),
   J Carruthers (Technical),
   A A Adeyeye,
   Alhaji M K Bayero,
   A H Bello,
   Dr S O Biobaku,
   Omo N'Oba Erediauwa,
   C S Stewart
Senior Executives: J E Olanipekun (Financial Controller),
   I F Buckle (Assistant General Manager, Northern Operations),
   Mrs C A Brown (Assistant General Manager, Pensions),
   A A Omiyale (Assistant General Manager, Production),
   G W Shaw (Consultant)

PRINCIPAL ACTIVITIES: Pensions consultants and insurance
   brokers
Branch Offices: 69 Akpakpava Street, Benin City; 1 Obiagu Rd,
   Enugu; Ileori Detu, 1 Shell Close, Onireke, Ibadan; Nigerian
   Standard Building (5th Floor), 5 Zaria Rd, Jos; 20A Airport
   Rd, Kano; 115 Wetheral Rd (1st Floor), Owerri; 24 Ikwerre Rd,
   Port Harcourt; NNDC New 6 Storey Building (1st Floor), Kanta
   Rd, Kaduna; Ahmadu Bello Way (Opposite ECWA Church),
   Sokoto; School Rd, Plot 10/75, Housing Estate, Calabar; 51
   Mubi Rd, Jimeta, Yola
Associated Companies: Hogg Robinson Nigeria; Nigerian
   Universities Pensions Management Company
Principal Bankers: United Bank for Africa
Financial Information:

	N'000
Authorised capital	1,000
Paid-up capital	1,000
Turnover	27,000
Profits	1,250

Principal Shareholders: Hogg Robinson Benefits Consultants
   Ltd; New Nigeria Development Company; Junior and Senior
   Staff; Thorburn Investments (Nigeria) Ltd
Date of Establishment: 1964
No of Employees: 150

NIGERIAN MACHINE TOOLS CO LTD (NMT)

126/130 Nnamdi Azikiwe St, Lagos

PRINCIPAL ACTIVITIES: Construction
Financial Information:
Authorised capital   N 500,000

Date of Establishment: September 1978

NIGERIAN MAPPING COMPANY LTD

22 Moore Rd, Yaba, Lagos
Tel: 861836

PRINCIPAL ACTIVITIES: Surveyors, photogrammetrists,
   cartographers

NIGERIAN MARITIME SERVICES LTD

13/15 Sapele Rd, PO Box 331, Apapa, Lagos
Tel: 875761, 875668, 875189
Telex: 21566 Heship Ng

Chairman: Professor A Ogunsheye
Senior Executives: A Adam (General Manager),
   Mr Adeyemi (Manager, Apapa Branch),
   A Oke (Manager, Ikeja Branch),
   G Ohaeri (Manager, Kaduna Branch),
   Mr Odunwole (Manager, Travel Bureau)

PRINCIPAL ACTIVITIES: Customs agents, freight forwarding, air
   cargo charter handling, shipping, packing and removal,
   warehousing, travel bureau
Branch Offices: 1 Swamp Rd, Warri; 14 Industry Rd, PO Box
   509, Port Harcourt, Tel 228389; Murtala Mohammed Airport,
   Ikeja, Tel 961359, N6/69A Oyo Rd, Mokola, Ibadan; PMB
   3212, Kano; 3 Katchia Rd, PO Box 321, Kaduna, Tel 243319;
   Travel Bureau; 170 Broad St, Lagos
Principal Bankers: Barclays Bank Nigeria Ltd
No of Employees: 700

NIGERIAN MATCH & CHEMICAL INDUSTRIES LTD

12 Independence Rd, Bompai Industrial Area, PO Box 13, Kano
Tel: 3695, 4556
Cable: Fedmatch
Telex: 77222 Nima Ng

Chairman: Alhaji M I Wada
Directors: Dr O Czerweny von Arland,
   Alhaji A Yaro,
   H Boellmann (Managing),
   W Putner,
   Dipo Faradoye,
   Alhaji Abba Gana,
   Alhaji Musa Aliyu,
   Alhaji Mustafa Danlami

PRINCIPAL ACTIVITIES: Manufacturers of matches; matchbox
   printers
Principal Bankers: United Bank for Africa Ltd
Principal Shareholders: Alhaji M I Wada; Dr O Czerweny von
   Arland; Alhaji A Yaro
Date of Establishment: 25th July 1968
No of Employees: 150

NIGERIAN MEDICAL SUPPLIES LTD

149/153 Broad St, PO Box 1732, Lagos
Tel: 630504

PRINCIPAL ACTIVITIES: Sales and servicing of medical and
   general scientific instruments

NIGERIAN MERCHANTS & PRODUCE SUPPLIERS

15 Harcourt St, PO Box 324, Calabar, Cross River State

PRINCIPAL ACTIVITIES: Manufacturers' representatives;
   suppliers of metal furniture and general merchandise
Principal Agencies: St Karasek & Co, Austria

NIGERIAN METAL FABRICATING LTD

91 Tafawa Balewa Rd, PO Box 23, Kano
Tel: 4031, 2496, 3258/9
Cable: Metalfab Kano
Telex: 77244 Nomkan Ng

PRINCIPAL ACTIVITIES: Manufacturers of light engineering
   aluminium utensils and silver ware
Branch Offices: Moloney St, PO Box 453, Lagos; Tel Lagos
   635672, 614335, 634782, Telex 21330 Nibrok Lagos

NIGERIAN METALS LTD

8 and 44 Zaria Rd, PO Box 481, Jos, Plateau State
Tel: 2758

PRINCIPAL ACTIVITIES: Metal ore mining

NIGERIAN MINERAL DEVELOPMENT COMPANY LTD

PO Box 394, Jos, Plateau State
Tel: 2329

PRINCIPAL ACTIVITIES: Metal ore mining
No of Employees: 200

NIGERIAN MINERAL WATER INDUSTRY LTD

PMB 1549, Onitsha, Anambra State
Tel: 205
Cable: Unity Onitsha

PRINCIPAL ACTIVITIES: Manufacturers of assorted brands of
mineral water and soft drinks
Branch Offices: Factory: Awka Rd, Along Enugu/Onitsha Rd,
Anambra State

NIGERIAN MINING CORPORATION

Federal Secretariat (7th Floor), PMB 2154, Jos, Plateau State
Tel: 53423, 52990
Cable: Niminco
Telex: 81139 Mining Ng

Directors: M M Maigandu,
 U Dan-Iya,
 Chief M O Aroyewun,
 M Kundu,
 I P Ubom,
 I Gombe,
 R Lukman (General Manager/Chief Executive)
Senior Executives: D T Pwajok (Deputy General Manager,
 Operations),
 G Magaji (Secretary/Deputy General Manager,
 Administration),
 M K Ibrahim (Deputy General Manager, Engineering),
 R K Adewale (Deputy General Manager, Finance),
 Dr S O Ford (Deputy General Manager, Exploration),
 S O Ajetunmobi (Assistant General Manager, Investments)

PRINCIPAL ACTIVITIES: Mining, mineral processing and
quarrying, tin prospecting
Branch Offices: 24 Samuel Manuwa Street, PMB 12668, Lagos;
Akegbe Ugwu, PMB 1405, Enugu; PMB 1467, Maiduguri
Subsidiary Companies: Amalgamated Tin Mines of Nigeria Ltd;
Ex-Lands Nigeria Ltd; Ririwai Mines; Bisichi-Jantar Nigeria
Ltd; Kaduna Prospectors Nigeria Ltd; Gold and Base;
Associated Companies: Makeri Smelting Co Ltd; Jakura
Marble Industries Ltd; Plateau Ceramic Industries Ltd;
Mfamosin Limestone Project; NESCO
Principal Bankers: Bank of the North Ltd; United Bank for Africa
Ltd

Principal Shareholders: Nigerian Government
Date of Establishment: November 1972
No of Employees: 1,800

NIGERIAN MODERN STORES LTD

43-47 Balogun St, Lagos
Tel: 21516 Haga Ng

PRINCIPAL ACTIVITIES: Importers and general trading

NIGERIAN MOTORS INDUSTRIES LTD

26 Wharf Rd, PMB 1032, Apapa, Lagos
Tel: 871124, 871121, 876518, 876629
Cable: Nigermot
Telex: 22349

Chairman: Alhaji K A Agabalogun
Directors: P Chavannaz, R Horner, Dr J Sodipo, Chief O K
 Lampejo
Senior Executives: P Grauwin (General Manager)

PRINCIPAL ACTIVITIES: Sales and after sales service of
industrial, construction and agricultural equipment
Principal Agencies: International Harvester (USA); Huster (USA,
UK); Barber Greene (USA, UK); PPM (France); Galion (USA);
Toyo (Japan); Hokwetsu (Japan); Petter (UK); CD (France);
Hunt (UK); Guinard (France); Penven (France); Otis (UK);
Denyo (Japan)
Branch Offices: 26 Wharf Rd, Apapa; Industrial Scheme Plot I,
Block D Amuwo Odofin, Lagos; 55A Tafawa Balewa Rd, Kano;
2 Kyarizoram Rd, Maiduguri; 21/27 Trans Amadi Layout, Port
Harcourt; 24 Okpara Avenue, Enugu
Principal Bankers: International Bank for West Africa Ltd; Union
Bank; International Merchant Bank; Icon

Financial Information:

	N'000
Authorised capital	4,500
Turnover	40,000

Principal Shareholders: CFAO (Nigeria) Ltd
Date of Establishment: 31st August 1957
No of Employees: 575

NIGERIAN NATIONAL FISH COMPANY LTD

31A Airport Rd, PMB 1427, Benin City, Bendel State
Tel: 242191, 240194
Cable: Statefish
Telex: 41375 Nafish Ng

Chairman: Chief Daniel N Oronsaye
Directors: Chief G O D Eneh, Rep of NBCI, Chief M O
 Ogunmola, Rep of Atlantic Triton Company, Norway, Prince
 H E Ogei, Rep of NACB, Managing Director, NNFC, Federal
 Ministry of Industries
Senior Executives: A Dale (Managing),
 E Nwaiku (Assistant General Manager),
 E Vindenes (Operations Manager),
 J E Nehikhare (Finance Controller),
 S O Eboikpomwen (Personnel Manager),
 F U Azeta (Company Secretary),
 S Saebjornsen (Chief, Ref Engineer),
 H Larsen (Superintendent Engineer),
 M P Gracias (Production Manager),
 Mr Saetervik (Training Officer)

PRINCIPAL ACTIVITIES: Trawling and distribution of fish and
fish products
Branch Offices: Operation Base; Koko Port, Bendel State; 74
D'Alberto Rd, Palmgrove Estate, PMB 21394, Ikeja, Lagos
Principal Bankers: International Bank for West Africa Ltd;
United Bank for Africa Ltd
Financial Information:

	N'000
Authorised capital	7,000
Paid-up capital	7,000

Principal Shareholders: Federal Government of Nigeria (66%)
Date of Establishment: October 1975
No of Employees: 300

NIGERIAN NATIONAL PAPER MANUFACTURING COMPANY LTD

2 Keffi St, SW Ikoyi, PMB 12569, Lagos

PRINCIPAL ACTIVITIES: Paper manufacturing
Branch Offices: Factory; Iwopin, Ogun State

NIGERIAN NATIONAL PETROLEUM CORPORATION (NNPC)

Falomo Office Complex, PMB 12701, Broad St, Opposite old
 Secretariat, Ikoyi, Lagos
Tel: 603100/30
Cable: Napetcor
Telex: 21126 Petref Ng

Chairman: Horatio Agebah
Directors: Lawrence Amu (Managing Director),
 Festus Marinho (Energy Advisor to President)

PRINCIPAL ACTIVITIES: Holds the federal governments share in
the oil companies and deals with oil exploration, production,
refining and transportation
Branch Offices: PMB 5103, Port Harcourt, Rivers State, Telex
61139 Petref Ng, Cables Napetcor
Financial Information: NNPC replaced the Federal Ministry of
Petroleum Resources and the Nigerian National Oil Company

NIGERIAN NATIONAL SHIPPING LINE LTD

Development House, 21 Wharf Rd, PO Box 326, Apapa, Lagos
Tel: 877262, 877121
Cable: Nigerline
Telex: 21253

A major study, in two volumes, of Nigeria's petroleum geology and resources, providing the only complete description available of the country's sedimentary rocks and growth fault structure.

NIGERIA: Its Petroleum Geology, Resources and Potential

ARTHUR WHITEMAN

Professor of Geology, Petroleum Exploration Studies, Aberdeen University, Scotland, and formerly Professor of Petroleum Geology, Ibadan University, Nigeria

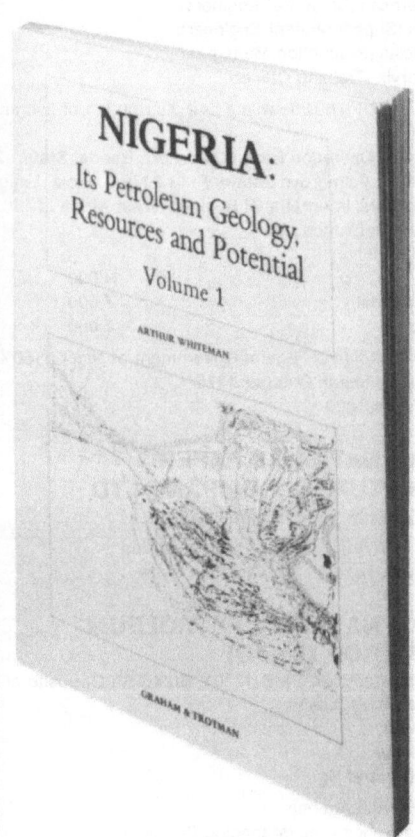

This important new reference work provides a comprehensive and authoritative account of the petroleum geology of Nigeria, a major oil producing country with enormous gas resources.

The book provides detailed coverage of the following key issues:

● Stratigraphy and structure of Nigeria's six major sedimentary basins, assessed from the point of view of petroleum exploration.

● General analysis of the hydrocarbon potential for each Nigerian basin, given by formation or major grouping.

● Plate tectonic studies, important for basin evaluation work.

● Oil and gas resources in the Niger Delta Complex — source, reservoir, migration and accumulation data, and case histories.

● Production and reserve data, and analysis of oil and gas prospects.

● Chronological review of selected exploration and production developments of Nigeria's petroleum industry.

● Exploration data and concession maps.

The book is illustrated with over 300 maps, diagrams, figures and tables to add a wealth of detailed information and statistics to the text.

Further details of this major reference work are available direct from: Marketing Department, Graham & Trotman Ltd, Sterling House, 66 Wilton Road, London SW1V 1DE. Telephone: 01-821 1123, Telex: 298878 Gramco G, Cables: Infobooks London.

Chairman: Alhaji Kam Selem
Directors: Prince P I Jegbefume, Mrs D I Olorunda, Chief J N Okpuruwu, Alhaji M I Jibrin
Senior Executives: E A Adeniyi (Assistant General Manager, Operations),
F C Oniah (Assistant General Manager, Owned Agencies),
C I U Ibia (Assistant General Manager, Technical),
I T A Bezi (Personnel Manager),
O Oladitan (General Manager),
A Falase (Assistant General Manager, Finance),
E O Sowade (Chief Internal Auditor)

PRINCIPAL ACTIVITIES: Shipping
Principal Agencies: Black Star Line of Ghana; 'K' Line of Japan
Branch Offices: Old Custom House, PO Box 425, Port Harcourt; PMB 1100, Warri; PO Box 48, Koko; PO Box 19, Marina, Calabar; Eastgate, 53-57 Leman St, PO Box 114, London E1 8ET; Oriel Chambers, 14 Water St, Liverpool L2 8TG
Subsidiary Companies: Nigerline (UK) Ltd
Principal Bankers: First Bank of Nigeria Ltd; United Bank for Africa Ltd; Bank of the North Ltd
Financial Information:

	N'000
Authorised capital	4,000
Paid-up capital	4,000
Turnover (approx)	45,000
Profits (approx)	2,500

Principal Shareholders: Federal Government of Nigeria
Date of Establishment: 5th February 1959
No of Employees: 1,300

NIGERIAN NATIONAL SHRIMP COMPANY LTD

PMB 4070, Sapeie, Bendel State
Tel: 60070
Cable: Natshrimp

Chairman: S E Aganbi
Directors: G C Akwaeze, R O Dosumu, B F Dada, J O Ajibola, F Bola Giwa, Chief Dr S F Okuru, N E Osayande, G G O Sonekan
Senior Executives: C O Akarue (Company Secretary),
R O Obanor (Production Manager),
Mr I Yelagha (Fleet Manager)

PRINCIPAL ACTIVITIES: Shrimping and fishing
Branch Offices: Plot 35 Western Nigeria Housing Estate, Off Adeniyi Jones Avenue, Ikeja, PO Box 6782, Lagos
Principal Bankers: Union Bank of Nigeria Ltd; African Continental Bank Ltd

Principal Shareholders: Federal Government of Nigeria; Bendel State Government; Nigerian Industrial Development Bank; Nigerian Bank for Commerce and Industry
Date of Establishment: 1976
No of Employees: 245

NIGERIAN NEWSPRINT MANUFACTURING COMPANY LTD

Oku Iboku, PMB 1045, ITU LGA, Cross River State
Tel: 684540, 684963
Cable: Newsprint
Telex: 21726

Chairman: Chief E U Okon
Directors: S T Hembah, A O Ekoh, Chief Dapo Daramola, S P Byrne, V S Inuaesiet, Alhaji M Muhammed
Senior Executives: C K Goddard (Managing Director),
E A Essien (Deputy Managing Director),
O O Eddie (Finance Controller/Secretary)

PRINCIPAL ACTIVITIES: Production of groundwood newsprint
Branch Offices: 2 Lalupon Rd, SW Ikoyi, PMB 12782, Lagos
Principal Bankers: African Continental Bank Ltd; Mercantile Bank of Nigeria Ltd; First Bank of Nigeria Ltd

Principal Shareholders: Federal Government of Nigeria; Cross River State
Date of Establishment: 27th August 1975
No of Employees: 1,000 when in full production

NIGERIAN OFFICE STATIONERY SUPPLY STORES LTD

Adebajo House, 25 Warehouse Rd, Apapa, PO Box 148, Lagos
Tel: 877144
Cable: Stationers Lagos

Chairman: Dr Arthur Nylander
Directors: Mrs Adunni Adebajo, Mrs Irene Adebajo, Adekunle Adebajo, Adetilewa Adebajo, E O O Mejule

PRINCIPAL ACTIVITIES: Suppliers of office and personal stationery, office equipment and furniture
Principal Agencies: Rotaprint offset printing machines; triumph typewriters and calculators
Branch Offices: 11 Kodesoh Street, Ikeja; 114 Broad Street, Lagos; 3 Broadcasting Rd, Kaduna; 56 Ibrahim Taiwo Rd, Kano; 37 Forestry Rd, Benin; 68A Warri/Sapele Rd, Warri; 63 Market Rd, Sapele; 57 Onireke Street, Ibadan
Subsidiary Companies: Nigerian Paper Converters Company
Principal Bankers: First Bank of Nigeria Ltd
Financial Information:

	N'000
Authorised capital	200
Paid-up capital	200

Principal Shareholders: Adebajo Family
Date of Establishment: 25th June 1947
No of Employees: 300

NIGERIAN OIL MILLS LTD

81/82 Tafawa Balewa Rd, PO Box 342, Kano
Tel: 3258/9
Cable: Nigomills Kano
Telex: 77244 Nomkan Ng

PRINCIPAL ACTIVITIES: Production of vegetable oil products
Branch Offices: 7A Eleke Crescent, PO Box 453, Victoria Island, Lagos, Tel 611939

NIGERIAN OIL SERVICES SHIPPING & EQUIPMENT CO LTD (NOSSEC)

14/16 Abibu-Oki St, Lagos
Tel: 632298
Cable: Nossec Lagos
Telex: 22626 Nossec

PRINCIPAL ACTIVITIES: Services for the oil industry

NIGERIAN PALM PRODUCE BOARD

Atlantic House, 20 Thomas Henshaw St, PMB 1264, Calabar, Cross River State
Tel: 522, 313, 262, 378
Cable: Pambod Calabar
Telex: 65107 Pambod Ng

Senior Executives: A Aielumo (Area Manager, Ogun State)

PRINCIPAL ACTIVITIES: Sole exporters of palm kernel, palm kernel oil, pellets, palm oil and copra; coconut oil; cakes and pellets
Branch Offices: Constanza House, 72 Campbell St, PMB 12760, Lagos, Tel 632692, Telex 22510, 22511

Date of Establishment: April 1977

NIGERIAN PAPER CONVERTERS COMPANY

25 Warehouse Rd, Apapa, PO Box 148, Lagos
Tel: 877144
Cable: Stationers

Chairman: Dr Arthur Nylander
Directors: Mrs Adunni Adebajo, Mrs Irene Adebajo, Adekunle Adebajo, Adetilewa Adebajo, E O O Mejule
Senior Executives: A I Odunlami (Factory Manager)

PRINCIPAL ACTIVITIES: Paper conversion, printer and book manufacturer
Subsidiary/Associated Companies: Nigerian Office Stationery Supply Stores Ltd
Principal Bankers: First Bank of Nigeria Ltd
Principal Shareholders: Abdebajo Family
Date of Establishment: November 1958
No of Employees: 100

NIGERIAN PAPER MILL LTD

118-120 Broad St, PO Box 1648, Lagos
Tel: 653346
Cable: Nigpaper
Telex: 21399 Paper Lagos

Directors: N K Mohatta (Managing),
  Alhaji M T Waziri,
  A O Ojediran,
  F L O Menkiti,
  T P Enodien,
  M Yahaya,
  H P Singhi

PRINCIPAL ACTIVITIES: Paper manufacturers
Branch Offices: Factory: PO Box 40, Jebba, Kwara State
Associated Companies: Central Packages (Nigeria) Ltd

No of Employees: 500

NIGERIAN PERFECTA SHOES LTD

PO Box 338, Ikeja, Ilupeju Industrial Estate, Ikeja, Lagos
Tel: 961009, 962183/4
Cable: Pershoes Lagos
Telex: 26272

Chairman: Chief I A S Adewale
Directors: G Freddi, C Galli, T A Oyebade, Chief D S Yaro,
  Chief O A Lampejo

PRINCIPAL ACTIVITIES: Manufacturers of footwear
Branch Offices: Onitsha; Warri; Ibadan; Lagos; Aba; Enugu
Date of Establishment: 1964

NIGERIAN PETROLEUM REFINING COMPANY LTD (NPRC)

PO Box 585, Alesa-Eleme, Port Harcourt, Rivers State
Tel: 21431/5, 228270
Cable: Refineries Port Harcourt

Directors: M A Talib, M B Yesufu, O E Ikpi, Brigadier G O Ejiga
Senior Executives: G B A Hamilton (General Manager),
  A Wishart (Refinery Manager),
  S A Ladipo

PRINCIPAL ACTIVITIES: Petroleum refining
Branch Offices: 2nd Floor, Investment House, 21/25 Broad, St, PO Box 2181, Lagos, Tel 657490, 657491, 636862

Principal Shareholders: Federal Government of Nigeria (NNPC); BP-Shell

NIGERIAN PETROLEUM TERMINALS LTD

PO Box 512, Lagos
Tel: 632003
Cable: NPT Lagos

Chairman: Ian Joseph Sims (also Managing Director)
Directors: J O Sheldon, T D Henshaw, J Poupeau, R N Tottenham-Smith, P J Bryers, G R K Warr
Senior Executives: G O Segun (Installation Manager),
  E O Olaleye (Finance and Accounts Manager)

PRINCIPAL ACTIVITIES: Petroleum marketing
Branch Offices: Installation, BP-Shell Rd, Apapa, Lagos
Principal Bankers: Union Bank of Nigeria Ltd

NIGERIAN PIPELINES LTD

Mandilas House, PO Box 5134, Lagos

PRINCIPAL ACTIVITIES: Manufacturing of gas and oil pipelines
Financial Information: Associate of Concord Carriers Ltd

NIGERIAN PORTS AUTHORITY (NPA)

26-28 Marina, PMB 12588, Lagos
Tel: 655020, 656786
Cable: Genports
Telex: 21500 Onponpa Ng

Chairman: Chief Akpata
Directors: Alhaji B M Tukur (General Manager),
  Chief Harold Sodipo,
  Felix Onyeahasi,
  L Ukom,
  S O Apetuje,
  Alhaji M Z Idris,
  Alhaji Bashir Dalhatu,
  Alhaji S O Mohammed,
  Chief S O Ukadike,
  Mallam Sule Jamso
Senior Executives: D P Opara (Assistant General Manager, Management Services and Develop),
  S O Ogundare (Assistant General Manager, Finance),
  A A Fowora (Assistant General Manager, Engineering),
  Chief J E Nkpang (Assistant General Manager, Port Operations/Marine Services),
  S A Amu (Assistant General Manager, Administration)

PRINCIPAL ACTIVITIES: Ports authority and related activities
Branch Offices: Port Harcourt; Bonny; Calabar; Delta Port; Port Offices at Warri, Sapele and Koko; London Office: Manfield House, 3rd Floor, 376/9 Strand, London WC2, Tel 01-240 5266
Principal Bankers: First Bank of Nigeria Ltd; National Bank of Nigeria Ltd; African Continental Bank Ltd; Bank of the North Ltd

Principal Shareholders: Federal Government of Nigeria
Date of Establishment: 1st April 1955
No of Employees: 30,000

NIGERIAN PRINTING & PUBLISHING COMPANY LTD

PO Box 139, Lagos

PRINCIPAL ACTIVITIES: Printing and publishing
Branch Offices: Port Harcourt

NIGERIAN PROCESSING COMPANY LTD

Maganda Rd, PO Box 342, Kano
Tel: 8258/9
Cable: Nigomills Kano

PRINCIPAL ACTIVITIES: Processors of hand-picked selected
groundnuts

NIGERIAN RAILWAY CORPORATION

PMB 1037, Ebute-Metta, Lagos State
Tel: 802000/9
Cable: Nigerail Lagos
Telex: 21020 Ebrail

Chairman: Alhaji Garba Ja Abdulkadir
Directors: Chief Mbazulike Amechi, Mamman Sule, Dennis
Afkawa, Chief E O Oke, Alhaji Kasimu Barau Auna, Alhaji
Abdu Tangaza, Chief W F Granville
Senior Executives: A F A Babatunde (Director, Civil Engineering),
N C U Okoro (Director, Operations),
I J Agbasi (Director Finance),
T O Griffin (Director, Mechanical Electrical Engineering),
Alhaji Mahe Dange (Director, Administration),
J O Mafeni (Director, New Lines),
M I Babalola (Secretary)

PRINCIPAL ACTIVITIES: Railways authority; transport
Branch Offices: Divisional Offices: Ebute-Metta Junction; Enugu;
Bauchi; Ibadan; Kafanchan
Principal Bankers: Central Bank of Nigeria; Union Bank of
Nigeria Ltd; National Bank of Nigeria Ltd; United Bank for
Africa; African Continental Bank; Bank of the North; First
Bank of Nigeria Ltd

Principal Shareholders: Statutory Corporation wholly owned by
the Federal Government of Nigeria
Date of Establishment: 1898
No of Employees: 35,000

NIGERIAN RAILWAY PRESS

Railway Compound, Ebute-Metta, Lagos

PRINCIPAL ACTIVITIES: Printing

NIGERIAN REMOVAL & STORAGE CO LTD (NIRSCO)

Km 10 Badagry Expressway, PO Box 2157, Apapa, Lagos
Tel: 880833

Directors: Mrs C M Abiona (Managing),
B A Abiona
Senior Executives: A F Afilaka (Operations Executive),
S O Yartey (Internal Co-ordinator),
Mrs K Oladunjoye (Packing Manager),
Billi Kashyap (Marketing Co-ordinator),
S A Omoaghe (Accountant)

PRINCIPAL ACTIVITIES: Transportation, clearing and
forwarding, etc
Principal Agencies: Vanpac Carriers Inc, USA; Aarid Enterprises
Corp, USA; Transcar Int, UK
Branch Offices: Old NPA Yard, PMB 156, Warri, Bendel State
Principal Bankers: United Bank for Africa Ltd
Financial Information:

	N'000
Authorised capital	100
Paid-up capital	100

Principal Shareholders: Directors as described
Date of Establishment: 1975
No of Employees: 50

NIGERIAN ROAD CONSTRUCTION LTD

PO Box 2008, Kano
Tel: 8498
Telex: 77134 NRC LTD

Chairman: Chief Okunowo
Directors: Chuka Okoli,
M Etseyatse,
J Idika,
F Douarin (Managing),
G Lessere

PRINCIPAL ACTIVITIES: Civil engineering
Branch Offices: 124 Awolowo Rd, SW Ikoyi, PO Box 2514, Lagos
Tel 683381
Principal Bankers: United Bank for Africa Ltd; International
Bank for West Africa Ltd; Societe General Bank; NAL
Financial Information:

	N'000
Authorised capital	1,000
Paid-up capital	820

NIGERIAN ROMANIAN WOOD INDUSTRIES LTD

Akure-Ondo Rd, PO Box 117, Ondo, Ondo State
Tel: 610583

Chairman: Mrs F M Ighodalo
Directors: J A Ajumobi, Dr A Papava, Chief J S Fagboyegun,
Alhaji G Gbadamosi, M O Ogunbiyi, G K Ajayi, J A Ajibola,
A M Oseni
Senior Executives: I G Margineanu (Acting Managing Director),
C A Adigun (Chief Accountant),
M A Adebayo (Acting Commercial Manager),
Major Edgar (Company Secretary/Administration Manager),
Ogunnaike (Senior Accountant),
A Ogunleye (Personnel Officer)

PRINCIPAL ACTIVITIES: Production of sawn timber, plywood
and furniture
Principal Bankers: First Bank of Nigeria Ltd; National Bank of
Nigeria Ltd
Financial Information:

	N'000
Authorised capital	12,000
Paid-up capital	10,143
Turnover	14,000
Profits	1,500

Principal Shareholders: Odu'a 30%; Forexim of Romania 30%;
Federal Government 25%; Ondo State; NIDB; NBCI
No of Employees: 1,000

NIGERIAN ROPES LTD

66/68 Eric Moore Rd, Iganmu, PO box 115, Apapa, Lagos
Tel: 831348, 831362, 836558, 835693
Cable: Nirop Lagos
Telex: 26630 Nirop Ng

Chairman: Alhaji Saadu Alanamu
Directors: C L Dean (Managing Director),
G J Beswick,
Alhaji Sani Bakori,
C C Ekwegh (Finance Director),
D Houghton,
Alhaji Mohammed Saadu
Senior Executives: John Brown (Technical Manager),
Colin Bryant (Archtectural Consultant)

PRINCIPAL ACTIVITIES: Manufacture and distribution of fibre
ropes, distribution of wire ropes, slings and fittings,
distribution of building products
Principal Agencies: British Ropes; George Taylor; Manville
Export Corporation; Tractel; Parsons Chains
Branch Offices: Offshore Division Wimpey-Brown & Root

Compound, Iwofe Base, PO Box 619, Port Harcourt; 23 Aliyu Makama Rd, PO Box 219, Kaduna
Subsidiary Companies: Wasco Ropes Ltd
Principal Bankers: First Bank of Nigeria Ltd; Chase Merchant Bank Nigeria Ltd
Financial Information:

	₦'000
Authorised capital	3,000
Paid-up capital	1,866
Turnover	6,717
Profits	887

Principal Shareholders: Bridon plc; Alhaji Saadu Alanamu
Date of Establishment: 8th March 1960
No of Employees: 105

NIGERIAN RUBBER BOARD

20 Iyobosa Street, New Benin, PMB 1084, Benin City, Bendel State
Tel: 200680, 200681
Cable: Nigrub Benin City
Telex: 41117 Nigrub Ng

PRINCIPAL ACTIVITIES: Marketing of natural rubber for the Federal Government. Sole authority to export natural rubber for Nigeria
Branch Offices: 72 Campbell Street, Lagos, Tel 631844, Cable Nigrub, Lagos, Telex 21250, 21251

Principal Shareholders: Federal Government of Nigeria
Date of Establishment: 1st April 1977
No of Employees: 420

NIGERIAN SAFETY INSURANCE COMPANY LTD

SW8/667 Lagos Bye-Pass, Ike-Ado, PO Box 2110, Ibadan, Oyo State
Tel: 413736
Cable: Safety

PRINCIPAL ACTIVITIES: Insurance
Branch Offices: Branches and accredited agencies in all main towns

NIGERIAN SECURITY PRINTING AND MINTING COMPANY LTD

PO Box 3053, 26 Ahmadu Bello Rd, Victoria Island, Lagos
Tel: 610790, 613021
Cable: Nigerprint

Chairman: Alhaji Abubakar Alhaji
Directors: A E Ekukinam (Managing Director & Chief Executive),
    Alhaji Shehu Abdulwahab (Executive Director, Administration),
    A B A Obilana (Executive Director, Finance & Commercial),
    P T Nicholson (Executive Director, Technical),
    Alhaji A Ahmed,
    A A Abdulkadir,
    E O Inyang,
    S E Odiete,
    C N Nwagu,
    P H Balmer,
    C G E Banks

PRINCIPAL ACTIVITIES: Printing and minting of currency and security documents
Principal Bankers: Union Bank of Nigeria Ltd; United Bank for Africa Ltd
Financial Information:

	₦'000
Authorised capital	9,600
Paid-up capital	9,600
Turnover	35,320
Profits	4,604

Principal Shareholders: Central Bank of Nigeria; Federal Ministry of Finance Incorporated; Thomas de la Rue International Ltd
Date of Establishment: 1963
No of Employees: 1,500

NIGERIAN SERVICES & SUPPLY COMPANY LTD (NISSCO)

PO Box 1169, Plot 298A Akin Olugbade St, Victoria Island, Lagos
Tel: 612406, 612419
Cable: Nissco
Telex: 21675 Nissco Ng

Chairman: R V Leriche
Directors: Chief J O Edewor, E C Akwiwu
Senior Executives: Dale Peterson (General Manager),
    C Kernech (Financial Controller),
    P Courbe (Operation Manager),
    J C Lecomre (Project Manager)

PRINCIPAL ACTIVITIES: Oil services. Construction of petroleum product storage depots. Offshore fabrication and construction
Branch Offices: Field Offices: PO Box 253, Port Harcourt, Tel 21485; Sapele Rd, Warri, Tel 388
Principal Bankers: Internaional Bank for West Africa Ltd
Financial Information:

	₦'000
Authorised capital	1,000
Paid-up capital	1,000
Turnover	70,000

Principal Shareholders: Chief J O Edewor; E C Akwiwu
Date of Establishment: 1963

NIGERIAN SEWING MACHINE MANUFACTURING COMPANY LTD

Plot 1 Block F Matori St, Mushin, PO Box 3000, Lagos
Tel: 846774, 845768
Cable: Singer Lagos
Telex: 21458 Ng

Chairman: Mallam Ahmadu Coomaise
Directors: B H Carlton,
    S S Rikhy (Financial),
    J A Solanke (Consumer Products),
    Chief M N Ugochukwu,
    Major General R A Adebayo,
    Chief C O Ogunbanjo,
    G J J Brunnbauer (Special Projects),
    J B Olaiya (Company Secretary),
    D N C Field (Managing)

PRINCIPAL ACTIVITIES: Manufacturing of sewing machine cabinets, TV cabinets, radiogram cabinets and assembling of sewing machines and refrigerators. Distribution of home appliances
Branch Offices: 11 Williams St, PO Box 3000, Lagos; Plot 3 Zaria Rd, PO Box 322, Kaduna; 81 New Court Rd, PO Box 1438, Ibadan; Oke-Fia St, PO Box 32, Oshogbo; 3 Mission Rd, PO Box 424, Benin City; May 28 Ave, PO Box 748, Enugu; 17 Harbour Rd, PO Box 528, Port Harcourt; 269 Agege Motor Rd, Mushin, Lagos State
Principal Bankers: First Bank of Nigeria Ltd
Financial Information:

	₦'000
Authorised capital	6,000
Paid-up capital	2,940
Turnover	15,000
Profits	2,000

Principal Shareholders: 60% Nigerians, Nigerian Sewing Machine Manufacturing Company Ltd; 40% Foreigners, The singer Company, New York USA
Date of Establishment: 1960
No of Employees: 700

NIGERIAN SHIPBUILDERS LTD

Registered Head Office, 11-13 Warehouse Rd, PO Box 356, Apapa, Lagos
Tel: 875151, 876200
Cable: Buildship Ph
Telex: 21476

Chairman: F Awomolo
Directors: G B O Sonekan, M W Zehm, P Holtappels, J Machl, A J Weber, D B Hart
Senior Executives: G Lischke (General Manager),
 H Braack (Technical Manager),
 W K Silva (Chief Accountant),
 Bon N Nkwocha (Marketing Manager),
 T Blau (Shipbuilding Engineer),
 W Heani (Civil Engineer)

PRINCIPAL ACTIVITIES: Shipbuilding, building of all inland waterway vessels. Ship repairs, slipping, derusting and painting, steel construction of all types. Building and installing of jetties, pontoons, steel and concrete, import and export of watercraft, machinery and equipment for water craft
Principal Agencies: Damen Shipyards of Holland; Hamstorf Shipyards, W Germany
Branch Offices: Shipyard: Reclamation Rd, PO Box 1887, Port Harcourt, Rivers State
Principal Bankers: United Bank for Africa Ltd
Financial Information:

	₦'000
Authorised capital	1,700
Paid-up capital	1,700

Principal Shareholders: Niteco; Schliching Werft GmbH; Rivers State Government of Nigeria
Date of Establishment: November 1975; Commenced operations December 1977

NIGERIAN SHOE & RUBBER PRODUCTS COMPANY LTD

PO Box 173, Ogbomosho, Oyo State
Tel: 83
Cable: Nishoe

PRINCIPAL ACTIVITIES: Manufacturers of shoes and handbags

NIGERIAN SMELTING & REFINING COMPANY LTD

PO Box 9644, Lagos
Tel: 680608

Chairman: S Dankaro
Directors: G I C Eneli, C K H Funcke, K P M Funcke, E K Hansen

PRINCIPAL ACTIVITIES: Smelting and refining of non-ferrous metals
Branch Offices: Ibeshe Rd, Ikorodu Division, Lagos State
Associated Companies: Paul Bergsoe & Sons A/S, Denmark
Principal Bankers: African Continental Bank Ltd
Financial Information:

	₦'000
Authorised capital	500
Paid-up capital	100

Date of Establishment: 1976

NIGERIAN SOFT DRINKS CO LTD

Isheri Rd, PO Box 164, Ikeja, Lagos
PRINCIPAL ACTIVITIES: Soft drinks

NIGERIAN SPANISH CEMENT CO LTD

13th Floor, 37 Marina, Lagos
PRINCIPAL ACTIVITIES: Suppliers of cement
Branch Offices: Factory: 27 Creek Rd, PO Box 1393, Apapa, Lagos, Tel 876928
Financial Information:
Registered capital ₦ 410,000

Date of Establishment: June 1976

NIGERIAN SPINNERS & DYERS LTD

6 Independence Rd, Bompai, PO Box 138, Kano
Tel: 2885
Cable: Spindye
Telex: 77101 Spindy

Chairman: Alhaji Shehu Ahmed
Directors: A J Akle (Alternate Managing),
 F A Akle (Managing Director),
 G A Akle,
 Alhaji Haruna Kassim

PRINCIPAL ACTIVITIES: Textile manufacturers, worsted yarn
Principal Bankers: Union Bank of Nigeria Ltd
Financial Information:

	₦'000
Authorised capital	1,500
Paid-up capital	800
Turnover	6,000

Date of Establishment: 1968
No of Employees: 480

NIGERIAN SPINNING AND WEAVING CO LTD (Newspin Ltd)

Plot 14, Iganmu Industrial Estate, PO Box 1013, Surulere, Lagos
Tel: 835219

Directors: D Dhaon (General Manager)

PRINCIPAL ACTIVITIES: Manufacturers of carpets and tarpaulins

NIGERIAN STARCH MILLS LTD

Ethiope House, PO Box 1, Ihiala, Anambra State
Tel: Ihiala 1

Chairman: Chief G E Okeke (also Managing Director)

PRINCIPAL ACTIVITIES: Production of gari, glucose custard and poultry feeds

Date of Establishment: September 1970
No of Employees: 395

NIGERIAN STEEL DEVELOPMENT AUTHORITY (NSDA)

138/146 Broad St, PMB 12015, Lagos

PRINCIPAL ACTIVITIES: Iron and steel projects; statutory corporation set up by the Federal Government

NIGERIAN STOCKBROKERS LTD

Bookshop House, 4th Floor, 50/52 Broad St, PO Box 4591, Lagos
Tel: 633222
Telex: 21505 Acepto Ng

Chairman: G O Onosode
Directors: Chief Dr C M Norman-Williams, O A Adeoshun

PRINCIPAL ACTIVITIES: Stockbroking
Branch Offices: Imam House, Ahmadu Bello Way, PMB 2172, Kaduna, Tel 213667, Telex 71328 Acepto Ng; 19 Onitsha Rd, 2nd Floor, Owerri, Imo State, Cable Acceptor Owerri

Date of Establishment: 24th September 1960

NIGERIAN SUGAR COMPANY LTD

Bacita Estate, PMB 65, Jebba, Kwara State
Tel: Bacita 1
Cable: Sugarcane Jebba
Telex: 21542

Chairman: Alhaji Muhammed Kaloma Ali
Directors: Alhaji Tanko Kuta, B O O Ugowe, Isa Tahir, M I Kusharki, Mrs D Daniyan, J F Taylor, J M Supran, E J Mol
Senior Executives: Alhaji Muhammed Shaaba Lafiagi (General Manager),
 Hammid Taju (Personnel Manager/Company Secretary),
 F A Dere (Factory Manager),
 H M Kpogho (Marketing Manager)

PRINCIPAL ACTIVITIES: Growing of sugar-cane and manufacturing of granulated sugar
Branch Offices: Investment House, 7th Floor, 21/25 Broad Street, PO Box 3936, Lagos, Tel 660081, 664870, Telex 21542
Associated Companies: Nigerian Yeast & Alcohol Manufacturing Company
Principal Bankers: Union Bank of Nigeria Ltd
Financial Information:

	₦'000
Authorised capital	10,000
Paid-up capital	10,000
Turnover	8,900

Principal Shareholders: Federal Ministry of Finance Inc; Imo & Anambra States; NNDC; NIDB; Cross River State; NNIL; Odua Investment Co; Kwara State Government
Date of Establishment: 1965
No of Employees: 4,000

NIGERIAN SUITING MANUFACTURING COMPANY LTD

Dantata Rd, PO Box 1135, Kano
Tel: 3346, 4441
Cable: Texma, Kano

Chairman: A A Dantata
Directors: E R Raccah (Managing Director)

PRINCIPAL ACTIVITIES: Textile manufacturers

NIGERIAN SWEETS AND CONFECTIONERY COMPANY LTD

155 Club Rd, PO Box 185, Kano
Tel: 2012, 2013, 2014
Cable: Nicco Kano
Telex: 77113 Nicco NG

PRINCIPAL ACTIVITIES: Manufacturers of sugar confectionery
Branch Offices: Lagos; Ibadan; Maiduguri; Jos

No of Employees: 900

NIGERIAN TECHNICAL CO LTD

11/13 Warehouse Rd, PO Box 356, Apapa, Lagos
Tel: 803190, 803191, 803192, 870596, 870602, 876200
Telex: 21476 Niteco NG

Chairman: F Awomolo
Directors: Alhaji I M Damcida, J A Koru, Alhaji M Bello, P Heibach, Dr H Dick
Senior Executives: P G Crowther (Director of Personnel & Finance),
J Kahl (Director of Sales),
G Kronschnabl (Director of Technical Service)

PRINCIPAL ACTIVITIES: Importers and distributors of vehicles, generators and construction equipment
Principal Agencies: Volkswagen, Steyr; King Trailer; Weeks Trailer; Parmiter Agric Implements; Deutz Generators; O&K; Wacker; Clark; Hella; Varta; Sunshine
Branch Offices: Apapa; Bauchi; Benin; Calabar; Enugu; Ibadan; Ikeja; Ilorin; Isolo; Kano; Maiduguri; Minna; Port Harcourt
Subsidiary Companies: African Lands Ltd; Associated Companies: Nigerian Shipbuilders Ltd; Steyr Nigeria Ltd
Principal Bankers: United Bank for Africa Ltd; First Bank of Nigeria Ltd; Union Bank of Nigeria Ltd; International Bank for West Africa Ltd
Financial Information:

	₦'000
Authorised capital	12,000
Paid-up capital	8,756
Turnover	115,000
Profits	2,500

Principal Shareholders: F Awomolo; Rivers State Government; Borno State Government; Steyr Daimler Puch AG; BGE Weber; A J Weber; D Schaudin
Date of Establishment: 1957
No of Employees: 1,600

NIGERIAN TELEVISION AUTHORITY

Television House, Ahmadu Bello Way, Victoria Island, Lagos
Chairman: Alhaji Aminu Tijani
Directors: Vincent I Maduka (Director General),
Adamu B Augie (Managing Director NTPC),
Ibrahim Mohammed (Managing Director News),
S I J Wigwe (Managing Director Zone A),
G C Ugwu (Managing Director Zone B),
Segun Olusola (Managing Director Zone C),
Abdulrahman Micika (Managing Director Zone D),
Madu Mailafiya (Managing Director Zone E),
Kere Ahmed (Managing Director Zone F)
Senior Executives: A N Onyia (Director of Engineering),
V Ezeokoli (Director of Programmes),
Bode Oluwole (Director of Finance),
Saidu Abubakar (Director Manpower Resources),
Olu Okunrinboye (Director of Operations),
E N Aniebona (General Manager Projects),
B O E Edebor (General Manager Operations),
D J Awoniyi (Director Abuja Projects),
Eddie-Brown Ayoghu (General Manager NTV Enugu),
Peter Olowo (General Manager, NTV Kaduna),
Dele Alli (General Manager, NTV Illorin),
Dipo H O Robbin (General Manager NTV Abeokuta),
Bayo Sanda (General Manager, NTV Ibadan),
Mallam Kere Ahmed (General Manager, NTV Sokoto),
Alhaji M Saidu (General Manager, NTV Yola),
Mallam Idi Jibrin (General Manager, NTV Jos),
Mallam Dahiru Ibrahim (General Manager, NTV Kano),
Bello M Tunau (General Manager NTV Minna),
Isaac Wakombo (General Manager, NTV Makurdi),
Mallam Yaya Abubakar (General Manager NTV Bauchi),
E Halliday (General Manager, NTV P/Harcourt),
Mazi A E Ukonu (General Manager, NTV Aba/Owerri),
Patrick I Ityohegh (General Manager, NTV Abuja),
Rowland O Ifidon (General Manager, NTV Benin),
Ayodele Bedu (General Manager, NTV Akure),
Alhaji Saka Fagbo (General Manager, NTV Ikeja),
Effiong M Etuk (General Manager, NTV Calabar),
Mallam Madu Maillafiya (General Manager, NTV Maiduguri)

PRINCIPAL ACTIVITIES: Federal Government owned national Television network
Branch Offices: Television House, PO Box 1480, Ibadan, Oyo State; PMB 2190, Abeokuta, Ogun State; Tejuosho Avenue, Surulere; West Circular Rd, PMB 1117, Benin City, Bendel State; PMB 7126, Aba, Imo State; PMB 5797, Port Harcourt, Rivers State; PMB 794, Oba Ile, Akure, Ondo State; Independence Layout, PMB 1530, Enugu, Anambra State; 105 Marina Rd Extension, PMB 1299, Calabar; PMB 2044, Makurdi, Benue State; PO Box 1347, Kaduna; PMB 2134, Jos, Plateau State; Bompai Rd, PMB 3343, Kano; PMB 1487, Maiduguri, Borno State; PMB 0146, Bauchi; Ahmadu Bello Way, Jimeta, Yola, Gongola State; PMB 2351, Sokoto; PMB 1478, Fate Rd, Ilorin, Kwara State; TV House, PMB 79, Minna, Niger State

Date of Establishment: 1st April 1977
No of Employees: 7,000

NIGERIAN TEXTILE MILLS LTD

PMB 21051, Industrial Estate, Oba Akran Avenue, Ikeja, Lagos State
Tel: 962011
Cable: Textile Lagos
Telex: 26206 Textil Ng

Chairman: Professor Saburi Biobaku
Directors: A A Gbadegesin, Dr Akin Ojo, Layiwola Olawo, S Solaja, L Palmer, G Oliver, R Francis, F Picciotto, E Picciotto
Senior Executives: Oludotun A Ilo (General Manager),
A A Ajao (Company Secretary/Legal Adviser),
A O Oshibo (Commercial Manager),
E O Akingbade (Financial Manager),
M S Ghorab (Technical Adviser)

PRINCIPAL ACTIVITIES: Spinners, weaver and finishers of textile goods
Principal Bankers: Union Bank of Nigeria Ltd; United Bank for Africa Ltd; First Bank of Nigeria
Financial Information:

	N'000
Authorised capital	6,560
Paid-up capital	6,560
Turnover	17,431

Principal Shareholders: Odu'a Investment Co Ltd; Amenital Holding Registered Trust; Chase International Investment Corporation; Nigerian Industrial Development Bank
Date of Establishment: 2nd February 1960
No of Employees: 3,000

NIGERIAN THERMOPLASTICS LTD

PO Box 178, Warri, Bendel State

Directors: Guido Zamblera

PRINCIPAL ACTIVITIES: Manufacturers of general steel products

No of Employees: 200

NIGERIAN TOBACCO COMPANY LTD

Western House, 8/10 Broad Street, PO Box 137, Lagos
Tel: 634504, 634574/5, 634644, 634715, 634789
Cable: Tobacco
Telex: 21561 Tobaccong

Chairman: Chief J O Udoji (Part-time)
Directors: E Brewis (Managing Director),
  I I Aig'Imoukhuede,
  A I Amenechi,
  C A Atoki,
  P Esiri,
  J C Downie,
  Alhaji Yahaya Gusau (Part-time),
  Alhaji M M Kyari
Senior Executives: M McWilliam (Chief Accountant),
  J Delany (General Sales Manager),
  N A J Kosoko (Asst. Company Secretary),
  B Nodroum (Technical Services Manager)

PRINCIPAL ACTIVITIES: Tobacco
Branch Offices: PO Box 6, Ibadan; PO Box 413, Zaria
Subsidiary Companies: Marina Investment Ltd; Nigerian Tobacco Management Pension Trust Ltd; Nigerian Tobacco Provident Fund Trust Co Ltd
Principal Bankers: United Bank for Africa Ltd; African Continental Bank Ltd; Union Bank of Nigeria Ltd; National Bank of Nigeria Ltd; First Bank of Nigeria Ltd
Financial Information:

	N'000
Authorised capital	25,000
Paid-up capital	25,000
Turnover	75,364
Profits (gross)	8,307
Total assets (1981)	122,665

Principal Shareholders: Percentage holding British American Tobacco (60%); Nigerians (40%)
No of Employees: 3,000

NIGERIAN TOYS MANUFACTURING COMPANY LTD (NITOMAC)

Benin/Sapele Rd, PMB 1082, Benin City, Bendel State
Tel: 240307
Cable: Nitomac Benin City

PRINCIPAL ACTIVITIES: Manufacturers of all types of wood and metal furniture, educational toys, and wooden boxes

NIGERIAN TRANSMISSION COMPANY LTD

6 Ireti St, PO Box 182, Yaba, Lagos

Directors: Florenzo Lombardo

PRINCIPAL ACTIVITIES: Suppliers of motor vehicles components

NIGERIAN TUBER & ROOT CROPS BOARD

PMB 2186, Makurdi, Benue State

PRINCIPAL ACTIVITIES: Producers and exporters of tuber and root crops

NIGERIAN URETHANE CO LTD

8 Uzama St, PO Box 444, Benin City, Bendel State
Tel: 241332

PRINCIPAL ACTIVITIES: Manufacturers of foam products
Financial Information: Part of Ribway Group of companies

NIGERIAN VICTORY ASSURANCE COMPANY LTD

15B Post Office Rd, PO Box 736, Kano
Tel: 2031, 2178
Cable: Vicassure

Chairman: Alhaji Sani Gezawa
Senior Executives: A O Sanni (Managing Director),
  Alhaji Abdu Umar (Assistant General Manager, Operations),
  Alhaji S I Ogunbekun (Company Accountant),
  Peter J Enaohwo (Underwriting Manager)

PRINCIPAL ACTIVITIES: Insurance business
Branch Offices: 8 Alli St, PO Box 8072, Lagos; Ahmadu Bello Way, PO Box 160, Sokoto; PMB 1103, Maiduguri
Principal Bankers: Bank of the North Ltd; Internationl Bank for West Africa Ltd; Union Bank of Nigeria Ltd
Financial Information:

	N'000
Authorised capital	400
Paid-up capital	340
Turnover	2,200

No of Employees: 150

NIGERIAN WATCH-MAKING INDUSTRY LTD

31 Fajuyi St, Ekotedo, PO Box 3123, Ibadan, Oyo State
Tel: 412452
Telex: 31226 Wachm

PRINCIPAL ACTIVITIES: Manufacturing of watches

NIGERIAN WEAVING & PROCESSING COMPANY LTD

100 Nnamdi Azikiwe St, Lagos
Tel: 900263/5

PRINCIPAL ACTIVITIES: Manufacturing of textiles, piece goods

NIGERIAN WEAVING, SPINNING & PRINTING COMPANY LTD (NEWSPIN LTD)

Plot 14, Iganmu Industrial Estate, Iganmu, PO Box 1013, Surulere, Lagos
Tel: 835219, 832432

Chairman: O Sonuga
Directors: H A Mansour, Mrs V Mansour, J Taher
Senior Executives: A O Shoyombo (Personnel Manager),
  J A Okandeji (Accounts Manager),
  F O B Adenuga (Sales Manager)

PRINCIPAL ACTIVITIES: Manufacturers of carpets and carpet tiles, upholstery material, tarpaulins, bags and wrapping materials
Principal Bankers: United Bank for Africa Ltd
Financial Information:

	N'000
Authorised capital	1,000
Paid-up capital	1,000

Principal Shareholders: O Sonuga; Mrs V Mansour; J Taher
Date of Establishment: 1975
No of Employees: 300

NIGERIAN WIRE INDUSTRIES LTD

PO Box 50, Ikeja, Lagos State
Tel: 963015, 963251
Cable: Niwind Lagos

Chairman: Alhaji Usman Dantata
Directors: M Nakano,
    S O Lambo,
    A C C Roose (Managing),
    G Halstead
Senior Executives: Y Adisa (Executive Commercial Director),
    M Forbes (Works Manager)

PRINCIPAL ACTIVITIES: Manufacture of wire and wire products
Branch Offices: Henry Carr St, Industrial Estate, Ikeja, Lagos
    State
Associated Companies: Nigerian Industrial Group Ltd, Kano
Principal Bankers: United Bank for Africa Ltd

Principal Shareholders: Bridon Ltd; Mitsui Co Ltd; Alhaji Usman
    Dantata; S O Lambo
No of Employees: 600

NIGERIAN YEAST & ALCOHOL MANUFACTURING COMPANY LTD

PMB 569, Jebba, Kwara State
Tel: Bacita 1 Ext 7
Cable: Niyamco Bacita

PRINCIPAL ACTIVITIES: Manufacturers of yeast and alcohol
Branch Offices: Factory: Pati Tunku Estate Ltd, Bacita, Kwara
    State
Associated Companies: Nigerian Sugar Co Ltd

NIGERIAN-AMERICAN MERCHANT BANK LTD

25 Boyle St, Onikan, Lagos

Chairman: Chief Dr Nabo Bekinbo Graham-Douglas
Directors: Alhaji Ibrahim Maina Damcida (Deputy Chairman),
    Rex I Alakija,
    Peter Graham Bates (Managing),
    George B Yurchyshyn

PRINCIPAL ACTIVITIES: Banking services

NIGERITE LTD (FORMERLY ASBESTOS CEMENT PRODUCTS LTD)

Oba Akran Ave, PMB 21032, Ikeja, Lagos
Tel: 900602/5
Cable: Asbcem
Telex: 26243

PRINCIPAL ACTIVITIES: Manufacturers of fibre cement roofing
    and ceiling sheets, moulded items, pressure and building
    pipes
Branch Offices: Ilorin, Kwara State
Principal Bankers: United Bank for Africa Ltd; Union Bank of
    Nigeria

Date of Establishment: April 1959
No of Employees: 870

NIGERLINK INDUSTRIES LTD

7th Floor, Western House, 8/10 Broad St, Lagos
Tel: 631022, 632061
Cable: Creative
Telex: 21107 Ojora Ng

Chairman: Chief Adekunle Ojora
Directors: Ojuolape Ojora, Adegboyega Ojora

PRINCIPAL ACTIVITIES: Importers and distributors of diesel
    generators and engines; Manufacturers representatives
Principal Agencies: Motoren-Werke Mannheim AG, West
    Germany; Cooper Energy Services International Inc
Subsidiary Companies: Nigerlink International Associates
Principal Bankers: United Bank for Africa Ltd

NIGERLINK INDUSTRIES LTD

7th Floor, Western House, 8/10 Broad Street, Lagos
Tel: 631022
Telex: 21107

PRINCIPAL ACTIVITIES: Manufacturers of plastics

NIGERPAK LTD

37 Warehouse Rd, PO Box 389, Apapa, Lagos
Tel: 875424, 877389
Cable: Nigerpak Apapa

Chairman: Alhaji Mogaji Dambatta
Directors: Anthony Adebayo Ibazebo, Christopher Adesanmi
    Atoki, Peter Esiri, Emmanuel Adagogo Jaja, Chief Abiola
    Adeniyi Ogundokun
Senior Executives: Rufus Ifedayo Orimolade (Deputy General
    Manager),
    Bolaji A Adeniran (Sales Manager),
    Joseph Jimoh Akano (Chief Accountant),
    George O Ogunleye (Chief Engineer),
    Gabriel O Osineye (Purchasing/Stores Manager),
    Emmanual A Onishile (Production Manager),
    J Tani-Olu (General Manager)

PRINCIPAL ACTIVITIES: Light-packaging designers and
    manufacturers
Branch Offices: ZZ4 Abubakar Kigo Rd, Kaduna; 3 Constitution
    Crescent, Aba, Imo State; 26 Rwang Pam St, Jos, Plateau
    State
Principal Bankers: First Bank of Nigeria Ltd; United Bank for
    Africa Ltd
Financial Information:

	N'000
Authorised capital	3,000
Paid-up capital	2,000

Principal Shareholders: Daily Times of Nigeria Ltd; Nigerian
    Tobacco Company Ltd
Date of Establishment: 1st April 1964
No of Employees: 1,000

NIGERPOOLS COMPANY LTD

PO Box 2453, 15 Ijora Causeway, Apapa, Lagos
Tel: 834928, 831728
Telex: 21417 Nipool Ng

PRINCIPAL ACTIVITIES: Manufacturers of swimming pools

NIGERSOL CONSTRUCTION CO LTD

PO Box 1423, Ibadan, Oyo State
Tel: 413334

PRINCIPAL ACTIVITIES: Building and civil engineering
    contractors

NIGERSTEEL COMPANY LTD

PMB 1229, Enugu, Anambra State
Tel: 254391
Cable: Nigersteel Enugu
Telex: 51106 Steel NG

Chairman: Chief B C Okwu
Directors: Chief R Ikwueke, Dr H I N Onoh, J Ayegba, Dr D
    Ewelukwa, E Hart, G C Akwaeze
Senior Executives: A Okpe (Acting Personnel Manager),
    G R Moorthy (Chief Engineer),
    N N Arya (General Manager),
    L O Otogbolu (Acting Financial Manager)

PRINCIPAL ACTIVITIES: Suppliers of building materials,
    manufacturing of mild steel rods and primary steel producers
Principal Bankers: African Continental Bank Ltd; United Bank for
    Africa Ltd; Cooperative Bank for Eastern Nigeria; Union Bank
    of Nigeria Ltd; International Bank for West Africa Ltd
Financial Information:

	N'000
Authorised capital	3,000
Paid-up capital	2,500
Turnover	4,000

Principal Shareholders: Nigerian Industrial Development Bank Ltd; Nigerian Bank for Commerce and Industries Ltd; Anambra State Government
No of Employees: 515

NIGERTAL INDUSTRIES LTD

18 Iya-Agan St, Ebute-Metta (West), PO Box 127, Apapa, Lagos
Tel: 834750
Cable: Nigertal Lagos

Chairman: A Ojora
Directors: S Ruffato, A Omololu, A Ojora

PRINCIPAL ACTIVITIES: Suppliers of furniture and building materials; engineering
Principal Bankers: United Bank for Africa Ltd
Financial Information:

	N'000
Authorised capital	405
Paid-up capital	405

No of Employees: 150

NIGER-TECHNO LTD

Plot 1019, Ologun Agbeje Street, Victoria Island, PO Box 5294, Lagos
Tel: 615980

Directors: A Zantedeschi, P G Cannata, Chief G F Appio, O Sotuminu
Senior Executives: Andrea Parboni Arquati (Area Manager)

PRINCIPAL ACTIVITIES: Planning and engineering consultants
Branch Offices: Lagos Office: Plot 1019, Ologun Agbeje St, Victoria Island, Lagos; PMB 1146, Calabar, Cross River State; PMB 1470, Enugu, Anambra State

Date of Establishment: August 1974

NIGERWEST STEEL COMPANY LTD

PMB 5288, Faleye Industrial Site, Lagos Rd, Ibadan, Oyo State
Tel: 410174
Cable: Nigertank
Telex: 31159 Nwsco Ng

Directors: G Zamblera

PRINCIPAL ACTIVITIES: Steel fabrication: Contractors

NIGUS PETROLEUM NIGERIA

Plot 1214, Victoria Island, Lagos

Senior Executives: R K Penny (General Manager)

PRINCIPAL ACTIVITIES: Oil exploration and production. An American-Nigerian joint venture

Date of Establishment: 1975

NIMESCO (NIGERIA) LTD

36 Balogun St, PO Box 577, Lagos
Tel: 633032, 683505
Telex: 21483 Dokebs Ng

PRINCIPAL ACTIVITIES: Sales and service of electrical and medical equipment

NIPOL LTD

Apata Ganga, Abeokuta Rd, PMB 5145, Ibadan, Oyo State
Tel: 412918, 412949
Cable: Nipolco Ibadan
Telex: 31136 Nipol Ng

Chairman: R O Odelusi
Directors: C A Ince,
   J E P Shaw (Managing),
   Mrs A O Adekanmbi,
   E O Elegbede
Senior Executives: R M Imoh (General Works Manager),
   W M Awotedu (Commercial Manager)

PRINCIPAL ACTIVITIES: Manufacturers of agricultural seedling bags and containers, industrial containers, industrial packaging materials and industrial components; household goods
Principal Bankers: First Bank of Nigeria Ltd
Financial Information:

	N'000
Authorised capital	961
Paid-up capital	960
Turnover	3,397
Profits	1,467

Principal Shareholders: Odu'a Investment Company; Public
Date of Establishment: 1957
No of Employees: 410

NIROTEC (A DIVISION OF NIGERIAN ROPES LTD)

66-68 Eric Moore Rd, Iganmu Industrial Estate, PO Box 115, Apapa, Lagos
Tel: 836558, 831348, 835693, 831362
Cable: Nirop Lagos
Telex: 26630 Nirop Ng

Chairman: Alhaji Saadu Alanamu, The Waziri of Ilorin
Directors: Alhaji Mohammed Saadu,
   Alhaji Sani Bakori,
   C C Ekwegh (Financial),
   C L Dean (Managing),
   G Halstead,
   A C C Roose
Senior Executives: J A Brown (Technical Manager),
   C J Bryant (Architectural Consultant)

PRINCIPAL ACTIVITIES: Sole distributors of Manville products in Nigeria; suppliers of air-conditioning, heating and refrigeration, insulation materials, filtration aids, celite, irrigation equipment and services, paint, plastics, etc
Principal Agencies: Manville Europe Corporation, France; Manville Int Corp, USA; Manville Italiana Corp, Italy; Nigerian Ropes Ltd, Lagos; Donn France SA, France; SABA, France; State Insulation Corp, USA; SGB Export Ltd, UK
Branch Offices: Lagos; Port Harcourt; Kaduna
Associated Companies: Bridon Ltd

Principal Shareholders: Bridon Ltd; Alhaji Saadu Alanamu; Alhaji Sani Bakori
Date of Establishment: March 1960 (Formerly Johns Manville Products)
No of Employees: 150

NISPAN CONSTRUCTION LTD

1 Ajoke Akinbami Street, PO Box 337, Ikeja, Lagos
Tel: 960364

PRINCIPAL ACTIVITIES: Civil engineering and construction

Date of Establishment: 1975
No of Employees: 450

NITOL LTD

10 Ijora Causeway, PO Box 397, Lagos
Tel: 835491

PRINCIPAL ACTIVITIES: Manufacturing of towels, towelling fabric, knitwear

NIYI IBIKUNLE (NIGERIA) LTD

40-56 Niyi Ibikunle Rd, Dada Estate, PO Box 220, Osogbo, Oyo State
Tel: 2167
Cable: Kunletex

Chairman: Chief Ademola Adeniyi Ibikunle
Directors: Mrs Tinuke Ibikunle, Popoola Bolarinwa, Richard Jimoh, Ibiyinka Adesoji Ibikunle, Fatai Akanni Asuni, John Ade Areoye Olawoye
Senior Executives: Chief A A Ibikunle (Managing Director/Chief Executive),
   Hiroshi Yoshimura (Factory Manager),

Olusola Olabode (Assistant Factory Manager),
Amisu Tiamiyu (Accountant)

PRINCIPAL ACTIVITIES: Manufacturers of polypropelene mats
Principal Bankers: Chase Merchant Bank Nigeria Ltd; National Bank of Nigeria Ltd
Financial Information:

	N'000
Authorised capital	600
Paid-up capital	600
Turnover	591
Profits	4

Principal Shareholders: Chief A A Ibikunle; Mrs Tinuke Ibikunle; Popoola Bolarinwa; Richard Jimoh; Ibiyinka Adesoji Ibikunle; Fatai Akanni Asuni
Date of Establishment: Commissioned 8th August 1981
No of Employees: 152

NIYI OFFICE STATIONERY SUPPLY STORES LTD

16 Johnson St, Ilupeju Industrial Estate, Lagos
Tel: 961773, 963775
Cable: Efficiency Lagos

Chairman: Daliat Adeniyi Obakoya
Directors: Risikat Adefolake Obakoya
Senior Executives: Elijah Shodiya (Account's Supervisor),
    E O Allum (Sales Manager),
    M O Busari (Administrative Officer),
    V O Sanni (Production Supervisor),
    O A Sonuga (Public Relations Officer)

PRINCIPAL ACTIVITIES: Manufacturers of office equipment, tapes, pens, etc; distributors of offset printing machines and inks
Branch Offices: 52 Tokunboh St, PO Box 1086, Lagos; 52 Shipe-Olu St, Palmgrove, Lagos; SW8/131, Lagos Bye Pass, Oke Ado, Ibadan, Oyo State
Associated Companies: Niyi Office Products Industries Ltd
Principal Bankers: Savannah Bank of Nigeria Ltd; United Bank for Africa Ltd
Financial Information:

	N'000
Authorised capital	100
Paid-up capital	100

Principal Shareholders: D A Obakoya; R A Obakoya; Jubril Tijani
Date of Establishment: October 1964

NKWONTA, D O, & SONS ENTERPRISES LTD

5 Railway Commercial Layout, Station Rd, PO Box 579, Enugu, Anambra State
Tel: 254607
Cable: Donkwonta

Chairman: Engineer Anayo A Nkwonta
Directors: Mrs F N Nkwonta
Senior Executives: Engineer S C Arora (Chief Electrical Engineer),
    Mr Nwokeforo (Administrative Manager),
    Henry Etche (Assistant Chief Engineer)

PRINCIPAL ACTIVITIES: Electrical and mechanical engineers, general contractors and manufacturers' representatives
Branch Offices: PO Box 8300, 77 Murtala Mohammed Way, Yaba, Lagos, Tel 861073
Principal Bankers: United Bank for Africa Ltd; African Continental Bank Ltd

Date of Establishment: 1952
No of Employees: 420

NMB MODERN BOOKSHOPS

16 Rwang Pam St, PO Box 262, Jos, Plateau State
Tel: 3230

PRINCIPAL ACTIVITIES: Suppliers of school textbooks, office equipment, stationery etc
Branch Offices: Kaduna; Bauchi; Kafanchan; Pankshin; Zonkwa

NOBGROUP OF COMPANIES

122 Zik Avenue, PO Box 773, Enugu, Anambra State
Tel: 333319
Cable: Nobgroup
Telex: 51312 Nobco Ng

Chairman: Chief S M Okeke
Directors: S J N Okoye,
    M U C Okoye,
    E E Ezekwe,
    B C Onwubuya,
    Prince A M Okoli,
    Ben N Nonyelu (Group Managing Director)
Senior Executives: Joe Anakwenze (Legal Adviser/Secretary),
    D C Eze (Group Accountant/Administration Manager),
    A B L Ezeilo (Sales Manager, Electronics),
    Chris Agu (Sales Manager, Motors),
    Joe Okoyeuzu (Service Manager)

PRINCIPAL ACTIVITIES: General merchants and contractors, motor dealers, transporters and distributors of electrical appliances
Principal Agencies: General Motors Overseas Distribution Corp, USA; Isuzu Motors Ltd, Japan; Advance Industries Ltd, USA
Branch Offices: PO Box 3004, Surulere, Lagos; PO Box 1728, Kaduna; PO Box 781, Jos; PO Box 419, Maiduguri; 110/111 Strand, London WC2, UK, Tel 8368918, Telex 24973
Subsidiary Companies: Nobgroup Enterprises Ltd; Nobgroup Electronics Ltd; Nobgroup Motors Ltd; Nobgroup International Ltd; A B Engineering Company; Pressmedia Ltd
Principal Bankers: African Continental Bank Ltd; Co-Operative & Commerce Bank Ltd; Union Bank of Nigeria Ltd
Financial Information:

	N'000
Authorised capital	500
Paid-up capital	390
Turnover	2,000

Principal Shareholders: Chairman and directors as described
Date of Establishment: Nobgroup Enterprises Ltd, 1971; Nobgroup Electronics Ltd 1975; Nobgroup Motors Ltd 1975; Nobgroup International Ltd 1982
No of Employees: 75

NORDIVE (WEST AFRICA) LTD

PO Box 7381, Lagos
Telex: 20117 Box No 708 Net Tds Ng

Chairman: I E Fraser
Directors: N O Oyesiku, J E Wey, A M Masaya, H Lints, T A Cardale
Senior Executives: D Evans (Technical Manager)

PRINCIPAL ACTIVITIES: Diving services

NORDMANN, RASSMANN & COMPANY (NIGERIA) LTD

40 Isaac John St, GRA Ikeja, PO Box 272, Ijeja, Lagos
Tel: 964433
Cable: Nordrascos Lagos
Telex: 26113 Noraco Ng

Directors: H M Ofurum, J Ugochukwu, K Wellinghausen
Senior Executives: G F Harder (General Manager)

PRINCIPAL ACTIVITIES: Technical and chemical consultants, generators; sales and service

NORDSTAHL (NIGERIA) LTD

7A Lishabi St, PMB 1138, Apapa, Lagos
Tel: 636147, 636218

Directors: B Neunkirchen

PRINCIPAL ACTIVITIES: General consultants and contractors

NOREN INDUSTRIES LTD (FORMERLY NIGERIAN SANDCRETE INDUSTRY LTD)

Km5 Ekenwan Rd, PO Box 718, Benin City, Bendel State
Tel: 242685, 244476
Cable: Nsil Benin
Telex: 41361 Noren

Chairman: M N Ozigbo-Esere (Managing)
Directors: M N Ozigbo
Senior Executives: R T Apraim (General Manager),
  B M Dutta (Production Manager),
  J A O Umoru (Administrative Manager),
  E O Adjemre (Accounts Manager),
  Har Bajan Singh (Factory Manager)

PRINCIPAL ACTIVITIES: Manufacturers and suppiers of building
  materials
Subsidiary Companies: Noren Construction Company Ltd
Principal Bankers: New Nigeria Bank Ltd

Date of Establishment: 4th December 1975

NORMAN INDUSTRIES LTD

PO Box 334, Isolo Industrial Estate, Ikeja, Lagos
Tel: 840058
Cable: Mannor
Telex: 21383

PRINCIPAL ACTIVITIES: Suppliers of electrical goods,
  air-conditioning equipment

NORMANN, C, INTERNATIONAL COMPANY

89 Aroloya St, Lagos

Chairman: C L Anpusim
Directors: C I Obiwulu (Managing),
  P Anapusim,
  E C Obiwulu,
  N Chiddy

PRINCIPAL ACTIVITIES: Importers, exporters, manufacturers
  representatives, general merchandise, suppliers of electrical
  equipment
Principal Bankers: First Bank of Nigeria Ltd

NORNIT LTD

PO Box 135, 18 Dantata Rd, Bompai, Kano
Tel: 2227
Cable: Nornit Kano
Telex: 77186 Nornit Ng

PRINCIPAL ACTIVITIES: Manufacturing of knitted fabrics and
  garments

Date of Establishment: 1963

NORSPIN LTD

PO Box 230, 11 Muhammed Ladan Rd, Kaduna South, Kaduna
  State
Tel: 213786, 243171
Cable: Norspin Kaduna
Telex: 71124 Norspin Ng

Chairman: L Hodgson
Directors: T H Pao, U Bonet, Y Hwa, J P Rauch, Mrs E O
  Daniyan, D D Leeming
Senior Executives: D H Heath (Financial Adviser),
  C W Sum (Technical Manager),
  J O Nnaji (Chief Accountant),
  A Akinbodewa (Personnel and Training Manager)

PRINCIPAL ACTIVITIES: Manufacturing of printed and woven
  textile fabrics and yarns
Branch Offices: Old Niger House, PO Box 6049, Lagos
Principal Bankers: Union Bank of Nigeria Ltd; First Bank of
  Nigeria Ltd

Financial Information:

	N'000
Authorised capital	7,000
Paid-up capital	7,000
Turnover	17,644
Profits	403

Principal Shareholders: UAC of Nigeria Ltd, Lagos
Date of Establishment: 1962
No of Employees: 3,000

NORTEX (NIGERIA) LTD

PO Box 276, Kaduna South, Kaduna
Tel: 211503

Directors: A M Inuwa (General Manager),
  M I Yusufu (Assistant General Manager),
  B Wood (Production Manager)

PRINCIPAL ACTIVITIES: Manufacturing of woven and printed
  cloth and shirts

Principal Shareholders: New Nigeria Development Company

NORTH BREWERY LTD

19-21 Dantata Rd, Bompai, Post Box 55, Kano
Tel: 5196, 5759
Cable: Northtop Kano
Telex: 77133 Norbru Ng

Chairman: Chief Inalegwu Entonu
Directors: Chief A O Lawson,
  O A Awoliyi,
  C Haythorn,
  Asama Ahinche,
  John Danfulani,
  L K Omosebi,
  March Abi,
  A B Fowowe (Managing)
Senior Executives: K H Tange (General Manager),
  A M G Mshelia (Assistant General Manager, Technical),
  F A Asuni (Assistant General Manager, Marketing),
  P E Okoronkwo (Assistant General Manager, Finance)

PRINCIPAL ACTIVITIES: Brewery, manufacturers of beer and
  stout
Branch Offices: Kaduna; Jos; Ilupeju; Maiduguri; Sokoto; Yola;
  Minna; Makurdi; Bauchi; Ibadan
Principal Bankers: First Bank of Nigeria Ltd; United Bank of
  Africa Ltd; Societe Generale Bank Ltd
Financial Information:

	N'000
Authorised capital	12,000
Paid-up capital	8,740
Turnover	65,000
Profits	5,500

Principal Shareholders: Federal Government of Nigeria (50%);
  West African Breweries Ltd (50%)
Date of Establishment: 12th May 1965
No of Employees: 948

NORTH EAST LINE CORPORATION

3/4 Kiri Kasama Rd, PO Box 27, Maiduguri, Borno State
Tel: 2460

PRINCIPAL ACTIVITIES: Bus services throughout the north and
  also inter-state services and to Lagos
Branch Offices: Kano; Bauchi Main Market; Gombe; Jos;
  Onitsha; Enugu; Kaduna; Lagos

NORTHCO CONSTRUCTION COMPANY LTD

10 Birnin Kebbi Rd, PO Box 91, Sokoto
Tel: 232031
Cable: Northco
Telex: 73113

Chairman: Alhaji Shehu Idris
Directors: Alhaji Malami Sarkin Pawa, Alhaji Ali Idris, Mallam Sanusi Ibrahim, Mallam Ahmadu Shehu, Mallam Isa Shehu, Mallam Garba Mallami
Senior Executives: L B Adigun (Technical Manager),
  Mr Qadir (Financial Controller),
  Alhaji Mohammed Kaoje (Purchasing Manager),
  Mr Oyinlola (Chief Quantity Surveyor),
  M Umam Yaro Daudare (Legal Adviser and Administrative Manager),
  Alhaji Musa Magaji (Purchasing Manager),
  Monawar Mannan (Mechanical Engineer)
PRINCIPAL ACTIVITIES: Civil engineering and construction, dam construction, water supplies undertakings and road construction
Branch Offices: 18 Odaliki St, Ebute-Metta (West), Lagos; Canteen Rd, PO Box 149, Gasau; PO Box 23, Kontagora; 1 Sulaimon Crescent, PO Box 2233, Kano
Subsidiary Companies: Engineering Services Agency Ltd (ESAL)
Principal Bankers: Bank of the North Ltd; Union Bank of Nigeria Ltd; First Bank of Nigeria Ltd
Financial Information:

	₦'000
Authorised capital	4,000
Paid-up capital	3,637
Sales turnover	8,555
Profits	443

Principal Shareholders: Alhaji Shehu Idris; Alhaji Malami Sarkin Pawa; Alhaji Ali Idris
Date of Establishment: 26th May 1971
No of Employees: 1,550

NORTHERN CABLE PROCESSING AND MANUFACTURING COMPANY LTD

Maichibi Rd, Kaduna South, Industrial Estate, PO Box 1423, Kaduna
Tel: 216746
Cable: Nocaco
Telex: 71376 Nocaco Ng

Chairman: D H Abdu
Directors: M Jeroch, S Y Kasimu, M I Shani, H D Berg, Deg-German Development Company, K H Hinrichs
Senior Executives: G Wilhelms (General Manager)

PRINCIPAL ACTIVITIES: Manufacturers of cable harnesses for the automobile industry, electrical wires, cables and conductors for power transmission
Branch Offices: Henry Carr Street, PMB 21253, Ikeja Industrial Estate, Ikeja
Associated Companies: Kabelmetal Nigeria Ltd
Principal Bankers: Bank of the North; United Bank for Africa; Icon Bank
Financial Information:

	₦'000
Authorised capital	2,000
Paid-up capital	2,000
Turnover (12 months to June 1982 estimated)	8,500

Principal Shareholders: Elmore's Metal Company Ltd; Kabelmetal Nigeria Ltd
Date of Establishment: 16th June 1978
No of Employees: 300

NORTHERN ENAMELWARE COMPANY LTD

25 Dantata Rd, Bompai, PO Box 24, Kano
Tel: 2723

PRINCIPAL ACTIVITIES: Manufacturing of enamelware

NORTHERN METAL WORKS CO LTD

PO Box 6461, 26 Dantata Rd, Bompai, Kano
Tel: 4050
Cable: Nnworks Kano
Telex: 77202 Trmph Ng

Chairman: H A Boukarroum
Directors: Alhaji Uba Dogo,
  M H Halawi (Managing)
Senior Executives: T O Aiyetan (Manager)

PRINCIPAL ACTIVITIES: Manufacturers of plastic crates, PVC pipes, polyethylene bags and sheets, jerry cans and domestic and industrial plastic products
Principal Bankers: Chase Merchant Bank of Nigeria Ltd; International Bank for West Africa
Financial Information:

	₦'000
Authorised capital	500
Paid-up capital	400

Principal Shareholders: H A Boukarroum
Date of Establishment: 4th July 1969
No of Employees: 130

NORTHERN NIGERIA FIBRE PRODUCTS LTD

PO Box 694, Old Airport Rd, Jos, Plateau State
Tel: 53333/4
Cable: Jutemill Jos
Telex: 81127 Nascos Ng

Chairman: Macido Dalhat
Directors: Alhaji Shehu Ahmed,
  Saleh I Nasreddin (Managing),
  Mrs M O Banigboye,
  Aaron Ako,
  A I Nasreddin
Senior Executives: Sallauddin Razaak (Chief Executive),
  A M Sallam (Deputy General Manager),
  A I Sani (Assistant General Manager, Production),
  K Brahmaji (Finance Manager),
  D P Ashu (Personnel Manager)

PRINCIPAL ACTIVITIES: Manufacturers of jute sacking, bags, hessian cloth, carpets, felts and wadding
Associated Companies: Household Products Ltd; Nasco Biscuits; Nasco Pack Ltd
Principal Bankers: Bank of the North; First Bank of Nigeria Ltd
Financial Information:

	₦'000
Authorised capital	7,300
Paid-up capital	4,648
Turnover	8,439
Profits	34

Principal Shareholders: A I Nasreddin; New Nigeria Development Company; Plateau Investments Company; Benue Investment Company
Date of Establishment: 1967

NORTHERN NIGERIA FLOUR MILLS LTD

PMB 3172, 15 Mai Malari Rd, Bompai Industrial Estate, Kano
Tel: 612070, 803370
Telex: 77114

Chairman: G S Coumantaros
Directors: Ali Umai Baba,
  Aminu Dantata,
  Saidu Yaya Kasuma,
  M Dantata,
  G S Missols,
  F G Jutzi,
  J G Sherey,
  A Ferguson,
  T A Oyeleke,
  A M Gashash,
  M S Nanono,
  C Fredericos (Managing)

PRINCIPAL ACTIVITIES: Manufacturers of flour wheat offals
Principal Bankers: United Bank for Africa Ltd

Date of Establishment: 29th October 1971

NORTHERN NIGERIA INVESTMENTS LTD

Nigerian Agricultural Bank Bldg, Hospital Rd, PO Box 138, Kaduna
Tel: 212528, 212573, 212980
Cable: Velop Kaduna
Telex: 71110 Norves Ng

Chairman: Alhaji Liman Ciroma
Directors: Abdu Abdulrahim, Tunji Olagunju, Hamman B Mohammed, S S Waniko, A Kollere, Baba Adi, Sule Kolo, Zakwai Zarma, Mahmud Tukur, Ali Al-Hakim
Senior Executives: S Y Kasimu (Acting Chief Executive), Stephen Adaji (Financial Controller), Edith O Daniyan (Head of Project Promotion), Babale Girei (Head of Investment Supervision), Alhaji F Bello (Acting Company Secretary)

PRINCIPAL ACTIVITIES: Provision of capital for the development and expansion of agricultural, mining, commercial and manufacturing industries
Principal Bankers: Union Bank of Nigeria Ltd; Bank of the North Ltd; United Bank for Africa Ltd
Financial Information:

	₦'000
Authorised capial	20,000
Paid-up capital	14,778
Investments (net)	23,823

Principal Shareholders: New Nigeria Development Company Ltd
Date of Establishment: 1959

NORTHERN NIGERIA PUBLISHING COMPANY LTD (NNPC)

Gaskiya Bldg, PO Box 412, Zaria, Kaduna State
Tel: 2087
Cable: Gasmac
Telex: 75243 Gasmac

Chairman: Alhaji M Mora
Directors: C R Harrison, Byam Shaw, Saidu Adamu, Muhtar Ahmad, Lamis Ibrahim
Senior Executives: John G Watson (Publishing Executive), Alhaji Mamman Maina (Sales Manager), Ms Ann Price (Managing Editor)

PRINCIPAL ACTIVITIES: Publishing
Principal Agencies: Macmillan Publishers, UK Ltd
Branch Offices: 79 Sharada Industrial Area, PMB 3027, Kano; Bauchi Rd, Dogon Dutse, PMB 902, Jos
Principal Bankers: Union Bank of Nigeria Ltd; Bank of the North Ltd

Principal Shareholders: Gaskiya Corporation Ltd; Macmillan Publishers Ltd, UK; NNDC Ltd
Date of Establishment: 1966

NORTHERN NIGERIA TEXTILE MILLS LTD

PO Box 131, Kaduna
Tel: 243329
Cable: Texweave
Telex: 71103 Kadtex

Chairman: Alhaji Abubakar Gum
Directors: Alhaji Yahaya Gusau, K F Moffatt, Ambros Feese, J A Smith
Senior Executives: K S Nilsson (General Manager)

PRINCIPAL ACTIVITIES: Bleachers, dyers and printers of woven textile piece-goods, on a commission basis
Principal Bankers: First Bank of Nigeria Ltd

Principal Shareholders: New Nigeria Development Company; Northern Nigeria Investments Ltd; Jama' Atu Nasril Islam; Kaduna Textiles Ltd
No of Employees: 350

NORTHERN NIGERIAN TECHNICAL SERVICE LTD

59 Tafawa Balewa Rd, PO Box 123, Kano
Tel: 3687
Cable: Nigerauto Kano
Telex: 77221

Chairman: Alhaji Usman Albishir
Directors: Alhaji Shehu Sanusi, Alhaji Baba Bukar, A J Dorman
Senior Executives: J Wilding (General Manager), G N Craze (Sales), J W Prentice (Technical)

PRINCIPAL ACTIVITIES: Sales of motor vehicle spares, agricultural machinery, spares, tools, workshop equipment, etc; manufacture of cotton dusters and mop-heads
Principal Agencies: Alvan Blanch Development Compahy Ltd; Olham Batteries Ltd; Holman Brothers Ltd
Principal Bankers: First Bank of Nigeria Ltd

Principal Shareholders: Alhaji Usman Albishir

NORTHERN SAWMILL & FURNITURE MANUFACTURING CO LTD

30A Kundila Rd, PO Box 147, Kano
Tel: 4739, 4794
Cable: Safumaco
Telex: 77141 Fast NG

Chairman: A K Fawaz
Directors: H K Fawaz, Alhaji M L Mohammed (Acting Managing Director), A E Fawaz, E H C Ward (Works Manager), Mallam Ali Umar Baba, Alhaji Kabiru Ahmed, Alhaji Amino Ibrahim

PRINCIPAL ACTIVITIES: Manufacturing of household furniture
Associated Companies: Fawaz Steelwood & Chemicals Ltd; Sokoto Furniture Factory
Principal Bankers: Bank of the North Ltd

Principal Shareholders: A K Fawaz; Kao State Investment Company
No of Employees: 200

NORTHERN STEEL WORKS LTD

PO Box 62, 181 Club Rd, Kano
Tel: 3057

PRINCIPAL ACTIVITIES: Manufacturing of metal doors and window frames
Associated Companies: Balmore Trading Company Ltd

NORTHERN TEXTILE MANUFACTURERS LTD

5 Independence Rd, Bompai, PO Box 116, Kano
Tel: 3088, 3087
Cable: Mantex Kano
Telex: 77220 Mantex NG

PRINCIPAL ACTIVITIES: Manufacturing of blankets

NORTHERN TIN COMPANY LTD

Gyel Village, PO Box 79, Bukuru, Jos, Plateau State
PRINCIPAL ACTIVITIES: Mining of metal ore
No of Employees: 200

NORTHERN TRANSPORTERS AND MERCHANTS SYNDICATE LTD

Dantata House, 66/67 Murtala Mohammed Way, PO Box 292, Kano
Tel: 4137
Cable: Syndicate Kano

PRINCIPAL ACTIVITIES: Transporters
Branch Offices: 4 Creek Rd, PO Box 130, Apapa, Lagos; Tel 841293, Cables Syndicate Apapa

NORTHERN WIRE & STEELWORKS LTD
26 Dantata Rd, PO Box 284, Kano

PRINCIPAL ACTIVITIES: Manufacturers of wire and steel products

NORWO TRADING COMPANY LTD
Kachia Rd, PO Box 308, Kaduna South
Tel: 243492, 213316
Cable: Norwo Kaduna
Telex: 71117 Nortco Ng

PRINCIPAL ACTIVITIES: Manufacturers' representatives; distributors of office stationery, technical drawing equipment, office furniture
Branch Offices: Kaduna; Kano; Jos; Sokoto; Maiduguri; Lagos

NOVACOKE BUILDERS LTD
135 Apapa Rd, PMB 1085, Apapa, Lagos
Tel: 830934

Directors: M Canova

PRINCIPAL ACTIVITIES: Construction

NOVELTY INDUSTRIAL COMPANY LTD (NOVIC)
Plot B Satellite Town Rd, Off Badagry Express Rd, Lagos

Chairman: Ossama M Oudeh (also Managing Director)
Directors: M A Buba, A G Azmeh, H Oudeh, A Ogunsanya

PRINCIPAL ACTIVITIES: Manufacturing of textiles, upholstery
Branch Offices: 77/79 Eric Moore Rd, Iganmu Industrial Estate, Lagos
Principal Bankers: United Bank for Africa Ltd; First Bank of Nigeria Ltd; Union Bank of Nigeria Ltd
Financial Information:

	N'000
Authorised capital	720
Paid-up capital	720
Turnover	6,000

Principal Shareholders: Chairman and directors as described
Date of Establishment: 4th August 1969
No of Employees: 190

NUBI TEXTILE MILLS (NIGERIA) LTD
Nubi Ave, Ifako, PO Box 124, Agege, Lagos
Tel: 931836

Chairman: Chief M Nubi (also Managing Director)
Directors: O O Nubi (General Manager)

PRINCIPAL ACTIVITIES: Textile manufacturers

NUCCON
1a Gwani Mukhtar Crescent, Kaduna

PRINCIPAL ACTIVITIES: Civil engineering consultants

NUCLEUS ELECTRONICS LTD
15 Ola-Ayeni St, PO Box 369, Ikeja, Lagos
Tel: 962018
Cable: Nucnics Lagos

Chairman: Jacob Kehinde Afolabi
Directors: John Taiwo Afolabi, Mrs Elizabeth Adejoke Afolabi
Senior Executives: Albert Tunde Afolabi (General Manager), G A Mohammed (Marketing Manager), A I Mordi (Project Engineer)

PRINCIPAL ACTIVITIES: Suppliers of electrical and electronic equipment, scientific instruments, telecommunications
Principal Agencies: Hyundai Corporation, South Korea; Eagle International, UK; Bouyer Electro-Acoustique, France; Telerep (Telephone Answering), Belgium
Branch Offices: 130 Broad St, Lagos; 3 Salvation Army Rd, Ibadan; 14 Hill Station Rd, Jos
Associated Companies: Radio Spares and Vision Parts (RSVP) Ltd; Flasks and Jugs (Nigeria) Ltd

Principal Bankers: Savannah Bank of Nigeria Ltd; Wema Bank Ltd

Principal Shareholders: Oloyede holdings

NUKOM ENGINEERING LTD
30 Oladipo Labinjo Crescent, PO Box 770, Surulere, Lagos
Tel: 833383
Telex: 26534 Nukeng Ng

Chairman: F A Ogbemi (also Chief Consulting Engineer)
Directors: Dr T Lawal (Associate Consultant)

PRINCIPAL ACTIVITIES: Engineering consultancy
Principal Bankers: First Bank of Nigeria Ltd
Financial Information:

	N'000
Authorised capital	100
Paid-up capital	80

Date of Establishment: July 1973

NWAEZU BUILDING COMPANY LTD
18 Iweka Rd, Onitsha, Anambra State

PRINCIPAL ACTIVITIES: Construction

NWANDU, D A, & SONS ENTERPRISES LTD
17 Ogui Rd, PO Box 648, Enugu, Anambra State
Tel: 252017, 252183, 252760, 254017
Cable: Dansons

PRINCIPAL ACTIVITIES: Building and civil engineering contractors, general merchants, consultants and hoteliers
Branch Offices: 11A Raymond St, Yaba, Lagos, Tel 861918

NWANKWU, J, & BROS LTD
Mile 3 Onitsha-Owerri Rd, PMB 1568, Onitsha, Anambra State
Tel: 210588, 210691
Cable: Nwabros Onitsha
Telex: 54328 Nwanqu

Chairman: Sir Joseph Ozoemena Nwankwu (also Managing Director)
Directors: Barrister C I Nwankwu, Mrs Regina O Nwankwu
Senior Executives: J K T Jayasinghe (Project Engineer), P J Emmanuel (Civil Engineer), M Srishanmuganathan (Civil Engineer), P Yogalingam (Structural Engineer), J C Udeagha (Company Secretary)

PRINCIPAL ACTIVITIES: Civil engineering, building construction and general merchants
Branch Offices: Enugu Sports Stadium Complex Site, Ogui Rd, Enugu; Federal Government Secretariat, Independence Layout, Enugu; ADCP Housing Site, Abuja; 50 Ayilara Street, Near Ojuelegba Roundabout, Surulere, Lagos
Associated Companies: Olympic Packers Ltd; Olympic Drinks Company Ltd; Petrogas Ltd
Principal Bankers: Union Bank of Nigeria Ltd
Financial Information:

	N'000
Authorised capital	1,000
Paid-up capital	1,000

Principal Shareholders: Chairman and directors as described
Date of Establishment: 9th December 1961 (Incorporated)
No of Employees: 250 staff (and over 2,000 casual workers)

NWEKE, J E, & SONS LTD
1 Ogui Rd, PO Box 733, Enugu, Anambra State
Tel: 255389, 254333
Cable: Jens Enugu
Telex: 51101 Jens NG

Directors: Jonas E Nweke
Senior Executives: T U Akalawu (Accountant)

PRINCIPAL ACTIVITIES: Manufacturers' representatives, importers, distributors and transporters
Principal Agencies: Nigercem Co Ltd; Nigeria; Lin Yuan Industrial Co Ltd, Taiwan, Republic of China
Principal Bankers: Standard Bank of Nigeria Ltd
Financial Information:

	N'000
Authorised capital	200
Paid-up capital	190

Principal Shareholders: Jonas E Nweke

NWONYE, I O M, & SONS COMPANY LTD

301 Agbani Rd, PMB 1508, Enugu, Anambra State
Tel: 3435 Enugu
Cable: Iomco

Chairman: Chief I O M Nwonye (also Managing Director)
Directors: Anthony Nwonye, Chukwuemeka O Nwonye, John Nwonye, I M Nwonye, C U Nwonye, C M Nwonye, E U Nwonye
Senior Executives: Anthony Nwobodo (Engineer),
    Simon Chukwurah (Engineer),
    Harrison C Igbo-Amalu (Senior Technical Officer),
    Peter Iro Iduma (Secretary)

PRINCIPAL ACTIVITIES: Building and civil engineering contractors; general importers; manufacturers' representatives; electrical engineering contractors; suppliers of building materials/cement; paint distributors and licensed buying agents
Principal Agencies: Ebony Paints (Nigeria) Ltd, Enugu; N V Steel Export Service, Belgium; Countryman Power Plant Ltd, UK
Branch Offices: 6b Alhaji Masha St, Lagos; PMB 1362, Owerri, Imo State; PO Box 170, Awgu, Anambra State; Makurdi, Benue State
Principal Bankers: Co-operative Bank of Eastern Nigeria Ltd; African Continental Bank Ltd; First Bank of Nigeria Ltd

O'BAHOR, J A, & COMPANY LTD

Susannah House, Near Federal Sub Post Office Buildings, PO Box 1700, Warri, Bendel State

Chairman: Chief J A O'Bahor
Directors: HRH Prince J A O'Bahor (Managing),
    W A O'Bahor,
    Mrs S O Bazunu-O'Bahor

PRINCIPAL ACTIVITIES: Architecture and town planning. Civil engineering and construction. Electrical and mechanical engineering; consultants
Principal Agencies: Dilinger Strasborg von Dusseldorf GmbH; Bilinger Berger Strasborg GmbH; Voest-Alpine AG; CSA GmbH (Eisen und Stahlwerke)
Branch Offices: 44 Lower Erejuwa Rd, Bazunu Layout, PO Box 1700, Warri, Bendel State; 1 Bazunu St, Warri, Bendel State
Associated Companies: First International Corporation of Japan
Principal Bankers: Union Bank of Nigeria Ltd
Financial Information:

	N'000
Authorised capital	3,000
Paid-up capital	1,500
Turnover	3,500
Profits	350

Principal Shareholders: Chairman and directors as described
Date of Establishment: 30th October 1978
No of Employees: 200

OBAN (NIGERIA) RUBBER ESTATES LTD

PO Box 236, Calabar-Ekang Rd, Calabar, Cross River State
Cable: Onrel

PRINCIPAL ACTIVITIES: Manufacturing of sheet and crepe rubber

Principal Shareholders: Nigerian Joint Agency Ltd

OBANLEARO TRADING COMPANY LTD

99 Ikorodu Rd, Igbodi, PO Box 49, Ebute-Metta, Lagos
Tel: 846704, 846802

PRINCIPAL ACTIVITIES: Suppliers of building materials

OBASKEKI, G I, & SONS LTD

134 Lagos St, PO Box 42, Benin City, Bendel State
PRINCIPAL ACTIVITIES: Sawmills

OBATRACO GROUP OF COMPANIES

99 Ikorodu Rd, Igbobi, PO Box 49, Ebute-Metta, Lagos
Tel: 846704, 846802
Cable: Obatraco Ebute Metta
Telex: 22652 Obatco NG

Chairman: Pastor S A Odunaiya
Directors: A W Odunaiya (Managing Director),
    Simi Odunaiya (Commercial Director)

PRINCIPAL ACTIVITIES: Distributors of agricultural equipment, building materials; ceramics, irrigation and power equipment, plastics; manufacturers' representatives
Principal Agencies: Lombardini Motori, Italy; Minex, Poland
Branch Offices: Matori Layout, Akinyemi St, Matori; NW4/133 Oke Padre, Ibadan, Oyo State; 2 and 28 Galadima Rd, Sabongari, Kano
Subsidiary Companies: (Wholly owned subsidiaries); Oba Nle Aro Trading Co Ltd; Oba Nle Aro Technical Co Ltd; Molubu Concrete Industries Ltd; Ceiling Tiles (Nigeria) Ltd; (subsidiary with major shareholding); Industrial and Farm Equipment Co Ltd (Ifeco)
Principal Bankers: Union Bank of Nigeria Ltd; United Bank for Africa Ltd
Financial Information:

	N'000
Authorised capital	500
Paid-up capital	500
Sales turnover	15,000

Principal Shareholders: Odunaiya family
No of Employees: 500

OBELAWO FARCHA FISHING INDUSTRIES LTD

1 Jetty Rd, Apapa, Lagos
Tel: 831660

PRINCIPAL ACTIVITIES: Fisheries

OBIOZO & PARTNERS POWER CONSTRUCTION COMPANY LTD

69 New Market Rd, Onitsha, Anambra State

PRINCIPAL ACTIVITIES: General electrical contractors, electrical designers

OCEAN INCHCAPE (NIGERIA) LTD

Leventis Bldg, 6 Azikiwe Rd, PO Box 1124, Port Harcourt, Rivers State
Tel: 333833, 334354
Telex: 61174 Hufras Ng

Directors: Captain I Farquhar (General Manager)

PRINCIPAL ACTIVITIES: Marine contracting and diving services
Branch Offices: 13/15 Wharf Rd, PO Box 155, Apapa, Lagos; PO Box 10, Bonny, Rivers State

Principal Shareholders: Oil UK (60%); Various Nigerian Businessmen and Company Employees (40%)
Date of Establishment: 1972
No of Employees: 350

OCEANIC & COASTAL MARINE LTD
114 Adeniyi Jones Avenue, Ikeja, Lagos
Tel: 901400/1/2
Cable: Oceehemes Lagos
Telex: 26724 Wbn Ng

Chairman: Ayomane Oladele Odimayo
Directors: John Nwuamaghyi,
  Wilfred Ighodaro (Managing),
  Olaseinde Odimayo,
  Saifudeen Ademola Edu,
  William A E George,
  Orekoya Odimayo,
  Peter F Cook
Senior Executives: Adesina Dawodu (Marketing Manager),
  O W Ajibola (Bills Manager),
  J O Chukwu (Technical Sales Manager)

PRINCIPAL ACTIVITIES: Buying, renting, leasing and servicing of
  boats (military, paramilitary, fishing and oil industry). Pleasure
  boats and yachts
Principal Agencies: Shipyard de Wiel BV, Netherlands; AMF
  Marine Products International, USA; Fairey Allday Marine Ltd,
  UK; Kappamarine, Italy
Branch Offices: Marine Base: Ibafon Village (Opposite Tin Can
  Island), PMB 1111, Apapa
Subsidiary/Associated Companies: Relmint Resources Co Ltd;
  Perkins Properties
Principal Bankers: Nigeria Acceptances Ltd; United Bank for
  Africa; International Bank for West Africa; International
  Merchant Bank
Financial Information:
Authorised capital   ₦ 1,000,000

Principal Shareholders: A O Odimayo; J Nwuamaghyi; W
  Ighodaro; O Odimayo
Date of Establishment: 29th May 1974
No of Employees: 73

OCEANNERING (NIGERIA) LTD
PO Box 3720, Plot 36 Adeniyi Jones Ave, Lagos
Tel: 680527
Cable: Nigdivcon Lagos

Directors: G A G C Parker (Regional Manager and Managing
  Director)

PRINCIPAL ACTIVITIES: Diving, construction and oceanographic
  services
Associated Companies: Divcon (Nigeria) Ltd

OCHUMBA PRESS LTD
3 O'Connor Street, PO Box 184, Asata, Enugu, Anambra Stae
Tel: 254172, 337371

Chairman: B B O Emeh
Directors: Kathlyn Ngozi, Lotanna Emeh, Osmond Obi
Senior Executives: Obi Emeh (General Manager),
  L U Onwuka (Marketing)

PRINCIPAL ACTIVITIES: Printing and publishing
Principal Agencies: Wiggins Teape (WA) Ltd
Branch Offices: Twopenny House, PO Box 7, Nnobi
Subsidiary/Associated Companies: Dozini Company Ltd
Principal Bankers: Union Bank of Nigeria Ltd
Financial Information:

	₦'000
Authorised capital	200
Paid-up capital	200
Turnover (at 31.12.81)	960

Principal Shareholders: B B O Emeh; K Ngozi; L Emeh; O Obi
Date of Establishment: 1972
No of Employees: 87

ODECO LTD
Km 8 Lagos Rd, Orita-Challenge, PO Box 1323, Ibadan, Oyo
  State
Chairman: Timothy O Odubanjo

Directors: T F Odubanjo (General Manager),
  B O Owolabi,
  Carlos M Berriz (Managing Director/Chief Engineer),
  B O Odubanjo (Techanical Director),
  Olatunde Onasanya
PRINCIPAL ACTIVITIES: Civil engineering and construction;
  agents & general trading Co; suppliers of agricultural
  equipment and services; building materials and cement;
  ceramics and sanitary fittings; construction plant; electrical
  and electronic equipment; industrial equipment and heavy
  machinery; livestock and animal feeds; machinery; plant hire;
  power equipment
Principal Agencies: Kuhl Intercontinental Inc, USA; Central Soya,
  USA; H C Davis Sons Manufacturing Co Inc; Chemical
  Engineering & Consulting (Chenco)
Branch Offices: Sonola Estate, Lisabi Elite Rd, Abeokuta, Ogun
  State; 32 Ondo Rd, Akure, Ondo State; 84 Cemetery St,
  Ebute-Metta, Lagos
Subsidiary/Associated Companies: Ingefisa, Spain (Associate);
  The International Corporation for Development; USA;
  (Associate); Odubanjo Engineering Construction Ltd; Ground
  Explorations Group Associates; Olatunde Electronics
  (Subsidiaries)
Principal Bankers: Co-Operative Bank Ltd; Societe Generale
  Bank (Nigeria) Ltd
Financial Information:

	₦'000
Authorised capital	250
Paid-up capital	250
Turnover	1,530

Principal Shareholders: T O Odubanjo; M O Odubanjo; T F
  Odubanjo; Carlos M Berriz; Olatunde Onasanya; B O Owolabi
Date of Establishment: 1979
No of Employees: 150

ODENG ENGINEERING COMPANY LTD
8 Adisa Bashua Street, Surulere, PO Box 2201, Lagos
Cable: Odecodeng Lagos

Chairman: Oluwole Dawodu
Directors: Mrs Olapeju Dawodu
Senior Executives: Joe Ijeoma (Chief Representative)

PRINCIPAL ACTIVITIES: Management consulting and project
  conception; automobile retailer; general traders, engineering
  consultants
Branch Offices: 19 Tejuoso St, Yaba; Abeokuta; Ibadan; Aba
Principal Bankers: First Bank of Nigeria Ltd

Principal Shareholders: Oluwole Dawodu

ODIBO AKHIGBE & CO LTD
See AKHIGBE, ODIBO, & CO LTD

ODU'A INVESTMENT COMPANY LTD
Cocoa House, (Floors 20-22), PMB 5435, Ibadan, Oyo State
Tel: 417515, 417710, 417540
Telex: 31225 Ng

Chairman: Chief (Dr) T A Oworu
Directors: A A Babalola,
  Duro Oyekane,
  Prof A A Ademosun,
  J D Onibon,
  C O S Oseni,
  M A Balogun,
  Dr G A Soyoye,
  F O Mogaji (Group Managing Director),
  O A Olawuyi (Director of Performance Measurement),
  S A Onadele (Director of Corporate Services/Company
    Secretary)
Senior Executives: T O Orenuga (Finance Manager),
  E A Akadiri (Planning & Development Manager),
  G A Oni (Financial Analyst),
  O O Akinnawo (Senior Investment Manager),
  E O Esho (Industrial Analyst)

PRINCIPAL ACTIVITIES: Holding company with diversified investments in commercial, industrial and other projects

Subsidiary/Associated Companies: There are 25 subsidiary companies and associated companies in the Group including National Bank of Nigeria Ltd, Wema Bank Ltd; Great Nigeria Insurance Company Ltd; Nigerian General Insurance Company Ltd; Glanvill Enthoven & Company (Nigeria), West African Portland Cement Company Ltd

Principal Bankers: National Bank of Nigeria Ltd; First Bank of Nigeria Ltd; United Bank for Africa (Nigeria) Ltd

Financial Information:

	₦'000
Authorised capital	12,000
Paid-up capital	12,000
Turnover	81,099
Profits	4,465

Principal Shareholders: Oyo; Ondo & Ogun State Governments
Date of Establishment: 1976
No of Employees: Over 20,000 in the Group

ODUS BAKERIES

77 Ojuelegba Rd, Surulere, Lagos

PRINCIPAL ACTIVITIES: Bakery

ODUS GLOBE & COMPANY LTD

23 Oba Akran Avenue, Industrial Estate, PO Box 5427, Ikeja, Lagos
Tel: 842493, 962791, 963289

Chairman: Johnson K Odusote

PRINCIPAL ACTIVITIES: Shipping; transporters; agents and general traders

Date of Establishment: 18th February 1974

ODUS INDUSTRIES (NIGERIA) LTD

22 Alaba St, Mushin, Lagos

PRINCIPAL ACTIVITIES: Manufacturing of soaps and soap powders

ODUTOLA NIGERIAN INDUSTRIES LTD

Adeola Industrial Estate, PO Box 52, Ijebu-Ode, Ojun State
Tel: 222, 300
Cable: Odunindus Ijebu-Ode
Telex: 21680 Rubber Ng

PRINCIPAL ACTIVITIES: Manufacturers of bicycle tyres and tubes

OFI LIVESTOCK INDUSTRIES LTD

Calabar, Cross River State

PRINCIPAL ACTIVITIES: Manufacturers of livestock feeds

OGHENEOVO VENTURES LTD

Odjevwedje Mansion, B34 Warri/Sapele Rd, PMB 1109, Warri, Bendel State
Tel: 233019

PRINCIPAL ACTIVITIES: Shipping agents, clearing and forwarding, warehousing, transportation, importing and exporting; registered customs agents

OGT GROUP OF COMPANIES LTD

44 Balogun St, PO Box 1444, Lagos
Tel: 662028, 662492, 662483, 660467
Cable: Ogtnations
Telex: 21389 OGT NG

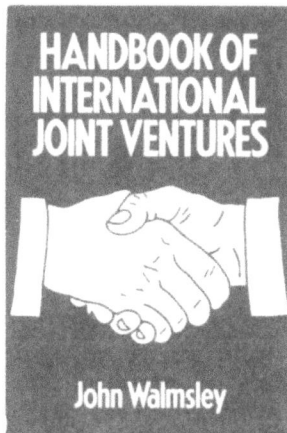

Chairman: Chief Okerentugba G Thompson
Directors: O O Okerentugba, B O Okerentugba, A A Okerentugba
Senior Executives: Dr Dejo Ogunlade (Group Administration Manager),
  O K Oji (Group Chief Accountant),
  Udo Edukere (Deputy Group Commercial Manager)
PRINCIPAL ACTIVITIES: A Holding Company to eight Subsidiary Limited Companies. Principal activities engaged in: agents and general trading; shipping; advertising; colour printing; public relations; oil and gas services; building and civil engineering contractors, etc
Branch Offices: Norjo International Company, 40/42 Oxford St, London WC1
Subsidiary Companies: OGT Contractors & Shipping Line Ltd; OGT Trading Company Ltd; OGT Promotions & Arts Ltd; OGT Block Industries Ltd; etc
Principal Bankers: African Continental Bank Ltd; United Bank for Africa Ltd
Financial Information:

	N'000
Authorised capital	500
Paid-up capital	500
Sales turnover	25,000

No of Employees: 100

OGUBULE INDUSTRIAL PRINTERS LTD
25 Apata St, Shomolu, Lagos
Tel: 846728

PRINCIPAL ACTIVITIES: Printing and packaging

OGUEJIOFOR, ALEX, COMPANY LTD
9 Fox Lane, PO Box 548, Enugu, Anambra State
Tel: 252022
Cable: Alexco
Telex: 51136 Alexco Ng

PRINCIPAL ACTIVITIES: Importers and exporters; building and civil engineering contractors; manufacturers' representatives; miners; general contractors

OGUINE BROTHERS
10/7 Bauchi Rd, PO Box 624, Jos, Plateau State
Tel: 3084

PRINCIPAL ACTIVITIES: Dealers in all electrical accessories and electrical contractors; importers of building materials
Branch Offices: 42 Rwang Pam St, Jos

OGUNMEFUN WORKS LTD
22 Jebba St (East), Ebute-Metta, PO Box 7899, Lagos
Tel: 861777

PRINCIPAL ACTIVITIES: Industrial electrical engineering and installation specialists

OGUNNIRE MODERN FURNITURE (NIGERIA) LTD
SW7/17 Old Barracks Rd, Oke-Bola, PO Box 1540, Ibadan, Oyo State
Tel: 413300

PRINCIPAL ACTIVITIES: Specialists in office equipment; metal works; interior design
Branch Offices: 201 Folagbade St, Ijebu-Ode, Ogun State; Tel 2366; Plot 176 Layi Oyekanmi St, Papa Ajao, Off Isolo Rd, PO Box 100, Ushodi Post Office, Mushin, Lagos

OHAKWE & ASSOCIATES (NIGERIA) LTD
27 Douglas Rd, Owerri, Imo State
Tel: 230215
Cable: Ohas

Chairman: Laz L A Ohakwe
Directors: Bartholomew Akwari, M C Ohakwe
Senior Executives: Innocent Onyenwere (Manager),
  C Onunogbo (Electrical Supervisor)

PRINCIPAL ACTIVITIES: Electrical and mechanical contractors, dealers in air-conditioners generators and electrical equipment
Principal Agencies: Sodik Asea Nigeria Ltd
Branch Offices: 26 Venn Rd, South Onitsha, Anambra State
Principal Bankers: First Bank of Nigeria Ltd
Financial Information:

	N'000
Authorised capital	50
Turnover	5,000
Profits	100

Date of Establishment: 23rd January 1978
No of Employees: 100

OHANENYE & SONS LTD
PO Box 510, Aba, Imo State
Tel: 322/3

PRINCIPAL ACTIVITIES: Transport contractors, supermarket, manufacturers' representatives

OHUKA BROTHERS LTD
5 Aba-Owerri Rd, PO Box 476, Aba, Imo State
Tel: 220237
Cable: Ohubros Aba

Chairman: A M Ohuka
Directors: Mrs M G N Ohuka, A O N N Ohuka
Senior Executives: J U Ngwakwe (Accountant)

PRINCIPAL ACTIVITIES: Manufacturers representatives
Principal Agencies: Brian Munro Ltd; Sphinx (Nigeria) Ltd
Subsidiary/Associated Companies: Genuinmack Ltd; Ohuka Cosmetics Industries Ltd
Principal Bankers: United Bank for Africa Ltd
Financial Information:

	N'000
Authorised capital	500
Paid-up capital	500
Turnover	4,911
Profits	190

Principal Shareholders: Directors as described
Date of Establishment: 27 October 1971
No of Employees: 52

OIL PALM COMPANY LTD
PMB 4063, Sapele, Bendel State
Tel: 41044

Directors: G E Izah (Managing Director)

PRINCIPAL ACTIVITIES: Palm oil processing and palm kernel
Branch Offices: 30 Ihama St, Benin, Bendel State

OIL SUPPLY CENTRE LTD (OSC)
95 Sapele Rd, Warri, Bendel State

Directors: Joseph Johnson (Manager)

PRINCIPAL ACTIVITIES: Equipment suppliers and servicers to the oil industry

OJENIYI, ADELEGAN, TRADING COMPANY NIGERIA
11 Ikorodu Rd, Mile 11 Ketu, Ikeja, Lagos

Chairman: S A Ojeniyi (also Managing Director)

PRINCIPAL ACTIVITIES: Importers, exporters, general merchants; suppliers of building materials, carpets, ceramics, glass, hardware, and paint; representatives
Principal Bankers: Wema Bank Ltd

Principal Shareholders: S A Ojeniyi

OJURI MARITIME SERVICES

8 Itapeju St, Apapa, Lagos
Tel: 876539, 874634
Telex: 22209

PRINCIPAL ACTIVITIES: Shipping, clearing, forwarding and transportation

OKADA BOTTLING COMPANY (NIGERIA) LTD

Plot 28, LSDPC Layout, Ikorodu, Lagos State

Chairman: Chief G O Igbinedion (also Managing Director)

PRINCIPAL ACTIVITIES: Manufacturers and bottlers of soft drinks
Financial Information:
Registered capital   ₦ 500,000

Date of Establishment: October 1979

O.K.C. (NIGERIA) LTD

8 Ikwerre Rd, PO Box 83, Port Harcourt, Rivers State
Tel: 331045, 331511
Telex: 61218 Oki Ng

Chairman: O K Isokariari
Directors: N K Isokariari
Senior Executives: E B Ryder (General Manager)

PRINCIPAL ACTIVITIES: Building and civil engineering contractors, storm water drainage contractors, precast concrete and concrete pipe manufacturers
Branch Offices: Plot 26, Trans-Amadi Industrial Estate, Port Harcourt, Tel 331067/330025, Telex 61108 KIO NG; 126 Bode Thomas St, Surulere, Lagos, Tel 837968; Suite 545, Chancery House, 53/64 Chancery Lane, London WC2, UK, Tel 8316925, Telex 21792
Associated Companies: O K Isokariari & Sons (Nigeria) Ltd
Principal Bankers: Pan African Bank
Financial Information:

	₦'000
Authorised capital	500
Paid-up capital	500
Turnover	7,500

Principal Shareholders: O K Isokariari
Date of Establishment: 2nd June 1980
No of Employees: 400

OKENABIRHIE ENTERPRISES LTD

PO Box 479, Warri, Bendel State
Tel: 280707, 233723

Chairman: J O Aaron-Okenabirhie
Directors: Otobo Okenabirhie
Senior Executives: F O Obi (Administrative Manager), N Ile (Assistant Production Manager), B G Arubayi (Procurement Manager)

PRINCIPAL ACTIVITIES: Venetian blinds manufacturers; suppliers of paper and paper products; electrical and electronic equipment
Branch Offices: 159A 2nd East Circular Rd, Benin City
Associated Companies: Glorylux Associated Industries (Nig) Ltd; Glorylux Venetian Blinds
Principal Bankers: First Bank of Nigeria Ltd
Financial Information:

	₦'000
Authorised capital	100
Paid-up capital	100
Turnover	600
Profits (after tax)	30

Date of Establishment: 1972

OKITIPUPA OIL PALM CO LTD

PMB 319, Okitipupa, Ondo State
Tel: 41129

Chairman: Chief C A Tewe
Senior Executives: D B A Longe (General Manager)

PRINCIPAL ACTIVITIES: Processing and production of palm produce
Principal Bankers: National Bank of Nigeria; First Bank of Nigeria
Financial Information:

	₦'000
Authorised capital	1,000
Paid-up capital	400
Turnover	4,800

Principal Shareholders: Ondo State Government
Date of Establishment: May 1976
No of Employees: 508 (Established), 2,181 (Casual)

OKPE MINING SYNDICATE

77 Cemetary St, PO Box 418, Jos, Plateau State

PRINCIPAL ACTIVITIES: Metal ore mining

OKUNOWO BROTHERS

139 Igbosere Rd, PO Box 143, Lagos
Tel: 636780

PRINCIPAL ACTIVITIES: General merchants, importers and exporters

OKWESA, JOHN, LTD

5 Onike Rd, PO Box 123, Yaba, Lagos
Tel: 861529, 860080

PRINCIPAL ACTIVITIES: Printers and stationers
No of Employees: 90

OKWUOSA MINING INDUSTRY

Isiagu Afikpo, PO Box 547, Enugu, Anambra State

PRINCIPAL ACTIVITIES: Metal ore mining

OLADAPO & COMPANY LTD

9 Aerodrome Rd, PO Box 436, Apapa, Lagos
Tel: 873360, 875167

PRINCIPAL ACTIVITIES: Exporters of timber, produce buyers, etc

OLAGBEMIRO, D O, & CO (NIGERIA) LTD

Ahmadu Bello St, PO Box 684, Jos, Plateau State
Tel: 55115

Chairman: D O Olagbemiro
Directors: D M Olagbemiro

PRINCIPAL ACTIVITIES: Importers and distributors of general merchandise
Principal Agencies: PZ; Cadbury; Lipton; A J Seward etc
Branch Offices: Ogbomosho, Oyo State
Principal Bankers: First Bank of Nigeria Ltd

OLAIYA FAGBAMIGBE LTD

See FAGBAMIGBE, OLAIYA, LTD

OLAOGUN ENTERPRISES LTD

Km 8 Old Ife Rd, Ibadan, Oyo State
Tel: 962199, 413620
Cable: Olaprises
Telex: 20311 TDS Box 043

Chairman: S O Bamgbose
Directors: S O Bamgbose Jnr, Mrs J E Bamgbose, Mrs A Y Bamgbose
Senior Executives: Mr Adedoja (Accountant), H W Lambert (Farm Manager), Mr Olaosebikan (Marketing Manager), Mr Ojayi (Administrative Manager)

PRINCIPAL ACTIVITIES: Agents and general trading company, agricultural equipment and services, food, food processing and livestock and animal feeds
Principal Agencies: Frank Wright Feeds Int Ltd, UK; L Danno, France; Ground Control Electronics, UK
Branch Offices: 2 Alhaji Shomade Alley, Obanikoro, Lagos; 56 Otukpo Rd, Makurdi; Anguldi, Jos; Idi-Iroko Rd, Sango Otta
Principal Bankers: Cooperative Rank Ltd; Societe Generale Bank Nigeria Ltd; United Bank for Africa
Financial Information:

	N'000
Authorised capital	300
Paid-up capital	300
Turnover	4,500

Principal Shareholders: S O Bamgbose; Mrs J E Bamgbose; Mrs A Y Bamgbose
Date of Establishment: 1960
No of Employees: : 200

OLASHINDE BROTHERS
PO Box 3133, Ibadan, Oyo State
Tel: 414094
Cable: Lash

Directors: S Ola Amoo (Managing)
PRINCIPAL ACTIVITIES: Importers, exporters, general merchants, agents
Principal Bankers: National Bank of Nigeria Ltd

OLATUNDE LALEYE AND PARTNERS
22 Rwang Pam Street, PO Box 189, Jos, Plateau State
Tel: 52846

Senior Executives: Olatunde Laleye (Licensed Surveyor), Drew Barlow (Business Manager)
PRINCIPAL ACTIVITIES: Licensed land surveyors; topographic, engineering and control surveys
Principal Bankers: First Bank of Nigeria Ltd

Date of Establishment: 1978

OLAU OLU MODERN BAKERY LTD
51 Lagos St, Ebute-Metta, Lagos
PRINCIPAL ACTIVITIES: Bakery

No of Employees: 200

OLAWALE ODELEYE ASSOCIATES
Plot 10 Jalupon Estate Extension, Off Bode Thomas Rd, Surulere, PO Box 4184, Lagos
Tel: 961821
Cable: Estetiks, Lagos

Chairman: Arc Dr O A Odeleye
Senior Executives: S Patel (Senior Architect/Planner),
O A Adebayo (Architect),
O Opoko (Architect),
B Egbe (Administrative Manager)

PRINCIPAL ACTIVITIES: Architecture, engineering and town planning
Branch Offices: Main Market Site, PO Box 1686, Jos; Emir Yahaya St, New Nigeria Building, PMB 2190, Sokoto; 5 Lalubu St, PO Box 2196, Oke-Ilewo, Ibara, Abeokuta, Ogun State; Plot 268 Trans-Amadi Layout, PO Box 417, Port Harcourt, Rivers State
Associated Companies: Arc-Models Company
Principal Bankers: United Bank for Africa Ltd

Date of Establishment: June 1975

OLDMAC SHIPPING LINES NIGERIA LTD
19 Nnamdi Azikwe St, 2nd Floor, PO Box 2635, Lagos
Tel: 664901
Telex: 21444 Oldmac Ng

Directors: O A Morakinyo (Managing)
PRINCIPAL ACTIVITIES: Shipping agents

OLEHSON BROTHERS COMPANY (NIGERIA) LTD

(Olehson's Agro Animal Kingdom)
39 Lafia Rd, Northbank, GPO Box 797, Makurdi, Benue State
Cable: Olehsonbrosco

Chairman: Igwe O Mbah
Directors: Martins U Chukwu, Williams O Chima, Alhaji D Yakamata
Senior Executives: Samuel Kalu Olehson (Managing Director/Principal Sales Executive)

PRINCIPAL ACTIVITIES: Distributors in Nigeria for veterinary medicines, vitamins, cosmetics, liquid soaps, agricultural chemicals, poultry, wiremesh, block making machines and assorted building blocks
Principal Agencies: Saint Torry Laboratories, Hong Kong; Euribrid BV, Holland; Rosa Cometta, Italy; Chu Chen-Pharmaco Ltd, Taiwan; IGV-Enterprise, Budapest; J L Hoffman, USA
Branch Offices: 18 Abiriba Street, Umuahia, Imo State; 29 Tenant Rd, Aba, Imo State; 7B Amuke Rd, Elu, Ohafia, Imo State
Subsidiary Companies: Unu Brosco (Nig); Olediuwanma Transport Co Ltd; Ukiwe International Co Ltd
Principal Bankers: Union Bank of Nigeria Ltd

Principal Shareholders: Uriem Odinma O O Olehson; Diana Njansi O O Olehson; Roseline A O O Olehson
Date of Establishment: 21st April 1978
No of Employees: 1,000 including local agents and sub distributors

OLLIVANT, G B, & CO (NIGERIA) LTD
PO Box 144, 182/184 Broad St, Lagos
Tel: 637216
PRINCIPAL ACTIVITIES: Suppliers of general merchandise

OLOKODANA GROUP OF COMPANIES
36 Balogun St, Lagos
Tel: 633032, 683505
Telex: 21483 Dokebs Ng
PRINCIPAL ACTIVITIES: General trading and contracting

OLORO PROPERTIES LTD
7th Floor, Investment House, Broad St, PO Box 5436, Lagos
Tel: 635240
Cable: Oloprop Lagos
Telex: 21113 Olopro Lagos

Directors: Adedayo A Adebiyi (General Manager)
PRINCIPAL ACTIVITIES: Legal consultants to the oil industry

OLU HOLLOWAY NIGERIA LTD
3 Araromi St, Onitira, Yaba, PO Box 3549, Lagos
Tel: 840317
Cable: Holly Lagos

PRINCIPAL ACTIVITIES: Industrial documentary films including cinema and television commercials

OLUFAWO ABAYOMI & PARTNERS
See ABAYOMI, OLUFAWO, & PARTNERS

OLUMO DUNWO COMMERCIAL ENTERPRISES LTD
6 Akanji St, Ikate, Surulere, Lagos
Tel: 861604
Cable: Odunwo
Telex: 61232 Ng

Chairman: M Ayo Shodeinde (also Managing Director)
Directors: Mrs B O Shodeinde, Z A Saunders, J P Shodeinde

PRINCIPAL ACTIVITIES: Shipping agents, importers, wholesalers and general trading
Principal Agencies: Grandpale Shipping Company Ltd, Greece
Branch Offices: 82 Aggrey Rd, Port Harcourt, Rivers State
Associated Companies: Odunwo Ltd
Principal Bankers: Pan African Bank Ltd

Principal Shareholders: M Ayo Shodeinde Z A Saunders
Date of Establishment: 1969

OLUTONE ELECTRONICS
112 Apapa Rd, Ebute-Metta, Lagos
Tel: 830762

PRINCIPAL ACTIVITIES: Importers and suppliers of electrical and electronic equipment

OLUWAKEMI MOTORS & FINANCE COMPANY LTD
SW8/91A Oke-Ado St, Mapo, PO Box 3316, Ibadan, Oyo State
Tel: 412296
Cable: Blessmotors Ibadan

Chairman: Alhaji Chief A A Suberu (also Managing Director)
Directors: Alhaji M A Suberu (Executive)

PRINCIPAL ACTIVITIES: Importers and exporters; dealers in all types of vehicles; electronics general contractors and industrial financiers; embroidery lace manufacturers
Branch Offices: 6 Adebayo Shopping Complex, Behind Kingsway Stores, Ibadan, Oyo State; Also at Lagos, Tel 637013; Warri and Kano
Principal Bankers: African Continental Bank Ltd; Union Bank of Nigeria Ltd
Financial Information:

	N'000
Authorised capital	500
Paid-up capital	500
Turnover (approx)	3,500

Principal Shareholders: Alhaji Chief A A Suberu; Alhaji M A Suberu
Date of Establishment: June 1972
No of Employees: 211

OLUWAKEMI (SWISS) NIGERIA EMBROIDERY INDUSTRIES LTD
Km 6 Old Ibadan-Lagos Rd, Oluwakemilayout, PO Box 599, Ibadan, Oyo State
Tel: 412296
Cable: KimiLace

Chairman: Alhaji Chief A A Seberu
Directors: Alhaji S Adelokun

PRINCIPAL ACTIVITIES: Manufacturers of lace and embroidery
Principal Bankers: African Continental Bank Ltd; Union Bank of Nigeria Ltd
Financial Information:

	N'000
Authorised capital	700
Paid-up capital	700

Date of Establishment: 1977

OLYMPIC GROUP LTD
4 Salako Crescent, Ifako, PMB 1083, Agege, Lagos

Chairman: Dr E A Okorie (also Managing Director)
Directors: Mrs A Okorie (Financial Director),
E C Okorie,
Dr W Ofili
Senior Executives: S O Fatusi (General Manager)

PRINCIPAL ACTIVITIES: Agents and general trading; suppliers of agricultural equipment, and produce, building materials, ceramics and sanitary fittings; electrical equipment, fertilisers, toiletries
Branch Offices: 12 branches; Lagos branch: 26 Olayemi St, Ikate, Lagos
Associated Companies: Olympic Stores; Olympic Farms

Financial Information:

	N'000
Authorised capital	2,000
Paid-up capital	1,200

Principal Shareholders: Dr E A Okorie; E C Okorie; Mrs A Okorie; Dr C E Obi; Dr W Ofili

OMENJOR & RAMSAUER ELECTRICAL COMPANY
1 Abule-Ijesha Rd, PMB 1154, Yaba, Lagos State

Directors: Werner Ramsauer, Joseph Omenjor
Senior Executives: J Schindele (Project Engineer),
Wilhelm Withof (Project Manager),
Albert Gruber (Project Engineer),
Francis Okpu (Project Manager)

PRINCIPAL ACTIVITIES: Electrical engineering consultants; power distribution, production, installation, maintenance; general contractors
Principal Agencies: Christian Geyer, West Germany; Gunther Spelsberg, West Germany; Albrecht Jung, West Germany
Principal Bankers: New Nigeria Bank Ltd; African Continental Bank
Financial Information:
Authorised capital N 400,000

OMO GROUP ORGANISATION
22 Commercial Ave, Yaba, Lagos
Tel: 844134, 862526

Chairman: Olusola Omoira (also Managing Director)

PRINCIPAL ACTIVITIES: Companies within the organisation are engaged in business consultancy, insurance, construction of furniture, boats; manufacturing of candles; supermarkets; agricultural produce

OMO-BARE & SONS (NIGERIA) LTD
Plot A18 Sapele Rd, PO Box 210, Benin City, Bendel State
Tel: 1184

Chairman: His Highness Timothy Omo-Bare
Directors: Mrs Florence Omo-Bare,
Adam Omobare,
Iren Omobare (Administrative Manager),
Attah Omobare (Production Manager),
Chief Ayo Omobare
Senior Executives: Richard Edogun (Company Accountant),
Moses Enetomeh (Factory Engineer)

PRINCIPAL ACTIVITIES: Manufacturing of nails
Branch Offices: Union Bank of Nigeria Ltd; New Nigeria Bank Ltd
Financial Information:

	N'000
Authorised capital	200
Paid-up capital	200

Principal Shareholders: Chairman and directors as described

OMOLE, LAWRENCE, & SONS LTD
B203, Okesha Benin Rd, PO Box 75, Ilesha, Oyo State
Tel: 2144, 2048
Cable: Felucca

Chairman: Lawrence Omole
Directors: Dr Akanni Omole,
Olajide Esan,
Dr Akintola Omole,
Ayoola Omole,
Gabriel Onipede,
Taiwo Omole,
Oladele Agbaje Williams (General Manager),
Obafemi Adeniyi (District Manager)

PRINCIPAL ACTIVITIES: Dealers in agricultural products and cement; transportation business
Principal Agencies: Nigerian Cocoa Board; Nigerian Palm Produce Board; West African Portland Cement Company Ltd
Branch Offices: PO Box 131, Ile-Ife, 5 Hospital Rd, Ondo
Associated Companies: Omole Motors Ltd; Omole Investments Ltd
Principal Bankers: First Bank of Nigeria Ltd

No of Employees: 165

OMOLE MOTORS LTD

B203 Okesha Benin Rd, PO Box 75, Ilesha, Oyo State
Tel: 2048, 2144
Cable: Felucca

Chairman: Lawrence Omole
Directors: Dr Akintola Omole, Abiodun Omole, Taiwo Omole, Ayoola Omole

PRINCIPAL ACTIVITIES: Buying and selling of motor vehicles and components
Principal Agencies: Intra Motors Nigeria Ltd; SCOA Motors Ltd; CFAO Motors Ltd; UTC Motors Ltd; Mandilas Ltd
Branch Offices: Ile-Ife; Ibadan; Lagos
Principal Bankers: First Bank of Nigeria Ltd

OMON STORES LTD

82 Mission Rd, PO Box 17, Benin City, Bendel State
Tel: 240945, 240726
Cable: Omostos Benin

Chairman: M E Omonzogie
Directors: M I Omon Appai, A E Omonzogie

PRINCIPAL ACTIVITIES: Agents and general trading company; wholesale and departmental stores and supermarkets
Principal Agencies: Nestles-Food Specialities (Nig) Ltd; Lever Brothers Nigeria Ltd; Tate & Lyle (Nig) Ltd; Lipton of Nigeria Ltd; Cadbury Nigeria Ltd; West African Distillers Ltd; West Africa Milk Co (Nig) Ltd, etc
Branch Offices: PO Box 120, Uromi; 22 New Lagos Rd, Benin City; 19 Murtala Mohammed Way, Benin City
Principal Bankers: African Continental Bank Ltd; First Bank of Nigeria Ltd; New Nigeria Bank Ltd
Financial Information:

	N'000
Authorised capital	100
Paid-up capital	100

Principal Shareholders: M E Omonzogie; M I Omon Appai; A E Omonzogie

OMOT FIRE PROTECTION ENGINEERING LTD

8 Agege Motor Rd, Opposite Shogunle Railway Station, PO Box 1551, Ikeja, Lagos
Tel: 961348

PRINCIPAL ACTIVITIES: Design, supply installation and service of automatic fire extinguishing systems
Branch Offices: E9/897G Iwo Rd (Opposite Army Barracks), Ibadan; 22 Ekere St, Off Aba Rd, Rumuobiakani, Port Harcourt, Rivers State

OMOTOSO PHARMACEUTICALS LTD

13-17 Breadfruit St, PO Box 4024, Lagos
Tel: 661898, 662366

PRINCIPAL ACTIVITIES: Suppliers of pharmaceuticals

Date of Establishment: 1976

OMUNA CONSTRUCTION COMPANY (NIGERIA) LTD

17 Trans-Amadi Industrial Layout, PO Box 184, Port Harcourt, Rivers State
Tel: 227180
Cable: Omunacon

Chairman: Chief Omunakwe Nyeche Nsirim (also Managing Director)
Directors: Aleruchi Etcheson Nsirim, Mrs Maureen Ebie Nsirim (Director, Cashier)
Senior Executives: Kevin J Connolly (General Manager), Manasseh O Ikpeoha (Project Manager), Clement W Ichegbo (Office Manager), Frank Hindley (Plant Manager)

PRINCIPAL ACTIVITIES: Civil engineering and construction
Subsidiary Companies: Nyeche Dredging Company (Nig) Ltd
Principal Bankers: Pan African Bank Ltd
Financial Information:
Authorised capital   N 200,000

No of Employees: 600

ONDO STATE INVESTMENT CORPORATION

Investment House, Parliament Rd, PMB 700, Akure, Ondo State
Tel: 2180

Chairman: Wunmi Adegbonmire
Senior Executives: E A Ogunode (General Manager)

PRINCIPAL ACTIVITIES: Promoters of agricultural and industrial projects
Principal Agencies: Crittal Hope Metal Products (Nigeria) Ltd; Pepsi Cola Company Ltd, Ibadan
Principal Bankers: First Bank of Nigeria Ltd; Union Bank of Nigeria Ltd; Co-Operative Bank Ltd; United Bank for Africa Ltd; National Bank of Nigeria Ltd; Wema Bank Ltd

Principal Shareholders: Ondo State Government
Date of Establishment: 1st July 1976
No of Employees: 2,500

ONI ERNST & WHINNEY LASEBIKAN & COMPANY

See ERNST & WHINNEY, ONI, LASEBIKAN & COMPANY

ONIBONOJE PRESS & BOOK INDUSTRIES (NIG) LTD

Felele Layout, PO Box 3109, Ibadan, Oyo State
Tel: 413956

Chairman: Gabriel Omotayo Onibonoje
Directors: Josephine Olufunmilayo Onibonoje, Jonathan Olusanija Onibonoje
Senior Executives: Mrs Florence Abike Onibonge (Administrative Manager), Gabriel Olusegun Dada (Editorial Manager), M A Mustapha (Senior Press Superintendent), T O Olatunji (Area Sales Manager)

PRINCIPAL ACTIVITIES: Printing and publishing
Branch Offices: SW8/77 Oke Ado, Ibadan; 23 Danbata St, Kano; 8 Ikorodu Rd, Lagos; 25A Tafawa Balewa St, Jos; 75 Beda Rd, Onitsha; 16 Iriemila St, by James Watts Rd, Benin City; PO Box 115, Sokoto
Subsidiary Companies: Onibonoje Agricultural Industries
Principal Bankers: Union Bank of Nigeria Ltd
Financial Information:

	N'000
Authorised capital	10
Paid-up capital	10
Turnover	1,836
Profits	419

Principal Shareholders: Chairman and directors as described
Date of Establishment: 1958
No of Employees: 180

ONIBUDO, A, & COMPANY LTD

13 Harbour Rd, PO Box 631, Port Harcourt, Rivers State
Tel: 228082
Cable: Budo
Telex: 61125 Onbudo Ng

PRINCIPAL ACTIVITIES: Suppliers of building materials; tile manufacturers
Associated Companies: Atlas Fishing Industries (Nigeria) Ltd; Budotiles Industries (Nigeria) Ltd

ONIGBINDE, M A, & SONS LTD
14 Ahmadu Bello Way, PO Box 854, Jos, Plateau State
Tel: 55513
Cable: Onigbinde Jos
Telex: 81361 Poboy

Chairman: M A Onigbinde
Directors: Z G Onigbinde, J O Onigbinde, B D Onigbinde

PRINCIPAL ACTIVITIES: Agents and general trading; manufacturers of confectionery; suppliers of optical and photographic equipment; supermarkets and wholesalers
Principal Agencies: Food Specialities Nigeria Ltd; A C Christlieb; Chesebrough Ponds International
Branch Offices: B5 Jos Rd, PO Box 19, Bukuru; 24 Sabo Line, Gombe; 2-4 Folarin St, Idi-Oro, Lagos
Subsidiary Companies: Nigeria Associated Best Foods Ltd, Jos
Principal Bankers: United Bank for Africa Ltd; First Bank of Nigeria Ltd; Union Bank of Nigeria Ltd

Principal Shareholders: M A Onigbinde and Sons
Date of Establishment: Established 1940; Incorporated 1963
No of Employees: 250

ONISE POLYWARE LTD
PO Box 356, Ijebu-Ode, Ogun State

PRINCIPAL ACTIVITIES: Manufacturers of woven polypropylene sacks
Financial Information:
Registered capital   ₦ 500,000

Date of Establishment: March 1978

ONO & PARTNERS
1 Chapel St, Yaba, Lagos State
Tel: 862531
Cable: Aequator
Telex: 21433

Chairman: Ajaro W O Ono
Directors: Okemute Ono
Senior Executives: John Taylor (General Manager)

PRINCIPAL ACTIVITIES: Business consultants; suppliers of food and beverages
Principal Agencies: United Commercial Agencies Ltd, UK; Seedburo, USA; Frederic Kirshman, USA; Emi Corp, Japan
Branch Offices: Benin; Sapele; Warri; Jos; Kano; Kaduna; Sokoto; Aba; Onitsha; Ibadan; Owo; Port Harcourt Calabar
Associated Companies: Pisces Aequator; Holiday Farms
Principal Bankers: African Continental Bank Ltd; Savannah Bank Ltd
Financial Information:
Sales turnover   ₦ 3,000,000

Principal Shareholders: Ajaro W Onokpanu Ono; Okemute Ono
No of Employees: 800

ONOCHIE BROTHERS & SONS COMPANY LTD
97 Zik Avenue, Uwani, PO Box 537, Anambra State
Tel: 3759

PRINCIPAL ACTIVITIES: General contractors and merchants for building materials

ONUSELOGU, C N, ENTERPRISES LTD
16 Nnaji St, Uwani, PO Box 272, Enugu, Anambra State
Tel: 255253, 255185
Cable: Carlsnogel Enugu
Telex: 51245 Cangel

Directors: C N Onuselogu, C U Onuselogu, A Ume

PRINCIPAL ACTIVITIES: General merchants and contractors; transporters, building materials stockists
Branch Offices: 11 Nottidge St, Osha; Makurdi; Oturkpo; Akwanga; Warehouse: 3 Edinburgh Rd, Enugu, Anambra State

ONWARD PAPER MILL LTD
Obagun Avenue, Matori Industrial Estate, Oshodi, PMB 21356, Ikeja, Lagos
Tel: 830889, 845953

PRINCIPAL ACTIVITIES: Manufacturers of paper and paper products

ONWARD STATIONERY STORES LTD
32 Lewis St, PO Box 2863, Lagos
Tel: 630154, 634326

PRINCIPAL ACTIVITIES: Suppliers of office stationery and printing materials

ONYENAKAZI, I N, & SONS COMPANY
104 Ehi Rd, PO Box 3227, Aba, Imo State

Chairman: Innocent Nnaechete Onyenakazi
Directors: Nnaecheta Onyenakazi
Senior Executives: B N Onyenakazi (Executive Director)

PRINCIPAL ACTIVITIES: Importers, exporters, manufacturers' representatives; general merchants
Branch Offices: 36 Danfodio Rd, Aba, Imo State
Principal Bankers: African Continental Bank Nigeria Ltd
Financial Information:

	₦'000
Paid-up capital	700
Turnover	1,810
Profits	300

Date of Establishment: 1976

OPUKIRI CONSTRUCTIONS COMPANY LTD
19 Harbour Rd, PO Box 839, Port Harcourt, Rivers State

PRINCIPAL ACTIVITIES: Building and civil engineering contractors
Branch Offices: Riverine Area Office: 1 Chief Ere St, Ogbopina Layout, Amassoma-Oporoma Division, Rivers State; 111 Ezeagu St, Ojo Rd, Ajegunle, Apapa, Lagos State

ORAZULIKE TRADING COMPANY LTD
14A Edinburgh Rd, PMB 1271, Enugu, Anambra State
Tel: 255153
Cable: Oratraco Ltd

Chairman: J O Orazulike
Directors: H E Orazulike, N T Orazulike, Mrs P A Orazulike
Senior Executives: J I Igboanugo (Chief Commercial Manager), R N Orji (Senior Commercial Manager), A O Akpunonu (Senior Commercial Manager), C I Madakor (Personnel Manager), P C Ndupu (Accountant)

PRINCIPAL ACTIVITIES: Dealers in building materials/cement, sanitary-ware and fittings, manufacturers' agents and distributors
Principal Agencies: Nigerian Foundries Ltd, Pilkinton Glass (Nig) Ltd; Plastex (Nig) Ltd; Modern Ceramics Industry Ltd; Crittall-Hope (Nig) Ltd; Turners Building Products (Emene) Ltd; Nigersteel Industry
Branch Offices: 83B and 22B Ngwa Rd, Aba-Imo State; 139 Agbani Rd, Enugu, Anambra State; 77 Douglas Rd, Owerri, Imo State; Ugwuolie Central Market, Ozubulu, Anambra State; 3A Jerico Rd, Otukpo, Benue State
Associated Companies: General Purpose Builders Ltd, Enugu
Principal Bankers: United Bank for Africa Ltd

Principal Shareholders: Directors as described above

OREDOLA OKEYA TRADING COMPANY LTD

68 Nnamdi Azikiwe St, PO Box 811, Lagos
Tel: 632322, 632272, 657146
Cable: Dolayat

Chairman: Alhaji A Adesanu Amodu
Directors: Alhaji Yusuf Alabi Amolegbe
Senior Executives: J O Adeyemo (Personnel/Administrative
    Manager),
    M A Akanmu (Sales Manager),
    Lanre Omoya (Accounts)

PRINCIPAL ACTIVITIES: Importers and exporters of general
    goods; suppliers of footwear and travelling equipment
Principal Agencies: Alpenvelour Amstetten, West Germany
Branch Offices: 22 Docemo St, Lagos; 9 Nnamdi Azikiwe St,
    Lagos; 24 Old Jebba Rd, Ilorin, Kwara State
Associated Companies: Nigeria Watch/Clock Industries
Principal Bankers: First Bank of Nigeria Ltd
Financial Information:

	N'000
Authorised capital	100
Paid-up capital	100
Turnover	1,000
Profits	58

Principal Shareholders: Alhaji A A Amodu; Alhaji Y A Amolegbe
Date of Establishment: February 1954

ORIWU COMMERCIAL AGENCY LTD

5 Okoya St, PO Box 208, Lagos
Tel: 630872

PRINCIPAL ACTIVITIES: Building materials and equipment
    suppliers

OROKE CONSTRUCTIONS NIGERIA LTD

10 Jefia Crescent, PO Box 2305, Warri, Bendel State
Tel: 232956, 233515

Chairman: Chief Fred U Oroke (also Managing Director)
Directors: Omiragwa Boss Oroke, Madam Ogba Rhiogbere
Senior Executives: Wilfred O Igbinomwanhia
    (Accountant/Administration Manager),
    A O Diafe (Senior Engineer),
    Olateru O Olagbegi (Senior Quantity Surveyor)

PRINCIPAL ACTIVITIES: Builders and civil engineering
    contractors
Principal Bankers: New Nigeria Bank Ltd
Financial Information:

	N'000
Authorised capital	500
Paid-up capital	500
Turnover	2,000
Profits	300

Principal Shareholders: Chairman and directors as described
Date of Establishment: 27th July 1974
No of Employees: 250

ORTHOPAEDIC SUPPLIES LTD

761 Kofar Mazugar Rd, PO Box 595, Kano
Tel: 5235
Cable: Orthosupply Kano

Directors: Alhaji Bala Hassan
Senior Executives: Alhaji Shaba Umar (Managing)

PRINCIPAL ACTIVITIES: Pharmaceutical and medical supplies
    and services, scientific instruments
Principal Agencies: Hugh Steeper (Roehampton) Ltd; J E
    Hanger; Pope Brace Company
Associated Companies: B H Organization Ltd, Kano
Principal Bankers: Union Bank of Nigeria Ltd; Bank of the North
    Ltd

ORUCHE, JOE, TRADING COMPANY LTD

4 Kano St, Ogbete, Enugu, Anambra State
Tel: 252072

PRINCIPAL ACTIVITIES: Importers of mechanical engineering
    equipment

ORUMOKPO & SONS (NIGERIA) LTD

12 Harbour Rd, PMB 5313, Port Harcourt, Rivers State
Tel: 228820

PRINCIPAL ACTIVITIES: Transporters; manufacturers'
    representatives; importers and exporters; general contractors;
    insurance agents and suppliers of motor accessories

OSA MARINE SERVICES (NIGERIA) LTD

PMB 12651, Lagos
Tel: 874583
Cable: Panalpina
Telex: 21347

PRINCIPAL ACTIVITIES: Boat services

OSBORNE, E, NIGERIA LTD

34 McCarthy St, PO Box 558, Lagos
Tel: 631403, 635667
Cable: Osbowa Lagos

Directors: Benjamin A Agim, Herman P Clayton, Aloysius O
    Ekechi, Raphael A Bademosi, Derek H Adams

PRINCIPAL ACTIVITIES: Manufacturers of hardware products
    and merchants for building materials
Principal Agencies: Nairn Floors Ltd, UK

OSCARTE (NIGERIA) LTD

1 Moorhouse St, Ogui-Enugu, PO Box 2450, Enugu, Anambra
    State
Tel: 253746
Cable: Oscanil

Chairman: Theo Okonkwo (also Managing Director)
Directors: Geraldine Roderique,
    Chief Albert Okonkwo,
    Charles Okonkwo (Administrative Manager)

PRINCIPAL ACTIVITIES: General contractors and business
    consultants; suppliers of safety and security equipment
Principal Agencies: Walter Kidde & Company Inc, New Jersey,
    USA; Koppers Company Inc, UK Ltd
Associated Companies: Afroequip (Nigeria) Ltd
Principal Bankers: Union Bank of Nigeria Ltd

Date of Establishment: 1977

OSENA SHIPPING COMPANY LTD

20 Payne Crescent, PMB 1058, Apapa, Lagos
Tel: 876207, 876756
Cable: Osenaship Lagos
Telex: 21584 Osena Ng

PRINCIPAL ACTIVITIES: Shipping agents, freight brokers,
    charterers
Principal Bankers: International Bank for West Africa

OSHINMI COMPANY LTD

40 Commercial Ave, Yaba, Lagos
Tel: 861025, 860968
Cable: Oshinsigns Lagos

Directors: Chief S O Odugbesan (Managing),
    Mrs C O Odugbesan
Senior Executives: G O Akinyemi (Administrative Manager)

PRINCIPAL ACTIVITIES: Manufacturer of school chalk and stationery, importer and distributor of building materials, distributors of engraving machinery and equipment, aluminium doors, windows and rail manufacturers, rubber stamp and marking devices manufacturers; commercial printers
Principal Agencies: Gravograph; Plextone; Invicta; Hermes Plastic; C Williams; Magiboard, Etc
Branch Offices: 99 Ijebu Byepass, Ibadan, Oyo State
Principal Bankers: Union Bank of Nigeria Ltd; Savannah Bank of Nigeria Ltd
Financial Information:

	₦'000
Authorised capital	100
Paid-up capital	100

Date of Establishment: 1945

OSHUE BROTHERS & COMPANY (NIGERIA) LTD
PO Box 1452, Ibadan, Oyo State
Tel: 414547

PRINCIPAL ACTIVITIES: Distributors of motor vehicles

OSHUNKEYE BROTHERS (NIGERIA) LTD
64 Glover St, PO Box 262, Ebute-Metta, Lagos
Tel: 861303, 860241
Cable: Oshunk
Telex: 21368 Chacom Ng

Chairman: S O Oshunkeye
Directors: Oluseyi Oshunkeye, Adeolu Oshunkeye
Senior Executives: O A Sowunmi (Secretary/Accountant), V Kadri (Factory Manager), Mrs R A Fadahunsi (Lithographic Manager)

PRINCIPAL ACTIVITIES: Commercial printers; importers of printing machines, board and paper; almanac producers
Principal Agencies: Milthorp Paper Sales Ltd, UK
Branch Offices: 14 Kano St, Ebute-Metta, Lagos
Principal Bankers: United Bank for Africa Ltd; First Bank of Nigeria Ltd
Financial Information:

	₦'000
Authorised capital	500
Paid-up capital	300
Turnover	977

Principal Shareholders: S O Oshunkeye
Date of Establishment: 1946

OSITADINMA INTERNATIONAL LTD
23 Nottidge Street, Top Floor, PO Box 3546, Onitsha, Anambra State
Tel: 210720
Cable: Assignment Onitsha

President: B O Obi
Directors: B I O Obi
Senior Executives: Ejike Obadike (General Manager), Basil Okafor (Commercial Director), Susan Okeke (Company Secretary/Public Relations Officer)

PRINCIPAL ACTIVITIES: Agents and general trading, defence and armaments, pharmaceutical and medical supplies and services, chemicals, office equipment and supplies, scientific instruments, building materials and cement, ceramics and sanitary fittings, hardware, optical and photographic equipment
Principal Agencies: A C Atonis Industries Ltd, Taiwan
Associated Companies: Union Drug and Surgical Co Nigeria Ltd; Cornbrough Products Nigeria Ltd
Principal Bankers: Pan African Bank Ltd
Principal Shareholders: B O Obi; B I O Obi
Date of Establishment: 19th July 1978

OSOSAMI, J F, & CO
PO Box 373, Ibadan, Oyo State
Tel: 412976
Cable: Osomsco
Telex: 31114 Osomco Ng
PRINCIPAL ACTIVITIES: Civil engineering

OSOT ASSOCIATES CONSULTING ENGINEERS
Prost Building, Polytechnic Rd, Opposite Polytechnic South Campus, Sango-Eleiyele Expressway, PO Box 4050 (UI), Ibadan, Oyo State
Tel: 411248
Cable: Osot Ibadan
Telex: 31137 Ledot Ng

Directors: A O Olumide (Managing), K A Segun (Partner), A Tokun (Partner)
Senior Executives: S K Das (Branch Manager, Kaduna), S M Shamsuddin (Principal Resident Engineer), A O A Fakorede (Senior Resident Engineer), K Nandakoban (Senior Highway Engineer), E O Bucknor-Smartt (Chief Structural Engineer), A P Ocampo (Principal Resident Engineer)

PRINCIPAL ACTIVITIES: Civil and structural engineering consultants
Branch Offices: 3 Ahmadu Bello Way, PO Box 472, Kaduna, Tel 242695; PO Box 130, Bauchi; Plot 37 Ranjan Shambo, PO Box 866, Sokoto
Principal Bankers: Co-operative Bank Nigeria Ltd; First Bank Ltd
Principal Shareholders: A O Olumide; K A Segun; A Tokun
Date of Establishment: 1968

OTIS OF NIGERIA LTD
38 Awolowo Rd, PO Box 3694, Lagos
Tel: 683032

Chairman: M E Shelton
Directors: Douglas R Parmley (General Manager)

PRINCIPAL ACTIVITIES: Oil and gas services and equipment and pipeline contractors
Principal Agencies: Otis Engineering Corporation, Dallas, USA
Branch Offices: PMB 1069, Warri; PO Box 462, Port Harcourt;
Principal Bankers: Union Bank of Nigeria Ltd
Financial Information:
Authorised capital ₦ 600,000

Principal Shareholders: M E Shelton; W V Traeger; R A Yancey; D Y Fisher

OTT-ATTAFUA, A, & COMPANY LTD
25 Maye Street, Yaba, PO Box 2376, Lagos
Tel: 861802
Cable: Tesco Books
Telex: 26390 Air Mail

Chairman: D O Ademuyiwa
Directors: O Oyewole, T W Ogude
Senior Executives: F Asubonteng (Accountant), S O Tella (Chief Storekeeper)

PRINCIPAL ACTIVITIES: Manufacturers' representative, paper and board merchants, stationers, paper converters and printers
Principal Agencies: John Dickinson & Company, UK; Redcliffe Ink, UK; J Arthur Dixon, Isle of Wight; D R G Hospital Supplies
Branch Offices: 198/200 Faulks Road, Aba, Imo State
Principal Bankers: United Bank for Africa Ltd; First Bank of Nigeria Ltd

Financial Information:

	N'000
Authorised capital	250
Paid-up capital	230
Turnover	2,500
Profits	50

Principal Shareholders: D O Ademuyiwa; O Oyewole; T W Ogude
Date of Establishment: 11th November 1969
No of Employees: 52

OTTO WOLFF (NIGERIA) & COMPANY LTD
See WOLFF, OTTO, (NIGERIA) & COMPANY LTD

OVALTINE (WEST AFRICA) LTD
Acme Road, Ogba Industrial Estate, PMB 21558, Ikeja, Lagos
Tel: 960526
Cable: Ovalwaf Lagos

Chairman: A O Rewane
Directors: D C Brown (Managing),
  A A Abiodun,
  Chief A E Enahoro,
  I O Hayble-Ohomele,
  W F Sandmeier,
  Y O A Sanni
Senior Executives: N Ryan-Evans (Factory Manager),
  Samuel Oke (Company Accountant),
  Colin Moore (Chief Engineer)

PRINCIPAL ACTIVITIES: Packing and marketing of food
  products. Manufacturers of metal containers
Principal Bankers: United Bank for Africa Ltd; Chase Merchant
  Bank
Financial Information: 1981

	N'000
Authorised capital	3,000
Paid-up capital	3,000
Turnover	13,892
Profits (net)	628

Principal Shareholders: Wander Ltd UK 40%; Beverages (Nigeria)
  Ltd 27%; Nigerian Public 33%
Date of Establishment: 18th August 1971
No of Employees: 125

OVE ARUP & PARTNERS NIGERIA LTD
25 Boyle St, 4th Floor, PO Box 2088, Lagos
Tel: 633583, 636648, 633654, 631060
Cable: Ovarpart Lagos
Telex: 21892 Ovarup Ng

Partners: F G Clarke (Lagos),
  W Haigh (Lagos),
  A O Oyemade (Lagos),
  F O Oduneye (Ibadan),
  M E Dunk (Kano),
  O O D Thomas (London),
  P Ahm,
  P Dunican
Senior Executives: R K Elms (Executive Partner),
  B R Ellis (Executive Partner),
  J M Jowett (Executive Partner)

PRINCIPAL ACTIVITIES: Civil and structural engineering
  consultants
Branch Offices: 6 Stones Rd, PO Box 571, Ibadan, Oyo State,
  Tel 410011/410102, Telex 31441 Ng, Cables Ovarpart; 16
  Audu Bako Way, PO Box 718, Kano, Tel 7240/5479, Telex
  71771 Ovarup Ng, Cables Ovarpart Kano
Principal Bankers: First Bank of Nigeria Ltd
Financial Information:

Turnover	N 5,000,000

Date of Establishment: 1955
No of Employees: 300

OVERSEAS COMMERCIAL AGENCY
9 Breadfruit St, Lagos
Tel: 633977
Telex: 21425 Ocomex Ng

PRINCIPAL ACTIVITIES: General traders and contractors

OVERSEAS TECHNICAL SERVICE (NIGERIA) LTD (OTS)
77 Ademola St, SW Ikoyi, PO Box 4998, Lagos
Tel: 683540
Cable: Overtex Lagos

Chairman: R Carton Tickell
Directors: Chief T O S Benson, S Olakunri, R K Clues
Senior Executives: George Burns (General Manager)

PRINCIPAL ACTIVITIES: Consultants, technical services for the
  oil and gas industry
Principal Agencies: Global Diving Services Ltd; A H Venison Ltd
Branch Offices: Field Office at Eket
Associated Companies: Overseas Technical Service (Harrow) Ltd

Date of Establishment: 1969

OWENA BANK (NIGERIA) LTD
Head Office: 17 Oyemekun Rd, Akure, Ondo State
Tel: 230710, 230241

Directors: Iwajomo C O N Javed Yusuf, T S Aliu, Chief S B
  Falegan, Chief F Afelumo, S I Hussain, D V Taneja
PRINCIPAL ACTIVITIES: Banking
Branch Offices: Central Office: 54 Warehouse Rd, PMB 1122,
  Apapa, Lagos, Tel 877901, 877903, 877905, 877907, 877887,
  Telex 22825 Owena Ng; SW7/3A Lagos Bye Pass, Oke-Bola,
  Ibadan, Tel 414534, 414613, Telex 31556; 17 Balogun Street,
  Lagos; 9 Odo Ijigbo Street, Ado Ekiti, Ondo State, Tel
  240723, 240823. Also opening shortly branches in Kano,

Ondo Town and Owo
Subsidiary/Associated Companies: Affiliated with Middle East
Bank Ltd, Dubai, UAE

OWOYEMI MOTORS & FINANCE COMPANY LTD

SW8/119 Lagos Bye-Pass, Oke-Ado, PO Box 186, Dugbe Post
Office, Ibadan, Oyo State
Tel: 415624
Cable: Ofinance
Telex: 31118 Omfcol Ng

Chairman: Chief (Alhaji) Y A S Adegbayi
Directors: Alhaji R A Sarumi, K Ossman
Senior Executives: A G Virjee (Spare Parts Manager),
    B R Patel (Workshop Manager),
    P S Iyer (Marketing Manager)

PRINCIPAL ACTIVITIES: Importers and distributors of motor
    vehicles, components and motorcycles
Principal Agencies: Isuzu Motors Ltd, Japan; Peugeot
    Automobiles Nigeria
Branch Offices: Old Lagos Rd, Podo, Ibadan; Oshodi/Apapa
    Expressway, Isolo, Mushin; Ikirun Rd, Osogbo
Subsidiary Companies: R C F Building Construction & Civil
    Engineering Co Ltd; IIGG Ltd
Principal Bankers: National Bank of Nigeria Ltd; Bank of Credit
    & Commerce (International) Nigeria Ltd; Arab Bank of Nigeria
    Ltd
Financial Information:

	N'000
Authorised capital	5,000
Paid-up capital	2,500

Principal Shareholders: Chief (Alhaji) Y A S Adegbayi; Alhaji
    Sanusi Adegbayi; Alhaja Moriamo Adegbayi
Date of Establishment: 9th July 1970
No of Employees: 75

OYEBANJI BUILDING MATERIALS STORES LTD

10a Adeniji Adele Rd, PO Box 315, Lagos
Tel: 630275

PRINCIPAL ACTIVITIES: Suppliers of building materials

OYENUGA, DEJI, & PARTNERS

66 Adeniran Ogunsanya St, Surulere, PO Box 2169, Lagos
Tel: 845927
Cable: Nigerarch

Directors: Deji Oyenuga (Principal Partner)

PRINCIPAL ACTIVITIES: Architecture and town planning
Branch Offices: University of Ife Campus Office, PO Box 1053,
    Ile Ife; c/o The Vice-Chancellor's Office, University of Ilorin,
    Red Cross Rd, Ilorin, Kwara State
Principal Bankers: Barclays Bank Nigeria Ltd; National Bank
    Nigeria Ltd; United Bank for Africa

OYEWUMI, J O, & CO (NIGERIA) LTD

PO Box 628, Jos, Plateau State
Tel: 53594
Cable: Wumco

Chairman: His Highness Oba J O Oyewumi
Senior Executives: J A Adeleke, R A Akingbade, S A Farinola

PRINCIPAL ACTIVITIES: Importers and distributors of general
    merchandise
Principal Agencies: Nigerian Breweries Ltd; North Brewery, Jos;
    International Breweries; West African Distillers Ltd;
    International Paints (WA) Ltd etc
Branch Offices: Ogbomoso, Oyo State; Oshogbo, Oyo State
Principal Bankers: Union Bank of Nigeria Ltd

Financial Information:

	N'000
Paid-up capital	100
Turnover	4,105
Profits	145

Principal Shareholders: Oba J O Oyewumie
Date of Establishment: June 1962

OYINDA ENTERPRISES LTD

PO Box 469, BZ 175 Junction Rd, Kaduna
Tel: 211121, 243504, 212120

PRINCIPAL ACTIVITIES: Building and civil engineering
    contractors; dealers in building materials

OYO STATE INVESTMENT AND CREDIT CORPORATION

PMB 5085, Ibadan, Oyo State
Tel: 462810/2, 461622
Cable: Oysicco Ibadan
Telex: 31122

PRINCIPAL ACTIVITIES: Initiates and finances industrial and
    agricultural projects
Financial Information: Statutory organisation of Oyo State
    Government

OYUN BREWERIES

Offa, Kwara State
PRINCIPAL ACTIVITIES: Breweries

OZO BROTHERS CABINET WORKS LTD

134 Hospital Rd, Aba, Imo State
PRINCIPAL ACTIVITIES: Furniture manufacturers
Branch Offices: 14 Liverpool Rd, Eket, Cross River State

P A IBEKWE LTD
See IBEKWE, P A, LTD

P BECCARELLI & CO LTD
See BECCARELLI, P, & CO LTD

P COMAZZI
See COMAZZI, P

P R SANDWELL & CO (NIGERIA) LTD
See SANDWELL, P R, & CO (NIGERIA) LTD

P S MANDRIDES & CO LTD
See MANDRIDES, P S, & CO LTD

P W NIGERIA LTD

40 Itohan Avenue, PO Box 1829, Ikeja, Lagos
Tel: 931337
Cable: Scraper Lagos
Telex: 26804 Civils Ng

Chairman: Chief Dr Charles Norman-Williams
Directors: H V Flinn (Managing),
    Alhaji M Armiyau,
    Chief E I O Akpata
Senior Executives: J Christie (General Manager),
    J Boyce (Chief Civil Engineer),
    I O Nze (Assistant to Managing Director),
    P McElroy (Financial Controller),
    D Hurley (Contracts Manager)

PRINCIPAL ACTIVITIES: Building and civil engineering contractors; construction of roads and bridges; irrigation work and water supply
Branch Offices: PO Box 49, Vom, Plateau State; PO Box 270, Minna, Niger State
Principal Bankers: First Bank of Nigeria Ltd
Financial Information:

	N'000
Authorised capital	1,000
Paid-up capital	697
Turnover (approx)	20,000
Profits (approx)	1,500

Principal Shareholders: Directors as described
Date of Establishment: 3rd December 1974
No of Employees: 650

PAAS INDUSTRIES (NIGERIA) COMPANY LTD

6 New Zaria Terrace Rd, PO Box 823, Jos, Plateau State
Tel: 3333

PRINCIPAL ACTIVITIES: Building and civil engineering contractors, general merchants, transporters
Branch Offices: PMB 1395, 39 Obioma St, Enugu, Anambra State, Tel 252721; 1 Stadium Lane, Owerri, Imo State

PABOD FINANCE & INVESTMENT COMPANY LTD

10 Ikwerre Rd, PMB 5166, Port Harcourt, Rivers State

PRINCIPAL ACTIVITIES: Financiers

PABOD SUPPLIES LTD

1 Azikiwe Rd, PMB 5162, Port Harcourt, Rivers State
Tel: 335770
Cable: Superbod
Telex: 61115

Chairman: M K Amakoromo
Directors: Chief F N Barika, L D Fiberesima, R Oboro, A F Okara, Chief S S Ogboka
Senior Executives: G B Itari (General Manager),
C A Egbunefu (Financial/Administration Controller),
A R Lolomari (Commercial Controller),
J D Angba (Pharmaceutical Marketing Manager)

PRINCIPAL ACTIVITIES: Importers of essential commodities, hospital and scientific equipment. Supermarket and pharmacy operation
Branch Offices: 206 Broad St, Lagos; Supabod Stores, 1 Azikiwe Rd, Port Harcourt; Pabod Pharmacy, 10 Harbour Rd, Port Harcourt; 35 Aba Rd, Port Harcourt, Rivers State
Principal Bankers: Pan African Bank Ltd; First Bank of Nigeria Ltd; African Continental Bank Ltd; National Bank of Nigeria Ltd
Financial Information:

	N'000
Authorised capital	400
Paid-up capital	400
Sales turnover	18,000

Principal Shareholders: Ministry of Finance Incorporated and Ministry of Trade & Economic Development Incorporated on behalf of Rivers State Government
Date of Establishment: December 1973
No of Employees: 250

PACIFIC PRINTERS LTD

38 Commercial Ave, PMB 1038, Yaba, Lagos
Tel: 860684, 860767
Cable: Pacific Yaba

Chairman: Prince C O Otubushin
Directors: Mrs Orija, Mrs A O Oshikanlu
Senior Executives: M O Okunade (Accountant),
Lawal Oduala (Works Manager),
M Abiodun Aregbe (Senior Supervisor),
N O Okanlawon (Assistant Works Supervisor)

PRINCIPAL ACTIVITIES: Printing; suppliers of plastic and leather products
Principal Agencies: Kurz Pragenafolien (Foils), Germany; Color Metal, Switzerland; G Schurfeld & Company, Hamburg; Germany; A Schwalbach, Hamburg, Germany
Branch Offices: 11 Sokoto Rd, Sabo-Oke, Ilorin, Kwara State
Associated Companies: Nigerian School of Printing & Graphic Arts; Pacific Plastic & Leathercraft Co Ltd; Pacific Marketing Co
Principal Bankers: Union Bank of Nigeria
Financial Information:

	N'000
Authorised capital	3,000
Paid-up capital	3,000
Sales turnover	8,500
Profits (after tax)	6,000

Principal Shareholders: Prince C O Otubushin
No of Employees: 350

PAKTANK NIGERIA LTD

Plot 1303 Akin Adesola Street, Victoria Island, PO Box 1785, Lagos
Tel: 615589, 612077
Cable: PO Box 1785 Lagos
Telex: 21978 Pt ng

Chairman: Chief M N Ugochukwu
Directors: Chief C Ogunbanjo,
Alhaji G J Abdulkadir,
Mr Chidi-Ofong,
D N A Verburg,
B A Seckel,
F J Thate (Managing)
Senior Executives: B Mill (Engineering Manager),
I T Turner (Financial Manager)

PRINCIPAL ACTIVITIES: Professional and technical advisers, designers, researchers, inspectors and managers to the oil industry
Principal Bankers: Union Bank of Nigeria Ltd
Financial Information:

	N'000
Authorised capital	100

Principal Shareholders: Pakraf BV 60%; Ugochukwu & Sons Ltd 20%; Chief C O Ogunbanjo 10%; Alhaji G J Abdulkadir 10%
Date of Establishment: June 1979
No of Employees: 35

PALM LINE AGENCIES (NIGERIA)

11 Wharf Rd, PO Box 531, Apapa, Lagos
Tel: 803800/7
Cable: Palmcon
Telex: 21246 Palmag Ng

Senior Executives: Chief Ayo Afolabi (General Manager)

PRINCIPAL ACTIVITIES: Shipping agents, clearing and forwarding, airfreight and lighterage

PAMOL (NIGERIA) LTD

PO Box 50, Sapele Rubber Estate, Sapele, Bendel State
Tel: 41005

PRINCIPAL ACTIVITIES: Manufacturing of sheet and crepe rubber

No of Employees: 1,000

PAN AFRICA GAS DISTRIBUTORS LTD

23 Creek Rd, PO Box 443, Apapa, Lagos
Tel: 875504

PRINCIPAL ACTIVITIES: Distributors of natural gas, hydrous ammonia and oxygen

PAN AFRICAN AIRLINES (NIGERIA) LTD

PMB 21054, Ikeja, Lagos
Tel: 963601, 963798, 963972
Cable: Pancharter

Chairman: Chief C O Ogunbanjo
Directors: T Espedalen (Managing),
   Chief A Ojora,
   Chief M N Ugochukwu,
   Chief Mene-Afejuku,
   D B Sittman,
   M L Evans

PRINCIPAL ACTIVITIES: Air transport, transportation equipment
Principal Agencies: Cessna Aircraft Co; Bell Helicopter; Teledyne Continental Motors; King Radio Corporation
Principal Bankers: United Bank of Africa Ltd; Union Bank of Nigeria

Principal Shareholders: Africair Inc, Chief A Ojora; Chief C Ogunbanjo; Chief M N Ugochukwu
Date of Establishment: 1961
No of Employees: 100

PAN AFRICAN BANK LTD

3 Azikiwe Rd, Port Harcourt, Rivers State
Tel: 333086
Cable: Panafbank 61157

Chairman: Barrister Samuel O Nwogu
Directors: K T Kia, Dr F C Eze, Dr B N Birabi, E B Kalango, E Tekena-Sackey, Alhaji Tijani Ramallam
Senior Executives: R F P Abbey (Assistant General Manager),
   J F Amachree (Secretary/Head of Legal Department),
   J F Isowo (Chief Accountant),
   A K Joffa (Advances Controller),
   C E Allen (Chief Inspector),
   J O Agbegha (Administration Manager),
   H M S Onwuka (Branches Controller),
   S A Obinna (Personnel Manager),
   N E Martyns-Yellowe (Public Relations Manager)

PRINCIPAL ACTIVITIES: Banking
Principal Agencies: Grindlays Bank Ltd, London; Chase Manhattan Bank NA, New York; Irving Trust Co, New York; Birmingham Trust National Bank, USA; Vereins Und West Bank, West Germany; Bank fur Gemeinwirtschaft, Frankfurt; Thomas Cook Bankers Ltd, England; Thomas Cook Inc, New York; Commerzbank, Frankfurt; Riyad Bank, Jeddah; Bankers Trust Co, New York; Citi Bank NA, New York; Chase Manhattan Bank, Japan; Deutsche Bank, West Germany
Branch Offices: 3 Club Rd, Port Harcourt; 51 Ikwerre Rd, Port Harcourt; Hospital Rd, Bori; Abua Rd, Ahoada; Marina, Bonny; 35/37 Martins Street, Lagos; 1A Galadima Rd, Kano; 16 Bright Street, Onitsha; 20 Asa Rd, Aba; 121 Azikiwe Rd, Owerri; Yenagoa Town, Yenagoa; Elele Town, Elele; Enugu Rd, Ogidi; Degema Town, Degema; Buguma Town, Buguma; 44 Creek Rd, Port Harcourt; Nembe Town, Nembe; Shopping Centre, University of Port Harcourt; Near Broadcasting House, Suleja/Abuja
Principal Bankers: Pan African Bank Ltd
Financial Information:

	N'000
Authorised capital	20,000
Paid-up capital	8,000
Turnover	187,990
Profits	1,261

Principal Shareholders: Rivers State Government of Nigeria through Ministries of Finance, Trade and Industry
Date of Establishment: 19th May 1971
No of Employees: 1,000 Approx

PAN AFRICAN CONSULTANCY SERVICES (NIGERIA) LTD

22 Idowu Taylor Street, Victoria Island, PO Box 6776, Lagos
Tel: 617310, 616472, 617308, 616474, 616473
Cable: Panafcons Lagos
Telex: 21003 Panaf Ng

Chairman: Alhaji Shehu Malami
Directors: Alhaji Aliyu Mai Sango,
   G P Birla,
   M Singh (Managing)
Senior Executives: H Vikram (Technical Manager),
   S K Somany (Contracts Manager),
   I Singh (Development Manager),
   A K Bhandari (Project Manager),
   B L Singhania (Financial Controller),
   Y K Jain (Manager Engineering Services),
   B S Joshan (Project Co-ordinator),
   G P Singh (Project Co-ordinator),
   C Mukerjea (Project Co-ordinator),
   N N Maheshwari (Planning Engineer),
   P K Gangopadhyay (Civil Engineer),
   A P Singh (Project Co-Ordinator)

PRINCIPAL ACTIVITIES: Industrial management; project co-ordination and management, technical assistance and training, techno-economic studies, environmental design
Principal Agencies: Projects and equipment corporation of India Ltd; Birla Brothers Private Ltd; Hildebrand Engineering Ltd; Hong Kong Commercial House; Gleno Industrial Consultants, UK; Euro-Plan
Branch Offices: Associate offices in Zug (Switzerland), London (UK), Delhi and Calcutta (India)
Associated Companies: Nigeria Pipes Ltd; Nigerian Asbestos Industries Ltd; Nigerian Industrial Complex Amalgamation Ltd; Steelfab (Nigeria) Ltd; Zaki Bottling Co (Nig) Ltd; Nigeria Engineering Works Ltd; Odin Biscuits Manufacturing Co; Osondu Bottling Co Ltd; Plastic and Plastic Ltd; Kainji Bottling Co
Principal Bankers: Allied Bank of Nigeria Ltd
Financial Information:

	N'000
Authorised capital	1,000
Turnover (approx)	10,000

Principal Shareholders: Alhaji Shehu Malami; Alhaji Aliyu Mai Sango; Birla Brothers Private Ltd, India
Date of Establishment: 1st July 1975
No of Employees: 100-150

PAN AFRICAN HOLDINGS (NIGERIA) LTD

17th Floor, Western House, 8/10 Broad St, PO Box 4554, Lagos
Tel: 655545

PRINCIPAL ACTIVITIES: Importers of general goods

PAN AFRICAN SUPPLY COMPANY LTD

130 Awolowo Rd, SW Ikoyi, Lagos
Tel: 681482, 655376, 611756
Telex: 21395 Pasco Ng

PRINCIPAL ACTIVITIES: General traders

PAN AFRICAN SURVEYS LTD

9 Oliyide Street, Off Unity Rd, Ikeja, Lagos
Tel: 962754

Directors: Suru J O Daramola (Managing),
   S A Oba

PRINCIPAL ACTIVITIES: Land surveyors
Branch Offices: Ibadan
Financial Information:

	N'000
Authorised capital	100
Paid-up capital	100

PAN ATLANTIC SHIPPING & TRANSPORT AGENCIES LTD

89/91 Kofo Abayomi Avenue, PMB 1204, Apapa, Lagos
Tel: 870510, 870514, 870516
Cable: Panat Lagos
Telex: 21038

Chairman: Edward I Aleyideino
Directors: Sunday Shehu, Alhaji S O Kassim, Alhaji Ibrahim
   Katune
Senior Executives: M S Siddiqi (General Manager),
   E E Ikeji (Head of Agenices),
   M Decalut (Head of Operations),
   M Stephenson (Area Manager),
   L S Akele (Administrative Manager)

PRINCIPAL ACTIVITIES: Shipping agencies, clearing, forwarding
Principal Agencies: Rhein Maas und see Schiffahrtskontor
   GmbH, Duisburg; Rijn Maas en Zee Scheepvaartkantoor NV,
   Antwerp; Compagnie Nationale Centraficaine de Navigation
   GmbH, Bremen; Baco Liner GmbH & Company KG, Emden;
   Orient Overseas Container Line Ltd, Hong Kong; Noga
   Commodities (Overseas) Inc, New York; Ideomar SA, Spain;
   Westgate Shipping Ltd, London
Branch Offices: 9 Njemanze Street, Port Harcourt; Jide House,
   Warri/Sapele Rd, Warri; 106 Murtala Mohammed Highway,
   Calabar
Associated Companies: Pan Atlantic Maritime Ltd; Pan Atlantic
   Clearing & Forwarding Agencies Ltd; Panatrade Ltd; Pan
   Atlantic Road Haulage Ltd
Principal Bankers: Bank of Credit & Commerce International Ltd;
   Societe Generale Bank (Nig) Ltd
Financial Information:

	N'000
Authorised capital	500
Paid-up capital	400
Turnover	2,500

Principal Shareholders: Edward I Aleyideino; Alhaji S O Kassim;
   Alhaji Ibrahim Katune; Sunday Shehu
Date of Establishment: 17th December 1976
No of Employees: 400

PAN ELECTRIC LTD

76/78 Murtala Mohammed Way, PO Box 7, Ebute Metta, Lagos
Tel: 860208, 860269

Senior Executives: A O Babatunde (Production Manager),
   K A Sodeinde,
   J W E Ilenre

PRINCIPAL ACTIVITIES: Manufacturers of domestic electrical
   equipment such as radios, televisions, etc
Financial Information: Division of UAC of Nigeria

PAN INDUSTRIAL ESTATE AGENCIES

43 Aggrey Rd, PO Box 422, Port Harcourt, Rivers State

PRINCIPAL ACTIVITIES: Importers and exporters; commission
   agents, manufacturers' representatives, general contractors
   and building materials suppliers

PAN NIGERIAN AGENCY

17/19 Durojaiye St, Ikate, Surulere, PO Box 2700, Lagos
Tel: 830293

PRINCIPAL ACTIVITIES: Dealers in agricultural and
   earth-moving equipment; heavy machinery

PAN OCEAN OIL CORPORATION (NIGERIA)

2/4 Adeola Odeku St, Victoria Island, PO Box 93, Lagos
Tel: 610494, 612633, 610906
Cable: Panoco Lagos
Telex: 21468

Directors: B E Yester (Managing Director),
   E B Maki (District Manager),
   I R Potter (Operations Manager)

PRINCIPAL ACTIVITIES: Exploration and production of crude oil;
   importers and oilfield equipment
Branch Offices: Field Office: PO Box 582, Warri, Bendel State
No of Employees: 100

PANALPINA WORLD TRANSPORT (NIGERIA) LTD

4 Creek Rd, PO Box 69, Apapa, Lagos
Tel: 803610/4, 803440/4
Cable: Panalpina
Telex: 21347

Chairman: Chief (Dr) N B Graham Douglas
Directors: Chief F R A Williams,
   Alhaji U S Dantata,
   W Ruoff,
   G Fischer (Managing),
   E W Ikomi (General Manager)

PRINCIPAL ACTIVITIES: International freight forwarding, general
   warehousing, customs brokerage, shipping agency, packing,
   transport and related services
Principal Agencies: Air Sea Broker Ltd, Zurich; Torm Line,
   Copenhagen; Seco Shipping, Rotterdam; Atlantic Africa Line,
   London
Branch Offices: 59 Tafawa Balewa Rd, PO Box 788, Kano, Tel
   2572, 5219, Telex 77119; Plot 463/467 Trans Amadi Ind.
   Layout, Port Harcourt, Box 170, Tel 331731, 331038, Telex
   61106; Warri/Sapele Rd, PO Box 135, Tel 233818, Telex
   42276; Local Airport Cargo Area, PO Box 84, Ikeja, Tel
   962026, 961690, 932728; 1 Cemetry Rd, PO Box 451, Sapele,
   Tel 42551, Telex 42276; 18/19 Ahmadu Bello Way, NNDC
   Building, PO Box 158, Kaduna, Telex 71109
No of Employees: 965

PANAV INTERNATIONAL LTD

A7 Junction Rd, Box 695, Kaduna
Tel: 213517

Chairman: Benjamin Erua
Directors: J O Anavhe, Godson Anavhe
Senior Executives: Frank Ileile, Ignatius Ozorma

PRINCIPAL ACTIVITIES: Building materials distributors, building
   and civil engineering contractors
Principal Agencies: G B Ollivant (Nigeria) Ltd; John Holt (Nigeria)
   Ltd; CFAO (Nigeria) Ltd
Branch Offices: 7 Nnamdi Azikiwe St, Lagos; 8 Iyamu St, Benin
   City, Bendel State; 1 Market Rd, Fugar, Bendel State
Subsidiary/Associated Companies: Panav Group, Maris
   Provision Department
Principal Bankers: Union Bank of Nigeria Ltd
Financial Information:

	N'000
Authorised capital	250
Paid-up capital	250
Turnover	1,950
Profits	165

Date of Establishment: 1970
No of Employees: 180

PANNEL FITZPATRICK & COMPANY

21/22 Marina, PMB 2047, Lagos
Tel: 636148, 636219
Telex: 77221 Lennap Ng Kano

PRINCIPAL ACTIVITIES: Chartered accountants

PAPER CONVERSION CORPORATION (NIGERIA) LTD

PMB 21219, Oregun Village Rd, Ikeja, Lagos
Tel: 37573, 34114

PRINCIPAL ACTIVITIES: Manufacturers of paper bags, folding
   boxes
No of Employees: 150

PAPER SACK (NIGERIA) LTD

PO Box 1138, Plot 44, Iganmu Industrial Estate, Iganmu, Lagos
Tel: 832027, 832272, 837762, 836865

Chairman: Chief Moyo Aboderin
Directors: S A Adeyemo

PRINCIPAL ACTIVITIES: Manufacturers of paper sacks
Principal Bankers: First Bank of Nigeria Ltd

Date of Establishment: 1965
No of Employees: 180

PAR EXCELLENCE (NIGERIA) LTD

Development House, 21 Wharf Rd, Apapa, Lagos
Tel: 876749
Cable: Pexnil

Chairman: Thomas C Dumzo-Ajufo (also Managing Director)
Directors: C O Dumzo-Ajufo

PRINCIPAL ACTIVITIES: Freight forwarding and customs agents;
  foreign shipping company's agents
Principal Agencies: International Housing Nigeria Ltd; Nigeria
  Produce Marketing Co Ltd
Associated Companies: Dumzo Farms Ltd; Trans Avon Agencies
Principal Bankers: Arab Bank Nigeria Ltd
Financial Information:

	N'000
Authorised capital	100
Paid-up capital	100

Principal Shareholders: T C Dumzo-Ajufo; C D Dumzo-Ajufo
No of Employees: 500

PARKE-DAVIS & COMPANY (NIGERIA) LTD

PO Box 2784, Apapa, Lagos
Tel: 21305 PdnLos Ng

Chairman: Chief A O Lawson
Directors: H C Graham,
  D Mountbatten (Managing),
  Chief J O Igwe,
  Chief F R A Williams

PRINCIPAL ACTIVITIES: Manufacturers and importers of
  pharmaceuticals
Branch Offices: Head Office Location: J102 Isaac John St, GRA,
  Ikeja, Lagos; Factories: Plot 57 Iganmu Industrial Estate,
  Iganmu, Lagos; Branches: Plot 3A & 3B Oladipo Oluwole St,
  Ikeja, Lagos; Plot 288 Bode Thomas St, Surulere, Lagos
Principal Bankers: First Bank of Nigeria Ltd; International
  Merchant Bank (Nigeria) Ltd

Date of Establishment: 18th December 1969

PARKES, JOSIAH, & SONS (NIGERIA) LTD

Plot 3 Block F, Ladipo St/Badejo Kalesanwo St, Mushin, PO Box
  382, Apapa, Lagos
Cable: Parklock, Lagos

Chairman: D S Maitland
Directors: P A Freeman, J A O Olopade, P T Rowlands, B A O
  Fisher, W O Adekoya, J T F Iyalla, J F McArthur, D F
  Langley
Senior Executives: A O Adekoya (Accounts Manager),
  T D A Jiboye (Sales Manager)

PRINCIPAL ACTIVITIES: Manufacturers of locks and builders
  hardware
Principal Bankers: Union Bank of Nigeria Ltd
Financial Information:

	N'000
Authorised capital	1,000
Paid-up capital	500

Principal Shareholders: Josiah Parkes & Sons (Holdings) Ltd; J A
  O Olopade; J T F Iyalla; B O A Fisher; S A O Olorunshola
Date of Establishment: February 1964
No of Employees: 216

PASSAT INDUSTRIES LTD

Plot 20 Iganmu Industrial Estate, PO Box 396, Apapa, Lagos
Tel: 834472/3
Cable: Passat Lagos

Chairman: Chief A O Amoje
Directors: Alhaji Fatai Uthman,
  G O Ogunlami,
  P Sauer,
  J Borle,
  O Meyn (Managing)
Senior Executives: A Alalade (Public Relations Manager),
  F Afolabi (Personnel Manager),
  K A Shobayo (Accountant),
  A Oguntowo (Production Manager),
  S Kofoworola (Maintenance Manager)

PRINCIPAL ACTIVITIES: Shoe manufacturing
Principal Bankers: First Bank of Nigeria Ltd
Financial Information:

	N'000
Authorised capital	1,000
Paid-up capital	839
Turnover	8,000

Principal Shareholders: Chief A O Omoje; Voss & Umlauft,
  Germany; CFAO Nigeria Ltd
Date of Establishment: December 1963
No of Employees: 609

PATERSON ZOCHONIS INDUSTRIES LTD

33 Planning Office Way, Ilupeju Industrial Estate, PMB 21132,
  Ikeja, Lagos
Tel: 962076/9
Cable: Bodyguard Lagos

Chairman: Alhaji Shehu Malami (Sarkin Sudan of Wurno)
Directors: J Giannopoulos (Vice-Chairman, Chief Executive),
  Th Grigoris (Managing Director),
  Chief O I Akinkugbe,
  D W Evans,
  P Giouras,
  V A Kushimo,
  Dr A Nnubia,
  G R E Obong,
  A Sideris,
  K B Jamodu

PRINCIPAL ACTIVITIES: Manufacturers of soap, detergents,
  perfumery, cosmetics, pharmaceuticals, and confectionery,
  and suppliers of technical equipment and general goods
Branch Offices: Ibadan; Kano; Port Harcourt; Margaret Ave, Aba
  and throughout Nigeria
Subsidiary/Associated Companies: Paterson Zochonis Nigeria
  Ltd (Subsidiary); Thermocol engineering Co Ltd (Associated)
Principal Bankers: First Bank of Nigeria Ltd; Union Bank of
  Nigeria Ltd; United Bank for Africa Ltd; Chase Merchant
  Bank Nigeia Ltd

Principal Shareholders: Nigerians (60%); Paterson Zochonis & Co
  Ltd; UK (40%)
Date of Establishment: 1948
No of Employees: 3,000

PATRICK GEORGE & SONS LTD

See GEORGE, PATRICK, & SONS LTD

PATY IMPORT COMPANY OF NIGERIA

76 Asa Rd, PO Box 675, Aba, Imo State

Chairman: O Mozie
Directors: Paty Mozie (Managing Director),
  Bernadine Ogbonna

PRINCIPAL ACTIVITIES: Confirming house agents, export
  shippers' agents; agents and general trading
Principal Bankers: African Continental Bank Ltd

Date of Establishment: 23rd May 1977

PEARL & DEAN (NIGERIA) LTD

25 Thorburn Ave, PO Box 15, Yaba, Lagos
Tel: 860489, 861674

PRINCIPAL ACTIVITIES: Production and distribution of
advertising and documentary films

PEAT MARWICK ANI, OGUNDE & COMPANY

Bolex House, Plot 33 Imam Dauda St, Iganmu Industrial Estate,
PO Box 549, Lagos
Tel: 830484, 830494, 830496, 830498, 830503, 830605
Cable: Veritatem Lagos
Telex: 1117 Tds No 270 UK Correspondents: 11117 No 270
Correspondents from other Countries

Senior Partner: Chief A A Ani
Partners: A O Ogunde, H A A Agbebiyi, P A Adeyemi, J K
Randle, M O Adeyeri, A O Ajayi, M A Popoola, F O
Akinbohun, C F G Akinwolemiwa, P K Asu, E U Isen
PRINCIPAL ACTIVITIES: Chartered accountants; auditors; tax
consultants
Branch Offices: Airport Rd, PO Box 103, Kano; Block B
Ahmadu Bello Way, PO Box 256, Kaduna; 14 Nnamdi Azikiwe
Rd, PMB 5615, Port Harcourt, Rivers State; Plot 13 Effanga
Nkpa St, PMB 1006, Calabar, Cross River State
Associated Companies: Ani, Ogunde, Sotinwa & Company
Principal Bankers: United Bank for Africa Ltd; First Bank of
Nigeria Ltd; Union Bank of Nigeria Ltd

Principal Shareholders: All the Partners
Date of Establishment: 1923
No of Employees: 390

PECCO LTD

Victoria Street, Ojota, Km 16 Ikorodu Rd, PO Box 672, Marina,
Lagos
Tel: 963243
Telex: 21113 Ng Attn AOA

Chairman: Chief A O Adenubi (also Chief Executive)
Directors: Dr J O Adenubi,
Mrs S O Adenubi (Commercial Director),
O K Atewologun (Public Relations Director)
Senior Executives: Soladoye Adenubi (Financial Controller)

PRINCIPAL ACTIVITIES: Building and civil engineering
construction; furnishers and furniture production; concrete
products; manufacturers of general merchandise and motor
dealership
Subsidiary/Associated Companies: Intercraft Furniture
Company; Kwikway Enterprises Ltd; AOA Motors Ltd
Principal Bankers: Union Bank Nigeria Ltd
Financial Information:

	₦'000
Authorised capital	500
Paid-up capital	500
Turnover	2,500
Profits (approx)	300

Principal Shareholders: Chief A O Adenubi; O K Atewologun;
Mrs S O Adenubi; Soladoye Adenubi
Date of Establishment: 4th September 1972
No of Employees: 200 (variable)

PEDRO LEE ASSOCIATES (NIGERIA) LTD

15 Oko-Baba St, Ebute-Metta, Lagos
Tel: 861768

Chairman: Oliver Ped Ukah
Directors: Ambrose Diala
Senior Executives: Leonard Ukah (General Manager),
Sunny Adibe (Personnel Officer),
Boniface Anyanwu (Office Manager)

PRINCIPAL ACTIVITIES: Building maintenance, painters,
chromatic/graphic designers, interior decorators
Branch Offices: 118 Douglas Rd, Owerri, Imo State
Principal Bankers: National Bank (Nigeria) Ltd

No of Employees: 145

PEDRO TRADING COMPANY LTD

4 Adeleke Adedoyin St, Victoria Island, Lagos
Tel: 655376
Telex: 21479 Pedro Ng

PRINCIPAL ACTIVITIES: General traders

PEEZONE FREIGHT SERVICE AGENCY

4 Creek Rd, Apapa, Lagos
PRINCIPAL ACTIVITIES: Customs brokers

PEGASUS INDUSTRIES (NIGERIA) LTD

Plot E Ikosi Rd, Oregun Industrial Estate, PO Box 1629, Ikeja,
Lagos
Tel: 612453
Cable: Pegasus
Telex: 20202/TDS Box 157

Directors: P K Mirchandani (Managing),
Alhaji Malilo,
Alhaji Ladan Zaria
Senior Executives: N L Narasimhan (Financial Controller),
M P Wadekar (Production Manager - Lagos),
Ashok Apte (Production Manager - Kano)

PRINCIPAL ACTIVITIES: Manufacturers of industrial and
domestic plastic packaging materials
Branch Offices: 9 Mai Malari Rd, Plot 9, Bompai Industrial
Estate, PO Box 6271, Kano
Principal Bankers: Nigerian American Merchant Bank Ltd;
Savannah Bank of Nigeria Ltd
Financial Information:

	₦'000
Authorised capital	400
Paid-up capital	200
Turnover	5,000

Principal Shareholders: P K Mirchandani; Alhaji Malilo; Alhaji
Karimu Ayinde; E I Lawore; Alhaji Malilo; Alhaji Adamu
Abubakar
Date of Establishment: 30th May 1977
No of Employees: 250 - 300

PEM LTD

29 New Lagos Rd, PO Box 540, Benin City, Bendel State
Tel: 241789

PRINCIPAL ACTIVITIES: Building materials merchants, general
suppliers, importers and transporters
Branch Offices: Benin City

PENCOL INTERNATIONAL (NIGERIA) LTD

10 Boyle St, Lagos Island, PO Box 6269, Lagos
Tel: 633657
Cable: Spencay Lagos
Telex: 21881 Penspn Ng

Directors: P R Buckley, M T Usman, I Balarabe
Senior Executives: M K White (Manager)

PRINCIPAL ACTIVITIES: Design consultants in oil, gas,
petrochemical, water and liquid waste. Project Managers and
Supervisors
Associated Companies: Pencol Engineering Consultants, London

Date of Establishment: 1976

PEPSI COLA

PMB 1084, Ikeja, Lagos

PRINCIPAL ACTIVITIES: Manufacturers of soft drinks

Date of Establishment: 1970
No of Employees: 500

PESTKILL NIGERIA LTD

40 Balogun St, PO Box 8190, Lagos
Tel: 655748
Cable: Pestkill Lagos

PRINCIPAL ACTIVITIES: Suppliers of spraying equipment for
pest control; insecticides, rodenticides

PETER HARRISON NIGERIA LTD
See HARRISON, PETER, NIGERIA LTD

PETRACO, DE, INDUSTRIES LTD
7 Apapa Rd, PO Box 259, Ebute Metta, Lagos
Tel: 862714
Cable: Petelenics
Telex: 26274 Petrac

Chairman: D A Peterside (also Managing Director)
Directors: G Brown Peterside, N J Nengia, D D Peterside
Senior Executives: A S Bell-Gam (Administration Manager)

PRINCIPAL ACTIVITIES: Stockists of office and security
   equipment, air conditioners, domestic appliances and home
   electronics
Principal Agencies: Glynwed Appliances Ltd, UK; Elba Spa,
   Italy; BSR (Houseware) Ltd, UK
Branch Offices: 4 Aggrey Rd, PO Box 1159, Port Harcourt,
   Rivers State; 111 Market Rd, Aba, Imo State
Principal Bankers: First Bank of Nigeria Ltd
Financial Information:

	N'000
Authorised capital	40
Paid-up capital	26

Date of Establishment: 2nd January 1969
No of Employees: 72

PETRA-MONK ENGINEERING & CONTRACTING COMPANY LTD
Airport Rd, Onigbagbo Village, PO Box 327, Ikeja, Lagos
PRINCIPAL ACTIVITIES: Civil engineering

PETROLEUM CONSULTANTS (NIGERIA) LTD
Unity House, 14th Floor, 37 Marina, Lagos Island, PO Box 4212,
   Lagos
Tel: 630512
Telex: 21173 Cosales Ng

Directors: O Abara (Managing Director)

PRINCIPAL ACTIVITIES: Consultants

PETRO-ORGANICO (NIGERIA) LTD
4 Ibikunle Street, Yaba, Lagos
Tel: 863893
Cable: Petoganic
Telex: 26773 Petro Ng

Directors: Kunle Ogunade (Managing),
   Doyin Ogunade
Senior Executives: Jide Junaid (Chemicals Manager)

PRINCIPAL ACTIVITIES: Chemicals, fertilizers, petrochemicals,
   plastics and rubber goods
Principal Agencies: Esso Chemicals (Exxon Corp); AMOCO
   Chemicals Europe; B F Goodrich
Branch Offices: Warehouse: Isolo Industrial Estate, Lagos
Subsidiary Companies: Churchill Construction Ltd; Western
   Polysacks (Nigeria) Ltd
Principal Bankers: Savannah Bank of Nigeria Ltd; Union Bank
   of Nigeria Ltd
Financial Information:

	N'000
Authorised capital	100
Paid-up capital	100

Principal Shareholders: K Ogunade
Date of Establishment: January 1980

PEUGEOT AUTOMOBILE NIGERIA LTD
PMB 2266, Turaki Ali House, 3 Kanta Rd, Kaduna
Tel: 201160/63
Telex: 71132 Peugnig

Chairman: Alhaji Abdu Abubakar
Directors: Chief C O Ogunbanjo, J Boillot, P Peugeot, F B O
   Olokun, Alhaji Sani Sambo, R E Peguignot, J Mahe
Senior Executives: Mr Mariot (General Manager, Finance),
   Mr Uzokwe (Deputy General, Manager Finance),
   Mr Baldeyroux (General Manager, Assembly Plant),
   Mr Battarel (General Manager, Commercial),
   Mr Suinner (Deputy General Manager, Commercial),
   Mr Osadebe (General Manager, Administration)

PRINCIPAL ACTIVITIES: Car assembling
Branch Offices: Eastern District Office, PMB 1553, Enugu, Tel
   258323; Northern District Office, PO Box 5341, Kano, Tel
   7034; Western District Office, PMB 12034, Lagos, Tel 613146
Principal Bankers: International Bank for West Africa Ltd;
   United Bank for Africa Ltd; Bank of the North Ltd
Financial Information:

	N'000
Authorised capital	15,000
Paid-up capital	14,500
Turnover (1981)	526,000
Profits	17,155

Principal Shareholders: Federal Government of Nigeria;
   Automobiles Peugeot France
Date of Establishment: 11th August 1972
No of Employees: 4,500

PFIZER PRODUCTS LTD
1 Henry Carr St, PMB 21111, Ikeja, Lagos State
Tel: 900371
Cable: Pfizer Ikeja

Chairman: J A Veitch
Directors: Chief G O Olukoya (Managing),
   Dr S B Olupitan (Medical Affairs),
   Cleve Aldenhoven (General Manager, Deputy Managing
   Director),
   A O Idufueko (Animal Health)
Senior Executives: S O Akingbala (Personnel Manager),
   R A Tade (Pharmaceutical Manager),
   Dr M Z Alam (Plant Manager),
   E A Onanuga (Controller/Secretary)

PRINCIPAL ACTIVITIES: Manufacturers of pharmaceuticals,
   animal health and nutritional products
Principal Agencies: Pfizer Pharmaceutical and Animal Health
   Products Division
Branch Offices: (Livestock Feeds) 12 Industrial Layout, PMB
   7119, Aba; Sapele Rd, PMB 1203, Benin City; Waziri Ibrahim
   Crescent, PMB 2115, Kaduna
Subsidiary/Associated Companies: Livestock Feeds Ltd
Principal Bankers: Union Bank of Nigeria Ltd
Financial Information:

	N'000
Authorised capital	8,000
Paid-up capital	5,625
Turnover	16,000
Profits	1,732

Principal Shareholders: Pfizer Corporation; Nigerian Citizens and
   Associations
Date of Establishment: 30th August 1957
No of Employees: 360

PGL GROUP LTD
43 Ibrahim Taiwo Rd, PO Box 2145, Kano
Tel: 4025
Cable: Pholog Kano

PRINCIPAL ACTIVITIES: Suppliers of audio-visual equipment
Branch Offices: Imo; Sokoto; Borno; Anambra and Benue States

PGN LTD
11 Creek Rd, PO Box 270, Apapa, Lagos
Tel: 874066/69/70

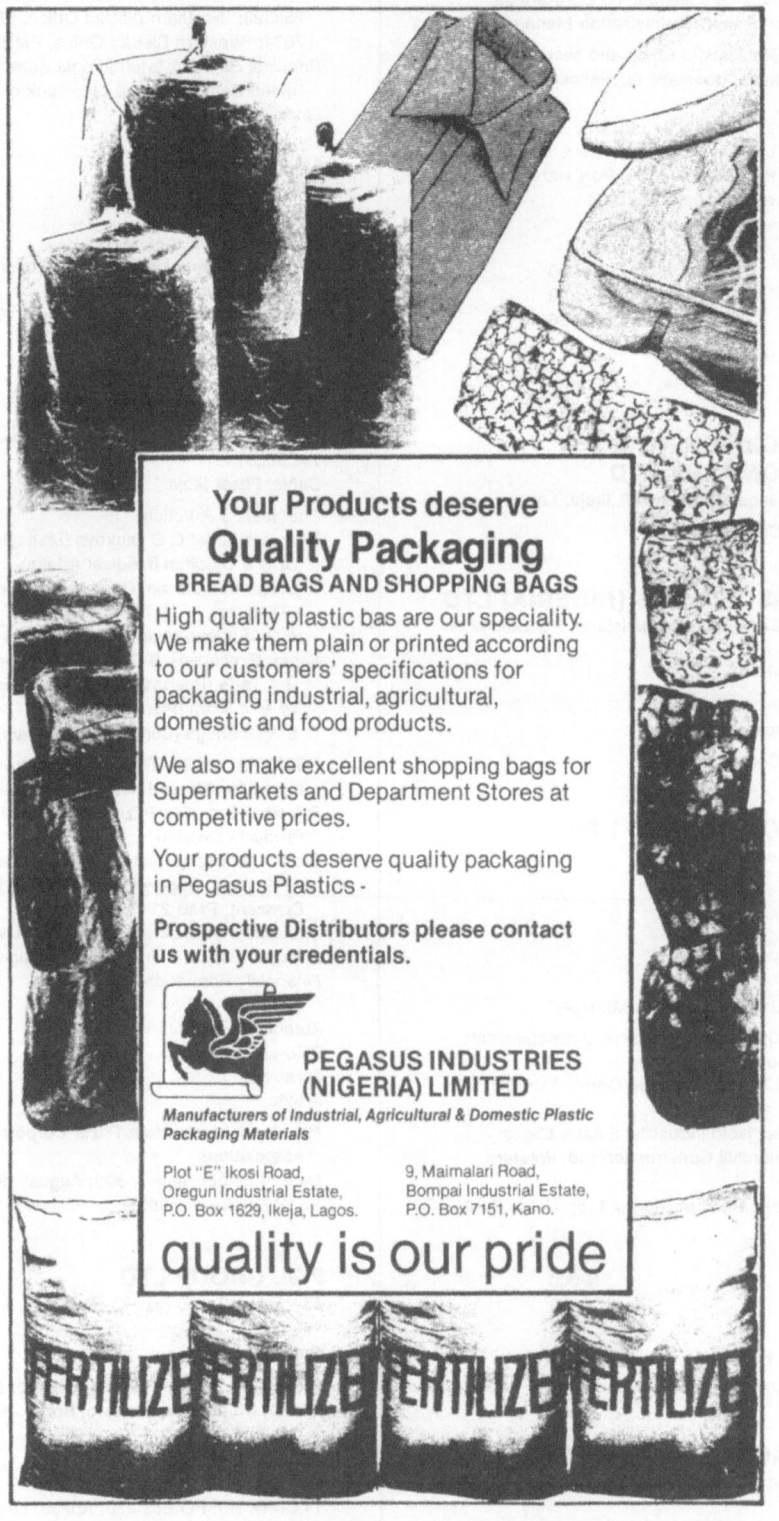

Chairman: A Rimmer
Directors: M T Mbu,
Chief J O Udoji,
E T Tunstall,
A C B Guild (Managing),
Alhaji S Idris (Emir of Zaria),
Alhaji A Mutallab,
R A Scholefield,
Professor I U W Osisiogu
Senior Executives: Chief A O Oduntan (Works Manager),
S A Sanya (Distribution Manager),
S O Adeoye (Company Accountant),
D O Fatoke (Personnel/Training Manager),
J B Padgett (Engineering Services Manager)

PRINCIPAL ACTIVITIES: Glass processors and merchants, fibreglass stockists
Principal Agencies: Fibreglass Ltd, Scott Bader
Branch Offices: 10A Park Rd, PO Box 214, Aba, Imo State; 157 Agbani Rd, PMB 1685, Enugu, Anambra State; Plot H Kaduna South, Off Katchia Rd, PO Box 183, Kaduna; 168 Beggar Lane, Kano; 29 New Lagos Rd, Benin City, Bendel State
Subsidiary Companies: Pilkington Brothers Ltd
Principal Bankers: First Bank of Nigeria Ltd
Financial Information:

	₦'000
Authorised capital	2,000
Paid-up capital	1,600
Turnover	7,000
Profits	540

Principal Shareholders: Pilkington Flat Glass Ltd
Date of Establishment: December 1964
No of Employees: 272

PHARCHEM INDUSTRIES LTD
Plot J Industrial Estate, Ilupeju, PMB 21211, Lagos
Tel: 963505, 961004

Joint Chairmen: G O Egabor, G O Philactou
Directors: S O Adebesin, Mrs D Dimitra

PRINCIPAL ACTIVITIES: Manufacturers of pharmaceutical products
Principal Bankers: United Bank for Africa Ltd

Date of Establishment: February 1968
No of Employees: 100

PHARCO (NIGERIA) LTD (PHARMACEUTICAL COMPANY OF WEST AFRICA)
290 Herbert Macaulay Street, PO Box 493, Yaba, Lagos
Tel: 861282, 862338
Cable: Pharimport

Chairman: Chief E O Ashamu
Directors: Chief S O Lambo,
Alhaji M K Bayero,
G G Uflerbaumer,
P Manlik,
E A Hentschel (Managing),
B O Alaka (Executive Director/General Manager)
Senior Executives: S O Abe (Chief Accountant),
Bade Adeniji (National Sales Manager)

PRINCIPAL ACTIVITIES: Importers of pharmaceuticals and chemicals; manufacturing of pharmaceuticals
Principal Agencies: E Merck, West Germany; Grunenthal, West Germany; E Scheurich, West Germany; Ravensberg, West Germany; Martinet, France
Branch Offices: SW4/406 Ekotedo Street, Ibadan; 73 New Lagos Rd, Benin-City; 17B Constitution Crescent, Aba; 24 Beirut Rd, Kano; V3/4 Maichibi St, Jenta, Jos
Principal Bankers: Union Bank of Nigeria Ltd; Societe Generale Bank

Financial Information:

	₦'000
Authorised capital	2,000
Paid-up capital	700
Turnoer	9,200

Principal Shareholders: Chief E O Ashamu; Mrs P D Ashamu
Date of Establishment: 4th February 1959
No of Employees: 200

PHARMA DYN CHEMICAL PRODUCTS
290 Herbert Macaulay St, PO Box 493, Yaba, Lagos
Tel: 835541

Directors: Africo Cagnani, Oslavio Damiani

PRINCIPAL ACTIVITIES: Suppliers of chemical products and pharmaceuticals

PHILIP MORRIS NIGERIA LTD
See MORRIS, PHILIP, NIGERIA LTD

PHILLIPS OIL COMPANY (NIGERIA) LTD
19 Bishop Aboyade-Cole Street, Victoria Island, PMB 12612, Lagos
Tel: 610021, 615641, 615638
Cable: Philag Lagos
Telex: 21390

Directors: Dr U J Itsueli
Senior Executives: M O Taiga (Chief Accountant),
T D Harding (Operations Manager)

PRINCIPAL ACTIVITIES: Petroleum exploration and production
Branch Offices: Plot 29D Airport Rd, PMB 1692, Benin City, Bendel State
Subsidiary/Associated Companies: Phillips Petroleum Company Europe-Africa
Principal Bankers: First Bank of Nigeria Ltd

Date of Establishment: 1965

PHOEBUS ECONOMIDES RUBBER INDUSTRY LTD
Ogba Village, Ogba Rubber Factory, Via Airport Rd, PO Box 374, Benin City, Bendel State
Tel: 243043

PRINCIPAL ACTIVITIES: Production of crepe rubber

PHOENIX MOTORS LTD
Ikosi Rd, Oregun, PMB 12011, Lagos
Tel: 861168, 861246, 860743

Senior Executives: M L G Amsden (General Manager)

PRINCIPAL ACTIVITIES: Sales and servicing of motor vehicles, agricultural equipment and generators
Principal Agencies: Universal Graders, UK; Mitsubishi
Branch Offices: Mokola Roundabout, PO Box 364, Ibadan, Oyo State, Tel 410186, 410350; 206 Barde Rd, PMB 3231, Kano, Tel 3359, 2726

PHOENIX OF NIGERIA ASSURANCE COMPANY LTD
96/102 Broad Street, PO Box 2893, Lagos
Tel: 661210, 661160
Cable: Phoenix Lagos
Telex: 21383

Chairman: Chief J B Mandilas
Directors: C R Harding, W C Harris, Alhaji Sir Kashim Ibrahim, Nnanna Kalu, A Ojora, Chief F R A Williams, Chief Dr Kole Abayomi
Senior Executives: J C D Nocher (General Manager),
Chief G F Wiggle (Assistant General Manager),
A Robertson (Technical Manager)

PRINCIPAL ACTIVITIES: Insurance
Branch Offices: 11 Station Rd, PO Box 795, Port Harcourt,
    Rivers State; Ring Rd, PO Box 1471, Ibadan, Oyo State;
    Edeinor Shopping Centre, Efurun, PO Box 473, Warri, Bendel;
    67 Maganda Rd, PO Box 5254, Kano
Principal Bankers: First Bank of Nigeria Ltd
Financial Information:

	₦'000
Authorised capital	750
Paid-up capital	750
Turnover	16,000
Profits	1,611

Principal Shareholders: Mandilas Trust Ltd, Lagos; Phoenix
    Assurance Company Ltd, London
Date of Establishment: 1964
No of Employees: 160

PHONOGRAM LTD

PO Box 2997, 6 Ijora Causeway, Lagos
Tel: 876147
Cable: Philrec
Telex: 21297

Directors: Peter Bond (Managing Director)

PRINCIPAL ACTIVITIES: Manufacturers of gramophone records,
    cassettes, cartridges

PICCADILLY INSURANCE COMPANY LTD

SW8/340 Lagos Bye-Pass, Oke-Ado, PO Box 637, Ibadan, Oyo
    State
Tel: 410779

PRINCIPAL ACTIVITIES: Commercial insurance
Branch Offices: Ibadan; Enugu; Warri; Kaduna; Port Harcourt;
    Ilorin; Benin City; Onitsha; Makurdi; Maiduguri etc

PIEDMONT PLYWOODS NIGERIA LTD

Ologbo Village, PO Box 284, Benin City, Bendel State
Tel: 680543
Cable: Piedco
Telex: 44306 Piedco Ng

Chairman: Chief Adeniran Ogunsanya
Directors: Prince Clifford Ogiesoba Eweka, Olufemi Osaze Uzzi,
    Adebiyi Adekeye, Emanuele Comoglio
Senior Executives: Dr Giorgio Tartaglino (Managing Director),
    High Chief Adedapo Adekeye (Director),
    Giuseppe Gardino (Director)

PRINCIPAL ACTIVITIES: Plywood and particle-board
    manufacturers. Sawmillers and general merchants
Principal Agencies: Forest & Sawmills Equipment (Engineers),
    UK
Branch Offices: 35b Maduike Street, Ikoyi, Lagos State
Principal Bankers: Union Bank of Nigeria Ltd; United Bank for
    Africa Ltd
Financial Information:

	₦'000
Authorised capital	2,000
Paid-up capital	2,000
Turnover (approx)	10,000
Profits	600

Principal Shareholders: Chief Adeniran Ogunsanya; High Chief
    Adedapo Adekeye; Dr Giorgio Tartaglino; Giuseppe Gardino
Date of Establishment: 27th March 1982
No of Employees: 1,500

PILGRIM BOOKS LTD

9 First Rd, Oluyole Estate, Ring Rd, PMB 5617, Ibadan, Oyo
    State

PRINCIPAL ACTIVITIES: See Entry for African Universities Press

PILLARS NIGERIA LTD

Bank Chambers, 7th Floor, 27/29 Martins St, PO Box 4581,
    Lagos
Tel: 636394

Directors: Chief G C Ikokwu, G I Ikokwu, P C Anaekwe

PRINCIPAL ACTIVITIES: Real estate
Branch Offices: 142 Ehi Rd, Aba, Imo State; 15 May 27th
    Avenue, Enugu, Anambra State; Agaga Layout, Warri, Bendel
    State; Isu Lodge, PO Box 9, Oba, Onitsha, Anambra State;
    134/136 Ikwere Rd, Port Harcourt, Rivers State; 134a Brent
    St, London NW4

PINTOPLANE NIGERIA LTD

17th Floor, Western House, 8-10 Broad St, PO Box 8015, Lagos
Tel: 636865
Cable: Pintoplane Lagos

Chairman: Michael Ojo Osomo (also Managing Director)
Directors: Morayo Osomo
Senior Executives: Osho Bankole (Administrative Manager)

PRINCIPAL ACTIVITIES: Agents and general trading company
Principal Agencies: Polish Foreign Trade Co
Associated Companies: Pintoplane (UK) Ltd
Principal Bankers: Union Bank of Nigeria Ltd

Principal Shareholders: M O Osomo

PIONEER BISCUIT FACTORY LTD

1 Bonny St, PO Box 305, Apapa, Lagos
Telex: 21531 Arakat Ng

PRINCIPAL ACTIVITIES: Manufacturing of biscuits

PIONEER CHEMICAL MANUFACTURING COMPANY (NIGERIA) LTD

Plot 9 Block A Ogba Scheme, End of Adeniyi Jones Industrial
    Estate, PMB 1158, Ikeja, Lagos
Tel: 934358, 961103, 961486, 963367, 961741

PRINCIPAL ACTIVITIES: Manufacturers of bicycle and
    motorcycle tyres and tubes, and other allied rubber products
Financial Information: Member of Sanusi Group of Companies

PIONEER METAL PRODUCTS COMPANY LTD

Oba Akran Ave, Ikeja Industrial Estate, PO Box 72, Ikeja, Lagos
Tel: 900531/2
Cable: Piometal Ikeja

Chairman: Ryozo Ochi
Directors: S B Akande, J Giannopoulos, S Malami, S Nishio
Senior Executives: H A Erinle (Financial Controller),
    M O Alabi (Works Manager)

PRINCIPAL ACTIVITIES: Manufacturing of galvanised iron
    sheets, corrugated iron roofing sheets
Principal Bankers: First Bank of Nigeria Ltd

Principal Shareholders: Nippon Kokan KK, Japan; Marubeni
    Corporation, Japan; PZ and Co Ltd, Manchester
Date of Establishment: 1962
No of Employees: 550

PIONEER STARCH INDUSTRIES (NIGERIA) LTD

3-7 Nnamdi Azikiwe St, PO Box 2975, Lagos

PRINCIPAL ACTIVITIES: Manufacturing of starch products

PIPES BELOW GROUND LTD

1 Railway Avenue, Kaduna South
Tel: 242505
Cable: PBG Kaduna
Telex: 71316 Songhai Ng

Chairman: Ahmadu Yakubu
Directors: Moreino Properties,
    H G Pepper (Managing)

PRINCIPAL ACTIVITIES: Water supply contractors; pipe supply and laying; complete water systems and technological installations
Principal Agencies: Thyssen Ductile Iron Pipes; Wanit AC Pipes; VAG Valves and Watermeters
Principal Bankers: First Bank of Nigeria Ltd
Financial Information: Member of Songhai Group of Companies

Date of Establishment: 1976

PLASCO SHEETS (NIGERIA) LTD

PO Box 1325, Ikeja, Lagos State
Tel: 901100/1/2
Cable: Plascolli
Telex: 26147 Plasco Ng

Chairman: G Collinetti
Directors: F Collinetti, A Giudici, Alhaji J O Adebambo, Miss O M Finnih

PRINCIPAL ACTIVITIES: Manufacturers of imitation leather, plastic sheeting and PVC tarpaulin
Branch Offices: 6 Ajisegiri Street, Shogunle, Lagos State
Principal Bankers: United Bank for Africa Ltd
Financial Information:

	N'000
Authorised capital	1,000
Paid-up capital	1,000

Principal Shareholders: Foreigners (60%); Nigerians (40%)
Date of Establishment: 28th March 1969
No of Employees: 300

PLASTEX NIGERIA LTD

Iju Rd, Ifako-Agege, PO Box 285, Ikeja, Lagos
Tel: 931627, 931506

PRINCIPAL ACTIVITIES: Plastics processing machinery suppliers

PLASTIC AND ENGINEERING WORKS LTD

PO Box 194, Ikeja, Lagos

PRINCIPAL ACTIVITIES: Manufacturing of metal and plastic wares

PLASTIC MANUFACTURING COMPANY LTD (PMC)

Plot 12A Iganmu Industrial Estate, Aminu Jinadu Close, PO Box 5171, Lagos
Tel: 834801
Cable: Susy-Plast Lagos
Telex: 11117 TDS Ng

Directors: Mauro Salvi, B Fiore

PRINCIPAL ACTIVITIES: Manufacturers of plastic products for cosmetic, pharmaceutical, drug, building and petroleum industries

PLASTO-CROWN (NIGERIA) LTD

1 Barracks Rd, PMB 1117, Calabar, Cross River State

Chairman: H W Akpan

PRINCIPAL ACTIVITIES: Manufacturers of plastic beer crates
Branch Offices: Factory: Ugo, Cross River State
Financial Information:
Registered capital   N 600,000

Principal Shareholders: NIDB 15%; DAH 20%; Investment Trust Company 50%; Utuks Motors Ltd 10%; Other Nigerians 5%
Date of Establishment: October 1976

PLATEAU CERAMICS INDUSTRY LTD (JOS)

3A Bukuru Rd, PO Box 1166, Jos, Plateau State
Tel: 55562

Chairman: A B Jatau
Directors: Bala Na'Anban,
A Z Nansoh,
Messrs Nigerian Mining Corporation (Jos),
Alhaji Gonto,
Mr Ayejime,
A Dasokot
Senior Executives: Dr Saidu Na'Allah (General Manager)

PRINCIPAL ACTIVITIES: Manufacturers of sanitary wares
Branch Offices: Factory under construction
Principal Bankers: Savannah Bank of Nigeria Ltd
Financial Information:
Authorised capital   N 6.6 million

Principal Shareholders: Plateau Investment Company Ltd; Nigerian Mining Corporation; Technical Foreign Partners
Date of Establishment: 1977
No of Employees: 30 (Projected 300 when production starts)

PLATEAU CONSTRUCTION LTD

5 Constitution Hill, PO Box 806, Jos, Plateau State
Tel: 3540
Cable: Plastruct
Telex: 81363

Directors: G Romersa

PRINCIPAL ACTIVITIES: Building and civil engineering contractors

PLATEAU FOODS PROCESSING COMPANY LTD

1 Miango Rd, PO Box 6169, Jos, Plateau State
Tel: 55001, 53388

PRINCIPAL ACTIVITIES: Food and food processing. Agricultural produce

PLATEAU HOTELS & TOURISM COMPANY LTD

PMB 2170, Zaria Rd, Jos, Plateau State
Tel: 55381
Telex: 81118 Platex Ng

Chairman: J K Tallen
Directors: J T Nimfa, Thomas Waje, Gamu Isheni, Habiba Bokkos, Mrs H Thomas, Rilwanu Yahaya, Mrs Dokotri
Senior Executives: A S Ahmed (General Manager),
S N Miri (Assistant General Manager),
Miss D Dareng (Assistant General Manager),
B J K Karingithi (Project Manager),
Alhaji A Bage (Company Secretary/Legal Adviser)

PRINCIPAL ACTIVITIES: Hoteliers
Branch Offices: Plateau Hotel, Tudun-Wada, PMB 2038, Jos, Tel 55740/55741; Jos Hotel, PMB 2170, Zaria Rd, Jos, Tel 55382; Keffi Hotel, PO Box 12, Keffi, Plateau State; Pankshin Hotel, PO Box 40, Pankshin, Plateau State; Shendam Hotel, Shendam, Plateau State; Lafia Hotel, PO Box 24, Lafia, Plateau State
Principal Bankers: Bank of the North Ltd; First Bank of Nigeria Ltd
Financial Information:

	N'000
Authorised capital	5,000
Paid-up capital	3,000
Turnover	3,000
Profits	500

Principal Shareholders: Plateau State Government
Date of Establishment: April 1976
No of Employees: 500

PLATEAU INVESTMENTS COMPANY LTD

PMB 2088, 19 Ahmadu Bello Way, Jos, Plateau State

PRINCIPAL ACTIVITIES: Investment banking and development finance company

Principal Shareholders: Plateau State Government

PLATEAU PUBLISHING COMPANY LTD

5 Zaria Rd, (Joseph Gom Walk House), PMB 2112, Jos, Plateau
  State
Tel: 55010, 53872, 54329
Cable: Otand Ng
Telex: 81113

Chairman: D D Dimka
Directors: J K N Waku, T J Davou, A Angibi, A Z Barde,
  Permanent Secretary/Information, Plateau State, A Oyebola,
  A Ibrahim, H Adamu, G Ironkwe
Senior Executives: S D Makama (General Manager/Chief
    Executive),
  D A Maina (Company Secretary/Legal Adviser),
  Richard Umaru (Editor),
  Michael Longhoom (Production Manager),
  A G Zaku (Chief Accountant)

PRINCIPAL ACTIVITIES: Printing and publishing
Branch Offices: 28 Abibu-Oki St, Lagos; Km 10 Chawai Rd,
  T/Wada, Kaduna; Peacock Hotel Rd, Yola, Gongola State;
  PPC, Opposite Bank Rd, Makurdi, Benue State; Custom Area,
  Along Bama Rd, Maiduguri; 12 Galadima St, Sabon Gari,
  Kano; 20 Edinburgh Rd, Enugu, Anambra State
Principal Bankers: Bank of the North Ltd
Financial Information:

	N'000
Authorised capital	3,000
Paid-up capital	3,000

Principal Shareholders: Plateau State Government; Plateau
  Investment Company
Date of Establishment: 1978
No of Employees: Over 700

PLATEAU TOURISM, DEVELOPMENT & TRANSPORT CO LTD

16/18 Murtala Mohammed Way, PMB 2067, Jos, Plateau State
Tel: 2585, 3354
Cable: Plabus
Telex: 81140 Ng

PRINCIPAL ACTIVITIES: Bus services all over Plateau State;
  inter-state services and services to Lagos. Hoteliers

PLESSCOMMS NIGERIA LTD (FORMERLY PLESSEY (NIGERIA) LTD)

Wesley House, 21/22 Marina, PO Box 3481, Lagos
Tel: 631790, 631859, 631931
Cable: Plessey Lagos
Telex: 21269 Xbar

Chairman: M T Mbu
Directors: O Oyewole, P J Kennedy, P D Parmella
Senior Executives: J Jeffrey (General Manager),
  F Florsheim (Deputy General Manager),
  M A Brown (Electronics Manager),
  A I Paul (Marketing Manager),
  S A Olajuyi (Chief Accountant),
  Chief Ibidapo-Obe (Personnel Manager),
  I Essien (Technical Manager)

PRINCIPAL ACTIVITIES: Suppliers of electrical and electronic
  equipment; telecommunications
Principal Agencies: Oki Electrical, Japan; Carl Zeiss, Jena;
  Plessey Company Ltd (all companies); Ringmaster,
  Intercomms, Norway; BICC; Simrad, Norway
Branch Offices: PMB 5274, Ibadan; PO Box 719, Enugu; PO
  Box 339, Kaduna; PMB 1201, Benin City
Principal Bankers: Union Bank of Nigeria Ltd; Chase Merchant
  Bank Ltd
Financial Information:

	N'000
Authorised capital	420
Paid-up capital	240
Turnover	3,500
Profits	380

Principal Shareholders: Plessey Company Ltd (40%); four
  institutions, eight individuals (60%)
Date of Establishment: 1972

PLISSON FISKO NIGERIA LTD

PO Box 8355, 8B Louis Solomon Close, Victoria Island, Lagos
Tel: 614656

Chairman: F I Osikoya
Directors: Alhaji M A Belo (Financial Director),
  Chief V O Onabanjo
Senior Executives: John Anthony Williamson (General Manager),
  Roger Vinatier (Accountant),
  Peter Beresford-May (Project Manager)

PRINCIPAL ACTIVITIES: Civil engineering and construction
Branch Offices: Area Office, Ilorin, Kwara State
Associated Companies: Fisko Engineering Co Ltd, Lagos
Principal Bankers: International Bank for West Africa Ltd;
  Societe Generale Bank (Nigeria) Ltd; Bank of the North Ltd
Financial Information:

	N'000
Authorised capital	400
Paid-up capital	400
Turnover	15,000
Profits	2,250

Principal Shareholders: Chairman (55%); Financial Director
  (25%); Chief Onabanjo (15%); Employees (5%)
Date of Establishment: 1975
No of Employees: 1,200

POCO CONTAINER REMOVALS LTD

281 Apapa Rd, PO Box 288, Surulere, Lagos
Tel: 876848

PRINCIPAL ACTIVITIES: Forwarding and clearing

POCO MINERALS LTD

Oguwashi-Uku, Bendel State

Directors: P O C Ozieh (Managing Director)

PRINCIPAL ACTIVITIES: Production of prefabricated houses and
  wharfs

POLAMP (NIGERIA) LTD

Okebola Street, Ikole Ekiti, PO Box 115, Ikole Ekiti, Ondo State
Tel: 664811
Cable: Polamp Lagos
Telex: Via 21262 Daltd Ng

Chairman: J S Ogunyemi (also Managing Director)
Directors: F O Ogunyemi, B Gendaj, A Fogg
Senior Executives: Henry Giezek (Technical Director),
  A A Moradeyo (Administrative Manager),
  N A Arhin (Accountant),
  Babatola Joel (Clerk)

PRINCIPAL ACTIVITIES: Manufacturers of electric bulbs,
  flourescent tubes and starters
Branch Offices: 109D Alakoro St, Marina, PO Box 8311, Lagos,
  Tel 831083
Subsidiary/Associated Companies: Dal International Trading
  Company; Unitra Foreign Trade Enterprise
Principal Bankers: National Bank of Nigeria Ltd
Financial Information:

	N'000
Authorised capital	1,000
Paid-up capital	708

Principal Shareholders: Chairman and directors as described
Date of Establishment: 26th September 1978

POLETTI BROTHERS & CO LTD

15 Burma Rd, PO Box 378, Apapa, Lagos State
Tel: 876991, 874807, 875881
Cable: Polbros Apapa

Chairman: Giuseppe Poletti
Directors: Q L Poletti, D Perazzi, W B Dawodu, Chief T O S Benson, U Poletti, S O Adesina
Senior Executives: K O Oyesile (Personnel Manager), Alhaji M O Banjo (Public Relations Manager), Alhaji S A Afoke (Chief Accountant), F A Odifa (Credit Controller)
PRINCIPAL ACTIVITIES: Building and civil engineering contractors
Branch Offices: 21 Ukpashia St, Benin City, Bendel State; Temidayo St, Oke-Ado, Ibadan, Oyo State
Principal Bankers: Union Bank of Nigeria Ltd; First Bank of Nigeria Ltd
No of Employees: 900

POLLACK, SHELDON L, (NIGERIA) LTD

2 Odutaye St, Surulere, Lagos
Tel: 842196

Directors: Victor Monyei

PRINCIPAL ACTIVITIES: Construction

POLLY PEN & INK COMPANY (NIGERIA) LTD

19 Burma Rd, PO Box 373, Apapa, Lagos
Tel: 874552
Cable: Pollypen, Lagos

PRINCIPAL ACTIVITIES: Manufacturers of ball-pens and other pens

POLONI & COMPANY LTD

PO Box 77, Ikeja, Lagos

Directors: D Poloni

PRINCIPAL ACTIVITIES: Consultants

POLY PRODUCTS (NIGERIA) LTD

Ikorodu Rd, Ilupeju Industrial Estate, PO Box 3511, Lagos
Tel: 963221, 964605
Cable: Polyproducts

Chairman: Alhaji Nuhu Bamali
Directors: Nari S Gwalani (Managing), T I Bhojwani, K J Gwalani, R I Bhojwani (Deputy Chairman)

PRINCIPAL ACTIVITIES: Manufacturers of plastic products, polythene bags and sheets
Branch Offices: Aba; Kaduna; Sango Otta, Ogun State
Principal Bankers: United Bank for Africa Ltd; Union Bank of Nigeria Ltd
Principal Shareholders: Nigerian Citizens & Associations; R I Bhojwani
Date of Establishment: May 1965
No of Employees: 400

POLYTHENE ENTERPRISES (NIGERIA) LTD

PMB 1057, 4 Obasa Rd, Ikeja, Lagos State
Tel: 963009, 961221

PRINCIPAL ACTIVITIES: Manufacturers of paper and PVC products
No of Employees: 150

PONTI & COMPANY LTD

PO Box 740, Ibadan, Oyo State
Tel: 410219

Directors: G Ponti, F Barberis

PRINCIPAL ACTIVITIES: Consultants
Branch Offices: Port Harcourt

PORT & MARINE SERVICES LTD

9 Creek Rd, PO Box 319, Apapa, Lagos
Tel: 875887, 875969, 874188, 833504, 874215
Telex: 21342 Imas Ng

PRINCIPAL ACTIVITIES: Inland waterways transportation, lighterage, shipbuilding, repairs and general engineering contractors
Branch Offices: Lagos

PORT EXPRESS SERVICES LTD

46 Sadiku St, Olodi-Apapa, PO Box 2774, Apapa, Lagos
Tel: 870751
Cable: Lizayecos
Telex: 20200 Net TDS Box 035

PRINCIPAL ACTIVITIES: Shipping, clearing and forwarding
Branch Offices: Port Harcourt, Warri, Kano

PORT HARCOURT FLOUR MILLS LTD

No 8 Industry Rd, PO Box 809, Port Harcourt, Rivers State
Tel: 333853
Cable: Rivgoc Nigeria
Telex: 61105

Chairman: R A George
Directors: Akandu Nwogu, Chief A Waobikeze-Woko, G R Chagoury
Senior Executives: W E O Oburu (Chief Accountant), A Ghani (Head Miller), Miss K O Adoki (Special Assistant to the Managing Director), J S Chidiac (Deputy Managing Director)

PRINCIPAL ACTIVITIES: Flour milling, production of semolina, wheat offal, pelletised wheat, etc
Principal Bankers: Savannah Bank of Nigeria Ltd
Financial Information:

	₦'000
Authorised capital	2,000
Paid-up capital	800
Turnover (approx)	16,600
Profits (after tax)	171

Principal Shareholders: Rivers State Government
Date of Establishment: April 1972

POULTRY & ANIMAL PRODUCTS (NIGERIA) LTD

55 Femi Ayantuga Crescent, Surulere, PO Box 50581, Falomo, Lagos
Tel: 835959
Telex: 26781 Pap Ng

Chairman: Michael J Cantle
Directors: F Asekun (Managing), A J G Watson (Project Director), R Asekun
Senior Executives: C J Eaves (Sales Manager), M Bettle (Technical Manager)

PRINCIPAL ACTIVITIES: Modern poultry projects of all types; poultry equipment, including cages and housing; day old chicks; feed and feed concentrates
Principal Agencies: Poultry & Animal Products Ltd, UK
Principal Shareholders: Poultry & Animal Products Ltd, UK; F Asekun
Date of Establishment: October 1979

POWER & COMMUNICATION ENGINEERING NIGERIA LTD

7 Henry Carr Street, Industrial Estate, PMB 21253, Ikeja, Lagos
Tel: 901140, 901141
Telex: 26100 Pcn Ng

Chairman: Chief Jerome Udoji
Directors: H D Berg (Managing),
 M Oluwa,
 D Nordmann,
 C Werse
Senior Executives: F Paproth (General Manager),
 Engr D O Uzoigwe (Chief Engineer/Sales Manager)
PRINCIPAL ACTIVITIES: Electrical and civil engineering
 contractor, power generation, transmission and distribution,
 telecommunications and general sales
Principal Agencies: Kabelmetal Nigeria Ltd; SAG, West
 Germany; S & S, Switzerland
Principal Bankers: International Bank for West Africa Ltd
Financial Information:

	N'000
Authorised capital	400
Paid-up capital	400
Turnover	494

Principal Shareholders: Kabelmetal Electro; SAG Frankfurt; Chief
 J Udoji; Mr Oluwa; Engr D Uzoigwe
Date of Establishment: 1977

POWERLINES LTD
Awosika St, Ikeja, PO Box 185, Lagos
Tel: 900233, 960085
Cable: Powerlines Lagos
Telex: 26636 Plines

Chairman: Chief C O Ogunbanjo
Directors: J I Harry, H O Omenai, C Colombo, F Pellicano

PRINCIPAL ACTIVITIES: Building and civil engineering
 contractors

Date of Establishment: 1959

PRACOTRADE (NIGERIA) LTD
40 Balogun St, PO Box 8190, Lagos
Tel: 655748

Directors: H Sebauder

PRINCIPAL ACTIVITIES: General trading and representation

PRC (NIGERIA) LTD
6 Kingsway Rd, PO Box 8536, Lagos
Tel: 682761

Chairman: Alhaji Mustapha B Wali
Directors: Ime J Ebong (Managing),
 Walt G Hansen,
 Steve C Lockwood

PRINCIPAL ACTIVITIES: Engineering consultants, city, regional
 planners
Branch Offices: 29 Kakawa St, c/o Etteh-Aro, Lagos
Associated Companies: Planning Research Corporation, USA

Date of Establishment: May 1979

PREMIER BREWERIES LTD
Industrial Layout, Bridge Head, PMB 1620, Onitsha, Anambra
 State
Tel: 210388
Cable: Prembrew Onitsha

Chairman: Chief S E Nnaji
Directors: Chief C N Ezea, Chief O Fejika, S Anyigor, S
 Azikiwe, G G O Sonekan, C E Okobi
Senior Executives: E I Anoliefo (General Manager),
 Engr I N Onwuegbusi (Chief Engineer),
 B C Nwonu (Marketing Manager),
 K Eidenchink (Brewmaster),
 L U Udaba (Financial Controller)

PRINCIPAL ACTIVITIES: Brewing
Branch Offices: Plot 306A Aba/Owerri Rd, Aba; 4 Ogoja Rd,
 Aba Kiliki; Awka: Amawbia/Awka; Benin/Asaba Rd, Benin; 65

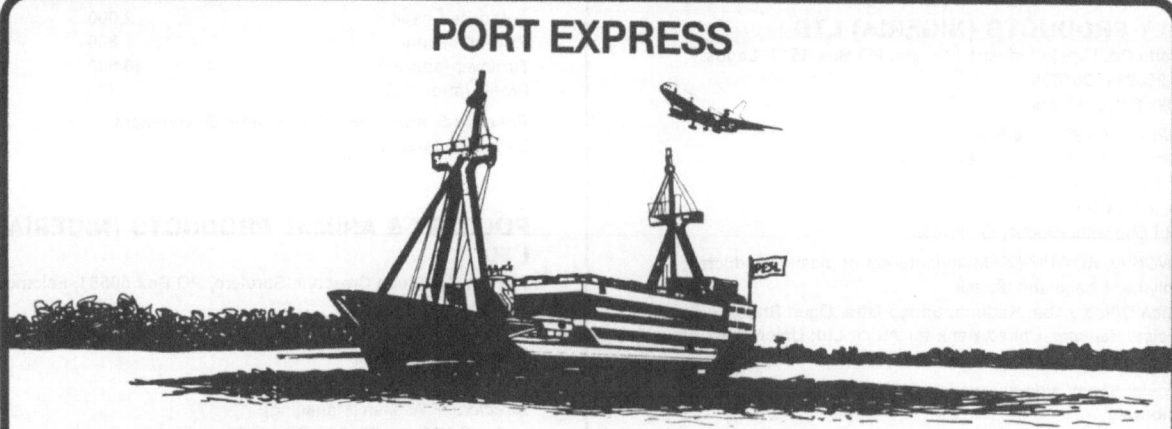
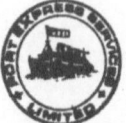

Chime Avenue, Enugu; 56 Oturkpo Rd, Makurdi; 2 Onuiyi Rd, Nsukica, Nsukka

Subsidiary/Associated Companies: Eastern Plastic Industry
Principal Bankers: First Bank of Nigeria Ltd; African Continental Bank Ltd
Financial Information:

	₦'000
Authorised capital	10,500
Paid-up capital	10,500
Turnover	85,434
Profits (after tax)	23,498

Principal Shareholders: Anambra State Government (80%); Nigerian Industrial Development Bank (NIDB) (10%); Nigerian Bank of Commerce and Industry (NBCI) (10%)
Date of Establishment: October 1977
No of Employees: 1,500

PREMIER ENGINEERING WORKS LTD

4/6 Oil Mill St, Lagos

Directors: Jacques Amaeka (Managing), Jean-Paul Etienne (Technical)

PRINCIPAL ACTIVITIES: Joint Nigerian and Swiss assembling of watches
Financial Information:
Registered capital   ₦ 150,000

Date of Establishment: 1979 Registered

PRESIDENT CLOTHING CO LTD

Plot F 221, Apapa Rd, PO Box 905, Lagos
Tel: 960071, 832123, 960073, 960037, 832153, 832373, 832265
Cable: President Lagos
Telex: 21143 Presit Ng

Chairman: S B Awoniyi
Directors: H A Lardner,
Malam I M Damcida,
H B Chaturvedi (Executive),
M E Ibie (Executive),
L C Chanrai (Managing)
Senior Executives: Y G Upadhye (Financial Controller), P M Prabakar Rao (Factory Manager)

PRINCIPAL ACTIVITIES: Manufacturer of textiles; cotton guinea brocades, shirting, suiting, bedsheeting and knitted fabrics
Branch Offices: Plot 12 Israel Adebajo Avenue; Ikeja Industrial Estate, Ikeja, Lagos
Principal Bankers: Union Bank of Nigeria Ltd; United Bank for Africa (Nig) Ltd; Societe Generale Bank (Nig) Ltd
Financial Information:

	₦'000
Authorised capital	3,500
Paid-up capital	2,187
Turnover	15,200

Principal Shareholders: Non Resident Shareholders (60%); Nigerians (40%)
Date of Establishment: June 1968
No of Employees: 1,100

PRESSED METAL INDUSTRY LTD

PMB 5358, Mile 5, Ibadan-Lagos Rd, Ibadan, Oyo State
Tel: 411180
Cable: Oscar Ibadan

PRINCIPAL ACTIVITIES: Metal products manufacturers, steel butt hinges; furniture springs; door bolts, etc

PRESSED METAL WORKS LTD

212 Apapa Rd, Iganmu, PO Box 110, Apapa, Lagos
Tel: 833897, 874838, 836069, 831341

Directors: S Gerino (Managing Director)

PRINCIPAL ACTIVITIES: Manufacturers of oil tanks and steel structures

PRESTIGE INDUSTRIES LTD

1 Adegunwa St, Yaba, PO Box 4258, Lagos
Tel: 860005, 860569, 862075

PRINCIPAL ACTIVITIES: Manufacturing of fabrics, clothing, footwear and stationery

PRESTIGE STORES NIGERIA LTD

28 Abibu Oki St, PO Box 1099, Lagos
Tel: 683555

PRINCIPAL ACTIVITIES: Distributors of leather goods, floor coverings, etc

PRESTREST LTD

PO Box 55, Abeokuta, Ogun State

PRINCIPAL ACTIVITIES: Building and civil engineering contractors

PREUSSAG DRILLING ENGINEERS NIGERIA LTD

1A Bida Rd, PO Box 4314, Kaduna
Tel: 216659
Telex: 71342

Chairman: Alhaji Aminu Dantata
Directors: Alhaji Mai Deribe, H Gerhard, W A Herold, H H Kruse

PRINCIPAL ACTIVITIES: Hydrogeological and geophysical services; borehole drilling, core drilling, industrial piping, water storage tank production, engineering and installation of water treatment plants. Engineering and sale of all types of fire-fighting equipment
Branch Offices: PMB 1372, 13 Monguno Rd, Maiduguri, Borno State; Canteen Rd, PO Box 935, Sokoto, Tel 232327; 19B Chief Okupe Estate, Maryland, PO Box 804, Oshodi, Lagos, Tel 960182, Telex 26737
Principal Bankers: International Bank for West Africa Ltd

Date of Establishment: Established 1977

PRICE WATERHOUSE

Plot 1 Western Avenue, Alaka Estate, PO Box 2419, Lagos
Tel: 837107, 837173
Cable: Pricewater
Telex: 26652 PW LOS Ng

Directors: M C Taylaur, C Amako, N Harrison

PRINCIPAL ACTIVITIES: Management consultants, chartered accountants

Date of Establishment: 1960

PRIDECO - PROJECTS & INDUSTRIAL EQUIPMENT CO (NIGERIA) LTD

3 Hospital Rd, PO Box 9289, Lagos
Tel: 631227
Cable: Prideco Lagos
Telex: 21046 Pridec Ng

Chairman: Chief S O Adebo
Directors: T Kiencke (Managing Director)

PRINCIPAL ACTIVITIES: Business and engineering consultants; suppliers of industrial equipment and heavy machinery. Execution/financing turnkey industrial plants
Principal Agencies: Ferrostaal Ag, W Germany
Subsidiary Companies: Ferrostaal Ag, West Germany
Principal Bankers: United Bank for Africa Ltd

Date of Establishment: 1978

PRIMARY STEEL (NIGERIA) LTD

Plot G Ikosi Rd, Oregun, Ikeja, PO Box 3262, Lagos
Tel: Primasteel

Chairman: M T Mbu
Directors: V Burhardt, V Parker, C Mercenier
Senior Executives: S A Badro (Financial Manager)

PRINCIPAL ACTIVITIES: Suppliers of building materials, steel importers
Associated Companies: Primary Industries Corporation, New York; Primary Industries Trading SA, Switzerland; Lonconex Ltd, London; Primary Steel Inc, Washington, Primary Industries (Far East) Corp, Tokyo; Primary Industries GmbH, West Germany; Primary Industries, Brazil
Principal Bankers: United Bank for Africa Ltd

Principal Shareholders: Nigerians 60%; Primary Steel SA, Belgium 40%
Date of Establishment: 1974

PRIME FEATHERS INTERNATIONAL SERVICES LTD
1 Ganikale Court, PMB 1092, Oshodi, Lagos
Tel: 960060, 932796
Cable: Prifinsel Lagos
Telex: 20200/032 Net-TDS-Ng

Chairman: J C Ezigbo (also Managing Director)
Directors: L C Ezigbo, S I Harrison
Senior Executives: P A Eluwa (Marketing Manager),
  Z O Nwosu (Chief Accountant),
  F A Onuoha (Company Secretary/Personnel),
  M I Akparajah (General Manager)

PRINCIPAL ACTIVITIES: Agents and general trading company; optical and photographic equipment; pharmaceutical and medical supplies; toiletries, cosmetics and allied products; office equipment supplies; educational equipment and training services; scientific instruments and chemicals; food products; household goods and appliances, brewing, soft drinks and wine
Principal Agencies: Mark IV International Company, USA
Branch Offices: Umuahia, Imo State; Bauchi, Bauchi State; Jos, Plateau State
Subsidiary Companies: Prime Constructions; Lozitete (Nigeria) Enterprises; Lawbecca Enterprises
Principal Bankers: Union Bank of Nigeria Ltd

Principal Shareholders: Chairman and directors as described
Date of Establishment: 1st December 1976

PRIMUS (NIGERIA) LTD
11 Aba Rd, 1st Floor, PO Box 668, Port Harcourt, Rivers State
Tel: 229559

PRINCIPAL ACTIVITIES: Transporters, freight forwarders

PRINCEGATE TRADING & CONTRACTING COMPANY LTD
22 Moor House St, PO Box 378, Ogui, Enugu, Anambra State
Tel: 252876
Cable: Princegate

Chairman: A N Nwamu
Directors: Dr P C Ofili,
  T N Nwamu (Secretary)

PRINCIPAL ACTIVITIES: Importers and exporters; civil engineering and construction contractors; manufacturers' representatives; supplies of textiles and household goods; electrical equipment, building materials
Principal Agencies: General Tire International Co Inc
Branch Offices: 14A Uda St, Asaba, Bendel State
Associated Companies: Eddide Inc Nigeria Ltd; P I Nwamu Associates Inc
Principal Bankers: Union Bank of Nigeria Ltd

Principal Shareholders: A N Nwamu; Dr P C Ofili; T N Nwamu

PRINCIPAL BOOKSHOP & COMMERCIAL STORES LTD
1 Maikano Dutse Rd, PO Box 1687, Kano
Tel: 3196

PRINCIPAL ACTIVITIES: Suppliers of books, stationery, office and sports equipment, general merchandise; printers and publishers
Branch Offices: Ahmadu Bello Way, PMB 2160, Sokoto, Tel 2341; A62 Dandal Way, Hausari Ward, PO Box 261, Maiduguri, Borno State, Tel 2748

PROFESSIONAL AND MANUFACTURING SERVICES (NIGERIA) LTD
Oregun Industrial Estate, (Off Clay Industry), PO Box 1225, Ikeja, Lagos
Cable: Promaserve

Chairman: E Young Owukiabo (Executive)
Directors: John H Hawkey, Tonye Y Owukiabo
Senior Executives: Gani Williams (Company Secretary),
  Babatunde Carew (Marketing Manager),
  I J Akpan (Executive Assistant to the Chairman)

PRINCIPAL ACTIVITIES: Manufacturers of carbon papers, typewriter and computer ribbons, duplicating ink and stencils
Associated Companies: Semfek Industrial Machinery & Chemicals Co (Nig) Ltd; Diversified Packaging UK Ltd
Principal Bankers: Savannah Bank of Nigeria Ltd
Financial Information:

	₦'000
Authorised capital	400
Paid-up capital	350
Turnover	1,800
Profits	350

Principal Shareholders: Diversified Packaging UK Ltd; E Yougn Owukiabo
Date of Establishment: December 1976
No of Employees: 180

PROGRESS CONTRACTS LTD
SW8/491 Lagos Bye-Pass, Oke-Ado, PO Box 788, Ibadan, Oyo State
Tel: 631227/631047

Directors: Alhaji A A Andu, Alhaji S A Andu

PRINCIPAL ACTIVITIES: Civil engineering and construction

PROGRESS ENTERPRISES
21 Wharf Rd, Apapa, Lagos
Tel: 874290
Telex: 21534 Minne Ng

PRINCIPAL ACTIVITIES: General traders and contractors

PROGRESSIVE INSURANCE COMPANY LTD
Akure/Owo Rd, Before Ado-Ekiti Junction, PO Box 17, Akure, Ondo State
Tel: 230496
Telex: 35361 Pogre Ng

PRINCIPAL ACTIVITIES: Insurance
Branch Offices: Throughout Nigeria

PROJECT MANAGEMENT LTD
Gidan Shehu Ahmed, Bank Rd, PO Box 422, Kano
Tel: 2557
Telex: 77221 Lennap

Chairman: Alhaji Aminu Dantata
Directors: A J Dorman (Managing Director),
  Alhaji U Albishir,
  Dr S Kumo,
  B Hassan
Senior Executives: I G Macleod (Consultant),
  A Idris (Consultant)

PRINCIPAL ACTIVITIES: Management consultants and project managers
Principal Bankers: United Bank for Africa Ltd

Principal Shareholders: A J Dorman; Alhaji A Dantata
Date of Establishment: July 1975

PROJECT TEXTILE MILL (NIGERIA) LTD
Industrial Estate, Ilorin, Kwara State
PRINCIPAL ACTIVITIES: Manufacturers of cotton yarn

PROMANA ASSOCIATES
291 Ikorodu Rd, PO Box 573, Lagos
Tel: 964939, 901310/2
Cable: Dimensions
Telex: 26345 Modelo Ng

Chairman: Arc Chief O O Balogun
Senior Executives: A A Ajibola (General Manager),
 Mrs S O Ajomo (Group Administrative Manager),
 A A Adeyemi (Personnel Manager),
 Kunle Balogun (Project Manager),
 Mrs R H Sodipo (Company Secretary/Legal Adviser),
 Arc U Shrestha (Chief Architect, Housing),
 R E Long (Principal Project Coordinator)

PRINCIPAL ACTIVITIES: Project management, turnkey projects,
 interior design and decoration
Principal Bankers: United Bank for Africa Ltd; Union Bank of
 Nigeria Ltd

Date of Establishment: 1980
No of Employees: 192

PROMEXPORT INTERNATIONAL (NIGERIA) LTD
76 Adetokunbo Ademola St, Victoria Island, PO Box 2468,
 Lagos
Tel: 613603
Cable: Promexport
Telex: 20117 Net

Chairman: R K Okudzeto
Directors: Ekow Awooner (Company Secretary),
 Lois Okudzeto,
 Ananth D Raman

PRINCIPAL ACTIVITIES: General trading
Subsidiary Companies: Lastra Construction; Eao Construction
Principal Bankers: Bank of the North

Principal Shareholders: R K Okudzeto (major shareholder)
Date of Establishment: 1970

PRUDENT FINANCE LTD
3rd Floor, Ebani House, 149/153 Broad Street, PO Box 9779,
 Lagos
Tel: 661754, 663889, 664647
Cable: Prudef Lagos
Telex: 22512 Prudef Lagos

Chairman: Chief Olu Akinkugbe
Directors: S O Ogundipe (Managing/Chief Executive),
 W J Anukpe,
 F A Wodi,
 Dr A Ajayi-Obe,
 E D Obademi (Finance Director)
Senior Executives: R A Aina (Assistant Commercial Manager),
 O Yusuff (Assistant Corporate Finance Manager),
 R F Shofuyi (Assistant Administration Manager)

PRINCIPAL ACTIVITIES: Finance house
Principal Bankers: Union Bank of Nigeria Ltd; United Bank of
 Africa; First Bank of Nigeria Ltd; New Nigeria Bank
Financial Information:

	N'000
Authorised capital	1,000
Paid-up capital	1,000

Principal Shareholders: Chief O I Akinkugbe; W J Anukpe; S O
 Ogundipe; Chief J O Udoji; Alhaji O A G Otiti; Arc G Y
 Aduku; Dr O Ajayi-Obe; Senator A A Ali; M Ade Ojo; T A
 Bakare; Alhaji A Abubakar
Date of Establishment: 3rd December 1979

PUKKE, HORST, & CO (NIGERIA) LTD
19 Obun Eko St, PO Box 3697, Lagos
Tel: 664910
Cable: Hopex Lagos

Chairman: Gabriel Ayoola Awe (also Managing Director)
Directors: Ojo Awe, Olu Awe
Senior Executives: Brimah Adio Jinadu (Personnel Officer),
 Kalu Agwu (Manager)

PRINCIPAL ACTIVITIES: Agents and general trading; suppliers
 of agricultural equipment and services; plastics
Principal Agencies: Horst Pukke GmbH & Co, West Germany
Branch Offices: 55 Jubilee Rd, PO Box 1314, Aba, Imo State;
 83 Obafemi Awolowo Way, Ikeja, Lagos; 2-4 Ikirun Bye Pass,
 Oshogbo; N6A/451 Adekunle Fajuyi Rd, Adamasingba,
 Ibadan, Oyo State
Principal Bankers: First Bank of Nigeria Ltd

Principal Shareholders: Gabriel Ayo Awe; Gabriel Olusola Awe

PUMP SERVICES NIGERIA LTD
Plot 14 Block A, Ogba Industrial Estate, Surulere Industrial Rd,
 Ogba, Ikeja
Tel: 664630, 664803

Chairman: T A Oke (also Managing Director)
Directors: Mrs R A Adams, J R Manger, P J Hardman
Senior Executives: T Everitt (Ag General Manager)

PRINCIPAL ACTIVITIES: Supplies and service of pumps and
 generating sets
Principal Agencies: Gilbarco Ltd, UK
Principal Bankers: Societe Generale Bank of Nigeria Ltd

PUNCH (NIGERIA) LTD
Kudeti Street, Agege Motor Rd, PMB 21204, Ikeja, Lagos
Tel: 963580
Cable: Skyway
Telex: 26277 Punch

Chairman: James Olubunmi Aboderin
Directors: Olu Aboderin, Oladimeji Akinwale, Sunday Dankaro,
 Lolu Foresythe, Sam Amuka-Pemu, Afolabi Sasegbon
Senior Executives: E C Igbokwe (General Manager),
 Sola Odunfa (Editor-in-Chief),
 M A Omokunga (AG Chief Accountant),
 J O Akinyemi (Personnel Manager),
 Ikem Ohia (Company/Legal Secretary)

PRINCIPAL ACTIVITIES: Printing and publishing of newspapers
 and magazines
Principal Agencies: All over Nigeria; 24 Bryanston Street,
 London W1A 7AE
Associated Companies: Skyway Press Ltd; Puski Travel Bureau
 Ltd; Puski Agencies Clearing & Forwarding Ltd
Principal Bankers: Savannah Bank of Nigeria Ltd; National Bank
 of Nigeria Ltd; Allied Bank of Nigeria Ltd

Date of Establishment: Incorporated 8th August 1970
No of Employees: 708

PUREWAY CORPORATION OF NIGERIA LTD
5 Mercy Eneli St, PMB 3058, Surulere, Lagos
Tel: 830791

Directors: Chief A Jones

PRINCIPAL ACTIVITIES: Construction
Branch Offices: Falomo Shopping Centre, C8 SW Ikoyi
 Showroom, Lagos, Tel 680732

PYRAMID PAPER PRODUCTS LTD
Plot 7 Block E, Matori Industrial Estate, PO Box 113, Yaba,
 Lagos
Tel: 830910

PRINCIPAL ACTIVITIES: Paper converters, stationery
manufacturers, tissue products
Branch Offices: 530 Lagos Rd, PO Box 353, Ibadan, Tel 61237;
16 Arakale St, Akure; 124 Murtala Mohammed Way, Benin
City; Plot 121 Niger Bridge Approach Rd, Onitsha; 209 Faulks
Rd, Aba, Imo State; 64 Faskari Rd, Tundun Wada, PO Box
1695, Kaduna; 18 Hausa Rd, Jos, Plateau State; 86 Egbe Rd,
PO Box 6365, Kano, Tel 8011; Ali Akilu Rd, Angwa Rogo
Junction, Sokoto; Maching Rd, Behind Borno Guest Inn,
Maiduguri; 155/107 Apapa Rd, Ebute - Metta; 102 Ogunlana
Drive, Surulere; 22c Ikorodu Rd, Ketu; 11 Simpson Street,
Lagos; 70 Araromi Street, Ijebu - Ode; 53 Goldie Street,
Calabar

R & A SERVICES (DIVISION OF UAC OF NIGERIA LTD)
1 Taylor Rd, Iddo, PMB 1015, Ebute Metta, Lagos
Tel: 800200/6
Cable: Raquip, Lagos

Chairman: Chief E A O Shonekan
Directors: H M Mathers, J P Rauch, His Highness Alhaji Shehu
Idris, Alhaji Bello Sanni, M C Thompson, J G A Clegg, S B
Daniyan, J C Egri-Okwaji, A C I Mbanefo, F M O Osifo, B
Foster, J O Omidiora, P D Tueart
Senior Executives: Chief J O Omidiora (General Manager),
S A Olarewaju (Marketing Manager),
J Dempsey (General Technical Manager),
S O Olasoji (Commercial Manager)

PRINCIPAL ACTIVITIES: Installation and service of refrigeration
and air-conditioning equipment. Suppliers of accessories and
tools to the trade, manufacture and sales of air conditioners
Principal Agencies: Qualitair (Air Conditioning) Ltd, UK; Keeprite
Products Ltd, Canada; Prestcold Searle Ltd, UK; Bally
Coldrooms, USA; Sadia Airofreeze Ltd, UK; Danfoss
Compressors, Denmark; International Airmonitors Ltd, UK;
L'Unite Hermetique SA, France
Branch Offices: 121/123 Broad Street, Lagos, Tel 662208; Bank
Rd, PO Box 2, Ibadan, Tel 410528; 120 Abdul Azeez Attah
Rd, Ilorin; 10 Awolowo Rd, PO Box 504, Port Harcourt, Tel
334251; 2 Sokoto Rd, PO Box 3818, Onitsha, Tel 211107;
143 Marine Rd, PO Box 46, Calabar, Tel 224659; Giden
Niger, Ahmadu Bello Way, PO Box 1687, Kaduna, Tel 243402;
9 Niger Street, PO Box 1171, Kano, Tel 4173; Kirikasama Rd,
PO Box 12, Maiduguri, Tel 232695; Danfodio Rd, PO Box 29,
Sokoto, Tel 232370; 67 Akpakpava Street, PO Box 2260,
Benin, Tel 244154; Delta House, Warri/Sapele Rd, PO Box
543, Warri, Tel 231137; 21B Adeola Rd, Junction of
Okpe/Adeola Rd, PMB 4131, Sapele, Tel 41428
Principal Bankers: United Bank For Africa Ltd; Union Bank of
Nigeria Ltd; First Bank of Nigeria Ltd

Principal Shareholders: 60% UACN; 40% CW Holdings
Date of Establishment: Over 25 years

R I ERHAHON & CO LTD
See ERHAHON, R I, & CO LTD

R RAJENDRAM AND ASSOCIATES
See RAJENDRAM, R, AND ASSOCIATES

R T BRISCOE (NIGERIA) LTD
See BRISCOE, R T, (NIGERIA) LTD

RAABE SANITARY AND WATER ENGINEERING
7A Fowler Rd, PO Box 50828, Ikoyi, Lagos
Tel: 684587

Chairman: W Raabe
Directors: K Meinhardt, K Pakull
Senior Executives: H Emmerich (Technical Manager)

PRINCIPAL ACTIVITIES: Suppliers of pipes and fittings, water
engineering and construction, chemicals

RABIU, ISIYAKU, & SONS LTD
73 Ibrahim Taiwo Rd, PO Box 582, Kano
Tel: 5011, 4489, 3173
Cable: Israbiu

PRINCIPAL ACTIVITIES: Importers of foodstuffs, especially rice,
groundnut oil and vegetable oil, building materials and
general goods
Associated Companies: Bagauda Textile Mill Ltd (see separate
entry); Kano Vehicle & Accessories Ltd; Kano Merchants
Trading Company Ltd; Rabiu Food Industries; Rabiu
Investments Ltd

RACCAFORM LTD
PO Box 434, Kundila Rd, Bompai, Kano
Tel: 4715

PRINCIPAL ACTIVITIES: Manufacturers of metal beds, wooden
furniture and steel structures

RACCAH & CHAKER FACTORY LTD
PO Box 434, Kano
Tel: 4715, 4472

PRINCIPAL ACTIVITIES: Manufacturing of steel beds, office
furniture, agricultural equipment

RADIATORS NIGERIA LTD
18th Floor, Western House, 8/10 Broad St, PO Box 3606, Lagos
Tel: 635004, 635076
Cable: Jurisconsult
Telex: 21164 Buguma

Chairman: Chief Godfrey K J Amachree
Directors: Major-General H U Katsina, Mrs G Ogbemi, Chief
Paul R Lanique, W R Ford
PRINCIPAL ACTIVITIES: Manufacturing of car and lorry
radiators
Branch Offices: Plot 75, Trans-Amadi Industrial Area, Port
Harcourt, Rivers State
Principal Bankers: International Bank for West Africa Ltd
Financial Information:

	N'000
Authorised capital	400
Paid-up capital	400
Sales turnover	3,000

Principal Shareholders: Delta Oil Nigeria Ltd; Chief G K J
Amachree
No of Employees: 100

RADIO COMMUNICATIONS (NIGERIA) LTD
362 Herbert Macaulay Street, Yaba, PO Box 7700, Lagos
Tel: 860538

Chairman: Alhaji Chief M K O Abiola (also Chief Executive)
Directors: Alhaja Chief Mrs S A Abiola,
Alhaja Mrs R A Y Adegboyega (Group Manager, Finance,
Administration, Personnel)
Senior Executives: A O Oyeniji (Personnel & Contracts Manager),
Alhaji R A Mustafa (Administrative Manager),
J O Ojo (Deputy Operations & Maintenance Manager),
M O Abiola (Field Services Manager),
R A Sunmonu (Network Operations Manager),
A Fawole (Deputy Depot Manager),
B M Sadiq (Technical Sales Manager)

PRINCIPAL ACTIVITIES: Telecommunications (domestic earth
satellite communications)
Branch Offices: All state capitals
Principal Bankers: United Bank for Africa Ltd

Date of Establishment: 18th July 1972
No of Employees: 400

RADIO VISION CENTRE (NIGERIA) LTD

15 Aggrey Rd, Port Harcourt, Rivers State
Tel: 226505

PRINCIPAL ACTIVITIES: Suppliers and servicers of electrical
equipment
Principal Agencies: Sony; JVC; National Panasonic; Akai etc
Branch Offices: 12 & 18 Aggrey Rd, Port Harcourt, Rivers State;
11 Liberation Drive, Port Harcourt, Tel 225916; 1/2 Park Rd,
Aba, Imo State, Tel 343

RAJENDRAM, R, AND ASSOCIATES

John Holt Compound, 149/153 Broad Street, PO Box 1989,
Lagos
Tel: 663096
Cable: Rajchart Lagos
Telex: 11117, 2017 UK only, Box No 467

Chairman: Arc Rasiah Rajendram
Directors: Arc R Rajendram, M O Johnson

PRINCIPAL ACTIVITIES: Architectural, civil engineering,
structural, electrical and mechanical engineering services.
Quantity surveying, town planning and surveying
Branch Offices: PO Box 4049, Maiduguri, Borno State; PO Box
524, Bauchi, Bauchi State
Principal Bankers: First Bank of Nigeria Ltd; United Bank for
Africa Ltd
Financial Information:

	₦'000
Authorised capital	500
Paid-up capital	100

Principal Shareholders: Arc R Rajendram; M O Johnson
Date of Establishment: Established 1963, Incorporated 1981

RAJI BAKERIES LTD

PO Box 11, 8 Ahmadu Bello St, Jos, Plateau State
Tel: 2828
Cable: Raji Bakeries, Jos

Directors: Y Y Raji

PRINCIPAL ACTIVITIES: Manufacturers of bread and
confectionery

RALEIGH INDUSTRIES (NIGERIA) LTD

11/12 Mai Malari Rd, Bompai Industrial Estate, PO Box 2043,
Kano
Tel: 5321/3
Cable: Ralind Kano
Telex: 77124 Raling Ng

Chairman: Alhaji Aminu Dantata
Directors: Alhaji Nababa Badamasi,
Alhaji Zakari Muhammad,
Alhaji Aliyu Daneji,
I H Phillips,
R A L Roberts,
J B Dunnill (Managing)
Senior Executives: P E Abbott (Works Manager),
C J Hoare (Financial),
E R K Mackay (Sales)

PRINCIPAL ACTIVITIES: Manufacturers of bicycles, bicycle
components and spare parts
Branch Offices: 17 Gbajuma (Breadfruit St), PO Box 1188,
Lagos, Cable Ralsale Lagos, Tel 662488; PO Box 11, Port
Harcourt, Rivers State, Tel 223530; PO Box 461, Sapele,
Bendel State
Principal Bankers: United Bank for Africa Ltd; First Bank of
Nigeria Ltd; Icon Ltd (Merchant Bankers)

Principal Shareholders: T I Raleigh Industries Ltd, UK
Date of Establishment: 1st October 1973
No of Employees: 350

RAMONU ALABI, S B, & COMPANY

34 Docemo St, Lagos
Chairman: Ramonu Alabi

Directors: Mukaila Ramonu, Bashiru Ramonu
Senior Executives: Yinusa Ibrahim (Sales Manager),
Rasaki Ibrahim (Sales)

PRINCIPAL ACTIVITIES: Suppliers of pharmaceuticals products
Principal Agencies: Sun High Trading Company Ltd, Taiwan;
Annelies Grunwald, West Germany
Branch Offices: 53 Iga-Idungaran St, Lagos
Subsidiary/Associated Companies: R Mikaila & Sons; R
Mickyson Industrial Company
Principal Bankers: First Bank of Nigeria Ltd
Financial Information:

	₦'000
Authorised capital	50
Paid-up capital	17
Profits	30

Principal Shareholders: Alhadji Ibrahim Alabi
Date of Establishment: 10th February 1950

RAMSON MELLAMBY & COMPANY LTD

3 Olabode Close, Ilupeju Estate, Mushin, PO Box 1065, Lagos
Tel: 653896, 842016
Cable: Meehar Lagos

Chairman: R M Laniyan (also Managing Director)
Directors: A A Alli, B Laniyan

PRINCIPAL ACTIVITIES: General traders, suppliers of
agricultural equipment, building materials, chemicals,
fertilisers, household goods, food, etc
Branch Offices: 37 Orile Rd, Tabon Tabon, Agege; 48
Ogbomosho Rd, Kaduna; 12 Pump St, Jos
Principal Bankers: Wema Bank Ltd

Principal Shareholders: Chairman and directors as described

RANK XEROX (NIGERIA) LTD

Block C Plot 3 Matori Scheme, Oshodi, PMB 21314, Ikeja, Lagos

Tel: 962421
Chairman: Professor A Ogunsheye
Directors: G Milton,
G P Thompson (Managing Director),
D A Thompson,
C O Lawson,
O Fajemirokun,
Dr N Graham-Douglas,
A Ade-Kaka

PRINCIPAL ACTIVITIES: Office equipment suppliers
Principal Agencies: Rank Xerox International
Branch Offices: 21/23 Odunlami St, Lagos; SW8/1488 Lagos
Bye-Pass, Molete, Ibadan; 15e Bello Rd, PO Box 6282,
Bompai, Kano; Afrinsure House, Zik Ave, Enugu; Atari
Chambers, 2 Ring Rd, Benin City; 6 Kachia Rd, Kaduna; 9
Moscow Rd, PMB 5979, Port Harcourt; Edewor Shopping
Centre, Warri/Sapele Rd, Warri
Principal Bankers: Chase Merchant Bank Nigeria Ltd; United
Bank for Africa Ltd; First Bank of Nigeria Ltd

Principal Shareholders: Rank Xerox Ltd; Henry Stephens Ltd
Date of Establishment: March 1974
No of Employees: 417

RAPID ELECTRICAL & MECHANICAL COMPANY NIGERIA LTD (REMCO)

58 Fosberry Rd, PO Box 29, Calabar, Cross River State
Tel: 222610
Cable: Remco

Chairman: Chief William E Ufot
Directors: Oboe A Umoh (Administraion),
Udoh H Unang-Ekong (Electrical Department Manager),
Chief Dr Okoi Arikpo (Vice-President),
Rex M A Udom,
M A Udom (President and Managing Director)
Senior Executives: Ramesh Shandilly (Project Manager),
U P Oton (Project Engineer, Electrical),

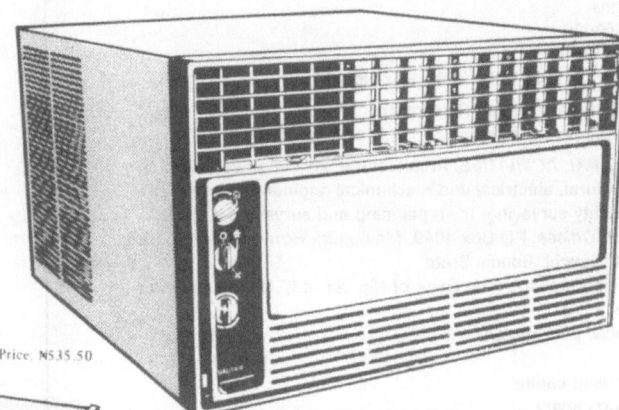
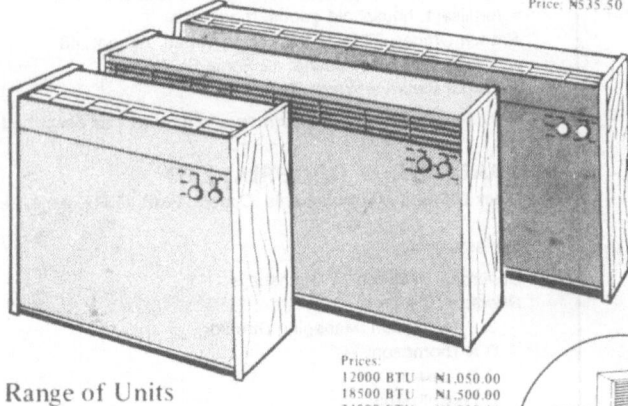
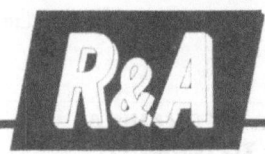

Magnus Akpan (PR Officer and Co-Ordinator),
Engr Danilo Araham Chua,
Engr Hendrik Mulder

PRINCIPAL ACTIVITIES: Building and civil engineering
contractors; electrical and mechanical engineering, suppliers
of building materials, and agricultural machinery;
transporters; consultants

Principal Agencies: AEI Nigeria Ltd; Gemco Engineers, Holland;
United Project Consultants, Holland; Kobe, Japan; ETTDC
Ltd, India, etc

Branch Offices: PO Box 219, Ikot Ekpene, Cross River State;
Okpoto Ete Town, Ikot Abasi, PO Box 44, Cross River State;
Lagos; Abuja; Ibadan; Port Harcourt; Aba; Ghana; Holland;
Philippines

Associated Companies: Concord International Design Partners &
Associates Groups (CIDPAD) Ltd; ETECO Ltd; Rian Ltd; AEI
Nigeria Ltd; UPC/Remco Ltd

Principal Bankers: Mercantile Bank Nigeria Ltd; First Bank of
Nigeria Ltd; United Bank for Africa Ltd

Financial Information:

	₦'000
Authorised capital	1,000
Paid-up capital	405
Sales turnover	2,200
Profits	800

Principal Shareholders: Chairman and directors as described
Date of Establishment: 18th May 1976
No of Employees: 1,240

RAYCON & COMPANY (NIGERIA) LTD

PO Box 568, Warri/Sapele Rd, Opposite Union Bank Efurun,
Warri, Bendel State
Tel: 230935

PRINCIPAL ACTIVITIES: Building and civil engineering
contractors

RAYMOND CONSTRUCTORS (NIGERIA) LTD

Investment House, Suite 213, 2 1/25 Broad Street, PO Box
10019, Lagos
Tel: 662956
Cable: Raymondint Lagos
Telex: 21818

Chairman: S O Akinwunmi
Directors: A A Akinwunmi (Executive Director),
J S K Macgregor,
Alhaji M S Malumfashi,
G Papayoti (Managing),
E M Draper (General Manager)
Senior Executives: Philip Cannell (Chief Engineer),
Brian Davies (Financial Controller),
Anthony Uche (Chief Geotechnical Engineer),
Olufemi Ogunmuyiwa (Foundation Engineer),
Olakekan Odubayo (Chief Accountant)

PRINCIPAL ACTIVITIES: Subsoil investigations, foundation piling
works, construction of jetties and marine facilities, heavy civil
engineering construction

Branch Offices: Port Harcourt Shipyard, Reclamation Rd, PO
Box 1887, Port Harcourt, Tel 331690/334313, Telex 61216

Subsidiary Companies: Raymond International Inc, USA; Kaiser
Engineers, USA

Principal Bankers: Societe Generale Bank (Nig) Ltd; Savannah
Bank (Nig) Ltd

Financial Information:
Authorised capital ₦ 1,000,000

Principal Shareholders: Sylokin Investments Ltd 60%; Raymond
International Builders Inc, 40%
Date of Establishment: 24th September 1979
No of Employees: 300

REA REAL PROPERTY INVESTMENTS (NIGERIA) LTD

New Africa House, 31 Marina, Lagos
Tel: 664431
Cable: Kennels

Chairman: Alhaji Ahmadu Coomassie
Directors: Alhaji S Ahmed (Madakin Kano),
D L C Hunt,
A V Caddick

PRINCIPAL ACTIVITIES: Property investment
Principal Bankers: International Bank for West Africa Ltd
Financial Information:

	₦'000
Authorised capital	1,500
Paid-up capital	800
Turnover (1981)	2,000
Profits (1981)	500

Principal Shareholders: Grea Real Property Investments Ltd
Date of Establishment: 1965

RECKITT & COLMAN (NIGERIA) LTD

PO Box 2157, 21-25 Broad St, Lagos
Tel: 654895
Cable: Mustard

Chairman: M O Falomo
Directors: G T Welch (Managing),
F D Lakanu,
M A Southern,
V A Kushimo
Senior Executives: J A Exley (Technical Services Manager)

PRINCIPAL ACTIVITIES: Manufactures of air fresheners, laundry
aids and polish; agents and general trading
Principal Agencies: Reckitt & Colman (Overseas) Ltd
Principal Bankers: First Bank of Nigeria

Principal Shareholders: Reckitt & Colman PLC

RECORD MANUFACTURERS OF NIGERIA LTD

Plot 13 Block A, Ogba Industrial Estate, PMB 1511, Ikeja, Lagos
Cable: Recordman

PRINCIPAL ACTIVITIES: Manufacturers of gramophone records,
cassettes and cartridges, record sleeves and labels

RECORD MARKET (NIGERIA) LTD

PO Box 6371, 89 Bamgbose St, Lagos
Tel: 657945
Cable: Rodpub

PRINCIPAL ACTIVITIES: Manufacturers, distributors and
importers of records and tapes

REGENCY (OVERSEAS) COMPANY LTD

PO Box 856, 13 Abebe Village Rd, Iganmu, Lagos
Tel: 833484

PRINCIPAL ACTIVITIES: Building and civil engineering
contractors and paint manufacturers

REGENT HOTEL

23/29 Abibu Oki St, PO Box 489, Lagos
Tel: 635787, 635858, 637609
Cable: Regotel

PRINCIPAL ACTIVITIES: Hoteliers

REGGIO BUILDERS LTD

4 Udoji St, Ogui New Layout, PMB 1647, Enugu, Anambra State
Tel: 252559
Cable: Reggio Enugu

PRINCIPAL ACTIVITIES: Building and civil engineering
contractors

Date of Establishment: 1976

REHAU PLASTIKS (NIGERIA) LTD

Plot 13 Iganmu Industrial Estate, Eric Moore Rd, PO Box 329,
  Apapa, Lagos
Tel: 837550

Chairman: Chief Y O Lawal
Directors: Ramal Lawal, Yaya Lawal, D O Fasami, E O Oke,
  Dr J Faniran
Senior Executives: E O Adebomi (Administrative
    Manager/Company Secretary),
  H Frischmann (Production Manager),
  'Wole Faniran (Office Manager),
  M O Oke (Accountant)

PRINCIPAL ACTIVITIES: Suppliers of plastic products;
  manufacturers of plastic waste pipes and pressure pipes
Associated Companies: Plastex Nigeria Ltd; Lopin Ltd
Principal Bankers: United Bank for Africa Ltd

Date of Establishment: 1976

RECORD MANUFACTURERS OF NIGERIA LTD.,

MUSIC

BY

THE LEADING NIGERIAN RECORD COMPANY

FOR NIGERIAN MUSIC AND INTERNATIONAL REPERTOIRE

MANUFACTURER OF RECORDINGS
MASTERS STAMPERS PRESSING
PRINTING LABELS AND COVER SLEEVES
RECORDING — MASTERS

R. M. N. L.
Plot 13 — Block "A" OGBA INDUSTRIAL ESTATE
ACME ROAD. OGBA. IKEJA
LAGOS — STATE
CABLE: RECORDMAN — IKEJA

REISS & CO (NIGERIA) LTD

PO Box 678, 71 Apapa Rd, Ebute-Metta, Lagos
Tel: 834215
Cable: Reico
Telex: 21161

Chairman: Chief Edward Adewole Adefusika
Directors: J C L Torenvlied (Managing),
  B M Jokoh,
  J A Petrus van Loon,
  N Nwakile Unigwe

PRINCIPAL ACTIVITIES: Building and civil engineering
  contractors
Principal Agencies: G & R Gilbert Ltd, UK; Stewart Wales, UK;
  N Foss Electric, Denmark; Mather & Platt Ltd, UK
Branch Offices: 82 Azikiwe Rd, PMB 7187, Aba, Imo State; 20
  Mission Rd, PO Box 455, Benin City, Bendel State; 28
  Bedwell St, PO Box 1115, Calabar, Cross River State; 63

Murtala Way, PMB 3174, Kano, Tel 4420; Plot 6, Kachia Rd,
  Kakuri, Kaduna South, PO Box 1439, Kaduna; 16 Iweka Rd,
  PO Box 1955, Onitsha, Anambra State, Tel 210779; 2A
  Robert Rd, PO Box 458, Warri, Bendel State; Reicotec
  Division: Wholesale Department and Distribution Centre, Plot
  7, House 32515, Isolo Industrial Layout, Lagos
Associated Companies: Adefusika Trading Co Ltd; Fusi
  Industrial Supplies
Principal Bankers: First Bank of Nigeria Ltd

RELIANCE BUSINESS CONSULTATIONS

Plot 3 Mile 12, Bus Stop, Ikorodu Rd, PO Box 2565, Lagos

PRINCIPAL ACTIVITIES: Business consultants

RELIANCE GROUP OF COMPANIES

R1 Lagos St, PO Box 1795, Kaduna
Tel: 211524, 213833
Telex: 71291 Remco Ng

Directors: M Yode Titiloye (Managing Director)

PRINCIPAL ACTIVITIES: Builder's merchants; distributors of
  paints, sanitary-ware, wall tiles, asbestos products, glass,
  flush doors and plywood; manufacturers of school and
  technical equipment; wholesalers
Branch Offices: Opposite Ilorin Grammar School, Ilorin; Abdu St,
  Minna; Factory: 5 Maiubi Close, Kaduna South
Subsidiary Companies: Reliance Investment & Supplies Ltd;
  Reliance Equipment Manufacturing Co Ltd; Reliance
  Contractors Ltd

RELIANCE INTERNATIONAL (NIGERIA) LTD

PO Box 647, 119 Agbani Rd, Enugu, Anambra State
Tel: 255494

PRINCIPAL ACTIVITIES: Building and civil engineering
  contractors; fire extinguisher engineers

RENAISSANCE ASSURANCE COMPANY LTD

3/5 Sulu Bolaji St, PO Box 4818, Lagos
Tel: 664079, 664008, 664150
Cable: Renaicon Lagos

Chairman: Chief R A Fani-Kayode
Directors: Chief B Olowofoyeku, Chief Sabo Sowemimo, V A
  Haffner, A O Duduyemi
Senior Executives: M A Akinsemoyin (Chief Executive),
  T O Balogun (Executive Director),
  E U N Okoye (Secretary/Accountant),
  J A Akindiya (Underwriting Manager)

PRINCIPAL ACTIVITIES: Insurance
Branch Offices: 21A Asa Rd, PO Box 459, Aba, Imo State; 136
  Akpakpava St, PMB 1516, Benin City, Bendel State; 63 New
  Market Rd, PO Box 759, Onitsha, Anambra State; Aje House,
  3rd Floor, PO Box 11387, Ibadan, Oyo State
Principal Bankers: National Bank of Nigeria Ltd; Societe
  Generale Bank (Nigeria) Ltd
Financial Information:

	N'000
Authorised capital	300
Paid-up capital	300

Principal Shareholders: The directors
Date of Establishment: 1970

RENAISSANCE MARBLE WORKS LTD

Km 1, Lagos/Badagry Rd, PO Box 1279, Lagos
Tel: 834451

Directors: E Castellani, E Biagini

PRINCIPAL ACTIVITIES: Marble products

RENDEZVOUS GROUP HOTELS (NIGERIA) LTD

1 Textile Rd, PMB 2136, Kaduna
Tel: 213502
Cable: Rendez Kaduna

Chairman: Chief L O Nnaji
Directors: Patrick C Nnaji, Emmanuel E Nnaji, Pauline U Nnaji, Felicia N Nnaji, Francisca O Nnaji, Felicia Nnaji, Jane Nnaji, Vivian Nnaji
Senior Executives: J A Nwagwu (Manager),
   G O L Anaejionu (Accountant/Secretary),
   A I Okoye (Rec Manager),
   G O Nzeh (Supervisor)

PRINCIPAL ACTIVITIES: Catering; civil engineering contractors
Branch Offices: Kaduna; Zaria
Principal Bankers: International Bank for West Africa Ltd; Standard Bank of Nigeria Ltd

No of Employees: 208

REX RADIO ELECTRONIC COMPANY LTD

54 and 83 Ogunmokun St, PO Box 184, Mushin, Lagos

PRINCIPAL ACTIVITIES: Suppliers of electronic equipment

REYNOLDS CONSTRUCTION COMPANY (NIGERIA) LTD

Plot 1300/A, Akin Adesola Street, Victoria Island, PO Box 5990, Lagos
Tel: 611437, 610186
Telex: 22498 Reynco Ng

Chairman: Chief S O Fadahunsi
Directors: E Porat,
   M Shawkan,
   D Gur (Managing)
Senior Executives: N Koerner (Branch Manager - Port-Harcourt),
   Y Gutstadt (Branch Manager - Calabar),
   E Sela (Branch Manager - Enugu),
   Y Diaz (Branch Manager - Enugu),
   E Klein (Branch Manager - Iwuru),
   M Rozanes (Chief Controller)

PRINCIPAL ACTIVITIES: Civil engineering, building, and general contractors: highways, hospitals, hotels, housing, public building infrastructure, mechanical - electrical works
Branch Offices: PO Box 97, Calabar; PO Box 815, Enceple; PO Box 5349, Port Harcourt; PO Box 206, Gboko
Principal Bankers: First Bank of Nigeria Ltd
Financial Information:

	N'000
Authorised capital	1,650
Paid-up capital	1,650
Turnover	70,000

Principal Shareholders: Reynolds Construction Company, New York Plus Nigerian Individual Shareholders
Date of Establishment: 1969
No of Employees: 6,000

RHINE-SCHELDE-VEROLME ENGINEERS

Midmotors Building, 4th Floor, 174 Broad St, Lagos Island, PO Box 18, Lagos
Tel: 634218
Telex: 21240 Holric

Directors: L Los (General Manager)

PRINCIPAL ACTIVITIES: Construction and design engineering

RIBWAY GROUP OF COMPANIES

95 Igbosere Rd, PO Box 3333, Lagos
Tel: 634558
Cable: Ribgroup Lagos

Chairman: Chief E E Eribo
Directors: Dr E O Eribo (Managing Director),
   Mrs Omosede Eribo
Senior Executives: M O Orhue (General Marketing Manager),
   R I Odenore (General Operation Manager),
   W G Bateson (General Production Manager),
   T P Baevski (General Manager Construction)

PRINCIPAL ACTIVITIES: Suppliers of carpets, textiles, foam, poly products, balloons and gloves, tyre retreading and road construction, commercial printing
Branch Offices: 1 Ribway Close, Oliha's Quarters PO Box 294, Benin City, Benin State
Subsidiary Companies: Nigerian Carpet Mfg Co Ltd (see separate entry); Ribway Printers Ltd; Ribway Tyre Retreading; Ribway Farm Estate Ltd; Ribway Construction Co Ltd; Edo Textile Mills Ltd; Nigerian Urethane Co Ltd (see separate entry)
Principal Bankers: African Continental Bank Ltd; New Nigeria Bank Ltd; Union Bank Ltd

No of Employees: 2,000

RIBWAY TYRE RETREADING CO LTD

PO Box 577, Benin City, Bendel State
Tel: 240654

PRINCIPAL ACTIVITIES: Retreading of tyres
Financial Information: Part of Ribway Group of Companies

RICHARD RIKO (NIGERIA) LTD

51 Edebiri St, Off Ekenwan Rd, Behind Hotel Joromi, PO Box 98, Benin City, Bendel State

PRINCIPAL ACTIVITIES: Cosmetics industry and soap

RICHAS ENGINEERING WORKS COMPANY LTD

79 Zik Ave, PO Box 1, Enugu, Anambra State
Tel: 2522244
Cable: Rixhas Enugu

Chairman: Engineer R C Agu
Directors: B O Okonkwo, J A Agunta
Senior Executives: C O Anozie

PRINCIPAL ACTIVITIES: Electrical/mechanical engineering contractors
Branch Offices: 25 Okigwe Rd, Owerri; 22 Lagos St, Umuahia; Lagos; Nsukka; Onitsha; Aba; Benin City; Makurdi
Principal Bankers: Co-operative Bank Ltd
Financial Information:

	N'000
Authorised capital	400
Paid-up capital	250

No of Employees: 100

RIDA CONSTRUCTION COMPANY LTD

Intra House, 16 Ijora Causeway, PO Box 2392, Lagos
Tel: 832173

Directors: M A Bohsoli (Managing Director)

PRINCIPAL ACTIVITIES: Construction

RIDA NATIONAL DISTRIBUTORS LTD

16 Ijora Causeway, Ijora, Lagos
Tel: 962771, 962773
Cable: Ridalab
Telex: 21391 Ridala

Chairman: Alhaji Sule Katagum
Directors: Alhaji I Owodunni, G Ade Owodunni, T A Agha, A G Sabbagh
Senior Executives: T A Agha (Managing Director)

PRINCIPAL ACTIVITIES: Vehicles and spare parts distributor, motor vehicles and components
Principal Agencies: Hino Motors Ltd, Japan; Intra Motors (Nig) Ltd, Lagos
Branch Offices: State Highway, Ilupeju Industrial Estate, GPO Box 1243, Lagos; 16 Umaru Babura Rd, Bompai, PMB 3154, Kano; 78 Lagos Bye-Pass, Oke-Ado, PMB 5243, Ibadan; PO Box 2371, Port Harcourt, Rivers State
Associated Companies: Intra Motors (Nigeria) Ltd
Principal Bankers: Bank of Credit and Commerce International Ltd
Financial Information:

	N'000
Authorised capital	10,000
Paid-up capital	2,000
Turnover	5,428
Profits	94

Principal Shareholders: Intra Motors (Nig) Ltd
Date of Establishment: January 1976
No of Employees: 95

RIDA NATIONAL PLASTICS LTD
PMB 1122, Ikeja, Lagos
Tel: 963113/6
Telex: 21391 Lagos

PRINCIPAL ACTIVITIES: Manufacturers of vinyl; vinyl asbestos floor tiles and polythene film

RIMAX COMPUTER SERVICES LTD
6 Adebiaye St, Off Tejuosho, Surulere, Lagos
Cable: Rimax Lagos

Chairman: Richard L Okwara
Directors: David Etakpofe
Senior Executives: C I Anwuna (Software/Hardware Co-ordinator),
E U Osakwe (Public Relations),
F N Ejieke (Chief Accountant),
Bola Jimoh (Administrative Manager),
Yemisi Olubi (Personnel Manager)

PRINCIPAL ACTIVITIES: Computer assembly and marketing, computer systems consultancy, computer training; printing and publishing
Principal Agencies: Computer Technology Ltd, UK; Metro Data Equipment Ltd, UK
Branch Offices: 35 Hawley St, Lagos; 142nd East Circular Rd, Benin; A216 Bakori Rd, Kaduna
Principal Bankers: Barclays Bank Nigeria Ltd; International Bank for West Africa

No of Employees: 200

RIOCO (NIGERIA) LTD
Plot 160, Oyadiran Estate, PMB 1013, Yaba-Lagos
Tel: 860119

Chairman: Anthony Chuks Iwenjiora
Directors: Rita Oyibo Iwenjiora
Senior Executives: Oliver Osadebey Anam (Pharmaceutical Manager),
Eko Udo Eko (Secretary),
Mfon William Mfon (Sales Representative)

PRINCIPAL ACTIVITIES: Suppliers of pharmaceuticals, natural health products, cosmetics, body care products and general goods: building and civil engineering contractors
Principal Agencies: Braswell Inc, USA; Cosvetics Laboratories, USA; Standard Research Laboratories, USA; GB International Inc, USA; American Health Products, USA; Quest Research Laboratories, USA; Peak Laboratories, USA
Branch Offices: 4 Tillingbourne Gardens, London N3 3IJ
Principal Bankers: Union Bank of Nigeria Ltd

Financial Information:

	N'000
Authorised capital	300
Paid-up capital	250
Turnover	500
Profits	75

Principal Shareholders: Anthony Chuks Iwenjiora; Rita Oyibo Iwenjiora
Date of Establishment: 15th December 1978
No of Employees: 25

RISONPALM LTD
35 Aba Rd, PMB 5236, Port Harcourt, Rivers State
Tel: 226856, 226871
Cable: Risonpalm

Chairman: Dr C Oyolu
Directors: L L Loolo,
B A Lawson,
T O Abigo,
G S Beke,
Permanent Secretary (Ministry of Economic Development),
Permanent Secretary (Ministry of Agriculture and Natural Resources)
Senior Executives: G D K Briggs (Acting General Manager),
M D Opuiyo (Acting Secretary),
G O Omereji (Senior Division Manager),
D N Onyebuenyi (Mills Superintendent),
J S A Pepple (Accountant)

PRINCIPAL ACTIVITIES: Production and processing of palm fruits
Principal Agencies: Ministry of Agriculture and Natural Resources
Branch Offices: Elele Oil Palm Estate, Elele, Rivers State
Principal Bankers: Pan African Bank Ltd

Principal Shareholders: Government-owned company
No of Employees: 2,000

RIVBANK INSURANCE COMPANY LTD
38 Ikwerre Rd, PO Box 177, Port Harcourt
Tel: 335100, 335102, 335462

Chairman: D D Obunge
Senior Executives: S A T Amukele (General Manager),
E S Tekena (Assistant General Manager),
T A K Wenah (Chief Accountant),
W G Inokoba (Company Secretary),
T N C Asiji (Life/Pensions Manager),
B A Aprekum (Fire/Accidents Manager),
J Krukru (Lagos Area Manager)

PRINCIPAL ACTIVITIES: Insurance business
Branch Offices: 35/37 Martins Street, PO Box 7220, Lagos, Tel 660859; 30 Oguta Street, Onitsha, Anambra State; 1 Station Rd, Ahoada, Rivers State; 115 Douglas Rd, Owerri, Imo State; 10 Hospital Rd, Bori, Rivers State; SW9/229B Ago-Taylor, PO Box 4880, Ibadan, Oyo State, Tel 411203; Ia Galadima Rd, Kano; 144 Trans Amadi Industrial Layout, Port Harcourt, Rivers State; Elele Roundabout, Elele, Port Harcourt, Rivers State
Principal Bankers: Pan African Bank Ltd
Financial Information:

	N'000
Authorised capital	2,000
Paid-up capital	800
Turnover (1981)	8,000

Principal Shareholders: Rivers State Ministry of Finance, Port Harcourt; Rivers State Ministry of Trade & Industry, Port Harcourt
Date of Establishment: 1972
No of Employees: 400

RIVERS STATE NEWSPAPER CORPORATION

4 Ikwerre Rd, Diobu, PMB 5072, Port Harcourt, Rivers State
Tel: 21773/4
Cable: Tide Port Harcourt
Telex: 61144 Tide Ng

Chairman: Reginald Furo
Directors: Chief J A Akon, Chief E O O Oriahwa, P Okosi, B
    Wifa, E Obonna, Chief R U Akigha, J Inko-Tariah, D J
    Dambo
Senior Executives: D Amucha (General Manager),
    M Bara-Hart (Editor-in-Chief),
    J Yekwe (Production),
    M Damboh,
    J Bakor (Chief Accountant)

PRINCIPAL ACTIVITIES: Lithographers; newpapers and
    calendars and letterpress printers
Branch Offices: Enugu; Owerri; Benin City; Kaduna
Subsidiary Companies: Nigerian Tide
Principal Bankers: First Bank of Nigeria Ltd; Pan African Bank
    Ltd

Principal Shareholders: Rivers State Government
No of Employees: 760

RIVERS STATE TOURIST & HOTEL CORPORATION

PMB 5004, 3 Olusegun Obasanjo Rd, Port Harcourt, Rivers
    State
Tel: 21754

PRINCIPAL ACTIVITIES: Hoteliers

RIVERS STATE TRANSPORT CORPORATION

PMB 5001, Port Harcourt, Rivers State
Tel: 228026, 22559

PRINCIPAL ACTIVITIES: Coach services from Port Harcourt to
    all the mainland area of Rivers State; water transport
    services

RIVERS VEGETABLE OIL COMPANY LTD

Reclamation Rd, Port Harcourt, Rivers State
Tel: 22177, 22243, 22196
Telex: 61153 Vegoil Ng

PRINCIPAL ACTIVITIES: Manufacturing of vegetable oil
Branch Offices: Factory: 80/84 Trans-Amadi Layout, Port
    Harcourt

ROAAG COMPANY (NIGERIA) LTD

Olapade Agoro Estate, Behind Govt College, Ibadan-Abeokuta
    Rd, PMB 5404, Ibadan, Oyo State
Tel: 412363
Cable: Roaagco
Telex: 31432 Roaag Ng

Chairman: Rev Prophet Roland Olapade Agoro
Directors: Olaitan Agoro, Omotunde Agoro, Olusola Agoro,
    Roland Olapade Agoro
Senior Executives: R O Agoro (Managing Director),
    S A Bolarinwa (Branch Manager Lagos/Ogun States),
    H A Oyeyemi (Plant Engineering Sales/Service Engineer),
    A Bakare (Electrical Engineer Sales/Service Engineer),
    O Michael (Branch Manager Ondo/Bendel States)

PRINCIPAL ACTIVITIES: Agents and general trading; suppliers
    of electrical equipment; power and industrial equipment;
    safety and security equipment; agricultural and irrigation
    equipment
Principal Agencies: Countryman Power Plants Ltd, UK;
    Dictaphone International AG, Switzerland; Identification
    Systems Inc, USA; Ello Power Plant Ltd, UK; Turner
    Machinery Ltd, UK
Branch Offices: 7 Balogun St, Anifowoshe, Off Awolowo Way,
    Ikeja, Lagos; Oba Adesida Rd, Akure, Ondo State; Olapade
    Agoro Estate, Behind Govt College, Apata, Ibadan
Principal Bankers: Cooperative Bank Ltd

Financial Information:

	₦'000
Authorised capital	100
Paid-up capital	100
Turnover (1980)	1,000

Principal Shareholders: Chairman and directors as described
Date of Establishment: 20th July 1973

ROAD AND GENERAL CONSTRUCTION COMPANY LTD

9 Goriola St, Victoria Island, PO Box 6070, Lagos
Tel: 610511, 614977

Directors: E Pacifici

PRINCIPAL ACTIVITIES: Civil engineering
Branch Offices: Eket

ROADS NIGERIA LTD

595 Club Rd, PO box 187, Kano,
Tel: 4469
Telex: 77231 Roanig

Chairman: Alhaji Musa Yar'Adua - Tafidan Katsina
Directors: Alhaji R A Aminu (Public Relations),
    J M Dansu (Administrative),
    P Kaura,
    Alhaji S M Jega,
    F Nienhuis (Managing),
    J Lucas,
    C B J Ribbert (Finance)
Senior Executives: O Ojetola (Chief Accountant),
    T O Jimoh (Purchase Manager)

PRINCIPAL ACTIVITIES: Construction of road, bridges, airfields
    and dams
Branch Offices: 2 Ashanti Rd, PMB 1053, Apapa; 10 Gombe Rd,
    PO Box 365, Bauchi; By Pass Rd, PO Box 24, Sokoto; Ikere
    Gorge Dam, PO Box 348, Iseyin; Mile 7, Zaria Rd, PMB 2090,
    Jos; Wuyo Biu Rd, PMB 528, Biu
Subsidiary Companies: Technical management agreement with
    Volker Stevin Roads a member of the Royal Volker Stevin, A
    Dutch Based International Construction Company
Principal Bankers: International Merchant Bank (Nigeria) Ltd;
    United Bank for Africa Ltd
Financial Information:

	₦'000
Authorised capital	15,000
Paid-up capital	7,500
Turnover (1982)	73,933
Profits after tax (1982)	2,936

Principal Shareholders: Royal Volker Stevin 40%; Sokoto
    Investment Company Ltd; Ministry of Finance Incorporated
Date of Establishment: 11th October 1974
No of Employees: 4,200

ROBERTS, T L, & COMPANY LTD

1 Alhaji Sikiru Otun Rd, Kuje Amuwo, Badagry Rd, PO Box
    2051, Lagos
Tel: 880384, 631336
Cable: Roberts Lagos

Directors: C W Shaw (Managing Director),
    Alhaji A A Kadiri,
    I B Degan

PRINCIPAL ACTIVITIES: Building and civil engineering
    contractors
Principal Agencies: Smid & Hollander, Holland
Principal Bankers: United Bank for Africa Ltd
Financial Information:

	₦'000
Authorised capital	200
Paid-up capital	200

Date of Establishment: 1959

ROBERTSON, H H, (NIGERIA) LTD
Emene Industrial Layout, PO Box 1590, Enugu, Anambra State
Tel: 255674/5
Telex: 51289 HHRNIG Ng

Directors: A G Aldwinckle (Managing)
Senior Executives: M J C Barlow (Sales Manager)

PRINCIPAL ACTIVITIES: Manufacturers of roofing and cladding, sheets together with ancillary ventilation equipment
Branch Offices: 28 Saka Tinubu Street, Victoria Island; Lagos, Tel 611584; A10 Lagos Street, Kaduna
Associated Companies: Robertson Construction (Nigeria) Ltd
Principal Bankers: Union Bank of Nigeria Ltd
Financial Information:

	N'000
Authorised capital	1,000
Paid-up capital	1,000

Date of Establishment: Incorporated 2nd March 1978

ROBINS, A H, INTERNATIONAL COMPANY LTD
PO Box 493, Yaba, Lagos
Tel: 861282

Senior Executives: Brian S Ulyatt

PRINCIPAL ACTIVITIES: Suppliers of pharmaceuticals and cosmetics

ROCHE (NIGERIA) LTD
PO Box 463, Ikeja, 31 Planning Way, Ilupeju, Lagos
Tel: 935109

Chairman: Chief C O Ogunbanjo
Directors: Alhaji A Mai-Sango,
    G O Onosode,
    Chief J O Udoji,
    R Piness (Managing),
    Dr M Altwegg,
    Dr W A Werner

PRINCIPAL ACTIVITIES: Suppliers of pharmaceuticals
Principal Agencies: C H Bohringer and Sohn, West Germany
Principal Shareholders: Swiss (40%); Nigerians (60%)
Date of Establishment: 1976

ROD PUBLICITY LTD
178 Palm Ave, PO Box 6371, Mushin, Lagos
Cable: Rodpub

Chairman: Chief Remi Adeoye (also Managing Director)
Directors: Chief Akin Davies (Public Relations),
    Chief Olu Falaiye (Creative Director),
    Mallam Turi Mohammed,
    Bode Senbanjo
Senior Executives: Ayo Abdul (General Manager),
    Wale Odewole (Client Service Group Head),
    Tunde Harrison (Public Relations Manager)

PRINCIPAL ACTIVITIES: Advertising and public relations
Associated Companies: Dewe Rogerson Ltd
Principal Bankers: United Bank for Africa Ltd; Bank of the North; Societe Generale Bank (Nigeria) Ltd
Financial Information:

	N'000
Authorised capital	200
Paid-up capital	99
Turnover	2,000

Principal Shareholders: Chief Remi Adeoye; Chief Olu Falaiye; Chief Akin Davies
Date of Establishment: 1971

ROKANA INDUSTRIES LTD
5 Akintola Cole Crescent, Ikeja, Lagos
Telex: 20202 Tds 038

PRINCIPAL ACTIVITIES: Manufacturers of toiletries
Principal Bankers: Union Bank of Nigeria Ltd

ROMAIN, H W, & SON LTD
17/18 Club Rd, PO Box 349, Kano
Tel: 2290, 2873
Cable: Romain Kano

PRINCIPAL ACTIVITIES: Manufacturers of steel products, steel structures, tanks, trailers, body works, etc

RON MINING AND DEVELOPMENT COMPANY LTD
Kuru 3 Hq, Jos, Plateau State

PRINCIPAL ACTIVITIES: Mining of metal ore

Principal Shareholders: Bisichi-Jantar (Nigeria) Ltd, Jos, Plateau State

RONKE COMMERCIAL ENTERPRISES
Tawaliu Bello St, PO Box 8378, Lagos
Tel: 650887, 680732

PRINCIPAL ACTIVITIES: Exporters and importers of textiles, cosmetics, and general goods

ROOMANS ENELI FLYNN & COMPANY
49 Awolowo Rd, Ikoyi, PO Box 1168, Lagos
Tel: 682303, 683137
Cable: Refinsure
Telex: 22307 Ng

Chairman: Sunday Dankaro
Directors: G I C Eneli,
    J J Roomans (Managing),
    H Flynn

PRINCIPAL ACTIVITIES: Insurance broking
Subsidiary/Associated Companies: Manlyn SA, Luxemburg
Principal Bankers: Union Bank of Nigeria Ltd
Financial Information:

	N'000
Authorised capital	24
Paid-up capital	24
Turnover	5,000

Principal Shareholders: S Dankaro; G I C Eneli; Manlyn SA
Date of Establishment: 4 December 1974

RORO TERMINAL COMPANY (NIGERIA) LTD
42/44 Warehouse Rd, PO Box 767, Apapa, Lagos
Tel: 876552
Telex: 21226 Lagos

Chairman: Chief Bode Akindele
Directors: A Grimaldi, J Maillier, P Meldal, B Midander, E Rothschild

PRINCIPAL ACTIVITIES: Roro operators
Branch Offices: Operations Office: Tincan Island Port, Berth 9
Date of Establishment: December 1978

ROSAAB INDUSTRIAL DESIGN LTD
11 Bashua St, Off Morocco Rd, Shomolu, PO Box 207, Lagos
Tel: 845180
Cable: Rosindes Lagos

Chairman: Abiodun Odojukan (also Managing Director)
Directors: Patience E Odojukan, Ibidapo A Odojukan
Senior Executives: Gerhard Bading (Production Manager),
    Mrs Ayo Adeyemi (Public Relations Manager),
    Ambrose Olisakwe (Maintenance Manager)

PRINCIPAL ACTIVITIES: Plastic welding and plastic designing, precision engraving, name plates and marking devices, lighted signs
Branch Offices: Car Number Plate Division, 18 Catholic Mission St, Lagos
Principal Bankers: United Bank for Africa Ltd
Date of Establishment: 1974

ROTAG ASSURANCE COMPANY LTD
1 Murtala Muhammed Way, PMB 2130, Jos, Plateau State
Tel: 3088
Cable: Rotag
Telex: 81137 Ng

Chairman: Prince Bolu Ademiluyi
Directors: R O Yussuff, T Ogunshuyi
Senior Executives: T Adenuga (General Manager)

PRINCIPAL ACTIVITIES: Insurance, life business planned
Branch Offices: 93 Oju-Elegbe Rd, Lagos; Ahmadu Bello Way, Sokoto; Ibrahim Taiwo St, Kano
Associated Companies: Rotag International Ltd
Principal Bankers: National Bank of Nigeria; Union Bank of Nigeria Ltd
Financial Information:

	N'000
Authorised capital	300
Paid-up capital	300
Turnover	1,000
Profits	100

No of Employees: 300

ROTIMI & SONS LTD
PO Box 1044, 78 Broad St, Lagos
Tel: 651587

PRINCIPAL ACTIVITIES: Building and civil engineering contractors

ROUSSEL (NIGERIA) LTD
5 Oba Adetona St, Ilupeju, PMB 1021, Mushin, Lagos
Tel: 962285

PRINCIPAL ACTIVITIES: Suppliers of pharmaceuticals

ROYAL EXCHANGE ASSURANCE (NIGERIA) LTD
New Africa House, 31 Marina, PO Box 112, Lagos
Tel: 663120, 663143
Cable: Foxhound

Chairman: Chief E J U Ndem
Directors: Alhaji S Ahmed, A Coomassie, Dr J Folayan, Dr S A Chuks-Orji, Alhaji S Idris, Alhaji S I Musa, A V Caddick, J D Brennan
Senior Executives: K A Onalaja (Managing Director), I O Oshosanya (General Manager)

PRINCIPAL ACTIVITIES: Insurance
Branch Offices: Apapa; Ibadan; Kano; Kaduna; Yola; Bauchi; Ikeja; Akure; Warri; Sokoto; Port Harcourt; Onitsha; Lagos; Maiduguri; Jos; Oshodi; Ilorin; Enugu; Benin; Aba
Principal Bankers: Union Bank of Nigeria Ltd
Financial Information:

	N'000
Authorised capital	2,000
Paid-up capital	1,200
Turnover	40,000
Profits	1,000

Principal Shareholders: Federal Government of Nigeria; Guardian Royal Exchange Assurance PLC; Bendel State Government; Bauchi State Government; Anambra State Government
Date of Establishment: 1921
No of Employees: 536

RUBERY OWEN FASTENERS (NIGERIA) LTD
Plot 3C Block A, Ilupeju Industrial Estate, Oshodi/Isolo Expressway, PMB 1155, Oshodi, Lagos
Cable: Ruberyfast Lagos
Telex: 21037 Dodco Ng

Directors: G S Eccleston (Managing Director), C E Dafinone, S A Onomakpome

PRINCIPAL ACTIVITIES: Distributors of industrial fasteners
Principal Agencies: Rubery Owen Fasteners, West Midlands, UK
Principal Bankers: First Bank of Nigeria Ltd

Date of Establishment: January 1977

RUNSEWE GROUP OF COMPANIES
45 Ibadan Rd, PO Box 277, Ijebu-Ode, Lagos
Cable: Runspares
Telex: 31169 Runst Ng

Chairman: A O Runsewe
Directors: Mrs C A Runsewe, A O Runsewe (Junior)
Senior Executives: T A Adenuga (Executive Director), M A Adenuga (Administrative Secretary), M A Olufeko (Group Co-ordinator), E I Akintaju (Service Engineer), O Okintoye (Accounts Supervisor), O A Luther (Acting Parts Manager)

PRINCIPAL ACTIVITIES: Agents and general trading; suppliers and servicers of agricultural equipment; civil engineering and construction; electrical and electronic equipment; hotels and catering; motor vehicles and components; suppliers of plastics, plastic products and safety equipment
Principal Agencies: Liechtech Ltd, Canada; Lockmasters of Alton, UK; Trustbuck, UK; L A Electronics, UK; Nissan Motor Co Ltd, Japan
Branch Offices: 32 Reclamation Rd, Lagos; 13 Ashogbon St, Lagos; 34A Great Bridge St, Lagos; Badagry Rd, Opposite 1st Gate to the Festac Village, Lagos; Abeokuta Rd, Ojota, Ikeja, Lagos; 42 New Court Rd, Ibadan; 20 Oba Adesida Rd, Akure, Ondo State
Subsidiary/Associated Companies: Afrotec Technical Services (Nigeria) Ltd; Onibu-Ore Industries Ltd; Amonat (Nigeria) Ltd; Afcon Engineering Co (Nigeria) Ltd; Model Electronics Co (Nigeria) Ltd; Aero Film Production Ltd
Principal Bankers: Union Bank of Nigeria Ltd; First Bank of Nigeria Ltd; United Bank for Africa; Co-operative Bank Ltd
Financial Information:

	N'000
Authorised capital	2,650
Paid-up capital	2,550
Turnover	25,000

Date of Establishment: 1949
No of Employees: 500

RUTAM LTD
225 Apapa Rd, PMB 1155, Apapa, Lagos
Tel: 836336, 836618

Chairman: Chief M C O Ibru
Directors: G M Ibru, A M Egoh, Chief A O Amuwo, A U Ibru
Senior Executives: Benson Akinola O Ogunlana (General Manager)

PRINCIPAL ACTIVITIES: Importers, distributors and servicers of automobiles and components, and heavy equipment
Principal Agencies: Peugeot Company of Nigeria Ltd, Kaduna
Principal Bankers: African Continental Bank Ltd; Union Bank of Nigeria Ltd; First Bank of Nigeria Ltd
Financial Information:

Paid-up capital	N 855,000

Principal Shareholders: Delta Freeze Ltd; Oteri Holdings Ltd; Ibru Sea Foods Ltd
No of Employees: 526

S & K ASBESTOS PRODUCTS LTD
PMB 1402, Ikeja, Lagos
Tel: Ota 25
Cable: Skasbestos Lagos

Chairman: Chief C M Smith
Directors: E B Odebunmi (Managing Director), Alhaji M O Owodunni, Chief O B Akin-Olugbade, Dr Klaus Bohnemann

Senior Executives: D Glaus (Factory Manager),
   O J Balogun (Controller of Finance/Administration),
   R B Osobemekun (Sales Manager),
   F A Odelola (Commercial Manager),
   G A Shobo (Administrative Manager)

PRINCIPAL ACTIVITIES: Manufacturers of asbestos cement
   products
Principal Bankers: United Bank for Africa Ltd
Financial Information:

	₦'000
Authorised capital	1,000
Paid-up capital	1,000
Sales turnover	5,200
Profits (gross)	800

Principal Shareholders: Keen Investors Nigeria Ltd; Impo &
   Expo Nigeria Ltd; M De Bank Transport Ltd; Wehrhahn
   Engineering, West Germany
No of Employees: 650

S A IJAGBEMI & SONS (NIGERIA) LTD
See IJAGBEMI, S A, & SONS (NIGERIA) LTD

S B BAKARE & BROTHERS LTD
See BAKARE, S B, & BROTHERS LTD

S B RAMONU ALABI & COMPANY
See RAMONU ALABI, S B, & COMPANY

S G BONOMI LTD
See BONOMI, S G, LTD

S N EZENNWA & SONS LTD
See EZENNWA, S N, & SONS LTD

S S ADEJORO & COMPANY LTD
See ADEJORO, S S, & COMPANY LTD

SABON SARA NIGERIA LTD
79 Sharala Industrial Area, PMB 3220, Kano
Tel: 4043

Directors: Alhaji Sani Abbas (Group Managing Director)

PRINCIPAL ACTIVITIES: Manufacturers of steel and wood
   furniture, metal doors and windows and also general steel
   construction

SAFA SPLINTS LTD
PO Box 1499, Eleiyele Industrial Layout, Ibadan, Oyo State
Tel: 410339, 410080
Cable: Safasplint, Ibadan
Telex: 31107 Nigmat

PRINCIPAL ACTIVITIES: Manufacturers of splints and skillets for
   match industry and particle boards

SAFNI LTD
17 Elsie Femi Pearse Street, Victoria Island, Lagos
Tel: 611757/9
Telex: 21855 Safni Ng

Chairman: Alhaji A D Rufai
Directors: R Vrebos,
   M Novakovic (Managing),
   Alhaji Musa Usman,
   Elias Khawam,
   Alhaji G Pokta,
   Mohamed Sallama
Senior Executives: V Videnovic (Plant Manager),
   H Cayet (Financial Controller),
   H Close (Business Development Manager),
   T A Babalola (Personnel Manager)

PRINCIPAL ACTIVITIES: Civil engineering and construction
Branch Offices: 101E Lamido Crescent, Kano; Udubo Branch,
   Bauchi State; Jebill Amba, Gongola State
Associated Companies: CFE International, Belgium
Principal Bankers: United Bank for Africa Ltd, ICON Ltd, Nal
   (Merchant Bank)

Date of Establishment: 12th December 1974
No of Employees: 875

SAGE CONSTRUCTIONS (NIGERIA) LTD
130 Broad St, Lagos
Tel: 633451

Directors: J Edozie (Director)

PRINCIPAL ACTIVITIES: Construction

SAIPEM NIGERIA LTD
PO Box 1909, Plot 1028 Ologun Agbaje St, Via Adeola Odeku,
   Victoria Island, Lagos
Tel: 682679
Telex: 21268 Agipoil Lagos

Directors: Luciano Imazio (General Manager)
Senior Executives: C Ornstein (District Manager, Port Harcourt)

PRINCIPAL ACTIVITIES: Engineering, construction, pipeline and
   drilling contractors
Branch Offices: 10 Nwobidike Nwanodi St, PO Box 5183, Port
   Harcourt, Tel 21856

SAKPOBA RUBBER ESTATE
Sakpoba, Via Sapele, Bendel State

PRINCIPAL ACTIVITIES: Production of crepe rubber

SALLEH, ALHAJI BABA M, & SONS (NIGERIA) LTD
Abbatoir Rd, Gamboru Ward, PO Box 178, Maiduguri, Borno
   State
Tel: 232818, 232535
Cable: Babasalleh Maiduguri

PRINCIPAL ACTIVITIES: Building/civil engineering contractors,
   transporters, suppliers of all building materials, dealers in all
   cotton and woollen materials
Branch Offices: Bauchi; Numan Gombe; Lagos; Kano; Kaduna

SALZGITTER (WA) LTD
Plot 105 Joel Ogunnaike St, Ikeja, PO Box 2115, Lagos
Tel: 961973
Cable: Sagstahl Lagos

Directors: G Bruch (General Manager)

PRINCIPAL ACTIVITIES: Designers, and suppliers of plant and
   equipment for metal industry

SAMMY & SONS CONTRACTS & STORES
PO Box 209, Kaduna

PRINCIPAL ACTIVITIES: General contractors and traders
Branch Offices: Uwani; Enugu; Apapa; Lagos

SAMS AGENCIES & MARITIME SERVICE (NIG)
42 St Michael's Rd, Aba, Imo State

Directors: S O Agomuoh

PRINCIPAL ACTIVITIES: Importation of motor vehicles and
   motorcycle spare parts and accessories, electrical
   accessories, building materials, freight forwarding and
   customs agents, manufacturers' and exporters'
   representatives
Principal Bankers: National Bank of Nigeria Ltd

SAMSUNG (NIGERIA) LTD

Plot 1303A Akin Adesola St, Victoria Island, PO Box 60394,
Ikoyi Secretariat, Lagos
Tel: 611060, 615051, 616365
Cable: Samsung Nigeria
Telex: 21808 Stars Ng; 22162 Stars Ng

Chairman: R K Okudzeto
Directors: Alhaji Abubakar Jibril, Alhaji Rabiu Bello, Raymond
K Okudzeto, Sae-Chang Song, Mu-Sung Yu, Sung-Rai Choi
Senior Executives: S H Hong (Manager),
C Bae (Manager),
J A Ojo (Accountant),
A N Ukaegbu (Assistant Manager)

PRINCIPAL ACTIVITIES: Importation, distribution, assembly and
service of agricultural equipment and communication
equipment. Exportation and importation and wholesale
distribution of general goods. Investment and financing
Principal Agencies: Samsung Company Ltd, Korea
Branch Offices: PO Box 509, Port Harcourt, Tel 333390
Principal Bankers: Union Bank of Nigeria Ltd; United Bank of
Africa; First Bank of Nigeria Ltd
Financial Information:

	N'000
Authorised capital	401
Paid-up capital	401
Turnover	10,000

Principal Shareholders: Promexport Int (Nig) Ltd; Samsung
Company Ltd, Korea
Date of Establishment: 14th December 1978

SANDOZ (NIGERIA) LTD

Plot 9 Block A, Gbagada Industrial Estate, PO Box 3873, Ikeja,
Lagos
Cable: Sandopharm/Sandocolour
Telex: 21531 via NET 070, Lagos

Chairman: Chief Alfred F Odulana
Directors: Bruno Stalder,
C M Pintaud,
Fred Egbe,
Chief Ade S Koleosho,
Oba Sikiru K Adetona,
His Highness Alhaji Ado Bayero,
W S Zerr (Managing Director)
Senior Executives: J Bielser (Manager, Dyes Division),
A J Zust/D. Skiadas (Marketing Adviser),
E A Aniatang (Head of Finance & Planning),
S C Okupa (Head of Accounts & Administration),
K Kryzsczyk (Technical Range Manager)

PRINCIPAL ACTIVITIES: Suppliers of dyestuffs, chemicals and
pharmaceuticals products
Principal Agencies: Sandoz Ltd, Switzerland; Biochemie MBH,
Austria; Sandoz (India) Ltd; Dianic, Greece; Meyhall; Sandoz
(Products) Ltd, London
Principal Bankers: Icon Ltd; First Bank of Nigeria Ltd; United
Bank for Africa Ltd; International Bank for West Africa Ltd
Financial Information:

	N'000
Authorised capital	600
Paid-up capital	600

Principal Shareholders: Sandoz Ltd, Basle
Date of Establishment: 11th August 1970

SANDWELL, P R, & CO (NIGERIA) LTD

PO Box 8374, 100 Olatunde Labinjo Ave, Obanikoro, Ikorodu
Rd, Lagos
Tel: 964284
Cable: Petrisand Lagos

Chairman: D G Hepburn
Directors: John M Rait (Managing),
O D S Olutimayin,
S B Ojo

PRINCIPAL ACTIVITIES: Engineering consultants, specialists in
pulp and paper, forest products etc
Branch Offices: Vancouver BC, Canada
Associated Companies: P R Sandwell and Co UK Ltd
Principal Bankers: Bank of Montreal, Canada

SANMI BREWERIES LTD

Z 211 Bolorunduro Street, Imelu, Ifewara Rd, PO Box 147,
Ilesha, Oyo State

PRINCIPAL ACTIVITIES: Brewing of beer and soft drinks

SANTA FE NIGERIA DEVELOPMENT COMPANY LTD

15A Waring Rd, Ikoyi, PO Box 878, Lagos
Tel: 684083
Cable: Santafe Lagos
Telex: 61107 Safeph Ng

Chairman: C L Elliott (also Managing Director)
Directors: Chief Dotun Okubanjo,
S C Okafor,
K K Beaty (Operations Manager),
Richard C Parsons
Senior Executives: A E W Watson (Directional Manager),
E A C Akuruka (Office Manager, Lagos)

PRINCIPAL ACTIVITIES: Onshore and offshore drilling
contractors
Branch Offices: Operations Office: PMB 5019, Port Harcourt
Principal Bankers: Savannah Bank of Nigeria Ltd; First Bank of
Nigeria Ltd

Date of Establishment: 1966
No of Employees: 350

SANTANA FURNITURE FACTORY LTD

13 Auno Rd, PO Box 172, Maiduguri, Borno
Tel: 232853
Cable: Santana Maiduguri
Telex: 82188

Directors: A U S Birma (Managing Director),
A U Kadafur,
A M P Garba,
M Tafida,
M S Birma

PRINCIPAL ACTIVITIES: Manufacturers of office, household,
hotel and school furniture
Principal Bankers: United Bank for Africa Ltd

No of Employees: 250

SANUSI BROTHERS (NIGERIA) LTD

Plot 9 Block A, Ogba Scheme, Ikeja Industrial Estate, PMB
1158, Ikeja, Lagos
Tel: 961103, 961486
Telex: 21462 Sanbro Ng

PRINCIPAL ACTIVITIES: Importers and suppliers of steel and
steel products
Principal Agencies: Sole agents for SGB Scaffolding Products
Branch Offices: 41 Ikorodu Rd, Yaba, Lagos, Tel 845775; 46
Ikorodu Rd, Mushin, Lagos, Tel 844496; SW7/250 Onireke St,
Old Ogunpa, Ibadan, Oyo State; Steel Factory Sales Office:
Oluyole Industrial Estate, Ring Rd, Ibadan, Tel 411228; 8
Independence Rd, PMB 3210, Kano, Tel 5728

SANYO (NIGERIA) LTD

PMB 78, U1, Post Office, Ibadan, Oyo State
Cable: Telerex Lagos

PRINCIPAL ACTIVITIES: Manufacturing and assemblying of
colour and black and white television sets, car audio
equipment, refrigerators, bottle coolers and radio cassette
recorders
Branch Offices: Factory: Ibadan-Ife Rd, Ibadan, Oyo State

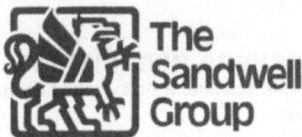
SAO ENGINEERING COMPANY LTD
PMB 21178, Airport Rd, Ikeja, Lagos
Tel: 962462
Cable: Sao Eng

Chairman: Engr S A Olukoya (also Managing Director)
Directors: B Olukoya, A O Shonibare
Senior Executives: D M Durohom (Project Enginer),
    C C Nwoke (Group Administrative Manager),
    A S Onafowora (Building Engineer)

PRINCIPAL ACTIVITIES: Building and civil engineering
    contractors
Subsidiary Companies: Lykoy Plant Hire
Principal Bankers: United Bank for Africa Ltd

Principal Shareholders: Engr S A Olukoya; B Olukoya; A O
    Shonibare
Date of Establishment: 28th August 1967
No of Employees: 200

SATT CONSTRUCTION (NIGERIA) LTD
134 Nnamdi Azikiwe St, Lagos
Tel: 846816, 846813

Chairman: George Ndu Obioha
Directors: Antonio Maglioni (Managing)

PRINCIPAL ACTIVITIES: Construction
Branch Offices: 139 Igbosere Rd, Lagos
Principal Bankers: United Bank for Africa
Financial Information:

	N'000
Authorised capital	500
Paid-up capital	500

Principal Shareholders: George Ndu Obioha; Ciro Rainone
Date of Establishment: 1976
No of Employees: 350

SAVANNA PRESS LTD
6 Zaria Rd, PMB 2122, Jos, Plateau State
Tel: 2217

PRINCIPAL ACTIVITIES: General offset and letterpress printers

SAVANNAH BANK OF NIGERIA LTD
19 Gbajumo St, PO Box 2317, Lagos State
Tel: 682522, 662663, 662941, 662954, 663284
Telex: 21274

Chairman: Alhaji Mahmud Aliyu
Directors: Jacob y Lot (Managing Director),
    E B Adegbite (Executive Director),
    Alhaji Mahmud Abubakar,
    Alhaji Bello Dange,
    Martin N Elechi,
    Stephen B Hunt (Vice Chairman),
    John D Hurd (Executive Director),
    David M McVeigh,
    J C Kearney

PRINCIPAL ACTIVITIES: Banking
Branch Offices: 138/146 Broad St, Lagos; Apapa; Kano; Port
    Harcourt; Jos; Kaduna; Ibadan
Financial Information: Affiliate of Bank of American NT and SA,
    USA

	N'000
Authorised capital	10,000
Paid-up capital	9,000
Net profit (1980)	3,389

No of Employees: 926

SAVANNAH PRECAST CONCRETE & TERRAZO INDUSTRIES LTD
Murtala Mohammed Rd, PMB 1430, Ilorin, Kwara State
Cable: Savannah Ilorin

Directors: J A Toye (Managing),
  J A Jetawo (Executive)
Senior Executives: S A Alamu (Secretary/Accountant),
  Amos Adeyemo (Senior Technical Officer)

PRINCIPAL ACTIVITIES: Manufacturers of building blocks,
  posts, prestressed concrete electronic poles, etc
Principal Bankers: First Bank of Nigeria Ltd; Bank of the North;
  Societe Generale Bank (Nig) Ltd
Financial Information:

	N'000
Authorised capital	500
Paid-up capital	400
Turnover	500
Profits	55

Date of Establishment: 10th November 1972
No of Employees: 100

SAVANNAH SUGAR COMPANY LTD

PO Box 93, Yola, Gongola State
Tel: Radio link with Lagos and Kano offices

Chairman: Elias Nathan
Directors: Dr S Aleyideino, G Boguslawski, D Byers, O F J
  Oyaide, M Udebiuwa, Alhaji Abba Kawu
Senior Executives: B Woodhead (General Manager)

PRINCIPAL ACTIVITIES: Sugar cane production and milling,
  sugar refining
Branch Offices: 13 Duala Rd, Lagos; 73 Lamido Crescent, Kano;
  Site: Near Numan, Gongola State
Principal Bankers: NAL Merchant Bank Ltd; Union Bank of
  Nigeria Ltd; Bank of the North Ltd
Financial Information:

	N'000
Authorised capital	65,000
Paid-up capital	62,500

Principal Shareholders: Federal Government of Nigeria
Date of Establishment: 1st August 1970 (Pilot Project)
No of Employees: 4,500

SAVOIA, A

10 Ikorodu Rd, PO Box 490, Yaba, Lagos
Tel: 843681

Directors: Antonio Savoia

PRINCIPAL ACTIVITIES: Building and civil engineering
  contractors

SAWYERR ENTERPRISES (NIGERIA) LTD

PO Box 7921, 1 Sawyerr Crescent, Opposite Corona School,
  Gbagada Estate, Ilupeju, Lagos
Tel: 963345

Chairman: G O Sawyerr
Directors: Janet Sawyerr
Senior Executives: Femi Orefejo (Partner),
  P O Kuforiji (Partner)

PRINCIPAL ACTIVITIES: Freight forwarding and custom's
  agents, warehousing
Branch Offices: Ibadan Ring Rd; Kano; Port Harcourt
Associated Companies: Kopf & Lubben GmbH, West Germany
Principal Bankers: United Bank for Africa Ltd

Principal Shareholders: Gladstone Olajide Sawyerr

SAYBOLT (NIGERIA) LTD

174 Broad St, 4th Floor, Lagos Island, PO Box 4998, Lagos
Tel: 630391
Telex: 21240 Holric Ng

Directors: M Stephenson (General Manager)

PRINCIPAL ACTIVITIES: Service company for the oil and gas
  industry, laboratory analysis services

SB SHIPPING & TRADING AGENCIES LTD

18-20 Rhodes Crescent, PMB 1018, Apapa, Lagos
Tel: 873102
Cable: Marserline
Telex: 21401 Lagos

PRINCIPAL ACTIVITIES: General traders and transporters

SCAN AFRICAN NIGERIA LTD

Asogun Village, Km 15 Badagry Rd, PO Box 1792, Lagos
Tel: 860054, 830227
Cable: Swedafrica Lagos

Chairman: L J Howes (also Managing Director)
Directors: W A Usuanlele (Administration),
  O O Somefun,
  B S Potter (Technical)
Senior Executives: P E Ijerhe (Manager, Accounts)

PRINCIPAL ACTIVITIES: Sales and service of banking and
  security equipment, reprographic equipment, prefabricated
  building and refuse disposal equipment
Principal Agencies: De La Rue Crossfields Ltd; John Tann Ltd;
  Scan Coin Ltd; System & Checker Co Ltd; Toshiba Ltd;
  Conder Exports Ltd; Rosengren Ltd
Branch Offices: 61 Broad St, Lagos; 1 Obiagu Rd, Enugu; 31
  Mission Rd, Benin City; 2 Civic Centre, Kano
Principal Bankers: Union Bank of Nigeria Ltd; Societe Generale
  Bank (Nigeria) Ltd
Financial Information:

	N'000
Authorised capital	1,500
Paid-up capital	1,500
Sales turnover	4,250

No of Employees: 200

SCANO (NIGERIA) ENTERPRISES LTD

1 Airport Rd, Rumuola Junction, PMB 5393, Port Harcourt,
  Rivers State
Tel: 334775
Cable: Scano Ph
Telex: 61271

Chairman: Reverend S C Nwachuku (also Managing Director)
Senior Executives: Cyril Nwosu (Works Engineer),
  Miss Beatrice N Oduda (Administrative Assistant)

PRINCIPAL ACTIVITIES: Manufacturers of metal, wood and
  plastic furniture
Branch Offices: Plot 36B Industrial Layout, Owerri, Imo State
Principal Bankers: Union Bank of Nigeria Ltd
Financial Information:

	N'000
Turnover	1,000
Profits	75

Principal Shareholders: S C Nwachuku; Mrs S C Nwachuku; G O
  Nwachuku
Date of Establishment: 18th November 1970
No of Employees: 200

SCANSILA CONTRACTING COMPANY LTD

5 Ahmed Talib Ave, PO Box 352, South Kaduna

Directors: Ugo Scandella

PRINCIPAL ACTIVITIES: General contractors

SCANTRAVEL LTD

37 Marina, Unity House, PO Box 1897, Lagos
Tel: 651776, 634954, 635289, 633178, 635218
Cable: Scantravel

Chairman: Chief Frank O Akinrele
Directors: I K Akinrele
Senior Executives: B C J Ezenekwe (General Manager)

PRINCIPAL ACTIVITIES: All aspects of air travel business, tourism, car hire, etc

Principal Bankers: United Bank for Africa Ltd; Union Bank of Nigeria Ltd; Arab Bank (Nigeria) Ltd

Principal Shareholders: Chief Frank O Akinrele; I K Akinrele

SCEI
11 Cappa Ave, Palmgrove, PO Box 2053, Lagos
Tel: 862552

PRINCIPAL ACTIVITIES: Building materials importers

Branch Offices: PO Box 405, Kaduna; PO Box 256, Port Harcourt

SCHLUMBERGER (NIGERIA) LTD
7 Ogalade Close, Victoria Island, PO Box 1625, Lagos
Tel: 680819, 680938
Cable: Spewaf Lagos
Telex: 21415 Spelag Ng

Directors: R Maestrati

PRINCIPAL ACTIVITIES: Service company to the oil industry, electric logging

Branch Offices: Field Offices: PMB 5095, Plot 267, Trans-Amadi Layout, Port Harcourt, Tel 21227, Cable Spewaf Lagos (for PHT), Telex 61124; Speport Ng (for PHT); PO Box 153, Warri, Tel 359

SCHROEDER, H F, (WA) LTD
Plot 3 Amuwo Odofin Scheme, Isolo Expressway, PO Box 1209, Lagos
Tel: 835216, 831989
Cable: Simex Lagos
Telex: 21454 Simex Ng

Directors: D Priess

PRINCIPAL ACTIVITIES: General trading and representation; industrial electrical installations, manufacturers of carbon brushes

Principal Agencies: Demac Chain Hoists

Branch Offices: PMB 5307, Port Harcourt, Rivers State; PMB 4934, Kano

SCOA IARD - A DIVISION OF SCOA NIGERIA LTD
Surulere Industrial Rd, Ogba, Ikeja, PO Box 7419, Lagos
Tel: 962052/3/4/5
Telex: 26708 Ng

Chairman: Mallam Ahmed Joda
Directors: Ph Duchemin, Chief R U Mbalewe, Chief O I Akinkugbe, J P Lucas, Lt Gen T Y Danjuma
Senior Executives: J P Cuissard (General Manager),
  J O Farinde (Chief Accountant),
  Alhaji L O Nurudeen (Staff Manager),
  J B Ogbeta (Admin Manager),
  A Bel (Air Conditioning S J Manager),
  C Oliver (Air Conditioning West Manager),
  P Blanchout (Plumbing/Catering Equipment Manager),
  C Renauld (After Sales Manager)

PRINCIPAL ACTIVITIES: Federal ministry of works registered mechanical, plumbing and airconditioning contractors; engineering - importation of equipment - local production of components and installation. Aftersales service

Branch Offices: Abuja; Benin City; Ibadan; Zaria
Principal Bankers: International Bank for West Africa Ltd
Financial Information: See Scoa Nigeria Ltd

No of Employees: 280

SCOA MOTORS (NIGERIA) LTD
241 Igbosere Rd, PO Box 2083, Lagos
Tel: 634191, 632289, 632360, 632432
Telex: 21376

PRINCIPAL ACTIVITIES: Distribution of motor vehicles
Principal Agencies: Peugeot; Austin; Suzuki
Branch Offices: PO Box 194, 1 Ali Akilu Rd, Kaduna, Tel 213788, Telex 77144 Torfyr Ng; Kano, Telex 77106 Torfyr Ng
Financial Information: A division of SCOA Nigeria Ltd
Sales turnover (approx)   ₦ 92,000,000

No of Employees: 1,600

SCOA NIGERIA LTD
11/13 Davies Street, PO Box 2318, Lagos
Tel: 661856, 663095, 661228, 664842
Cable: Torfyrdep Lagos
Telex: 21017 Scoa Nig

Chairman: Ahmed Joda
Directors: J P Lucas (Managing),
  Chief O J Akinkugbe,
  P L Duchemin,
  LT Gen T Y Danjuma,
  Eze R U Mbalewe,
  M Picot
Senior Executives: R Pequignot (General Manager, Scoa Motors),
  L Williamson (General Manager, Scoatrac),
  J P Quissard (General Manager, Equip Iard),
  Mr Dexters (General Manager, Assembly Plant),
  L Boyard (Heavy Industrial Development Manager),
  F Gori (General Manager, Equip Home),
  P Butel (General Manager, Equip Pro)

PRINCIPAL ACTIVITIES: Motor vehicle assembly. Distribution and servicing of motor and commercial vehicles, earthmoving, construction and technical equipment; installation and servicing of air conditioners and refrigeration equipment
Principal Agencies: Pan (Kaduna); Lyland Ibadan; Pan Spares; Fiat Allis; Cummins Engine; Bernard Meuters
Branch Offices: Lagos; Apapa; Apapa Kirikiri; Isolo-Ikeja; Ogba-Ikeja; Abeokuta; Abuja; Ibadan; Ondo; Benin; Warri; Onitsha; Enugu; Aba; Port Harcourt; Kano; Kaduna; Makurdi; Bauchi; Jos; Minna; Maiduguri; Gusau; Sokoto; Yola; Zaria
Subsidiary/Associated Companies: Tanarewa Nigeria Ltd; Agbara Plastic Industry Ltd; Brume Mechanical Industry Ltd
Principal Bankers: United Bank for Africa Ltd; Union Bank of Nigeria Ltd; International Bank for West Africa Ltd; First Bank of Nigeria Ltd; Societe Generale Bank; WEMA Bank; ICON Ltd; Nigerian - American Merchant Bank
Financial Information: As at 30th September 1981

	₦'000
Authorised capital	24,000
Paid-up capital	24,000
Turnover	361,540
Profits (before tax)	11,610

Principal Shareholders: SCOA Paris; Dr Majeko Duam; Alhaji Dantata
Date of Establishment: Incorporated 24th June 1969
No of Employees: 3,621

SCOAGRI
6A Randle Close, PO Box 142, Apapa, Lagos
Tel: 876546

PRINCIPAL ACTIVITIES: Suppliers of agricultural machinery

SCOATRAC (A DIVISION OF SCOA (NIGERIA) LTD)
Dual Carriage Way, Isolo Industrial Estate, PMB 21108, Ikeja, Lagos
Tel: 848144, 845249
Cable: Torfytrac
Telex: 21376

Chairman: Alhaji A Joda
Directors: Lt Gen T Y Danjuma,
  J P Lucas (Managing),
  Ph Duchemin,
  Chief Mbalewe,

O I Akinkugbe,
M Picot
Senior Executives: L Williamson (General Manager),
P Thisse (Finance Controller),
P I Olumhense (Administration Personnel Manager)

PRINCIPAL ACTIVITIES: Suppliers of heavy machinery to civil
engineers and contractors in Nigeria, earthmoving equipment
etc
Principal Agencies: Fiat Allis; Ingersoll-Rand; Cummins Engine
Ltd; Ermont Cresot-Loire; Ateliers Bergeaud Macon; Diesel
Energie
Branch Offices: Dual Carriage Way, Isolo, PMB 21108, Ikeja; 44
Trans-Amadi Industrial Layout, Port Harcourt; Airport Rd,
Emene, Box 1361, Enugu; Kawo Industrial Estate, Kaduna;
Maiduguri; Bauchi; Yola; Sokoto
Principal Bankers: First Bank of Nigeria Ltd
Financial Information:
Turnover (approx)   ₦ 45,000,000

Principal Shareholders: A division of SCOA (Nigeria) Ltd
Date of Establishment: 1974
No of Employees: 600

SCOBI ASSOCIATES
PO Box 52751, Ikoyi, Lagos

President: Sam Chudi Obi

PRINCIPAL ACTIVITIES: Business and financial consultants,
training; business newsletter publishers, training
Principal Agencies: Alexander Norton Publishers, USA;
Resources for Education and Management Inc, USA; Torrk
Research and Development, USA; Center for Entrepreneurial
Management, USA
Principal Bankers: Union Bank of Nigeria Ltd; Bank of Credit &
Commerce International Ltd

SEA DANTAINER LINES LTD
Gidan Shehu Ahmed, Bank Rd, Kano
Tel: 2557

Directors: Alhaji Aminu Dantata, Alhaji Hamza Ahmed, Hugh
David R Walford, G Ingram Ward-Willis

PRINCIPAL ACTIVITIES: Shipping sevices
Branch Offices: PO Box 323, 176 Warri/Sapele Rd, Warri,
Bendel State

SEA TRUCKS (NIGERIA) LTD
49 Awolowo Rd, Ikoyi, PO Box 1168, Lagos
Tel: 683144, 680808
Cable: Seatruck
Telex: 22307 Seatru Ng

Chairman: Sunday Dankaro
Directors: Gen T Y Danjuma, J Roomans, H Flynn

PRINCIPAL ACTIVITIES: Marine oil service company
Branch Offices: ACM Yard, Trans Amadi Industrial Area, Port
Harcourt Tel 332205; Enerhen/Effurun Rd, Warri, Bendel
State, Tel 234098; Nigerian Army Marine Base, Calabar, Tel
221502
Subsidiary Companies: Manlyn SA Luxembourg; Sea Trucks
Offshore Ltd
Principal Bankers: First Bank of Nigeria Ltd; International
Merchant Bank (Nigeria) Ltd
Financial Information:

	₦'000
Authorised capital	1,000
Paid-up capital	875
Turnover	4,000

Principal Shareholders: S Dankaro; Gen T Y Danjuma; Manlyn
SA
Date of Establishment: 16th September 1977
No of Employees: 450

SEBO TECHNICAL INDUSTRIES NIGERIA LTD
SW9/714 Adeniran Oyinlola Ave, Ring Rd, PMB 5495, Ibadan,
Oyo State
Cable: Sebotech

Chairman: B A Effiong
Directors: S O Aiyedun, S A Akinsola
Senior Executives: A O Sonaike (Engineer),
F O Fakunle (Accountant),
A Ogundola (Supervisor, Electrical Department)

PRINCIPAL ACTIVITIES: Suppliers of electrical equipment
Principal Agencies: Hussmann Refrigeration Company, USA; J D
Marshall International Inc, USA
Principal Bankers: Co-operative Bank Ltd
Financial Information:
Sales turnover   ₦ 500,000

SECOM LTD
132 Broad Street, PO Box 6577, Lagos
Tel: 662621
Telex: Scograph

Chairman: Chief Zacchaeus Olafenwa Osiberu
Directors: Mrs J O Osiberu, Solomon Olusegun Osiberu,
Afolabi Osiberu, Olukayode Osiberu
Senior Executives: J O Asani (Secretary),
F A Arowogbokun (Office Manager)

PRINCIPAL ACTIVITIES: Business consultants, trustees,
company formation
Principal Agencies: African Newspapers of Nigeria Ltd; John
West Group of Companies; Kesington and Company Ltd;
Temitope Bakery & Catering Services Ltd; Aduragbemi &
Sons Industries Ltd; Face to Face Million Dollars
Branch Offices: 88 Akarigbo Street, PO Box 60, Sagamu; 15th
Floor, Cocoa House, Ibadan
Associated Companies: Lafenwa Osiberu and Company
(Chartered Accountants)
Principal Bankers: Union Bank of Nigeria Ltd; National Bank of
Nigeria Ltd; Wema Bank Ltd
Financial Information:

	₦'000
Authorised capital	100
Paid-up capital	42
Turnover	116
Profits	8

Principal Shareholders: Janet Oluwalambe Osiberu; Solomon
Olusegun Osiberu; Olukayode Osiberu
Date of Establishment: 21st June 1973

SEDCO NIGERIA LTD
PO Box 7906, 13 Norman Williams St, SW Ikoyi, Lagos
Tel: 680993, 683581, 681504
Telex: 21485 Sedco Ng

Chairman: Kerner J Barras
Directors: L F Newton, G E Burch, Mrs T Madarikan, S C
Mahood
Senior Executives: Michael J Thibodeaux (Deputy Manager),
Porter F Pearson (Dredge Manager),
Jay Thibodeaux (General Superintendent),
Anthony X Pinheiro (Project Manager),
Joseph I Obi (Government Relations Manager)

PRINCIPAL ACTIVITIES: Pipeline construction, dredging, and
drilling
Branch Offices: PMB 737, Port Harcourt, Rivers State; Udu Rd,
Warri, Bendel State
Associated Companies: Sedco-Bean Constructors
Principal Bankers: Savannah Bank of Nigeria

SEEPC (NIGERIA) LTD
1 Abimbola Awoniyi Close, Off Kasumu Ekemode St, Victoria
Island, PO Box 9911, Lagos
Tel: 610714, 615878
Telex: 21862

Chairman: Alhaji M G Lawan

Directors: L Monange, Dr B S Oloruntoba, Alhaji Bata Mai, B Portal, G Quelia

PRINCIPAL ACTIVITIES: Fertilizers, animal feeds and chemicals

Principal Agencies: EMC Group; Kaliexport; Complexport; Sanders

Subsidiary Companies: Amo Sanders

Principal Bankers: International Bank for West Africa Ltd; Societe Generale Bank (Nigeria) Ltd

Financial Information:

	N'000
Authorised capital	1,000
Paid-up capital	800
Turnover	10,000

Principal Shareholders: SCPA (EMC Group); Alhaji Lawan

Date of Establishment: 1978

No of Employees: 100

SEGUN INTERNATIONAL GROUP LTD

Plot 74/78, Segun Industrial Estate, PMB 1233, Apapa, Lagos

Tel: 830026

Cable: Morin

Telex: 44179

Chairman: Chief Richardson Okeowo Smith

Directors: Alex F Morin, Alhaji Hassan Mohammed, Mrs B S Gupta, Jonnie Koehler, Dr S L Gomez

Senior Executives: S Smith (Chief Executive, Administrative Division),
R Canne (General Manager),
O Popoola (Group Marketing Controller),
C D Nnamdi (Group Chief Accountant)

PRINCIPAL ACTIVITIES: General importers and exporters; buying agents; business confirming house representatives; industrial and agricultural consultants; building and electrical contractors; shipping and airfreight agents; transporters; travel agents; stores and wholesale depots; manufacturers of plastics and toys

Principal Agencies: Lisle Corporation, Clarinda, Iowa, USA; Frank'sche GmbH, Dillenbury, West Germany; Samsung International Corp, Tokyo, Japan

Branch Offices: Nigeria: Lagos; Enugu; Aba; Kano; Kaduna; Ilorin; Ibadan and Akure; Ghana; Accra; Kumasi and Tamale; Republic of Benin; Cotonuo; Porto Novo

Subsidiary Companies: Seven Sea Enterprises (Nigeria) Ltd, Lagos; Greenham Breweries Ltd, Aba; Dennis & Morin Cold Storages Ltd; Apapa; Morin International (Sales) Ltd, Apapa

Principal Bankers: First Bank of Nigeria Ltd; Savannah Bank of Nigeria Ltd

Date of Establishment: 1st April 1972

No of Employees: 865

SEHL INTERNATIONAL

PO Box 50828, Ikoyi, Lagos

Tel: 684887

Chairman: W Raabe

Directors: K Meinhardt, H Emmerich, G O Sodipo

PRINCIPAL ACTIVITIES: General trading company; importers of chemicals, fertilizers, sanitary equipment and plant equipment

SEISMOGRAPH SERVICE (NIGERIA) LTD (SSL)

2 Alhaji Ribadu Rd, Ikoyi Island, PO Box 3320, Lagos

Tel: 682323, 681226

Directors: M I Oduah (Managing),
B O Madubunyi,
J K Smith,
R C Anderson,
E R Wolf

PRINCIPAL ACTIVITIES: Geophysical survey contractors to the oil industry

Branch Offices: 144 Margaret Ave, PO Box 937, Aba, Imo State; 11 Alhaji Ribadu Rd, PO Box 3320, Ikoyi Island, Lagos, Tel 681226

SELWOOD PUMPS

Apapa Rd, Iganmu, PO Box 391, Apapa, Lagos

Tel: 844027

PRINCIPAL ACTIVITIES: Suppliers of technical equipment, pumps

Branch Offices: 12 Lagos St, PO Box 18, Kano; 8 Liberation Drive, PMB 5130, Port Harcourt, Rivers State

SEM STEELS (NIGERIA) LTD

Plot 719A Adetokunba Ademola St, Victoria Island, PMB 1063, Apapa, Lagos

Tel: 614205

Cable: Semsteinig Lagos

Telex: 21537

Directors: A Fleischhauer

PRINCIPAL ACTIVITIES: Importers of steel products

SEM-EDO WIRE INDUSTRIES LTD

Oregbeni, Ikpoba Hill, Agbor Rd, PMB 1396, Benin City, Bendel State

Tel: 242432

PRINCIPAL ACTIVITIES: Suppliers of steel products; reinforcing fabric, wire mesh, etc

SENN-SOUND (WEST AFRICA) LTD

PO Box 1262, 37 Adeniran Ogunsanya Street, Surulere, Lagos

Tel: 830857

Cable: 'Senn-Sound'

Telex: 26349 Ng (Senn-KA)

Chairman: Kaye A Abraham (Senior)

Directors: Mrs Y A Abraham,
K A Abraham (Junior),
A O Abraham

Senior Executives: C N Ohajuba (General Manager),
Charles Otudoh (Administrative Executive),
Okon Akpan (Workshop Manager),
Henry Okeowo (Sales & Marketing Executive),
Ms Kate Esin (Sales Supervisor)

PRINCIPAL ACTIVITIES: Import and distribution of electronic and communication equipment. Local assembly of Hi-fi stereo, colour television sets

Principal Agencies: Voxsons, Italy; Cybernet, Japan; Barco, Belgium; Nakamichi, Japan; Fisher, West Germany; Tandberg, Norway

Branch Offices: Service Center: 77 St Finbarrs Rd, Akoka, Yaba, Lagos; Assembly Plant: 80 St Finbarrs Rd, Akoka, Yaba, Lagos

Subsidiary Companies: Grapevine Ltd

Principal Bankers: International Bank for West Africa Ltd; Bank of the North Ltd

Financial Information:

	N'000
Authorised capital	1,250
Paid-up capital	1,000
Turnover	4,200
Profits	200

Principal Shareholders: K A Abraham (Senior)

Date of Establishment: 31st March 1973

No of Employees: 64

SENTINEL ASSURANCE COMPANY LTD

126 Broad St, PO Box 3003, Lagos

Tel: 663116, 662776

Chairman: Chief F A Nzeribe

Directors: Chief O Aina, Chief F S Giwa-Osagie

PRINCIPAL ACTIVITIES: Insurance
Branch Offices: Aba; Benin City; Enugu; Ibadan
Financial Information:

	N'000
Authorised capital	500
Paid-up capital	500

Date of Establishment: 1970
No of Employees: 100

SENTRYCOM ALARMS (NIGERIA) LTD
360 Herbert Macaulay St, Yaba, Lagos
Tel: 862599, 862024
Telex: 21443 Sentry Ng

PRINCIPAL ACTIVITIES: Suppliers of alarm systems
Branch Offices: Plot 139A Aina George St, Ilupeju, Lagos, Tel 963071

SEPI ESTERO CONSULTANTS (NIGERIA) LTD
8/10 Broad St, Lagos
Tel: 636559

Directors: Dr D O Ekesi

PRINCIPAL ACTIVITIES: Consultants

SERA PRINTING LTD
Kilometer 11, Lagos/Badagry Express Rd, Opp Satellite Town, PO Box 678, Apapa, Lagos
Tel: 880235

Chairman: Chief S N Ebinum
Directors: Alhaji R A O Najekodunmi, Chief S O Ossai (Managing), C Kruegel
Senior Executives: Manfred Jung (General Manager)

PRINCIPAL ACTIVITIES: Commercial printing and light packaging, annual reports, brochures, calenders, labels, light cartons for cigarettes and pharmaceuticals
Principal Agencies: Pfizer; Bayer; Hoechst; Farmex; NTC
Principal Bankers: Savannah Bank of Nigeria Ltd
Financial Information:

	N'000
Authorised capital	750
Paid-up capital	500

Principal Shareholders: Chairman and directors as described
Date of Establishment: 17th January 1977 Production began 1st April 1979
No of Employees: 70

SERVICE & SUPPLY COMPANY OF WEST AFRICA LTD (SASCO)
Plot 52 Trans-Amadi Industrial Area, PO Box 387, Port Harcourt, Rivers State
Tel: 21455/7, 21440
Cable: Sasco Port Harcourt
Telex: 61128

Directors: Eric G Schofield

PRINCIPAL ACTIVITIES: Suppliers of equipment for oil and gas industry
Principal Agencies: Demco Inc; Mattco/TTE; Smith Tools; Weatherford Oil Tools
Branch Offices: Field Office: PO Box 346, Warri, Bendel State

SERVO NIGERIAN ENTERPRISES LTD
Km 7, Lagos Rd, PO Box 76, Ibadan, Oyo State
Tel: 412792
Telex: 31164 Servon Ng

Chairman: Sam Oshinowo
Directors: Mrs Elizabeth Oshinowo (Deputy Managing Director), Miss Adenike A Oshinowo, Obafemi O Oshinowo

PRINCIPAL ACTIVITIES: General suppliers of building materials and electronics
Branch Offices: 46 Oba Akran Ave, Ikeja Industrial Estate, PO Box 7905, Marina, Lagos, Tel 964626, 934716
Associated Companies: Diesel Generating Company Ltd
Principal Bankers: Standard Bank of Nigeria Ltd
Financial Information:

	N'000
Authorised capital	100
Sales turnover (approx)	700
Profits (approx)	188

SESWA, STEEL AND ENGINEERING SERVICES (WA) LTD
29 Burma Rd, Apapa, Lagos
Tel: 871434, 871436, 871352
Cable: Tradeseswa

PRINCIPAL ACTIVITIES: Suppliers of iron and steel products
Branch Offices: Trans Amadi Layout, Plot C, Port Harcourt, Rivers State, Tel 333693, 334180; 58 Lamido Crescent, Kano

SEVEN-UP BOTTLING COMPANY LTD
PO Box 134, 237 Ijora Rd, Apapa, Lagos
Tel: 803420/1/2/3
Cable: Sevenupco Lagos
Telex: 21304 Sevnup

Chairman: M El Khalil
Directors: Chief Dr N B Grahame Douglas, Chief Dr C M Norman Williams, Mr Samuel Adedoyin, Alhaji Ahmaou Yaru, E O Okorafor, A El Khalil, Fr El Khalil, Fj El Khalil
Senior Executives: P G Crabb (Financial Controller)

PRINCIPAL ACTIVITIES: Bottlers of carbonated beverages; franchises of Seven-Up International and Crush International
Branch Offices: Bottling plants: 247 Apapa Rd, Ijora; New Secretariat Way, Oregun, Lagos; Oluyole Extension Estate, PO Box 92, Ibadan; Depots: Abeokuta; Akure; Benin; Ijebu-Ode; Oshogbo and Shagamu
Financial Information:

	N'000
Authorised capital	3,375
Turnover (1982 estimated)	32,000
Profits (1982 estimated)	3,000

Principal Shareholders: 60% Nigerian Public
Date of Establishment: 1960
No of Employees: 1,800

SEWARD, A J, (A DIVISION OF UAC OF NIGERIA LTD)
Billingsway, Oregun Industrial Estate, PO Box 1063, Ikeja, Lagos

Tel: 901030/9
Cable: Worksward Ikeja

Senior Executives: P R Batchelor (General Manager)

PRINCIPAL ACTIVITIES: Manufacture and distribution of toiletries and proprietary medicines
Branch Offices: Aba; Benin; Enugu; Ibadan; Jos; Kaduna; Kano; Lagos; Maiduguri; Onitsha; Zaria; Sokoto

Principal Shareholders: UAC of Nigeria Ltd
No of Employees: 1,200

SGE NIGERIA LTD
PO Box 7314, 180 Awolowo Rd, Ikoyi, Lagos
Tel: 685537, 680907
Telex: 21758

PRINCIPAL ACTIVITIES: Building and civil engineering contractors

SHALHOUB BROTHERS LTD

PO Box 377, Lagos Rd, Ibadan, Oyo State
Tel: 411192
Cable: Mirroglass Ibadan
Telex: 31110 Shalub

PRINCIPAL ACTIVITIES: Manufacturers of mirrors and glass
Branch Offices: Benin

SHAWMONT NIGERIA LTD

19A Awolowo Rd, South West Ikoyi, PO Box 7106, Lagos
Tel: 683752
Telex: 21655

Directors: H W D Armstrong,
 G Yomi Legunsen (Executive),
 G A Tonolawi,
 R M King

Senior Executives: A Salau (Office Manager)

PRINCIPAL ACTIVITIES: Consulting engineers
Branch Offices: Doma Dam Project Office, Doma, Plateau State;
 Dadin Kowa Dam Project Office, Dadin Kowa, Banchi State;
 Zobe Dam Project, Dustin-Ma, Kaduna
Associated Companies: Shawinigan Engineering Co Ltd;
 Montreal Engineering Co Ltd, Canada
Principal Bankers: Bank of Credit Commerce & Industry; First
 Bank of Nigeria Ltd

Date of Establishment: 1973

SHEKONI INDUSTRIES NIGERIA LTD

55 Igbosere Rd, PO Box 7075, Lagos
Tel: 633740
Telex: 21985 Ng

PRINCIPAL ACTIVITIES: Suppliers of security equipment, safes
 etc
Branch Offices: 30 Coker Rd, Opposite Awaye Motors, Badagry
 Express Rd, Lagos State

Date of Establishment: 1977

SHELDON L POLLACK (NIGERIA) LTD

See POLLACK, SHELDON L, (NIGERIA) LTD

SHELL PETROLEUM DEVELOPMENT COMPANY OF NIGERIA LTD

Freeman House, 21/22 Marina, Lagos Island, PMB 2418, Lagos
Tel: 601600/17
Cable: Shell, Lagos
Telex: 21235 Shell Ng

Directors: David Richard Welham (Managing),
 N J van Dijk,
 Chief Francis Edo Osagie,
 Alhaji Yahaya Gusau,
 Godwin Eyarubere Omene,
 Henry Ibhade Kwame Omenai,
 Nnaemeka Alfred Achebe,
 Jack Lucas (Secretary)
Senior Executives: G E Omene (Manager, Western Division),
 N A Achebe (Manager, Eastern Division)

PRINCIPAL ACTIVITIES: Oil exploration and production
Branch Offices: Field Offices: PO Box 263, Port Harcourt, Rivers
 State; PO Box 230, Warri, Bendel State

SHEVA (WA) LTD

96 Zik Ave, PO Box 21, Enugu, Anambra State
Tel: 252374
Telex: 51136 Nigeria

PRINCIPAL ACTIVITIES: Manufacturers' representatives, general
 traders
Branch Offices: Lagos; Jos; Kaduna; Maiduguri

SHITTU, ALHAJI M R, & SONS LTD

PO Box 157, Yaba, 6 Shifawu St, Surulere, Lagos
Tel: 834191

PRINCIPAL ACTIVITIES: Building and civil engineering
 contractors
Branch Offices: 41 Oguntola St, Shomoly, Lagos

SHO'S ENGINEERING COMPANY LTD

Plot 40-41 Bamigboye St, Lagos
Tel: 843282

PRINCIPAL ACTIVITIES: Suppliers of heavy diesel engine
 crankshafts, industrial and locomotive shafts etc
Branch Offices: Stores: 26 Alafia St, Mushin, Lagos; 2A Offin
 Canal, Lagos State; Works: 87 Ibadan St, Ebute Metta; 2
 Adesola Close, Near Cocoa Industry, Ogba Agege; 3 Asajeun
 Close, Idi Aba Rd, Abeokuta, Ogun State

SHOUR INDUSTRIAL ENTERPRISES LTD

5 Bompai Rd, PO Box 220, Kano
Tel: 2255, 5205, 4548, 5586
Cable: Alishour Kano
Telex: 77208 Ashour Nig

PRINCIPAL ACTIVITIES: General contractors, transporters

SIAB ENGINEERING COMPANY NIGERIA LTD

Plot 10 Emina Street, PMB 21233, Ikeja, Lagos
Tel: 935205
Telex: 26664 Siab Ng

Chairman: Friedrich Stetzler
Senior Executives: E H Lemprecht (Managing Director)

PRINCIPAL ACTIVITIES: Building, construction and civil
 engineering, telecommunications, power generation, water
 resources engineering, harbour and dredging works,
 consultancy services - architectural and engineering,
 industrial projects, turn-key industrial, health and education
 projects
Associated Companies: Friedrich Stetzler, West Germany; Siab
 Pforzheim, West Germany; ATP Pforzheim, West Germany;
 BWP Betonwerk Pforzheim, West Germany; Zentro-Elekrik,
 West Germany; Silverball Integrated Engineering Nigeria Ltd;
 SIAB United Arab Emirates, Abu Dhabi, Dubai, Sharjah;
 SIAB-Iraq
Principal Bankers: United Bank for Africa Ltd
Financial Information:

	N'000
Authorised capital	420
Paid-up capital	420

Date of Establishment: 15th November 1974
No of Employees: 456

SIEJ AGENCIES

84-5 Market Rd, PO Box 808, Aba, Imo State
Tel: 481

PRINCIPAL ACTIVITIES: Importers of building materials,
 electrical appliances, chemicals

SILVERBALL INTEGRATED ENGINEERING CO NIGERIA LTD

Plot 10 Emina Street, PMB 21233, Ikeja, Lagos
Tel: 935205
Telex: 26664 Siab Ng

Chairman: Friedrich Stetzler (also Managing Director)

PRINCIPAL ACTIVITIES: Building, construction and civil
 engineering
Associated Companies: Friedrich Stetzler, West Germany; Siab
 Pforzheim, West Germany; ATP Pforzheim, West Germany;
 BWP Betonwerk Pforzheim, West Germany; Zentro-Elekrik;
 Siab Engineering Co Nigeria Ltd; Siab United Arab Emirates,
 Abu Dhabi, Dubai, Sharjah; Siab-Iraq
Principal Bankers: United Bank for Africa Ltd

Financial Information:

	N'000
Authorised capital	410
Paid-up capital	410

Date of Establishment: 29th June 1976
No of Employees: 250

SIRAM INDUSTRIAL PRODUCTS LTD

129 Oladeinde Coker Street, (Off Sadiku St), Ilasamaja, Mushin, Lagos State
Tel: 833108
Cable: Siras Lagos

Directors: Bernard N Onyene (Managing Director)

PRINCIPAL ACTIVITIES: Suppliers of industrial and car care products
Principal Bankers: African Continental Bank Ltd

SKETCH PUBLISHING COMPANY LTD

PMB 5067, Oba Adebimpe Rd, Ibadan
Tel: 414851, 414922, 414983, 411852, 412988
Cable: Sketch Ibadan
Telex: 31591

Chairman: Chief V A Olayanju
Directors: Segun Osoba (Managing Director/Chief Executive),
Tony Adefuye,
Prof T O Bamkole,
Arc Tunde Ogunniyi,
Dr Wale Oyemakinde,
Olu Olofin,
Akin Oluwakuyide
Senior Executives: Peter Ajayi (General Manager),
J O Fashola (Chief Accountant),
L O Fajuyitan (Administrative Manager),
O Oladele (Marketing Manager),
Sola Oyegbemi (Daily Editor),
M A Okulaja (Company/Legal Secretary),

O Afolabi (Production Manager),
M A Oyekan (Commercial Printing Manager)

PRINCIPAL ACTIVITIES: Newspaper publishing
Branch Offices: Banuso House, 88/92 Broad Street, PMB 12025, Lagos
Principal Bankers: National Bank of Nigeria Ltd

Principal Shareholders: Oyo, Ogun and Ondo State Governments
Date of Establishment: 1964
No of Employees: 564

SKOUP & CO LTD

45 Martins St, Lagos
Tel: 658316
Telex: 21497

Chairman: Dr P N C Okigbo
Directors: Dr S U Ugoh, K U Kalu
Senior Executives: L C Okigbo (Chief Consultant),
Mr Onuoha (Chief Consultant)

PRINCIPAL ACTIVITIES: Business consultants
Branch Offices: 2 Ogui Rd, Enugu, Anambra State; Ibadan
Principal Bankers: First Bank of Nigeria Ltd; African Continental Bank Ltd

SMEATON LTD

PO Box 4131, 106/110 Lewis St, Lagos
Tel: 630691, 654398
Cable: Eddistone Lagos

Chairman: Harry M Osha
Directors: S A Ademilehin (Managing),
J A Aina,
Dr E A Akinleye,
Y O Giwa
Senior Executives: John Hughes (General Manager),
S G Izokpu (Company Secretary)

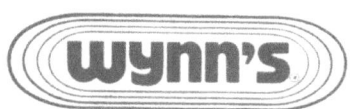
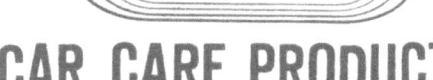
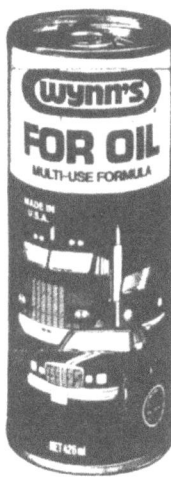
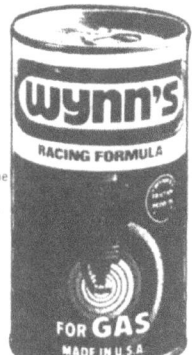
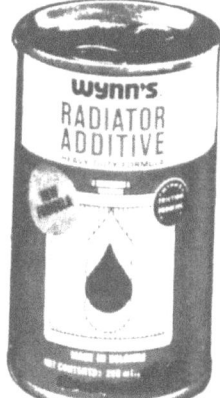

PRINCIPAL ACTIVITIES: Mechanical and electrical engineering contractors; suppliers of air-conditioning equipment
Branch Offices: PMB 2115, Jos, Plateau State; PO Box 321, Calabar, Cross River State; PO Box 3368, Kano
Principal Bankers: First Bank of Nigeria Ltd
Financial Information:

	₦'000
Authorised capital	1,000
Paid-up capital	140
Sales turnover	6,500

No of Employees: 600

SMITH KLINE & FRENCH NIGERIA LTD
PMB 599, Ikeja, Lagos State
Cable: Eskayef Lagos

Directors: E A Drake (General Manager)

PRINCIPAL ACTIVITIES: Suppliers of pharmaceuticals and cosmetics

SNAMPROGETTI
16 Louis Solomon Close, Victoria Island, PMB 12589, Lagos
Tel: 612006, 611532
Telex: 22607 Snamprong

Senior Executives: L Bertele (General Manager), C Sampaolo (Construction Manager)

PRINCIPAL ACTIVITIES: Design engineers and construction of oil refineries; petrochemical plants and pipelines
Branch Offices: PMB 1117, Warri, Bendel State, Tel 234544, Telex 43296
Principal Bankers: United Bank for Africa Ltd

Date of Establishment: November 1975
No of Employees: 230

SNC (NIGERIA) LTD
148 Mission Rd, PMB 1255, Benin City, Bendel State
Tel: 242280
Telex: 41109 Michem Ng

PRINCIPAL ACTIVITIES: Engineering consultants; contractors
Branch Offices: PO Box 8390, Western House, 7th Floor, 8/10 Broad St, Lagos, Telex 21543 Bekbek Ng

SOBAT LTD
14 Itapeju St, PO Box 740, Apapa, Lagos
Tel: 874920, 875803
Cable: Sobat Apapa
Telex: 21351 Sobat Lagos; 77113 Kano

Senior Executives: John Linardos, A M Bedri (Managing), Anthony Eguwe (Administrative Manager), Abu Bakr Ali (Operations Manager)

PRINCIPAL ACTIVITIES: Farming; suppliers of frozen foods; cold storage; shipping
Branch Offices: Ijora; Kano; Port Harcourt; Maiduguri; Onitsha; Benin
Associated Companies: NICCO Sweets Ltd, Kano; Global Chemical Agencies Ltd, Kano; Usman Eltayeb & Brother Ltd, Kano
Principal Bankers: Nigeria Arab Bank Ltd

Date of Establishment: 1979

SOCCER CHEWING GUM ENTERPRISES LTD
155 Club Rd, PO Box 185, Kano
PRINCIPAL ACTIVITIES: Manufacturers of confectionery
No of Employees: 500

SOCEA (NIGERIA) LTD

22 Herbert Macaulay Crescent-Gra, Ikeja, PO Box 50595,
  Falomo, Lagos
Tel: 961508
Telex: 26209 Socea Ng

PRINCIPAL ACTIVITIES: Pipelaying for water, sewage and
  irrigation networks. Treatment of urban wastes
Principal Bankers: United Bank for Africa

SOCIETE GENERALE BANK (NIGERIA) LTD

PMB 12741, 126/128 Broad St, Lagos
Tel: 660315, 660386
Cable: Sogeni Lagos
Telex: 21379 Sogeni Ng; 21022 Sogeni Ng

Chairman: N A B Kotoye
Directors: Charles Louis Buttay (Vice-Chairman),
  Alhaji Mohammed Hayatuddini,
  R Gely,
  Alhaji Muhammadu King,
  J de Maleville,
  Chief Gregory Ishong Ayim
Senior Executives: Michel E Barat (Managing Director),
  J A Sauzier (Head Office Manager)

PRINCIPAL ACTIVITIES: Banking
Branch Offices: Nasco House, 29 Burma Rd, Apapa, Lagos; 89
  Ibrahim Taiwo Rd, Ilorin, Kwara State; 8 Bompai Rd, Kano; 2
  Makare Rd, Kaduna South, Kaduna; 9 Alhaji Jimoh Odutola
  Rd, Ibadan

Principal Shareholders: Private Nigerians (60%); Societe
  Generale, Paris (40%)
Date of Establishment: 16th December 1976
No of Employees: 360

SODANGI ENTERPRISES

15 Waff Rd, PO Box 200, Zaria, Kaduna State

PRINCIPAL ACTIVITIES: Distributors of beverages, spirits,
  paints and building materials

SODIK-ASEA (NIGERIA) LTD

Kirikiri Industrial Estate, Off Isolo-Apapa Expressway, PO Box
  728, Ikeja, Lagos
Telex: 21898 Eric Ng

Chairman: S Dike Odogwu
Directors: S Lindberg (Managing),
  V C Odogwu (Executive),
  Per Ranvall
Senior Executives: I A Ndubuisi (General Sales Manager),
  J E Uzoma (Head of Economy Department),
  B Skrufve (Product Manager)

PRINCIPAL ACTIVITIES: Sales, manufacture, supply, erection
  and service of electrical and electro mechanical equipment
Principal Agencies: Asea AB, Sweden; Asea A/S, Denmark;
  Asea Lepper, West Germany; Asea Kabel, Stockholm
Branch Offices: Port Harcourt; Owerri; Enugu; Warri; Calabar;
  Kaduna
Principal Bankers: Union Bank of Nigeria Ltd; Societe General
  Bank (Nig) Ltd; United Bank for Africa Ltd
Financial Information:

	₦'000
Paid-up capital	400
Turnover	400
Profits	4,000

Principal Shareholders: Asea-AB, Sweden
Date of Establishment: 1st January 1978
No of Employees: 200

SODIPO, HAROLD, & CO LTD

19 Alaka St, PO Box 213, Yaba, Lagos
Tel: 860775, 862756

PRINCIPAL ACTIVITIES: Building and civil engineering
  contractors

SOINTECO (NIGERIA) LTD

13 Daniya Street, Off Oniwaya Rd, Agege, Lagos State
Tel: 862079
Cable: Sointeco Lagos

Chairman: Chief A A Sobitan
Directors: B O Sobitan, A O Sobitan, 'Wale Sobitan
Senior Executives: Mrs A O Ogundium (Administration Manager),
  Mr David (Accounting Officer),
  J Esomije (Sales Executive),
  B O Ojo (Technical Manager)

PRINCIPAL ACTIVITIES: Suppliers of lubricating pumps,
  petroleum equipment and electrical generating plants
Principal Agencies: The Armaturenfabrick Ernst Horn GmbH,
  West Germany; Busin & Stephenson Ltd, UK; Friese
  Import/Export, Germany; Dunlop Ltd, UK; D J J Sullivan (Fire
  Extinguishers) Ltd, UK; English Abrasives, UK;
  Franken-Industrie-Werk, Germany; New Jersey Inc, USA
Branch Offices: 1 Abeokuta Street (Anifowoshe) Ikeja; 40 Ilugun
  Rd, Abeokuta; 4 UU4 Kazaure Rd, Kaduna
Subsidiary Companies: 'Wale, Lekan & Brothers; Ajayi &
  Brothers; Soji Associates; Wennok Wilson & Sons
Principal Bankers: Bank of the North Ltd; Wema Bank (Nigeria)
  Ltd

Principal Shareholders: Chief A A Sobitan; B O Sobitan; A O
  Sobitan
Date of Establishment: 1980

SOKOTO FURNITURE FACTORY LTD

Furniture Factory Rd, PMB 2170, Sokoto
Tel: 232204, 232539
Cable: Sokofur
Telex: 73124 Sokfur

Directors: A K Fawaz (Managing Director)
Senior Executives: M Shalakani (Works Manager)

PRINCIPAL ACTIVITIES: Manufacture of steel and wood
  furniture
Associated Companies: Fawaz Steelwood & Chemicals (Kano)
  Ltd

SOLEL BONEH (NIGERIA) LTD

Opposite University of Ibadan, Oyo Rd, PMB 5131, Ibadan, Oyo
  State
Tel: 417733, 417230
Cable: Solelboneh Ibadan
Telex: 31580 Solelb Ng

Chairman: Chief G Akin Deko
Directors: E Porat,
  G B Egbe,
  A Brown,
  E Leible (Managing)
Senior Executives: J Levenberg (Deputy Managing Director),
  R Barkan (Chief Engineer, Roads),
  J Levy (Operations Manager),
  S Ophir (Operations Manager, Administration),
  Y Feldhay (Resident Manager, Buildings),
  A Hadar (Chief Accountant),
  E Nadiv (Plant Manager)

PRINCIPAL ACTIVITIES: Civil engineering and construction
Branch Offices: 30 Sura Mogaji St, Ilupeju, PO Box 1729,
  Mushin, Lagos; Tel: 962136, 962138, 935254, 935267, Telex
  26433 Solelb Ng; 32 Ofumwegbe Street, Off Sapele Rd, PMB
  1085, Benin City, Bendel State, Tel: 242744, 240387
Principal Bankers: First Bank of Nigeria Ltd; International Bank
  for West Africa Ltd
Financial Information:

	₦'000
Authorised capital	2,734
Paid-up capital	2,734
Turnover	70,000

Principal Shareholders: Solel Boneh International Ltd; Chief

Gabriel Akin-Deko; Odu'a Investment Company Ltd
Date of Establishment: 8th November 1969
No of Employees: 6,000

SOLUS SCHALL (NIGERIA) LTD
39 Norman Williams St, South West Ikoyi, PO Box 8596, Lagos
Tel: 681243, 682999, 680781
Cable: Soluschall Lagos

Directors: V A Allum

PRINCIPAL ACTIVITIES: Diving services, inspection, cathodic protection design, installation and maintenance; materials

SOMIT (NIGERIA) LTD (FORMERLY UNITED ASIAN TRADERS (NIGERIA) LTD)
17 Ijaiye St, PO Box 761, Lagos
Tel: 637679
Cable: Mahboob
Telex: 11117

Chairman: I L Adeoye
Directors: L J Mahboobani,
  J L Mahboobani (Managing Director),
  JS Agboighale (Executive),
  P L Mahboobani,
  Mrs G J Mahboobani
Senior Executives: S A Egberongbe (General Manager),
  T Okonji (Head Salesman),
  R Otun (Stores Manager)

PRINCIPAL ACTIVITIES: Agents and general trading company
Principal Agencies: Lijempf BV, Holland; Holland Food Products BV, Holland; W M McKinney & Sons Ltd, Ireland
Associated Companies: Halken Trading Co (Nigeria)
Principal Bankers: Bank of India (Nigeria) Ltd; United Bank for Africa Ltd

Principal Shareholders: I L Adeoye; J L Mahboobani; Mrs G J Mahboobani; P L Mahboobani; J S Agboighale
Date of Establishment: 18th August 1978

SONA BREWERIES LTD
94 Broad St, Lagos

PRINCIPAL ACTIVITIES: Brewing of beer and soft drinks
Branch Offices: Otta; Ogun State
Financial Information:

	₦'000
Authorised capital	6,000
Paid-up capital	6,000

Principal Shareholders: 40% BSN Gervais Danone; 60% Nigerians
Date of Establishment: 1977 Registered
No of Employees: 500 when in production

SONGHAI CONSTRUCTION LTD
Railway Ave, Kaduna South, PO Box 362, Kaduna
Tel: 242505
Telex: 71316 Songhai Ng

Chairman: Alhaji Isa Kaita
Directors: G A Yakubu, J A Laing
Senior Executives: K Blake (Accountant),
  L H Craig (Company Plant Manager)

PRINCIPAL ACTIVITIES: Civil engineering and construction
Branch Offices: PO Box 343, Maiduguri, Borno State; PMB 1026, Ankpa, Benue State
Associated Companies: Songhai Ltd; Songhai Airlines Ltd
Principal Bankers: Union Bank of Nigeria Ltd
Financial Information: Member of the Songhai Group of Companies

	₦'000
Authorised capital	400
Paid-up capital	300

Principal Shareholders: G A Yakubu; Moreino Properties Ltd
Date of Establishment: January 1976
No of Employees: 150

SONGHAI GROUP OF COMPANIES
5 Station Rd, PO Box 326, Kaduna North
Tel: 213432
Telex: 71112 Ferkad Ng

Chairman: Ahmadu Yakubu
Directors: Alhaji Isa Kaita

PRINCIPAL ACTIVITIES: Industrial holding company with subsidiaries involved in building and road construction in Northern States, electrical power supply, the provision of administrative services, general trading, agriculture, aircraft sales and service, water roticulation and treatment, quarrying, pipe manufacture, electrical engineering and contracting
Branch Offices: Kaduna; Kano; Maiduguri; Gusau
Subsidiary Companies: Songhai Ltd (see separate entry); Songhai Construction Ltd (see separate entry); Songhai Airlines Ltd (air charters and sales agency); Soncrete Ltd (Building materials /cement, irrigation equipment); Ahmadu Yakubu & Associates (Agents and general trading, suppliers of agricultural equipment); Prime Power Ltd, 1 Railway Ave, Kaduna South, Tel 42505 (Electrical engineering and contracting; sales and service of electricity generators); Kaduna Farms Ltd (Agricultural produce, animal feeds); Moreino Properties Ltd (Real estate); Agplan Ltd (Suppliers of agricultural equipment and services); Associate: Unisteel Works Ltd (see separate entry)
Principal Bankers: United Bank for Africa Ltd; Union Bank of Nigeria Ltd; First Bank of Nigeria Ltd
Financial Information:

	₦'000
Authorised capital	2,251
Paid-up capital	1,520
Sales turnover	16,000

No of Employees: 1,200

SONGHAI LTD
5 Station Rd, PO Box 326, Kaduna
Tel: 213432
Telex: 71112 Ferkad Ng

Chairman: Ahmadu Yakubu

PRINCIPAL ACTIVITIES: Building and civil engineering contractors
Branch Offices: 7 Bompai Rd, Kano; Baga Rd, Maiduguri; Gusau
Principal Bankers: United Bank for Africa
Financial Information: Member of the Songhai Group of Companies

	₦'000
Authorised capital	1,000
Paid-up capital	1,000
Sales turnover	8,500

No of Employees: 1,200

SOPROG CONSTRUCTION LTD
38 Town Planning Way, Ilupeju, Ikeja, PO Box 4220, Lagos
Tel: 964530, 960054

Chairman: Prince Yemi Eweka (also Managing Director)
Directors: J K Pinheiro,
  Ernest A Obasuyi (Executive Director),
  E Dosu Eluyemi (Finance/Administration Controller),
  Basil A Adu (Legal Advisor/Secretary)
Senior Executives: Neville L Scott (Project Co-ordinator),
  O A Cisbani (Project Manager),
  Antonio Duccati (Technical Co-Ordinator)

PRINCIPAL ACTIVITIES: Civil engineering and construction
Associated Companies: Sellsoman Ltd; Ernestco Ltd; Sinco Real Estate & Investment Co Ltd
Principal Bankers: United Bank for Africa Ltd
Financial Information:

	₦'000
Authorised capital	1,000
Paid-up capital	750
Sales turnover	1,247

Principal Shareholders: Sinco Real Estate & Investments Company Ltd; Prince Yemi Eweka; Ernest A Obasuyi; J K Pinheiro
Date of Establishment: July 1974
No of Employees: 2,000

SOUTH CHAD LTD
Sir Kashim Ibrahim Way, PMB 1213, Maiduguri, Borno State
Tel: 2367
Telex: 82102 Mintek Ng

PRINCIPAL ACTIVITIES: Building contractors
Branch Offices: 46 Balogun St, PO Box 67, Lagos; Yola Bye-Pass, PMB 2075, Yola, Gongola State

SOUTH PACIFIC CHEMICAL & PLASTICS ENGINEERING COMPANY LTD
Ayodele Diya St, PO Box 173, Ikeja, Lagos
Tel: 932385, 932657, 933495

PRINCIPAL ACTIVITIES: Manufacturers of plastic products; shoes

Date of Establishment: 1971

SOUTHEASTERN DRILLING CO (NIGERIA) LTD (SEDCO)
13 Norman Williams St, SW Ikoyi, PO Box 7906, Lagos
Tel: 680993, 681504, 683581
Telex: 21485 Sedco Ng

Directors: R Gentles (Managing Director),
A O Pinheiro (Financial),
J I Obi (Manager Government Relations),
J R Cross (Base Manager, Port Harcourt),
J Gauslin (Base Manager, Warri)

PRINCIPAL ACTIVITIES: Construction and drilling contractors
Principal Agencies: Sedco, USA
Branch Offices: PO Box 737, Port Harcourt, Rivers State, Cable Sedco Port Harcourt; PMB 1145, Udu Rd, Warri, Bendel State

SPECIAL STRUCTURES & COMPANY LTD
PMB 2147, 26 Ahmadu Bello Way, Kaduna
Tel: 211928

PRINCIPAL ACTIVITIES: Building and civil engineering contractors

SPECO MILL TEXTILES LTD
PO Box 149, Awosika Ave, Industrial Estate, Ikeja, Lagos
Tel: 963617, 964567
Cable: Specomill Lagos
Telex: 21466 Speco Ng

PRINCIPAL ACTIVITIES: Textile manufacturers

SPEED-BIRD CLEARING AND FORWARDING AGENCY LTD
71 Murtala Muhammed Way, PO Box 306, Kano
Tel: 4442
Telex: 77183 Speed Ng

PRINCIPAL ACTIVITIES: Clearing and forwarding agency for all air-freight
Branch Offices: 39 Bornu Crescent, PO Box 112, Apapa, Lagos, Tel 874977
Associated Companies: John Sutcliffe & Son (Grimsby) Ltd, UK

SPICERS (NIGERIA) LTD
89 Murtala Muhammed Way, PO Box 481, Yaba, Lagos
Tel: 862421, 861830
Cable: Spigram Lagos
Telex: 26228 or 11117 TDS 096 Spicer Ng

Chairman: T A Doherty
Directors: Theodore Adesanya Doherty, Simon U Shango
Senior Executives: David Hamilton Simpson (General Manager), Ronald Hobbs (Technical Services Manager)

PRINCIPAL ACTIVITIES: Suppliers of paper, graphic materials, machinery and technical services to the printing, packaging and paper converting industries
Principal Agencies: E I Dupont Photoproducts; Ishida Company Ltd; Sulby; Miller-Johannis-Berg; Stephenson Blake; Nebiolo SpA; Vickers Ltd; Kolbus; Hunter Penrose Littlejohn; AM International; Linotype-Paul; Shoei Star; Kovo; Rockwell-Gos; Timson; Bobst SA; Bielomatik Leuze; Schneider-Senator
Branch Offices: 1/Z Jos Rd, Kaduna
Principal Bankers: First Bank of Nigeria Ltd
Financial Information:

	N'000
Authorised capital	1,000
Paid-up capital	816

Date of Establishment: 1955
No of Employees: 100

SPIROPOULOS, F G, & COMPANY LTD
PO Box 57, Sapele, Bendel State

PRINCIPAL ACTIVITIES: Crepe rubber production

SPORTY FANCY & GENERAL STORES LTD
PO Box 1748, 51 Iga-Idunganran St, Lagos
Tel: 634165, 631659
Cable: Sporty Lagos Nigeria

Chairman: Chief J A Ola Ewuoso (also Managing Director)
Directors: C A Ewuoso, J A Ewuoso, B A Ewuoso, M O Mayomi

PRINCIPAL ACTIVITIES: Importers of sports goods; general merchandise, mostly household electrical appliances, house hold goods, decorations and Christmas decorations; baby products; motor vehicle accessories
Principal Agencies: Cannon Rubber Ltd; OCE Commercial Export Ltd; Burgess Power Tools Ltd; Pifco Ltd; The M H Berlyn Co Ltd; G Weil Ltd; Penguin Plate Ltd
Branch Offices: 7 Ibara Rd, Imo, Abeokuta; 26 Idumagbo Ave, Lagos; N3/915 Oniyanrin Rd, Ibadan, Oyo State
Associated Companies: Oluwo United Company
Principal Bankers: Union Bank of Nigeria Ltd; United Bank for Africa Ltd
Financial Information:

	N'000
Authorised capital	100
Paid-up capital	100
Turnover	1,500

Principal Shareholders: Directors as described
Date of Establishment: 1958

SQUIBB (NIGERIA) LTD
1 Kolawole Shonibare Street, (Off Coker Rd), Ilupeju Industrial Estate, Ilupeju, PMB 12732, Lagos
Tel: 931204
Cable: Ersquibb Lagos
Telex: 26895

Directors: Chief F S Giwa-Osagie,
C O Aniyi (Managing),
M A Kitchen,
E G O Kuye,
H N Ezeudo,
A M Rowsell

PRINCIPAL ACTIVITIES: Suppliers of pharmaceuticals and cosmetics
Principal Agencies: E R Squibb & Sons Inc, USA; E R Squibb & Sons Ltd, UK; Squibb AEBE, Greece, Squibb, Egypt
Branch Offices: 93 Francis Okediji Street, Bodija Estate, PO Box 9850, UI Post Office, Ibadan, Oyo State
Principal Bankers: International Bank for West Africa Ltd; Nigerian Merchant Bank Ltd

Date of Establishment: 8th June 1971

STABILINI & VISINONI LTD
10 Oyabiyi St, Surulere, PO Box 43, Yaba, Lagos
Tel: 836850

Directors: T Visinoni, L Visinoni, V Visinoni

PRINCIPAL ACTIVITIES: Building and civil engineering
contractors

STABILINI, B, & COMPANY LTD
Plot C Makera Rd, Kaduna South, PO Box 245, Kaduna
Tel: 213423

Chairman: E Stabilini
Directors: B Stabilini, B A Ajibola, Alhaji L Baloni, Alhaji
Mohammed Bello
Senior Executives: G Cuffini (General Manager),
L Stabilini (Project Manager)

PRINCIPAL ACTIVITIES: Building and civil engineering
contractors and wholesale distributors
Principal Agencies: Genoa Techno Trade SRL, Italy
Branch Offices: 36 Liverpool Rd, PO Box 104, Zaria, Kaduna
State
Principal Bankers: Union Bank of Nigeria Ltd; United Bank for
Africa Ltd
Financial Information:

	N'000
Authorised capital	600
Paid-up capital	600
Turnover	5,000
Profits	240

Principal Shareholders: B Stabilini; E Stabilini; B A Ajibola;
Alhaji L Baloni
Date of Establishment: 1956
No of Employees: 600

STAG ENGINEERING NIGERIA LTD
PO Box 353, 18 Hamed Jimoh Close, Surulere, Lagos
Tel: 830328
Cable: Engstag Lagos

PRINCIPAL ACTIVITIES: Suppliers of industrial machinery,
precision optical instruments, engineering hand tools, power
generating plants, hospital equipment, etc
Principal Bankers: United Bank for Africa

STANDARD BREWERIES (NIGERIA) LTD
Alomaja Village, Ibadan, Oyo State

Chairman: Chief Labode Oladimeji Akindele

PRINCIPAL ACTIVITIES: Brewing
Financial Information:
Registered capital   N 200,000

Date of Establishment: April 1971

STANDARD CONSTRUCTION LTD
Sharada Industrial Area, PO Box 2029, Kano
Tel: 4068
Cable: Stancol Kano
Telex: 77263 Stacon Ng

Chairman: Alhaji Sani Buhari
Directors: U Peraldo (Managing),
Alhaji Shuiab Kazaure (Executive),
Alhaji Buhari Sani (Executive)
Senior Executives: Claudio Piccinelli (Contracts Manager),
Colin Cummings (Financial Controller),
Cornelio Moda (Project Manager, Civil),
Enrico Massaza (Project Manager, Building)

PRINCIPAL ACTIVITIES: Civil engineering and construction
Branch Offices: Bauchi

No of Employees: 2,000

STANDARD INDUSTRIAL DEVELOPMENT COMPANY LTD
Plot D17, Ogba Industrial Estate, PMB 21350, Ikeja, Lagos
Tel: 962377
Cable: Essayedee
Telex: 21569 Msklgs Ng

Chairman: C F Hsu (also Managing Director)
Directors: Alhaji Inuwa Wada,
K Sekiguchi (General Manager),
John Tung,
D J Rosenberg,
T Urano,
M Tagai,
E B Onifade,
C Ade Atoki,
O A Adeosun
Senior Executives: J P Y Yang (Financial Controller),
Philip Lee,
Dixon Oyekan

PRINCIPAL ACTIVITIES: Manufacturers of building materials;
steel pipes for water and gas systems; furniture
Associated Companies: I-Feng Co Ltd
Principal Bankers: International Bank for West Africa Ltd; Icon
Ltd (Merchant Bank); NAL Merchant Bank

Principal Shareholders: Great Nigerian Insurance Co; Mitsubishi
Corporation (Japan); John Tung; Kobe Steel (Japan) Ltd; C F
Hsu; John Holt Holdings Ltd
Date of Establishment: 1969
No of Employees: 130

STAR MATCH COMPANY LTD
1 Queens Barracks Rd, PO Box 404, Apapa, Lagos
Tel: 836314, 877672
Cable: Bestmatch

PRINCIPAL ACTIVITIES: Manufacturers of book and box
matches
Branch Offices: Factory: 39, Warehouse Rd, Apapa, Lagos

STAR SWEETS CO LTD
172 Mission Rd, PO Box 1230, Kano
Tel: 4162, 7111, 7112, 7113, 7114
Cable: Starco Kano
Telex: 77246 Starco Ng

Chairman: M R Jabr
Directors: Alhaji Mudi Salisu,
Alhaji Almu Inwa,
A M Jabr (Managing),
Alhaji Jimoh Illufoye
Senior Executives: Rasheed Jabr (General Manager),
S Arnaout (Production Manager),
A M Nabahan (Chief Engineer)

PRINCIPAL ACTIVITIES: Manufacturers of boiled sweets, toffees
etc
Financial Information:

	N'000
Authorised capital	1,000
Paid-up capital	1,000
Turnover	9,000

Principal Shareholders: Alhaji Mudi Salisu; Alhaji Almu Inwa; A
M Jabr; M R Jabr
Date of Establishment: 1967
No of Employees: 450

STARLINE NIGERIA LTD
106 Azikiwe Rd, PO Box 562, Aba, Imo State
Tel: 384
Telex: 63107 Starnig Ng

Chairman: P S Owunna

PRINCIPAL ACTIVITIES: Manufacturers of pharmaceuticals
Principal Bankers: Union Bank of Nigeria Ltd

Date of Establishment: 1973
No of Employees: 500

STATE PLASTICS DESIGN COMPANY
West End Rd, Opposite Murtala Muhammed Sq, Mafoni Ward,
   Maiduguri, Borno State
Tel: 9160, 9134
Telex: 82135

Directors: L A Okeh (Managing Director)

PRINCIPAL ACTIVITIES: Suppliers of plastic products

STEEL WORKS LTD
SW7/18 Lagos Bye-Pass, Oke Bola, Ibadan, Oyo State
Tel: 412984, 461430
Telex: 31147

PRINCIPAL ACTIVITIES: Suppliers of steel structures

STEINER, F, & COMPANY LTD
150 Broad Street, PO Box 602, Lagos
Tel: 660723, 66128
Cable: Steiner or Precision

Chairman: Mrs E N Ibru
Directors: G M Ibru,
   A U Ibru,
   Dr E E Essien (Executive),
   J A Balogun

PRINCIPAL ACTIVITIES: Precision engineering, optical and
   photographic equipment
Principal Agencies: Wild Heerbrugg Ltd; Patek Philippe; SSIH
   (Omega Tissot & Lanco); Looping; Junghans; Maurice Lipkin;
   Benzing, Alfred Dunhill; Caran D'Ache
Branch Offices: 19 Burma Rd, Apapa; 79 Mission Rd, PO Box
   731, Benin
Associated Companies: Jewellers Company (Nigeria) Ltd
Principal Bankers: Union Bank of Nigeria Ltd
Financial Information:

	N'000
Authorised capital	1,000
Paid-up capital	200
Turnover	5,000

Principal Shareholders: Ibru Organisation
Date of Establishment: 1949
No of Employees: 200

STEPHENS, HENRY, ENGINEERING COMPANY LTD
2 Ilupeju Bye Pass, PMB 21386, Ikeja, Lagos
Tel: 901460-4
Cable: Hensenco
Telex: 21286, 21256

Directors: Professor Ayo Ogunseye, J E Aldridge, Oladele
   Fajemirokun, S A Oyemakinde
Senior Executives: G Olu Fajemirokun (Executive Director),
   Fred A Akinsanmi (Deputy General Manager),
   A Akintoye (Chief Credit Controller),
   B K Adejuyigbe (Assistant General Manager, Finance),
   Chief A Bakare (Assistant General Manager),
   S A Fagoyinbo (Assistant General Manager)

PRINCIPAL ACTIVITIES: Dealers in construction machinery and
   mechanical engineering plant
Principal Agencies: Allis Chalmers Corporation; Alvan Blanch
   Development Company Ltd; Eaton International Corporation;
   Mannesmann Demag Baumaschinen; Winget (Babcock
   Construction Equipment Ltd); Enfield Ltd, India;
   Steyr-Nigeria Ltd
Branch Offices: Akure/Owo Highway, PMB 715, Akure, Ondo
   State; 5 Ali Akilu Rd, PO Box 1216, Kaduna; Aba Rd/Rumola
   Junction, PMB 5386, Port-Harcourt
Principal Bankers: First Bank (Nigeria) Ltd

STEPHENS, HENRY, GROUP OF COMPANIES
90 Awolowo Rd, SW Ikoyi, PO Box 2480, Lagos
Tel: 655090, 680721, 655092
Telex: 21286

PRINCIPAL ACTIVITIES: Industrial group with diversified
   activities, for specific details see below under associated
   companies
Associated Companies: Henry Stephens & Sons Ltd, 90
   Awolowo Rd, SW Ikoyi, PO Box 2480, Lagos, Activities:
   Importers and exporters, petroleum prospecting; exporters of
   agricultural products; Adriatic Company (Nigeria) Ltd, 40
   Balogun St, PO Box 2480, Lagos, Activities: Estate and
   property Development; Henry Stephens Shipping Company
   Ltd, 13/15 Sapele Rd, PO Box 1013, Apapa, Lagos, Activities:
   Shipping; Nigerian Maritime Services Ltd, 13/15 Sapele Rd,
   PO Box 331, Apapa, Lagos, Activities: Packing, removals,
   storage, airfreight, clearing and forwarding; Nigmarship
   Agencies Ltd, 13/15 Sapele Rd, PMB 1027, Apapa, Lagos,
   Activities: Shipping agency; Gilco (Nigeria) Ltd (see separate
   entry); Henry Stephens Building Materials Co Ltd, 20 Creek
   Rd, PO Box 331, Apapa, Lagos, Tel 875761, Telex 21566
   Henship, Cables Hensbuild Apapa; Henry Stephens
   Engineering Co Ltd (see separate entry); NMS Travel Bureau
   Ltd; 170 Broad St, PO Box 4243, Lagos, Activities: Travels
   and car hire

STERLING PRODUCTS (NIGERIA) LTD
Plot A, D and K Ilupeju Industrial Estate, Mushin, PO Box 3199,
   Lagos
Tel: 964300/4
Cable: Sterlprod Lagos
Telex: 21419 Stern Ng

Directors: David R Weir (Managing Director),
   M J Lusher (General Manager),
   Alhaji Kurami,
   J M Gammon

PRINCIPAL ACTIVITIES: Manufacturers of pharmaceuticals and
   cosmetics
Branch Offices: Ibadan; Aba; Kano; Kaduna

Date of Establishment: 21st February 1969
No of Employees: 800

STEYR NIGERIA LTD
Industrial Estate, PMB 0135, Bauchi
Tel: 42204
Telex: 83325 Stn-Bh-Ng

Chairman: Rtd Brigadier A S Wali
Directors: I Odoe,
   Y D Hassan,
   Alhaji Y B Musawa,
   Alhaji I Damcida,
   H M Malzacher,
   J J Feichtinger,
   E Wengersky,
   F Nisslmueller (Managing)
Senior Executives: B M Gadzama (Company Secretary),
   M Weber (Financial Manager),
   K Mahringer (Commercial Manager),
   B G Stacey (Logistics Manager),
   Mr Triebell (Technical Manager)

PRINCIPAL ACTIVITIES: Assembly and production of
   commercial vehicles, trucks agricultural tractors and
   implements
Principal Bankers: United Bank for Africa Ltd; Union Bank of
   Nigeria Ltd; International Bank for West Africa Ltd; First Bank
   of Nigeria Ltd
Financial Information:

	N'000
Authorised capital	21,100
Paid-up capital	16,000
Turnover	21,529

Principal Shareholders: Nigerian Government; Bauchi State
  Government; Borno State Government; Gongola State
  Government; Plateau State Government; NIDB; Steyr Daimler
  Puch AG; Nigerian Technical Company
Date of Establishment: 22nd November 1976
No of Employees: 750

STIRLING CIVIL ENGINEERING NIGERIA LTD

12 Creek Rd, PO Box 40, Apapa, Lagos
Tel: 875127
Cable: Roller Lagos
Telex: 21331 Roller Ng

Chairman: Alhaji M A Muhammed
Directors: G Vianello (Managing),
  M Baraya,
  D Camerini,
  V K Dangin,
  Mallam Masa'Abu Mohammed,
  M Possenti,
  B Lattanzi,
  Mallam Ibrahim Madaki,
  Alhaji Yahaya Ali (Executive Director),
  Alhaji Kyari Sandabe (Executive Director),
  P Di Costanzo (Executive Director),
  G Facchini (Alternate Director),
  G M Valentini (Alternate Director)
Senior Executives: C A Egede (Assistant to Managing Director)

PRINCIPAL ACTIVITIES: Building and civil engineering
  contractors
Principal Bankers: Union Bank of Nigeria Ltd; First Bank of
  Nigeria Ltd; United Bank for Africa Ltd; Bank of the North
  Ltd; International Bank for West Africa Ltd
Financial Information:

	N'000
Authorised capital	3,000
Paid-up capital	3,000
Turnover	90,000

Principal Shareholders: Benue; Plateau; Kano; Kaduna; Bauchi;
  Borno; Gongola States; Nigerian Employees (60%); Stirling
  International Civil Engineering Ltd (40%)
Date of Establishment: 27th August 1960
No of Employees: 6,000

STOKVIS (NIGERIA) LTD

1 Dawodu Lane, PO Box 136, Ebute-Metta, Lagos
Tel: 834609, 833391

Chairman: B O Benson
Directors: B Binoche, L Dashorst, B Lamigny, Mrs O M
  Benson, Mrs V Onyia, Alhaji Waziri Bagudu
Senior Executives: S A Odoffin (Deputy General Manager),
  Chief J B Oduwale (Chief Accountant),
  M K Osinowo (Product Manager),
  A Amaliku (Product Manager),
  O Ikuomola (Product Manager)

PRINCIPAL ACTIVITIES: Importers and distributors of technical
  equipment, generating sets, surface and submersible pumps
  and hand tools
Principal Agencies: Stahlwille, Germany; Dale Electric, UK;
  Stork Pumps; Guinnard
Branch Offices: Ibadan; Apapa; Warri; Benin; Port Harcourt;
  Kano; Kaduna; Jos; Minna
Principal Bankers: International Bank for West Africa; United
  Bank for Africa; Societe Generale Bank
Financial Information:

	N'000
Authorised capital	2,500
Paid-up capital	1,450
Turnover	9,000
Profits	500

Principal Shareholders: Optorg France; B O Benson; Financial
  Institutions
Date of Establishment: 1957
No of Employees: 320

STORM (NIGERIA) LTD

PO Box 1236, Lagos

PRINCIPAL ACTIVITIES: Offshore drilling contractors
Branch Offices: Plot 714 Adetokunbo Ademola St, Victoria
  Island, Lagos

STRABAG CONSTRUCTION (NIGERIA) LTD

Plot 12 Adeniyi Jones Avenue, PO Box 6025, Ikeja, Lagos
Tel: 960432, 960267
Telex: 26488 Straco Ng

Chairman: Professor O A Seriki
Directors: K John (Managing),
  D N Offor,
  Alhaji Halilu Mandawari,
  H Barrow
Senior Executives: Engr K Sperlich (Chief Engineer),
  G Heidler (Financial Controller),
  M A Shafau (Administrative Manager)

PRINCIPAL ACTIVITIES: Building and civil engineering
  contractors
Branch Offices: PO Box 20, Abuja, Niger State; Ibadan Site,
  Oyo State
Principal Bankers: United Bank for Africa Ltd; Union Bank of
  Nigeria Ltd; First Bank of Nigeria Ltd; Icon Ltd
Financial Information:

	N'000
Authorised capital	1,000
Paid-up capital	1,000

Principal Shareholders: Strabag Construction Nigeria Ltd;
  Strabag Overseas, Nigerians
Date of Establishment: 1977
No of Employees: Approx 2,000

STRONGHOLD (NIGERIA) LTD

Plot 17, Oba Akran Ave, Industrial Estate, PMB 21060, Ikeja,
  Lagos
Tel: 961719, 962476
Cable: Clareng Ikeja
Telex: 26590 Strhld Ng

Chairman: Alhaji Z Muhammed
Directors: R V Parker,
  W T Collison (Managing),
  H A Mohammed,
  A Bello,
  A E Odulesi

PRINCIPAL ACTIVITIES: Importers and distributors of
  construction machinery; manufacturers, sales and service of
  handy angles and accessories
Principal Agencies: Coles Cranes Ltd; Simon Engineering Co
  Ltd; Link 51 Ltd; Chubb Fire Export; Lancer Boss Ltd
Branch Offices: 6 Trans-Amadi Industrial Layout, Oginigba
  Village, PO Box 3437, Port Harcourt, Rivers State; Plot 1304,
  Isa Wali Rd, Tundun Wada, PO Box 806, Kano
Associated Companies: Jambo Holdings Ltd; Benue Electrical
  Co Nigeria Ltd, Kaduna; Distran (Nigeria) Ltd
Principal Bankers: First Bank of Nigeria Ltd
Financial Information:

	N'000
Authorised capital	1,000
Paid-up capital	563
Turnover	8,000

Principal Shareholders: S M Jambo
Date of Establishment: 1974
No of Employees: 176

STRUCTEC

Amuwo Odofin Industrial Layout, Block D Plot 2/4, Isolo Express
  Way, Lagos
Tel: 834027, 834439
Cable: Senafrica Lagos
Telex: 21438 Senafr NG

Senior Executives: G J Bour (Manager for Nigeria),
J Picherot (Manager North)

PRINCIPAL ACTIVITIES: Civil engineering and construction,
suppliers of construction plant, water supply and treatment
tanks, plants and pipes, sewage pipes, plants and pumps,
irrigation equipment

Principal Agencies: Acrow Engineers; Horseley Bridge Water
Tanks; Sambron Dumper and Jack Lifts; Pont-A-Mousson
Halberger Hutte; Flygt Pumps; Selwood Pumps; Laho
Concrete Mixers; Acrow Automation; Pierron Prefabricated
Building; ITT Marlow Pumps & Loewe Pumps; Ductile Cast
Iron Pipes and Products

Branch Offices: 134 Murtala Mohammed Way, PO Box 2024,
Kano, Tel 3853, 3854, 7546, Telex 77156 CFAO KN NG; Plot
9 Trans Amadi Rd, PO Box 58, Port Harcourt, Tel 334350,
331392, Cable Senafrica P/H, Telex 61118 CFAO PH NG

Principal Bankers: First Bank of Nigeria Ltd; United Bank for
Africa Ltd; International Bank for West Africa

Principal Shareholders: A branch of CFAO (Nigeria) Ltd
No of Employees: 190

STRUCTENG ASSOCIATES

318 Murtala Muhammed Way, PMB 1015, Yaba, Lagos
Tel: 863035, 862363

President:
Partners: A J U Osuji, G H Carpenter
Associate Partners: L A Osho, P O Ikezue

PRINCIPAL ACTIVITIES: Civil and structural engineering
consultants

Branch Offices: 15A Dipcharima Crescent, GRA PMB 1549,
Maiduguri, Borno State; 11 Okigwe Rd, PMB 1323, Owerri,
Imo State; NF4 Maiduguri Rd, PO Box 5357, Kaduna, Kaduna
State

Principal Bankers: Union Bank of Nigeria Ltd

Date of Establishment: 1972
No of Employees: 102

STRUCTOR

1 Aerodrome Rd, PO Box 391, Apapa, Lagos
Tel: 877384, 877455

PRINCIPAL ACTIVITIES: Distributors of plywood

STRUCTURAL STEEL WORKS LTD

229/231 Apapa Rd, Iganmu, PO Box 2420, Apapa, Lagos
Tel: 831005, 830215
Cable: Melchimpresse Lagos

Directors: G Cava, C Vegezzi

PRINCIPAL ACTIVITIES: Manufacturers of lorry bodies and
tanks

STUDIO PRESS (NIGERIA) LTD

30 Henry Carr St, PO Box 102, Ikeja, Lagos
Tel: 964007, 964785
Cable: Studiopres
Telex: 26104 Studio Ng

Chairman: Chief M Okoya Thomas
Directors: B J Williams (Managing),
Alhaji F Uthman,
CFAO Nigeria Ltd,
O Lijadu,
Interpart Stuttgart,
D E G Cologne

PRINCIPAL ACTIVITIES: Lithographic printers and
manufacturers of cartons and light packaging materials;
labels

Principal Agencies: Interpart Gesellschaft fur Internationale
Beleiligungen mbH & Co KG, West Germany; Ernst Klett,
West Germany

Principal Bankers: United Bank for Africa Ltd; International Bank
for West Africa Ltd

Financial Information:

	N'000
Authorised capital	2,245
Paid-up capital	2,245
Turnover	8,000

Principal Shareholders: Interpart, Stuttgart, West Germany;
Ernst Klett Verlag, Stuttgart, West Germany; DEG, Cologne,
West Germany; CFAO (Nigeria) Ltd, Lagos
Date of Establishment: 1965
No of Employees: 320

SUBETRA NIGERIA INDUSTRIES LTD

Km 6 Old Ibadan-Lagos Rd, Oluwakemi Layout, PO Box 599,
Ibadan, Oyo State
Tel: 412296

Chairman: Alhaji Chief A A Suberu
Directors: Alhaji S Adelokun

PRINCIPAL ACTIVITIES: Manufacturers of PVC pipes, plastics
and accessories

Principal Bankers: African Continental Bank Ltd; Union Bank of
Nigeria Ltd

Financial Information:

	N'000
Authorised capital	600
Paid-up capital	600

Principal Shareholders: Alhaji Chief A A Suberu; Alhaji S
Adelokun
Date of Establishment: January 1978

SUN INSURANCE OFFICE (NIGERIA) LTD

16th Floor Unity House, 37 Marina, PO Box 2694, Lagos
Tel: 660551, 661318
Cable: Sunallco Lagos
Telex: 21994 Ng

Chairman: Alhaji Baba Danbappa
Directors: Michael H Black (Managing),
E O Enwerem,
Chief J A Akintoba,
R A G Neville,
D S Onyamom,
A J Everest
Senior Executives: E O Kushanu (Accountant/Secretary),
F C Jibunoh (Agency Manager),
M O Dibia (Administration Manager),
A J Adeniji (Underwriting Manager)

PRINCIPAL ACTIVITIES: Insurance
Branch Offices: 242 Herbert Macaulay St, Yaba, Lagos, Tel
862243; Zard Building, 2nd Floor, 6 Lagos Bye Pass, PMB
5290, Ibadan, Oyo State, Tel 413564; 16B Post Office Rd,
PMB 3127, Kano, Tel 4563; 112 Douglas Rd, 1st Floor, PO
Box 408, Owerri, Imo State, Tel 230814; 5 Murtala
Mohammed Rd, PMB 1504, Ilorin, Kwara State, Tel 5445,
5465; 16E Ahmadu Bello Way, PO Box 3603, Kaduna
Subsidiary Companies: Sun Alliance Group, London
Principal Bankers: United Bank for Africa Ltd

Principal Shareholders: Nigerian Participation 60%; Foreign
Ownership 40%
Date of Establishment: Incorporated 1970
No of Employees: 200

SUNFLAG KNITTING MILLS (NIGERIA) LTD

3 Plateau Rd, PO Box 320, Apapa, Lagos
Tel: 836039, 833340
Cable: Sunflag

PRINCIPAL ACTIVITIES: Manufacturing of cotton and synthetic
fabrics

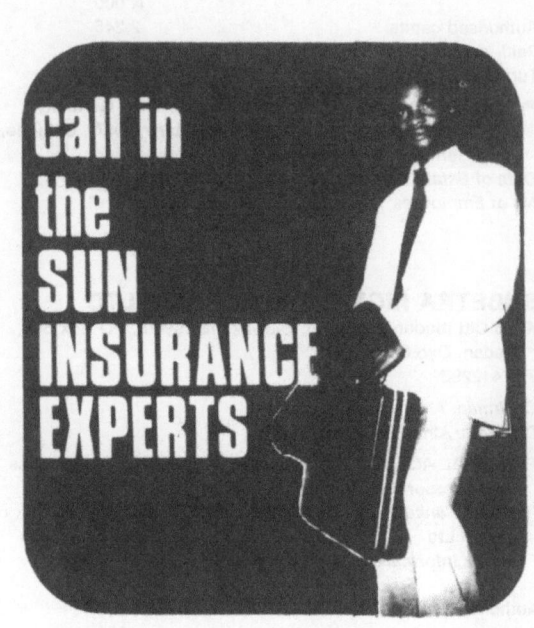

SUNFRESH BREWERY COMPANY NIGERIA LTD

PO Box 248, Warri Rd, Sapele, Bendel State
Tel: 42034
Cable: Oghene Sapele

PRINCIPAL ACTIVITIES: Manufacturers of squashes, and soda

SUNGAS COMPANY LTD

1 Obasa Rd, Ikeja, PO Box 1563, Lagos
Tel: 963070

Chairman: S O Oyewole
Directors: Prince Y O Olagunju, J A Olowolaju, J O Ogunsusi, Prince M O Oluyomi, Chief S A Oladipupo, Chief D O Asolo
Senior Executives: S O Dundun (Operations Manager), E R Ufot (Sales Manager), T O Ologuro (Personnel & General Services Manager)

PRINCIPAL ACTIVITIES: Sales of liquified petroleum gas and domestic applicances
Principal Agencies: Zanusi Grandi Impianti Spa, Italy
Branch Offices: 1 Malu Rd, Apapa; PO Box 527, Ibadan; PO Box 693, Port Harcourt; PMB 1176, Benin City; PO Box 686, Zaria; PO Box 5018, Maiduguri
Principal Bankers: First Bank of Nigeria Ltd
Financial Information:

	N'00
Authorised capital	800
Paid-up capital	800
Turnover	2,590

Principal Shareholders: Odu'a Investment Company Ltd
Date of Establishment: 7th June 1962
No of Employees: 80

SUNNY STATIONERY SUPPLY & BOOKSHOP

37 Daddy Alaja St, PO Box 8320, Lagos State
Tel: 636296

PRINCIPAL ACTIVITIES: Stationery and office equipment supplies

SUNSHINE BATTERIES MANUFACTURING COMPANY

1A Barracks Rd, PMB 1117, Calabar, Cross River State

PRINCIPAL ACTIVITIES: Under construction. When completed, manufacturing of batteries for cars, trucks, tractors and telecommunication equipment
Branch Offices: Factory: Ukana Ikot Ide, Ikot Ekpene, Cross River State
Financial Information:
Registered capital   N 100,000

Date of Establishment: January 1980 Registered
No of Employees: 500 when in full production

SUPERBRU LTD

Agbarha-Otor, PMB 43, Ughelli, Bendel State

PRINCIPAL ACTIVITIES: Brewing

Date of Establishment: 1974 Registered

SUPERFINE FURNITURE & TRADING COMPANY LTD

Airport Rd, PO Box 633, Jos, Plateau State
Tel: 3302, 3060
Cable: Superfine
Telex: 81147 Sufine Nigeria

Chairman: P G Korinjoh
Directors: Mrs R M Korinjoh, T K Korinjoh, C G Korinjoh
Senior Executives: L R Akure, A Irodubar

PRINCIPAL ACTIVITIES: Furniture manufacturing, departmental stores (supermarket, etc)
Branch Offices: PMB 2135, Makurdi, Benue State
Principal Bankers: First Bank of Nigeria Ltd
Financial Information:

	N'000
Authorised capital	500
Paid-up capital	500
Sales turnover	800

Principal Shareholders: Chairman and directors as described
Date of Establishment: 1971
No of Employees: 150

SUPERFORM AFRICA COMPANY LTD
7 Bode Thomas St, Surulere, PO Box 3565, Lagos
Tel: 834360

Chairman: T A Adenekan
Directors: Dapo Adenekan

PRINCIPAL ACTIVITIES: Business and engineering consultants; transporters
Branch Offices: 11 First Ave, Ogun State Housing Corporation Estate, Abeokuta, Ogun State
Associated Companies: Misso Services Corporation & Associates
Principal Bankers: Union Bank of Nigeria Ltd

Principal Shareholders: T A Adenekan
Date of Establishment: August 1978

SUPERIOR SYSTEMS INTERNATIONAL LTD
3 Joseph St, PMB 12699, Lagos
Tel: 634096, 630399, 846343
Cable: Supsysint Lagos

Chairman: David F George

PRINCIPAL ACTIVITIES: Sale of audio-visual items, teaching aid equipment; distributors of public address equipment
Principal Agencies: Buhl Incorporated, USA; Special Instruments Laboratory, USA
Branch Offices: 14 Mission Rd, PO Box 112, Benin City, Bendel State
Associated Companies: Bayajida Educational Supplies Ltd, Kano; Newbroom Enterprises, Cross River State; Labware, Kware State
Principal Bankers: Union Bank of Nigeria Ltd; United Bank for Africa Ltd
Financial Information:

	N'000
Authorised capital	250
Paid-up capital	200

SUTHERLAND, B K, & COMPANY LTD
6 Labinjo Lane, PO Box 3648, Lagos
Tel: 633996, 612800
Telex: 21332 Weline Ng

PRINCIPAL ACTIVITIES: Exporters of timber

SVERDRUP & PARCEL & ASSOCIATES
5 Taslim Elias Close, Victoria Island, (Opposite King Solomon), PO Box 4073, Lagos

Directors: Carl E Tiller (Director)

PRINCIPAL ACTIVITIES: Engineering consultants

SWENIG FURNITURE COMPANY LTD
Block F Ladipo Street, Oshodi Industrial Estate, PMB 21328, Ikeja, Lagos
Tel: 964600
Cable: Mico
Telex: 26232 Manda Ng

Chairman: Chief Adedokun Adeyemi
Directors: Chief E O Adeniyi, Justice S D Adebiyi, Stephen Cheng, Raymond Cheng, Eric Hon
Senior Executives: C K Hon (Plant Engineer)

PRINCIPAL ACTIVITIES: Production of furniture
Branch Offices: Accra Rd, Port-Harcourt
Principal Bankers: Icon Merchant Bank; Savannah Bank of Nigeria Ltd
Financial Information:

	N'000
Authorised capital	400
Paid-up capital	100
Turnover	2,600
Profits	263

Principal Shareholders: Nigerians 60%; Chiap-Hua Timbers Ltd of Hongkong 40%
Date of Establishment: Business commenced on 1st June 1980
No of Employees: 120

SWISS NIGERIAN CHEMICAL COMPANY LTD
287 Agege Motor Rd, PO Box 4310, Ikeja, Lagos
Tel: 963408

Chairman: Alhaji Inua Wada
Directors: P S Dawson, Chief Dr M A Majekodunmi, B Nwankwo, Dr J Walvogel, A M Ferguson (Alternate)

PRINCIPAL ACTIVITIES: Distribution of pharmaceuticals, dyes and chemicals, photochemicals, agrochemical products; agricultural research and technical services; plastics and pigments
Principal Agencies: Ciba Geigy, Basle, Switzerland; Ciba Geigy, Duxford
Branch Offices: 9 Sultan Bello Way, Kaduna; PO Box 4710, Kano; 47 Anawbia St, Enugu; PO Box 1907, Ibadan
Principal Bankers: Union Bank of Nigeria Ltd; International Bank for West Africa; United Bank for Africa Ltd

Principal Shareholders: Ciba Geigy Basle 40%; Nigerians 60%
Date of Establishment: 1964
No of Employees: 250

SWISS NIGERIAN WOOD INDUSTRIES LTD
PMB 1009, Epe, Lagos State

PRINCIPAL ACTIVITIES: Production of sawn timber, plywoods and veneers
Branch Offices: 10/14 Calcutta Crescent, Apapa, Lagos, Tel 47425

SYNDIVEL PLASTIC INDUSTRY NIGERIA LTD
33 Awka Rd, Nkpor, PO Box 4148, Onitsha, Anambra State
Tel: 212651
Cable: PO Box 4148, Onitsha

Chairman: Chief Silas Anakpe
Directors: Anthony Mann, David Mann
Senior Executives: Mrs Beth Mann (Executive Secretary)

PRINCIPAL ACTIVITIES: Plastics and plastic products
Branch Offices: 33 Enu-Owa St, PO Box 5042, Lagos
Principal Bankers: African Continental Bank Ltd
Financial Information:

	N'000
Authorised capital	440
Paid-up capital	440

Principal Shareholders: Directors as described above
Date of Establishment: 28th February 1980

T A BRAITHWAITE (INSURANCE BROKERS) & CO
See BRAITHWAITE, T A, (INSURANCE BROKERS) & CO

T A HAMMOND PROJECTS LTD
See HAMMOND, T A, PROJECTS LTD

T L ROBERTS & COMPANY LTD
See ROBERTS, T L, & COMPANY LTD

TABANSI MOTORS LTD
15A Oguta Rd, PMB 1641, Onitsha, Anambra State
Tel: 547

Senior Executives: Prince R N Tabansi (Managing),
O M Obiegbunem,
Prince F O Tabansi,
J I Obiegbunem,
Prince V C Tabansi,
E C O Okoye

PRINCIPAL ACTIVITIES: Transporters and motor vehicle agents
Branch Offices: 148 Murtala Mohammed Way, Lagos, Tel
842145; 18A Aba/Owerri Rd, Aba, Imo State, Tel 540; 32
Chukwuani St, Enugu, Anambra State; 136 Akpakpava St,
Benin City, Bendel State; 61 Aba Rd, Port Harcourt, Rivers
State

TADAT ENGINEERING COMPANY LTD
9 Lagos University Rd, Akoka, Yaba, Lagos
Tel: 835677

PRINCIPAL ACTIVITIES: Building and civil engineering
contractors

TAIKE & BROTHERS LTD
4/6 Boyle St, Shomolu, PO Box 1115, Surulere, Lagos
Tel: 846260, 962883

Chairman: Rueben Babatunde Osunkoya
Directors: Mrs Julianah Adejumoke Osunkoya, Thomas
Olunlade Osunkoya
Senior Executives: J O Osunkoya (Sales Manager),
Mrs N Ogunwale (Office Manageress)

PRINCIPAL ACTIVITIES: Building contractors and merchants
Branch Offices: 5 Taike St, Ikosi-Ketu, Lagos
Principal Bankers: Union Bank of Nigeria Ltd
Financial Information:

	N'000
Sales turnover	2,500
Profits	800

Principal Shareholders: Directors as described above
Date of Establishment: 1974
No of Employees: 450

TAIWO AJAI COMMUNICATIONS
28 Akinwonmi St, Ire Akari Estate, Isolo, PMB 1133, Oshodi,
Lagos
PRINCIPAL ACTIVITIES: Sales and service of motor vehicles

TAKE YOUR CHOICE RECORD STORES LTD
182 Obafemi Awolowo Way, PO Box 1979, Ikeja, Lagos
Tel: 960029

PRINCIPAL ACTIVITIES: Suppliers and manufacturers of
gramophone records, cassettes and cartridges

Principal Shareholders: Member of the Bolarinwa Abioro
Organisation

TAKKO ENGINEERING LTD
Yandoko Rd, PO Box 39, Bauchi
Tel: 42256

Directors: Alhaji Mohammed B Takko (Managing),
Mallam Abubakar Luji
PRINCIPAL ACTIVITIES: Civil engineering and construction;
stationers, poultry farming etc

Date of Establishment: 1977

TAMACO LTD
15 Martins St, PO Box 195, Lagos
Tel: 632827

PRINCIPAL ACTIVITIES: Importers, exporters, caterers,
hoteliers, etc

TARA CONSULTING NIGERIA LTD
25 Bishop Oluwole Street, Plot 1136, Victoria Island, PO Box
9144, Lagos
Tel: 614898
Cable: Taraconnig, Lagos

Directors: Michael Olutunde Olowu,
James J Sheehy (Managing)
PRINCIPAL ACTIVITIES: Computer consultancy

TARMAC ENGINEERING COMPANY LTD
PO Box 491, Plot 28, Iganmu Industrial Estate, Apapa, Lagos
Tel: 835625

PRINCIPAL ACTIVITIES: Building and civil engineering
contractors

TARPAULIN INDUSTRIES (WA) LTD
8 Burma Rd, Apapa, PO Box 2227, Lagos
Tel: 876470, 876024
Cable: Tarpind Lagos

Chairman: Chief I A S Adewale
Directors: A M Ferguson,
Chief D S Yaro,
S Mamman,
C O Eguntola,
D S B Webster (Managing)
Senior Executives: R A Popoola (Deputy General
Manager/Secretary),
A Agudah (Commercial Manager),
Mr Cathro (Technical Service/Training Manager)

PRINCIPAL ACTIVITIES: Manufacturers of tarpaulins, tents,
vehicle covers, mail bags, manufacturers' representatives.
Distributors of power equipment, woodworking equipment and
terrapin steel clad accommodation units
Principal Agencies: Bonar Textiles PLC
Principal Bankers: First Bank of Nigeria Ltd

Date of Establishment: 1956
No of Employees: 200

TASIUS NIGERIA LTD
106 Nnamdi Azikiwe St, 2nd Floor, PO Box 4749, Lagos
Tel: 630742
Cable: Reward
Telex: 20117 UK Correspondent; 11117 Tds Box 233 Lagos
Other Countries

Chairman: A A K Ibeh
Directors: E O Ibeh, M O Ibeh
Senior Executives: F B O Emenyonu (Sales Manager)

PRINCIPAL ACTIVITIES: Suppliers of industrial safety
equipment; office equipment suppliers
Principal Agencies: Martindale Protection Ltd, UK;
Industriservice GmbH, West Germany; A Werner GmbH, West
Germany
Branch Offices: 138 Wetheral Rd, PO Box 335, Owerri, IMO
State; 188 Agege Motors Rd, Mushin, Lagos
Principal Bankers: First Bank of Nigeria Ltd
Financial Information:

	N'000
Authorised capital	100
Paid-up capital	100
Turnover	1,000

Principal Shareholders: Directors as described
Date of Establishment: 1975

TATE & LYLE (NIGERIA) LTD
47/48 Eric Moore Rd, Iganmu Industrial Estate, PO Box 1240,
Lagos
Tel: 837364, 837582, 834874, 830097
Telex: 21258, 21087

Chairman: Dr A Liman Ciroma
Directors: Alhaji Isa Tahir (Vice Chairman & Managing Director),
  G H Maingot (Deputy Managing Director),
  L C Arukwe (Marketing Director),
  B O Osibo (Works Director),
  M A Salako (Finance Director),
  Mrs M R A Adeleke (Director/Secretary),
  J E Wright,
  M J L Attfield,
  Mallam M Z Idris
Senior Executives: E A Akinsiwaju (General manager, Plastics),
  Mrs T O Oreagba (Marketing Manager, Sugar),
  J O U Abiri (Personnel Manager),
  Y O Odutola (Manufacturing Manager)

PRINCIPAL ACTIVITIES: Manufacturing and distribution of cube and granulated sugar, ridgways tea and UPVC pipes
Principal Agencies: Hepworth Plastics International Ltd; Tate & Lyle Industries Ltd; General Sucriere; Beghin Say; Ridgways Tea
Branch Offices: Commercial Avenue, PO Box 2589, Yaba; PO Box 611, 18/19 Ahmadu Bello Way, Kaduna; PO Box 308, Niger House, Onitsha; PO Box 124, Aba; C/O MDS, PO Box 342, Calabar; PO Box 482, Port Harcourt; PO Box 96, Offa Rd, Ilorin; Fagboun Building, Oke-Bola Street, PO Box 1453, Ibadan; Akpakpava Street; Ikpoba Slope; PO Box 86, Benin-City; 18B Post Office Rd, 27/32 Beirut Rd, PO Box 175, Kano; PMB 1534, Maiduguri; The Beach Rd, PMB 1386, Jos
Principal Bankers: First Bank of Nigeria Ltd; Union Bank of Nigeria Ltd; United Bank for Africa Ltd; International Bank for West Africa Ltd
Financial Information:

	₦'000
Authorised capital	4,000
Paid-up capital	3,180
Turnover	91,540
Profits	2,620

Principal Shareholders: Nigerian Public
Date of Establishment: 1st March 1962
No of Employees: 876

TAYLOR WOODROW OF NIGERIA LTD

10 Abebe Village Rd, Iganmu, PO Box 138, Lagos
Tel: 837290, 837468, 837407, 834828, 832335
Cable: Tayrow Lagos
Telex: 21544

Chairman: Chief Adebayo A Ogunsanya
Directors: F A B Shepherd (Managing),
  Alhaji Sani Zangon Duara,
  E A L Webber,
  Tanko Kuta,
  R W Pitfield,
  Chief T A Iwajomo,
  Dr L A Shonubi,
  M K Abinde
Senior Executives: Y O K Garuba (Company Secretary),
  R J Gilbert (Commercial Manager),
  J B Oduyela (Administration Manager),
  A L Holmes (Contracts Manager)

PRINCIPAL ACTIVITIES: Building, civil engineering and mechanical contractors: well drilling contractors
Branch Offices: PO Box 2041, 48 Lamido Crescent, Kano; PO Box 247, Minna, Niger State; PO Box 177, Sokoto; PO Box 34, 719 Bank Rd, Kaduna
Principal Bankers: First Bank of Nigeria Ltd

Principal Shareholders: Ogunsanya Investments Company Ltd; Taylor Woodrow International Ltd; Taylor Woodrow Ltd; Sokoto State Government; Niger State Government
Date of Establishment: 1946
No of Employees: 4,000

TAYLORBIRD FABRIC & DESIGN LTD

10 Harbour Rd, PO Box 57, Lagos

PRINCIPAL ACTIVITIES: Manufacture of textiles

TECHINT ENGINEERING (NIGERIA) LTD

23 Musa Yaradua Street, Plot 210, Victoria Island, PO Box 51135, Falomo, Lagos
Tel: 617392/3/4
Telex: 21340 Rexco Nig or Net 20117 TDS Box 218

Chairman: Chief O Oyewole
Directors: S B Adegbayibi, P B Oyebolu, P L Tesei
Senior Executives: D Rondinone (Managing Director),
  V Tocco (Contract Manager)

PRINCIPAL ACTIVITIES: Consulting engineers, project management, oil, gas facilities and pipeline design and engineering; construction work supervision
Associated Companies: Techint Engineering SA, Switzerland; Techint Overseas Ltd, UK
Principal Bankers: United Bank for Africa Ltd

Date of Establishment: 1977

TECHJOB ASSOCIATES

12 Rosamond St, PO Box 3272, Surulere, Lagos State
Tel: 848447

Chairman: Isaac Adebisi Olaiya
Senior Executives: J O J Ademulegun, M A Ojejinmi

PRINCIPAL ACTIVITIES: Civil and structural engineering consultants
Principal Bankers: Co-operative Bank Ltd; Union Bank of Nigeria Ltd

TECHNAE (NIGERIA) LTD

PO Box 199, Apapa, Lagos
Tel: 873897

Chairman: I A S Adewale
Directors: C D P Papanastiou (Managing)

PRINCIPAL ACTIVITIES: Importers and suppliers of electrical equipment and neon signs
Date of Establishment: 1958

TECHNICAL & BUILDING MATERIALS LTD

PO Box 470, Waff Rd, Zaria, Kaduna State
Tel: 2059

PRINCIPAL ACTIVITIES: Building and civil engineering contractors

TECHNICAL CONSTRUCTIONS (NIGERIA) LTD

PMB 2378, 6 Ijora Causeway, Ijora, Lagos
Tel: 831053, 831387
Cable: Nigtelco

Chairman: Brigadier E E Ikwue
Directors: Dr E O Ogbu, J T F Iyalla, Mrs M Papadopoulos, C P Leventis, Federal Ministry of Finance Inc
Senior Executives: N Roy (General Manager),
  J C Onwuka (Financial Controller),
  R W Wilson (Contracts Manager),
  J L Olota (Projects Manager),
  Olu Adenodi (Commercial Officer)

PRINCIPAL ACTIVITIES: Electrical engineering contractors
Branch Offices: Sir Kashim Ibrahim Rd, PMB 1095, Maiduguri, Borno State
Principal Bankers: United Bank for Africa Ltd
Financial Information:

	₦'000
Authorised capital	500
Paid-up capital	200
Turnover	5,000
Profits	200

Principal Shareholders: Chairman and directors as described
Date of Establishment: 1959
No of Employees: 250

TECHNOPHON ELECTRICAL ENTERPRISES COMPANY LTD

2 Sunday St, Palm Grove, PO Box 291, Ebute Metta, Lagos
Tel: 841546, 861116

PRINCIPAL ACTIVITIES: Suppliers of electrical equipment

TEDDY CONTINENTAL COMPANY

Plot 26 Adetola Street, Aguda, PO Box 3819, Surulere, Lagos State
Cable: Teddycon Lagos

President: Christopher I Tedela
Senior Executives: Simeon Ojo Tedela (Sales Manager), Charlotte Olusola Ajayi (Miss) (Public Relations Officer)

PRINCIPAL ACTIVITIES: Safety and security equipment; industrial plants and machinery; general importers and agents
Principal Agencies: ABC Europ Production GmbH, West Germany; Hashmira Security Co Ltd, Israel
Principal Bankers: Union Bank of Nigeria ltd
Financial Information:
Turnover   ₦ 30,000,000

Date of Establishment: 8th June 1978

TEJU INDUSTRIES LTD

10/12 Ilupeju Bye-Pass, Industrial Estate, Ilupeju, PMB 1191, Ikeja, Lagos
Tel: 964493, 964421, 964420, 964164
Cable: Tejufoam Lagos

PRINCIPAL ACTIVITIES: Manufacturers of foam mattresses, cushions, pillows, etc; assemblying of radios and televisions
Branch Offices: Kano; Warri; Onitsha; Aba; Ibadan

TELEREX ELECTRONICS LTD

Plot D Industrial Crescent, Ilupeju, PO Box 1806, Lagos
Tel: 963624
Cable: Telerex Lagos

PRINCIPAL ACTIVITIES: Assemblying of radios, radiograms and television sets
Branch Offices: Odo-Oba Elere Village, Oke-Oluokun, Ibadan, Oyo State

TELOTA COSMETICS COMPANY NIGERIA LTD

13 Ogundare Street, Aguda Surulere, PO Box 2638, Marina, Lagos
Tel: 830067
Cable: Darkelota Lagos

Chairman: Frederick Sigismund McEwen
Directors: Anthony K Onipede (Managing), F Olatunji Onipede

PRINCIPAL ACTIVITIES: Manufacturers of cosmetics
Principal Bankers: United Bank for Africa Ltd
Financial Information:

	₦'000
Authorised capital	40
Paid-up capital	40

Principal Shareholders: Chairman and directors as described
Date of Establishment: Registered 1975

TEMPLAR AFRIQUE (NIGERIA) LTD

PO Box 445, Apapa, Lagos

PRINCIPAL ACTIVITIES: Wholesale books and stationery

TENIMASUNWON AGENCY

37/39 Smith St, PO Box 4615, Lagos
Tel: 657386

Chairman: S A Ogunsanya
Directors: Mrs Olufolake Opesanwo, Olufemi Ogunsanya
Senior Executives: Martin Oduwole (General Manager), Akim Ogunsanya (Operations Manager, Printing), Miss Abiola Ayodele (Sales Executive), Michael Ajayi (Secretary, Accountant), Tajudeen Alimi (Public Relations Officer)

PRINCIPAL ACTIVITIES: Importation of stationery, printing materials and office equipment; agro-allied supplies, transporters and haulage agents
Principal Agencies: Wiggins Teape (WA) Ltd; Uni-Nigeria (International) Company
Branch Offices: 83 Old Yaba Rd, Ebute-Metta, Lagos; 1 Odubote Lane, Omu-Ijebu, Ogun State
Associated Companies: Ayo Ogunsanya Brothers
Principal Bankers: Savannah Bank of Nigeria Ltd; African Continental Bank Ltd

TENNECO OIL COMPANY OF NIGERIA

Western House, 13th Floor, 8/10 Broad St, Lagos Island, PO Box 2119, Lagos
Tel: 657790/1, 656585, 630931
Cable: Tenni Ng
Telex: 21328 Tenni Ng

PRINCIPAL ACTIVITIES: See Mobil Producing Nigeria

TETENGI, ALHAJI USMAN, & SONS LTD

604 Bukuru Bye Pass, PO Box 222, Jos, Anambra State
Tel: 3076

PRINCIPAL ACTIVITIES: General contractors, importers and exporters of general goods, transporters

TEXACO NIGERIA LTD

PO Box 166, 241 Igbosere Rd, Lagos
Tel: 630577, 632076

Chairman: H C Minor
Directors: J O Sheldon, Chief E Ade Ojo (Administration), Alhaji G A Adegboyega (Finance/Accounts), E I Nwizu (General Manager), G E Smith (Managing), J Poupeau, Chief M O Feyide, A M Ferguson
Senior Executives: S C O Ahuchogu (General Operations Manager), J A Southey (Manager, Commercial Department), A I Ohomele (Manager, Planning and Development), A S T Danmole (Manager, Resale Department)

PRINCIPAL ACTIVITIES: Marketing of petroleum products, petrochemicals
Branch Offices: Yaba; Ibadan; Kano; Jos; Enugu; Port Harcourt; Warri
Principal Bankers: Union Bank of Nigeria Ltd; International Bank for West Africa; Unity Bank for Africa Ltd; International Merchant Bank (Nigeria) Ltd
Financial Information:

	₦'000
Authorised capital	13,607
Paid-up capital	13,606
Turnover	163,765
Profits (after tax)	13,216

Principal Shareholders: Texas Petroleum Company New York 60%; Nigerian Citizens 40%
Date of Establishment: 12th August 1969
No of Employees: 416

TEXAS OVERSEAS (NIGERIA) PETROLEUM CO (TOPCON)

Western House, 6th Floor, 8/10 Broad St, Lagos Island, PO Box 1986, Lagos
Tel: 636770, 656544, 657176
Cable: Topcon Lagos
Telex: 21293 Topcon Ng

Directors: J E Robinson (General Manager),
  R K Helms (Operations Manager),
  T C Iloabachie (Accounts Manager)
Senior Executives: Dallas R Staples (Production Supt)

PRINCIPAL ACTIVITIES: Petroleum exploration and production
Branch Offices: Field Office: PO Box 467, Warri, Bendel State

No of Employees: 193

TEXTILE COMMODITIES LTD

149 Club Rd, PO Box 1238, Kano
Tel: 4404, 3467
Cable: Socfa Kano

PRINCIPAL ACTIVITIES: Manufacturers of shoe laces and hosiery

TEXTILE UTILITIES MANUFACTURING LTD

Ayodele Diyan Rd, PO Box 184, Ikeja, Lagos

PRINCIPAL ACTIVITIES: Spinning, weaving and finished textile products

THEO & THEO PAINTS COMPANY (NIGERIA) LTD

Plot 58 Adeola Ave, Ifako, PO Box 297, Ikeja, Lagos

PRINCIPAL ACTIVITIES: Manufacturers of paint

Date of Establishment: December 1972

THERMOCOOL ENGINEERING COMPANY LTD

33 Planning Office Way, Ilupeju, PMB 21132, Ikeja, Lagos
Tel: 901110/9

Chairman: J Giannopoulos
Directors: Th Grigoris (Managing),
  A Mariolis,
  G R E Obong,
  K B Jamodu

PRINCIPAL ACTIVITIES: Refrigeration

Date of Establishment: 9th July 1971
No of Employees: 450

THERMOSTEIN LTD

Plot F Block 6 Industrial St, Ilupeju Industrial Estate, PMB 1124, Apapa, Lagos
Tel: 964259
Cable: Steinertec Lagos
Telex: 21324 Ibru Ng

PRINCIPAL ACTIVITIES: Suppliers of air conditioning equipment

THINGS INTERNATIONAL (NIGERIA) LTD

33 Modupe Johnson Crescent, Surulere, Lagos

PRINCIPAL ACTIVITIES: Distribution of chemical products
Principal Agencies: Crain Chemical Company, USA

THOMADE ENTERPRISES (NIG) LTD

Ac 254, Ahmadu Bello Way, PO Box 67, Maiduguri, Borno State
Tel: 232115, 232514
Cable: Thomade

Chairman: Thomas A Popoola (also Managing Director)
Directors: Suleiman A Salawu
Senior Executives: Adamu Alhaji Usman (Acting General Manager),
  Samual F Kadir (Branch Manager)

PRINCIPAL ACTIVITIES: Suppliers of educational equipment, electrical and electronic equipment, office equipment and supplies, paper/paper products
Principal Agencies: Thomas Wyatt Nigeria Ltd; Nigeria Paper Mills; Continental Office Products; Leventis Technical Ltd; Oxford University Press; Longman Nigeria Ltd; Evans Brothers Ltd, etc
Branch Offices: 20 Anjorin Rd, PO Box 439, Kwara State; Block 10 Jimeta New Market, PO Box 502, Yola, Gongola State, Tel 24024; CMS Cathedral Rd, PO Box 182, Offa, Kwara State
Principal Bankers: Union Bank of Nigeria Ltd

Principal Shareholders: Thomas A Popoola; Suleiman A Salawu

THOMAS ADEMOLA & CO LTD

See ADEMOLA, THOMAS, & CO LTD

THOMAS FURNITURE COMPANY LTD

PMB 5156, Factory Mile 85, Lagos Rd, Ibadan, Oyo State
Tel: 461267
Cable: Tomfurn
Telex: 31131 Tomfur Ng

Chairman: Chief O I Akinkugbe
Directors: O O Fawehinmi
Senior Executives: G J F Mesker (General Manager, Furniture/Sawmill Division),
  Hans Naerebout (Production Manager, Furniture Division),
  M M Branly (Operation Manager, Sawmill Division)

PRINCIPAL ACTIVITIES: Wooden furniture manufacturers and sawmilling
Branch Offices: Sawmill Factory, Agbabu via Ore, Ondo State
Principal Bankers: United Bank for Africa Ltd

Principal Shareholders: Nigerians
Date of Establishment: 1957
No of Employees: 335

THOMAS, J A, RUBBER ESTATES LTD

Awadagin Port, Jamieson River, PO Box 1, Sapele, Bendel State

Tel: 40280
Cable: Speedwell

Chairman: Chief B J A Uku
Directors: A David, C Ogbuagu, P Ajuyah, V T Uku, V Abido, V A Thomas
Senior Executives: W M Omatsone (Manager),
  G A Bello (Engineer),
  J O Igalah (Accounting Officer),
  Walter Brownridge (Electrical Engineer)

PRINCIPAL ACTIVITIES: Production of sheet and crepe rubber; sawmills
Principal Agencies: Nigerian Rubber Board
Associated Companies: Timber and Sawmills
Principal Bankers: New Nigeria Bank Ltd
Financial Information:

	N'000
Authorised capital	200
Paid-up capital	200

Principal Shareholders: Children of Founder - Late James Awadagin Thomas
Date of Establishment: 1899; Incorporated 1959

THOMAS MECHANICAL PLUMBING

PO Box 2933, 6 McNeil Rd, Yaba, Lagos
Tel: 860351

PRINCIPAL ACTIVITIES: Building and civil engineering contractors

THOMPSON DICKSON TECHNICAL CO LTD

24 Efosa St, Uzebu Quarters, Off Ekenwan Rd, PO Box 142, Benin City, Bendel State
Tel: 241888, 242823
Telex: 41137 Tomdic Ng

PRINCIPAL ACTIVITIES: Suppliers of refrigerators, air-conditioners, sewing machines, televisions, stereo and office equipment; building materials
Branch Offices: 5 Aba Rd, Port Harcourt, Rivers State, Tel 229684; 23 Bassey Duke St, PO Box 177, Calabar, Cross River State, Tel 2345; 20 Cooke Rd, Forestry Rd, Benin City, Bendel State; 9 Warri/Sapele Rd, Warri, Bendel State; 6 Robert Rd, Warri, Bendel State

THORESEN & COMPANY (NIGERIA) LTD

Plot 44, Iganmu Industrial Estate, Iganmu, PO Box 114, Apapa, Lagos
Tel: 837762, 836865
Cable: Papover Lagos

Chairman: Chief Moyo Aboderin
Directors: Chief Franco Olugbake, Ajibola O Ogunsola, Solomon O Adeyemo, Miss Olufunmilola Aboderin
Senior Executives: O Sjolie (Managing Director),
    T A Ogunrinola (Executive Director, Marketing and Corporate Affairs),
    G A Olayode (Finance Manager)

PRINCIPAL ACTIVITIES: Paper conversion, importation of printing papers and boards, printing machines and related products for the printing trade, sales of power tools and graphic systems
Principal Bankers: First Bank of Nigeria Ltd
Financial Information:

	N'000
Authorised capital	500
Paid-up capital	200
Sales turnover	2,515
Profits	30

No of Employees: 120

TIDEX NIGERIA LTD

PO Box 5542, 105 Awolowo Rd, Ikoyi, Lagos State
Tel: 682792, 683003
Cable: Tiwadex Lagos
Telex: 21104

Directors: Bill Ramey (Managing Director),
    W R Croyle,
    Chief Esiso,
    G Ogunlami,
    R Gates
Senior Executives: D Hart (Operations Manager),
    A Barley (Operations Manager)

PRINCIPAL ACTIVITIES: Shipping services; transport; oil and gas services
Branch Offices: Tidewater Marine Inc, PO Box 61117, New Orleans, USA; Field offices: PMB 5187, Port Harcourt; PO Box 280, Warri, Bendel State
Principal Bankers: First Bank of Nigeria Ltd

No of Employees: 500

TILBURY CONTRACTING CO (NIGERIA) LTD

Orogun Village, Oyo Rd, PO Box 474, Ibadan, Oyo State
Tel: 411641, 411672, 411723
Telex: 31133

Directors: M W Reed (Managing),
    D A Carey,
    D W J Savage,
    S A Osobamiro,
    A O Runsewe

PRINCIPAL ACTIVITIES: Civil engineering contractors
Branch Offices: United Bank for Africa Ltd
Financial Information:
Registered capital   N 1,200,000

Date of Establishment: 1976
No of Employees: 1,000

TILLA INTERNATIONAL LTD

18 Eric Moore Rd, Surulere, Lagos
Tel: 831198

Chairman: Alhaji Mohammed Mamman Biu
Directors: Ibrahim Mohammed Biu

PRINCIPAL ACTIVITIES: Civil engineering and construction
Branch Offices: Throughout Nigeria
Principal Bankers: Bank of the North Ltd; First Bank of Nigeria Ltd
Financial Information:
Paid-up capital   N 500,000

Date of Establishment: 1974 Tilla International, 1976 Ahar-Tilla Construction
No of Employees: 150

TILLEY GYADO GROUP OF COMPANIES

Tilley Gyado House, PO Box 452, Jos, Plateau State
Tel: 54322
Cable: Tilleysons Jos
Telex: 81145 Tilley Ng

Chairman: Tilley Gyado
Directors: Jacob Tilley-Gyado, Joseph Tilley-Gyado
Senior Executives: Anthony Chikwendu (Group Financial Controller)

PRINCIPAL ACTIVITIES: Hoteliers, hardware suppliers, exporters and importers of general merchandise, real estate owners
Subsidiary Companies: Tilley Gyado Assurance (Nigeria) Ltd; Tilley Gyado Motors (Nigeria) Ltd; Tilley Gyado Colleges; Gyado-Steers (Nigeria) Ltd

TIMES LEISURE SERVICES LTD

Plot 32 Imam Dauda St, Off Eric Moore, PO Box 1211, Surulere, Lagos

PRINCIPAL ACTIVITIES: Suppliers of electrical goods, television sets, cookers, etc, car hire services, travel agency
Financial Information: Part of Daily Times Group

TIMES PRESS LTD

9 Warehouse Rd, PO Box 306, Apapa, Lagos
Tel: 875942, 875547

Chairman: Alhaji Magaji Dambata
Directors: O Oyerinde, E A Jaja, S U Shango
Senior Executives: O Oyerinde (Director/General Manager),
    C Ghomorai (Deputy General Manager),
    D B Ajibade (Chief Accountant),
    O Sonubi (Commercial Manager)

PRINCIPAL ACTIVITIES: Commercial printing; calenders, labels, posters, stationery, diaries, magazines, books, stationery forms, etc
Principal Bankers: United Bank for Africa Ltd; First Bank of Nigeria Ltd; Union Bank of Nigeria Ltd

Principal Shareholders: Daily Times of Nigeria
Date of Establishment: 1963
No of Employees: 600

TIMMY PRINTING PRESS

35 Apapa Rd, Ebute Metta, Lagos
Tel: 833249

PRINCIPAL ACTIVITIES: Printing

TIN & ASSOCIATED MINERALS LTD

PO Box 462, Jos, Plateau State
PRINCIPAL ACTIVITIES: Tin mining

TOMAX-BETON CONSTRUCTION COMPANY LTD

1 Femi Ayantuga Crescent, Surulere, PO Box 4277, Lagos
Tel: 876898, 877105
Cable: Tobecon

Chairman: Alhaji Ibrahim Tako Galadima Bida
Directors: Chief O Uwadibie (Managing Director),
　Major M B Deinsah,
　H Krahmer,
　G Will,
　H J Stieringer,
　Mallam Shehu Sanusi
Senior Executives: F C Delaon (General Manager),
　David G Joaquin (Controller of Operations),
　Mrs R Brebonia (Finance Manager)

PRINCIPAL ACTIVITIES: Building and civil engineering;
　architectural designers
Branch Offices: Kaduna; Abuja; Benin City; Issele-Uku
Associated Companies: Ututu Holding Company Ltd, Lagos;
　Interocean Seahorse Ltd, Lagos; Omado Industrial Ventures
　Ltd
Principal Bankers: New Nigeria Bank Ltd
Financial Information:

	₦'000
Authorised capital	400
Paid-up capial	325
Turnover	30,000
Profits	3,000

Principal Shareholders: Chief O Uwadibie
Date of Establishment: April 1976
No of Employees: 600

TOMMY BUILDING & CONSTRUCTION COMPANY LTD

PO Box 142, 24 Efosa St, Off Ekenwan Rd, Benin City, Bendel
　State
Tel: 240510, 241888, 242823
Telex: 41137 Tomdic Ng

PRINCIPAL ACTIVITIES: General contractors, construction;
　distribution of building materials, electrical appliances, office
　equipment and furniture

TOPAZ (NIGERIA) LTD

94 Griffith St, PMB 1063, Ebute-Metta, Lagos State
Tel: 847146
Cable: Topaz Lagos

Chairman: Emmanuel A Ogunade
Directors: Ebenezer Ogunade (Printer),
　Timothy Ogunade (Printer)
Senior Executives: V A Bangbelu (Accountant),
　G A Ajayi (Secretary),
　Isaac Obe (Production Manager)

PRINCIPAL ACTIVITIES: Agents and general trading; suppliers
　of office equipment/supplies and industrial equipment and
　heavy machinery; printing, etc
Principal Agencies: Drem Offset; Mercedes; Minmetal Swiss;
　Jac; Mecanorma Industries and Plastic Maschinen
Branch Offices: 9 Ajiwun St, Bariga, Lagos State
Principal Bankers: First Bank of Nigeria Ltd

Principal Shareholders: Directors as described above
Date of Establishment: 21st September 1973

TOPIC LTD

PO Box 1274, Ibadan, Oyo State

PRINCIPAL ACTIVITIES: Building and civil engineering
　contractors

TORONTO ORGANISATION (NIGERIA) LTD

Head Office, 1 Ometan St, Warri, Bendel State

PRINCIPAL ACTIVITIES: Dealers in various types of furniture;
　designers and general contractors
Branch Offices: 14 Warri/Sapele Rd, Warri, Bendel State;
　Workshop; 3 Ometan St, Warri, Bendel State

TOTAL NIGERIA LTD

New Africa House, PMB 2143, 31 Marina, Lagos
Tel: 664821, 664892, 664750
Cable: Dispetrof
Telex: 21334 Total Ng

Chairman: J Goubeau
Directors: J C Boilon (Managing),
　Chief H O Davies,
　Olateju Oyeleye,
　Alhaji Y Garba Ali,
　G E Mbonu,
　S Jegede

PRINCIPAL ACTIVITIES: Marketing of petroleum products
Principal Bankers: Union Bank of Nigeria Ltd; United Bank for
　Africa Ltd; International Bank for West Africa Ltd

Date of Establishment: 1st June 1956

TOURIST COMPANY OF NIGERIA LTD

Ahmadu Bello Rd, Victoria Island, PO Box 1000, Lagos
Tel: 610031, 610082, 610134, 610175, 610206, 610247
Cable: Palace Lagos
Telex: 21432 Palace Ng

Chairman: Alhaji Musa Kazir
Directors: Alhaji Bunu Bala,
　Alhaji A Maje Adananu,
　Alhaji Hassan S Ibeto,
　Dr G A Adeosun,
　Mrs V C Omenukor,
　W O Obeten,
　Chief C N Ijeoma,
　Solomon Lipdo,
　Alhaji B O Owolowo (Managing)
Senior Executives: A A Idowu (Finance Controller),
　N T A Ogundipe (Chief Engineer),
　M O Oyebola (Group Personnel Manager),
　M O Dada (Group Operations Manager),
　S K Awoniyi (Chief Internal Auditor),
　Alhaji R G A Oyekan (Company Secretary)

PRINCIPAL ACTIVITIES: Hotels and catering; Federal Palace
　and Federal Palace Suites Hotels
Principal Bankers: Union Bank of Nigeria Ltd

Principal Shareholders: Federal Government of Nigeria
Date of Establishment: 1964
No of Employees: 955

TOWER ALUMINIUM (NIGERIA) LTD

Oba Akran Avenue, PO Box 9, Ikeja, Lagos
Tel: 962801, 960490/3
Cable: Tower Lagos
Telex: 26408

Chairman: A M Ferguson
Directors: C T David (Managing),
　Alhaji Y A Salami,
　E A Adegoke,
　Comcraft Services Ltd
Senior Executives: K P Venugopal (Chief Engineer),
　R S Venkataraman (Technical Manager),
　M U Kuriakose (Production Manager),
　S Sankaran (Financial Controller)

PRINCIPAL ACTIVITIES: Manufacture of aluminium holloware,
　aluminium collapsible tubes, aluminium roof sheets and
　accessories, and aluminium extrusions, and future production
　of aluminium coils and circles
Branch Offices: 22 Ahmadu Bello Way, PO Box 1870, Kaduna,
　Tel 242352
Subsidiary Companies: Tower Galvanised Products (Nig) Ltd;
　Midland Galvanising Products (Nig) Ltd; Intermatch Company
　Ltd; Metoxide (Nigeria) Ltd; Apex Paints Ltd; Asaba
　Aluminium Company Ltd; Kolorkote Nigeria Ltd
Principal Bankers: Union Bank of Nigeria Ltd

Financial Information:

	US$'000
Authorised capital	5,100
Paid-up capital	4,700
Turnover	23,369
Profits	1,860

Date of Establishment: September 1959
No of Employees: 912

TOYIN RISING BAKERY

10 Shokunbi St, PO Box 360, Mushin, Lagos
Tel: 841142

PRINCIPAL ACTIVITIES: Baking and confectionery

TOYO MENKA KAISHA LTD

31-33 Martins St, PO Box 1178, Lagos
Tel: 682125
Cable: Tomen Lagos
Telex: 21336 Tomen Ng

PRINCIPAL ACTIVITIES: Importers of all types of steel products

TRACTOR & EQUIPMENT

Billingsway (Off Lagos/Ibadan Expressway), Oregun Industrial
   Estate, PMB 21480, Ikeja, Lagos
Tel: 900840 (10 lines), 901080 (10 lines)
Cable: Unatrac Lagos

Chairman: Chief E A O Shonekan
Senior Executives: E A Scott (General Manager),
   R A Bello (Commercial Manager),
   R A Chinnock (General Parts Manager),
   R L Colquhoun (General Service Manager),
   S P Adams (General Sales Manager),
   A C Atiomo (Personnel Manager),
   U P Okudo (Marketing Manager)

PRINCIPAL ACTIVITIES: Sales and service of agricultural,
   earthmoving, and material handling equipment; engines and
   generator sets
Principal Agencies: Caterpillar Tractor Co, USA; Caterpillar
   Overseas, SA Geneva; Albaret, France; Rome Corporation,
   USA; Fleco Corporation, USA
Branch Offices: Apapa; Kaduna; Kano; Maiduguri; Warri; Port
   Harcourt; Yola; Enugu; Ilorin; Ibadan; Sokoto; Shiroro
Principal Bankers: Union Bank of Nigeria Ltd; First Bank of
   Nigeria Ltd; United Bank for Africa
Financial Information: Division of UAC of Nigeria Ltd

No of Employees: 1,700

TRACTORS UNDER-CARRIAGE INDUSTRY NIGERIA LTD

17/19 Durojaiye St, Ikate, Surulere, PO Box 5108, Lagos
Tel: 830293

PRINCIPAL ACTIVITIES: Suppliers and servicers of agricultural
   and heavy machinery; spare parts
Principal Agencies: Tek Rubber & Plastics Ltd, UK

TRADEV LTD

Aliyu Jodi Rd, PO Box 142, Sokoto
Tel: 232530, 232958
Cable: Tradev
Telex: 73106

Directors: Abdullahi Bayero (Managing),
   I Dasuki,
   A Tumay,
   Ministry of Finance,
   Ministry of Trade

PRINCIPAL ACTIVITIES: State Government bulk purchasing
   organisation; department stores
Principal Agencies: A G Leventis & Co; Bewac; Brian Munro; R &
   A Services; Sanyo etc
Branch Offices: Aliya Jodi Rd, Sokoto; Canteen Rd, Gusau;
   Bida; Talata Mafara
Principal Bankers: Bank of the North Ltd; Union Bank of Nigeria
   Ltd

Principal Shareholders: Government of Sokoto State; General
   Public
Date of Establishment: 1972
No of Employees: 400

TRADEWINDS EXPRESS (NIGERIA) LTD

PO Box 2672, Old Domestic Terminal Area, Murtala Mohammed
   International Airport, Ikeja, Lagos
Tel: 960800

Chairman: Dr A E Ikomi
Directors: N J King, W J Ejuetami, R D Parmenter
Senior Executives: D Fagan (General Manager)

PRINCIPAL ACTIVITIES: International and domestic air courier
   services
Principal Agencies: Tradewinds Express (UK) Ltd; Cargosave
   (UK) Ltd
Branch Offices: 9c Station Rd, Port Harcourt, Rivers State, Kano
Principal Bankers: United Bank for Africa Ltd

Principal Shareholders: Dr A E Ikomi; W T Ejuetami; Tradewinds
   Express (UK) Ltd
Date of Establishment: May 1981

TRADON NIGERIA LTD

2/4 Arochuku St, Rumuomasi, Obio, PMB 5558, Port Harcourt,
   Rivers State
Tel: 334726
Cable: Tradon Ng
Telex: 61297 Tradon Ng

Chairman: Tim Edoka Okah
Directors: Abraham Thomas (Operations),
   Mrs Diana Omo-Igho Okah
Senior Executives: Chief J F U Onuotu (Procurement Director),
   Mrs Patience Okonko (Secretary),
   Silas Ugboaja (Staff Manager)

PRINCIPAL ACTIVITIES: Engineering and industrial services;
   consultants and merchants; shipping and trade
Principal Agencies: M C Seong Moolsan Corporation, Korea;
   Tae Chang Ind Co Ltd, USA; Kolon International Corp, Korea
Branch Offices: 60A Nekpenekpen Str, PO Box 806, Benin City;
   Plot 7, Pogconsult House, Emede/Oleh Rd, Emede P A
   Emede, Bendel State
Subsidiary/Associated Companies: Diana Tradon Internationl
   Agencies; Pogconsult Nig Engineers; Estate Services and
   Maintenance; Posteff Steel and Aluminium Products Mfg Co
Principal Bankers: First Bank Nigeria Ltd; Mercantile Bank
   Nigeria Ltd; New Nigerian Bank Ltd; African Continental Bank
   Ltd
Financial Information:

	N'000
Authorised capital	200
Paid-up capital	200

Date of Establishment: 1974, Incorporated 15th July 1976
   (Formerly Pogconsult Holdings Ltd)
No of Employees: 36 (excluding casuals)

TRANS ATLANTIC SHIPPING AGENCY LTD

25 Creek Rd, Apapa, PO Box 4890, Lagos
Tel: 832292, 873074, 873065
Cable: Tasal Lagos
Telex: 22266 Tasal Ng

Chairman: Alhaji R A Bello
Directors: Azad Shivdasani,
   Alhaji A Aliyu,
   Lalit Malhotra (Managing)

Senior Executives: Captain K Sharma (Shipping Manager),
   T A Alabi (Freight Manager),
   B R Sarda (Financial Controller),
   C Punjabi (Clearing Manager)

PRINCIPAL ACTIVITIES: Shipping, clearing and forwarding
Principal Agencies: Jeco Shipping BV, Rotterdam; Golden
   Liberty Lines, Hamburg; Armada Line Aps, Copenhegen
Branch Offices: NPA Yard, PO Box 2122, Warri; Leanto Shed 6,
   PMB 6180, Port Harcourt; 9A Post Office Rd, PO Box 11548,
   Kano
Principal Bankers: United Bank for Africa Ltd
Financial Information:

	N'000
Authorised capital	200
Paid-up capital	200

Date of Establishment: 1st October 1979
No of Employees: 250

TRANS NIGERIA ROAD HAULAGE LTD

Kilometer 11.5 Badagry Expressway, Opposite Constitutuent
   Assembly Village, Satelite Town, PMB 1064 or PMB 1185,
   Apapa, Lagos
Tel: 880426, 870812
Telex: 21122, 22318

Chairman: Alhaji R A O Majekodunmi
Directors: Chief S N Ebinum,
   C Kruegel (Technical),
   J A S Fidgett (General Manager)
Senior Executives: A A A Okene (Assistant General Manager),
   N J Butt (Workshop Manager),
   B Sutcliffe (Transport Engineer)

PRINCIPAL ACTIVITIES: Specialist road transporters with
   equipment and experience in hauling oversize, overweight
   project consignments
Principal Agencies: Triana Ltd; Trianon Ltd; Make Ltd; Nigerian
   Marine Services; Nigerian Forwarders Ltd; Nigerian Bottling
   Company; Casman Ltd
Branch Offices: Calabar; Kaduna; Kano; Port Harcourt; Warri
Subsidiary Companies: Triana; Trianon; Casman; Make Ltd
Principal Bankers: United Bank for Africa Ltd; Societe Generale
   Bank (Nigeria) Ltd
Financial Information:

	N'000
Authorised capital	750
Paid-up capital	750

Principal Shareholders: Alhaji R A O Majekodunmi; Chief S N
   Ebinum
Date of Establishment: 1975
No of Employees: 190

TRANS NIGERIA TRADING AND INDUSTRIAL CO LTD

13th Floor, 8/10 Broad St, Western House, Lagos
Tel: 630858, 657790/1

PRINCIPAL ACTIVITIES: Importers and exporters, wholesale
   distributors of general merchandise

TRANS-AFRICA ENGINEERING LTD

PO Box 851, 57 Trans-Amadi Industrial Layout, Port Harcourt,
   Rivers State
Tel: 21040, 21324
Cable: Esecor Ng
Telex: 61147

Directors: E C Schofield (Managing Director),
   L Scott-Lowe (Finance Manager),
   B Duran (Operations Manager),
   A Cutmore (Operations Manager, Warri),
   M J Dominques (General Sales Manager)

PRINCIPAL ACTIVITIES: Equipment suppliers and services for
   the oil and gas industry
Branch Offices: Field Office: Edewor Complex, Enerhen Rd, PO

Box 313, Warri, Bendel State; Investment House, Suite 918,
   21/25 Broad St, Lagos Island, PO Box 3651, Lagos; Tel
   23973, 23986, 21857, 52049

TRANSCAP LTD

28 Burma Rd, PMB 1095, Apapa, Lagos
Tel: 874161, 875537, 875628
Cable: Transcap Apapa
Telex: 21272 Trscap Ng

Chairman: P Chavannaz
Directors: Alhaji S A Bello, P Chavannaz, R Horner, Chief M
   Okoya-Thomas, Alhaji F Uthman
Senior Executives: D Exshaw (General Manager)

PRINCIPAL ACTIVITIES: International freight forwarders,
   shipping and travels agents; warehousing
Principal Agencies: Transcap Network, France
Branch Offices: 8 Nnamdi Azikiwe Rd, Port Harcourt, Rivers
   State
Principal Bankers: International Bank for West Africa Ltd; First
   Bank of Nigeria Ltd; Societe Generale Bank (Nigeria) Ltd
Financial Information:

	N'000
Authorised capital	400
Paid-up capital	400

Principal Shareholders: CFAO (Nigeria) Ltd
Date of Establishment: 24th October 1958
No of Employees: 317

TRANSELEK NIGERIA LTD

47 Hospital Rd, PO Box 1374, Aba, Imo State
Tel: 220689, 222041

Chairman: C O Maduako
Directors: Dr B D Acholonu,
   A G Ozumba (Managing Director),
   E C Dillibe (Executive),
   A O Tangban (Executive),
   A Ozumba

PRINCIPAL ACTIVITIES: Electrical engineers and contractors
Principal Bankers: United Bank for Africa Ltd
Financial Information:

	N'000
Authorised capital	1,000
Paid-up capital	1,000

Principal Shareholders: Chairman and directors as described
Date of Establishment: December 1971

TRANSEX & COMPANY LTD

PMB 1011, Ebute Metta Post Office, Lagos

PRINCIPAL ACTIVITIES: Sales and service of air conditioning,
   plumbing and electrical installations
Branch Offices: Office Location: Transex House, 20 Okusaga St,
   Ilupeju, Lagos

TRANSMARCO AGENCIES (NIGERIA) LTD

182 Kirikiri Rd, Olodi, PO Box 7341, Apapa, Lagos
Tel: 877286, 870337
Cable: Leeway Lagos
Telex: 20200/TDS 060

Chairman: Chief M O Etim
Directors: E O Etim, A O Etim
Senior Executives: J D Ufot (Operations Manager),
   O P Umana (Forwarding Manager),
   F X E Nkuda (Administrative Manager),
   S A Boglo (Accountant)

PRINCIPAL ACTIVITIES: Shipping, clearing, forwarding, ship
   chartering, air freighting, transportation, warehousing, import,
   export and general contractors
Principal Agencies: Milestone Enterprises Ltd; Paper Sack
   (Nigeria) Ltd; Polfa (Nigeria) Ltd; Commind (Nigeria) Ltd;
   Wiggins Teape (WA) Ltd; Camber Brothers Enterprises; Etico
   Construction & Eng Co Ltd; Macknell Engineering Co Ltd
Branch Offices: 5A Murtala Highway, PO Box 670, Calabar; 45

Okponung Street, Oron, Cross River State
Subsidiary Companies: Etico Construction & Engineering
  Company Ltd; Etico Farms Enterprises; Etico Records &
  Promotion Company
Principal Bankers: Mercantile Bank of Nigeria Ltd
Financial Information:

	N'000
Authorised capital	100
Paid-up capital	100
Turnover	1,700
Profits	55

Principal Shareholders: Chairman and directors as described
Date of Establishment: 24th February 1978
No of Employees: 50

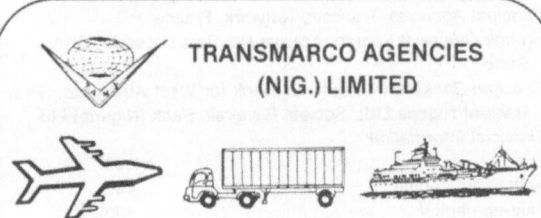

TRANSMARCO AGENCIES (NIG.) LIMITED

*Air Freighting   *Transportation   *Shipping Clearing   *Ship Chartering

WE ARE PROFESSIONALS IN SHIPPING, CLEARING, FORWARDING, SHIP-CHARTERING & TRANSPORTATION, AND OUR NUMEROUS CUSTOMERS WOULD BE GLAD TO CONFIRM TO OUR SERVICES AND RATE.

LET US TAKE THAT PROBLEM OFF YOUR HEAD AND YOU HAVE TIME TO ATTEND OTHER PROBLEMS.

CONTACT US TODAY AT:

TRANSMARCO AGENCIES (NIG.) LIMITED

HEAD OFFICE:
182 KIRIKIRI ROAD
OLODI, APAPA
PO BOX 7341, LAGOS
TEL: 870337/877286
TELEX: 21619 NACC NG

5A, MURTALA HIGHWAY
PO BOX 670, CALABAR
TEL: 221398

UNITED KINGDOM
I.F.A. (SHIPPING) LIMITED
UNIT B5, MOTHERWELL WAY
WEST THURROCK, GRAYS, ESSEX
RM16 1XD

TRANSWORLD DRILLING COMPANY LTD
PO Box 635, 21-25 Broad St, Lagos
Tel: 634622, 634638
Cable: Esecor
Telex: 21335 Esecor

Directors: John R Irwin (Managing Director)
Senior Executives: B Skaggs (Drilling Superintendent Warri)

PRINCIPAL ACTIVITIES: Offshore drilling contractors
Branch Offices: PO Box 221, Warri, Bondel State, Tel 229

TREBOR (NIGERIA) LTD
35/39 Creek Rd, PO Box 392, Apapa, Lagos
Tel: 803100, 803101/2
Cable: Trebor Apapa
Telex: 22378 Accnl Ng

Directors: I R Marks, J G Marks, A S Marinho, A K A
  Ogunnuga, P F Adepo
Senior Executives: A O Ogundiran (Company Secretary),
  D K Onanuga (Factory Manager),
  F W Baker (Group Technical Adviser),
  H A Momoh (Group Financial Controller)

PRINCIPAL ACTIVITIES: Food and food processing, specialising
  in confectionery products
Principal Agencies: Trebor Ltd, UK
Branch Offices: Plot 82 Sharada Industrial Area, Kano; 50
  Enugu/Awka Rd, Nkpor Junction, Onitsha
Associated Companies: Danafco Nigeria Ltd; A C Christlieb
  (Nigeria) Ltd
Principal Bankers: First Bank of Nigeria Ltd
Financial Information:

	N'000
Authorised capital	500
Paid-up capital	500
Turnover	19,000
Profits	323

Principal Shareholders: Wholly owned subsidiary of A C
  Christlieb (Nigeria) Ltd
Date of Establishment: 1962
No of Employees: 1,250

TREVI FOUNDATIONS NIGERIA LTD
5 Gbolade Adebanjo St, Ilupeju, PMB 1189, Oshodi, Lagos

PRINCIPAL ACTIVITIES: Piling and foundation specialists

TRIANA LTD
18/20 Commercial Rd, PMB 1064, Apapa, Lagos
Tel: 803040, 803041, 876693
Cable: Triana
Telex: 21122

Chairman: Chief S N Ebinum
Directors: C Kruegel (Managing),
  Alhaji Rao Majekodunmi,
  A I Dasuki,
  J A S Fidgett,
  M Emmenegger (Financial),
  B Mustapha,
  Mrs C Imevbore
Senior Executives: E N Ugoji (Company Sec/Legal Adviser),
  W G Thomas (Special Projects Manager),
  W F Ullrich (Operations Controller)

PRINCIPAL ACTIVITIES: Freight forwarding (sea, land and air)
  and customs agents; industrial, domestic packing; shipping
  and shipping services; transport
Principal Agencies: Kranos AG, Switzerland
Branch Offices: SW9/1405A Elekuku Layout, Ring Rd, PMB
  5427, Ibadan, Tel 412841/2; Airfreight: 26A Adeshina St,
  PMB 21201, Ikeja, Tel 933440, 933456; 83 Tafawa Balewa Rd,
  PMB 3146, Kano, Tel 3701, (Airport Office 5163), Telex
  77157; 1440 Kachia Rd, PO Box 4043, Kaduna, Tel 243307; 10
  Harbour Rd, PMB 5116, Port Harcourt, Tel 22388; 32B
  Warri-Sapele Rd, PMB 1105, Warri; 117 Odukpani Rd, PMB
  1285, Calabar
Associated Companies: Trianon Shipping & Chartering Ltd;
  Trans-Nigeria Road Haulage Ltd; Nigerian Removal & Storage
  Company Ltd
Principal Bankers: United Bank for Africa Ltd; Societe Generale
  Bank Nigeria Ltd
Financial Information:

	N'000
Authorised capital	1,000
Paid-up capital	700
Turnover	20,000

Principal Shareholders: C Kruegel; R A O Majekodunmi; Chief S
  N Ebinum; S O Odugbesan; A I Dasuki; B Mustapha; J A S
  Fidgett; Mrs C Imevbore; M Emmeneger
Date of Establishment: 10th March 1970
No of Employees: 270

TRIANON SHIPPING & CHARTERING LTD
6 Kofo Abayomi Avenue, PO Box 237, Apapa, Lagos
Tel: 874120/870817
Cable: Trustchart
Telex: 22297 Triano Ng

Directors: Chief M Ihem Alaike, C Kruegel, Chief S N Ebinum, Alhaji R A O Majekodunmi
Senior Executives: Capt K R Keswani (General Manager), A M Enu (Chief Accountant)
PRINCIPAL ACTIVITIES: Shipping, chartering, brokerage, slipway, engineering and offshore services
Branch Offices: 10 Harbour Rd, PMB 5118, Port Harcourt; 117 Odukpani Rd, PMB 1285, Calabar; 32b Warri-Sapele Rd, PMB 918, Effurun-Warri
Principal Bankers: United Bank for Africa Ltd
Financial Information:
Authorised capital ₦ 100,000

Date of Establishment: 13th November 1975
No of Employees: 84

TRINDEL (NIGERIA) LTD
983A Sakajojo St, Victoria Island, PO Box 60381, Ikoyi Secretariat, Lagos
Tel: 610662, 610643
Telex: 21735 Tnl Ng

Chairman: F A Ogbemi
Directors: R Ayme (Managing), A Ferry
PRINCIPAL ACTIVITIES: Mechanical and electrical engineering services
Principal Bankers: United Bank for Africa Ltd; International Bank for West Africa
Principal Shareholders: Travaux Industriels pour l'Electricite, Paris; Roje Holdings Ltd, Lagos
Date of Establishment: July 1978

TRIPLEX SAFETY GLASS (NIGERIA) LTD
KM 9 Iwo Rd, PMB 64 Agodi BO, Ibadan, Oyo State
Telex: 31463 Tsgn Ib

Chairman: G Nightingale
Directors: E Gatti (Managing), Chief O I Akinkugbe, D B M Johnston, Chief M T Mbu
PRINCIPAL ACTIVITIES: Production of laminated and toughened safety glass for the motor trade: windscreens, side and back lights, etc
Principal Bankers: First Bank of Nigeria Ltd
Financial Information:

	₦'000
Authorised capital	6,000
Paid-up capital	5,400

Principal Shareholders: Pilkington Bros PLC (60%); Nigerian Private Investors (40%)
Date of Establishment: May 1977
No of Employees: 235

TRIUMPH (NIGERIA) LTD
26 Dantata Rd, Bompai, PO Box 423, Kano
Tel: 5021, 2536
Cable: Triumph
Telex: 77202

PRINCIPAL ACTIVITIES: Manufacturers of corrugated cartons and cardboard boxes

TROPICAL TARPAULIN INDUSTRY (NIGERIA) LTD
PO Box 193, 167 Mission Rd, Kano
Tel: 3634
Cable: Canvas Kano

PRINCIPAL ACTIVITIES: Manufacturers of tarpaulin and other canvas products

TSMPE (TSVETMETPROMEXPORT)
Ikorodu-Shagamu Rd, Construction Site, PO Box 99, Ikorodu, Lagos State

President: R I Kuprevich
Directors: V M Shtefan (General Director), B P Kozintsev (Commercial Director), V I Tsherbakov (Technical Director), R M Shakirov (Construction Director), V P Bobylev (Administration Manager)
Senior Executives: O S Komissarov (Commercial Department Manager), A V Sereda (Production Department Manager), A A Duhanin (Supply Department Manager), V N Chernyivsky (Technical Department Manager)
PRINCIPAL ACTIVITIES: Oil services and equipment and pipeline contractors
Principal Agencies: V/O Tsvetmetpromexport, Moscow
Principal Bankers: Union Bank of Nigeria Ltd

TSTC COASTAL AGENCY
3 Karimu St, Surulere, Lagos
Tel: 837055

PRINCIPAL ACTIVITIES: Clearing and forwarding agents

TUDOR BATTERIES (NIGERIA) LTD
9 Breadfruit St, PO Box 3064, Lagos
Tel: 662532, 610575, 616988

Directors: Adetayo Amusan
PRINCIPAL ACTIVITIES: Manufacturers of batteries for cars and trucks, generators, hospital plants and ocean vessels
Financial Information:
Registered capital ₦ 500,000

Date of Establishment: June 1980

TUNTARIC NIGERIA LTD
21 Oyekan Rd, Apapa, PO Box 50180, Lagos
Tel: 873167

Chairman: J B Olatunde
Directors: A S Adigun, A A U Erikhuemen, C O Olatunde, Mary Williams
PRINCIPAL ACTIVITIES: Shipping, clearing and forwarding

TURNERS BUILDING PRODUCTS (AREWA) LTD
PO Box 347, Kakuri Industrial Estate, Kaduna South, Kaduna
Tel: 211739
Cable: Turners Kaduna
Telex: 71131 Turners Ng

Chairman: R K Day
Directors: C J M Rankin (General Manager), J R Stedman, Alhaji Mohammed Hayatuddini, Alhaji D Adamu, Alhaji Hassan Mu'Azu, Alhaji Shehu Wunti
Senior Executives: S K Ajulo (Commercial Manager/Company Secretary), H M Abdul (Sales Manager), E B Alley (Chief Accountant), M J Turner (Works Manager)
PRINCIPAL ACTIVITIES: Manufacturers of products for the construction industry, pipes, corrugated sheets, etc
Branch Offices: 19 Niger St, PO Box 1383, Kano, Tel 4788; 56 Dogon Karfe St, Jos; Ahmadu Bello Way, Bulabulin Ward, PMB 1415, Maiduguri; 13 Yakubu Lame Rd, PO Box 487, Minna
Principal Bankers: Union Bank of Nigeria Ltd
Financial Information:

	₦'000
Authorised capital	3,000
Paid-up capital	1,983

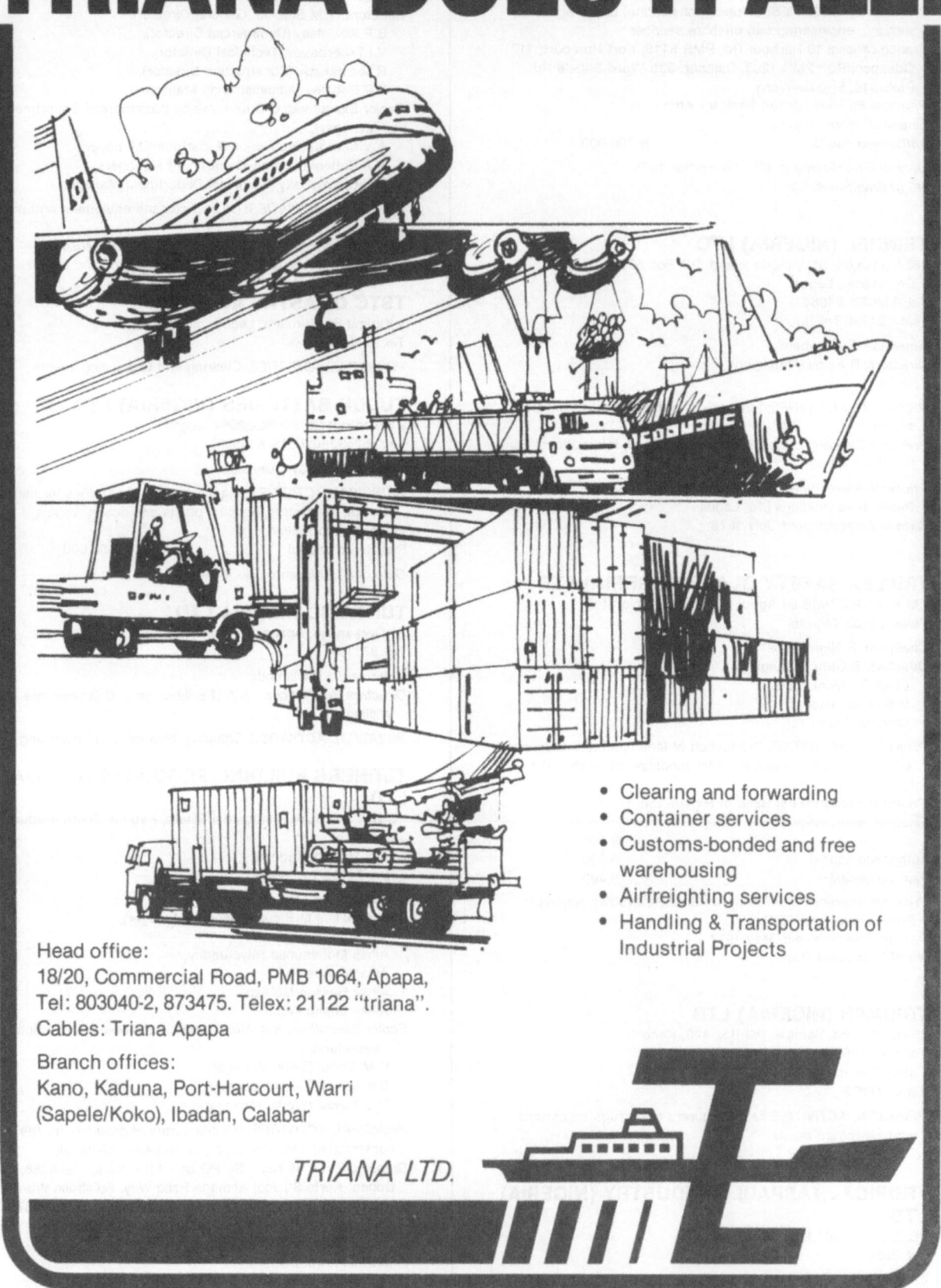

Principal Shareholders: Turner & Newall International Ltd; New Nigerian Development Company Ltd; KIC Ltd
Date of Establishment: 1963
No of Employees: 255

TURNERS BUILDING PRODUCTS (EMENE) LTD

7 Abakaliki Rd, Emene, PO Box 646, Enugu, Anambra State
Tel: 253553/4, 253568
Cable: Turners Enugu
Telex: 51146 Bigsix Ng

Chairman: R K Day
Directors: J R Stedman (General Manager),
C Ezenaya,
O C Ememe
Senior Executives: S I Egbuka (Sales Manager),
U U Anyalechi (Works Manager),
C E Oleka (Chief Accountant)

PRINCIPAL ACTIVITIES: Manufacturers of asbestos cement roofing and cladding materials, pressure pipes for water distribution, sewage and drainage
Principal Bankers: Union Bank of Nigeria Ltd; First Bank of Nigeria Ltd
Financial Information:

	N'000
Authorised capital	6,000
Paid-up capital	4,500

Principal Shareholders: Turner and Newall International Ltd; Anambra State Government; Imo State Government
Date of Establishment: 6th October 1961
No of Employees: 980

TURNERS ENGINEERING PRODUCTS (NIGERIA) LTD

PMB 5722, Ibadan, Oyo State

Chairman: R K Day
Directors: J C T Fell, C J M Rankin, J O Emanuel, Chief N O Idowu, C P Obusez

PRINCIPAL ACTIVITIES: Manufacturers of brake linings, disc brake pads and gaskets
Branch Offices: Factory: Lagos Road Industrial Estate, Behind Methodist High School, Ibadan
Principal Bankers: Union Bank of Nigeria Ltd
Financial Information:

	N'000
Authorised capital	500
Paid-up capital	500

Principal Shareholders: Turner & Newall International Ltd; Nigerians
Date of Establishment: 17th June 1976
No of Employees: 200

TWILIGHTS NIGERIA LTD

1 Nwakoby St, PO Box 627, Enugu, Anambra State
Cable: Twilight

Chairman: Margaret A Molokwu
Directors: M A Ochei, Chinwe Ochei, Joe Bel-Molokwu, Benedicter Molokwu
Senior Executives: Paul Ona (Secretary),
Chris Molokwu (Sales Manager)

PRINCIPAL ACTIVITIES: Agents, suppliers and distributors of laboratory chemicals; shelving; teaching aids etc
Principal Agencies: LABM, UK; RAACO, Denmark; ESL, UK
Branch Offices: 83 Zik Ave, PO Box 627, Enugu; 3 Convent Ave, PO Box 627, Enugu
Principal Bankers: Union Bank of Nigeria Ltd

TWZ (NIGERIA) LTD

1 Babatola Drive, PMB 1147, Ikeja, Lagos
Tel: 963992

PRINCIPAL ACTIVITIES: Building and civil engineering consultants and contractors

U MADUKA ENTERPRISES (NIGERIA) LTD
See MADUKA, U, ENTERPRISES (NIGERIA) LTD

UAC OF NIGERIA LTD

PO Box 2216, Niger House, 1/5 Odunlami St, Lagos
Tel: 663010, 660650, 660655
Cable: UNAREP
Telex: 21596 UNAREP NG; 21233 UNASUP NG

Chairman: E A O Shonekan (also Managing Director)
Directors: Chief S O Adebo,
His Highness Alhaji Shehu Idris,
M G Bloomer (Deputy Chairman and Deputy Managing Director),
A C I Mbanefo,
Chief S B Daniyan,
Chief J O Omidiora,
Alhaji I Kaita,
F M O Osifo,
J P Rauch,
H T Mathers,
P D Tueart,
M C Thompson,
A P Graham

PRINCIPAL ACTIVITIES: General traders, chain stores; suppliers of agricultural equipment, electrical goods, building materials, food, hardware, household goods, motor vehicles and components, office supplies and machinery, pharmaceuticals; plant hire, etc. Manufacturers
Branch Offices: Manufacturing Divisions; Foods Division; Bordpak Premier Packaging; A J Seward/Kingsway Chemists; Federated Motor Industries; African Timber & Plywood; Pan Electric; Technical Divisions; Niger Motors; Business Equipment & Manufacture; Tractor & Equipment; Machinery & Electrical Equipment; Refrigeration & Airconditioning Services; Palm Line Agencies (Nigeria); Computer Centre; Property Division; Manufacturers' Delivery Services; Trading; Group Textiles; GB Ollivant; Kingway Stores; Gottschalcks; Building Materials; Electrical Materials Supplies; Greenham Plant Hire
Principal Bankers: United Bank for Africa Ltd; Union Bank of Nigeria Ltd; First Bank of Nigeria Ltd; Savannah Bank of Nigeria Ltd; International Bank for West Africa Ltd; National Bank of Nigeria Ltd
Financial Information:

	N'000
Authorised capital	148,500
Paid-up capital	148,500
Sales turnover	707,292
Profits (after tax)	27,692

Principal Shareholders: Nigerian Public and CWA Holdings Ltd
Date of Establishment: 1931
No of Employees: 20,000

UBA, C, & BROTHERS TRADING COMPANY (WA) LTD

7 Affar St, PMB 1714, Onitsha, Anambra State
Tel: 490, 218, 333
Cable: Ubabros

PRINCIPAL ACTIVITIES: Manufacturers' representatives, confirming house, transporters, general merchants and estate agents
Principal Agencies: Leventis Motors Ltd; Continental Textiles Nigeria Ltd; Neweco Ltd; Honda Motorcycles etc
Branch Offices: 95A Iweka Rd, Onitsha, Anambra State; 16 Olayeni St, Ikeja, Lagos

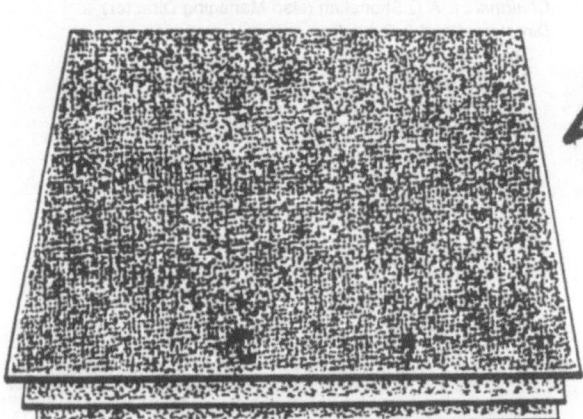
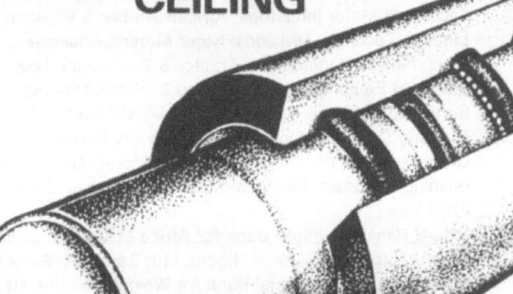
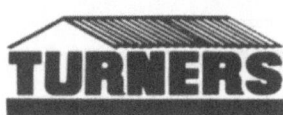
298

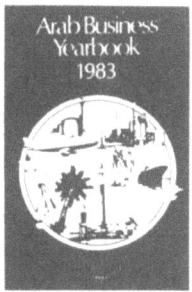
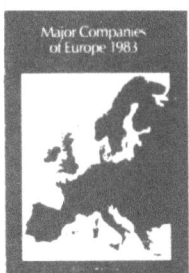 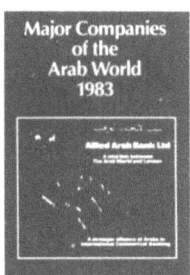 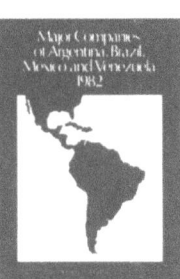
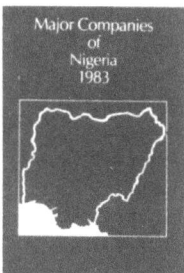 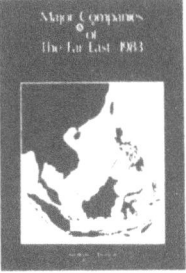
UCHE, A O, & SONS (NIGERIA) LTD

12 Damfodio Rd, Aba, Imo State

Chairman: Kalu A O Uche
Senior Executives: J U Uche

PRINCIPAL ACTIVITIES: Importers, exporters, general merchants, clearing, shipping, forwarding
Principal Agencies: Nigerian National Supply Company Ltd; Pioneer Chemical Company Ltd, Lagos; C Moore and Company, Aba; Ekonite Trading Co Ltd, Aba
Associated Companies: J Ohaks and Brothers, Aba, Oniuche Fam
Principal Bankers: African Continental Bank Ltd; Mercantile Bank of Nigeria Ltd; First Bank of Nigeria Ltd

UGBABE FURNITURE & CONSTRUCTION COMPANY LTD

Bukuru Bye Pass, PO Box 787, Jos, Plateau State
Telex: 52538

Chairman: Isaac Ugbabe
Directors: Daniel Ugbabe, Mrs A I Ugbabe, Aako Ugbabe, Onyum I Ugbabe
Senior Executives: Miss Yemisi (Production Manager), T O Igwe (General Manager), S Okam (Senior Accountant), Douglas Otoble (Accountant)

PRINCIPAL ACTIVITIES: Manufacturing of furniture; building and civil engineering contracting
Branch Offices: Otkpo, Makurdi, Benue State
Principal Bankers: African Continental Bank Ltd; Bank of the North Ltd

Principal Shareholders: Chairman and directors as described
No of Employees: 180

UGOCHUKWU AND SONS LTD

Industrial Layout, Umunze, PO Box 344, Onitsha, Anambra State

Tel: Onitsha 397
Cable: Destiny Onitsha
Telex: 21238 c/o Lagos

Chairman: Chief Mathias Nwafo Ugochukwu
Directors: Chief B O Ofu (Managing), R I Ugochukwu, J A Ugochukwu, P O Ugochukwu, Mrs H M Ugochukwu, Mrs C M Ugochukwu, Mrs A N Ugochukwu, Mrs M M Ugochukwu, G I Okafor
Senior Executives: J C Emezie (General Manager), A I Selkirk (Financial Controller), V A Egemonye (Accountant)

PRINCIPAL ACTIVITIES: Agents and general trading company; investment/holding company; property and real estate
Principal Agencies: Ford Motor Company; Biscuit Manufacturing Company of Nigeria Ltd
Branch Offices: 17 Calcutta Crescent, PO Box 162, Apapa, Lagos, Tel 875390; 15 Ogui Rd, Enugu, Anambra State
Associated Companies: Ugochukwu Chemical Industries Ltd; Biscuit Manufacturing Company of Nigeria Ltd; Aladdin Construction Co Ltd; Ugo Motors Ltd; Central Finance Co Ltd; Nimpex Ltd; Continental Building & Engineering Ltd
Principal Bankers: Savannah Bank Ltd; African Continental Bank Ltd
Financial Information:

	₦'000
Authorised capital	7,000
Paid-up capital	7,000
Sales turnover	5,500

Principal Shareholders: Chief M N Ugochukwu; P O Ugochukwu; J A Ugochukwu; Mrs H M Ugochukwu; Mrs C M Ugochukwu;

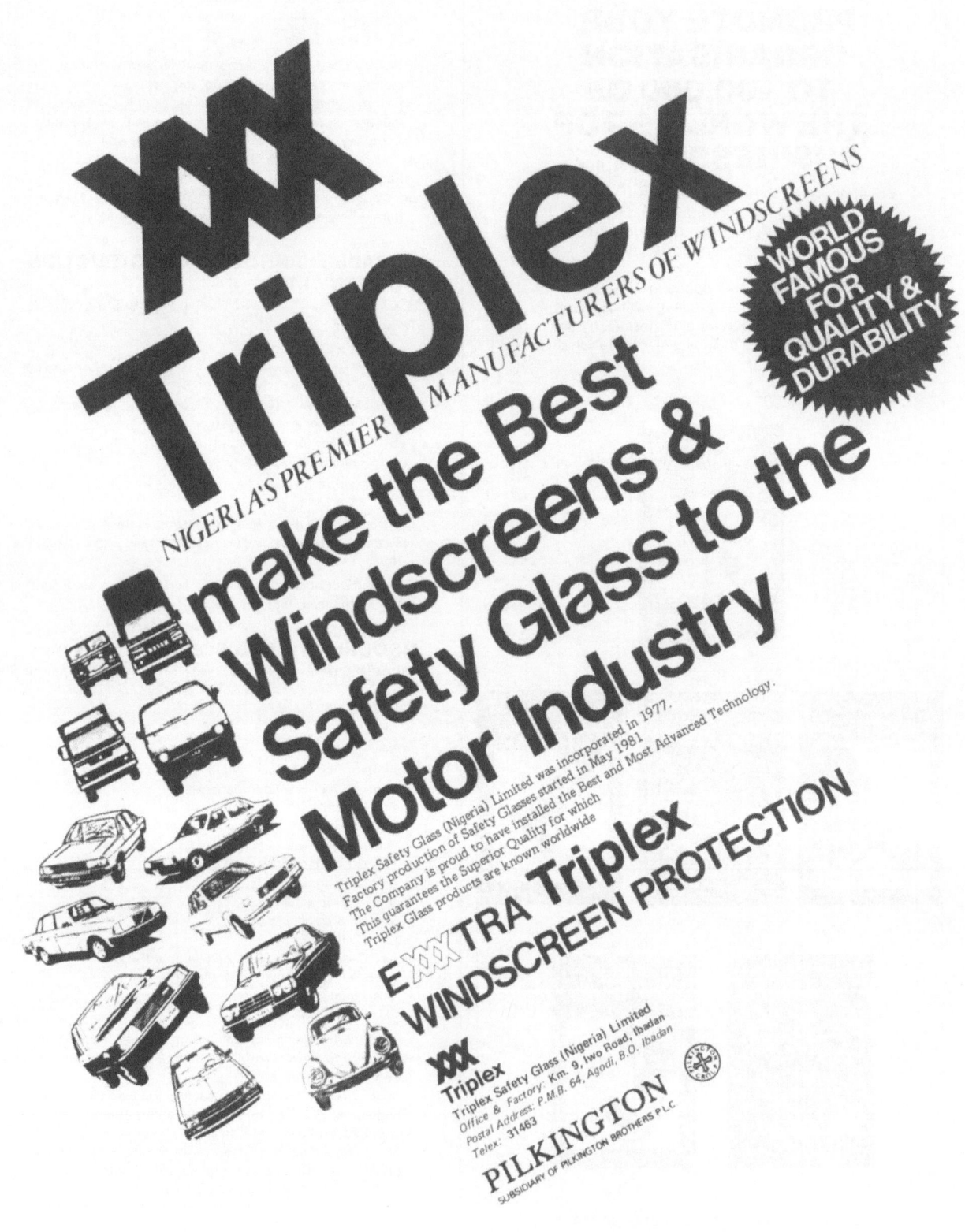

Mrs A N Ugochukwu; Mrs M M Ugochukwu
Date of Establishment: 1955
No of Employees: 200

UGOCHUKWU CHEMICAL INDUSTRIES LTD

Umunze, Aguata Local Government Area, PO Box 344, Onitsha,
Anambra State
Tel: 397
Cable: Ugochemical Onitsha

Chairman: Chief Mathias Nwafo Ugochukwu (also Managing
Director)
Directors: P O Ugochukwu, Mrs H M Ugochukwu, Mrs C M
Ugochukwu, A N Ugochukwu, Mrs M M Ugochukwu, R I
Ugochukwu
Senior Executives: John P Goodier (General Manager),
B S C Nweke (Deputy General Manager),
A A Ugwumadu (Business Manager),
E A Igwiloh (Accountant),
R A Opara (Personnel Manager),
E Uko (Sales Manager)

PRINCIPAL ACTIVITIES: Manufacturers of furniture
(polyurethane foam)
Branch Offices: Aba; Apapa; Akure; Benin; Enugu; Jos; Kaduna;
Onitsha; Owerri
Principal Bankers: African Continental Bank Ltd; First Bank of
Nigeria Ltd
Financial Information:

	₦'000
Authorised capital	1,000
Paid-up capital	500

Principal Shareholders: Ugochukwu & Sons Ltd; Mrs Helen
Ugochukwu; Mrs Christiana Ugochukwu; Mrs Agnes
Ugochukwu; Mrs Monica Ugochukwu; Obiora Ugochukwu
No of Employees: 800

UKAWOODS ENTERPRISES NIGERIA LTD

PMB 1650, Onitsha, Anambra State
Tel: 210023, 210025
Cable: Ukawoods

Chairman: Chief J O Udoji
Directors: J O Ukachukwu (Managing),
J A Ukachukwu,
Mrs F E Ukachukwu,
F J Ukachukwu
Senior Executives: Matthew U Okeke (Deputy Manager,
Administration),
Michael Udokwu (Production Manager),
Boniface Ifetu (Administrative Assistant),
Mrs Justina Ukachukwu (Financial Controller)

PRINCIPAL ACTIVITIES: Wooden/metal furniture manufacturing,
house decoration; building and civil engineering
Branch Offices: 126 Tetlow Rd, Owerri; 9 Oji St, Uwani, Enugu
Principal Bankers: First Bank of Nigeria
Financial Information:

	₦'000
Authorised capital	400
Paid-up capital	322
Turnover	580

Principal Shareholders: J O Ukachukwu; J A Ukachukwu; F E
Ukachukwu; F J Ukachukwu
Date of Establishment: 13th March 1973
No of Employees: 120

UKPILLA CEMENT COMPANY LTD

PO Box 35, Km 164, Benin-Okene Rd, Okpella, Benin City,
Bendel State
Tel: 243388
Cable: Rhinocem
Telex: 41109 Ucefac Ng

PRINCIPAL ACTIVITIES: Manufacturing of cement
Financial Information:
Authorised capital   ₦ 2,200,000

Date of Establishment: June 1964

UMARCO (NIGERIA) LTD

PO Box 94, 5 Creek Rd, Apapa, Lagos
Tel: 874646, 874207
Cable: Umarco
Telex: 21226 Mafric Lagos

Chairman: Chief L O Akindele
Directors: Alhaji Ahmed Joda,
Prince A Haastrup,
A C I Mbanefo,
G Sabouret,
Eric De Rothschild,
J P Maillier (Managing),
Ph Duchemin,
M Fiemeyer

PRINCIPAL ACTIVITIES: Shipping and forwarding agents
Principal Agencies: Farrell Lines Int Ltd; Lloyds Brasileiro; Jeco
Shipping
Branch Offices: Maiduguri; Sapele; Warri; 11 Industry Rd, PO
Box 253, Port Harcourt

Date of Establishment: 1969
No of Employees: 640

UMARU, LAWAN & SONS LTD

PO Box 208, Shehu Laminu Way, Maiduguri, Borno State
Tel: 232178
Cable: Umarlawan

Directors: Alhaji Umaru,
Alhaji Lawan (Managing)

PRINCIPAL ACTIVITIES: Manufacturers of blocks, general
contractors, distributors, suppliers of textiles, building
materials, licensed buying agents and transporters

UMERAH COMMERCIAL AGENCY LTD

PMB 1149, 43 Commercial Ave, Yaba, Lagos State
Tel: 843557, 861747
Cable: Umecom Yaba
Telex: 21553 Umecom Ng

PRINCIPAL ACTIVITIES: Suppliers of animal health products,
agricultural chemicals, pharmaceuticals, hospital equipment

UNCLE FADO AND SONS FURNITURE FACTORY LTD

Kaga Rd, PO Box 56, Maiduguri, Borno State
Tel: 2224

Directors: F T Bagula (Managing Director)

PRINCIPAL ACTIVITIES: Manufacturers of furniture and general
contractors

UNIBUILDER INDUSTRIES LTD

Dakar Rd, PO Box 157, Apapa, Lagos

Directors: P Boeri

PRINCIPAL ACTIVITIES: Construction

UNICO STORES

70 and 83 Old Yaba Rd, Yaba, Lagos
Tel: 862818

PRINCIPAL ACTIVITIES: Distributors of spare parts for motor
vehicles

UNIGWE, FRED BALONWU, GROUP OF COMPANIES

1 Amagbo Lane, Uwani, Enugu, Anambra State
Tel: 253236

PRINCIPAL ACTIVITIES: Building and civil engineering
  contractors; importers and distributors of chemical and
  scientific equipment, building materials and electrical goods
Associated Companies: Fees Brothers Nigeria, Unifess Ltd

UNIJE, B C, & SONS LTD

2 Zik Ave, PO Box 288, Enugu, Anambra State
Tel: 2788

PRINCIPAL ACTIVITIES: Importers and distributors of electrical
  equipment

UNION BANK OF NIGERIA LTD

Head Office, 40 Marina, PMB 2027, Lagos
Tel: 661810
Cable: Unionhead
Telex: 21222

Chairman: Alhaji Shehu Malami
Directors: P A Ogwuma (Managing Director and Chief Executive),
  A O Akinrimisi (Executive),
  S Allwell-Brown,
  E C Cade (Executive),
  W L Cockburn,
  W Duncan,
  J Eakin,
  Alhaji A S Maiyaki (Executive),
  Alhaji Y D Mohammed,
  Alhaji M A Muhammed (Executive),
  Mrs Anne Obi,
  Dr Eze Ogueri II,
  Alhaji Yakubu Wanka,
  J H C Whicker (Alternate),
  D Payne (Alternate)
Senior Executives: M A Ajomale (Assistant General Manager),
  I U Iwe (Assistant General Manager),
  F U S Jarikre (Assistant General Manager),
  A Jibueze (Assistant General Manager),
  W A Kinnear (Assistant General Manager),
  Alhaji M A Usman (Assistant General Manager),
  R D Archer (Advances Controller),
  G J Evans (Chief Inspector),
  G A Odunlami (Regional Controller),
  J C Ezegbu (Lagos Island, Area Manager),
  G B O Asiru (Lagos Mainland, Area Manager),
  A M Scott (40 Marina, Lagos, Area Manager),
  S O Babayemi (Ibadan, Area Manager),
  F B Peters (Benin, Area Manager),
  C G Ihe (Port Harcourt, Area Manager),
  K O Kalu (Enugu, Area Manager),
  Alhaji A Sadauki (Kano, Area Manager),
  Alhaji G A Yakasai (Kaduna, Area Manager)
PRINCIPAL ACTIVITIES: Commercial Banking
Branch Offices: Branches throughout Nigeria
Associated Companies: Barclays Bank International Ltd
Financial Information: As at 30th September 1981

Liabilities	₦'000	Assets	₦'000
Share capital (authorised)	50,000	Cash & Bank	2,549,50
Share capital (issued and fully paid)	36,288	Investments, loans & other assets	2,281,655
Reserves	68,630	Fixed assets	30,561
Deposits and other liabilities	2,462,248		
	2,567,166		2,567,166

Principal Shareholders: Ministry of Finance Incorporated
  (51.67%); Nigerian Citizens and Associations (28.33%);

Barclays Bank International (20%)
Date of Establishment: 1917
No of Employees: 7,517

UNION BEVERAGES LTD

PMB 1057, Mile 7 Agege Motor Rd, Mushin, Lagos
Tel: 960597, 960606
Telex: 21644

PRINCIPAL ACTIVITIES: Manufacturers of pepsi-cola
Branch Offices: Ibadan

UNION BUILDERS COMPANY LTD

1/7 Abule Nla Rd, Ebute-Metta, PMB 1056, Yaba, Lagos
Tel: 831854

Directors: C Barazzotto, F Poletti

PRINCIPAL ACTIVITIES: Building and civil engineering
  contractors

UNION CARBIDE (NIGERIA) LTD

Sharada II Industrial Estate, Plots 50-55, PO Box 4736, Kano
Cable: Nioncarb Lagos

Chairman: Alhaji M M Gashash
Directors: M W Bankhead (Managing),
  Alhaji R Gambo,
  Alhaji T Ismar,
  N J Moden,
  Alhaji S Nanono,
  J K Parkey,
  P H Rees (Financial Director, Kano),
  B Sokoloff Jr,
  F T Wood (Project Co-ordinator, Lagos)
Senior Executives: B K Ng (Commercial Development Manager,
  Kano),
  S Opare-Obisaw (Plant Manager, Kano)
PRINCIPAL ACTIVITIES: Manufacturers of batteries and battery
  products
Branch Offices: 59 Bode Thomas St, Surulere, PO Box 8414,
  Lagos

UNION CONSTRUCTION COMPANY LTD

29A Oguta Rd, PMB 1765, Onitsha, Anambra State
Cable: Civenco

Chairman: Chief Dr G C Mbanugo
Directors: Uzor Nwobi (Managing),
  Ezemeka Ifezue,
  N O Ekpunobi,
  Dr D O Ekwulugo,
  Dr J C O Iewenofu
PRINCIPAL ACTIVITIES: Building and civil engineering
  contractors

UNIPETROL NIGERIA LTD

4th Floor, Western House, 8/10 Broad Street, PO Box 176,
  Lagos
Tel: 601290/1/2/3
Cable: Unipetnig Lagos

Chairman: Alhaji Adamu Suleiman
Directors: Alfred O Olatokun (Managing),
  Alhaji A Mohammed,
  Dr Felix Okoye,
  R A Fayose,
  S M Akpe
Senior Executives: C B Oruche (Assistant General Manager -
  Special Duties),
  G J Amadi (Assistant General Manager - Lubes & Projects),
  E O Oladipo (Operations & Planning Manager),
  Miss N A Chibututu (Staff Administration Manager/Company
    Secretary),
  J S O Kadiri (Accounts & Finance Manager),
  M U N Obiofuma (Assistant to the Managing Director),
  Chief V O Odofin-Belo (Public Relations Manager),
  C C Ikemefuna (Engineering Manager),

A E Okoroh (Sales Manager)

PRINCIPAL ACTIVITIES: Petroleum products marketing; dealers in motor gasoline, diesel oil, kerosine, lubricants, tyres, batteries and accessories; cooking gas and insecticides

Principal Agencies: Firestone Tyres, Spain; Champion Spark Plug Company; Nigerian National Petroleum Corporation; Gulf, London

Branch Offices: PO Box 848, Ibadan; PO Box 441, Benin City; PO Box 424, Port Harcourt; PO Box 255, Kaduna; PO Box 1733, Jos; PO Box 1434, Enugu; PO Box 653, Kano; 2 Kofo Abayomi St, Apapa, Lagos

Principal Bankers: First Bank of Nigeria Ltd; Union Bank of Nigeria Ltd; Societe General Bank (Nigeria) Ltd; United Bank for Africa Nigeria Ltd

Financial Information:

	₦'000
Authorised capital	7,000
Paid-up capital	6,100
Turnover	154,835
Profits	6,123

Principal Shareholders: Nigerian National Petroleum Corporation
Date of Establishment: 1956
No of Employees: 600

UNIQUE TRADING CO LTD

7c Waff Rd, Commercial Area, PO Box 430, Zaria, Kaduna State

Tel: 2033, 2415
Cable: Unique Zaria

Chairman: John Oye Idowu
Directors: Nunasu Amosu (Managing),
   Samson Oye Idowu,
   Francis Segun Idowu,
   Mrs Comfort Ajani,
   Alhaji Aliyutafida
Senior Executives: Joseph Ofon (Group Accountant),
   J B Agyeman (Assistant Group Accountant),
   V B Idowu (Commercial Manager, Trading Division),
   W A Ayorinde (Administrative/Commercial Manager, Printing Division),
   I M Wogu (Works Manager),
   Betty Nwosu (Public Relations/Sales Executive)

PRINCIPAL ACTIVITIES: Booksellers, stationers and printers; importers, general merchants, manufacturers' representatives

Principal Agencies: Oxford University Press; Longman Nigeria Ltd; Evans Educational Publishers; Heineman Educational Publishers; Wiggins Teape (WA) Ltd, Nigeria

Branch Offices: B340 Wunti St, PMB 47, Bauchi; 33 Hospital Rd, PO Box 430, Zaria

Associated Companies: Cosmos (Nigeria) Enterprises; Sam-Franco (Nigeria) Co; Joid International Agencies; Hansteman Cosmetics Co (Nigeria) Ltd; Unique Printing Press Ltd

Financial Information:

	₦'000
Authorised capital	100
Paid-up capital	100

Principal Shareholders: John Oye Idowu; Mrs Comfort Ajani; Samson Idowu; Francis Idowu; Nunasu Amosu

UNISTEEL WORKS LTD

PO Box 4004, Kaduna South
Tel: 242213

Directors: G A Yakubu, G Pizzinat

PRINCIPAL ACTIVITIES: Steel fabrication, and erection of steel structures; building of oil tankers, tippers, trailers and water tanks
Principal Bankers: United Bank for Africa
Financial Information: Associate of Songhai Group pf Companies

UNITED AFRICAN DRUG CO (NIG) LTD

1 Abimbola Shodipe St, PO Box 1180, Surulere, Lagos
Tel: 837744, 836695, 836698
Cable: Unidrug Lagos
Telex: GMOCO 22148 Ng

Chairman: Chief J O Igwe
Directors: Chief G E Chikeluba, Chief M O Arinze, R C Azubike, N C Nzewi
Senior Executives: S N Okechukwu (Pharmacist/Manager),
   O O Salako (Marketing Manager),
   B C Aralu (Accountant),
   G C Okafor (Medical Technologist),
   C I Eze (Sales Manager, North),
   M O Eruchalu (Sales Manager, East)

PRINCIPAL ACTIVITIES: Distribution of pharmaceutical products
Principal Agencies: Instituto Biochemico Italiano; Lagap SA; Gruppo Lepetit; Cupal Ltd; New Asiatic Chemical Works Ltd
Branch Offices: 3 Eziukwu Rd, Aba, Tel 220892; 61B Bida Rd, Onitsha, Tel 212830; LL14 Wushishi Rd, Kaduna, Tel 212638
Subsidiary Companies: Ciana Agencies Ltd; Hero Engineering Constructions Ltd
Principal Bankers: United Bank for Africa Ltd; Union Bank of Nigeria Ltd
Financial Information:

	₦'000
Authorised capital	120
Paid-up capital	120
Turnover	8,200

Principal Shareholders: Chairman and directors as described
Date of Establishment: 1964
No of Employees: 160

UNITED AREWA CHEMISTS LTD

66/67 Fagge Ta Gabas (Murtala Muhammed Way), PO Box 1106, Kano
Tel: 4895, 4182, 4703
Cable: Unichem

PRINCIPAL ACTIVITIES: Importers of pharmaceuticals, toiletries and cosmetics
Branch Offices: 10A Galadima Rd, Kano

UNITED BANK FOR AFRICA LTD

97/105 Broad St, PO Box 2406, Lagos
Tel: 664866, 664010, 664740, 661224, 664980
Cable: Mindobank Lagos
Telex: 21241, 21580

Chairman: Alhaji Audu Buba
Directors: Alhaji U A Mutallab (Managing Director and Chief Executive),
   H M Byington III,
   P Fenichel (Alternate to H M Byington III),
   E Finot,
   C Domercq (Alternate to E Finot),
   M L Berger,
   E Mouterde,
   M Deveze (Alternate of E Mouterde),
   F Vincent (Executive Director),
   O Ogunsulire (Executive Director),
   Professor B O Nwabueze (Executive Director),
   E O Ebiefie (Executive Director),
   Alhaji Abubakar Tunau,
   Alhaji Usman S Dantata,
   Alhaji Hassan Kwai,
   B Doria,
   M O Anibaba
Senior Executives: O Ogunsulire (Deputy General Manager, Administration),
   J Woodhead (Assistant General Manager, Administration),
   A R Hawkins (Assistant General Manager, Personnel),
   W O'Byrne (Assistant General Manager, Finance),
   Prof B O Nwabueze (Company Secretary)

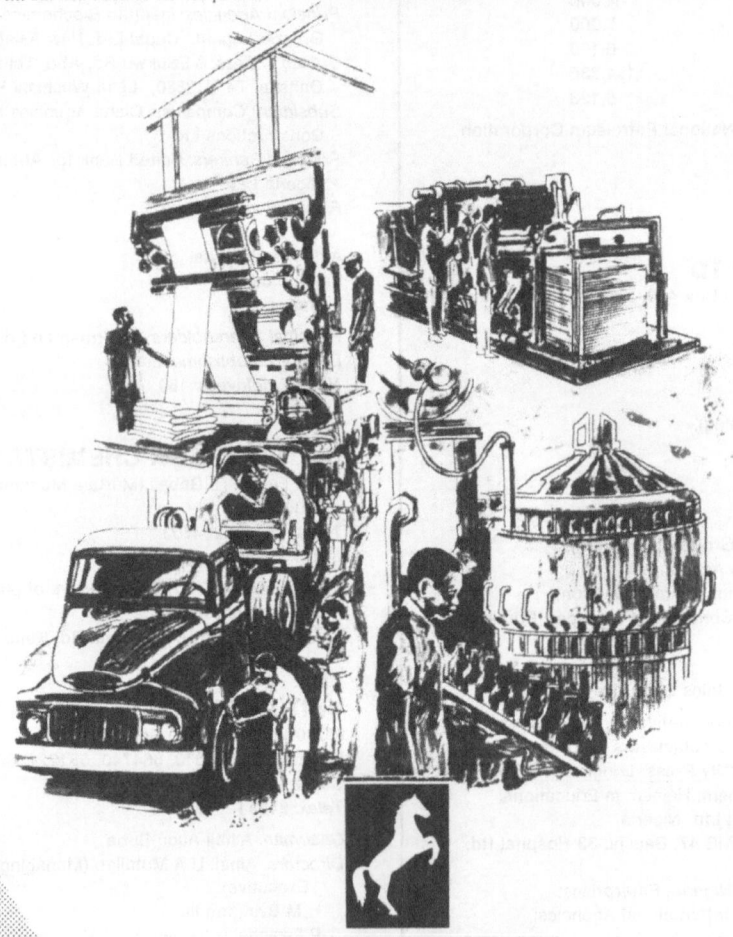

PRINCIPAL ACTIVITIES: Commercial banking
Branch Offices: Branches throughout Nigeria
Financial Information: As at 31st March 1982

Liabilities	₦'000	Assets	₦'000
Capital	65,000	Cash & banks	1,079,823
Reserves	78,239	Investments	79,210
Deposits, etc	2,548,230	Loans and discounts	1,532,436
Contra A/cs	976,650	Contra A/cs	976,650
Total	3,668,119	Total	3,668,119

Principal Shareholders: Federal Government (48.89%); Nigerian Public (11.11%); Banque Nationale de Paris, France (5.20%); Banque Nationale de Paris Ltd, UK (25.50%); Bankers Trust Company, USA (4.50%); Banca Nazionale del Lavoro, Italy (2.40%); Monte dei Paschi di Siena, Italy (2.40%)

UNITED CONSOLIDATED INDUSTRIES LTD

24A Ja'afaru Rd, PO Box 661, Kano
Tel: 4333, 3637
Cable: Unilco
Telex: 77143

PRINCIPAL ACTIVITIES: Manufacturers of toilet soap, kettles, kerosene tins, ball-point pens, plastic containers

UNITED DEVELOPMENT TRADING COMPANY LTD

PO Box 541, Ibadan, Oyo State
Tel: 410181
Cable: Undetraco

Chairman: Richard Oladipo Makanjuola
Directors: Abimbola Oladipo Makanjuola
Senior Executives: A O Makanjuola (Managing Director), E A Abiodun (Legal Adviser)

PRINCIPAL ACTIVITIES: Exportation of raw materials (crushed bones, cattle horns, kola nuts, hooves); plastics; products; photographic equipment; automatic accessories. Real estate
Principal Agencies: Wells Fargo Alarm Services, USA; Unicolor, Photo Division, Dexter, USA; STP, Florida, USA
Branch Offices: Emir's Rd, Ilorin, Kwara State
Subsidiary Companies: A R O Makanjuola and Sons Ltd, Ibadan
Principal Bankers: Union Bank of Nigeria Ltd
Financial Information:
Authorised capital ₦ 100,000

Principal Shareholders: R O Makanjuola; Dr R O Makanjuola; A O Makanjuola; Mrs D O Adebisi S O Makanjuola
Date of Establishment: Established 1933; Incorporated 1963

UNITED EDUCATIONAL SUPPLIES LTD

1 Ibadan Rd, PMB 3220, Kano
Tel: 5732, 5748

PRINCIPAL ACTIVITIES: Suppliers of stationery, and office equipment

UNITED GEOPHYSICAL (NIGERIA) LTD

73A Tinubu Rd, Palm Grove Estate, PO Box 286, Ikeja, Lagos State
Tel: 964281, 964301
Cable: Unitedgeo Lagos
Telex: 26300 Unigeo Ng

Directors: H Morley (Managing),
    J Onikute (Company Secretary),
    G Onwuchekwa,
    B Kehinde
Senior Executives: J A Carter (Manager),
    J M Harwood (Manager, Warri)

PRINCIPAL ACTIVITIES: Geophysical services for the oil industry
Branch Offices: PO Box 258, Warri
Principal Bankers: Savannah Bank of Nigeria Ltd

UNITED MATCH COMPANY OF NIGERIA LTD

17 Liverpool Rd, Apapa, PO Box 941, Lagos
Tel: 610429, 873185
Telex: 21507 Match Ng

PRINCIPAL ACTIVITIES: Manufacturers of safety matches
Branch Offices: Factory: Offa Rd, PO Box 180, Ilorin, Kwara State

UNITED NIGERIA INSURANCE COMPANY LTD (THE)

53 Marina, PO Box 588, Lagos
Tel: 663130, 663153, 663201, 663229, 663253
Cable: Unance

Chairman: Arc Gabriel Yakubu Aduku
Directors: F C Nwokolo (Managing),
    J A C Amos,
    C O Rowe,
    O Dike,
    Mrs H A Folakan,
    A C Uzokwe,
    Alhaji A A Hassan,
    J C Onwubuya
Senior Executives: Chief E O A Adetunji (Assistant General Manager, Finance),
    A O Degun (Assistant General Manager, Claims),
    Alhaji M K Laguda (Assistant General Manager, Underwriting),
    A A Obakeye (Assistant General Manager, Administration/Company Secretary),
    Chief J C Onwubuya (Deputy Managing Director)

PRINCIPAL ACTIVITIES: Insurance, all classes except life
Branch Offices: PO Box 1470, Ibadan, Oyo State; PO Box 350, Benin City, Bendel State; PO Box 278, Yola, Gongola State; PO Box 318, Kaduna; PO Box 400, Jos, Plateau State; PO Box 667, Enugu, Anambra State; 131 Calabar Rd, Calabar, Cross River State; PMB 1162, Maiduguri, Borno State; PO Box 381, Kano; Onitsha; Sokoto; Aba; Abeokuta; Ilorin; Makurdi
Associated Companies: The United Nigeria Life Insurance Company Ltd; Commercial Union Assurance Co Ltd; UAC of Nigeria Ltd
Principal Bankers: First Bank of Nigeria Ltd; Union Bank of Nigeria Ltd
Financial Information:

	₦'000
Authorised capital	5,000
Paid-up capital	5,000
Turnover	56,377
Profits	8,155

Principal Shareholders: Northern Assurance Co Ltd; Federal Ministry of Finance Incorporated; CWA Holdings Ltd; CFAO; Kaduna State Investment Co Ltd; Kano State Investment and Properties Ltd; Ministry of Finance Incorporated Imo State; K Sofola
Date of Establishment: 2nd April 1965
No of Employees: 760

UNITED NIGERIA MOTORS LTD

SW8/117 Ijebu Bye Pass, PO Box 1754, Ibadan, Oyo State
Telex: 31161

PRINCIPAL ACTIVITIES: Wholesale suppliers; distributors of motor vehicles, construction equipment machinery

UNITED NIGERIAN TEXTILES LTD

Plot 0 Industrial Area, PO Box 365, Kaduna
Tel: 201060, 201063
Cable: Uniontex
Telex: 71140

Chairman: Cha Chi Ming
Directors: Alhaji Mamman Daura,
    Payson Cha,
    Richard Young (Managing),
    Laurence S Fong,

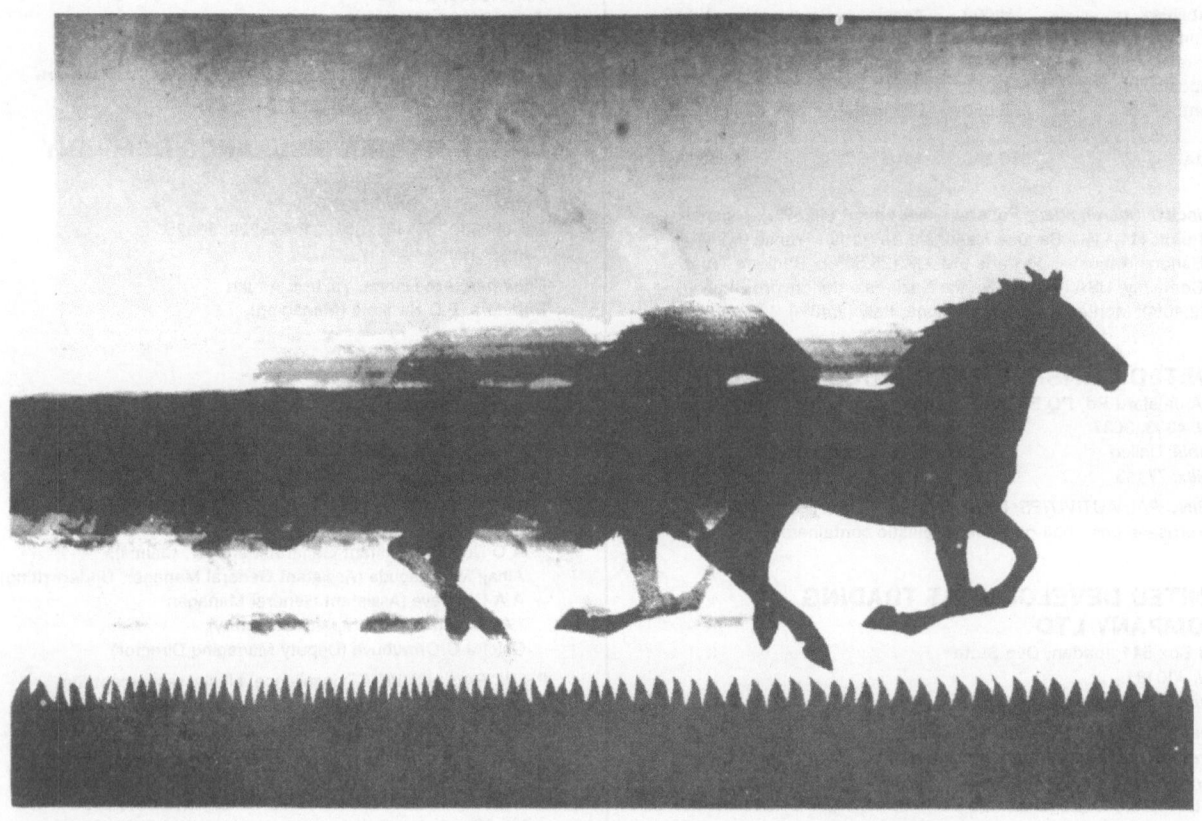

Walter Sannemann,
Chief S B Daniyan,
M A Sanusi,
Sandy S T Pan,
M D Yusufu,
S Y Kasimu
Senior Executives: L S Fong (General Manager),
 M Abubakar (Assistant General Manager, Personnel),
 Y S Wong (Assistant General Manager, Production),
 T Inn (Assistant to General Manager, Sales),
 Alhaji F Abdullahi (Company Secretary/Assistant General
 Manager, Administration)

PRINCIPAL ACTIVITIES: Manufacturers of textiles
Branch Offices: PO Box 2990, Lagos; 20 Unity Rd, PO Box 552,
 Kano; 35 New Market Rd, PO Box 1701, Onitsha
Associated Companies: Zamfara Textile Industries Ltd; Funtua
 Textiles Ltd; Unitex Ltd
Principal Bankers: First Bank of Nigeria Ltd; Union Bank of
 Nigeria Ltd; Bank of the North Ltd; Co-operative Bank Nigeria
 Ltd
Financial Information:

	N'000
Authorised capital	17,000
Paid-up capital	17,000
Turnover	106,845
Profits	8,972

Principal Shareholders: Maritime Atlantic Holding Ltd; Northern
 Nigeria Investments Ltd; New Nigerian Development Co Ltd
Date of Establishment: July 1964
No of Employees: 6,909

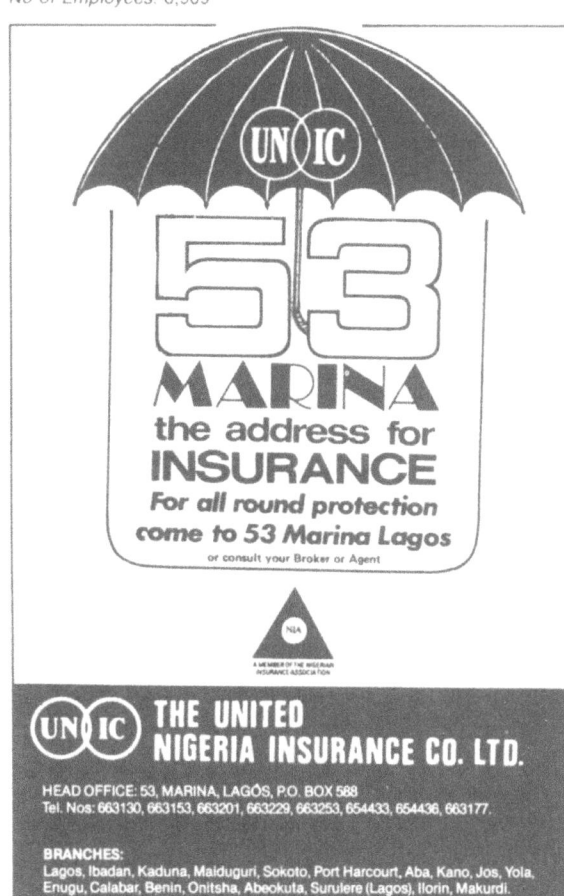

UNITED TECHNOLOGY (NIGERIA) LTD
12 Abimbola Shodipe Street, Suru-Lere, Yaba, Lagos
Tel: 834725

Chairman: Aderemi Abdul
Directors: Oladunni Abdul, Adeyemi Abdul

Senior Executives: S Fujie (General Manager),
 R Ogunnaike (Plant Manager),
 K Miyamoto (Marketing Manager),
 P Siabour (Administrative Manager),
 H Ando (Production Engineer),
 M Ayoola (Accountant)

PRINCIPAL ACTIVITIES: Assembly and marketing of air
 conditioning and refrigeration equipment
Principal Agencies: Licensee of daikin Industries Ltd, Japan
Branch Offices: 20 Bola Tiyamiyu Street, Molipa Layout,
 Ijebu-Ode, Ogun State
Subsidiary/Associated Companies: H O Abdul Trading Company
 Ltd
Principal Bankers: Savannah Bank of Nigeria Ltd
Financial Information:

	N'000
Authorised capital	1,000
Paid-up capital	1,000
Turnover	6,000
Profits	400

Principal Shareholders: Aderemi Abdul; Alhaja H O Abdul; Alhaji
 G A Abdul
Date of Establishment: September 1978
No of Employees: 80

UNITY LIFE AND FIRE INSURANCE COMPANY LTD
9 Nnamdi Azikiwe St, PO Box 3681, Lagos
Tel: 662388, 662783
Cable: Unilife
Telex: 21657 Unity Ng

Chairman: Henry Osime Omenai
Directors: Chief P M C Ebigbo,
 Chief F S Yesufu,
 Dr V G Ene,
 A Adejumo,
 A S Guobadia,
 F A Nzeribe,
 J O Irukwu (Managing)

PRINCIPAL ACTIVITIES: Insurance
Branch Offices: Throughout Nigeria
Principal Bankers: First Bank of Nigeria Ltd; United Bank for
 Africa Ltd; African Continental Bank Ltd; National Bank of
 Nigeria Ltd

Date of Establishment: 30th August 1965

UNITY SOAP MANUFACTURERS LTD
PO Box 308, Kano
PRINCIPAL ACTIVITIES: Manufacturing of soap and detergents

UNIVERSAL DISTRIBUTORS LTD
The Bestseller, Falomo Shopping Centre, Awolowo Rd, Ikoyi, PO
 Box 7036, Lagos
Tel: 684867

Chairman: Mrs I Fatayi-Williams
Directors: B Fatayi-Williams (Managing),
 Dr A Fatayi-Williams,
 Mrs O Williams (General Manager)
Senior Executives: Oladele Fatayi-Williams (Special Projects
 Manager),
 Rotimi John (Publicity Manager),
 Mrs Y Ogunlari (Manager, Lagos Bookshop),
 Mrs T A Ajayi (Manager, Kaduna Bookshop),
 Mrs C Onyeacholam (Manager, Benin City Bookshop)

PRINCIPAL ACTIVITIES: Booksellers
Branch Offices: Durbar Hotel, Kaduna; 18 Mission Rd, Benin
 City, Bendel State
Associated Companies: Nigerian Card Suppliers Ltd; Nigerian
 Book Suppliers Ltd
Principal Bankers: Union Bank of Nigeria Ltd; United Bank for
 Africa Ltd

UNIVERSAL EDUCATIONAL SUPPLIES LTD (MORISON ARNOLD LTD)
3 Bompai Rd (Opposite Central Hotel), PO Box 251, Kano
Tel: 4856 Kano
Cable: Clipper Kano

Chairman: Alhaji Usman Nagado
Directors: Alhaji Usman Abubakar (Managing Director),
   Alhaji Tijjani Hashim,
   Alhaji U S Birma,
   Alhaji A Musa,
   Alhaji Z Tela,
   Alhaji B Rabiu,
   Alhaji Balarabe Jega
Senior Executives: Mallam Idris Audu (Administrative Manager),
   Olayiwola Bolaji (Accountant)

PRINCIPAL ACTIVITIES: Suppliers of educational equipment, textbooks, sports, office and audio-visual equipment, and stationery supplies
Principal Agencies: E J Arnold (International) Ltd, UK; C P J Overseas Ltd, UK; Thomas Wyatt Nigeria Ltd; Oxford University Press; Longmans, Evans Nigeria Ltd, etc
Branch Offices: Borno State College of Basic Studies, Maiduguri; Kano State Polytechnic; Sultan Abubakar Rd, Sokoto
Principal Bankers: Union Bank of Nigeria Ltd
Financial Information: Formerly Morison Arnold Ltd

Principal Shareholders: Alhaji Maikano Gwarzo (Durbin Kano); Alhaji Haruna Galdimare; Chairman and Directors as described

UNIVERSAL FISHING COMPANY LTD
13 Ijora Causeway, PO Box 1383, Ijora, Lagos
Tel: 831081
Cable: Mackerels Lagos
Telex: 21591 Priuni Ng

Chairman: H K Kamlesh
Directors: M L Mansukhani (Managing),
   H K Ram,
   A O Adewunmi,
   Miss H O Agoro
Senior Executives: D T Gurbani (Operations Controller),
   B M Thawani (Operations Controller),
   F O Oladipo (Chief Accountant)

PRINCIPAL ACTIVITIES: Fishing and fish processing
Branch Offices: Plot No 7 Amaigbo St, PMB 5280, Port Harcourt, Rivers State
Principal Bankers: Savannah Bank of Nigeria Ltd; United Bank for Africa Ltd; International Merchant Bank (Nigeria) Ltd; Bank of India (Nigeria) Ltd
Financial Information:

	₦'000
Authorised capital	1,800
Paid-up capital	900
Turnover (approx)	19,000

Date of Establishment: October 1971

UNIVERSAL INSURANCE COMPANY LTD
Corner of Ridgeway/Station Rd, PO Box 360, Enugu, Anambra State
Tel: 255038, 255056
Cable: Unisure Enugu
Telex: 51227 Unisur Ng

Chairman: Dr D N Nwatu
Directors: Dr C Umezurike,
   Dr J Onah,
   B O Asiegbunam,
   S B Ogujawa,
   C N E Olieh,
   O E Amaonwu (General Manager)
Senior Executives: Mrs L Obienu (Company Secretary),
   V A Obiozor (Chief Accountant)

PRINCIPAL ACTIVITIES: Insurance/Reinsurance
Branch Offices: 27/29 Martins St, PO Box 2623, Lagos, Tel

660557; 95 Upper New Market Rd, PMB 1624, Onitsha, Tel 509; 21A Asa Rd, PMB 7149, Aba, Tel 446; 97 Aba Rd, PMB 5282, Port Harcourt, Rivers State, Tel 22199; ACB Building, 2 Maikano Dutse Rd, PMB 3320, Kano; Uyo, Cross River State; Owerri; Abakaliki; Awka; Umuahia; Okigwe; Orlu; Nnewi; Nsukka
Subsidiary/Associated Companies: Ridgeway Properties Ltd; Premier Brokers
Principal Bankers: African Continental Bank Ltd; United Bank for Africa Ltd; Co-operative Bank of Eastern Nigeria
Financial Information:

	₦'000
Authorised capital	1,000
Paid-up capital	800
Sales turnover	6,500
Profits	500

Principal Shareholders: Government of Imo State; Government of Anambra State; African Continental Bank Ltd
Date of Establishment: 1961
No of Employees: 340

UNIVERSAL MONOLITHIC BEARING STRUCTURE LTD
Plot 33 and 34, Sharada Industrial Area Phase II, PO Box 283, Kano
Tel: 2456
Cable: UMBS Ltd
Telex: 77131 UMBS Ng

Chairman: Kassim S K Hammoud
Directors: V Cavallo (Managing Director),
   Alhaji Tijjani Hashim,
   Evan Enewerem

PRINCIPAL ACTIVITIES: Manufacturers of prefabricated houses, schools, offices; manufacturers of fibreglass vans and refrigerated bodies for vehicles
Principal Bankers: African Continental Bank Ltd
Financial Information:

	₦'000
Authorised capital	500
Paid-up capital	250

No of Employees: 140

UNIVERSAL PACKAGING (NIGERIA) LTD
Kilometer 16 Ikorodu Rd, PO Box 1516, Ikeja, Lagos State
Cable: Unipac Lagos
Telex: 22371 Mellos Ng

Chairman: J Adetunji Cole
Directors: Ram S Agrawal (Managing),
   Alhaji Kam Selem,
   Dr Mahmud Tukur,
   Harish L Chulani,
   Fred Egbe,
   Ravi Kapur

PRINCIPAL ACTIVITIES: Packaging, production of corrugated cardboard boxes
Associated Companies: Ranbaxy Montari (Nigeria) Ltd; Milestone Enterprises Ltd; Nigerian Industrial Auxiliaries Ltd; Zodiac Auto Industries (Nig) Ltd; Iddo Plastics Ltd; International Plastics Ltd
Principal Bankers: United Bank for Africa Ltd; International Bank for West Africa Ltd

Date of Establishment: November 1977
No of Employees: 150

UNIVERSAL STEELS LTD
Israel Adebajo Rd, PO Box 144, Ikeja, Lagos
Tel: 964185, 963145, 961028
Cable: Usteels Ikeja

Chairman: S Dankaro
Directors: R K C Lee (Vice-Chairman),
   Alhaji H H T Wong,
   Mustapha Aliyu (Emir of Biu),

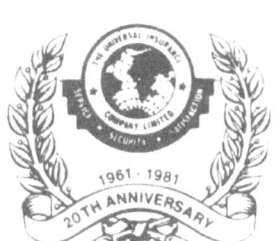

Olisa Chukura,
David Dankaro,
C C Lee,
Alhaji S F Cheung,
F S Tu,
Mallam I Damci
Senior Executives: H H T Wong (General Manager)

PRINCIPAL ACTIVITIES: Manufacturers of mild steel rods, flats
and angle bars; household enamelware

UNIVERSAL TEXTILE INDUSTRIES LTD
PO Box 2243, Bompai Industrial Estate, Kano

Directors: C A Jaafar

PRINCIPAL ACTIVITIES: Manufacturers of towels and other
textile goods

UNIVERSAL VULCANIZING COMPANY
NIGERIA LTD
SW9/989 Idi-'Roko Challenge, PMB 5201, Ibadan, Oyo State
Tel: 413582
Cable: Univulco, Ibadan
Telex: 31170 Univul Ng

Chairman: Chief Amos Olasupo Adegoke
Directors: Kehinde Adegoke, Miss Taiwo Adegoke
Senior Executives: J F Alagbada (General Manager),
O B Akinwande (Chief Accountant),
M O Odeyemi (Area Manager, North)

PRINCIPAL ACTIVITIES: Distributors of tyres, conveyor belts,
automobile and other types of tyres, vulcanizing equipment
and materials, workshop tools and garage equipment
Principal Agencies: Semperit AKG, Austria; Bridgestone Rubber
Company, Japan; Banner Batterien, Austria; Carl Walter
Tools, Austria; National Rubber Company, Canada
Branch Offices: 10 Olofin Street, PMB 1079, Apapa, Lagos;
32/34 Calcutta Crescent, Apapa, Lagos; 63 Uselu Lagos Rd,
Benin City, Bendel State; PMB 1466, Opposite Iloring
Grammar School, Ilorin; KM 20 Ibrahim Taiwo Rd,
Tundunwada, Kaduna; 1008G Yanbalangu Way, Gwagwarwa
Quarters, Kano
Associated Companies: Adegoke Motors Ltd; Adecentro Nigeria
Ltd
Principal Bankers: Savannah Bank of Nigeria Ltd; United Bank
for Africa Ltd
Financial Information:

	₦'000
Authorised capital	500
Paid-up capital	300
Turnover	4,500
Profits	207

Principal Shareholders: Chief A O Adegoke; Kehinde Adegoke;
Miss Taiwo Adegoke
Date of Establishment: 1967
No of Employees: 140

UNIVERSAL WELDING & CONSTRUCTION
COMPANY LTD
PO Box 407, Warri, Bendel State
Tel: 231863
Telex: 41101

PRINCIPAL ACTIVITIES: Welding and construction

UNIVERSITY OF IFE PRESS LTD
University of Ife, Ile-Ife, Oyo State
Tel: 2291/9
Cable: Press Ifevarsity

Chairman: Professor O S Adegoke
Directors: B O Iluyomade, W O Funmilayo, J O Dipeolu, I
Ademokun, I O Agbaje, Prince Olu Joshua
Senior Executives: Dr 'Sola Soile (Publishing Manager),
Akin Fatokun (Editor),
Miss A Adeyanju (Editor),
J O Agbe (Senior Sales Representative),

'Leke Odeyemi (Sales Representative)

PRINCIPAL ACTIVITIES: Publishing, specialists in African law and local government

Principal Bankers: National Bank of Nigeria Ltd

Principal Shareholders: University of Ife

Date of Establishment: 1968

UNIVERSITY PRESS LTD

Three Crowns Building, PMB 5095, Jericho, Ibadan, Oyo State

Tel: 413117, 412056, 411356

Cable: Oxonian Ibadan

Telex: 31121

Chairman: Professor H A Oluwasanmi

Directors: M O Akinleye (Managing),
   A Butcher,
   J A Hemingway,
   V C Ike,
   Alhaji H R Zayyad,
   W R Andrewes

Senior Executives: R A Popoola (Financial Controller/Company Secretary),
   B O Adeleke (Publishing Services Manager),
   Chief O Bankole (Marketing Manager),
   J A Fawibe (Trade Manager),
   V Olayemi (Editorial Manager)

PRINCIPAL ACTIVITIES: Book pulishing and distribution

Principal Agencies: Cassell Ltd, London; Collier Macmillan Ltd, London; Intercontinental Book Production Ltd, UK; Prentice Hall International, UK; WAEC; ABU; UNN Press

Branch Offices: Depots: Kano; Owerri; Jos; Zaria; Showrooms: Lagos; Benin City; Enugu; Akure

Associated Companies: Oxford University Press, UK

Principal Bankers: United Bank for Africa Ltd; International Bank for West Africa Ltd; Chase Merchant Bank; Nigeria Merchant Bank

Financial Information: (Formerly Oxford University Press Nigeria Ltd)

	N'000
Authorised capital	4,000
Paid-up capital	4,000
Turnover	14,000
Profits	2,500

Principal Shareholders: Oxford University Press, Oxford (40%); Nigerian Shareholders (60%)

Date of Establishment: 1978

No of Employees: 253

UOO TRADING COMPANY LTD

4 Balogun Sq, PO Box 2556, Lagos

Tel: 652166

Cable: Uoos Lagos

PRINCIPAL ACTIVITIES: Textile merchants

Branch Offices: 9a Abibu Oki St, Lagos, Tel 635126; 73 Broad St, Lagos; 15 Lebanon St, Ibadan, Oyo State; 47 Onireke St, Ibadan, Oyo State

UPJOHN NIGERIA PTY LTD

Plot 1 Block F, Oshodi Industrial Estate, PMB 1182, Oshodi, Lagos State

Tel: 933520, 933606

Cable: Togamix, Lagos

Chairman: Chief J E Ukueku

Directors: K L Neumueller (Managing),
   J Y Gbefwi,
   P Omo-Dare,
   J Gauthier

Senior Executives: L Hellemans (Project Manager),
   P A Ogunlowo (Financial Controller),
   A G Bello (Marketing Manager),
   R A Oduwole (Marketing Planning Manager),
   O Adesanya (Sales Manager)

PRINCIPAL ACTIVITIES: Suppliers of pharmaceuticals and medical supplies

Branch Offices: 19 Chief Sam Mbakwe Rd, PMB 7077, Aba, Imo State

Principal Bankers: Union Bank of Nigeria Ltd; Icon Ltd (Merchant Bankers); Nal Merchant Bank Ltd

Principal Shareholders: Upjohn International, Panama (40%); Nigerian Citizens (60%)

Date of Establishment: 12th November 1973

No of Employees: 100

URBAHN, MAX O, INTERNATIONAL LTD

2/4 Adeola Odeku St, 2nd Floor, Victoria Island, Pan Ocean Building, PMB 12734, Lagos

Tel: 612633, 610494

Telex: 21468 Panaco Ng

Directors: J M Danels (Managing Director),
   J Burrows (Deputy Managing Director)

PRINCIPAL ACTIVITIES: Management consultants

Branch Offices: PO Box 1026, Kaduna; PMB 5589, Ibadan; PMB 1504, Enugu

URBAN ENGINEERS

41 Sura Mogaji/Coker Rd, Ilupeju, PO Box 2298, Lagos

Tel: 961068

PRINCIPAL ACTIVITIES: Construction

UREN CONSTRUCTION ENGINEERING COMPANY LTD

26 Aina Rd, Isolo, PO Box 1135, Mushin, Lagos

Tel: 840002

Chairman: Engineer Olusesan Adebajo (also Managing Director)

Directors: Kolawole Oronti (Finance)

Senior Executives: Rtd Major P R Shinde (Contracts Manager),
   Y R Vohra (Chief Engineer),
   B G K Ariyaratna (Chief Engineer),
   Chief D O Solesi (Office Manager),
   Tai Akinola (Marketing Manager)

PRINCIPAL ACTIVITIES: Specialists in water distribution networks, sewerage systems, pressure lines and pumping stations, reinforced concrete reservoirs, drinking and industrial water facilities and sewerage purification works, road construction and ancilliary civil engineering works

Branch Offices: 36 New Court Rd, PO Box 1201, Ibadan; Laminga Dam Rd, PO Box 6097, Anglo-Jos

Associated Companies: Uren Tissues Ltd; Adebajo Structures

Principal Bankers: United Bank for Africa Ltd; National Bank of Nigeria

Financial Information:

	N'000
Authorised capital	250
Paid-up capital	250

Principal Shareholders: Engr Olusesan Adebajo; Kolawole Oronti

Date of Establishment: 15th November 1972

No of Employees: 497

UROBO AGENCIES (NIGERIA) LTD

Head Office, 101 Market Rd, PMB 7253, Aba, Imo State

Cable: Urobo

PRINCIPAL ACTIVITIES: General merchants and contractors; importers and distributors of all types of building materials, electronic equipment; scientific, hospital, laboratory and educational equipment; all types of chemicals

Branch Offices: 175 Zik Ave, PMB 1151, Enugu

UTAGBA-UNO RUBBER ESTATES LTD

Utagba-Uno, 52 Warehouse Rd, PMB 1082, Apapa, Lagos

PRINCIPAL ACTIVITIES: Crepe rubber production

UTC NIGERIA LTD (FORMERLY UNION TRADING COMPANY OF NIGERIA LTD)

139 Broad St, PO Box 572, Lagos
Tel: 656720/9
Cable: Uniontrade
Telex: 21232 Unitra Ng

Chairman: Alhaji Laman Ciroma
Directors: S B Awoniyi (Vice Chairman),
K Wegmueller (Managing),
Alhaji H Abdullahi,
Adekunle Ojora,
A E Sarasin,
T C M Eneli,
F Mohr (Finance Director),
Dr G A Jawando (Administration & Development),
J Zumstein,
Major General J J Oluleye (Rtd)

PRINCIPAL ACTIVITIES: Main activities of each Division:- Motor Division - Sale and service of heavy commercial trucks, light commercial vehicles, Komatsu earth-moving equipment, agricultural tractors, Peugeot cars and spare parts, etc; Technical Division - Sale, installation and service of technical equipment, diesel engine generators, agricultural, construction machinery, welding supplies, hospital equipment, schindler lifts; Hardware Division - Distributes and services quality tools, equipment, machinery building supplies, agrochemicals, crop spraying equipment and fertilizers; Department Stores & Supermarkets - including meat processing factory and biscuits/dry bakery goods, office equipment, opthalmic optician, etc; Textile Division - Designing and wholesale distribution of real handblock wax print and other textile piece goods; Engineering Division - Sale, installation and service of electric power generation, water purification and sewage treatment and irrigation equipment all on turnkey projects, swimming pools and weir pumps; Business Promotion - Indenting, confirming, importing, distribution representing, stocking and warehousing of all types of merchandise for and/or on behalf of Nigerian traders, manufacturers, clients, government departments, corporations and authorities
Branch Offices: Ijebu Bye Pass, PO Box 1381, Ibadan, Telex 31184 Unitra Ng; 28 Sapele Rd, PO Box 316, Benin, Telex 41119 Unitra Ng; 7 Doka Crescent, PO Box 101, Kaduna, Telex 71133 Unitra Ng; 17-18 Bello Rd, PO Box 365, Kano, Telex 77111 Unitra Ng; Colliery Ave, PO Box 306, Enugu, Telex 51103 Unitra Ng; 16 Liberation Drive, Port Harcourt, Telex 61110 Unitra Ng
Associated Companies: Nigerian Hardware Industries Ltd
Principal Bankers: Union Bank of Nigeria Ltd; First Bank of Nigeria Ltd; United Bank for Africa; International Bank for West Africa Ltd; Icon Ltd
Financial Information: As at March 1982

	₦'000
Authorised capital	40,000
Paid-up capital	39,167
Turnover	396,396
Profits (before tax)	39,664
Profits (after tax)	22,664

Principal Shareholders: Nigerians 60.51%; Non-Nigerians 39.49%
No of Employees: 5,900

UTILGAS NIGERIAN AND OVERSEAS GAS COMPANY LTD

34 Nnamdi Azikiwe Street, PO Box 2735, Lagos
Tel: 657446, 658595
Cable: Utilgas
Telex: 21883 Utlgas Ng

Chairman: Chief Adeniran Ogunsanya
Directors: R Fradis, Mrs A Adeniji, S Moriel, Mrs T Ibironke, F Brunschwig
Senior Executives: M Kovacs (General Manager)
PRINCIPAL ACTIVITIES: Marketers of LP gas for domestic and industrial cooking, catering equipment, air conditioners and refrigerators installation and service
Principal Agencies: T I Creda International Ltd, UK; Foster Refrigeration (UK), Ltd; Thorn Gas International, UK
Branch Offices: 2 Market Rd, PO Box 437, Enugu; 14 Aggrey Rd, PO Box 598, Port Harcourt; 2 Ali Akilu Rd, PO Box 426, Kaduna; N6/474 Oyo Rd, PO Box 766, Ibadan; 135 Lagos Street, PO Box 244, Benin-City
Principal Bankers: Savannah Bank of Nigeria Ltd; United Bank for Africa Ltd; Union Bank of Nigeria Ltd
Financial Information:

	₦'000
Authorised capital	150
Paid-up capital	150

Principal Shareholders: Chief Adeniran Ogunsanya; Overgaz SA, Switzerland; Chief T O S Benson; S Moriel Overseas Econ Ent Ltd; B E Ogbuagu
Date of Establishment: 20th February 1961
No of Employees: 175

UWAI AND SONS ENTERPRISES

PO Box 28, Ikot Abasi, Cross River State

Chairman: Francis Uwai (also Managing Director)
Directors: Raymond Uwai (Consultant)

PRINCIPAL ACTIVITIES: General traders, importers and exporters, manufacturers' representatives, hotels and catering, transporters
Branch Offices: Ossissa via Kwale; Koko via Sapele
Principal Bankers: First Bank of Nigeria Ltd

Principal Shareholders: Francis Uwai; Raymond Uwai; Rosaline Uwai; John Uwai

VALID ASSURANCE COMPANY LTD

12/14 Broad Street, PO Box 5715, Lagos
Tel: 651226, 631296, 631353
Cable: Valassure Lagos

Chairman: Chief R C Nwakoby
Directors: Professor C O Ekwueme, P O Nwakoby, Chief J A Ekwueme, Dr E O Ogbu, Alhaji I M Damcida, J N D Ubanwa, Aneto Okeke
Senior Executives: G I Osude (General Manager/Chief Executive),
L O Iwegbu (Assistant General Manager),
V U Ogbunuju (Financial Controller),
P M Ozor (Marketing Manager)

PRINCIPAL ACTIVITIES: Insurance
Branch Offices: 1 Unity Rd, Ikeja, Lagos State; 3A Colliery Avenue, PO Box 240, Enugu, Anambra State; Giban Badamasi, 25 Niger Street, PMB 3201, Kano State; 47 St Micheal's Street, PO Box 2168 Aba, Imo State; 74 Christ Church Street, Owerri, Imo State; 42 New Market Rd, Onitsha, Anambra State; 3 Emir Yahaya Rd, Sokoto, Sokoto State
Principal Bankers: United Bank for Africa Ltd
Financial Information:

	₦'000
Authorised capital	1,000
Paid-up capital	400
Turnover	4,500

Date of Establishment: 12th September 1977
No of Employees: 94

VALLEY FOODS NIGERIA LTD

Iddo House, PO Box 159, Lagos

PRINCIPAL ACTIVITIES: Food production and processing
Branch Offices: Ejiba, Kwara State; Mopa, Kwara State
Financial Information:
Registered capital ₦ 400,000

Principal Shareholders: A G Leventis; Nigerians
Date of Establishment: December 1978

VAN LEER CONTAINERS (NIGERIA) LTD

VAN LEER CONTAINERS (NIGERIA) LTD
1 Alapata Rd, Off Dockyard Rd, PO Box 16, Apapa, Lagos State

Tel: 873007, 877024, 877085
Cable: Metaconta Lagos
Telex: 22257 Valecn Ng

Chairman: Dr J E Andriessen
Directors: A Jolles (Managing),
  D O Ogungbemi (Technical),
  G O Onosode,
  Dr M Tukur,
  G A Sangosanya (Financial),
  J Van Den Burg,
  Akintola Williams
Senior Executives: G D Mordi (Marketing Manager),
  A O Bedford (Personnel Manager)

PRINCIPAL ACTIVITIES: Manufacturers of metal containers for petroleum products, chemicals and paints, vegetable oils etc
Principal Agencies: N V Van Leer SA, Belgium; Van Leer Nederland BV, Holland
Branch Offices: 1 Reclamation Rd, PO Box 858, Port Harcourt; 205A Barde Rd, PO Box 4957, Kano; Total Blending Plant Site, PO Box 43, Koko
Associated Companies: Industrial Gases Ltd; Gas Producers Ltd
Principal Bankers: United Bank for Africa Ltd; Chase Merchant Bank; International Merchant Bank (Nigeria) Ltd
Financial Information:

	N'000
Authorised capital	7,000
Paid-up capital	5,330
Turnover (approx)	25,000

Principal Shareholders: Royal Packaging Industries Van Leer BV, Holland; Van Leer Nigeria Education Trust; Nigerian Citizens and Associations
Date of Establishment: 1940
No of Employees: 475

VANNI HOLDINGS LTD
25 Adeniyi Jones Avenue, Industrial Estate, Ikeja, Lagos State
Tel: 961918, 962264
Telex: 21048 N

Chairman: Joseph Adeola
Directors: Victor Vanni (Managing),
  Rt Rev Adenrele
Senior Executives: Chief M O Idowu (Director of Administration),
  M O Adamu (Chief Accountant),
  B O Kuboye (Group Legal Adviser/Secretary),
  T O Oparaugo (Internal Auditor)

PRINCIPAL ACTIVITIES: Security systems, alarms, safety equipment, operation of airlines and travel agencies
Principal Agencies: Brinley Vickers Ltd, UK; Armoured Money Trucks, West Germany; Atlas Aircraft Corp, USA; Charlotte Aircraft Corp, USA; Chubb Integrated Systems Ltd, UK
Branch Offices: 24 Fiddlers Walk, Wargrave, Berks, UK; all 19 State Capitals of Nigeria
Subsidiary/Associated Companies: Vanni International Security Systems Ltd; Inter-Continental Airlines Ltd; Chubb Alarms Ltd; Hobkarn Holidays Ltd
Principal Bankers: United Bank for Africa Ltd; Savannah Bank of Nigeria Ltd; Union Bank of Nigeria Ltd; International Bank for West Africa Ltd
Financial Information:

	N'000
Authorised capital	2,500
Paid-up capital	700
Turnover	5,000
Profits	100

Principal Shareholders: Chief Victor Oje Vanni
Date of Establishment: 1975
No of Employees: 2,000

VARAMAN INDUSTRIES (NIGERIA) LTD
PO Box 4661, Lagos
Tel: 862194
Cable: Varaman

Chairman: A P Vashi
Directors: H B Mangho, Alhaji A Yusuff, A H Hemnani, J O Adebayo
Senior Executives: A P Hajani, A U Nnebe, C C Madueke
PRINCIPAL ACTIVITIES: Manufacturing of textile piece goods

VEGETABLE & FRUIT PROCESSING LTD
Plot 3/4 21 Abebe Village Rd, Iganmu Industrial Estate, Iganmu, PO Box 4610, Lagos
Tel: 835575, 855509, 835174
Cable: Vegfru
Telex: 26763 Sona Ng

Chairman: Alhaji Ibrahim Damcida
Directors: H G Makhijani, M N Dhamdhere, Alhaji Sule Katagum, Azad Shivdasani, V Uttamchandani, Alhaji Magaji Bello, Zana Sheshu Usman, S C Chadda, B B Parikh
Senior Executives: S C Chadda (General Manager),
  G K Ramachandra

PRINCIPAL ACTIVITIES: Processing of tomato paste, tomato juice, mango juice, and other fruit and vegetable products
Branch Offices: 10 Iddo Railway Compound, Iddo, Lagos State; Jourgarga; Borno State
Subsidiary Companies: Inlaks Ltd
Principal Bankers: United Bank for Africa Ltd
Financial Information:

	N'000
Authorised capital	2,000
Paid-up capital	2,000
Turnover	9,000

Date of Establishment: 11th July 1970
No of Employees: 400

VEGETABLE OILS (NIGERIA) LTD
Kilometer 16, Ikorodu Rd, Ojota, PO Box 121, Ikeja, Lagos State

Tel: 963680, 900500
Cable: Westvon Ikeja

Chairman: Lati Okunola
Directors: S I Afun, Deacon T O Ogundare, Chief Olu Majekodunmi, Chief G O Oduwole, Chief D O Ogunleye
Senior Executives: V O Ola (Managing),
  J T Talabi (Chief Accountant/Company Secretary),
  Mrs B F Adebayo (Production Manager)

PRINCIPAL ACTIVITIES: Oil millers and exporters; manufacturers of palm kernel oil and palm kernel cake
Principal Bankers: National Bank of Nigeria Ltd
Financial Information:

	N'000
Authorised capital	800
Paid-up capital	800
Turnover (2 year average)	2,400
Profits (3 year average)	665

Principal Shareholders: Fully owned by Odu'a Investment Company Ltd
Date of Establishment: 1964
No of Employees: 250

VEN HOTELS LTD
21 Potts Johnson St, PO Box 1136, Port Harcourt, Rivers State
Tel: 228266

PRINCIPAL ACTIVITIES: Hoteliers

VENTURES, COOPERS BENLY, & COMPANY LTD (THE)

11/13 William St, 1st and 2nd Floor, PO Box 250, Onitsha, Anambra State
Tel: 210515, 211267
Cable: Coopers Group

Chairman: Ben Obiora Ezeibe
Directors: Joe O Ezibe, Jim O C Ezibe, K C Okoli
Senior Executives: Mathew Ezeibe (General Sales Manager), Benjamin Ogbaji (Marketing Manager)

PRINCIPAL ACTIVITIES: Importers and exporters of building materials, hardware, hand tools, brushware, crash helmets, industrial headwear, machine tools, spare parts for motor vehicles, sports equipment, household goods, agricultural implements, ceramics and sanitary fittings etc
Principal Agencies: Thetford Moulded Products, UK; Wirminghaus & Funcke, West Germany; Briton Chadwick Ltd, UK; Arthur Rinke & Sohne, West Germany; Wing Wah Enterprises Ltd, Hong Kong; Wing On Securities, Hong Kong; Moritz Industries Group Inc, Taiwan; China National Machinery Import v Export Corporation, China
Branch Offices: Warehousing/Wholesales/Bulk Transactions Department; Nkwo Main Market, PO Box 128, Nnewi 32 Reclamation St, Lagos
Subsidiary/Associated Companies: Coopers Benly Industrial Ventures (Nigeria) Ltd; J O Obiamalunweze Merchandise Company; Joint Industrial & Commercial Company Ltd
Principal Bankers: First Bank of Nigeria Ltd; Union Bank of Nigeria Ltd; Co-operative Bank of Eastern Nigeria Ltd

Date of Establishment: May 1966 (Formerly Ben C O Ezibe Merchandise Company Ltd)

VERCON (NIGERIA) LTD

PO Box 572, 24/26 Strachan St, Igbosere Rd, Lagos
Tel: 656720

PRINCIPAL ACTIVITIES: Building and civil engineering contractors

VERITAS INSURANCE COMPANY LTD

19 Martins St, PO Box 2056, Lagos
Tel: 635173
Cable: Verinsure Lagos

Directors: Simon N Okoro (General Manager), Trevor Cole (Managing Director), Raymond Temple (Deputy General Manager), Joseph O Offor (Assistant General Manager), Musa B Wahuyini (Assistant General Manager, Nothern Operation), John O Nsofor (Chief Accountant)

PRINCIPAL ACTIVITIES: Insurance
Branch Offices: 36 Balogun Sq, Lagos, Tel 636185; 7 Agege Motor Rd, Yaba, Lagos; 3 Olowu St, Ikeja, Lagos; 2 Galadima Rd, PMB 3255, Kano; 35 Asa Rd, PO Box 1357, Aba, Imo State; Sator House, SW7/3A Oke Bola, Lagos Bye Pass, PO Box 594, Ibadan, Oyo State

Date of Establishment: 31st October 1973 Incorporated
No of Employees: 220

VERSATA ENTERPRISES & MERCHANTS TRUST LTD

70 Murtala Mohammed Way, PMB 3139, Kano
Cable: Vemtrust

PRINCIPAL ACTIVITIES: General merchants and contractors; importers and exporters

VIC-ADUN & SONS LTD

10 Oroyinyin St, Lagos
Tel: 631397

PRINCIPAL ACTIVITIES: Importers and exporters, distributors of general merchandise

VICINANZA CONSTRUCTION LTD

1 Bida Rd, PO Box 82, Kano
Tel: 2488, 3278, 4422

Directors: F Vicinanza
PRINCIPAL ACTIVITIES: Construction

VICKINS (NIGERIA) ASSOCIATES

PO Box 471, Warri, Bendel State
Tel: 231985
Cable: Vickings

Chairman: Victor Ezeji
Directors: H O Ezuma, R A Iwe, B O Ezeji

PRINCIPAL ACTIVITIES: Suppliers of educational equipment and training services, books, magazines and periodicals
Branch Offices: Lagos; Aba
Associated Companies: Vickings International Services
Principal Bankers: Union Bank of Nigeria Ltd

Date of Establishment: 1975

VIKTORS, N, INTERNATIONAL AGENCIES

12 Awkuzu St, PO Box 1681, Enugu, Anambra State
Cable: Intervik

Chairman: Victor N Nwagbogu (also Managing Director)
Directors: Mrs N J Nwagbogu, Dr Fema Obi, Chief J E Okeiyi
Senior Executives: Jackson Nmbodo (Accountant), D Ufondu (Sales Manager)

PRINCIPAL ACTIVITIES: General merchants, general contractors, importers, exporters, manufacturers' representatives, building materials merchants
Principal Agencies: Mikasa Trading Company Ltd, Japan
Branch Offices: Imo State
Principal Bankers: First Bank of Nigeria Ltd

Date of Establishment: 5th December 1977

VILLAGE GATE & COMPANY LTD

233A Kirikiri Rd, Apapa, Lagos

PRINCIPAL ACTIVITIES: Importers of photographic materials and cosmetics

VINBEN (NIGERIA) LTD

115B Akpakpava Rd, PO Box 245, Benin City, Bendel State
Tel: 243216
Cable: Vinben Benin

PRINCIPAL ACTIVITIES: Building contractors; importers, suppliers of building materials; plastic products manufacturers
Branch Offices: 8 Mission Rd, PO Box 151, Uromi, Bendel State

VINCENTI ENGINEERING LTD

PO Box 1526, 198 Clifford St, Yaba, Lagos
Tel: 862363

PRINCIPAL ACTIVITIES: Building and civil engineering contractors

VITAFOAM NIGERIA LTD

Oba Akran Avenue, Industrial Estate, PMB 21092, Ikeja, Lagos State
Tel: 900170/1
Cable: Vitafoam Ikeja

Chairman: Dr C E Abebe
Directors: S O Bolarinde, O A Ogunlewe, G Blunt, A G C Hunt, Chief G O Dike, Alhaji Turi Muhammadu
Senior Executives: P G Dudeney (Managing Director)

PRINCIPAL ACTIVITIES: Manufacturing of polyurethane foam for mattresses, cushions, pillows and sheetings; carpet underlay and polyurethane insulating panels
Branch Offices: PO Box 870, Industrial Rd, Aba, Imo State; PO Box 6135, Mai-Malari Rd, Bompai Estate, Kano; Warri Rd, Sapele; Plot 35, Industrial Area, Jos
Principal Bankers: First Bank of Nigeria Ltd
Financial Information:

	N'000
Authorised capital	13,650
Paid-up capital	13,650
Turnover	29,836
Profits	2,988

Principal Shareholders: Vita International Ltd; C W A Holdings Ltd, UK
Date of Establishment: August 1962
No of Employees: 880

VITALINK PHARMACEUTICAL INDUSTRIES LTD

1st Commercial Rd, Oluyole Industrial Estate, Ring Rd, PMB 5613, Ibadan, Oyo State
Tel: 416635
Telex: 31127 Linkup

Chairman: Chief O I Akinkugbe
Directors: Mrs J Akinkugbe,
  H Postema,
  P M Towns (Managing)
Senior Executives: E J Pilcher (Factory Manager),
  Mrs L T Taylor (Financial Controller),
  J P C Obi (Marketing Manager)
PRINCIPAL ACTIVITIES: Manufacturers of pharmaceuticals, toiletries and cosmetics
Principal Agencies: Richardson-Vicks Ltd, UK
Branch Offices: 17A Commercial Avenue, Yaba, Lagos; 23 Oguta Rd, Onitsha; 1 Sarkin Yaki Rd, Kano
Principal Bankers: Union Bank Nigeria Ltd
Financial Information:

	N'000
Authorised capital	1,000
Paid-up capital	1,000

Principal Shareholders: Link-up Investments Ltd; FMO Netherland
Date of Establishment: December 1972
No of Employees: 200

VK PLASTIKS & MARBLE CO

54 Sam Shonibare Street, Surulere, Lagos
Tel: 962181/2
Cable: Vikeplastiks
Telex: 21511 Elapat

President: Bayo Akinyemi

PRINCIPAL ACTIVITIES: Manufacture of plastic shopping bags, pallet shrink wrappers, marble sanitary ware and slabs; aluminium windows and sanitary ware
Branch Offices: Factory: 50/54 Alimosho Rd, Off Ipaja Rd, Off Abeokuta Expressway, Agege, Lagos State
Principal Bankers: Nigeria-Arab Bank Ltd

Date of Establishment: 1976

VOLKSWAGEN OF NIGERIA LTD

Km 17 Badagry Highway, PMB 12663, Lagos
Tel: 880763, 880765, 880771/4
Telex: 21145

Chairman: H Babs Akerele
Directors: H Denfeld,
  M D Galadima,
  G Hartwich,
  Chief N B Kole-James,
  Chief J B Mandilas,
  W Nadebusch (Managing),
  K Vacano

Senior Executives: Alade A Akesode (Division Manager, Legal),
  K von Bothmer (Division Manager, Finance),
  D Effertz (Division Manager, Marketing),
  J Mayer (Division Manager, Supply),
  B Staschinski (Division Manager, Production),
  B D Tschorn (Division Manager, Quality Control)
PRINCIPAL ACTIVITIES: Car assembly
Principal Agencies: Volkswagenwerk AG, Germany; Volkswagen do Brazil; Audi Nsu Auto Union, West Germany
Principal Bankers: African Continental Bank Ltd; Union Bank of Nigeria Ltd; First Bank of Nigeria Ltd; United Bank for Africa Ltd
Financial Information:

	N'000
Authorised capital	23,000
Paid-up capital	17,150
Turnover (1981)	133,221

Principal Shareholders: Federal Ministry of Industries (Rep of the Federal Government of Nigeria); Volkswagenwerk Ag, Germany; Lagos State Government; BHF-Industrie Beteiligungs-Gesellschaft, Germany; Mandilas Ltd (Nigeria); New Century Motors Ltd (Nigeria)
Date of Establishment: 21st March 1974
No of Employees: 3,246

VOLVO LTD

47 Marina, Lagos

PRINCIPAL ACTIVITIES: Distributors of motor vehicles
Principal Agencies: AB Volvo, Sweden

VONO PRODUCTS LTD

248 Agege Motor Rd, PO Box 382, Mushin, Lagos
Tel: 841807, 841809
Cable: Vonpro Mushin

Chairman: S G Laoye
Directors: E O Elegbede,
  O Osanyin,
  P A Fashole,
  J N Bridson,
  D B Genders (Managing)
Senior Executives: S O Olasoji (Financial Manager),
  B O Thomas (Commercial Manager),
  V A Soares (General Sales Manager),
  M A Okorodudu (Chief Engineer),
  J O Ajayi (Personnel Services Manager)

PRINCIPAL ACTIVITIES: Manufacturing of metal furniture, mattresses, pillows, etc
Branch Offices: PO Box 688, Onitsha; PO Box 152, Kano; Benin City; Kaduna; Jos
Principal Bankers: United Bank for Africa Ltd
Financial Information:

	N'000
Authorised capital	4,535
Paid-up capital	4,533
Turnover	15,736
Profits (before tax)	1,328

Principal Shareholders: Vono Ltd, UK; CWA Holdings
Date of Establishment: 1962
No of Employees: 750

VOSS & UMLAUFT NIGERIA LTD

3 First Rd, Iganmu, Apapa, PO Box 63, Lagos
Tel: 831215
Cable: Voss
Telex: 21463 Voslos Ng

Directors: R F Roenz (Managing)

PRINCIPAL ACTIVITIES: Business and engineering consultants
Branch Offices: 9 Dawaki Rd, Nassarawa, PO Box 4489, Kano Tel 7118 Telex 77197
Principal Bankers: First Bank of Nigeria Ltd

Date of Establishment: 1965

VP (NIGERIA) LTD

25B Niger St, PO Box 56, Kano
Tel: 5731

PRINCIPAL ACTIVITIES: Manufacturers' representatives, and technical equipment suppliers

VYB (NIGERIA) LTD

13/15 Wharf Rd, PO Box 155, Apapa, Lagos
Tel: 803700/6
Cable: Vybond Apapa
Telex: 21344 Lagos

Chairman: Chief (Alhaji) I A S Adewale
Directors: Mrs D B A Kuforiji (Managing),
    E Gbeworo,
    D A Edmonds,
    M O Areh,
    K O Shaibu
Senior Executives: E Gbeworo (Manager Repro Division),
    S G Budd (Factory Manager),
    A A Odukoya (Engineering Manager),
    A K Boglo (Manager, Bearing/Transmission Division),
    A O Adebanjo (Personnel Manager),
    M A O Kuye (Chief Accountant),
    S J Ndubueze (Administrative Manager),
    E A Salami (Planning Manager),
    R A Breeze (General Service Manager)

PRINCIPAL ACTIVITIES: Suppliers of electrical and electronic equipment; printing equipment and materials; mechanical and allied engineering products; manufacturers of polythene bags and wrappers
Principal Agencies: Agfa Gaevert NV; Color Metal AG; Ozalid Company Ltd; Nashua Corporation, USA; Auto Diesels Braby Ltd; J A Crabtree Ltd; General Electric Co Ltd, USA; T I Transport Services Equipment; Ransome Hoffmann Polland Ltd; Fenner International Ltd; Tucker Fasteners Ltd; Hitachi Ltd; Perkin Boiler Ltd; Danks International Ltd
Branch Offices: 10 Club Rd, PO Box 1707, Kano; 102 Marian Rd, Extension, PO Box 479, Calabar, Cross River State; 37 Zik Ave, PMB 1155, Enugu, Anambra State; Ahmadu Bello Way, PO Box 183, Kaduna; 18 Aba Rd, PO Box 522, Port Harcourt; 118 Tetlow Rd, PMB 1127, Owerri, Imo State; 148 Uselu Lagos Rd, PMB 1181, Benin City, Bendel State; 1 Obosi Village Rd, PO Box 1561, Onitsha, Anambra State; 176 Warri/Sapele Rd, PO Box 394, Warri, Bendel State; N5B/2052 Giant House, Plot 13 Iwo Rd, Ibadan, Oyo State; 34 Murtala Mohammed Way, PO Box 504, Jos, Plateau State; 15B Agege Motor Rd, Maboju, Ikeja, Lagos State
Subsidiary/Associated Companies: Intercotra; Plant Sales & Hire (Nigeria) Ltd; Getflex (Nigeria) Ltd (Subsidiaries); Naco Nigeria Ltd (Associated)
Principal Bankers: Union Bank Nigeria Ltd; First Bank of Nigeria Ltd; Societe Generale Bank (Nigeria) Ltd
Financial Information: Member of the Inchcape Group of Companies

	N'000
Authorised capital	2,000
Paid-up capital	2,000
Turnover	18,094
Profits (after tax)	669

Principal Shareholders: Bewac Ltd
Date of Establishment: 1955
No of Employees: 600

W F CLARKE (NIGERIA) LTD

See CLARKE, W F, (NIGERIA) LTD

W J BUSH & COMPANY (NIGERIA) LTD

See BUSH, W J, & COMPANY (NIGERIA) LTD

W W WHYTE & CO LTD

See WHYTE, W W, & CO LTD

WAHLER, JOSEF, (NIG) LTD

102 Ikorodu Rd, Igbobi, PO Box 76, Yaba, Lagos
Tel: 844803, 845909
Telex: 31145 Motorba

Chairman: R A Olashoju
Directors: J O Falana, Chief L O Lawal, Franz Kugel
Senior Executives: P R Roever (Managing Director)

PRINCIPAL ACTIVITIES: Civil engineering and contruction
Associated Companies: Farmland Industries (Nig) Ltd
Principal Bankers: Barclays Bank (Nig) Ltd
Financial Information:

	N'000
Authorised capital	400
Paid-up capital	400
Sales turnover	15,000

Principal Shareholders: Josef Wahler KG Munich, West Germany; Motorways (Nig) Ltd
No of Employees: 350

WALTER CLARKE & SONS (OVERSEAS) LTD

See CLARKE, WALTER, & SONS (OVERSEAS) LTD

WALTON SOLOMON & ASSOCIATES

132 Broad St, 3rd Floor, PO Box 4397, Lagos
Tel: 664271

PRINCIPAL ACTIVITIES: Management and business consultants
Branch Offices: Enugu; Kano

WARD, ASHCROFT & PARKMAN (NIGERIA) LTD

9 Nnamdi Azikwe St, PO Box 4373, Lagos
PRINCIPAL ACTIVITIES: Engineering consultants

WARMAC PRODUCTS LTD

PO Box 135, Ikeja, Lagos
PRINCIPAL ACTIVITIES: Plastics manufacturers

WARRI MINING SYNDICATE

H16 Monedic St, PO Box 110, Jos, Plateau State
Tel: 3081

Chairman: F E Chunu
Directors: D I Okarevu,
    T U Ogaga,
    M E Ikpe (Managing Director),
    P I Iweriebor

PRINCIPAL ACTIVITIES: Metal ore mining
Principal Bankers: First Bank of Nigeria Ltd
No of Employees: 200

WASCO ROPES LTD

4 Henry Carr Street, Industrial Estate, PO Box 50, Ikeja, Lagos
Tel: 963015, 963251
Cable: Niwind Lagos
Telex: 26849 Niwil Ng

Chairman: Alhaji Sa'Adu Alanamu
Directors: G Halstead, A C C Roose, Alhaji Mohammed Sa'Adu, Alhaji Sani Bahori
Senior Executives: A C Lang (General Manager),
    N A Ibraheem (Office Manager),
    A McKenna (Production Manager)

PRINCIPAL ACTIVITIES: Manufacturers of steel wire ropes, strands and prestressed concrete strands
Distributor: Nigerian Ropes Ltd
Principal Bankers: United Bank for Africa Ltd
Principal Shareholders: Bridon Ltd, UK (60%); Nigerian Shareholders (40%)
Date of Establishment: September 1971
No of Employees: 65

WATA TIMBER COMPANY LTD
Oghareki via Sapele, PO Box 304, Sapele, Bendel State
Tel: Oghara 11
Telex: 42269

Directors: M Thiele, Chief A K Oladapo, Chief S L Edu, H R H
Oba N'Oba Erediauwa, W Thies, K G Dahms

PRINCIPAL ACTIVITIES: Timber merchants; sawmill;
manufacturers of equipment for the timber industry
Branch Offices: 25 Liverpool Rd, Apapa, Lagos, Tel 877110,
874383; Ijebu Ode; Ibadan; Ondo Ado Ekiti; Benin City; Warri;
Sapele; Enugu; Aba; Calabar

WATERGLASS BOATYARD & STEEL CONSTRUCTION LTD
PO Box 683, Port Harcourt, Rivers State
Tel: 224310, 227094
Cable: Watboat Port Harcourt

PRINCIPAL ACTIVITIES: Manufacturers of fibreglass boats, life
buoys, roofing sheets, steel structures, and steel frame
buildings, storage tanks, lorry bodies
Branch Offices: Factory: Marine Base Rd, Port Harcourt

WATSON & SONS (ELECTRO-MEDICAL) NIGERIA LTD
26 Creek Rd, PO Box 133, Apapa, Lagos
Tel: 870192, 870194, 875869
Cable: Skiagram Apapa

Chairman: Major-General (Dr) Henry E O Adefope
Directors: U N Okezie (Chief Executive),
T S Gilmour (Technical),
Dr O A Banjo,
J I Ediale,
K Hughes
Senior Executives: E U Uzodike (Finance Manager),
C E Umeh (Sales Manager),
E A N Efiong (Administration Manager)

PRINCIPAL ACTIVITIES: Sales and service of diagnostic medical
and hospital equipment
Principal Agencies: Picker International; GEC Medical Equipment
Ltd; E I Du Pont de Nemours - Photo Products Division;
Sybron Corporation's Dental Equipment Group; Ritter;
Baisch; Reco
Branch Offices: PO Box 363, Kaduna; PMB 01375, Enugu; PO
Box 10330, Ibadan; C/O X-Ray Department, UBTH, PMB
1111, Benin City
Associated Companies: GBC of England Ltd
Principal Bankers: First Bank of Nigeria Ltd; Savannah Bank of
Nigeria Ltd
Principal Shareholders: Nigerian Equity Shareholding (60%);
British (40%)
Date of Establishment: May 1955
No of Employees: 60

WAYNE (WEST AFRICA) LTD
20 Creek Rd, PO Box 103, Apapa, Lagos State
Tel: 876760, 876644
Cable: Wayne Oil
Telex: 21576 Wayne Ng

Chairman: Meye M Ottah
Directors: O A Alakija,
D J Moreton,
J O Tomisin,
A O Sardella,
M M Ottah (Managing),
A G Okeowo
Senior Executives: Moses O Ogunbayo (Company
Secretary/Controller),
Geoffrey N Iku (Sales Manager)

PRINCIPAL ACTIVITIES: Equipment suppliers and servicers to
the oil and gas industries; petroleum dispensing pumps,
meters, generating plants etc
Principal Agencies: Dresser Industries Inc; Petroleum Equipment
Group, USA; Tecalemit Garage Equipment Co, UK;
Geosource Inc, UK; Geosource GmbH, West Germany; Emco
Wheaton, UK; Suntester Ltd, UK; Sun Electric Corp, USA;
Amsterdam, Austria
Branch Offices: PO Box 219, Benin City; PO Box 701, Enugu;
PMB 5212, Ibadan; PO Box 97, Jos; PO Box 1240, Kano; PO
Box 651, Port Harcourt; PO Box 608, Kaduna; PO Box 977,
Warri
Associated Companies: Dresser Europe SA, UK; Dresser
Industries Inc, USA; Dresser Europe SA, West Germany;
Dresser Industries E Comercio Ltda, Brazil
Principal Bankers: First Bank of Nigeria Ltd
Financial Information:

	₦'000
Authorised capital	1,200
Paid-up capital	1,050
Turnover	7,100
Profits	948

Principal Shareholders: Symington Wayne Overseas Ltd; Alakija
Holdings Ltd, Ibadan; Tominco Investment Ltd, Lagos
Date of Establishment: 18th June 1962
No of Employees: 300

WEATHERFORD (NIGERIA) LTD
66 Awolowo Rd, SW Ikoyi, Lagos
Tel: 681706
Telex: 21312

PRINCIPAL ACTIVITIES: Technical equipment suppliers to the oil
and gas industry

WEIDE & CO (GROUP OF COMPANIES) LTD
PO Box 239, 17/19 Abebe Village Rd, Iganmu, Lagos
Tel: 831813
Cable: Weiconi
Telex: 21407

Chairman: Sir Mobolaji Bank-Anthony
Directors: Mrs J O Senbanjo,
O A Braithwaite,
Dr Ohu Onagoruwa (Managing)

PRINCIPAL ACTIVITIES: Manufacturers of electronic equipment,
refrigerators and air-conditioners
Principal Agencies: Northmende, West Germany; Taisei
Industries, Japan; Riello, Italy; Thorn Electrics, UK
Branch Offices: 20e Bello Rd, Kano; 11 Ahmadu Bello Rd,
Kaduna; 2 Mjemanze St, Port Harcourt
Subsidiary/Associated Companies: Universal Electronics
Principal Bankers: National Bank of Nigeria; Union Bank of
Nigeria Ltd; Savannah Bank of Nigeria Ltd

Date of Establishment: 1960
No of Employees: 600-700

WELFARE PHARMACEUTICALS LTD
L4 Ahmadu Bello Way, PO Box 522, Kaduna
Tel: 243637
Cable: Bomajid Kaduna
Telex: 71119 Wechem Ng

PRINCIPAL ACTIVITIES: Suppliers of pharmaceuticals
Branch Offices: Lagos

WELLCOME NIGERIA LTD
Oba Akran Ave, PMB 21099, Ikeja, Lagos
Tel: 962671, 961628, 961745
Cable: Tabloid Lagos
Telex: 26746 Tablod Ng

Chairman: N A Khwaja
Directors: O I Akinkugbe, P I Aladetoynbo, Prof Olumbe Bassir,
H Mitchel, K Gay, J G Martin

PRINCIPAL ACTIVITIES: Manufacturers of drugs and medicines
Principal Bankers: Union Bank of Nigeria Ltd; United Bank for Africa Ltd; Bank of Credit & Commerce International (Nigeria) Ltd

Date of Establishment: 27th December 1962
No of Employees: 200

WELLYPLATES

3/5 Adebambo St, PO Box 3664, Mile 7 Ikorodu Rd, Obanikoro, Lagos State
Tel: 964498
Cable: De-Welley Lagos

Chairman: M O Badmus-Wellington
Directors: Mrs M A Badmus-Wellington
Senior Executives: Segun Dada (General Manager)

PRINCIPAL ACTIVITIES: Vehicle number plate, house numbering and road markings manufacturers
Principal Agencies: Bestplate Ltd, UK; Zell-Em Ltd, UK; James Crowe Traders International Ltd, UK
Branch Offices: 315 Folagbade St, Ijebu-Ode, Ogun State; 28 Durosimi Etti St, Shomolu, Lagos State
Associated Companies: Wellington Motors Ltd; Motor Parts International; Honey Enterprises
Principal Bankers: Union Bank of Nigeria Ltd

Principal Shareholders: Mr and Mrs M O Badmus-Wellington

WEMA BANK LTD

52/54 Murtala Muhammed Way, PMB 1033, Ebute-Metta, Lagos
Tel: 861634, 863110, 862686
Cable: Wemabank
Telex: 21546

Chairman: Professor I O Agbede
Directors: Alhaji R G Fetuga,
    O O Olurankinse,
    S O Folayan,
    J A Okunola,
    O Ogunbo,
    A O Olatokun,
    J A Court (Managing)
Senior Executives: S I Adegbite (Executive Director, Bank Operations),
    D A Aklinrelere (Executive Director, Finance & Administration),
    A A Elias (Secretary/AG Chief Legal Officer),
    S S Soyemi (Chief Inspector),
    O Ajiboye (Chief Credit Controller),
    B Maradesa (Overseas Manager),
    F O Phillips (Senior Accountant)

PRINCIPAL ACTIVITIES: Banking, finance and investment
Branch Offices: Throughout Nigeria
Financial Information:

	N'000
Authorised capital	8,000
Paid-up capital	4,800

Principal Shareholders: Odu'a Investment Company Ltd
Date of Establishment: 1970
No of Employees: 797

WEMABOD ESTATES LTD

Western House, 8/10 Broad St, PO Box 1164, Lagos
Tel: 635577, 635509

PRINCIPAL ACTIVITIES: Estate agents, planners and valuers

Date of Establishment: September 1962
No of Employees: 270

WEST AFRICA HOUSEHOLD UTILITIES MANUFACTURING COMPANY (NIGERIA) LTD

PMB 1096, Ikeja, Lagos
Tel: 931768, 931801, 961838, 963207
Cable: Wahum
Telex: 21487 Wahum Ng

Directors: Z M Chen

PRINCIPAL ACTIVITIES: Manufacturing of household goods and appliances
Associated Companies: Battery Manufacturing Co (Nigeria) Ltd

WEST AFRICA MILK COMPANY (NIGERIA) LTD

Plot 7B Ogba Scheme, PMB 21319, Ikeja, Lagos
Cable: Wafmilco Lagos

PRINCIPAL ACTIVITIES: Manufacturers of evaporated milk

WEST AFRICA OFFSHORE LTD

B38 Warri-Sapele Rd, Warri, Bendel State
Tel: 232901
Cable: Waoff Warri
Telex: 43288 Waoff Ng

Chairman: Captain D Duindam (also Managing Director)

PRINCIPAL ACTIVITIES: Service company to the offshore oil and gas industry; marine transportation, aids to navigation

WEST AFRICAN ALUMINIUM PRODUCTS (NIGERIA)

Abeokuta, Ogun State

Chairman: Chief S O A Bankole

PRINCIPAL ACTIVITIES: Manufacturing of aluminium windows, doors and furniture

WEST AFRICAN AUTOMOBILE & ENGINEERING COMPANY LTD (WAATECO)

217/219 Apapa Rd, Iganmu, PO Box 3237, Lagos State
Tel: 831883, 841914, 833037
Cable: Waateco Lagos
Telex: 21423 Waarec Ng

PRINCIPAL ACTIVITIES: Distributors of motor vehicles, tractors, generators, water pumps, etc
Branch Offices: 1 Sunday St, Palmgrove, Lagos; Ibadan; Benin; Jos; Kano; Maiduguri; Sokoto; Katsina; Kaduna; Enugu

WEST AFRICAN BATTERIES LTD

Iwo Rd, PMB 5299, Ibadan, Oyo State

PRINCIPAL ACTIVITIES: Automobile battery manufacturers

WEST AFRICAN BREWERIES LTD

121/123 Western Ave, PO Box 2246, Lagos
Tel: 832595/6
Cable: Topbeer

Directors: Chief A O Lawson (Managing Director),
    C Haythorn (General Manager and Director),
    A B Fowowe (Director of Finance),
    H P J Walsh (Director of Production),
    S M Akinwale (Director of Marketing)
Senior Executives: A Ibironke (Assistant General Manager, Administration),
    O Roberts (Assistant General Manager, General Manager's Office),
    S O Edwin-Cole (General Sales Manager),
    J Sorunke (Publicity Manager),
    O Ajayi (Area Sales Manager for Benin/Akure)

PRINCIPAL ACTIVITIES: Lager beer brewing
Branch Offices: Abeokuta; Ibadan; Benin; Akure; Oshogbo; Ijebu-Ode; Ilorin
Associated Companies: Associated Breweries & Co Ltd
Principal Bankers: First Bank of Nigeria Ltd
Financial Information:

	N'000
Authorised capital	5,000
Sales turnover (approx)	25,000

No of Employees: 900

WEST AFRICAN CHEMICAL COMPANY LTD (WACHEM)

Pest Control Service, 15 Ijora Causeway, PO Box 2806, Lagos
Tel: 832276, 836136

PRINCIPAL ACTIVITIES: Suppliers of industrial, agricultural and
domestic pest control, and general crop protection; suppliers
of agro-chemicals

WEST AFRICAN COLD STORAGE CO OF NIGERIA LTD

230 Apapa Rd, PO Box 177, Lagos

PRINCIPAL ACTIVITIES: Importers of foodstuffs

WEST AFRICAN DISTILLERS LTD

21 Warehouse Rd, PO Box 383, Apapa, Lagos
Tel: 964222

PRINCIPAL ACTIVITIES: Distillery
Branch Offices: Plot 9, Block C, Ogba Industrial Scheme, Ikeja,
Lagos; Kano; Aba; Ibadan; Benin

No of Employees: 250

WEST AFRICAN DRUG COMPANY LTD

21 Wharf Rd, Development House, PO Box 434, Apapa, Lagos
Tel: 876257, 876350
Cable: Wesafdrug

Chairman: Chief M N Ugochukwu
Directors: C E J Allanson,
  H B S Gemmel,
  D J C Wood (Managing),
  P Best,
  G M Onyiuke,
  L O Anyafulu (General Manager),
  E A Adesioye (Chief Accountant),
  N O Onwuanyi (National Sales Manager)

PRINCIPAL ACTIVITIES: Retailers and dispensers of
pharmaceutical and medical supplies, toiletries and cosmetics
Principal Agencies: Cupal Ltd; DDD Ltd; B Braun; 3m/Riker
Laboratories; A/S Gea; Sterling Winthrop; Bayer AG; Frisolac;
Pampas (Procter and Gamble)
Branch Offices: Apapa; Ibadan; Benin; Warri; Onitsha; Enugu;
Aba; Kano; Kaduna; Jos
Principal Bankers: First Bank of Nigeria Ltd
Financial Information:

	N'000
Authorised capital	900
Paid-up capital	900

Principal Shareholders: Wholly owned subsidiary of John Holt
Ltd
Date of Establishment: 1924
No of Employees: 324

WEST AFRICAN ENGINEERING COMPANY NIGERIA LTD (WAECO)

30 Wharf Rd, PO Box 388, Apapa, Lagos
Tel: 877463, 877468
Cable: Electrical Apapa
Telex: 22281

Chairman: J O Emanuel
Directors: T Crawford (Managing),
  D H Parker,
  Dr L Emanuel,
  C O A Smith
Senior Executives: E O Koleoso (Technical Manager),
  E A Abidogun (National Sales Manager),
  S A Ojurongbe (Commercial Manager)

PRINCIPAL ACTIVITIES: Electrical, power and construction
equipment importers and suppliers; manufacturers'
representative
Principal Agencies: Evershed & Vignoles Ltd (Meggers
Instrument Division); BICC Group Ltd; Bill Switchgear Ltd;
Chloride Gent Ltd; Claude Lyons Ltd; GEC Walsall Ltd; Kent

Meters Ltd; Thorn Lighting Ltd; Arc Tap and Die Co Ltd;
Attwater and Sons Ltd; Avo Ltd; H W Sullivan Ltd; Bonar
Long and Co Ltd; British Lightning Preventor Ltd; Kent
Meters Ltd; Ferranti Meters Ltd; Watford Control Instruments
Ltd; Herbert Morris Ltd; Newton Derby Ltd; Crabtree
Electrical Industries Ltd; Moorlite Industries; N Greenings Ltd
Branch Offices: 22 Aba Rd, PO Box 595, Port Harcourt, Tel
227200; 24 Upper New Lagos Rd, PMB 1107, Uselu, Benin,
Tel 244478; 55E Ado Bayero Rd, PO Box 392, Kano, Tel 4178
Principal Bankers: United Bank for Africa Ltd; Union Bank of
Nigeria Ltd
Financial Information:

	N'000
Authorised capital	900
Paid-up capital	400
Turnover	4,000
Profits	250

Principal Shareholders: Expatriate, Agar Cross (40%); Nigerians
(20%); J O Emanuel (40%)
Date of Establishment: 1953
No of Employees: 100

WEST AFRICAN GLASS INDUSTRY LTD

PO Box 642, Trans-Amadi Industrial Layout, Port Harcourt,
Rivers State
Tel: 21611/2, 21036, 22103
Cable: Rivglass Port Harcourt
Telex: 61121 Glahak Ng

PRINCIPAL ACTIVITIES: Manufacturers of glass

WEST AFRICAN PORTLAND CEMENT COMPANY LTD

Elephant House, KM 12 Ikorodu Rd, PO Box 1001, Lagos
Tel: 901060-3
Cable: Wapcemco
Telex: 26695

Chairman: S O Ige
Directors: C S O Akande (Vice Chairman/Chief Executive),
  C J Roots (Managing Director),
  O N E Nwaozuzu (Finance Director),
  P Mosley (Technical Director),
  D A Stirling,
  J K Shepherd,
  C Nwaekwu,
  Chief P A O Adeleye,
  Chief A Rotimi,
  Chief K Oduguwa,
  A A Oniyitan
Senior Executives: E A Ogunleye (Sales/Marketing Executive),
  D A Adeyemo (Commercial Executive),
  B T Oluokun (Personnel Executive),
  R J Hughes (General Manager/PPD),
  R A Bald (General Works Manager),
  J S A Otubaga (General Works Manager)

PRINCIPAL ACTIVITIES: Manufacturers and distributors of
cement and building materials
Subsidiary/Associated Companies: Cheecolite System Building
Ltd; Nigerian Kraft Bags Ltd
Principal Bankers: First Bank of Nigeria Ltd; United Bank of
Nigeria Ltd; Union Bank of Nigeria Ltd; National Bank of
Nigeria Ltd; Nigerian Industrial Development Bank Ltd;
African Continental Bank Ltd
Financial Information:

	N'000
Authorised capital	30,500
Paid-up capital	30,150
Turnover	95,081
Profits (before tax)	10,110

Principal Shareholders: Odu'a Investment Company Ltd;
Federal Government of Nigeria; Associated International
Cement (Nig) Ltd
Date of Establishment: 1958
No of Employees: 2,500

WEST AFRICAN PROVINCIAL INSURANCE COMPANY LTD

Wesley House, 21 Marina, PO Box 2103, Lagos
Tel: 653690/1
Cable: Insurprove Lagos
Telex: 21613

Directors: H V Walker,
    R B Johnson (General Manager),
    Chief M N Ugochukwu,
    Chief G U Eyewumi,
    Alhaji Ahmed Sani,
    Mallam Carpenter
Senior Executives: S A Odeleye (Assistant General Manager),
    A A Akintunde (Assistant General Manager, Technical)

PRINCIPAL ACTIVITIES: Insurance and reinsurance
Branch Offices: 1 Beach Rd, PO Box 384, Jos, Tel 2731; 36 Ibrahim Taiwo Rd, PO Box 545, Kano, Tel 2553; Imaro House, 93b Sapele Rd, Benin, Tel 222084; N6/50E Sabo Rd, Mokola Roundabout, PO Box 4328, Ibadan, Oyo State; 65 Old Yaba Rd, Yaba, Lagos; Ahmadu Bello Way, PO Box 716, Sokoto; 24 Ikwere Rd, Port Harcourt
Principal Bankers: Union Bank of Nigeria Ltd
Financial Information:

	₦'000
Authorised capital	300
Paid-up capital	300

Principal Shareholders: Nigerian Government; Ministry of Finance Inc; Sokoto State Government; Provincial Insurance Company Ltd; Kendal, UK
Date of Establishment: 1958

WEST AFRICAN SHIPPING AGENCY (NIGERIA) LTD

21 Warehouse Rd, PO Box 235, Apapa, Lagos
Tel: 873801
Cable: Nautik
Telex: 21223 Nautik

PRINCIPAL ACTIVITIES: Shipping agents; travel bureau
Principal Agencies: Soc Navale Chargeurs Delmas-Vieljeux; Woermann Line, West Germany
Branch Offices: PO Box 204, Sapele, Tel 280, Cable Nautik Sapele

WEST AFRICAN SHRIMPS LTD

PO Box 547, Sapele, Bendel State
Tel: 42590
Cable: Washrimp
Telex: 42270 Lifeco Ng; 26816 Lflour Ng

Chairman: Chief A O Rewane
Directors: O N Rewane,
    H Bresky,
    R G Myers,
    J E Rodrigues (Managing),
    S B Babajide,
    A Ede,
    R I Fleming,
    Chief A E Enahoro
Senior Executives: D Harbaum (Operations Manager),
    D T M Greening (Controller)

PRINCIPAL ACTIVITIES: Fish and shrimp fishing, processing, importation and sales of fish, other sea foods, poultry and meat
Branch Offices: Ogorode, Near Sapele, (main production and sales); 11 Idita St, Surulere, PO Box 7008, Lagos, Tel 834467
Associated Companies: Life Flour Mill Ltd; Top Feeds Ltd
Principal Bankers: United Bank for Africa Ltd
Financial Information:

	₦'000
Authorised capital	410
Paid-up capital	410

Principal Shareholders: Private companies - Nigerian (69%); Bermuda (40%)
Date of Establishment: 1973

WEST AFRICAN SURVEYS LTD

PMB 5120, Port Harcourt, Rivers State
Tel: 335686

Senior Executives: J E Piper (General Manager),
    A Fadero (Manager, Lagos)

PRINCIPAL ACTIVITIES: Geophysical surveying and services for the oil and gas industry. Distributors and service agents of electronic surveying, positioning and radar equipment
Principal Agencies: Racal Decca Survey; Racal Decca Marine Radar; Brocks Seafarer
Branch Offices: PMB 21002, 45 Opebi Rd, Ikeja, Lagos State

WEST AFRICAN THREAD COMPANY LTD

16/17 Burma Rd, PO Box 105, Apapa, Lagos
Tel: 875866, 875788
Cable: Stitching Apapa
Telex: 22275 Sewing

Directors: G F Herring (Managing),
    I Hartley,
    F O Adenubi,
    A D McConachie,
    H K Offonry,
    B S Thompson

PRINCIPAL ACTIVITIES: Manufacturers of domestic and industrial sewing thread and cord

No of Employees: 350

WEST AFRICAN TRADES CORPORATION LTD

110 Nnamdi Azikiwe St, Lagos

PRINCIPAL ACTIVITIES: Timber exporters and merchants

WEST AFRICAN TYRE RETREADING COMPANY LTD

5-7 Jimoh Odutola Rd, PO Box 39, Ibadan, Oyo State

PRINCIPAL ACTIVITIES: Tyre retreading

WEST CONSTRUCTION COMPANY LTD

43 Siluko Rd, PO Box 417, Benin City, Bendel State
Tel: 241448

Directors: B Rondi

PRINCIPAL ACTIVITIES: Construction

WEST, JOHN, PUBLICATIONS LTD

Plot A Block 2 Acme Rd, PMB 21001, Ikeja, Lagos
Telex: 26446

Chairman: Alhaja Abimbola Jakande
Directors: Bayo Fadoju (Executive Director),
    Alhaji S A O Ajala,
    Lekan Otubu
Senior Executives: Jimi Taiwo (Chief Accountant),
    Dele Olamiyi (Assistant General Manager),
    Femi Mabogunje (Administrative Manager)

PRINCIPAL ACTIVITIES: Publishing and distribution of books, importers of printing materials
Principal Agencies: McGraw-Hill Books Co (UK) Ltd; Allied Publishers; Bantam Publishing Company
Associated Companies: Labsco Supplies Ltd; John West Packaging Ltd; Technical Magazines Ltd
Principal Bankers: United Bank for Africa Ltd; First Bank of Nigeria Ltd
Financial Information:
Turnover   ₦ 1,650,000

Principal Shareholders: Alhaji Lateef Kayode Jakande; Alhaja Abimbola Jakande; Bayo Fadoju

WESTEND ENGINEERING LTD

140 2nd East Circular Rd, PO Box 718, Benin City, Bendel State
Tel: 241890

PRINCIPAL ACTIVITIES: Electrical engineering,
telecommunications; airconditioning, refrigeration and
ventilation specialists
Branch Offices: 73A Siluko Rd, Benin City, Bendel State; 17
Sumola St, PO Box 4875, Okupe Estate, Ikeja, Lagos

WESTERN NIGERIA TARPAULIN INDUSTRIES LTD

PO Box 576, SW9/480 Ago-Tailor, Abeokuta Rd, Ibadan, Oyo
State
Tel: 462803

PRINCIPAL ACTIVITIES: Manufacturers of tarpaulin; coin bags
and canvas items

WESTERN NIGERIAN TECHNICAL CO LTD

Fajuyi St, PMB 5148, Ibadan, Oyo State
Tel: 411291, 411442
Cable: Wenitra
Telex: 31111 Wentec

Directors: R O Nau (Joint Managing),
E O Ojurongbe (Joint Managing)

PRINCIPAL ACTIVITIES: Manufacturing of machinery for
agricultural processing and building industries; poultry
equipment; workshop services
Principal Bankers: Standard Bank of Nigeria Ltd
Financial Information:
Sales turnover   N 1,000,000

Principal Shareholders: R Nau; E Ojurongbe
No of Employees: 100

WESTERN STEEL WORKS

Blind Centre Rd, Matori, PO Box 650, Oshodi, Lagos
Tel: 964904
Telex: 26120

PRINCIPAL ACTIVITIES: Steel fabricators
Financial Information:
Registered capital   N 2,000,000

Date of Establishment: April 1977

WESTERN TEXTILE INDUSTRIES COMPANY LTD

PMB 5337, Iyin Rd, Ado-Ekiti, Ondo State
Tel: 2231/32

Senior Executives: M F Abajingin (Chief Executive),
S A Obayemi (Sales Manager)

PRINCIPAL ACTIVITIES: Manufacturing of piece goods and
cotton fabrics

WESTERN TEXTILE MILLS LTD

Plot 1 Block A, Gbagada Industrial Estate, PO Box 2800, Lagos
Tel: 964611/3
Cable: Westextile

Chairman: Alhaji Y Jega
Directors: L D Vaswani (Managing),
P D Vaswani,
Chief A A Oyedipe,
H G Lakhani
Senior Executives: S V Chandorkar (Production Manager),
C W A Akiri (General Manager, Administration),
P Thangam (Financial Controller)

PRINCIPAL ACTIVITIES: Textile goods manufacturers and
spinners
Branch Offices: Weaving Mill: Plot A1 Block 1X Ilupeju Industrial
Estate, Lagos; Spinning Mill and Administrative Office: Plot 1
Block A Gbagada Industrial Estate, Lagos
Principal Bankers: Chase Merchant Bank Nigeria Ltd; United
Bank for Africa Ltd; First Bank of Nigeria Ltd

Financial Information: 1981

	N'000
Authorised capital	5,000
Paid-up capital	4,950
Turnover	12,000
Profits (before tax)	217

Principal Shareholders: L D Vaswani; Alhaji Yusufu Jega; E B
Odebunmi; P D Vaswani; Chief A A Oyedipe
Date of Establishment: 11th January 1969
No of Employees: 918

WESTMINSTER DREDGING (NIGERIA) LTD

Westminster House, Obafon Yard, Kirikiri, PO Box 1518, Lagos
Tel: 875439
Cable: Nidredge Lagos
Telex: 21451 Dredge Ng

Chairman: Chief M N Ugochukwu
Directors: Th M Leijnse (General Manager),
Chief Dr M A Majekodunmi,
P Teijema,
S B Fasan,
M T Boustead

PRINCIPAL ACTIVITIES: Dredging and reclamation, deepening
ports and waterways, dredging access slots for oil exploration
rigs, dredging trenches for pipelines, dredging canals,
reclaiming land for industry, housing, port developments etc
Branch Offices: 1 Ihiala Street, Gborokiri, PMB 5096, Port
Harcourt, Rivers State; Ogunu Yard, PO Box 145, Warri,
Bendel State
Principal Bankers: Union Bank of Nigeria Ltd; United Bank for
Africa Ltd; National Bank of Nigeria Ltd; First Bank of Nigeria
Ltd; Societe Generale Bank (Nigeria) Ltd; Savannah Bank of
Nigeria Ltd
Financial Information:

	N'000
Authorised capital	8,000
Paid-up capital	3,800
Turnover	65,000
Profits (before tax)	2,150

Principal Shareholders: Bos Kalis Westminster Ltd; Imo State;
Lagos State; Kwara State; Bauchi State; Ugochukwu & Sons
Ltd; Employees in Trust and Others
Date of Establishment: 11th February 1970
No of Employees: 1,700

WESTMINSTER OFFSHORE (NIGERIA) LTD

Westminster House, Opposite Shell Police Barracks, Ogunu, PO
Box 799, Warri, Bendel State
Tel: 233159

PRINCIPAL ACTIVITIES: Terminal operations and services on
land and offshore

Principal Shareholders: Member of the Bos Kalis Westminster
Group

WHESSOE ENGINEERING LTD

PO Box 256, Aba Rd, Port Harcourt, Rivers State
Tel: 224621
Telex: 61249

Chairman: W Smart
Directors: G J Metcalfe (Managing),
S L Edu,
J Nwankwu,
R W Phillips,
G Renwick

PRINCIPAL ACTIVITIES: Engineers, designers, fabricators and
contractors of capital plant and process equipment for the
petroleum, chemical, gas, offshore, iron, steel, cement and
newsprint industries including complete 'turnkey' process
plant, with a capability embracing construction of process
and storage installations, civil and building works, pipework
design and implementation, electrical installation, mechanical
services of all types and refinery maintenance

Branch Offices: Iwafe Base, Rumuolumeni, PO Box 256, Port Harcourt, Rivers State; 78 Airport Rd, Ikeja, PO Box 6523, Lagos, Tel 963969
Principal Bankers: Union Bank of Nigeria Ltd

Date of Establishment: Registered in Nigeria 1960
No of Employees: 300

WHIPSTOCK (NIGERIA) LTD

Plot 268 Kofo Abayomi St, Victoria Island, PO Box 4413, Lagos
Tel: 654064
Cable: Whipco Lagos

Directors: Red Brown (Managing Director)

PRINCIPAL ACTIVITIES: Directional drilling
Branch Offices: Field Office: PO Box 31, Port Harcourt, Rivers State, Tel 705

WHITE, JOHNSON, UNITED LTD

58B Aderiran Ogunsanya St, Surulere, Lagos
Tel: 835083
Cable: Johnywhite

Chairman: Johnson Sakutu
Directors: Sonny P Adidi
Senior Executives: Goran Rolling (General Manager), Anthony Noyes (Project Director)

PRINCIPAL ACTIVITIES: Civil engineering and building construction
Principal Bankers: Pan African Bank Ltd
Financial Information:
Authorised capital   N 405,000

Principal Shareholders: Johnson Sakutu; Sonny P Adidi
No of Employees: 1,000

WHYTE, W W, & CO LTD

7 Aba Rd, PO Box 220, Port Harcourt, Rivers State
Tel: 227029, 227130
Cable: Wilit

Chairman: W W Whyte (also Managing Director)
Directors: L K Jombo (Project Engineer), S A Effiong (Accountant), Mrs I R Douglas (Transport Manager)

PRINCIPAL ACTIVITIES: Building and civil engineering contractors and transporters
Associated Companies: Silver Line Laundry & Dry Cleaning Services; Nyemoni Enterprises Ltd
Principal Bankers: Pan African Bank; International Bank for West Africa; United Bank for Africa Ltd

No of Employees: 350

WIDNELL AND TROLLOPE NIGERIA

39 Campbell Street, PO Box 2107, Lagos
Tel: 636290, 636358
Cable: Widtroll Lagos
Telex: 21162 Beques Ng

Partners: Olutade O Ismail, Michael A H Savage, David G Lain
Senior Executives: John Tuffrey (Manager, Kano), Terrance Lazarus (Manager, Warri), Y A Alaka (Manager, Ibadan)

PRINCIPAL ACTIVITIES: Chartered quantity surveyors, building and civil engineering cost consultants
Branch Offices: 27 Awolowo Avenue, Bodija Estate, Ibadan; 24A Club Rd, PO Box 1078, Kano

Date of Establishment: 1950
No of Employees: 50

WIEDEMANN & WALTERS (NIGERIA) LTD

24 Warehouse Rd, Apapa, Lagos
Tel: 876721
Telex: 21369 Wiwa Ng

Chairman: Konsul Arthur Habicht
Directors: S B Williams, Jibril Isa, C Habicht (Managing)
Senior Executives: W Weigl (General Manager)

PRINCIPAL ACTIVITIES: Importation, assemblying, sales and servicing of various types of industrial and agricultural machinery and equipment
Principal Agencies: Lindenberg; Zenith; Harrison & Sons Ltd; Atika; Demag; Dalex; Farymann; Homelite; Stetter; EBG; AC-Crane; Attendorner; Boge-Kompressoren; DWU-Belzer; Kläger; Klinett; Malsbury; Susemihl; Schwing; Kelvin Diesels etc
Branch Offices: PO Box 2107, Kano; PO Box 493, Port Harcourt; PO Box 260, Warri; PO Box 260, Maiduguri; PO Box 1666, Kaduna; PO Box 399, Yola; PO Box 1477, Sokoto; PO Box 2226, Makurdi
Subsidiary Companies: Export Union Düsseldorf GmbH, West Germany
Principal Bankers: First Bank of Nigeria Ltd

Date of Establishment: 1960
No of Employees: 250

WIGGINS TEAPE WEST AFRICA LTD

23 Burma Rd, PO Box 95, Apapa, Lagos
Tel: 803260/2
Cable: Gateway Apapa
Telex: 22157 Wigtip

Chairman: Chief J O Udoji
Directors: B J M Evans (Managing), F O Odeleye (Financial Controller), Y A Sokoya (Director/Secretary), Chief M T Mbu, Dr C E Abebe, B F Coupland, G W M Grose
Senior Executives: K O Oniwinde (Division Manager, Converting), E F Ekejuba (Divisional Manager, Graphic Supplies)

PRINCIPAL ACTIVITIES: Paper converters, paper merchants, graphics suppliers
Principal Agencies: Wiggins Teape Overseas Sales Ltd; Howson Algraphy; Adana; Pivano SPA, Italy; GBC; Tuckers Products Ltd
Branch Offices: 2b/4b Niger Rd, Kano; Kachia Rd, Kaduna; 37 Milverton Ave, Aba; Plot D Block E, Oluyole Industrial Estate, Ring Rd, Ibadan
Associated Companies: Wiggins Teape Overseas Ltd
Principal Bankers: First Bank of Nigeria Ltd
Financial Information:

	N'000
Authorised capital	3,000
Paid-up capital	3,000
Turnover	13,950
Profits	1,647

Principal Shareholders: Wiggins Teape Overseas Holdings Ltd, UK
Date of Establishment: 11th February 1957
No of Employees: 352

WILLIAMS INTERNATIONAL (NIG) LTD

6 Elsie Femi Pearse, Victoria Island, PO Box 1057, Lagos
Tel: 614877
Cable: Boncon
Telex: 21115

Senior Executives: Bill Messec (Managing Director), J P Duggan (General Manager), T B Reilly (Contracts Manager)

PRINCIPAL ACTIVITIES: Construction of crude oil, gas and petroleum products pipelines and related facilities
Branch Offices: PO Box 649, Port Harcourt, Rivers State, Tel

285

Date of Establishment: 1969
No of Employees: 480

WILMER INDUSTRIES NIGERIA LTD

268 Herbert Macaulay St, Yaba, Lagos
Tel: 861888

Directors: Chief E S B Wilkey (Managing)

PRINCIPAL ACTIVITIES: Production of melamine tableware.
Large expansion programme is underway

WIMPEY, GEORGE, & CO (NIGERIA) LTD

PMB 21483, Oregun Village Rd, Ikeja, Lagos State
Tel: 683707
Cable: Wimpeyco Lagos

Chairman: Alhaji A M Joda
Directors: Lady K Ademola,
T K Audifferen,
A A Egunjobi,
F H Archer (Managing),
J Kinloch,
P A Ryalls,
Alhaji A M Joda

PRINCIPAL ACTIVITIES: Building and civil engineering
contractors
Associated Companies: Wimpey-Brown and Root (Nigeria) Ltd
Principal Bankers: First Bank of Nigeria Ltd; Union Bank of
Nigeria Ltd
Financial Information:

	N'000
Authorised capital	1,000
Paid-up capital	1,000
Sales turnover (Approx)	70,000

Principal Shareholders: George Wimpey & Co, London; TAW
Construction Co Ltd, Nigeria; A A Egunjobi; Alhaji A M Joda
Date of Establishment: 20th August 1969

WIMPEY-BROWN & ROOT (NIGERIA) LTD

Rumuolumeni Waterside, PO Box 619, Port Harcourt, Rivers
State
Tel: 22
Cable: Wimbrown

Directors: P F Cook, T T Candlish, Chief C O Ogunbanjo
Senior Executives: Fred Cockerill (Manager),
B U Okpala (Administrative Manager)

PRINCIPAL ACTIVITIES: Contractors, fabrication, shipping and
oil service base
Principal Agencies: NNOC; Gulf Oil Company; Mobil Producing
Nigeria; Med-Africa Lines Ltd and Jeco Shipping Lines
Principal Bankers: Standard Bank of Nigeria Ltd
Financial Information:

	N'000
Authorised capital	410
Paid-up capital	410

Principal Shareholders: George Wimpey & Co (Nigeria) Ltd;
Brown & Root (Nigeria) Ltd; Chris Ogunbanjo
No of Employees: 300

WITT & BUSCH (SHIPYARD) LTD

PO Box 571, Reclamation Rd, Port Harcourt, Rivers State
Tel: 333358

Chairman: Chief Adeniran Ogunsanya
Directors: Samam Egunema, Chief J T S Faafa, G N Hatch, B
O Beredugo
Senior Executives: E Notoma (Liaison Officer)

PRINCIPAL ACTIVITIES: Shipbuilding: construction of pipelaying
barges for oil companies, passenger launches: tugs,
rivercraft: bridges, jetties, floating jetties; machine shops
Principal Bankers: United Bank for Africa Ltd

Financial Information:

	N'000
Authorised capital	405
Paid-up capital	400

Principal Shareholders: Rivers State Government (40%); IAC
Amsterdam (40%); Other Nigerians (20%)
Date of Establishment: 1964
No of Employees: 200

WOCLIF (NIGERIA) VENTURES

14 Trans-Amadi Industrial Layout, PO Box 675, Port Harcourt,
Rivers State
Tel: 21241

PRINCIPAL ACTIVITIES: Buidong and civil engineering
contractors, importers, exporters, estate owners and agents

WOERMANN, C, (NIGERIA) LTD

31a Association Ave, PO Box 318, Ilupeju, Lagos
Tel: 960603, 962410
Cable: Woerman Lagos

Chairman: A O Abudu
Directors: H Woerman,
F Schaffler (General Manager)

PRINCIPAL ACTIVITIES: Suppliers of technical and engineering
equipment, chain saws, etc
Branch Offices: 18a Yaba St, Ondo; 98 Okigwe Rd, Aba
Principal Bankers: United Bank for Africa Ltd; Savannah Bank of
Nigeria; National Bank of Nigeria Ltd

No of Employees: 150

WOLFF, OTTO, (NIGERIA) & COMPANY LTD

9A Marine Rd, PMB 1153, Apapa, Lagos
Tel: 876559, 876978
Cable: OWEX Lagos
Telex: 22653 Ownig Ng

Chairman: Chief M A Balogun
Directors: D Doorduyn (Managing),
Alhaji Sani Bakori,
W Robie,
G I C Eneli
Senior Executives: G Focke (Technical Co-Ordinator),
B A Ogunlewe (Chief Accountant),
S Hoecht (Northern Area Manager),
K H Schmitz (Branch Manager)

PRINCIPAL ACTIVITIES: Distributors of steel products and
building materials, metals, steel and metal processing and
fabrication, distributors of tools and machine tools and
suppliers of machinery, plant and equipment
Principal Agencies: Otto Wolff Handelsgesellschaft mbH, W
Germany; Otto Wolff Indag, W Germany; Hommel Handel, W
Germany; Otto Wolff Benelux, Belgium
Branch Offices: 3 Independence Rd, PO Box 1004, Kano; 147
Transamadi Layout, PMB 5595, Port Harcourt; 23 Aliyu
Makama Rd, PO Box 6441, Kaduna South, Kaduna
Subsidiary/Associated Companies: All Otto Wolff Companies
Principal Bankers: Union Bank of Nigeria Ltd; First Bank of
Nigeria Ltd; Societe Generale Bank (Nigeria) Ltd
Financial Information:

	N'000
Authorised capital	1,000
Paid-up capital	1,000
Turnover	16,000

Date of Establishment: April 1961
No of Employees: 120 (approx)

WOOLLEN & SYNTHETIC TEXTILE MANUFACTURING LTD

88 Oba Akran Ave, Industrial Estate, PO Box 507, Ikeja, Lagos
State
Tel: 962903, 964804
Cable: Woolsuit

Chairman: Chief H B Chanrai
Directors: M N Sadhwani,
    G G Assomull (Managing Director),
    Mrs R H Chanrai,
    Mr Ochi
Senior Executives: K K Dosi (Technical Adviser),
    S B Panjwani (Financial Controller),
    C Obasi (Marketing Manager),
    O A Ogun (Assistant General Manager, Administration)
PRINCIPAL ACTIVITIES: Manufacturers of textile piece goods
Principal Bankers: United Bank for Africa Ltd; Allied Bank of (Nigeria) Ltd
Financial Information:

	N'000
Authorised capital	1,500
Paid-up capital	800
Turnover	6,000
Profits	250

Principal Shareholders: Nigerian Industrial Development Bank Ltd; J T Chanrai (PH) Ltd; Sadhwanis (Nigeria) Ltd; Doulatram (Nigeria) Ltd; Kuraray Co (Japan); Marubeni (Japan); Chief H B Chanrai
No of Employees: 350

WORLD COURIER NIGERIA LTD

15 Commercial Ave, Yaba, Lagos
Tel: 860897, 860889
Telex: 26665 Wcnl

Chairman: Chief F R A Williams
Directors: James R Berger,
    Enoma Agbontaen (General Manager),
    Edwin Ditchfeild Agboh
Senior Executives: Mrs Marion Ezedima, Deji Adenuga

PRINCIPAL ACTIVITIES: Courier service, business consultants
Principal Agencies: World Courier Management Consultant
Branch Offices: All state capitals
Principal Bankers: Union Bank of Nigeria Ltd
Financial Information:

	N'000
Authorised capital	20
Paid-up capital	20

Principal Shareholders: James Berger; Chief Fra Williams; Enoma Agbontaen; Edwin Ditchfield Agboh
Date of Establishment: 30th November 1978
No of Employees: 50

WOVEN TEXTILES LTD

PO Box 1238, Kano

PRINCIPAL ACTIVITIES: Manufacture of woven textiles

WOZABETH TRADING COMPANY

24 Efosa St, Uzebu Quarters, Off Ekenwan Rd, Benin City, PO Box 142, Bendel State
Tel: 241888, 242823, 240510
Telex: 41137 Tomdic Ng

PRINCIPAL ACTIVITIES: Manufacturers' representatives; distributors of general merchandise, building materials, electronic equipment and stationery

WROUGHT IRON (NIGERIA) LTD

Ilupeju Industrial Estate, Agege Motor Rd, PO Box 132, Mushin, Lagos
Tel: 964147, 963324, 963286
Cable: Winig

PRINCIPAL ACTIVITIES: Manufacturers of metal furniture for hospitals and schools
Branch Offices: Ibadan

Principal Shareholders: Odua Investment Co Ltd
Date of Establishment: 1957
No of Employees: 200

WYATT, THOMAS, NIGERIA LTD

Apex Mill, 2/4 Abebe Village Rd, Iganmu, PMB 1006, Ebute-Metta, Lagos
Tel: 833086/8
Cable: Apex Lagos
Telex: 21452 Apex Ng

Chairman: Chief G K J Amachree
Senior Executives: T A B Adekunle (Managing Director)

PRINCIPAL ACTIVITIES: Manufacturing of stationery and envelope makers
Branch Offices: Sales Depot, Obosi Rd, PO Box 750, Onitsha; Sales Depot, Ring Rd, PMB 5445, Ibadan
Subsidiary/Associated Companies: Thomas Wyatt & Son (Northern Nigeria) Ltd (Subsidiary); Apex (Eastern Nigeria) Ltd (Associate)
Principal Bankers: First Bank of Nigeria Ltd
Financial Information:

	N'000
Authorised capital	10,500
Paid-up capital	10,500

Date of Establishment: 18th March 1948
No of Employees: 1,650

WYETH NIGERIA LTD

Mile 7 Ikorodu Rd, PMB 21324, Ikeja, Lagos
Tel: 961594
Cable: Wyethical Lagos

Directors: V H Townsend (Managing Director)

PRINCIPAL ACTIVITIES: Suppliers of pharmaceuticals and infant formulae

YASSIN CONFECTIONERY & SWEET COMPANY LTD

116 Zaria Ave, PO Box 1118, Kano
Tel: 4857
Cable: Yassinco Kano

PRINCIPAL ACTIVITIES: Manufacturers of sweets and confectionery

No of Employees: 400

YERIMA HAMMAN WABI, ALHAJI, & SONS

15 Ahmadu Bello Way, PO Box 311, Maiduguri, Borno State
Tel: 232054
Cable: Yerima Wabi
Telex: 82116 Yerima Ng

PRINCIPAL ACTIVITIES: General contractors; transporters and licensed buying agents; general merchants
Branch Offices: Workshop: Mubi

YINKUS BOOK CENTRE LTD

5 Alli St, Lagos
Tel: 657876

PRINCIPAL ACTIVITIES: Suppliers of school textbooks, wholesale and retail
Branch Offices: 72 Broad St, Lagos, Tel 625604; 48 Bedwell St, Calabar, Cross River State, Tel 406

Principal Shareholders: Member of the Yinkus Group of Companies Ltd

YODESONS (NIGERIA) LTD

Plot 19 Badejo Kalesanwo Street, Matori Industrial Estate, Matori, PO Box 1930, Mushin, Lagos
Tel: 837913, 861464
Cable: Yoasociate Lagos

Chairman: Solomon Kayode Onafowokan
Directors: Miss Olubunmi Onafowokan, Matthew Olukayode Odunukan
Senior Executives: A I Towose (General Manager),
    C Uzoechi (Branch Manager, Rivers State),
    M O Kafaru (Operations Manager),
    A Akinwole (Sales Manager),

B Ogunbanjo (Sales Engineer),
I Nwabuko (Administration Manager/Accountant),
Mrs R Ohorogu (Office Manager)

PRINCIPAL ACTIVITIES: Business consultants, suppliers of electrical and electronics equipment, building materials, welding equipment/power tools, communication cables and installation, manufacturers' representatives

Principal Agencies: Kabelmetal (Nigeria) Ltd; K Chellaram & Sons (Nigeria) Ltd; A G Leventis; Kaycee (Nigeria) Ltd; UAC of Nigeria Ltd; Kenwil Electrical Distributors Ltd, UK; Eribridge Ltd, UK

Branch Offices: 9 Ondo Street (West) Ebute-Metta, Lagos; Shop C8 Adenitan Ogunsanya Shopping Centre, Surulere; 120 Herbert Macaulay St, Ebute-Metta, Lagos; 169 Aba Rd, Port Harcourt; 71 Okere Rd, Warri, Bendel State; SW/999 Lodge St, Ibadan; 58 Middle Rd, Kano

Associated Companies: Yodesons & Associates; Solomon & Solomon Building Products Co; Coleman Technical Industries Ltd; A M International Ltd; Kypton Maritime Agencies; Federation Products Mfg Ltd; Eskay Investments Ltd; Hopkins Insurance Brokers

Principal Bankers: First Bank of Nigeria Ltd; Nal Merchant Bank Ltd

Financial Information:

	N'000
Authorised capital	200
Paid-up capital	200
Turnover	1,200
Profits (approx)	80-100

Principal Shareholders: S K Onafowokan
Date of Establishment: November 1972
No of Employees: 120

YONDAV PETROCOMPLEX LTD
1 Aro Omoba Crescent, PO Box 79, Ikeja, Lagos
Tel: 961274, 961302
Cable: Yessir Lagos

Chairman: A G Yon da Kolo (also Managing Director)

PRINCIPAL ACTIVITIES: Oilfield engineering

YOUNG, ARTHUR, OSINDERO & CO
12th Floor, Mandilas House, 96/102 Broad St, PO Box 916, Lagos
Tel: 636429, 634026

Directors: E A Osindero (Managing Director)

PRINCIPAL ACTIVITIES: Chartered accountants

YUSUFU MODERN INDUSTRIES CO
PO Box 65, 13 Middle Rd, Sabongari, Kano
Tel: 5266, 2082

Chairman: Alhaji Baita Yusuf
Directors: Alhaji B Jamilu Baita, Alhaji Bashiru Baita, Alhaji Kabiru Baita

PRINCIPAL ACTIVITIES: Furniture manufacturers
Branch Offices: 29E Ado Bayero Rd, Kano
Principal Bankers: Union Bank of Nigeria Ltd; Bank of the North Ltd

ZABADNE & COMPANY LTD
93 Broad St, PO Box 736, Lagos
Tel: 663030, 664305
Telex: 21625

Chairman: Chief Michael C O Ibru
Directors: W J Zabadne, A U Ibru, Chief S K T Aiyegoro

PRINCIPAL ACTIVITIES: Wholesale and retail distribution and manufacture of electronics, audio and video equipment, cameras, watches, home appliances, light fittings and lampshades

Branch Offices: 34 New Court Rd, PO Box 1494, Ibadan, Oyo State Tel 21134; 68E Bello Rd, PO Box 325, Kano, Tel 3744
Principal Bankers: Savannah Bank (Nigeria) Ltd

Financial Information:

	N'000
Authorised capital	500
Paid-up capital	500

Principal Shareholders: Oteri Holdings Ltd; Chief M C O Ibru
No of Employees: 176

ZAMFARA TEXTILE INDUSTRIES LTD
PO Box 365, Kaduna

PRINCIPAL ACTIVITIES: Manufacturing of cotton piece goods

ZANG, D B
Gyet Village, PO Box 79, Bukuru, Plateau State

PRINCIPAL ACTIVITIES: Mining of metal ore

ZAPATA MARINE SERVICE (NIGERIA) LTD
1 Swamp Rd, PO Box 502, Warri, Bendel State
Tel: 233088
Cable: Marineserv Warri

Senior Executives: G W Poarch (Manager)

PRINCIPAL ACTIVITIES: Marine services

ZARD, C, & COMPANY LTD
184 Adeniji Adele Rd, PO Box 818, Lagos
Tel: 630358, 830430, 634779
Cable: Returning Lagos

PRINCIPAL ACTIVITIES: Importers and distributors of building materials, tyres, hand tools, machinery and electrical goods
Principal Agencies: Busi & Stephenson Ltd, UK
Associated Companies: Busi Stephenson Ltd, Ghana

ZARMAGANDA TIN MINES LTD
PO Box 564, Jos, Plateau State

PRINCIPAL ACTIVITIES: Tin mining

ZARTECH LTD
6 Lagos Bye-Pass, PO Box 516, Ibadan, Oyo State
Tel: 410440
Telex: 31120

PRINCIPAL ACTIVITIES: Suppliers of agricultural implements, irrigation systems, pumps and generating sets
Financial Information:
Registered capital   N 100,000

Date of Establishment: December 1978

ZAWANG MINING COMPANY
PO Box 61, Bukuru, Plateau State

PRINCIPAL ACTIVITIES: Metal ore mining

ZELAN MINING COMPANY LTD
2 Vom Rd, PO Box 10, Bukuru, Plateau State

PRINCIPAL ACTIVITIES: Metal ore mining

ZENITH CONTAINERS COMPANY LTD
Plot 31 Trans-Amadi Industrial Estate, PO Box 18, Port Harcourt, Rivers State

PRINCIPAL ACTIVITIES: Manufacturers of enamelware, and plastic buckets

ZEROLAS BATTERIES COMPANY LTD
68 Shyllon St, PO Box 4327, Palmgrove, Lagos
Tel: 841762

PRINCIPAL ACTIVITIES: Manufacturers of lead acid batteries

Alphabetical Index

158 Baresel Ltd 3
A A Balogun & Sons (Nigeria) Ltd 3
A B Chami & Co Ltd 3
A C Christlieb (Nigeria) Ltd 3
A C E Jimona Ltd 3
A D Green & Co Ltd 3
(A Division of UAC of Nigeria Ltd) 13
A Ekerete Ltd 3
A G Leventis & Company (Nigeria) Ltd 3
A G S Barma Ltd 3
A H Robins International Company Ltd 3
A I Chiakwelu & Brothers 3
A J Missri & Co Ltd 3
A J Seward (A Division of UAC of
Nigeria Ltd) 3
A M Faltas (West Africa) Ltd 3
A Micheletti 3
A O Adesanya Nigeria Ltd 3
A O Karunwi Ltd 3
A O Uche & Sons (Nigeria) Ltd 3
A Onibudo & Company Ltd 3
A Ott-Attafua & Company Ltd 3
A Savoia 3
A W Cross Ltd 3
A W Ibe & Co Ltd 3
ABA Textiles Mills Ltd 3
Abayomi, Olufawo, & Partners 3
Abbas Organisation Nigeria Ltd 4
Abbey Group of Insurance Brokers,
Life & Pensions Consultants 4
Abbott Laboratories Nigeria Ltd 4
Abdul Azeez Electrical Centre 4
Abdullai Group of Companies Nigeria
Ltd 4
Abebiyi Sonaike & Company 4
Abereoje (Nigeria) Ltd 4
Aboderin & Glahé Nigeria Ltd 5
Abukon Nigeria Ltd 5
Academy Press Ltd 5
(ACC Ltd) 22
Ace Builders & Building Material
Stockists (The) 5
ACE Metal Construction (Nigeria) Ltd 5
Acim 6
ACM of Nigeria Ltd 6
Acme Builders Ltd 6
Acrow Ltd 6
Adamu Management International 6
Adarice Company Ltd 6
Addis Engineering Ltd 6
Adebowale Electrical Industries Ltd 6
Adecentro Nigeria Ltd 6
Adefusika Trading Company Ltd 7
Adejobi, Adeoye, Trading Stores Ltd 7
Adejoro, S S, & Company Ltd 7
Adejumo Fam (Nigeria) Ltd 7
Ademola, Thomas, & Co Ltd 8
Adeola Babafunke Overseas Trading
Company 8
Adeome Company Ltd 8
Adeoye Adejobi Trading Stores Ltd 8
Adesanya, A O, Nigeria Ltd 8
Adetona Awe (Nig) Enterprises 8
Adetunji, Madebayo, & Sons Ltd 8
Adetunji Olokodana & Co 8
Adewale Bello Constructions Ltd 8
Adeyemi Commercial Syndicate
Sawmills Ltd 8
Admark (Nigeria) Ltd 8
Adobi Organisation 8
Adoks Engineering Ltd 8
Advance (Nig) Ltd 8
Aero Contractors Company of Nigeria
Ltd 8
Aeromaritime (Nigeria) Ltd 9
Aeronutronic Ford Overseas Systems 9
Afa Gateway Construction Company
Ltd 9
Afprint Nigeria Ltd 9

African Alliance Insurance Co Ltd 9
African Continental Bank Ltd 9
African Designs Development Centre
Ltd 11
African Era and Company Ltd 11
African Glass Company Ltd (Formerly
Central Glass (Nigeria) Ltd) 11
African Industrial Timber Co Ltd 11
African Insurance Company Ltd 11
African Ivory Insurance Company Ltd 11
African Newspapers of Nigeria Ltd 11
African Paints (Nig) Ltd 11
African Petroleum Ltd 12
African Prudential Insurance Company
Ltd (The) 12
African Reinsurance Corporation 13
African Timber & Plywood 13
African Universities Press 13
Afro Arab Techni-Chemicals Ltd 13
Afro Commerce (WA) Ltd 13
Afro Continental Nigeria Ltd 13
Afro Elektro Konsult Ltd 13
Afro International Construction
Company 13
Afro Nigerian Import & Export Co Ltd 14
Afroguard Publications 14
Afromedia Plastics & Engineering Ltd 14
Afrotec Technical Services Nigeria Ltd 14
Agbara Estates Ltd 14
Agbenor Mining Syndicate 14
Agip (Nigeria) Ltd 14
Agribuild Nigeria Ltd 14
Agricultural Development Corporation
(Anambra State) 14
Agro Industries & Development
Schemes Co (Nig) Ltd 15
Agroline (Nigeria) Ltd 15
Agrotec Services Ltd 15
Aircool Metal Industries (Nigeria) Ltd 15
Airegin Enterprises & Agencies Ltd 15
Airoe Construction & Civil Engineering
Co Ltd 15
Aisa Trading Company Ltd 15
Ajanga International Agency 15
Ajao, J A, Brothers 15
Ajaokuta Steel Company Ltd 16
Ajirotutu (Nigeria) Ltd 16
Ajosi Oilfields Supply Company Ltd 16
Aka and Sons (Nigeria) Ltd 16
Akande Trading Co Nigeria Ltd 16
Akanji Commercial Enterprises Ltd 16
Akanji, D L, & Co (Nig) Ltd 16
Akanji Transport 16
Akarolo Technical Company Nigeria
Ltd 16
Akhigbe, Odibo, & Co Ltd 16
Akija Hotel Ltd 16
Akin Martins (Nigeria) Ltd 16
Akinadod Akinloye Aboderin Ltd 16
Akin-George, J, & Company 16
Akpenlamen Co Ltd 17
Akutu Structures Ltd 17
Akwiwu Motors Ltd 17
Aladaire Export Ltd 18
Aladdin Construction Nigeria Ltd 18
Alakija & Alakija Contracting Services
Ltd 18
Alalade Group of Companies 18
Alban Pharmacy Ltd 18
Albishir, Alhaji, & Sons 18
Alcan Aluminium of Nigeria Ltd 18
Alcan Aluminium Products Ltd 18
Alex L M Davou Fom & Sons
Enterprise Ltd 18
Alex Oguejiofor Company Ltd 18
Alex Travel Agency Ltd 18
Alfa-Laval (Nigeria) Ltd 19
Algadama (Holdings) Ltd 19
Algadama Nigeria Film Distributors Ltd 19

Alhaji Albishir & Sons 19
Alhaji Audu Bida & Sons United
Company Ltd 19
Alhaji Baba M Salleh & Sons (Nigeria)
Ltd 19
Alhaji M R Shittu & Sons Ltd 19
Alhaji Madu Mala Sheriff Gamboru 19
Alhaji Mai Deribe & Sons Ltd 19
Alhaji Mustapha Haruna & Sons 19
Alhaji Nata'Ata and Sons 19
Alhaji Sani Mashall Estates 19
Alhaji Sani Musa & Sons 19
Alhaji Usman Tetengi & Sons Ltd 19
Alhaji Yerima Hamman Wabi & Sons 19
Alhaji Zanna K Mala & Sons Company 19
Alhassan Dantata & Sons Ltd 19
Alheri Mining Co Ltd 19
Alinaco (Nigeria) Ltd 19
All Purpose Nigeria Ltd 20
All-African Woodworking Industry Ltd 20
Allen, J, Co Ltd 20
Allgemein Business Associates 20
Allied Architects 20
Allied Bank of Nigeria Ltd 20
Allied Bendix Ltd 20
Allied Biscuit Company Ltd 20
Allied Electronics &
Telecommunications Services Ltd 20
Allied Metal & Chemical Works Ltd 20
Allied Oilfield Services (Nigeria) Ltd
(AOS) 20
Allied Trading Co Ltd 21
Allscope Communications (Nigeria) Ltd 21
Allwell Brown and Company 21
Alpha Industries (Nigeria) Ltd 21
Alraine (Nigeria) Ltd 21
ALUMACO 21
Aluminium Manufacturing Company of
Nigeria Ltd 21
Alusteel Construction Ltd 21
Amagra International Music House 21
Amagroup Engineers Ltd 21
Amalgamated Industries Ltd 22
Amalgamated Tin Mines of Nigeria Ltd 22
Amalighterage & Timber Exporting Co
Ltd 22
Amana Construction Co (Nigeria) Ltd 22
Amana Consulting Engineers 22
Amari Mines Ltd 22
Amarillo Umbrella Company (Nigeria)
Ltd 23
Amass Nigeria Ltd 23
Amatemeso Shipping Agencies Ltd 23
Ambrosini, L, Ltd 23
Amcord Nigeria Ltd 23
Amdumac Group (Nigeria) Ltd 23
Ameniger Construction Company Ltd 23
American International Insurance 24
Americo Ltd 24
Amey Roadstone Company (Nigeria)
Ltd 24
Amicable Assurance Company Ltd 24
Aminci International Co Ltd 24
Analex Group Ltd 24
Anamapharmaceutical Industries Ltd 24
Anambra Motor Manufacturing Co Ltd 24
Anambra Vegetable Oils Products
Nigeria Ltd 24
(ANAMMCO) 24
Anasoro Builders 25
Anbar Enterprises Ltd 25
Anglo-French Trading Co Ltd 25
Anglo-German Company
(Intercontinental) Ltd 25
Anglo-Norman Shipping (Nigeria) Ltd 25
Anombem Mokwunye, Twigg, Brown &
Partners 25
Anopit Ltd 25
ANSIL 25

Apapa Chemical Industries Ltd	25
Aparaki Enterprises	25
APC International Nigeria Ltd	25
Apex (Eastern Nigeria) Ltd	26
Apex Paints Ltd	26
Aprofim Engineering Construction Company (Nigeria) Ltd	26
Aratah, Josman, Trading Company	26
Arax Airlines Ltd	26
Arbico Ltd	26
Arbor Services Nigeria Ltd	26
(ARC (NIG) Ltd)	24
Arcee Textile Industries Ltd	26
Architechniques	26
Architectural Metal Products Ltd	26
ARC-Models Company	27
Arcus Consultant Ltd	27
Arewa Advancement Enterprises Ltd	27
Arewa Construction Ltd	27
Arewa Hotels (Developments) Ltd	27
Arewa Metal Containers Ltd	27
Arewa Steel Works Company (Nig) Ltd	27
Arewa Textiles Ltd	28
Arewa Tradewinds (Nig) Co Ltd	28
Arewa United Stores Ltd	28
Aridi Industries (Nigeria) Ltd	28
Arigas Construction Company Nigeria Ltd	28
Ark Stewart Wrightson	28
(ARMECO)	27
Aromolaran Publishers Nigeria Ltd	28
Aronaout Communications Ltd	28
Arroways of Nigeria	28
Arrowhead Insurance Co (Nig) Ltd	29
Arthur Andersen & Company	29
Arthur Young Osindero & Co	29
Asaboro, Joseph	29
Asagba, M A, & Sons	29
Asani (Nigeria) Trading Co	29
Asape (Nigeria) Company Ltd	29
Asemota Motors (Nigeria) Ltd	29
Ashaka Cement Company Ltd	29
Ashamu, E O, & Sons (Holdings) Ltd	29
Ashland Oil (Nigeria) Company	29
Asian African Container (Nigeria) Ltd	30
Asiatic Industries Ltd	30
Asiatic Industries Ltd	30
Askar of Nigeria Ltd	30
Aspect Construction Engineering Group (Nig) Ltd	30
Aspesi Ltd	30
Asphalt Company of Nigeria Ltd	30
Asra Seafoods (Nigeria) Ltd	30
Associated Battery Manufacturers (Nigeria) Ltd	30
Associated Breweries & Company Ltd	30
Associated Drug Company (Nig) Ltd	30
Associated Electronic Products (Nigeria) Ltd	31
Associated Exports (W.A.) Ltd	31
Associated Laboratory Supplies Ltd	31
Associated Metal & Allied Works Ltd	31
Associated Ores Mining Company Ltd	31
Associated Pharmaceutical Products Ltd	31
Associated Textile Manufacturers Co Ltd	32
Association of Nigerian Co-Operative Exporters Ltd	32
Aswani Textile Industries Ltd	32
Aticon Ltd	32
Atlantic Mercantile Co Ltd	32
Atlantic Textile Manufacturing Co Ltd	32
Atlas Nigeria Ltd	32
Atoki, Fred, Publishing Company Ltd	32
Atssco Abbey Office Machine Service Stationery (Nig) Ltd	32
Atta, M O, & Sons (Nigeria) Ltd	33
Audu Lukat Motors Ltd	33
August Reiners Nigeria Ltd	33
Aurora Produce & Shipping Co Ltd	33
Auto Components Ltd	33
Avery Nigeria Ltd	33
Avon Crowncaps and Containers (Nigeria) Ltd	33
(AVOP)	25
Awaye Continental Motors Co Ltd	33
Awosanmi & Sons Engineering Works	33
Ayana Mining Syndicate	33
Aye Marble & Terrazzo Industrial Works	33
Ayo, Lawrence, & Sons Ltd	34
B & C Autopanel Engineering Ltd	34
B & F Nigeria Ltd	34
B B C Brown Boveri (Nigeria) Ltd	34
B C Unije & Sons Ltd	34
B K Sutherland & Company Ltd	34
B Stabilini & Company Ltd	34
Babafunke, Adeola, Overseas Trading Company	34
Baertle, J, & Co (Nig) Ltd	34
Bafco Ltd	34
Bagauda Textile Mill Ltd	34
Bakare, S B, & Brothers Ltd	34
Baker Nigeria Ltd	34
Bakrin Enterprises Ltd	35
Balakhany (Nigeria) Ltd	35
Balin Builders & Aluminium Industries Ltd	35
Balmore Trading Company Ltd	35
Balogun, A A, & Sons (Nigeria) Ltd	35
Balogun, J A, Works	35
Bamgboye Engineering Ltd	35
Bana Consultants Nigeria Ltd	35
Banbury Systems (Nigeria) Ltd	35
Banjoko Firesafety Ltd	35
Banjoko, L A O, & Co Ltd	35
Bank of Credit & Commerce International (Nigeria) Ltd	36
Bank of the North Ltd	36
Bao Nigeria Ltd	36
Baraka Press & Publishers Ltd	36
Barlow Mines Ltd	36
Barma, A G S, Ltd	36
Baroid of Nigeria Ltd	36
Barshall, F M, (West Africa) Ltd	37
Basf (Nigeria) Ltd	37
Bata Nigeria Ltd	37
Battery Manufacturing Co (Nig) Ltd	37
Bayajida Group of Companies	37
Bayer (Nigeria) Ltd	37
Bayer Pharmaceuticals (Nigeria) Ltd	37
BEC Freres (Nigeria) Ltd	37
Beccarelli, P, & Co Ltd	37
Beciciti Construction Ltd	37
Becker-Voigt, H	37
Bedkana (Nig) Ltd	38
Beecham Ltd	38
Beggmatic Automations Ltd	38
Ben Agency Service	38
Bendel Brewery Ltd	38
Bendel Chemical Industries Ltd	38
Bendel Hotels Board	38
Bendel Insurance Company Ltd	38
Bendel Line	38
Bendel Newspapers Corporation	39
Bendel Pharmaceuticals Ltd	39
Bendel Plastic Industries Ltd	39
Bendel Steel Structures Ltd	39
Benjamin Nabena Nabenson Promotions	39
Bennett-Sasore-Dunn Ltd (Nigeria)	39
Benora Instruments & Company	39
Bentworth Finance (Nigeria) Ltd (BFN)	39
Benue Cement Company Ltd	39
Benue Plateau Rice Company Ltd	40
Bepco (Nig) Ltd	40
Berec Nigeria Ltd	40
Berenshot Moret Bosboom	40
Berg Geotechnical Engineering (Nigeria) Ltd	40
Berger, Julius, Nigeria Ltd	40
Berger Paints (Nigeria) Ltd	41
Berif International Company	41
Berliet Nigeria Ltd	41
Bestform Industries Co Ltd	41
Bewac Automotive Products Ltd	41
Bewac Ltd	41
Bhandari & Company (Nigeria) Ltd	42
Bhojsons & Company (Nigeria) Ltd	42
Bhojsons Industries Ltd	42
Bibson Associates Ltd	42
BICC Construction (Nigeria) Ltd	42
Bida, Alhaji Audu, & Sons United Company Ltd	42
Bidat Sportswear Company Ltd	42
Bideco (Nigeria) Ltd	43
Bimbotech (Nigeria) Ltd	43
Binatone Electronics	43
Biobaku Faber & Partners	43
Biode Pharmaceutical Industries Ltd	43
Biomedical Services Company Ltd	43
Birma General Supplies Ltd	43
Birom Mines Ltd	43
Bisceglia Brothers & Associates Construction Co (Nigeria) Ltd	43
Biscuit Manufacturing Company of Nigeria Ltd	43
Bisichi-Jantar (Nigeria) Ltd	44
Bisiolu Enterprises Ltd	44
Bisrod Furniture Company Ltd	44
BKI Building & Civil Engineering Co Ltd	44
Black & Decker Nigeria Ltd	44
Blackwood Hodge (Nigeria) Ltd	44
Blessed Furniture Enterprises	44
Blue Straps Ltd	44
Bodax Instruments & Tools Ltd	44
Bode International Nig Agencies (BOGI)	45
Boladele Brothers & Co Ltd	45
Bolex Enterprises	45
Bolingo Organisation	45
Bolokor MK Ltd	45
Bolori Brothers & Co Ltd (Bolbros)	45
Boma Associates (WA) Ltd	45
Bonny Lng Ltd	45
Bonny Oil & Gas Industries (Nigeria) Ltd	45
Bono International Ltd	45
Bonomi, S G, Ltd	45
Boots Company (Nigeria) Ltd (The)	46
Bordpak Premier Packaging	46
Borini Prono & Co Ltd	46
Borno Engineering & Steel Manufacturers Ltd	46
Bosag Builders	46
Boskalis Nigeria Ltd	46
Botam (Nigeria) Ltd	46
Boulos Enterprises Ltd	47
Boulos Enterprises Ltd	47
Bouygues (Nigeria) Ltd	47
Bozgomero of Nigeria Ltd	47
Braithwaite, T A, (Insurance Brokers) & Co	47
Brand Clay Works Ltd	47
Breckwoldt & Co (Nigeria) Ltd	47
Bremen Nnachetam Construction Company (Nigeria) Ltd	47
BRGM (Nigeria) Ltd	49
Brian Munro Ltd	49
Bright Aluminium Products Co Ltd	49
Bright Steel Structures Co Ltd	49
Brightstar Industries Ltd	49
Briscoe, Frank	49
Briscoe, R T, (Nigeria) Ltd	49
Bristol Hotel	49
Bristol Myers Company	49
Bristow Helicopters (Nigeria) Ltd	49
British India General Insurance Co (Nigeria) Ltd	49
British-American Insurance Company (Nigeria) Ltd	49
(BRMC)	51
Bronik Motors Ltd	50
Brossette (Nigeria) Ltd	50
Brown & Root Nigeria Ltd	50
Brunelli Construction Company	50
BSM Ltd	50
BT International (Nigeria) Ltd	50
Building & Civil Engineering Contractors Company Nigeria Ltd	50
Bulk Oil Plants of Nigeria Ltd	50
Buromat Data System Ltd	50
Bush, W J, & Company (Nigeria) Ltd	50
Business & Industrial Consultants	50
Business Equipment & Machinery Ltd (BEAM) (Division of UAC of Nigeria Ltd)	50
Business Research Management Center	51
C C Daniel Mining Industry	51
C C Ezeilo	51
C Funcke & Co (Nigeria) Ltd	51
C I F Construction Nigeria Ltd	51
C Itoh & Co Ltd	51
C Moore Obioha Sons & Company Ltd	51
C N Onuselogu Enterprises Ltd	51
C Normann International Company	51
C O Iguh and Sons Trading Co (Nigeria) Ltd	51
C Uba & Brothers Trading Company (WA) Ltd	51
C Woermann (Nigeria) Ltd	51
C Zard & Company Ltd	51
Caaso Constructional Works Ltd	51
Cadbury Nigeria Ltd	51
Calabar Cement Company Ltd	52
Calabar Veneer & Plywood Ltd	52
Calaro Oil Palm Estate Ltd	52
Caleb Bovis Johnson Construction Co Ltd	52

Caleb Brett & Son (Nigeria) Ltd 52
Camco Ltd 52
Cameron Iron Works (Nigeria) Ltd 52
Camplant Engineering Sales & Service Ltd 52
Candles & Polish Works Ltd 53
Cansult Ltd 53
Capital Trust Brokers Ltd 53
Cappa and D'Alberto Ltd 53
Cappa, G, Ltd 53
Caprihans Industries Ltd 53
Carl-Ploetner (Nigeria) Ltd 54
Carpet Royal (Nigeria) Ltd 54
Carrara Marble Co Ltd 54
Casting Nigeria Ltd 54
Cave Plastics Ltd 54
Caxton Press (West Africa) Ltd 54
CEC & Co (Nigeria) Ltd 54
CECA (Nigeria) Ltd 54
Cement Company of Northern Nigeria Ltd 54
Central Bank of Nigeria 54
Central Hotel 55
Central Investment Company Ltd 55
Central Packages of Nigeria Ltd 55
Central Water Transportation Company Ltd 55
Century Insurance Co (Nigeria) Ltd 55
CEP 55
Cepuz International Agencies 55
Cetaconsult (Nigeria) Ltd 55
CFAO (Nigeria) Ltd 56
CFC Furniture Co (En) Ltd 56
CFC Furniture Co (WC) Ltd 56
CGG Nigeria Ltd 56
Challenge Bookshops 56
Chami, A B, & Co Ltd 57
Champion Confectionery Co (Nigeria) Ltd 57
Chanrai, J T, & Co (Nigeria) Ltd 57
Charlie and Franco Ltd 57
Charlton Trading Company (Nigeria) Ltd 57
Chase Merchant Bank Nigeria Ltd 57
Chattalas Brothers Ltd 57
Chellaram, K, & Sons (Nigeria) Ltd 57
Chemdyes Nigeria Ltd 58
Chemex Nigeria Ltd 58
Chemical & Allied Products Ltd 58
Chesebrough Ponds Industries Ltd 59
Chiakwelu, A I, & Brothers 59
Chidiebere Transport Ltd 59
Chiyoda Chemical Engineering & Construction Co 59
Chrislow Associated Nigeria Ltd 59
Chrisray Nigeria Ltd 59
Christela Chemical Works Ltd 59
Christlieb, A C, (Nigeria) Ltd 59
Chukwurah Agriculture Industries Ltd 61
Chuwang Gyang & Sons Ltd 61
Ciba-Geigy Ltd 61
Cimeco Enterprises (Nigeria) Ltd 61
Cinsere Sewing Machine Industrial Company Ltd 61
Cistar (Nigeria) Ltd 61
City Group Organization 62
City Securities Ltd 62
Citymark (West Africa) Ltd 62
Claretta Maritime Services Ltd 62
Clarke, W F, (Nigeria) Ltd 62
Clarke, Walter, & Sons (Overseas) Ltd 62
Clay Industry (Nigeria) Ltd 63
Clyde Dial Construction (Nigeria) Ltd 63
Cneico (Nigeria) Ltd 63
CNMD Co 63
Coast Timber Co Ltd 63
Coastal Services (Nigeria) Ltd 63
Coates Brothers (WA) Ltd 63
Cocoa Industries Ltd 63
Cocoa Producers Alliance 63
Cogemat (Nigeria) Ltd 63
Coksee Engineering Works Ltd 63
Colodense Nigeria Ltd 63
Comazzi, P 64
Combined Maritime Agencies (Nigeria) Ltd 64
Commerce Assurance Ltd 64
Commercial Medicine Stores Ltd 64
Commind Nigeria Ltd 64
Commonwealth Commodity Company International 64
Communications Associates of Nigeria Ltd 64
Communications Consultants Nigeria Ltd 65

Compagnie Francaise de l'Afrique Internationale 65
Compass Trading Co Ltd 65
Complete Home Enterprises (Nig) Ltd 65
Comprehensive Engineering Consultants 65
COMSAC 64
Concorde Furniture Manufacturing Co Ltd 65
Concrete Building Contractors & General Works Ltd 65
Concrete Poles Industries (Nigeria) Ltd 65
Concrete Structures Ltd 66
Consolidated Structures 66
Construction & Support Services Nigeria Ltd 66
Construction Management Services 66
Containers (Nigeria) Ltd 66
Contex Nigeria Ltd 66
Continental & General Merchants Ltd 66
Continental Iron & Steel Co Ltd 66
Continental Lines (Africa) Ltd 66
Continental Medical Complex Ltd 66
Continental Pharmaceuticals Ltd 66
Continuous Printing Industry (Nigeria) Ltd 66
Controlled Plastics Ltd 67
Conveyancer (Nigeria) Ltd 67
Co-operative and Commerce Bank (Nigeria) Ltd 67
Co-Operative Bank Ltd 67
Co-Operative Bank of Kaduna State 67
Co-Operative Bank of Kano 67
Co-Operative Investment & Trust Society 68
Co-Operative Supply Association Ltd 68
Coopers & Lybrand Associates Ltd 68
Coopers Benly Ventures & Company Ltd (The) 68
Cope Builders' Supplies Ltd 68
Copiers (Nigeria) Ltd 68
Cornbrough Products (Nigeria) Ltd 69
Cornerstone Organisation Ltd 69
Corpio Constructions (Nigeria) Ltd 69
Cosmos Metal & Electrics Ltd 69
Costain (West Africa) Ltd 69
Cotsgas (Nigeria) Ltd 69
Coutinho, Caro & Co (Nigeria) Ltd 69
CPI-Moore (Nigeria) Ltd 69
Crittall-Hope Nigeria Ltd 70
Crocodile Matchets (Nigeria) Ltd 70
Cross, A W, Ltd 70
Cross Lines Ltd 70
Cross River Breweries Ltd 70
Cross River Estate Ltd 70
Cross River State Agricultural Development Corporation 71
Cross River State Newspaper Corporation 71
Crown Agents For Overseas Governments and Administrations 71
Crown Cork and Seal Company (Nigeria) Ltd 71
Crusader Insurance Co (Nigeria) Ltd 71
CSS Bookshops 71
CSS Press (Nigeria) Ltd 71
(CTC) 57
Cubitts (Nigeria) Ltd 71
Cunix Industrial & Commercial Co Ltd 71
Cutler-Hammer Nigeria Ltd 71
Czechoslovak Nigerian Minerals Development Co Ltd 63
Czechs (Nigeria) Ltd 72
D A Jideofo Enterprises Ltd 72
D A Nwandu & Sons Enterprises Ltd 72
D B Zang 72
D K Ejukorlem & Co Ltd 72
D L Akanji & Co (Nig) Ltd 72
D O Nkwonta & Sons Enterprises Ltd 72
D O Olagbemiro & Co (Nigeria) Ltd 72
Daboul Travel Office 72
Dada-Obe Industries (Nigeria) Ltd 72
Daddo International (Nigeria) Ltd 72
DAE International (Nigeria) Ltd 72
Dafinasi Enterprises Ltd 72
Dagazau International Ltd 72
Daily Need Chemists Ltd 72
Daily Soap Ltd 73
Daily Times of Nigeria 73
Dala (Nigeria) Ltd 73
Dalamal Textile Mills Ltd 73
D'Alberto, E, & Giampaoli Ltd 73
D'Alberto, L, & Co Ltd 73
Daltrade (Nigeria) Ltd 73

Dambiyowu Nigeria Ltd 73
Damdavy & Company 74
Damen Shipyards Nigeria Ltd 74
Daniel, C C, Mining Industry 74
Daniel Marryat (Nigeria) Ltd 74
Daniksi Ltd 74
Danlon Associates 74
Dantata Land and Sea Company Ltd 74
Danwawu Shipping Cargo Handling & Transport Co Ltd 74
Dapo Allied Industries (Nigeria) Ltd 75
Dar Al-Handasah Consultants & Partners 75
Data Processing Maintenance and Services Ltd 75
Data Sciences (Nigeria) Ltd 75
Dauphin (Nigeria) Ltd 75
De Facto Bakeries & Catering Ltd 76
De Petraco Industries Ltd 76
Deazula Trading Company (Nigeria) Ltd 76
Debs Modern Industries Ltd 76
Decca (West Africa) Ltd 76
Defence Industries Corporation of Nigeria 76
Deji Oyenuga & Partners 76
Delco (Nig) Ltd 76
Della Group Ltd 76
Delta Boatyard Ltd 76
Delta Freeze Ltd 76
Delta Furniture & Furnishing Ind Ltd 76
Delta Glass Company Ltd 76
Delta Hotels Ltd 77
Delta Oil Nigeria Ltd 77
Delta Pioneer Company Ltd 77
Delta Property Development Co Ltd 77
Delta Scientific & Technical Co Ltd 77
Delta Steel Company Ltd 77
Deltaplast Company (Nigeria) Ltd 77
Dema Engineering Ltd 78
Denchukwu Group of Companies 78
Deribe, Alhaji Mai, & Sons Ltd 78
Desam Development Company Ltd 78
Design Group Nigeria 78
Deutsche Kaiser Gruppe (Interkontinental) 78
Dexso Furniture Factory Ltd 78
Dhanamall & Co (Nigeria) Ltd 78
DHL International Nigeria Ltd 78
DHV Consultants Nigeria Ltd 79
Diamond Plastics Ltd 79
Diborsons Business Enterprises 79
Diesel Generating Company Ltd 79
Diesel Sales and Service (Nigeria) Ltd 79
Dipenta Nigeria Ltd 79
Disscol Ltd 79
Dixilyn (Nigeria) Ltd 79
Dizengoff West Africa (Nigeria) Ltd 79
DLP Pharmaceuticals Ltd 80
Doal Enterprises Ltd 80
DOF Chemicals Ltd 80
Dokunmu, M A, & Sons Ltd 80
Dolmech Engineering (Nig) Ltd 80
Dolphin Dive West Africa 80
Dolphin Properties Ltd 80
Domino Stores Ltd 80
Don International Ltd 80
Dorman Long & Amalgamated Engineering Ltd 80
Dornier-Nigeria Aeronautical Engineering 81
Dotun Okubanjo & Associates Ltd 81
Dowell Schlumberger (Nigeria) Ltd 81
Doyin Investments Nigeria Ltd 81
DPMS Ltd 81
Dr Pepper Bottling Company of Nigeria Ltd 81
Dragages Nigeria Ltd 81
Drake & Scull (Nigeria) Ltd 81
(Dresser Magcobar Minerals Ltd) 82
Dresser Nigeria Ltd 82
Drug Houses Nigeria Ltd 82
Drug Specialities (Nigeria) Ltd 82
DSD Nigeria Ltd 82
Dubic Breweries Ltd 82
Dubic Industries Ltd 83
Dubic International Ltd 83
Dubosh Plastics (Nigeria) Ltd 83
Dumex Pharmaceuticals Ltd 83
Dumez (Nigeria) Ltd 83
Dunlop Nigerian Industries Ltd 83
Dunon Furniture Industry Ltd 83
Duro International (Nigeria) Ltd 84
Dynamic Industries Ltd 84

Dys Trocca Valsesia & Company Ltd 84
E Osborne Nigeria Ltd 84
E A O Constructors (Nigeria) Ltd 84
E D'Alberto & Giampaoli Ltd 84
E M Micheletti & Son (Nigeria) Ltd 84
E Mocci Associates 84
E O Ashamu & Sons (Holdings) Ltd 84
Eagle Group Ltd 84
Earth Sciences Ltd 84
Eastern Bulkcem Company Ltd 84
Eastern Enamelware Factory Ltd 84
Eastern General Contractors Ltd 85
Eastern (Overseas) Agencies Ltd 85
Eastern Wrought Iron Ltd 85
Ebel Bau Nigeria Ltd 85
Ebun Oluwa Group of Companies 85
Eburutu Mining Syndicate 85
ECWA Productions Ltd 85
Eddymay Enterprises 85
Eddy's Electronics 85
Edemscot Engerprises Nigeria Ltd 85
Edewor International Ltd 86
Edilit Ltd 86
Edison Group & Parnters 86
Edmund & Edmund (Nigeria) Ltd 86
Edo Textile Mills Ltd 86
Edok-Eter-Mandilas Ltd 86
Edokpolo, John, & Co Ltd 86
Edrita & Company Ltd 86
Edun Commercial Agency 86
Efbiko Engineering Ltd 86
Egbema Enterprises Ltd (EEL) 86
Egbon Mining Syndicate 87
Egbor and Associates 87
Ejinaka and Thornber Ltd 87
Ejinkeonye, L E, Brothers Trading Co
  Ltd 87
Ejire Halleluih Trading Co Ltd 87
Ejukorlem, D K, & Co Ltd 87
Ekerete, A, Ltd 87
Ekisola Electrical Works Ltd 87
Ekman Construction Co Ltd 87
Eko Holiday Inn 87
Eko Leatherware Factory 87
Eksons (Nig) Ltd 87
Ekwueme Associates 89
Elder Dempster Agencies (Nigeria) Ltd 89
Eldorado (Nigeria) Ltd 89
Electrical Material Supplies (EMS) 89
Electricare Ltd 89
Electro Technologies Nigeria Ltd
  (ELTEC) 89
Electrode Nigeria Ltd 89
Electronics Industrial Company
  (Nigeria) Ltd 90
Electronics Instrumentations Ltd 90
Eleiyele Cashew Factory 90
Elettro Engineering 90
ELF Nigeria Ltd 90
El-Kalil, M, Transport Ltd 90
Emanento Company Agency 90
Embechem Ltd (Formerly May & Baker
  (Nigeria) Ltd) 90
EMI (Nigeria) Ltd 91
Emidson Nigeria Ltd 91
Emirate Technical Services 91
Emos Dynamics Co (Nigeria) Ltd 91
Endurance Ltd 92
Engineering Construction Co Ltd
  (ECC) 92
ENO Industries Ltd 92
Enomah Office Equipment Ltd 92
Enpee Industries Ltd 92
Envelope & File Co of Nigeria 92
Eom Construction Co Ltd 92
Epe Plywood Industries Ltd 92
Eppellion International Ltd 92
Equatorial Lines 92
Equity & General Accident Insurance
  Company Ltd 92
Erhahon, R I, & Co Ltd 93
Ernestco Ltd 93
Ernst & Whinney, Oni, Lasebikan &
  Company 93
Eslon Nigeria Ltd 93
Essdee Food Products Nigeria Ltd 93
Estate Electrical Industries (Nigeria)
  Ltd 93
ETAM 95
Etco-Engineering & Technical
  Company (Nigeria) Ltd 93
Eterna Electrical Engineering Works
  Ltd 94
Eternit Ltd 94

Ethiope Food Industries Ltd 94
Ethiope Publishing Corporation 94
Etuk Motors Technical Company Ltd 94
Eurotrade (Nigeria) Ltd 94
Evans Brothers (Nigeria) Ltd 95
Evans Medical (Nigeria) Ltd 95
Everett Trading & Manufacturing Co
  Ltd 95
Evian Africa Co Ltd 95
Excel Plastic Industries Ltd 95
Excelsior Garment Factory Ltd 95
Eximport & Company Nigeria Ltd 95
Ex-Lands Nigeria Ltd 95
Express Insurance Company Ltd 95
Express International Maritime Ltd 95
Eze, I O, & Sons Ltd 95
Ezeilo, C C 96
Ezennwa, S N, & Sons Ltd 96
F G Spiropoulos & Company Ltd 96
F M Barshall (West Africa) Ltd 96
F Steiner & Company Ltd 96
Fado Engineering Co Ltd 96
Fagbamigbe, Olaiya, Ltd 96
Falcon Nigeria Ltd 96
Fallad Commercial Enterprises Ltd 96
Faltas, A M, (West Africa) Ltd 96
Fan Milk Ltd 96
Fanz Holdings Ltd 96
Far East Mercantile Co Ltd 97
Farawametz Construction Co Ltd 97
Farrell Lines International (Nigeria) Ltd 97
Fas Brothers Ltd 97
Fashion Shoe Company (Nigeria) Ltd 97
Fatmok Associates 97
Fatsports Industries Ltd 97
Fawaz Steelwood & Chemicals (Kano)
  Ltd 97
Fawehinmi Furniture Factory Ltd 98
Fedco Foam (Nigeria) Ltd 98
Federal Ministry of Industries 98
Federal Mortgage Bank of Nigeria 98
Federal Radio Corporation of Nigeria 98
Federated Cork & Seal Company Ltd 98
Federated Motor Industries 98
Federation Products (Nigeria) Ltd 98
Felicity Engineering Co Ltd 98
Felico Industries Nigeria 98
Femce Marketing Company 98
Femina Hygienical Products (Nigeria)
  Ltd 99
Femo (West Africa) Ltd 99
Femope Marketing Company 99
Ferdinand Enterprises (Nigeria) Ltd 99
Ferrero, A G, & Co Ltd 99
Feso Mirror and Glass Works Ltd 99
Fibreglass Reinforced Plastics Co Ltd 100
Fidelity Mining Syndicate 100
Fimcon Ltd 100
Financial Trust Company Nigeria Ltd 100
Fire Protection Services Ltd 100
First Bank of Nigeria Ltd (Formerly
  Standard Bank Nigeria Ltd) 100
First Chicago Nigeria Ltd 100
First City Investment Company Ltd 100
Fisayo Holdings Ltd 100
Fisco-Chemicals (Nigeria) Ltd 100
Fisko Construction Engineering Co Ltd 101
Five Star Industries Ltd 101
Flag Aluminium Products Ltd 101
Flopetrol Nigeria Ltd 102
Flour Mills of Nigeria Ltd 102
Folam International Trading Company 102
Food Specialities (Nigeria) Ltd 102
Foods Division of UAC of Nigeria Ltd 102
Foremost Dairies (Nigeria) Ltd 102
Forex Neptune of Nigeria Ltd 103
(Formerly Akutu Construction
  Company Nigeria Ltd) 17
(Formerly Bartoletti (Nigeria) Ltd 131
Formerly Benue Piateau Biscuits Co
  Ltd 180
Formerly Benue Plateau Packages Ltd 180
(Formerly Haden (Nigeria) Ltd 117
(Formerly IBM Nig Ltd) 81
Formerly John Holt Investment
  Company Ltd 138
Formerly Johnson & Johnson (Nigeria)
  Ltd 121
(Formerly Merck Sharp & Dohme
  (Nigeria) Ltd) 31
Formerly Mitsui & Co (Nigeria) Ltd 166
(Formerly Nigerian Amicable
  Assurance Company Ltd) 24
(Formerly Oscar Faber (Nigeria)) 43

(Formerly Philips (Nig) Ltd) 31
(Formerly Polyplast Industrial Co Ltd) 67
Foster Wheeler (Nigeria) Ltd 103
Fougerolle Nigeria Ltd 103
Foundation Construction Ltd 103
Foundation Engineering (Nigeria) Ltd 103
Francis Goodwill Ltd 103
Franco Builders Ltd 103
Frank Briscoe 103
(FRCN) 98
Fred Atoki Publishing Company Ltd 103
Fred Balonwu Unigwe Group of
  Companies 103
Fredano Trading Co Ltd 103
Freedom Development Company Ltd 105
Freyssinet Nigeria Ltd 105
Fuason Industries (Nigeria) Ltd 105
Fubara Enterprises Ltd 105
Funcke, C, & Co (Nigeria) Ltd 105
Funtua Brickworks Ltd 105
Funtua Cottonseed Crushing Company
  Ltd 105
Furniture House Ltd 105
Fusi Industrial Supplies Co Ltd 105
G B Ollivant & Co (Nigeria) Ltd 105
G Cappa Ltd 105
G I Obaskeki & Sons Ltd 105
G Kewalram & Sons (Nigeria) Ltd 106
G N A Hamzer & Co (Nigeria) Ltd 106
G Ndah & Sons Foundation 106
Gaby and Company (Nigeria) 106
Galenika Nigeria Ltd 106
Galvanizing Industries Ltd 106
Gamboru, Alhaji Madu Mala Sheriff 106
Gas & Welding (Nigeria) Ltd 106
Gas Producers Ltd 106
Gaskiya Corporation Ltd 106
Gauff Consultants (Nigeria) Ltd 107
Gazal Industrial Enterprises Ltd 107
GDM Textiles Manufacturing Ltd 107
GEC (Telecommunications) Nigeria Ltd 107
Geco Engineering Co (Nigeria) Ltd 107
Gem Fasteners Industry (Nigeria) Ltd 107
General Appliances Company Ltd 108
General Contractors (Nigeria) Ltd 108
General Cosmetics Company Ltd 108
General Electric USA of Nigeria Ltd 108
General Metal Products Ltd 108
General Metalware Company Nigeria
  Ltd 108
General Technology Nigeria Ltd 108
Geocomsa & Co (Nigeria) Ltd 108
Geodetic Surveys Ltd 108
George Cohen (Nigeria) Ltd 108
George Engineering Co Ltd 109
George Hunters & Company Ltd 109
George Koku & Sons Ltd 109
George, Patrick, & Sons Ltd 109
George Wimpey & Co (Nigeria) Ltd 109
Geoservices Nigeria Ltd 109
German-Nigerian Engineering
  Company Ltd (Gernig) 110
Giampaoli Construction (Nigeria) Ltd 110
Gicen Technical Services Ltd 110
Gida Technical Enterprises Company 110
Gilco Nigeria Ltd 110
Gindiri Concrete Products Ltd 110
Gion (Nigeria) Ltd 110
Glanvill Enthoven & Company (Nigeria) 110
Glaxo (Nigeria) Ltd 111
Glendora Enterprises 111
Global Pharmaceutical and Chemical
  Agencies Ltd 111
Global Stars (Nigeria) Ltd 111
Globe Fishing Industries Ltd 111
Globestar Engineering Co (Nigeria) Ltd 111
Gloede & Hoff (Nigeria) Ltd 111
Goas Agencies Ltd 111
Gobecco Trading Company Ltd 111
GOCON 115
Godbless Motors Nigeria Ltd 111
Gold & Base Metal Mines of Nigeria
  Ltd 112
Gold Star Industries Ltd 112
Golden Furniture & Construction Co
  Ltd 112
Golden Guinea Breweries Ltd 112
Good-Name Stationery Stores 112
Goodwill, Francis, Ltd 112
Goodwill Press & Bookshop 113
Goodyear Midwest Rubber Processing
  Co (Nigeria) Ltd 113
Goswin & Co 113
Gottschalcks Buildings Materials 113

INDEX: Alphabetical

Grace Bakeries   113
Grand Industrial Company Ltd   113
Grandi Lavori (Nigeria) Ltd   113
Gränges Nigeria Ltd   113
Grant Advertising International (Nigeria) Ltd   113
Great Basins Petroleum Co (Nigeria) Ltd   113
Great Nigeria Insurance Company Ltd   113
Great Northern Tanning Co Ltd   113
Green, A D, & Co Ltd   114
Green Light Industries Ltd   114
Greenham Plant Hire   114
Greens Engineering Ltd   114
Gregson Trading Company Ltd   114
Grenigas Ltd   114
Group Elektro Power Nigeria Ltd   114
GTE Nigeria Ltd   114
Guffanti (Nigeria) Ltd   114
Guinea Insurance Company Ltd   114
Guinness (Nigeria) Ltd   115
Gulf Oil Company (Nigeria) Ltd   115
Gumo Mining Syndicate   115
Guobadia Furniture & Construction Company (Nigeria) Ltd   115
Guthrie (Nigeria) Ltd   115
Gyartagere Explosives & Chemicals Co Ltd   117
H B & Sons   117
H Becker-Voigt   117
H Clarkson Edu & Partners   117
H F Schroeder (WA) Ltd   117
H H Robertson (Nigeria) Ltd   117
H W Romain & Son Ltd   117
Habis Travels Ltd   117
Haco Ltd   117
Hademec Ltd   117
Haffar Industrial Co Ltd   117
Hagemeyer (Nigeria) Ltd   119
Halcon Engineering Associates Ltd   119
Halliburton Nigeria Ltd   119
Ham Dredging Nigeria Ltd   119
Hammond, Michael, Engineering Ltd   119
Hammond, T A, Projects Ltd   119
Hamzer, G N A, & Co (Nigeria) Ltd   119
Hanein & Solomons Ltd   120
Hans Mehr (Nigeria) Ltd   120
Hansen, Jos & Soehne (Nigeria) Ltd   120
Hapel Nigeria Ltd   120
Harboni Ltd   120
Harmony House Furniture Co Ltd   120
Harmony Insurance Co (Nigeria) Ltd   120
Harold Sodipo & Co Ltd   120
Harris International Telecommunications   120
Harrison, Peter, Nigeria Ltd   120
Harriteds International Company (Nigeria) Ltd   121
Haruna, Alhaji Mustapha, & Sons   121
Haskoning Nigeria Ltd (Formerly Nedeco)   121
Hassan Furniture & Joinery Company Ltd   121
Hassan Transport (Nigeria) Ltd   121
Haven Nigeria Computer Co Ltd   121
Hay, Barry, Odunsi & Associates   121
Health Care Products (Nigeria) Ltd   121
Heinemann Educational Books (Niger.a) Ltd   121
Henkel Chemicals Nigeria Ltd   122
Henry Stephens Engineering Company Ltd   122
Heplac Nigeria Ltd   122
Herbst & Ndusco Constructions Ltd   122
Herwa Insurance Ltd   122
Herwa Ltd   122
Higrade Construction & Engineering Company Ltd   122
Hilson Nigeria Ltd   122
Hitech (Nigeria) Ltd   122
Hoegh Line (Nigeria) Ltd   122
Hoek (Nig) Ltd   123
Hoesch Pipe Mills (Nig) Ltd   123
Hogg Robinson Nigeria   123
Holex Timber (Nigeria) Ltd   123
Holman Brothers (Nigeria) Ltd   123
Holt, John, Ltd   123
Holt's Nigerian Tanneries Ltd   123
Home & Overseas Trading Company Ltd   123
Home Charm Paints (Nigeria) Ltd   125
Honda Motors Nigeria Ltd   125
Horst Pukke & Co (Nigeria) Ltd   125
Hospital Equipment and Orthopaedic Supplies Ltd   125

Household Products Ltd   125
Howard Construction Co of Nigeria Ltd   125
Hulls Services Ltd   125
Hunting Surveys (Nigeria) Ltd   125
Huttig-Schmucker Construction (Nig) Ltd   125
I I Commercial Services (IICS)   125
I N Onyenakazi & Sons Company   126
I O Eze & Sons Ltd   126
I O M Nwonye & Sons Company Ltd   126
IAS Cargo Airlines   126
Ibadan City Motors (Nigeria) Ltd   126
Ibe, A W, & Co Ltd   126
Ibekwe, P A, Ltd   126
Ibile Properties Ltd   126
Ibru Organisation (Ibru Ltd)   126
Ibru Sea Foods Ltd   126
Ibukun Transport Ltd   126
Ibukun-Olu Enterprises   127
Icon Ltd (Merchant Bankers)   127
Iddo Plastics Ltd   127
Idechemists Ltd   127
Idehen, J I, & Sons (Nigeria) Ltd   127
Idehen Poultry Farm   127
Idem Consultants   127
Iffna Co Ltd   127
Igbomina Investment Co Nigeria Ltd   128
Iguh, C O, and Sons Trading Co (Nigeria) Ltd   128
Igwe Brothers & Co Ltd   128
Ijagbemi, S A, & Sons (Nigeria) Ltd   128
Ijomah International Co Ltd   128
Ikeja Retreads (Nigeria) Ltd   128
Ikorodu Trading Company Ltd   128
Ilonex Pharmaceutical Company   128
IMNL   133
Imo Newspapers Ltd   129
Impresit Bakolori (Nigeria) Ltd   129
Inaco Ltd   129
Incar (Nigeria) Ltd   129
Inco Consultants (Nigeria) Ltd   129
Incontra Nigeria Ltd   129
Indian Bazaar (Nigeria) Ltd   129
Indo Mining Co (Nigeria) Ltd   129
Industrial & Safety Equipment (Nigeria) Ltd   129
Industrial Clays Nigeria Ltd   129
Industrial Gases Ltd   130
Inlaks Ltd   130
Inland Containers (Nigeria) Ltd   130
Innocent Hope Overseas Company   130
INPLECON   133
Insumma (Nigeria) Ltd   130
Insurance Brokers of Nigeria   130
Integrated Consultants (Nigeria) Ltd   130
Inter Continental Fishing (Nigeria) Ltd   131
Inter Designs Partnership   131
Interbasic Products Co Ltd   131
Interbeton Nigeria Ltd   131
Intercare Ltd   131
Intercontractors (Nigeria) Ltd   131
Intermark Associates Ltd   131
International Agencies Ltd   131
International Bank for West Africa Ltd   131
International Beer & Beverages Industries Ltd   131
International Biscuits Ltd   132
International Breweries Ltd   132
International Cigarette Company Ltd   176
International Computers (Nigeria) Ltd   132
International Contact Centre   132
International Contractors Agency (ICA)   132
International Contracts & Consultancy Services Ltd   132
International Enamelware Industry Ltd   132
International Housing (Nigeria) Ltd   133
International Maritime Services   133
International Merchant Bank (Nigeria) Ltd   133
International Messengers (Nigeria) Ltd   133
International Packing Industries of Nigeria Ltd   133
International Paints (WA) Ltd   133
International Planning & Environmental Consultants (Nigeria) Ltd   133
International Planning Associates   134
International Plastics (Nigeria) Ltd   134
International Steel Industry Ltd   134
International Tanners Ltd   134
International Trade (WA) Ltd   134
International Yettco (Nigeria) Ltd   134
Interstate Architects   135
Interworld Enterprises Nigeria Ltd   135

Intra Motors (Nigeria) Ltd   135
Intra Tobacco Manufacturing Co Ltd   135
Investment Promotions Ltd   135
Irede Properties and Investment Company Ltd   135
Iron Products Industries Ltd   135
Ises Ltd   135
Isiyaku Rabiu & Sons Ltd   135
Isokariari, O K & Sons (Nigeria) Ltd   135
Itager (Nigeria) Ltd   135
Italafro Builders   136
Itidal-Epid Enterprises of Nigeria   136
Itiku & Co Ltd   136
Itoh, C, & Co Ltd   136
ITT Nigeria Ltd   136
Ivory Products Ltd   136
J & H International Agency   137
J A Ajao Brothers   137
J A Balogun Works   137
J A Jones (Nigeria) Ltd   137
J A O'Bahor & Company Ltd   137
J A Thomas Rubber Estates Ltd   137
J Akin-George & Company   137
J Allen Co Ltd   137
J Baertle & Co (Nig) Ltd   137
J E Nweke & Sons Ltd   137
J F Ososami & Co   137
J I Idehen & Sons (Nigeria) Ltd   137
J L Morison Sons & Jones (Nigeria) Ltd   137
J Morin & Co   137
J Nwankwu & Bros Ltd   137
J O Oyewumi & Co (Nigeria) Ltd   137
J T Chanrai & Co (Nigeria) Ltd   137
Jac-Ogho (Nigeria) Enterprises   137
Jafco Impex Ltd   137
James Kilpatrick (Nigeria) Ltd   137
Jammal Engineering (Nigeria) Ltd   137
Jarmakani Industries (Nig) Ltd   137
Jas Builders Ltd   137
Jaybee Industries (Nigeria) Ltd   138
JBL Star Trading Company   138
Jecima Mining Syndicate   138
Jemine Enterprises Ltd   138
Jeph International (Nigeria) Ltd   138
JHI Ltd   138
Jideofo, D A, Enterprises Ltd   138
Jimona, A C E, Ltd   138
Jire Engineering Ltd   138
JLGT Construction Company Nigeria Ltd   138
Joart United Construction & Engineering Ltd   138
Joas Electrical Industries Ltd   139
Jobba Trading Company   139
Joe Oruche Trading Company Ltd   139
Joe Oyegoke Associates   139
Joelson & Sons Holdings   139
John Edokpolo & Co Ltd   139
John Holt Ltd   139
John Holt Shipping Services   139
John Okwesa Ltd   139
John West Publications Ltd   139
Johnson Foluso International Enterprises (JOFI)   139
Johnson Products of Nigeria Ltd   140
Johnson Wax Nigeria Ltd   140
Johnson White United Ltd   140
Joint Design Partnership   140
JOKI (Nigeria) Ltd   140
Jolliters Chemists Nigeria Ltd   140
Jones Homes International Nigeria Ltd   140
Jones, J A, (Nigeria) Ltd   140
Jos Alluvials Ltd   140
Jos International Breweries Ltd   140
Josef Wahler (Nig) Ltd   140
Joseph Asaboro   140
Josiah Parkes & Sons (Nigeria) Ltd   140
Josman Aratah Trading Company   140
Juli Importers & Exporters Enterprises   140
Juli Pharmacy and Stores Ltd   140
Julius Berger Nigeria Ltd   141
K Chellaram & Sons (Nigeria) Ltd   141
Kabba Co-Operative Credit & Marketing Union Ltd   141
Kabelmetal Nigeria Ltd   141
Kabo Blocks Ltd   141
Kaduna Co-Operative Bank Ltd   141
Kaduna Hotels Co Ltd   141
Kaduna Investments Co Ltd   141
Kaduna Prospectors (Nigeria) Ltd   142
Kaduna Textiles Ltd   142
Kaeler (West Africa) Ltd   142
Kagho Industrial Enterprises Ltd   143

Kailash Industries (Nigeria) Ltd	143
Kailash Weaving & Garment Manufacturing Co (Nigeria) Ltd	143
Kandara Palace Hotel Ltd	143
Kano Citizens Trading Company Ltd	143
Kano Confectionery Ltd	143
Kano Cooperative Bank Ltd	143
Kano Dyeing and Printing Co Ltd	143
Kano Merchants Trading Co Ltd	143
Kano Oil Millers Ltd	143
Kano Residential Hotel	144
Kano State Hotels Management Board	144
Kano State Investment & Properties Ltd	144
Kano Sugar Industry Nigeria Ltd	144
Kano Suit and Packing Cases Factory Ltd	144
Kano Welding & Steel Construction Co Ltd	144
Kanotex Ltd	144
Kapital Insurance Company Ltd	144
Karopharm Laboratories Ltd	145
Karunwi, A O, Ltd	145
Kassa Mines Ltd	145
Kaura Biscuit and Macaroni Factory Ltd	145
Kay Industries Nigeria Ltd	145
Kaycee (Nigeria) Ltd	145
Kayson Company Ltd	145
KCA Drilling (Nigeria) Ltd	145
Kedam Holdings (Nigeria) Ltd	145
Kennedy Transport (Nigeria) Ltd	145
Kent Engineering Nigeria Ltd	146
Kenting Africa Resource Services Ltd	146
Keppler Hausbau (Nigeria) Ltd	146
Kesington Industries Ltd	146
Kewalram, G, & Sons (Nigeria) Ltd	146
Keydril Nigeria Ltd	146
Khalil & Dibbo Transport Ltd	146
Kikachukwu Agricultural Enterprises Ltd	146
Kilpatrick, James, (Nigeria) Ltd	146
King Carpet Manufacturing Co Ltd	147
Kingston Ltd	147
Kingsway Chemists Ltd	147
Kingsway Stores of Nigeria Ltd	147
KLF Ltd	147
Klifco (Nigeria) Ltd	148
Kloeckner Ina Nigeria Ltd	148
Knight, Frank & Rutley (Nigeria)	148
Kojusola Foam Industries Ltd	148
Koku, George, & Sons Ltd	148
Kole-James & Co Ltd	148
Kolinah Industries Nigeria Ltd	148
Kolinton Technical Industries Ltd	148
Koloko Imports & Exports Co Ltd	149
Kolynson Co Ltd	149
Kosm (West Africa) Ltd	149
Kpohraror & Sons Group of Companies	149
Krabo Nigeria Ltd	149
Kragha & Associates	149
Kramer-Italo Ltd	149
Kucena-Damian (Nigeria) Ltd	149
Kueppers (Nigeria) Ltd	149
Kufena Trading Co Ltd	150
Kunza Heed (W.A.) Enterprises	150
Kuru Ltd	150
Kusba Shipping Agencies Ltd	150
Kwa Falls Oil Palm Estate Ltd	150
L A O Banjoko & Co Ltd	150
L Ambrosini Ltd	150
L D'Alberto & Co Ltd	150
L E Ejinkeonye Brothers Trading Co Ltd	150
L R Nabena & Sons Ltd	150
Laas Ltd	150
Labstock (Nigeria) Ltd	150
Lacon Nigeria Ltd	151
Ladejobi Products Nigeria Ltd	151
Ladgroup Ltd	151
Lafa Soap & Cosmetic Industry	151
Lafia Canning Factory	151
Lago (Nigeria) Ltd	151
Lagos & Niger Shipping Agencies Ltd	151
Lagos Airport Hotel Ltd	151
Lagos Plant Hire Services (Nigeria) Ltd	151
Lagos State Development & Property Corporation	152
Lagos State Transport Corporation	152
Laing Construction Ltd	152
Lakati Construction & Company	152
Lake Concrete Industries Ltd	152
Landmark Industrial Supplies Ltd	152
Lanlek (Nigeria) Associates	152
Lanray & Sons	152
Lanre Bhadmus Industries Ltd	152
Las & Co Ltd	153
Lastra Construction (Nigeria) Ltd	153
Latadek Construction Company Ltd	153
Latderma Enterprises	153
Lavalin Nigeria Ltd	153
Law Union and Rock Insurance Co of Nigeria Ltd	153
Lawal Araromi Commercial Stores	153
Lawan Schutte & Co (Nigeria) Ltd	153
Lawrence Ayo & Sons Ltd	153
Lawrence Omole & Sons Ltd	153
Leadway Assurance Company Ltd	153
Leather Tanning Industry Nigeria Ltd	154
Lecco Engineering Construction Co Ltd	154
Leman Industries (Kaduna) Ltd	154
Lennards Nigeria Ltd	154
Leo-Jimbus Mercantile Agencies (Nigeria)	154
Leo's Group of Companies Ltd	154
Lever Brothers Nigeria Ltd	154
Levitt Industries	154
Lewis & Peat (NRI) Ltd	155
Leyland Nigeria Ltd	155
Life Flour Mill Ltd	155
Light Industries (Nigeria) Ltd	155
Lilleshall (Nigeria) Ltd	155
Limson & Co Ltd	156
Linbolsen Multi-Lingual Services Ltd	156
Link Group International Ltd	156
Lion of Africa Insurance Co Ltd	156
Lipton of Nigeria Ltd	156
Lisabi Mills (Nigeria) Ltd	156
Lisabi Mining Association Ltd	156
Lister Motors (Nigeria) Ltd	156
Litigo Enterprises (Nigeria) Ltd	157
Littleways International Ltd	157
Livestock Feeds Ltd	157
Lodigiani (Nigeria) Ltd	157
Lombard Insurance Co Ltd	157
London & Kano Trading Co Ltd	157
London Africa & Overseas Ltd	157
Longman Nigeria Ltd	157
Lonogu Enterprises Ltd	157
Louis Berger Inc Nigeria	158
Lovell Stewart Nigeria Ltd	158
Lowu International (Nigeria) Ltd	158
Luncheon Vouchers Nigeria Ltd	158
M A Asagba & Sons	158
M A Dokunmu & Sons Ltd	158
M A Onigbinde & Sons Ltd	158
M El-Kalil Transport Ltd	158
M O Atta & Sons (Nigeria) Ltd	158
Maachi-Valle and Associates	158
Maas (Nigeria) Ltd	158
Maasarant Industries Ltd	158
McDermott (Nigeria) Ltd	158
Macgregor & Ojutalayo	159
Maclisle Complex Ltd	159
Macmillan Nigeria Publishers Ltd	159
Macpon Engineering and Construction Company Ltd	159
Madebayo Adetunji & Sons Ltd	159
Madona Organisation Ltd	159
Madras Manufacturing Co Ltd	159
Maduka, U, Enterprises (Nigeria) Ltd	159
Mag Furniture and Interior Designs Ltd	159
Maiden Electronics Works Ltd	159
Maiden Maritime (Nigeria) Ltd	160
Mai-Nasara & Sons Ltd	160
Mainland Bros Ltd	160
Mainland Hotel	160
Maintenance Building Contractors Ltd	160
Mais Tyres Service (City Retreading Service)	160
Majand & Company	160
Majek Soetan Industries Enterprises	160
Majem Trading Company	160
Major & Company (Nigeria) Ltd	160
Make Ltd	160
Makella & Partners	161
Makeri Smelting Company Ltd	161
Makin Ltd	161
Makira Kwarin Mabuga Metal Wood Manufacturing Company Ltd	161
Mala, Alhaji Zanna K, & Sons Company	161
Management Enterprises Ltd	161
Manatec Company Ltd	161
Mandarin Industries Company Ltd	161
Mandilas Ltd	162
Mandrides, P S, & Co Ltd	162
Manila Construction Co (Nigeria) Ltd	162
Manilla Insurance Company Ltd	162
Mansa Construction Co Ltd	162
Manufacturers Agencies	162
Manufacturing & Marketing Co (Nig) Ltd	162
Mapcotec (Nigeria) Ltd	163
Marbs Furniture Industry Ltd	163
Mareen Industries Ltd	163
Marghi Enterprises Ltd	163
Marine and General Assurance Company Ltd	164
Marini Group	164
Maritime Associates (International) Ltd	164
Maritime Stores Ltd	164
Markdealers (Nigeria) Ltd	164
Marketing and Shipping Enterprises Ltd	165
Marryat, Daniel, (Nigeria) Ltd	165
Martin Mukoro Construction Company	165
Martins, Akin, (Nigeria) Ltd	165
Marubeni Engineering (WA) Ltd	165
Mas-Chrisco and Associates	165
Mascot I Abali & Brothers Ltd	165
Mashall, Alhaji Sani, Estates	165
Mass Stationery Stores Co (Nigeria)	165
Matco Agencies	165
Matef Ltd	166
Matson & Company (Nigeria) Ltd	166
Matsons (Nigeria) Enterprises	166
Mattem (Nigeria) Enterprises	166
Matuwo Electronics Co	166
Matzen & Timm (Nigeria) Ltd	166
Maurice Project Centre Ltd	166
Max O Urbahn International Ltd	166
Mbanejo Brothers Ltd	166
Mbata, Sam, & Company Ltd	166
MBC	160
MBK Nigeria Ltd	166
MBTG	168
Medac (Nigeria) Ltd	167
Medal Brothers Co Ltd	167
Mehr, Hans, (Nigeria) Ltd	167
Memco Steel Co Ltd	167
Memudu Arowolo & Brothers	167
Mentholatum (Nigeria) Ltd	167
Mercantile Bank of Nigeria Ltd	167
Merchant Banking Corporation Nigeria Ltd (MBC)	167
Mercury Assurance Co Ltd	167
Mereoleh Brothers Co (Nigeria) Ltd	168
Mesacom Electronics Instrumentations Ltd	168
Mesterom (Nigeria) Ltd	168
Metal & Wood Furniture Construction Company Ltd	168
Metal Box Nigeria Ltd	168
Metal Box Toyo Glass Nigeria Ltd	168
Metal Construction (WA) Ltd	169
Metal Fabricator (Nigeria) Ltd	169
Metal Furniture (Nigeria) Ltd	169
Metalloplastica (Nigeria) Ltd	169
Metals & Minerals (Nigeria) Ltd	169
Metalum Ltd	169
Metoxide (Nigeria) Ltd	169
Metra Nigeria	169
Metriscope Nigeria Ltd	169
Metrocom International Ltd	170
Metropol Management Consulting Services Ltd	170
Metropolitan Distributors Ltd	170
Metropolitan Industries (Nig) Ltd	170
Miccom Engineering Works Ltd	170
Michael Hammond Engineering Ltd	171
Micheletti, A	171
Micheletti, E M, & Son (Nigeria) Ltd	171
Michelin (Nigeria) Ltd	171
Micheljohnson Ltd	171
Middleton River Brothers (Nigeria) Ltd	171
Mid-Land Bottling Company Ltd	171
Midland Galvanizing Products Ltd	171
Midland Supplies Ltd	171
Mid-Motors Nigerian Company Ltd	171
Midwest Textile Mills Ltd	172
Midwestern Timber Manufacturers Syndicate	172
Mifi (Nigeria) Ltd	172
Mike Merchandise Co Ltd	172
Millet Nigeria Ltd	172
Minarfol Transport Co Ltd	172
Mingi Mining Co Ltd	172
Minister Technical Services	172
Minnesota Nigeria Ltd	172

Misr (Nigeria) Ltd 172
Missri, A J, & Co Ltd 172
Misting Everhot 173
Mitsubishi Shoji Kaisha (Nigeria) Ltd 173
Mitton Refrigeration Service 173
MMCS Ltd 170
Mobil Oil Nigeria Ltd 173
Mobil Producing Nigeria (MPN) 173
Mocci, E, Associates 173
Modearo (Nigeria) Ltd 173
Modelor Design Aids Ltd 174
Modern Ceramics Industries Ltd 174
Modern Domus Ltd 174
Modern Foundry Products Ltd 174
Modern Industries Ltd 174
Modern Shoe Industry Ltd 174
Modulor Group 174
Mofat Engineering Company Ltd 175
Mogaji Osona Enterprises Ltd 175
Moneme & Sons Bookshops 175
Monier Construction Company (Nig) Ltd 175
Monotype Nigeria Ltd 175
Montubi 175
Moon Confectionery Ltd 175
Moone Construction Co Ltd 175
Moore Obioha, C, Sons & Company Ltd 176
Morin International Group Ltd 176
Morin, J, & Co 176
Morison, J L, Sons & Jones (Nigeria) Ltd 176
Morpol Industrial Corporation Ltd 176
Morris, Philip, Nigeria Ltd 176
Mosheshe Group of Companies 176
Mothercat Overseas (Nigeria) Ltd 177
Motor and General Insurance Company 177
Motor Parts Industry Ltd 177
Motorola 177
Motorways Nigeria Ltd 177
Moukarim Industries Ltd 177
Moukarim Metalwood Factory Ltd 177
Mouldex Ltd 177
MRT Consulting Engineers (Nigeria) Ltd 177
Mukoro, Martin, Construction Company 178
MULMACO 178
Multi Aluminium Manufacturing Company Ltd 178
Multimalt Ltd 178
Munro, Brian, Ltd 178
Musa, Alhaji Sani, & Sons 178
N Viktors International Agencies 178
Naafco (Scientific Supplies) Ltd 178
Nabena, Benjamin, Nabenson Promotions 178
Nabena, L R, & Sons Ltd 179
Naco Nigeria Ltd 179
Nagarta Drug Company Ltd 179
Nails & General Steel Manufacturing Industry Ltd 179
NAL Merchant Bank Ltd 179
Namco Nigeria Ltd 179
Napak Services (Nigeria) Ltd 179
Narumal & Sons (Nigeria) Ltd 180
Nasco Biscuits (Nigeria) Ltd 180
Nasco Estate Company (Nigeria) Ltd 180
Nasco Pack Ltd 180
Nasreddin Group International (Nigeria) Ltd 180
Nassar, S, & Sons (Nigeria) Ltd 180
Nata'Ata, Alhaji, and Sons 180
National Bank of Nigeria Ltd 180
National Cash Register (WA) Ltd 181
National Electric Power Authority (NEPA) 181
National Freight Company 181
National Grains Production Company Ltd 181
National Insurance Corporation of Nigeria 181
National Motors (Nigeria) Ltd 183
National Oil and Chemical Marketing Company Ltd 183
National Road Construction Company of Nigeria Ltd 183
National Root Crops Production Company Ltd 183
National Salt Company of Nigeria Ltd 183
National Trucks Manufacturers Ltd 185
National Veterinary Research Institute 185
Navarro International (Nigeria) Ltd 185

NCIE Ltd 185
NCO Merchants Brothers Company 185
NCR 181
Ndah, G, & Sons Foundation 185
Nedlloyd Lines 185
Neital Nigeria Ltd 185
Nelson, Thomas (Nigeria) Ltd 185
NEM Insurance Company (Nigeria) Ltd 185
Neptune Constructions Ltd 186
Neptune Transport Services Ltd 186
Netarcomms Nigeria Ltd 186
Netherlands Harbourworks (Nigeria) Ltd 187
Nevlon Pharmaceutical (Revlon) Ltd 187
New Africa Development Company Ltd 188
New African Industries Ltd 188
New Agency of Nigeria 188
New Breed Organisation Ltd 188
New Independent Rubber Company Ltd 188
New India Assurance Company (Nigeria) Ltd 188
New Insurance Company (Nigeria) Ltd 188
New Nigeria Bank Ltd 188
New Nigeria Construction Company Ltd 189
New Nigeria Development Company Ltd 189
New Nigeria Insurance Company Ltd 189
New Nigeria Merchants Ltd 189
New Nigeria Press 189
New Nigeria Salt Company Ltd 189
New Nigerian Newspapers Ltd 189
New-Gate Insurance Co Ltd 190
Newmark Electric Co Ltd 190
Newmark Electric Company Ltd (Newspin Ltd) 217
NFS (Food and Cold Storage) Ltd 190
Nichedos and Company Ltd 190
Nichemtex Industries Ltd 190
Nichimen Company (Nigeria) Ltd 190
Nicholas Laboratories Nigeria Ltd 191
NICON 181
Nidanconsult 191
Nidoco Ltd 191
Nidogas Company Ltd 191
Nifeipiri Poultries Ltd 191
Niger Agencies International (Nigeria) Ltd 191
Niger Biscuits Company Ltd 191
Niger Construction Ltd 191
Niger Consultants Ltd 192
Niger Delta Shipping Agencies Ltd 192
Niger Insurance Company Ltd (The) 192
Niger Match Company Ltd 192
Niger Motors Ltd 192
Niger Oil Resources Ltd (Norco) 192
Niger Petroleum Co Ltd 192
Niger Raw Materials Ltd 192
Niger River Transport Ltd 192
Niger Sanitary Industry Ltd 192
Niger Sea Foods Ltd 192
Nigercare International Company (Nigeria) Ltd 193
Nigerchin Electrical Development Company Ltd 193
Nigergas Ltd 193
Nigergrob Ceramics Ltd 193
Nigerguards Ltd 193
Nigeria Airways Ltd 193
Nigeria Candle Stick Manufacturing Company Ltd 194
Nigeria Coach Construction Ltd 194
Nigeria Cold Stores Ltd 194
Nigeria Construction and Furniture Company Ltd (NCFC) 194
Nigeria Distilleries Ltd 194
Nigeria Drilling Company Ltd 195
Nigeria Engineering Works Ltd 195
Nigeria Fibre Industry Company Ltd (NIFINCO) 195
Nigeria General Motors Ltd 195
Nigeria Green Lines Ltd 195
Nigeria Group Four Construction Company Ltd 195
Nigeria Hotels Ltd 195
(Nigeria Hotels Ltd) 55
Nigeria Industrial Group Ltd 196
Nigeria Kraft Bags Ltd 196
Nigeria Marine & Trading Company Ltd 196
Nigeria Merchant Bank Ltd 196
Nigeria National Fish Company Ltd 196
Nigeria National Supply Company Ltd 197

Nigeria Publishers Services Ltd 197
Nigeria Reinsurance Corporation 197
Nigeria Reliance Furniture Company 197
Nigeria Steel Products Ltd 197
Nigeria Teijin Textiles Ltd 197
Nigeria-Arab Bank Ltd 198
Nigerian & Overseas Products Ltd 198
Nigerian Agip Oil Company Ltd 198
Nigerian Agricultural and Cooperative Bank Ltd 199
Nigerian Agricultural Promotions Company Ltd 199
Nigerian Alluvials Ltd 199
Nigerian Aluminium Development Co Ltd (NADECO) 199
Nigerian Aluminium Engineering Company Ltd (NAECO) 199
Nigerian Aluminium Extrusions Ltd (NIGALEX) 199
Nigerian American Merchant Bank Ltd 199
Nigerian Asbestos Industries Ltd 199
Nigerian Aviation Handling Company Ltd 200
Nigerian Bag Manufacturing Company Ltd 200
Nigerian Ball-Point Ben Industries Ltd 200
Nigerian Bank for Commerce and Industry (NBCI) 200
Nigerian Book Suppliers Ltd 200
Nigerian Bottling Company Ltd 200
Nigerian Breweries Ltd 201
Nigerian Bricks & Clay Products Ltd 201
Nigerian Cards Ltd 201
Nigerian Carpet Manufacturing Co Ltd 201
Nigerian Carton & Packaging Manufacturing Company Ltd 201
Nigerian Caterers & Supermarkets Ltd 201
Nigerian Cement Company Ltd (Nigercem) 201
Nigerian Cementation & Drilling Co Ltd 201
Nigerian Cereals Processing Company Ltd 202
Nigerian Chemical Services Ltd (NCS) 202
Nigerian Coal Corporation 202
Nigerian Cocoa Board 202
Nigerian Commercial & Industrial Enterprises Ltd 202
Nigerian Commercial Factory Ltd 202
Nigerian Commercial Press 202
Nigerian Company for Energy Engineering Ltd (NICOGEN) 202
Nigerian Concrete Industries Ltd 203
Nigerian Consolidated Food Producers Ltd 203
Nigerian Construction & Holding Co Ltd 203
Nigerian Construction and Water Resources Development Ltd 203
Nigerian Cotton Board 203
Nigerian Cutlery Ltd 203
Nigerian Diversified Investments Ltd 204
Nigerian Diving Service Ltd 204
Nigerian Door Fabrication Company Ltd 204
Nigerian Dredging and Marine Ltd 204
Nigerian Electric Fitting Ltd 204
Nigerian Electricity Supply Corporation (Nigeria) Ltd 204
Nigerian Electronics Company Ltd 204
Nigerian Embel Tin Smelting Company 204
Nigerian Enamelware Company Ltd (NEWCO) 204
Nigerian Engineering and Construction Company Ltd (NECCO) 205
Nigerian Enterprises Promotion Board (NEPB) 205
Nigerian Explosives & Plastics Co Ltd 205
Nigerian External Telecommunications Ltd 205
Nigerian Far East Company Ltd (NIFECO) 205
Nigerian Fibre Industries Company Ltd 206
Nigerian Food Company Ltd 206
Nigerian Foundries Ltd 206
Nigerian Gas Industries 206
Nigerian General Insurance Company Ltd (The) 206
Nigerian General Security & Safety Company Ltd 207
Nigerian General Superintendence Co Ltd 207
Nigerian Glass Containers & Metal Manufacturers Ltd 207
Nigerian Groundnut Board 207

Nigerian Hardware Industries Ltd 208
Nigerian Hardwood Company Ltd 208
Nigerian Hoechst Ltd 208
Nigerian Hollowblock Industries Ltd 208
Nigerian Industrial Auxiliaries Ltd 208
Nigerian Industrial Complex
  Amalgamation Ltd 208
Nigerian Industrial Development Bank
  Ltd 209
Nigerian Institute of Management 209
Nigerian International Construction
  Company Ltd 209
Nigerian International Exchange Ltd 209
Nigerian Investigation and Safety
  Company Ltd 209
Nigerian Iron & Wood Factory Ltd 209
Nigerian Joint Agencies Ltd 209
Nigerian Leather Works Company Ltd 209
Nigerian Life & Pensions Consultants 210
Nigerian Machine Tools Co Ltd (NMT) 210
Nigerian Mapping Company Ltd 210
Nigerian Maritime Services Ltd 210
Nigerian Match & Chemical Industries
  Ltd 210
Nigerian Medical Supplies Ltd 210
Nigerian Merchants & Produce
  Suppliers 210
Nigerian Metal Fabricating Ltd 210
Nigerian Metals Ltd 210
Nigerian Mineral Development
  Company Ltd 210
Nigerian Mineral Water Industry Ltd 211
Nigerian Mining Corporation 211
Nigerian Modern Stores Ltd 211
Nigerian Motors Industries Ltd 211
Nigerian National Fish Company Ltd 211
Nigerian National Paper Manufacturing
  Company Ltd 211
Nigerian National Petroleum
  Corporation (NNPC) 211
Nigerian National Shipping Line Ltd 211
Nigerian National Shrimp Company
  Ltd 213
Nigerian Newsprint Manufacturing
  Company Ltd 213
Nigerian Office Stationery Supply
  Stores Ltd 213
Nigerian Oil Mills Ltd 213
Nigerian Oil Services Shipping &
  Equipment Co Ltd (NOSSEC) 213
Nigerian Palm Produce Board 213
Nigerian Paper Converters Company 213
Nigerian Paper Mill Ltd 214
Nigerian Perfecta Shoes Ltd 214
Nigerian Petroleum Refining Company
  Ltd (NPRC) 214
Nigerian Petroleum Terminals Ltd 214
Nigerian Pipelines Ltd 214
Nigerian Ports Authority (NPA) 214
Nigerian Printing & Publishing
  Company Ltd 215
Nigerian Processing Company Ltd 215
Nigerian Railway Corporation 215
Nigerian Railway Press 215
Nigerian Removal & Storage Co Ltd
  (NIRSCO) 215
Nigerian Road Construction Ltd 215
Nigerian Romanian Wood Industries
  Ltd 215
Nigerian Ropes Ltd 215
Nigerian Rubber Board 216
Nigerian Safety Insurance Company
  Ltd 216
Nigerian Security Printing and Minting
  Company Ltd 216
Nigerian Services & Supply Company
  Ltd (NISSCO) 216
Nigerian Sewing Machine
  Manufacturing Company Ltd 216
Nigerian Shipbuilders Ltd 216
Nigerian Shoe & Rubber Products
  Company Ltd 217
Nigerian Smelting & Refining Company
  Ltd 217
Nigerian Soft Drinks Co Ltd 217
Nigerian Spanish Cement Co Ltd 217
Nigerian Spinners & Dyers Ltd 217
Nigerian Spinning and Weaving Co Ltd 217
Nigerian Starch Mills Ltd 217
Nigerian Steel Development Authority
  (NSDA) 217
Nigerian Stockbrokers Ltd 217
Nigerian Sugar Company Ltd 217
Nigerian Suiting Manufacturing
  Company Ltd 218

Nigerian Sweets and Confectionery
  Company Ltd 218
Nigerian Technical Co Ltd 218
Nigerian Television Authority 218
Nigerian Textile Mills Ltd 218
Nigerian Thermoplastics Ltd 219
Nigerian Tobacco Company Ltd 219
Nigerian Toys Manufacturing Company
  Ltd (NITOMAC) 219
Nigerian Transmission Company Ltd 219
Nigerian Tuber & Root Crops Board 219
Nigerian Urethane Co Ltd 219
Nigerian Victory Assurance Company
  Ltd 219
Nigerian Watch-Making Industry Ltd 219
Nigerian Weaving & Processing
  Company Ltd 219
Nigerian Weaving, Spinning & Printing
  Company Ltd (NEWSPIN Ltd) 219
Nigerian Wire Industries Ltd 220
Nigerian Yeast & Alcohol
  Manufacturing Company Ltd 220
Nigerian-American Merchant Bank Ltd 220
Nigerite Ltd (Formerly Asbestos
  Cement Products Ltd) 220
Nigerlink Industries Ltd 220
Nigerlink Industries Ltd 220
Nigerpak Ltd 220
Nigerpools Company Ltd 220
Nigersol Construction Co Ltd 220
Nigersteel Company Ltd 220
Nigertal Industries Ltd 221
Niger-Techno Ltd 221
Nigerwest Steel Company Ltd 221
Nigus Petroleum Nigeria 221
Nimesco (Nigeria) Ltd 221
Nipol Ltd 221
Nirotec (A Division of Nigerian Ropes
  Ltd) 221
Nispan Construction Ltd 221
Nitol Ltd 221
Niyi Ibikunle (Nigeria) Ltd 221
Niyi Office Stationery Supply Stores
  Ltd 222
Nkwonta, D O, & Sons Enterprises Ltd 222
NMB Modern Bookshops 222
Nobgroup of Companies 222
Nordive (West Africa) Ltd 222
Nordmann, Rassmann & Company
  (Nigeria) Ltd 222
Nordstahl (Nigeria) Ltd 222
Noren Industries Ltd (Formerly
  Nigerian Sandcrete Industry Ltd) 223
Norman Industries Ltd 223
Normann, C, International Company 223
Nornit Ltd 223
Norspin Ltd 223
Nortex (Nigeria) Ltd 223
North Brewery Ltd 223
North East Line Corporation 223
Northco Construction Company Ltd 223
Northern Cable Processing and
  Manufacturing Company Ltd 224
Northern Enamelware Company Ltd 224
Northern Metal Works Co Ltd 224
Northern Nigeria Fibre Products Ltd 224
Northern Nigeria Flour Mills Ltd 224
Northern Nigeria Investments Ltd 225
Northern Nigeria Publishing Company
  Ltd (NNPC) 225
Northern Nigeria Textile Mills Ltd 225
Northern Nigerian Technical Service
  Ltd 225
Northern Sawmill & Furniture
  Manufacturing Co Ltd 225
Northern Steel Works Ltd 225
Northern Textile Manufacturers Ltd 225
Northern Tin Company Ltd 225
Northern Transporters and Merchants
  Syndicate Ltd 225
Northern Wire & Steelworks Ltd 226
Norwo Trading Company Ltd 226
Novacoke Builders Ltd 226
Novelty Industrial Company Ltd
  (NOVIC) 226
Nubi Textile Mills (Nigeria) Ltd 226
Nuccon 226
Nucleus Electronics Ltd 226
Nukom Engineering Ltd 226
Nwaezu Building Company Ltd 226
Nwandu, D A, & Sons Enterprises Ltd 226
Nwankwu, J, & Bros Ltd 226
Nweke, J E, & Sons Ltd 226
Nwonye, I O M, & Sons Company Ltd 227

O'Bahor, J A, & Company Ltd 227
Oban (Nigeria) Rubber Estates Ltd 227
Obanlearo Trading Company Ltd 227
Obaskeki, G I, & Sons Ltd 227
Obatraco Group of Companies 227
Obelawo Farcha Fishing Industries Ltd 227
Obiozo & Partners Power Construction
  Company Ltd 227
Ocean Inchcape (Nigeria) Ltd 227
Oceanic & Coastal Marine Ltd 228
Oceannering (Nigeria) Ltd 228
Ochumba Press Ltd 228
Odeco Ltd 228
Odeng Engineering Company Ltd 228
Odibo Akhigbe & Co Ltd 228
Odu'a Investment Company Ltd 228
Odus Bakeries 229
Odus Globe & Company Ltd 229
Odus Industries (Nigeria) Ltd 229
Odutola Nigerian Industries Ltd 229
Ofi Livestock Industries Ltd 229
Ogheneovo Ventures Ltd 229
OGT Group of Companies Ltd 229
Ogubule Industrial Printers Ltd 230
Oguejiofor, Alex, Company Ltd 230
Oguine Brothers 230
Ogunmefun Works Ltd 230
Ogunnire Modern Furniture (Nigeria)
  Ltd 230
Ohakwe & Associates (Nigeria) Ltd 230
Ohanenye & Sons Ltd 230
Ohuka Brothers Ltd 230
Oil Palm Company Ltd 230
Oil Supply Centre Ltd (OSC) 230
Ojeniyi, Adelegan, Trading Company
  Nigeria 230
Ojuri Maritime Services 231
Okada Bottling Company (Nigeria) Ltd 231
O.K.C. (Nigeria) Ltd 231
Okenabirhie Enterprises Ltd 231
Okitipupa Oil Palm Co Ltd 231
Okpe Mining Syndicate 231
Okunowo Brothers 231
Okwesa, John, Ltd 231
Okwuosa Mining Industry 231
Oladapo & Company Ltd 231
Olagbemiro, D O, & Co (Nigeria) Ltd 231
Olaiya Fagbamigbe Ltd 231
Olaogun Enterprises Ltd 231
Olashinde Brothers 232
Olatunde Laleye and Partners 232
Olau Olu Modern Bakery Ltd 232
Olawale Odeleye Associates 232
Oldmac Shipping Lines Nigeria Ltd 232
Olehson Brothers Company (Nigeria)
  Ltd 232
(Olehson's Agro Animal Kingdom) 232
Ollivant, G B, & Co (Nigeria) Ltd 232
Olokodana Group of Companies 232
Oloro Properties Ltd 232
Olu Holloway Nigeria Ltd 232
Olufawo Abayomi & Partners 232
Olumo Dunwo Commercial Enterprises
  Ltd 232
Olutone Electronics 233
Oluwakemi Motors & Finance
  Company Ltd 233
Oluwakemi (Swiss) Nigeria Embroidery
  Industries Ltd 233
Olympic Group Ltd 233
Omenjor & Ramsauer Electrical
  Company 233
Omo Group Organisation 233
Omo-Bare & Sons (Nigeria) Ltd 233
Omole, Lawrence, & Sons Ltd 233
Omole Motors Ltd 234
Omon Stores Ltd 234
Omot Fire Protection Engineering Ltd 234
Omotoso Pharmaceuticals Ltd 234
Omuna Construction Company
  (Nigeria) Ltd 234
Ondo State Investment Corporation 234
Oni Ernst & Whinney Lasebikan &
  Company 234
Onibonoje Press & Book Industries
  (Nig) Ltd 234
Onibudo, A, & Company Ltd 234
Onigbinde, M A, & Sons Ltd 235
Onise Polyware Ltd 235
Ono & Partners 235
Onochie Brothers & Sons Company
  Ltd 235
Onuselogu, C N, Enterprises Ltd 235
Onward Paper Mill Ltd 235

Onward Stationery Stores Ltd 235
Onyenakazi, I N, & Sons Company 235
Opukiri Constructions Company Ltd 235
Orazulike Trading Company Ltd 235
Oredola Okeya Trading Company Ltd 236
Oriwu Commercial Agency Ltd 236
Oroke Constructions Nigeria Ltd 236
Orthopaedic Supplies Ltd 236
Oruche, Joe, Trading Company Ltd 236
Orumokpo & Sons (Nigeria) Ltd 236
OSA Marine Services (Nigeria) Ltd 236
Osborne, E, Nigeria Ltd 236
Oscarte (Nigeria) Ltd 236
Osena Shipping Company Ltd 236
Oshinmi Company Ltd 236
Oshue Brothers & Company (Nigeria) Ltd 237
Oshunkeye Brothers (Nigeria) Ltd 237
Ositadinma International Ltd 237
Ososami, J F, & Co 237
Osot Associates Consulting Engineers 237
Otis of Nigeria Ltd 237
Ott-Attafua, A, & Company Ltd 237
Otto Wolff (Nigeria) & Company Ltd 238
Ovaltine (West Africa) Ltd 238
Ove Arup & Partners Nigeria Ltd 238
Overseas Commercial Agency 238
Overseas Technical Service (Nigeria) Ltd (OTS) 238
Owena Bank (Nigeria) Ltd 238
Owoyemi Motors & Finance Company Ltd 239
Oyebanji Building Materials Stores Ltd 239
Oyenuga, Deji, & Partners 239
Oyewumi, J O, & Co (Nigeria) Ltd 239
Oyinda Enterprises Ltd 239
Oyo State Investment and Credit Corporation 239
Oyun Breweries 239
Ozo Brothers Cabinet Works Ltd 239
P A Ibekwe Ltd 239
P Beccarelli & Co Ltd 239
P Comazzi 239
P R Sandwell & Co (Nigeria) Ltd 239
P S Mandrides & Co Ltd 239
P W Nigeria Ltd 239
Paas Industries (Nigeria) Company Ltd 240
Pabod Finance & Investment Company Ltd 240
Pabod Supplies Ltd 240
Pacific Printers Ltd 240
Paktank Nigeria Ltd 240
Palm Line Agencies (Nigeria) 240
Pamol (Nigeria) Ltd 240
Pan Africa Gas Distributors Ltd 240
Pan African Airlines (Nigeria) Ltd 241
Pan African Bank Ltd 241
Pan African Consultancy Services (Nigeria) Ltd 241
Pan African Holdings (Nigeria) Ltd 241
Pan African Supply Company Ltd 241
Pan African Surveys Ltd 241
Pan Atlantic Shipping & Transport Agencies Ltd 242
Pan Electric Ltd 242
Pan Industrial Estate Agencies 242
Pan Nigerian Agency 242
Pan Ocean Oil Corporation (Nigeria) 242
Panalpina World Transport (Nigeria) Ltd 242
Panav International Ltd 242
Pannel Fitzpatrick & Company 242
Paper Conversion Corporation (Nigeria) Ltd 242
Paper Sack (Nigeria) Ltd 243
Par Excellence (Nigeria) Ltd 243
Parke-Davis & Company (Nigeria) Ltd 243
Parkes, Josiah, & Sons (Nigeria) Ltd 243
Passat Industries Ltd 243
Paterson Zochonis Industries Ltd 243
Patrick George & Sons Ltd 243
Paty Import Company of Nigeria 243
Pearl & Dean (Nigeria) Ltd 244
Peat Marwick Ani, Ogunde & Company 244
Pecco Ltd 244
Pedro Lee Associates (Nigeria) Ltd 244
Pedro Trading Company Ltd 244
Peezone Freight Service Agency 244
Pegasus Industries (Nigeria) Ltd 244
Pem Ltd 244
Pencol International (Nigeria) Ltd 244
Pepsi Cola 244
Pestkill Nigeria Ltd 244
Peter Harrison Nigeria Ltd 245

Petraco, De, Industries Ltd 245
Petra-Monk Engineering & Contracting Company Ltd 245
Petroleum Consultants (Nigeria) Ltd 245
Petro-Organico (Nigeria) Ltd 245
Peugeot Automobile Nigeria Ltd 245
Pfizer Products Ltd 245
PGL Group Ltd 245
PGN Ltd 245
Pharchem Industries Ltd 247
Pharco (Nigeria) Ltd (Pharmaceutical Company of West Africa) 247
Pharma Dyn Chemical Products 247
Philip Morris Nigeria Ltd 247
Phillips Oil Company (Nigeria) Ltd 247
Phoebus Economides Rubber Industry Ltd 247
Phoenix Motors Ltd 247
Phoenix of Nigeria Assurance Company Ltd 247
Phonogram Ltd 248
Piccadilly Insurance Company Ltd 248
Piedmont Plywoods Nigeria Ltd 248
Pilgrim Books Ltd 248
(Pilgrim Books Ltd) 13
Pillars Nigeria Ltd 248
Pintoplane Nigeria Ltd 248
Pioneer Biscuit Factory Ltd 248
Pioneer Chemical Manufacturing Company (Nigeria) Ltd 248
Pioneer Metal Products Company Ltd 248
Pioneer Starch Industries (Nigeria) Ltd 248
Pipes Below Ground Ltd 248
Plasco Sheets (Nigeria) Ltd 249
Plastex Nigeria Ltd 249
Plastic and Engineering Works Ltd 249
Plastic Manufacturing Company Ltd (PMC) 249
Plasto-Crown (Nigeria) Ltd 249
Plateau Ceramics Industry Ltd (Jos) 249
Plateau Construction Ltd 249
Plateau Foods Processing Company Ltd 249
Plateau Hotels & Tourism Company Ltd 249
Plateau Investments Company Ltd 249
Plateau Publishing Company Ltd 250
Plateau Tourism, Development & Transport Co Ltd 250
Plesscomms Nigeria Ltd (Formerly Plessey (Nigeria) Ltd) 250
Plisson Fisko Nigeria Ltd 250
Poco Container Removals Ltd 250
Poco Minerals Ltd 250
Polamp (Nigeria) Ltd 250
Poletti Brothers & Co Ltd 250
Pollack, Sheldon L, (Nigeria) Ltd 251
Polly Pen & Ink Company (Nigeria) Ltd 251
Poloni & Company Ltd 251
Poly Products (Nigeria) Ltd 251
Polythene Enterprises (Nigeria) Ltd 251
Ponti & Company Ltd 251
Port & Marine Services Ltd 251
Port Express Services Ltd 251
Port Harcourt Flour Mills Ltd 251
Poultry & Animal Products (Nigeria) Ltd 251
Power & Communication Engineering Nigeria Ltd 251
Powerlines Ltd 252
Pracotrade (Nigeria) Ltd 252
PRC (Nigeria) Ltd 252
Premier Breweries Ltd 252
Premier Engineering Works Ltd 253
President Clothing Co Ltd 253
Pressed Metal Industry Ltd 253
Pressed Metal Works Ltd 253
Prestige Industries Ltd 253
Prestige Stores Nigeria Ltd 253
Prestrest Ltd 253
Preussag Drilling Engineers Nigeria Ltd 253
Price Waterhouse 253
Prideco - Projects & Industrial Equipment Co (Nigeria) Ltd 253
Primary Steel (Nigeria) Ltd 253
Prime Feathers International Services Ltd 254
Primus (Nigeria) Ltd 254
Princegate Trading & Contracting Company Ltd 254
Principal Bookshop & Commercial Stores Ltd 254
Professional and Manufacturing Services (Nigeria) Ltd 254

Progress Contracts Ltd 254
Progress Enterprises 254
Progressive Insurance Company Ltd 254
Project Management Ltd 254
Project Textile Mill (Nigeria) Ltd 255
Promana Associates 255
Promexport International (Nigeria) Ltd 255
Prudent Finance Ltd 255
Pukke, Horst, & Co (Nigeria) Ltd 255
Pump Services Nigeria Ltd 255
Punch (Nigeria) Ltd 255
Pureway Corporation of Nigeria Ltd 255
Pyramid Paper Products Ltd 255
R & A Services (Division of UAC of Nigeria Ltd) 256
R I Erhahon & Co Ltd 256
R Rajendram and Associates 256
R T Briscoe (Nigeria) Ltd 256
Raabe Sanitary and Water Engineering 256
Rabiu, Isiyaku, & Sons Ltd 256
Raccaform Ltd 256
Raccah & Chaker Factory Ltd 256
Radiators Nigeria Ltd 256
Radio Communications (Nigeria) Ltd 256
Radio Vision Centre (Nigeria) Ltd 257
Rajendram, R, and Associates 257
Raji Bakeries Ltd 257
Raleigh Industries (Nigeria) Ltd 257
Ramonu Alabi, S B, & Company 257
Ramson Mellamby & Company Ltd 257
Rank Xerox (Nigeria) Ltd 257
Rapid Electrical & Mechanical Company Nigeria Ltd (REMCO) 257
Raycon & Company (Nigeria) Ltd 259
Raymond Constructors (Nigeria) Ltd 259
REA Real Property Investments (Nigeria) Ltd 259
Reckitt & Colman (Nigeria) Ltd 259
Record Manufacturers of Nigeria Ltd 259
Record Market (Nigeria) Ltd 259
Regency (Overseas) Company Ltd 259
Regent Hotel 259
Reggio Builders Ltd 259
Rehau Plastiks (Nigeria) Ltd 260
Reiss & Co (Nigeria) Ltd 260
Reliance Business Consultations 260
Reliance Group of Companies 260
Reliance International (Nigeria) Ltd 260
Renaissance Assurance Company Ltd 260
Renaissance Marble Works Ltd 260
Rendezvous Group Hotels (Nigeria) Ltd 261
Rex Radio Electronic Company Ltd 261
Reynolds Construction Company (Nigeria) Ltd 261
Rhine-Schelde-Verolme Engineers 261
Ribway Group of Companies 261
Ribway Tyre Retreading Co Ltd 261
Richard Riko (Nigeria) Ltd 261
Richas Engineering Works Company Ltd 261
Rida Construction Company Ltd 261
Rida National Distributors Ltd 261
Rida National Plastics Ltd 262
Rimax Computer Services Ltd 262
Rioco (Nigeria) Ltd 262
Risonpalm Ltd 262
Rivbank Insurance Company Ltd 262
Rivers State Newspaper Corporation 263
Rivers State Tourist & Hotel Corporation 263
Rivers State Transport Corporation 263
Rivers Vegetable Oil Company Ltd 263
Roaag Company (Nigeria) Ltd 263
Road and General Construction Company Ltd 263
Roads Nigeria Ltd 263
Roberts, T L, & Company Ltd 263
Robertson, H H, (Nigeria) Ltd 264
Robins, A H, International Company Ltd 264
Roche (Nigeria) Ltd 264
Rod Publicity Ltd 264
Rokana Industries Ltd 264
Romain, H W, & Son Ltd 264
Ron Mining and Development Company Ltd 264
Ronke Commercial Enterprises 264
Roomans Eneli Flynn & Company 264
Roro Terminal Company (Nigeria) Ltd 264
Rosaab Industrial Design Ltd 264
Rotag Assurance Company Ltd 265
Rotimi & Sons Ltd 265
Roussel (Nigeria) Ltd 265
Royal Exchange Assurance (Nigeria) Ltd 265

Rubery Owen Fasteners (Nigeria) Ltd 265
Runsewe Group of Companies 265
Rutam Ltd 265
S & K Asbestos Products Ltd 265
S A Ijagbemi & Sons (Nigeria) Ltd 266
S B Bakare & Brothers Ltd 266
S B Ramonu Alabi & Company 266
S G Bonomi Ltd 266
S N Ezennwa & Sons Ltd 266
S S Adejoro & Company Ltd 266
Sabon Sara Nigeria Ltd 266
Safa Splints Ltd 266
Safni Ltd 266
Sage Constructions (Nigeria) Ltd 266
Saipem Nigeria Ltd 266
Sakpoba Rubber Estate 266
Salleh, Alhaji Baba M, & Sons (Nigeria) Ltd 266
Salzgitter (WA) Ltd 266
Sammy & Sons Contracts & Stores 266
Sams Agencies & Maritime Service (Nig) 266
Samsung (Nigeria) Ltd 267
Sandoz (Nigeria) Ltd 267
Sandwell, P R, & Co (Nigeria) Ltd 267
Sanmi Breweries Ltd 267
Santa Fe Nigeria Development Company Ltd 267
Santana Furniture Factory Ltd 267
Sanusi Brothers (Nigeria) Ltd 267
Sanyo (Nigeria) Ltd 267
SAO Engineering Company Ltd 268
Satt Construction (Nigeria) Ltd 268
Savanna Press Ltd 268
Savannah Bank of Nigeria Ltd 268
Savannah Precast Concrete & Terrazo Industries Ltd 268
Savannah Sugar Company Ltd 269
Savoia, A 269
Sawyerr Enterprises (Nigeria) Ltd 269
Saybolt (Nigeria) Ltd 269
SB Shipping & Trading Agencies Ltd 269
Scan African Nigeria Ltd 269
Scano (Nigeria) Enterprises Ltd 269
Scansila Contracting Company Ltd 269
Scantravel Ltd 269
SCEI 270
Schlumberger (Nigeria) Ltd 270
Schroeder, H F, (WA) Ltd 270
Scoa lard - a Division of Scoa Nigeria Ltd 270
Scoa Motors (Nigeria) Ltd 270
Scoa Nigeria Ltd 270
Scoagri 270
Scoatrac (A Division of Scoa (Nigeria) Ltd) 270
Scobi Associates 271
Sea Dantainer Lines Ltd 271
Sea Trucks (Nigeria) Ltd 271
Sebo Technical Industries Nigeria Ltd 271
Secom Ltd 271
Sedco Nigeria Ltd 271
Seepc (Nigeria) Ltd 271
Segun International Group Ltd 272
Sehl International 272
Seismograph Service (Nigeria) Ltd (SSL) 272
Selwood Pumps 272
Sem Steels (Nigeria) Ltd 272
Sem-Edo Wire Industries Ltd 272
Senn-Sound (West Africa) Ltd 272
Sentinel Assurance Company Ltd 272
Sentrycom Alarms (Nigeria) Ltd 273
Sepi Estero Consultants (Nigeria) Ltd 273
Sera Printing Ltd 273
Service & Supply Company of West Africa Ltd (SASCO) 273
Servo Nigerian Enterprises Ltd 273
Seswa, Steel and Engineering Services (WA) Ltd 273
Seven-up Bottling Company Ltd 273
Seward, A J, (A Division of UAC of Nigeria Ltd) 273
SGE Nigeria Ltd 273
Shalhoub Brothers Ltd 274
Shawmont Nigeria Ltd 274
Shekoni Industries Nigeria Ltd 274
Sheldon L Pollack (Nigeria) Ltd 274
Shell Petroleum Development Company of Nigeria Ltd 274
Sheva (WA) Ltd 274
Shittu, Alhaji M R, & Sons Ltd 274
Sho's Engineering Company Ltd 274
Shour Industrial Enterprises Ltd 274

Siab Engineering Company Nigeria Ltd 274
Siej Agencies 274
Silverball Integrated Engineering Co Nigeria Ltd 274
Siram Industrial Products Ltd 275
Sketch Publishing Company Ltd 275
Skoup & Co Ltd 275
Smeaton Ltd 275
Smith Kline & French Nigeria Ltd 276
Snamprogetti 276
SNC (Nigeria) Ltd 276
Sobat Ltd 276
Soccer Chewing Gum Enterprises Ltd 276
Socea (Nigeria) Ltd 277
Societe Generale Bank (Nigeria) Ltd 277
Sodangi Enterprises 277
Sodik-Asea (Nigeria) Ltd 277
Sodipo, Harold, & Co Ltd 277
Sointeco (Nigeria) Ltd 277
Sokoto Furniture Factory Ltd 277
Solel Boneh (Nigeria) Ltd 277
Solus Schall (Nigeria) Ltd 278
Somit (Nigeria) Ltd (Formerly United Asian Traders (Nigeria) Ltd) 278
Sona Breweries Ltd 278
Songhai Construction Ltd 278
Songhai Group of Companies 278
Songhai Ltd 278
Soprog Construction Ltd 278
South Chad Ltd 279
South Pacific Chemical & Plastics Engineering Company Ltd 279
Southeastern Drilling Co (Nigeria) Ltd (SEDCO) 279
Special Structures & Company Ltd 279
Speco Mill Textiles Ltd 279
Speed-Bird Clearing and Forwarding Agency Ltd 279
Spicers (Nigeria) Ltd 279
Spiropoulos, F G, & Company Ltd 279
Sporty Fancy & General Stores Ltd 279
Squibb (Nigeria) Ltd 279
Stabilini & Visinoni Ltd 280
Stabilini, B, & Company Ltd 280
Stag Engineering Nigeria Ltd 280
Standard Breweries (Nigeria) Ltd 280
Standard Construction Ltd 280
Standard Industrial Development Company Ltd 280
Star Match Company Ltd 280
Star Sweets Co Ltd 280
Starline Nigeria Ltd 280
State Plastics Design Company 281
Steel Works Ltd 281
Steiner, F, & Company Ltd 281
Stephens, Henry, Engineering Company Ltd 281
Stephens, Henry, Group of Companies 281
Sterling Products (Nigeria) Ltd 281
Steyr Nigeria Ltd 281
Stirling Civil Engineering Nigeria Ltd 282
Stokvis (Nigeria) Ltd 282
Storm (Nigeria) Ltd 282
Strabag Construction (Nigeria) Ltd 282
Stronghold (Nigeria) Ltd 282
Structec 282
Structeng Associates 283
Structor 283
Structural Steel Works Ltd 283
Studio Press (Nigeria) Ltd 283
Subetra Nigeria Industries Ltd 283
Sun Insurance Office (Nigeria) Ltd 283
Sunflag Knitting Mills (Nigeria) Ltd 283
Sunfresh Brewery Company Nigeria Ltd 284
Sungas Company Ltd 284
Sunny Stationery Supply & Bookshop 284
Sunshine Batteries Manufacturing Company 284
Superbru Ltd 284
Superfine Furniture & Trading Company Ltd 284
Superform Africa Company Ltd 285
Superior Systems International Ltd 285
Sutherland, B K, & Company Ltd 285
Sverdrup & Parcel & Associates 285
Swenig Furniture Company Ltd 285
Swiss Nigerian Chemical Company Ltd 285
Swiss Nigerian Wood Industries Ltd 285
Syndivel Plastic Industry Nigeria Ltd 285
T A Braithwaite (Insurance Brokers) & Co 285
T A Hammond Projects Ltd 285
T L Roberts & Company Ltd 285

Tabansi Motors Ltd 286
Tadat Engineering Company Ltd 286
Taike & Brothers Ltd 286
Taiwo Ajai Communications 286
Take Your Choice Record Stores Ltd 286
Takko Engineering Ltd 286
Tamaco Ltd 286
Tara Consulting Nigeria Ltd 286
Tarmac Engineering Company Ltd 286
Tarpaulin Industries (WA) Ltd 286
Tasius Nigeria Ltd 286
Tate & Lyle (Nigeria) Ltd 286
Taylor Woodrow of Nigeria Ltd 287
Taylorbird Fabric & Design Ltd 287
Techint Engineering (Nigeria) Ltd 287
Techjob Associates 287
Technae (Nigeria) Ltd 287
Technical & Building Materials Ltd 287
Technical Constructions (Nigeria) Ltd 287
Technophon Electrical Enterprises Company Ltd 288
Teddy Continental Company 288
Teju Industries Ltd 288
Telerex Electronics Ltd 288
Telota Cosmetics Company Nigeria Ltd 288
Templar Afrique (Nigeria) Ltd 288
Tenimasunwon Agency 288
Tenneco Oil Company of Nigeria 288
Tetengi, Alhaji Usman, & Sons Ltd 288
Texaco Nigeria Ltd 288
Texas Overseas (Nigeria) Petroleum Co (TOPCON) 289
Textile Commodities Ltd 289
Textile Utilities Manufacturing Ltd 289
Theo & Theo Paints Company (Nigeria) Ltd 289
Thermocool Engineering Company Ltd 289
Thermostein Ltd 289
Things International (Nigeria) Ltd 289
Thomade Enterprises (Nig) Ltd 289
Thomas Ademola & Co Ltd 289
Thomas Furniture Company Ltd 289
Thomas, J A, Rubber Estates Ltd 289
Thomas Mechanical Plumbing 289
Thompson Dickson Technical Co Ltd 289
Thoresen & Company (Nigeria) Ltd 290
Tidex Nigeria Ltd 290
Tilbury Contracting Co (Nigeria) Ltd 290
Tilla International Ltd 290
Tilley Gyado Group of Companies 290
Times Leisure Services Ltd 290
Times Press Ltd 290
Timmy Printing Press 290
Tin & Associated Minerals Ltd 290
Tomax-Beton Construction Company Ltd 290
Tommy Building & Construction Company Ltd 291
Topaz (Nigeria) Ltd 291
Topic Ltd 291
Toronto Organisation (Nigeria) Ltd 291
Total Nigeria Ltd 291
Tourist Company of Nigeria Ltd 291
Tower Aluminium (Nigeria) Ltd 291
Toyin Rising Bakery 292
Toyo Menka Kaisha Ltd 292
Tractor & Equipment 292
Tractors Under-Carriage Industry Nigeria Ltd 292
Tradev Ltd 292
Tradewinds Express (Nigeria) Ltd 292
Tradon Nigeria Ltd 292
Trans Atlantic Shipping Agency Ltd 292
Trans Nigeria Road Haulage Ltd 293
Trans Nigeria Trading and Industrial Co Ltd 293
Trans-Africa Engineering Ltd 293
Transcap Ltd 293
Transelek Nigeria Ltd 293
Transex & Company Ltd 293
Transmarco Agencies (Nigeria) Ltd 293
Transworld Drilling Company Ltd 294
Trebor (Nigeria) Ltd 294
Trevi Foundations Nigeria Ltd 294
Triana Ltd 294
Trianon Shipping & Chartering Ltd 294
Trindel (Nigeria) Ltd 295
Triplex Safety Glass (Nigeria) Ltd 295
Triumph (Nigeria) Ltd 295
Tropical Tarpaulin Industry (Nigeria) Ltd 295
TSMPE (Tsvetmetpromexport) 295
TSTC Coastal Agency 295

Tudor Batteries (Nigeria) Ltd   295
Tuntaric Nigeria Ltd   295
Turners Building Products (Arewa) Ltd   295
Turners Building Products (Emene) Ltd   297
Turners Engineering Products (Nigeria) Ltd   297
Twilights Nigeria Ltd   297
Twz (Nigeria) Ltd   297
U Maduka Enterprises (Nigeria) Ltd   297
UAC of Nigeria Ltd   297
Uba, C, & Brothers Trading Company (WA) Ltd   297
Uche, A O, & Sons (Nigeria) Ltd   299
Ugbabe Furniture & Construction Company Ltd   299
Ugochukwu and Sons Ltd   299
Ugochukwu Chemical Industries Ltd   301
Ukawoods Enterprises Nigeria Ltd   301
Ukpilla Cement Company Ltd   301
Umarco (Nigeria) Ltd   301
Umaru, Lawan & Sons Ltd   301
Umerah Commercial Agency Ltd   301
Uncle Fado and Sons Furniture Factory Ltd   301
Unibuilder Industries Ltd   301
Unico Stores   301
Unigwe, Fred Balonwu, Group of Companies   302
Unije, B C, & Sons Ltd   302
Union Bank of Nigeria Ltd   302
Union Beverages Ltd   302
Union Builders Company Ltd   302
Union Carbide (Nigeria) Ltd   302
Union Construction Company Ltd   302
Unipetrol Nigeria Ltd   302
Unique Trading Co Ltd   303
Unisteel Works Ltd   303
United African Drug Co (Nig) Ltd   303
United Arewa Chemists Ltd   303
United Bank for Africa Ltd   303
United Consolidated Industries Ltd   305
United Development Trading Company Ltd   305
United Educational Supplies Ltd   305
United Geophysical (Nigeria) Ltd   305
United Match Company of Nigeria Ltd   305
United Nigeria Insurance Company Ltd (The)   305
United Nigeria Motors Ltd   305
United Nigerian Textiles Ltd   305
United Technology (Nigeria) Ltd   307
Unity Life and Fire Insurance Company Ltd   307
Unity Soap Manufacturers Ltd   307
Universal Distributors Ltd   307
Universal Educational Supplies Ltd (Morison Arnold Ltd)   308
Universal Fishing Company Ltd   308
Universal Insurance Company Ltd   308
Universal Monolithic Bearing Structure Ltd   308
Universal Packaging (Nigeria) Ltd   308
Universal Steels Ltd   308
Universal Textile Industries Ltd   309
Universal Vulcanizing Company Nigeria Ltd   309
Universal Welding & Construction Company Ltd   309
University of Ife Press Ltd   309
University Press Ltd   310
Uoo Trading Company Ltd   310
Upjohn Nigeria Pty Ltd   310
Urbahn, Max O, International Ltd   310
Urban Engineers   310
Uren Construction Engineering Company Ltd   310
Urobo Agencies (Nigeria) Ltd   310
Utagba-Uno Rubber Estates Ltd   310
UTC Nigeria Ltd (Formerly Union Trading Company of Nigeria Ltd)   311
Utilgas Nigerian and Overseas Gas Company Ltd   311
Uwai and Sons Enterprises   311
Valid Assurance Company Ltd   311
Valley Foods Nigeria Ltd   311
Van Leer Containers (Nigeria) Ltd   312
Vanni Holdings Ltd   312
Varaman Industries (Nigeria) Ltd   312
Vegetable & Fruit Processing Ltd   312
Vegetable Oils (Nigeria) Ltd   312
Ven Hotels Ltd   312
Ventures, Coopers Benly, & Company Ltd (The)   313
Vercon (Nigeria) Ltd   313

Veritas Insurance Company Ltd   313
Versata Enterprises & Merchants Trust Ltd   313
Vic-Adun & Sons Ltd   313
Vicinanza Construction Ltd   313
Vickins (Nigeria) Associates   313
Viktors, N, International Agencies   313
Village Gate & Company Ltd   313
Vinben (Nigeria) Ltd   313
Vincenti Engineering Ltd   313
Vitafoam Nigeria Ltd   313
Vitalink Pharmaceutical Industries Ltd   314
VK Plastiks & Marble Co   314
Volkswagen of Nigeria Ltd   314
Volvo Ltd   314
Vono Products Ltd   314
Voss & Umlauft Nigeria Ltd   314
VP (Nigeria) Ltd   315
VYB (Nigeria) Ltd   315
W F Clarke (Nigeria) Ltd   315
W J Bush & Company (Nigeria) Ltd   315
W W Whyte & Co Ltd   315
Wahler, Josef, (Nig) Ltd   315
Walter Clarke & Sons (Overseas) Ltd   315
Walton Solomon & Associates   315
Ward, Ashcroft & Parkman (Nigeria) Ltd   315
Warmac Products Ltd   315
Warri Mining Syndicate   315
Wasco Ropes Ltd   315
Wata Timber Company Ltd   316
Waterglass Boatyard & Steel Construction Ltd   316
Watson & Sons (Electro-Medical) Nigeria Ltd   316
Wayne (West Africa) Ltd   316
Weatherford (Nigeria) Ltd   316
Weide & Co (Group of Companies) Ltd   316
Welfare Pharmaceuticals Ltd   316
Wellcome Nigeria Ltd   316
Wellyplates   317
Wema Bank Ltd   317
Wemabod Estates Ltd   317
West Africa Household Utilities Manufacturing Company (Nigeria) Ltd   317
West Africa Milk Company (Nigeria) Ltd   317
West Africa Offshore Ltd   317
West African Aluminium Products (Nigeria)   317
West African Automobile & Engineering Company Ltd (WAATECO)   317
West African Batteries Ltd   317
West African Breweries Ltd   317
West African Chemical Company Ltd (WACHEM)   318
West African Cold Storage Co of Nigeria Ltd   318
West African Distillers Ltd   318
West African Drug Company Ltd   318
West African Engineering Company Nigeria Ltd (WAECO)   318
West African Glass Industry Ltd   318
West African Portland Cement Company Ltd   318
West African Provincial Insurance Company Ltd   319
West African Shipping Agency (Nigeria) Ltd   319
West African Shrimps Ltd   319
West African Surveys Ltd   319
West African Thread Company Ltd   319
West African Trades Corporation Ltd   319
West African Tyre Retreading Company Ltd   319
West Construction Company Ltd   319
West, John, Publications Ltd   319
Westend Engineering Ltd   320
Western Nigeria Tarpaulin Industries Ltd   320
Western Nigerian Technical Co Ltd   320
Western Steel Works   320
Western Textile Industries Company Ltd   320
Western Textile Mills Ltd   320
Westminster Dredging (Nigeria) Ltd   320
Westminster Offshore (Nigeria) Ltd   320
Whessoe Engineering Ltd   320
Whipstock (Nigeria) Ltd   321
White, Johnson, United Ltd   321
Whyte, W W, & Co Ltd   321
Widnell and Trollope Nigeria   321

Wiedemann & Walters (Nigeria) Ltd   321
Wiggins Teape West Africa Ltd   321
Williams International (Nig) Ltd   321
Wilmer Industries Nigeria Ltd   322
Wimpey, George, & Co (Nigeria) Ltd   322
Wimpey-Brown & Root (Nigeria) Ltd   322
Witt & Busch (Shipyard) Ltd   322
Woclif (Nigeria) Ventures   322
Woermann, C, (Nigeria) Ltd   322
Wolff, Otto, (Nigeria) & Company Ltd   322
Woollen & Synthetic Textile Manufacturing Ltd   322
World Courier Nigeria Ltd   323
Woven Textiles Ltd   323
Wozabeth Trading Company   323
Wrought Iron (Nigeria) Ltd   323
Wyatt, Thomas, Nigeria Ltd   323
Wyeth Nigeria Ltd   323
Yassin Confectionery & Sweet Company Ltd   323
Yerima Hamman Wabi, Alhaji, & Sons   323
Yinkus Book Centre Ltd   323
Yodesons (Nigeria) Ltd   323
Yondav Petrocomplex Ltd   324
Young, Arthur, Osindero & Co   324
Yusufu Modern Industries Co   324
Zabadne & Company Ltd   324
Zamfara Textile Industries Ltd   324
Zang, D B   324
Zapata Marine Service (Nigeria) Ltd   324
Zard, C, & Company Ltd   324
Zarmaganda Tin Mines Ltd   324
Zartech Ltd   324
Zawang Mining Company   324
Zelan Mining Company Ltd   324
Zenith Containers Company Ltd   324
Zerolas Batteries Company Ltd   324

Index to Business Activities

Accountants & Lawyers

Allwell Brown and Company	21
Arthur Andersen & Company	29
Ernst & Whinney, Oni, Lasebikan & Company	93
Pannel Fitzpatrick & Company	242
Peat Marwick Ani, Ogunde & Company	244
Price Waterhouse	253
Young, Arthur, Osindero & Co	324

Agents and general trading companies

Adefusika Trading Company Ltd	7
Adejobi, Adeoye, Trading Stores Ltd	7
Adejumo Fam (Nigeria) Ltd	7
Adetona Awe (Nig) Enterprises	8
Adetunji, Madebayo, & Sons Ltd	8
Adetunji Olokodana & Co	8
Afro Continental Nigeria Ltd	13
Aka and Sons (Nigeria) Ltd	16
Akande Trading Co Nigeria Ltd	16
Akanji, D L, & Co (Nig) Ltd	16
Akinadod Akinloye Aboderin Ltd	16
Akpenlamen Co Ltd	17
Akwiwu Motors Ltd	17
Alalade Group of Companies	18
Alex L M Davou Fom & Sons Enterprise Ltd	18
Allied Trading Co Ltd	21
Amass Nigeria Ltd	23
Americo Ltd	24
Anglo-French Trading Co Ltd	25
Anglo-German Company (Intercontinental) Ltd	25
Aparaki Enterprises	25
Aratah, Josman, Trading Company	26
Arbor Services Nigeria Ltd	26
Arewa United Stores Ltd	28
Asani (Nigeria) Trading Co	29
Associated Exports (W.A.) Ltd	31
Atlantic Mercantile Co Ltd	32
Atssco Abbey Office Machine Service Stationery (Nig) Ltd	32
B & F Nigeria Ltd	34
Babafunke, Adeola, Overseas Trading Company	34
Bakrin Enterprises Ltd	35
Balogun, A A, & Sons (Nigeria) Ltd	35
Bao Nigeria Ltd	36
Barshall, F M, (West Africa) Ltd	37
Bayer (Nigeria) Ltd	37
Bode International Nig Agencies	45
Bolex Enterprises	45
Boma Associates (WA) Ltd	45
Bono International Ltd	45
Botam (Nigeria) Ltd	46
Breckwoldt & Co (Nigeria) Ltd	47
Business & Industrial Consultants	50
Business Equipment & Machinery Ltd (BEAM) (Division of UAC of Nigeria Ltd)	50
Cepuz International Agencies	55
Chami, A B, & Co Ltd	57
Charlie and Franco Ltd	57
Chellaram, K, & Sons (Nigeria) Ltd	57
Chemdyes Nigeria Ltd	58
Chiakwelu, A I, & Brothers	59
Christlieb, A C, (Nigeria) Ltd	59
Citymark (West Africa) Ltd	62
Clarke, W F, (Nigeria) Ltd	62
Clarke, Walter, & Sons (Overseas) Ltd	62

Commonwealth Commodity Company International	64
Compagnie Francaise de l'Afrique Internationale	65
Contex Nigeria Ltd	66
Continental & General Merchants Ltd	66
Conveyancer (Nigeria) Ltd	67
Cornbrough Products (Nigeria) Ltd	69
Cunix Industrial & Commercial Co Ltd	71
Daltrade (Nigeria) Ltd	73
Damdavy & Company	74
Deazula Trading Company (Nigeria) Ltd	76
Desam Development Company Ltd	78
Deutsche Kaiser Gruppe (Interkontinental)	78
Dhanamall & Co (Nigeria) Ltd	78
Dokunmu, M A, & Sons Ltd	80
Domino Stores Ltd	80
Dubic International Ltd	83
Eagle Group Ltd	84
Eastern General Contractors Ltd	85
Ebun Oluwa Group of Companies	85
Eddymay Enterprises	85
Edemscot Engerprises Nigeria Ltd	85
Egbema Enterprises Ltd (EEL)	86
Ejinkeonye, L E, Brothers Trading Co Ltd	87
Ejire Halleluih Trading Co Ltd	87
Electronics Instrumentations Ltd	90
Emanento Company Agency	90
Emos Dynamics Co (Nigeria) Ltd	91
Endurance Ltd	92
Erhahon, R I, & Co Ltd	93
ETAM	95
Evian Africa Co Ltd	95
Fanz Holdings Ltd	96
Far East Mercantile Co Ltd	97
Fas Brothers Ltd	97
Fatmok Associates	97
Femce Marketing Company	98
Ferdinand Enterprises (Nigeria) Ltd	99
Fisayo Holdings Ltd	100
Folam International Trading Company	102
Formerly Mitsui & Co (Nigeria) Ltd	166
Fredano Trading Co Ltd	103
Fubara Enterprises Ltd	105
Gaby and Company (Nigeria)	106
Gloede & Hoff (Nigeria) Ltd	111
Gobecco Trading Company Ltd	111
H B & Sons	117
Harrison, Peter, Nigeria Ltd	120
Harriteds International Company (Nigeria) Ltd	121
Hoek (Nig) Ltd	123
Holt, John, Ltd	123
Home & Overseas Trading Company Ltd	123
Ibadan City Motors (Nigeria) Ltd	126
Ibe, A W, & Co Ltd	126
Ibekwe, P A, Ltd	126
Iguh, C O, and Sons Trading Co (Nigeria) Ltd	128
Ijagbemi, S A, & Sons (Nigeria) Ltd	128
Inaco Ltd	129
Indian Bazaar (Nigeria) Ltd	129
Inlaks Ltd	130
International Agencies Ltd	131
International Trade (WA) Ltd	134
Itidal-Epid Enterprises of Nigeria	136
Jafco Impex Ltd	137
JBL Star Trading Company	138
Jemine Enterprises Ltd	138
Jobba Trading Company	139
Joelson & Sons Holdings	139
Johnson Foluso International Enterprises (JOFI)	139
Kano Merchants Trading Co Ltd	143
Kole-James & Co Ltd	148

Koloko Imports & Exports Co Ltd	149
Kunza Heed (W.A.) Enterprises	150
Lanlek (Nigeria) Associates	152
Lanray & Sons	152
Lawal Araromi Commercial Stores	153
Lawan Schutte & Co (Nigeria) Ltd	153
Lilleshall (Nigeria) Ltd	155
Litigo Enterprises (Nigeria) Ltd	157
Lonogu Enterprises Ltd	157
Lowu International (Nigeria) Ltd	158
Maas (Nigeria) Ltd	158
Madona Organisation Ltd	159
Maduka, U, Enterprises (Nigeria) Ltd	159
Mai-Nasara & Sons Ltd	160
Mainland Bros Ltd	160
Majek Soetan Industries Enterprises	160
Majem Trading Company	160
Makella & Partners	161
Mala, Alhaji Zanna K, & Sons Company	161
Management Enterprises Ltd	161
Manufacturing & Marketing Co (Nig) Ltd	162
Marghi Enterprises Ltd	163
Maritime Associates (International) Ltd	164
Maritime Stores Ltd	164
Markdealers (Nigeria) Ltd	164
Mas-Chrisco and Associates	165
Matco Agencies	165
Matsons (Nigeria) Enterprises	166
Mbata, Sam, & Company Ltd	166
MBK Nigeria Ltd	166
Medac (Nigeria) Ltd	167
Medal Brothers Co Ltd	167
Memudu Arowolo & Brothers	167
Mereoleh Brothers Co (Nigeria) Ltd	168
Midland Supplies Ltd	171
Misr (Nigeria) Ltd	172
Missri, A J, & Co Ltd	172
Misting Everhot	173
Mocci, E, Associates	173
Morin International Group Ltd	176
Morin, J, & Co	176
Nabena, Benjamin, Nabenson Promotions	178
New Africa Development Company Ltd	188
NFS (Food and Cold Storage) Ltd	190
Nichedos and Company Ltd	190
Niger Agencies International (Nigeria) Ltd	191
Niger Raw Materials Ltd	192
Nigerian Merchants & Produce Suppliers	210
Nigerian Modern Stores Ltd	211
Nigerian Ropes Ltd	215
Nkwonta, D O, & Sons Enterprises Ltd	222
Nobgroup of Companies	222
Nordstahl (Nigeria) Ltd	222
Normann, C, International Company	223
Nwandu, D A, & Sons Enterprises Ltd	226
Nweke, J E, & Sons Ltd	226
Odeco Ltd	228
Odeng Engineering Company Ltd	228
Odus Globe & Company Ltd	229
OGT Group of Companies Ltd	229
Oguejiofor, Alex, Company Ltd	230
Ohanenye & Sons Ltd	230
Ohuka Brothers Ltd	230
Ojeniyi, Adelegan, Trading Company Nigeria	230
Okunowo Brothers	231
Olagbemiro, D O, & Co (Nigeria) Ltd	231
Olaogun Enterprises Ltd	231
Olashinde Brothers	232
Olehson Brothers Company (Nigeria) Ltd	232
(Olehson's Agro Animal Kingdom)	232
Ollivant, G B, & Co (Nigeria) Ltd	232
Olokodana Group of Companies	232

Olumo Dunwo Commercial Enterprises
Ltd 232
Olympic Group Ltd 233
Omon Stores Ltd 234
Onigbinde, M A, & Sons Ltd 235
Onochie Brothers & Sons Company
Ltd 235
Onuselogu, C N, Enterprises Ltd 235
Onyenakazi, I N, & Sons Company 235
Orazulike Trading Company Ltd 235
Oredola Okeya Trading Company Ltd 236
Orumokpo & Sons (Nigeria) Ltd 236
Ositadinma International Ltd 237
Ott-Attafua, A, & Company Ltd 237
Overseas Commercial Agency 238
Oyewumi, J O, & Co (Nigeria) Ltd 239
Paas Industries (Nigeria) Company Ltd 240
Pan African Consultancy Services
(Nigeria) Ltd 241
Pan African Holdings (Nigeria) Ltd 241
Pan African Supply Company Ltd 241
Pan Industrial Estate Agencies 242
Panav International Ltd 242
Paty Import Company of Nigeria 243
Pedro Lee Associates (Nigeria) Ltd 244
Pedro Trading Company Ltd 244
Fem Ltd 244
Piedmont Plywoods Nigeria Ltd 248
Pintoplane Nigeria Ltd 248
Pracotrade (Nigeria) Ltd 252
Prime Feathers International Services
Ltd 254
Princegate Trading & Contracting
Company Ltd 254
Progress Enterprises 254
Promexport International (Nigeria) Ltd 255
Pukke, Horst, & Co (Nigeria) Ltd 255
Rabiu, Isiyaku, & Sons Ltd 256
Ramson Mellamby & Company Ltd 257
Reckitt & Colman (Nigeria) Ltd 259
Roaag Company (Nigeria) Ltd 263
Ronke Commercial Enterprises 264
Runsewe Group of Companies 265
Sammy & Sons Contracts & Stores 266
Sams Agencies & Maritime Service
(Nig) 266
Samsung (Nigeria) Ltd 267
SB Shipping & Trading Agencies Ltd 269
Scansila Contracting Company Ltd 269
Schroeder, H F, (WA) Ltd 270
Scoa Nigeria Ltd 270
Segun International Group Ltd 272
Sheva (WA) Ltd 274
Shour Industrial Enterprises Ltd 274
Somit (Nigeria) Ltd (Formerly United
Asian Traders (Nigeria) Ltd) 278
Songhai Group of Companies 278
Sporty Fancy & General Stores Ltd 279
Stephens, Henry, Group of Companies 281
Stronghold (Nigeria) Ltd 282
Tamaco Ltd 286
Tetengi, Alhaji Usman, & Sons Ltd 288
Topaz (Nigeria) Ltd 291
Tradon Nigeria Ltd 292
Trans Nigeria Trading and Industrial
Co Ltd 293
Uba, C, & Brothers Trading Company
(WA) Ltd 297
Uche, A O, & Sons (Nigeria) Ltd 299
Ugochukwu and Sons Ltd 299
Umaru, Lawan & Sons Ltd 301
Unique Trading Co Ltd 303
United Development Trading Company
Ltd 305
Urobo Agencies (Nigeria) Ltd 310
Uwai and Sons Enterprises 311
Versata Enterprises & Merchants Trust
Ltd 313
Vic-Adun & Sons Ltd 313
Viktors, N, International Agencies 313
VP (Nigeria) Ltd 315
Wayne (West Africa) Ltd 316
Wiedemann & Walters (Nigeria) Ltd 321
Woclif (Nigeria) Ventures 322
Wozabeth Trading Company 323
Yerima Hamman Wabi, Alhaji, & Sons 323
Yodesons (Nigeria) Ltd 323

Agricultural equipment and services

Acim 6
Adamu Management International 6
Adebowale Electrical Industries Ltd 6
Adefusika Trading Company Ltd 7
Adejumo Fam (Nigeria) Ltd 7
Advance (Nig) Ltd 8
Afro Commerce (WA) Ltd 13
Afrotec Technical Services Nigeria Ltd 14
Agribuild Nigeria Ltd 14
Agricultural Development Corporation
(Anambra State) 14
Agrotec Services Ltd 15
Ajao, J A, Brothers 15
Alfa-Laval (Nigeria) Ltd 19
Aparaki Enterprises 25
Ashamu, E O, & Sons (Holdings) Ltd 29
B & F Nigeria Ltd 34
Bedkana (Nig) Ltd 38
Berliet Nigeria Ltd 41
Bewac Automotive Products Ltd 41
Blackwood Hodge (Nigeria) Ltd 44
Briscoe, R T, (Nigeria) Ltd 49
Camplant Engineering Sales & Service
Ltd 52
CFAO (Nigeria) Ltd 56
Chukwurah Agriculture Industries Ltd 61
Compagnie Francaise de l'Afrique
Internationale 65
Conveyancer (Nigeria) Ltd 67
Co-Operative Supply Association Ltd 68
Crocodile Matchets (Nigeria) Ltd 70
Cross River State Agricultural
Development Corporation 71
Daniksi Ltd 74
Desam Development Company Ltd 78
Diesel Generating Company Ltd 79
Disscol Ltd 79
Dizengoff West Africa (Nigeria) Ltd 79
Dolphin Dive West Africa 80
Emanento Company Agency 90
Folam International Trading Company 102
Gobecco Trading Company Ltd 111
Godbless Motors Nigeria Ltd 111
Guthrie (Nigeria) Ltd 115
Hamzer, G N A, & Co (Nigeria) Ltd 119
Holt, John, Ltd 123
J & H International Agency 137
Kikachukwu Agricultural Enterprises
Ltd 146
Kolinah Industries Nigeria Ltd 148
Lisabi Mills (Nigeria) Ltd 156
Louis Berger Inc Nigeria 158
Maclisle Complex Ltd 159
Major & Company (Nigeria) Ltd 160
Management Enterprises Ltd 161
Motorways Nigeria Ltd 177
National Trucks Manufacturers Ltd 185
Nigeria General Motors Ltd 195
Nigerian Agricultural Promotions
Company Ltd 199
Nigerian Motors Industries Ltd 211
Northern Nigerian Technical Service
Ltd 225
Obatraco Group of Companies 227
Odeco Ltd 228
Olaogun Enterprises Ltd 231
Olympic Group Ltd 233
Omole, Lawrence, & Sons Ltd 233
Ondo State Investment Corporation 234
Pan Nigerian Agency 242
Pestkill Nigeria Ltd 244
Phoenix Motors Ltd 247
Poultry & Animal Products (Nigeria)
Ltd 251
Pukke, Horst, & Co (Nigeria) Ltd 255
Raccah & Chaker Factory Ltd 256
Ramson Mellamby & Company Ltd 257
Rapid Electrical & Mechanical
Company Nigeria Ltd (REMCO) 257
Roaag Company (Nigeria) Ltd 263
Runsewe Group of Companies 265
Samsung (Nigeria) Ltd 267
Scoa Nigeria Ltd 270
Scoagri 270
Scoatrac (A Division of Scoa (Nigeria)
Ltd) 270
Seepc (Nigeria) Ltd 271
Sointeco (Nigeria) Ltd 277
Songhai Group of Companies 278
Stephens, Henry, Engineering
Company Ltd 281

Stephens, Henry, Group of Companies 281
Steyr Nigeria Ltd 281
Swiss Nigerian Chemical Company Ltd 285
Tenimasunwon Agency 288
Tractor & Equipment 292
Tractors Under-Carriage Industry
Nigeria Ltd 292
UAC of Nigeria Ltd 297
Umerah Commercial Agency Ltd 301
Ventures, Coopers Benly, & Company
Ltd (The) 313
West African Chemical Company Ltd
(WACHEM) 318
Western Nigerian Technical Co Ltd 320
Wiedemann & Walters (Nigeria) Ltd 321
Zartech Ltd 324

Agricultural produce

Adamu Management International 6
Adarice Company Ltd 6
Afro Continental Nigeria Ltd 13
Agricultural Development Corporation
(Anambra State) 14
Alhassan Dantata & Sons Ltd 19
Association of Nigerian Co-Operative
Exporters Ltd 32
Aurora Produce & Shipping Co Ltd 33
Calaro Oil Palm Estate Ltd 52
Commonwealth Commodity Company
International 64
Cross River Estate Ltd 70
Dauphin (Nigeria) Ltd 75
Deribe, Alhaji Mai, & Sons Ltd 78
Dokunmu, M A, & Sons Ltd 80
Eurotrade (Nigeria) Ltd 94
Hamzer, G N A, & Co (Nigeria) Ltd 119
Haruna, Alhaji Mustapha, & Sons 121
Ibru Organisation (Ibru Ltd) 126
Kabba Co-Operative Credit &
Marketing Union Ltd 141
Kano Oil Millers Ltd 143
Kano Sugar Industry Nigeria Ltd 144
Kolinah Industries Nigeria Ltd 148
Kwa Falls Oil Palm Estate Ltd 150
Lafia Canning Factory 151
Life Flour Mill Ltd 155
Management Enterprises Ltd 161
Mandrides, P S, & Co Ltd 162
Mogaji Osona Enterprises Ltd 175
Nabena, L R, & Sons Ltd 179
National Grains Production Company
Ltd 181
National Root Crops Production
Company Ltd 183
Nidoco Ltd 191
Nigerian Cereals Processing Company
Ltd 202
Nigerian Cocoa Board 202
Nigerian Groundnut Board 207
Nigerian Palm Produce Board 213
Nigerian Rubber Board 216
Nigerian Sugar Company Ltd 217
Nigerian Tuber & Root Crops Board 219
Northern Nigeria Flour Mills Ltd 224
Oil Palm Company Ltd 230
Okitipupa Oil Palm Co Ltd 231
Olympic Group Ltd 233
Omo Group Organisation 233
Plateau Foods Processing Company
Ltd 249
Port Harcourt Flour Mills Ltd 251
Poultry & Animal Products (Nigeria)
Ltd 251
Ribway Group of Companies 261
Risonpalm Ltd 262
Savannah Sugar Company Ltd 269
Sobat Ltd 276
Vegetable Oils (Nigeria) Ltd 312

Air conditioning, heating and refrigation

Addis Engineering Ltd 6
Adebowale Electrical Industries Ltd 6

Adejobi, Adeoye, Trading Stores Ltd 7
African Era and Company Ltd 11
Agrotec Services Ltd 15
Aircool Metal Industries (Nigeria) Ltd 15
Allen, J, Co Ltd 20
Bewac Ltd 41
Bozgomero of Nigeria Ltd 47
CFAO (Nigeria) Ltd 56
Corpio Constructions (Nigeria) Ltd 69
Daddo International (Nigeria) Ltd 72
Delta Freeze Ltd 76
Dolmech Engineering (Nig) Ltd 80
Drake & Scull (Nigeria) Ltd 81
Edmund & Edmund (Nigeria) Ltd 86
Ekisola Electrical Works Ltd 87
Etco-Engineering & Technical Company (Nigeria) Ltd 93
Eterna Electrical Engineering Works Ltd 94
General Appliances Company Ltd 108
George, Patrick, & Sons Ltd 109
Hulls Services Ltd 125
Ibru Organisation (Ibru Ltd) 126
Inlaks Ltd 130
International Contracts & Consultancy Services Ltd 132
International Yettco (Nigeria) Ltd 134
Johnson Foluso International Enterprises (JOFI) 139
Kent Engineering Nigeria Ltd 146
Leo's Group of Companies Ltd 154
Lonogu Enterprises Ltd 157
Mandilas Ltd 162
Mitton Refrigeration Service 173
Moukarim Industries Ltd 177
New Africa Development Company Ltd 188
Newmark Electric Company Ltd 190
Nigeria Engineering Works Ltd 195
Nigerian Electronics Company Ltd 204
Nirotec (A Division of Nigerian Ropes Ltd) 221
Nobgroup of Companies 222
Norman Industries Ltd 223
Ohakwe & Associates (Nigeria) Ltd 230
Petraco, De, Industries Ltd 245
R & A Services (Division of UAC of Nigeria Ltd) 256
Sanyo (Nigeria) Ltd 267
Scoa Iard - a Division of Scoa Nigeria Ltd 270
Scoa Nigeria Ltd 270
Smeaton Ltd 275
Technae (Nigeria) Ltd 287
Thermocool Engineering Company Ltd 289
Thermostein Ltd 289
Thompson Dickson Technical Co Ltd 289
Transex & Company Ltd 293
UAC of Nigeria Ltd 297
United Technology (Nigeria) Ltd 307
Utilgas Nigerian and Overseas Gas Company Ltd 311
Weide & Co (Group of Companies) Ltd 316
Westend Engineering Ltd 320

Architecture and town planning

African Designs Development Centre Ltd 11
Allied Architects 20
Ameniger Construction Company Ltd 23
Anombem Mokwunye, Twigg, Brown & Partners 25
Architechniques 26
ARC-Models Company 27
Becker-Voigt, H 37
Cetaconsult (Nigeria) Ltd 55
Citymark (West Africa) Ltd 62
Egbor and Associates 87
Ekwueme Associates 89
INPLECON 133
Insumma (Nigeria) Ltd 130
Integrated Consultants (Nigeria) Ltd 130
Inter Designs Partnership 131
International Planning & Environmental Consultants (Nigeria) Ltd 133
Interstate Architects 135
Joe Oyegoke Associates 139
Joint Design Partnership 140
Lagos State Development & Property Corporation 152

Louis Berger Inc Nigeria 158
Marubeni Engineering (WA) Ltd 165
Modulor Group 174
Nidanconsult 191
Niger Consultants Ltd 192
O'Bahor, J A, & Company Ltd 227
Olawale Odeleye Associates 232
Oyenuga, Deji, & Partners 239
Pan African Consultancy Services (Nigeria) Ltd 241
Rajendram, R, and Associates 257
Safni Ltd 266
Tomax-Beton Construction Company Ltd 290

Banks, finance and investment companies

A G Leventis & Company (Nigeria) Ltd 3
Abebiyi Sonaike & Company 4
African Continental Bank Ltd 9
Ajanga International Agency 15
Allied Bank of Nigeria Ltd 20
Bank of Credit & Commerce International (Nigeria) Ltd 36
Bank of the North Ltd 36
Bentworth Finance (Nigeria) Ltd (BFN) 39
BT International (Nigeria) Ltd 50
Capital Trust Brokers Ltd 53
Central Bank of Nigeria 54
Central Investment Company Ltd 55
Chase Merchant Bank Nigeria Ltd 57
City Group Organization 62
City Securities Ltd 62
Co-operative and Commerce Bank (Nigeria) Ltd 67
Co-Operative Bank Ltd 67
Co-Operative Bank of Kaduna State 67
Co-Operative Bank of Kano 67
Co-Operative Investment & Trust Society 68
Crown Agents For Overseas Governments and Administrations 71
Dubic International Ltd 83
Federal Mortgage Bank of Nigeria 98
Financial Trust Company Nigeria Ltd 100
First Bank of Nigeria Ltd (Formerly Standard Bank Nigeria Ltd) 100
First Chicago Nigeria Ltd 100
First City Investment Company Ltd 100
Formerly John Holt Investment Company Ltd 138
Icon Ltd (Merchant Bankers) 127
International Bank for West Africa Ltd 131
International Merchant Bank (Nigeria) Ltd 133
Investment Promotions Ltd 135
Irede Properties and Investment Company Ltd 135
JHI Ltd 138
Kaduna Co-Operative Bank Ltd 141
Kaduna Investments Co Ltd 141
Kano Cooperative Bank Ltd 143
Kano State Investment & Properties Ltd 144
Kedam Holdings (Nigeria) Ltd 145
Mercantile Bank of Nigeria Ltd 167
Merchant Banking Corporation Nigeria Ltd (MBC) 167
NAL Merchant Bank Ltd 179
Nassar, S, & Sons (Nigeria) Ltd 180
National Bank of Nigeria Ltd 180
New Nigeria Bank Ltd 188
New Nigeria Development Company Ltd 189
Nigeria Merchant Bank Ltd 196
Nigeria-Arab Bank Ltd 198
Nigerian Agricultural and Cooperative Bank Ltd 199
Nigerian American Merchant Bank Ltd 199
Nigerian Bank for Commerce and Industry (NBCI) 200
Nigerian Diversified Investments Ltd 204
Nigerian Industrial Development Bank Ltd 209
Nigerian Stockbrokers Ltd 217
Nigerian-American Merchant Bank Ltd 220
Northern Nigeria Investments Ltd 225
Odu'a Investment Company Ltd 228

Oluwakemi Motors & Finance Company Ltd 233
Owena Bank (Nigeria) Ltd 238
Oyo State Investment and Credit Corporation 239
Pabod Finance & Investment Company Ltd 240
Pan African Bank Ltd 241
Plateau Investments Company Ltd 249
Prudent Finance Ltd 255
Samsung (Nigeria) Ltd 267
Savannah Bank of Nigeria Ltd 268
Societe Generale Bank (Nigeria) Ltd 277
Ugochukwu and Sons Ltd 299
Union Bank of Nigeria Ltd 302
United Bank for Africa Ltd 303
Wema Bank Ltd 317

Brewing, soft drinks and wine

A G Leventis & Company (Nigeria) Ltd 3
Abukon Nigeria Ltd 5
Associated Breweries & Company Ltd 30
Bendel Brewery Ltd 38
Clarke, W F, (Nigeria) Ltd 62
Cross River Breweries Ltd 70
Dr Pepper Bottling Company of Nigeria Ltd 81
Dubic Breweries Ltd 82
Essdee Food Products Nigeria Ltd 93
Fanz Holdings Ltd 96
Federated Cork & Seal Company Ltd 98
Golden Guinea Breweries Ltd 112
Guinness (Nigeria) Ltd 115
Hulls Services Ltd 125
Ibru Organisation (Ibru Ltd) 126
International Beer & Beverages Industries Ltd 131
International Breweries Ltd 132
Joelson & Sons Holdings 139
Jos International Breweries Ltd 140
Ladejobi Products Nigeria Ltd 151
Lever Brothers Nigeria Ltd 154
Mid-Land Bottling Company Ltd 171
Morison, J L, Sons & Jones (Nigeria) Ltd 176
Multimalt Ltd 178
Nigeria Distilleries Ltd 194
Nigerian Bottling Company Ltd 200
Nigerian Breweries Ltd 201
Nigerian Mineral Water Industry Ltd 211
Nigerian Soft Drinks Co Ltd 217
Nigerian Yeast & Alcohol Manufacturing Company Ltd 220
North Brewery Ltd 223
Okada Bottling Company (Nigeria) Ltd 231
Oyun Breweries 239
Pepsi Cola 244
Premier Breweries Ltd 252
Prime Feathers International Services Ltd 254
Sanmi Breweries Ltd 267
Seven-up Bottling Company Ltd 273
Sodangi Enterprises 277
Sona Breweries Ltd 278
Standard Breweries (Nigeria) Ltd 280
Sunfresh Brewery Company Nigeria Ltd 284
Superbru Ltd 284
Union Beverages Ltd 302
West African Breweries Ltd 317
West African Distillers Ltd 318

Building materials and cement

Ace Builders & Building Material Stockists (The) 5
Adefusika Trading Company Ltd 7
Adejumo Fam (Nigeria) Ltd 7
Adetona Awe (Nig) Enterprises 8
Afro Continental Nigeria Ltd 13
Akanji Commercial Enterprises Ltd 16
Akanji, D L, & Co (Nig) Ltd 16
Alcan Aluminium Products Ltd 18
Alex L M Davou Fom & Sons Enterprise Ltd 18

Algadama (Holdings) Ltd — 19
Aparaki Enterprises — 25
Arewa Steel Works Company (Nig) Ltd — 27
Arewa Tradewinds (Nig) Co Ltd — 28
Ashaka Cement Company Ltd — 29
Askar of Nigeria Ltd — 30
Aye Marble & Terrazzo Industrial
  Works — 33
Balin Builders & Aluminium Industries
  Ltd — 35
Banbury Systems (Nigeria) Ltd — 35
Bayajida Group of Companies — 37
Bedkana (Nig) Ltd — 38
Benue Cement Company Ltd — 39
Bestform Industries Co Ltd — 41
Bibson Associates Ltd — 42
Bodax Instruments & Tools Ltd — 44
Bolori Brothers & Co Ltd (Bolbros) — 45
Bosag Builders — 46
Brand Clay Works Ltd — 47
Brossette (Nigeria) Ltd — 50
Bulk Oil Plants of Nigeria Ltd — 50
Calabar Cement Company Ltd — 52
Caprihans Industries Ltd — 53
Carrara Marble Co Ltd — 54
Cement Company of Northern Nigeria
  Ltd — 54
CFAO (Nigeria) Ltd — 56
Charlie and Franco Ltd — 57
Charlton Trading Company (Nigeria)
  Ltd — 57
Chrisray Nigeria Ltd — 59
City Group Organization — 62
Citymark (West Africa) Ltd — 62
Clay Industry (Nigeria) Ltd — 63
Commind Nigeria Ltd — 64
Complete Home Enterprises (Nig) Ltd — 65
Concrete Building Contractors &
  General Works Ltd — 65
Concrete Poles Industries (Nigeria) Ltd — 65
Concrete Structures Ltd — 66
Co-Operative Supply Association Ltd — 68
Cope Builders' Supplies Ltd — 68
Crittall-Hope Nigeria Ltd — 70
(CTC) — 57
Cunix Industrial & Commercial Co Ltd — 71
Dambiyowu Nigeria Ltd — 73
Dapo Allied Industries (Nigeria) Ltd — 75
Deazula Trading Company (Nigeria)
  Ltd — 76
Deltaplast Company (Nigeria) Ltd — 77
Denchukwu Group of Companies — 78
Deribe, Alhaji Mai, & Sons Ltd — 78
Desam Development Company Ltd — 78
Dizengoff West Africa (Nigeria) Ltd — 79
Eastern Bulkcem Company Ltd — 84
Endurance Ltd — 92
Epe Plywood Industries Ltd — 92
Ernestco Ltd — 93
Eslon Nigeria Ltd — 93
Eternit Ltd — 94
Eurotrade (Nigeria) Ltd — 94
Fanz Holdings Ltd — 96
Fawaz Steelwood & Chemicals (Kano)
  Ltd — 97
Flag Aluminium Products Ltd — 101
Flour Mills of Nigeria Ltd — 102
Fredano Trading Co Ltd — 103
Freedom Development Company Ltd — 105
Freyssinet Nigeria Ltd — 105
Fuason Industries (Nigeria) Ltd — 105
Funtua Brickworks Ltd — 105
Galvanizing Industries Ltd — 106
Gamboru, Alhaji Madu Mala Sheriff — 106
General Metal Products Ltd — 108
General Technology Nigeria Ltd — 108
George, Patrick, & Sons Ltd — 109
Gindiri Concrete Products Ltd — 110
Goas Agencies Ltd — 111
Gottschalcks Buildings Materials — 113
Gregson Trading Company Ltd — 114
Guthrie (Nigeria) Ltd — 115
Hamzer, G N A, & Co (Nigeria) Ltd — 119
Hapel Nigeria Ltd — 120
Hoesch Pipe Mills (Nig) Ltd — 123
Holex Timber (Nigeria) Ltd — 123
Hulls Services Ltd — 125
Ibekwe, P A, Ltd — 126
Industrial & Safety Equipment (Nigeria)
  Ltd — 129
Innocent Hope Overseas Company — 130
International Contracts & Consultancy
  Services Ltd — 132
JBL Star Trading Company — 138

Joart United Construction &
  Engineering Ltd — 138
Juli Importers & Exporters Enterprises — 140
Kabo Blocks Ltd — 141
Kaycee (Nigeria) Ltd — 145
Koku, George, & Sons Ltd — 148
Kolinah Industries Nigeria Ltd — 148
Lacon Nigeria Ltd — 151
Lake Concrete Industries Ltd — 152
Leman Industries (Kaduna) Ltd — 154
Lilleshall (Nigeria) Ltd — 155
Maclisle Complex Ltd — 159
Madona Organisation Ltd — 159
Make Ltd — 160
Management Enterprises Ltd — 161
Manufacturing & Marketing Co (Nig)
  Ltd — 162
Mascot I Abali & Brothers Ltd — 165
Mbata, Sam, & Company Ltd — 166
Medal Brothers Co Ltd — 167
Metrocom International Ltd — 170
Midland Galvanizing Products Ltd — 171
Mifi (Nigeria) Ltd — 172
Mike Merchandise Co Ltd — 172
Mosheshe Group of Companies — 176
Musa, Alhaji Sani, & Sons — 178
Nabena, Benjamin, Nabenson
  Promotions — 178
Nabena, L R, & Sons Ltd — 179
Nigeria Industrial Group Ltd — 196
Nigerian Aluminium Development Co
  Ltd (NADECO) — 199
Nigerian Aluminium Engineering
  Company Ltd (NAECO) — 199
Nigerian Aluminium Extrusions Ltd
  (NIGALEX) — 199
Nigerian Asbestos Industries Ltd — 199
Nigerian Bricks & Clay Products Ltd — 201
Nigerian Cement Company Ltd
  (Nigercem) — 201
Nigerian Commercial & Industrial
  Enterprises Ltd — 202
Nigerian Concrete Industries Ltd — 203
Nigerian Door Fabrication Company
  Ltd — 204
Nigerian Foundries Ltd — 206
Nigerian Hardware Industries Ltd — 208
Nigerian Hollowblock Industries Ltd — 208
Nigerian Industrial Complex
  Amalgamation Ltd — 208
Nigerian Romanian Wood Industries
  Ltd — 215
Nigerian Ropes Ltd — 215
Nigerian Spanish Cement Co Ltd — 217
Nigerite Ltd (Formerly Asbestos
  Cement Products Ltd) — 220
Nigersteel Company Ltd — 220
Nigertal Industries Ltd — 221
Nirotec (A Division of Nigerian Ropes
  Ltd) — 221
Nobgroup of Companies — 222
Noren Industries Ltd (Formerly
  Nigerian Sandcrete Industry Ltd) — 223
Northern Steel Works Ltd — 225
Nwonye, I O M, & Sons Company Ltd — 227
Obanleoro Trading Company Ltd — 227
Obatraco Group of Companies — 227
Odeco Ltd — 228
Oguine Brothers — 230
Ojeniyi, Adelegan, Trading Company
  Nigeria — 230
O.K.C. (Nigeria) Ltd — 231
Olehson Brothers Company (Nigeria)
  Ltd — 232
(Olehson's Agro Animal Kingdom) — 232
Olympic Group Ltd — 233
Omole, Lawrence, & Sons Ltd — 233
Onibudo, A, & Company Ltd — 234
Onochie Brothers & Sons Company
  Ltd — 235
Onuselogu, C N, Enterprises Ltd — 235
Orazulike Trading Company Ltd — 235
Oriwu Commercial Agency Ltd — 236
Osborne, E, Nigeria Ltd — 236
Oshinmi Company Ltd — 236
Ositadinma International Ltd — 237
Oyebanji Building Materials Stores Ltd — 239
Oyinda Enterprises Ltd — 239
Pan Industrial Estate Agencies — 242
Panav International Ltd — 242
Parkes, Josiah, & Sons (Nigeria) Ltd — 243
Pecco Ltd — 244
Pem Ltd — 244
Piedmont Plywoods Nigeria Ltd — 248

Pioneer Metal Products Company Ltd — 248
Primary Steel (Nigeria) Ltd — 253
Princegate Trading & Contracting
  Company Ltd — 254
Raabe Sanitary and Water Engineering — 256
Rabiu, Isiyaku, & Sons Ltd — 256
Ramson Mellamby & Company Ltd — 257
Rapid Electrical & Mechanical
  Company Nigeria Ltd (REMCO) — 257
Rehau Plastiks (Nigeria) Ltd — 260
Reliance Group of Companies — 260
Renaissance Marble Works Ltd — 260
Robertson, H H, (Nigeria) Ltd — 264
Rubery Owen Fasteners (Nigeria) Ltd — 265
S & K Asbestos Products Ltd — 265
Sabon Sara Nigeria Ltd — 266
Salleh, Alhaji Baba M, & Sons (Nigeria)
  Ltd — 266
Sams Agencies & Maritime Service
  (Nig) — 266
Savannah Precast Concrete & Terrazo
  Industries Ltd — 268
Scan African Nigeria Ltd — 269
SCEI — 270
Scoa Nigeria Ltd — 270
Servo Nigerian Enterprises Ltd — 273
Siej Agencies — 274
Socea (Nigeria) Ltd — 277
Sodangi Enterprises — 277
Standard Industrial Development
  Company Ltd — 280
Stephens, Henry, Group of Companies — 281
Structor — 283
Subetra Nigeria Industries Ltd — 283
Syndivel Plastic Industry Nigeria Ltd — 285
Thompson Dickson Technical Co Ltd — 289
Tommy Building & Construction
  Company Ltd — 291
Tower Aluminium (Nigeria) Ltd — 291
Tradon Nigeria Ltd — 292
Turners Building Products (Arewa) Ltd — 295
Turners Building Products (Emene) Ltd — 297
UAC of Nigeria Ltd — 297
Ukpilla Cement Company Ltd — 301
Umaru, Lawan & Sons Ltd — 301
Unigwe, Fred Balonwu, Group of
  Companies — 302
Universal Monolithic Bearing Structure
  Ltd — 308
Urobo Agencies (Nigeria) Ltd — 310
UTC Nigeria Ltd (Formerly Union
  Trading Company of Nigeria Ltd) — 311
Ventures, Coopers Benly, & Company
  Ltd (The) — 313
Viktors, N, International Agencies — 313
Vinben (Nigeria) Ltd — 313
VK Plastiks & Marble Co — 314
Waterglass Boatyard & Steel
  Construction Ltd — 316
West African Aluminium Products
  (Nigeria) — 317
West African Portland Cement
  Company Ltd — 318
Western Nigerian Technical Co Ltd — 320
Wolff, Otto, (Nigeria) & Company Ltd — 322
Wozabeth Trading Company — 323
Yodesons (Nigeria) Ltd — 323
Zard, C, & Company Ltd — 324

Carpets

Alex L M Davou Fom & Sons
  Enterprise Ltd — 18
Birma General Supplies Ltd — 43
Carpet Royal (Nigeria) Ltd — 54
Emanento Company Agency — 90
Ernestco Ltd — 93
George, Patrick, & Sons Ltd — 109
King Carpet Manufacturing Co Ltd
  (Newspin Ltd) — 147
Nigerian Carpet Manufacturing Co Ltd — 201
Nigerian Spinning and Weaving Co Ltd — 217
Nigerian Weaving, Spinning & Printing
  Company Ltd (NEWSPIN Ltd) — 219
Northern Nigeria Fibre Products Ltd — 224
Ojeniyi, Adelegan, Trading Company
  Nigeria — 230
Promana Associates — 255
Ribway Group of Companies — 261

Ceramics and sanitary fittings

African Era and Company Ltd	11
Alex L M Davou Fom & Sons Enterprise Ltd	18
Bisiolu Enterprises Ltd	44
Chrisray Nigeria Ltd	59
Cimeco Enterprises (Nigeria) Ltd	61
Clay Industry (Nigeria) Ltd	63
Deazula Trading Company (Nigeria) Ltd	76
Diborsons Business Enterprises	79
Ernestco Ltd	93
George, Patrick, & Sons Ltd	109
Goswin & Co	113
Interbasic Products Co Ltd	131
Kolinah Industries Nigeria Ltd	148
Management Enterprises Ltd	161
Metrocom International Ltd	170
Metropolitan Distributors Ltd	170
Modern Ceramics Industries Ltd	174
Nigergrob Ceramics Ltd	193
Obatraco Group of Companies	227
Odeco Ltd	228
Ojeniyi, Adelegan, Trading Company Nigeria	230
Olympic Group Ltd	233
Onibudo, A, & Company Ltd	234
Orazulike Trading Company Ltd	235
Ositadinma International Ltd	237
Plateau Ceramics Industry Ltd (Jos)	249
Reliance Group of Companies	260
Sehl International	272
Ventures, Coopers Benly, & Company Ltd (The)	313
VK Plastiks & Marble Co	314

Chain stores

Bhojsons & Company (Nigeria) Ltd	42
Chanrai, J T, & Co (Nigeria) Ltd	57
Chellaram, K, & Sons (Nigeria) Ltd	57
Domino Stores Ltd	80
H B & Sons	117
Kaycee (Nigeria) Ltd	145
Kewalram, G, & Sons (Nigeria) Ltd	146
Kingsway Stores of Nigeria Ltd	147
Koku, George, & Sons Ltd	148
Kolinah Industries Nigeria Ltd	148
Marketing and Shipping Enterprises Ltd	165
Ohanenye & Sons Ltd	230
Omo Group Organisation	233
Omon Stores Ltd	234
Onigbinde, M A, & Sons Ltd	235
Pabod Supplies Ltd	240
Segun International Group Ltd	272
Superfine Furniture & Trading Company Ltd	284
Tradev Ltd	292
UAC of Nigeria Ltd	297
UTC Nigeria Ltd (Formerly Union Trading Company of Nigeria Ltd)	311

Chemicals

Adejumo Fam (Nigeria) Ltd	7
Advance (Nig) Ltd	8
Agroline (Nigeria) Ltd	15
Agrotec Services Ltd	15
Alban Pharmacy Ltd	18
Apapa Chemical Industries Ltd	25
Associated Battery Manufacturers (Nigeria) Ltd	30
Associated Laboratory Supplies Ltd	31
Basf (Nigeria) Ltd	37
Battery Manufacturing Co (Nig) Ltd	37
Bendel Chemical Industries Ltd	38
Berec Nigeria Ltd	40
Brightstar Industries Ltd	49
CECA (Nigeria) Ltd	54
Chemdyes Nigeria Ltd	58
Chemical & Allied Products Ltd	58

Christela Chemical Works Ltd	59
Chukwurah Agriculture Industries Ltd	61
Commind Nigeria Ltd	64
Co-Operative Supply Association Ltd	68
Daily Need Chemists Ltd	72
Daniksi Ltd	74
Dizengoff West Africa (Nigeria) Ltd	79
DOF Chemicals Ltd	80
Dolphin Dive West Africa	80
Edmund & Edmund (Nigeria) Ltd	86
Embechem Ltd (Formerly May & Baker (Nigeria) Ltd)	90
Fanz Holdings Ltd	96
Felico Industries Nigeria	98
Fisco-Chemicals (Nigeria) Ltd	100
Gas Producers Ltd	106
Global Pharmaceutical and Chemical Agencies Ltd	111
Gobecco Trading Company Ltd	111
Greenham Plant Hire	114
Gyartagere Explosives & Chemicals Co Ltd	117
Henkel Chemicals Nigeria Ltd	122
Household Products Ltd	125
Industrial Gases Ltd	130
Labstock (Nigeria) Ltd	150
Ladejobi Products Nigeria Ltd	151
Lever Brothers Nigeria Ltd	154
Major & Company (Nigeria) Ltd	160
Metoxide (Nigeria) Ltd	169
Minnesota Nigeria Ltd	172
National Oil and Chemical Marketing Company Ltd	183
Nigerian Chemical Services Ltd (NCS)	202
Nigerian Explosives & Plastics Co Ltd	205
Nigerian Hoechst Ltd	208
Nigerian Urethane Co Ltd	219
Nordmann, Rassmann & Company (Nigeria) Ltd	222
Olehson Brothers Company (Nigeria) Ltd	232
(Olehson's Agro Animal Kingdom)	232
Ositadinma International Ltd	237
Pan Africa Gas Distributors Ltd	240
Pestkill Nigeria Ltd	244
Petro-Organico (Nigeria) Ltd	245
Pharma Dyn Chemical Products	247
Prime Feathers International Services Ltd	254
Raabe Sanitary and Water Engineering	256
Ramson Mellamby & Company Ltd	257
Sandoz (Nigeria) Ltd	267
Seepc (Nigeria) Ltd	271
Sehl International	272
Siej Agencies	274
Sunshine Batteries Manufacturing Company	284
Swiss Nigerian Chemical Company Ltd	285
Things International (Nigeria) Ltd	289
Tudor Batteries (Nigeria) Ltd	295
Twilights Nigeria Ltd	297
Ugochukwu Chemical Industries Ltd	301
Ukawoods Enterprises Nigeria Ltd	301
Umerah Commercial Agency Ltd	301
Unigwe, Fred Balonwu, Group of Companies	302
Union Carbide (Nigeria) Ltd	302
Unipetrol Nigeria Ltd	302
United African Drug Co (Nig) Ltd	303
Unity Soap Manufacturers Ltd	307
Urobo Agencies (Nigeria) Ltd	310
UTC Nigeria Ltd (Formerly Union Trading Company of Nigeria Ltd)	311
West African Batteries Ltd	317
West African Chemical Company Ltd (WACHEM)	318
Zerolas Batteries Company Ltd	324

Civil engineering and construction

158 Baresel Ltd	3
A G Leventis & Company (Nigeria) Ltd	3
Abereoje (Nigeria) Ltd	4
(ACC Ltd)	22
Ace Builders & Building Material Stockists (The)	5
ACE Metal Construction (Nigeria) Ltd	5
Acme Builders Ltd	6
Adecentro Nigeria Ltd	6

Adejoro, S S, & Company Ltd	7
Ademola, Thomas, & Co Ltd	8
Adewale Bello Constructions Ltd	8
Afa Gateway Construction Company Ltd	9
Afro International Construction Company	13
Airoe Construction & Civil Engineering Co Ltd	15
Akarolo Technical Company Nigeria Ltd	16
Akinadod Akinloye Aboderin Ltd	16
Akutu Structures Ltd	17
Aladdin Construction Nigeria Ltd	18
Alakija & Alakija Contracting Services Ltd	18
Albishir, Alhaji, & Sons	18
Alex L M Davou Fom & Sons Enterprise Ltd	18
Algadama (Holdings) Ltd	19
Alhassan Dantata & Sons Ltd	19
Alinaco (Nigeria) Ltd	19
Alusteel Construction Ltd	21
Amagroup Engineers Ltd	21
Amana Construction Co (Nigeria) Ltd	22
Amana Consulting Engineers	22
Amcord Nigeria Ltd	23
Ameniger Construction Company Ltd	23
Amey Roadstone Company (Nigeria) Ltd	24
Aminci International Co Ltd	24
Analex Group Ltd	24
Anasoro Builders	25
Anbar Enterprises Ltd	25
Anglo-German Company (Intercontinental) Ltd	25
Aprofim Engineering Construction Company (Nigeria) Ltd	26
Arbico Ltd	26
(ARC (NIG) Ltd)	24
Arcus Consultant Ltd	27
Arewa Construction Ltd	27
Arigas Construction Company Nigeria Ltd	28
Aspect Construction Engineering Group (Nig) Ltd	30
Aspesi Ltd	30
Asphalt Company of Nigeria Ltd	30
Aticon Ltd	32
Atta, M O, & Sons (Nigeria) Ltd	33
August Reiners Nigeria Ltd	33
B & F Nigeria Ltd	34
B B C Brown Boveri (Nigeria) Ltd	34
Bafco Ltd	34
Bakare, S B, & Brothers Ltd	34
Balakhany (Nigeria) Ltd	35
Balin Builders & Aluminium Industries Ltd	35
Balogun, J A, Works	35
Bamgboye Engineering Ltd	35
Banbury Systems (Nigeria) Ltd	35
Banjoko, L A O, & Co Ltd	35
Barma, A G S, Ltd	36
Bayajida Group of Companies	37
BEC Freres (Nigeria) Ltd	37
Beccarelli, P, & Co Ltd	37
Beciciti Construction Ltd	37
Bendel Steel Structures Ltd	39
Bennett-Sasore-Dunn Ltd (Nigeria)	39
Bepco (Nig) Ltd	40
Berger, Julius, Nigeria Ltd	40
BICC Construction (Nigeria) Ltd	42
Bida, Alhaji Audu, & Sons United Company Ltd	42
Bideco (Nigeria) Ltd	43
Bimbotech (Nigeria) Ltd	43
Bisceglia Brothers & Associates Construction Co (Nigeria) Ltd	43
BKI Building & Civil Engineering Co Ltd	44
Bolingo Organisation	45
Bonomi, S G, Ltd	45
Borini Prono & Co Ltd	46
Bosag Builders	46
Boskalis Nigeria Ltd	46
Bouygues (Nigeria) Ltd	47
Bremen Nnachetam Construction Company (Nigeria) Ltd	47
Briscoe, Frank	49
Brunelli Construction Company	50
BSM Ltd	50
Building & Civil Engineering Contractors Company Nigeria Ltd	50
C I F Construction Nigeria Ltd	51

Caaso Constructional Works Ltd	51	Holman Brothers (Nigeria) Ltd	123	Nigeria Construction and Furniture Company Ltd (NCFC)	194
Caleb Bovis Johnson Construction Co Ltd	52	Holt, John, Ltd	123	Nigeria Group Four Construction Company Ltd	195
Cappa and D'Alberto Ltd	53	Howard Construction Co of Nigeria Ltd	125	Nigerian Cementation & Drilling Co Ltd	201
Cappa, G, Ltd	53	Huttig-Schmucker Construction (Nig) Ltd	125	Nigerian Company for Energy Engineering Ltd (NICOGEN)	202
Chiyoda Chemical Engineering & Construction Co	59	Igwe Brothers & Co Ltd	128	Nigerian Construction & Holding Co Ltd	203
Cimeco Enterprises (Nigeria) Ltd	61	Impresit Bakolori (Nigeria) Ltd	129	Nigerian Construction and Water Resources Development Ltd	203
Cistar (Nigeria) Ltd	61	Integrated Consultants (Nigeria) Ltd	130	Nigerian Diving Service Ltd	204
City Group Organization	62	Interbeton Nigeria Ltd	131	Nigerian Dredging and Marine Ltd	204
Citymark (West Africa) Ltd	62	Intercontractors (Nigeria) Ltd	131	Nigerian Engineering and Construction Company Ltd (NECCO)	205
Clyde Dial Construction (Nigeria) Ltd	63	International Contractors Agency (ICA)	132	Nigerian Far East Company Ltd (NIFECO)	205
Comazzi, P	64	International Housing (Nigeria) Ltd	133	Nigerian International Construction Company Ltd	209
Complete Home Enterprises (Nig) Ltd	65	International Planning Associates	134	Nigerian Machine Tools Co Ltd (NMT)	210
Consolidated Structures	66	Isokariari, O K & Sons (Nigeria) Ltd	135	Nigerian Road Construction Ltd	215
Construction & Support Services Nigeria Ltd	66	Itager (Nigeria) Ltd	135	Nigerian Ropes Ltd	215
Contex Nigeria Ltd	66	Italafro Builders	136	Nigersol Construction Co Ltd	220
Corpio Constructions (Nigeria) Ltd	69	Itoh, C, & Co Ltd	136	Nigertal Industries Ltd	221
Costain (West Africa) Ltd	69	Jac-Ogho (Nigeria) Enterprises	137	Nirotec (A Division of Nigerian Ropes Ltd)	221
Coutinho, Caro & Co (Nigeria) Ltd	69	Jammal Engineering (Nigeria) Ltd	137	Nispan Construction Ltd	221
Cross, A W, Ltd	70	Jas Builders Ltd	137	Nobgroup of Companies	222
Cubitts (Nigeria) Ltd	71	Jemine Enterprises Ltd	138	Northco Construction Company Ltd	223
Dagazau International Ltd	72	Jeph International (Nigeria) Ltd	138	Novacoke Builders Ltd	226
D'Alberto, E, & Giampaoli Ltd	73	Jideofo, D A, Enterprises Ltd	138	Nwaezu Building Company Ltd	226
D'Alberto, L, & Co Ltd	73	Jimona, A C E, Ltd	138	Nwandu, D A, & Sons Enterprises Ltd	226
Daniksi Ltd	74	JLGT Construction Company Nigeria Ltd	138	Nwankwu, J, & Bros Ltd	226
Dantata Land and Sea Company Ltd	74	Joart United Construction & Engineering Ltd	138	O'Bahor, J A, & Company Ltd	227
Delco (Nig) Ltd	76	Joe Oyegoke Associates	139	Odeco Ltd	228
Dema Engineering Ltd	78	Jones Homes International Nigeria Ltd	140	OGT Group of Companies Ltd	229
Deribe, Alhaji Mai, & Sons Ltd	78	Jones, J A, (Nigeria) Ltd	140	Oguejiofor, Alex, Company Ltd	230
Desam Development Company Ltd	78	Karunwi, A O, Ltd	145	O.K.C. (Nigeria) Ltd	231
Deutsche Kaiser Gruppe (Interkontinental)	78	Kedam Holdings (Nigeria) Ltd	145	Olawale Odeleye Associates	232
Dipenta Nigeria Ltd	79	Kenting Africa Resource Services Ltd	146	Omuna Construction Company (Nigeria) Ltd	234
Dokunmu, M A, & Sons Ltd	80	Kilpatrick, James, (Nigeria) Ltd	146	Opukiri Constructions Company Ltd	235
Dolphin Properties Ltd	80	Klifco (Nigeria) Ltd	148	Oroke Constructions Nigeria Ltd	236
Dorman Long & Amalgamated Engineering Ltd	80	Kloeckner Ina Nigeria Ltd	148	Ososami, J F, & Co	237
Dragages Nigeria Ltd	81	Kosm (West Africa) Ltd	149	Oyinda Enterprises Ltd	239
DSD Nigeria Ltd	82	Kpohraror & Sons Group of Companies	149	P W Nigeria Ltd	239
Dumez (Nigeria) Ltd	83	Kramer-Italo Ltd	149	Paas Industries (Nigeria) Company Ltd	240
Dys Trocca Valsesia & Company Ltd	84	Kueppers (Nigeria) Ltd	149	Pan African Consultancy Services (Nigeria) Ltd	241
E A O Constructors (Nigeria) Ltd	84	Lago (Nigeria) Ltd	151	Panav International Ltd	242
Edilit Ltd	86	Laing Construction Ltd	152	Pecco Ltd	244
Edok-Eter-Mandilas Ltd	86	Lakati Construction & Company	152	Petra-Monk Engineering & Contracting Company Ltd	245
Efbiko Engineering Ltd	86	Las & Co Ltd	153	Pipes Below Ground Ltd	248
Ekman Construction Co Ltd	87	Lastra Construction (Nigeria) Ltd	153	Plateau Construction Ltd	249
Eksons (Nig) Ltd	87	Latadek Construction Company Ltd	153	Plisson Fisko Nigeria Ltd	250
Eom Construction Co Ltd	92	Levitt Industries	154	Poco Minerals Ltd	250
Eze, I O, & Sons Ltd	95	Lilleshall (Nigeria) Ltd	155	Poletti Brothers & Co Ltd	250
Ezennwa, S N, & Sons Ltd	96	Lodigiani (Nigeria) Ltd	157	Pollack, Sheldon L, (Nigeria) Ltd	251
Fanz Holdings Ltd	96	Longou Enterprises Ltd	157	Power & Communication Engineering Nigeria Ltd	251
Farawametz Construction Co Ltd	97	Louis Berger Inc Nigeria	158	Powerlines Ltd	252
Fas Brothers Ltd	97	Lovell Stewart Nigeria Ltd	158	Prestrest Ltd	253
Ferrero, A G, & Co Ltd	99	Macpon Engineering and Construction Company Ltd	159	Preussag Drilling Engineers Nigeria Ltd	253
Fisko Construction Engineering Co Ltd (Formerly Akutu Construction Company Nigeria Ltd)	101	Maintenance Building Contractors Ltd	160	Princegate Trading & Contracting Company Ltd	254
Formerly Bartoletti (Nigeria) Ltd	17	Manatec Company Ltd	161	Progress Contracts Ltd	254
Formerly Haden (Nigeria) Ltd	131	Mandilas Ltd	162	Promana Associates	255
Foster Wheeler (Nigeria) Ltd	117	Manila Construction Co (Nigeria) Ltd	162	Pureway Corporation of Nigeria Ltd	255
Fougerolle Nigeria Ltd	103	Mansa Construction Co Ltd	162	Raabe Sanitary and Water Engineering	256
Foundation Construction Ltd	103	Marghi Enterprises Ltd	163	Rajendram, R, and Associates	257
Foundation Engineering (Nigeria) Ltd	103	Marubeni Engineering (WA) Ltd	165	Rapid Electrical & Mechanical Company Nigeria Ltd (REMCO)	257
Franco Builders Ltd	103	Mas-Chrisco and Associates	165	Raycon & Company (Nigeria) Ltd	259
Gamboru, Alhaji Madu Mala Sheriff	106	Mascot I Abali & Brothers Ltd	165	Raymond Constructors (Nigeria) Ltd	259
Geco Engineering Co (Nigeria) Ltd	107	Mashall, Alhaji Sani, Estates	165	Regency (Overseas) Company Ltd	259
General Contractors (Nigeria) Ltd	108	MBC	160	Reggio Builders Ltd	259
George, Patrick, & Sons Ltd	109	Mesterom (Nigeria) Ltd	168	Reiss & Co (Nigeria) Ltd	260
Giampaoli Construction (Nigeria) Ltd	110	Metal Construction (WA) Ltd	169	Reliance International (Nigeria) Ltd	260
Gindiri Concrete Products Ltd	110	Micheletti, A	171	Rendezvous Group Hotels (Nigeria) Ltd	261
Globestar Engineering Co (Nigeria) Ltd	111	Micheletti, E M, & Son (Nigeria) Ltd	171	Reynolds Construction Company (Nigeria) Ltd	261
Golden Furniture & Construction Co Ltd	112	Middleton River Brothers (Nigeria) Ltd	171	Rhine-Schelde-Verolme Engineers	261
Gottschalcks Buildings Materials	113	Mifi (Nigeria) Ltd	172	Ribway Group of Companies	261
Greens Engineering Ltd	114	Monier Construction Company (Nig) Ltd	175	Rida Construction Company Ltd	261
Guffanti (Nigeria) Ltd	114	Moone Construction Co Ltd	175	Rioco (Nigeria) Ltd	262
Guobadia Furniture & Construction Company (Nigeria) Ltd	115	Morpol Industrial Corporation Ltd	176	Road and General Construction Company Ltd	263
Hademec Ltd	117	Mothercat Overseas (Nigeria) Ltd	177	Roads Nigeria Ltd	263
Halcon Engineering Associates Ltd	119	Mukoro, Martin, Construction Company	178	Roberts, T L, & Company Ltd	263
Ham Dredging Nigeria Ltd	119	Nabena, Benjamin, Nabenson Promotions	178	Rotimi & Sons Ltd	265
Hammond, T A, Projects Ltd	119	National Road Construction Company of Nigeria Ltd	183	Runsewe Group of Companies	265
Hamzer, G N A, & Co (Nigeria) Ltd	119	Navarro International (Nigeria) Ltd	185	Safni Ltd	266
Hanein & Solomons Ltd	120	Neptune Constructions Ltd	186		
Haruna, Alhaji Mustapha, & Sons	121	Netherlands Harbourworks (Nigeria) Ltd	187		
Hassan Furniture & Joinery Company Ltd	121	New Nigeria Construction Company Ltd	189		
Heplac Nigeria Ltd	122	Niger Construction Ltd	191		
Herbst & Ndusco Constructions Ltd	122	Nigercare International Company (Nigeria) Ltd	193		
Herwa Ltd	122				
Higrade Construction & Engineering Company Ltd	122				

Sage Constructions (Nigeria) Ltd 266
Saipem Nigeria Ltd 266
Salleh, Alhaji Baba M, & Sons (Nigeria)
  Ltd 266
SAO Engineering Company Ltd 268
Satt Construction (Nigeria) Ltd 268
Savoia, A 269
Scoa Nigeria Ltd 270
Sedco Nigeria Ltd 271
Segun International Group Ltd 272
SGE Nigeria Ltd 273
Shittu, Alhaji M R, & Sons Ltd 274
Siab Engineering Company Nigeria Ltd 274
Silverball Integrated Engineering Co
  Nigeria Ltd 274
Snamprogetti 276
SNC (Nigeria) Ltd 276
Sodipo, Harold, & Co Ltd 277
Sointeco (Nigeria) Ltd 277
Solel Boneh (Nigeria) Ltd 277
Songhai Construction Ltd 278
Songhai Group of Companies 278
Songhai Ltd 278
Soprog Construction Ltd 278
South Chad Ltd 279
Southeastern Drilling Co (Nigeria) Ltd
  (SEDCO) 279
Special Structures & Company Ltd 279
Stabilini & Visinoni Ltd 280
Stabilini, B, & Company Ltd 280
Standard Construction Ltd 280
Stirling Civil Engineering Nigeria Ltd 282
Strabag Construction (Nigeria) Ltd 282
Structec 282
Tadat Engineering Company Ltd 286
Takko Engineering Ltd 286
Tarmac Engineering Company Ltd 286
Taylor Woodrow of Nigeria Ltd 287
Techint Engineering (Nigeria) Ltd 287
Technical & Building Materials Ltd 287
Thomas Mechanical Plumbing 289
Tilbury Contracting Co (Nigeria) Ltd 290
Tilla International Ltd 290
Tomax-Beton Construction Company
  Ltd 290
Tommy Building & Construction
  Company Ltd 291
Topic Ltd 291
Tradon Nigeria Ltd 292
Trevi Foundations Nigeria Ltd 294
Twz (Nigeria) Ltd 297
Ugbabe Furniture & Construction
  Company Ltd 299
Ukawoods Enterprises Nigeria Ltd 301
Unibuilder Industries Ltd 301
Unigwe, Fred Balonwu, Group of
  Companies 302
Union Builders Company Ltd 302
Union Construction Company Ltd 302
Universal Welding & Construction
  Company Ltd 309
Urban Engineers 310
Uren Construction Engineering
  Company Ltd 310
Vercon (Nigeria) Ltd 313
Vicinanza Construction Ltd 313
Vinben (Nigeria) Ltd 313
Vincenti Engineering Ltd 313
Wahler, Josef, (Nig) Ltd 315
West Construction Company Ltd 319
Westminster Dredging (Nigeria) Ltd 320
Whessoe Engineering Ltd 320
White, Johnson, United Ltd 321
Whyte, W W, & Co Ltd 321
Widnell and Trollope Nigeria 321
Williams International (Nig) Ltd 321
Wimpey, George, & Co (Nigeria) Ltd 322
Wimpey-Brown & Root (Nigeria) Ltd 322
Woclif (Nigeria) Ventures 322

Commercial and industrial institutes and associations

Formerly Mitsui & Co (Nigeria) Ltd 166
MBK Nigeria Ltd 166
Nigerian Institute of Management 209

Computers

Anglo-German Company
  (Intercontinental) Ltd 25
Buromat Data System Ltd 50
Business Equipment & Machinery Ltd
  (BEAM) (Division of UAC of Nigeria
  Ltd) 50
Continuous Printing Industry (Nigeria)
  Ltd 66
CPI-Moore (Nigeria) Ltd 69
Data Processing Maintenance and
  Services Ltd 75
Data Sciences (Nigeria) Ltd 75
DPMS Ltd 81
DSD Nigeria Ltd 82
Earth Sciences Ltd 84
Electronics Instrumentations Ltd 90
Envelope & File Co of Nigeria 92
Eppellion International Ltd 92
Fanz Holdings Ltd 96
(Formerly IBM Nig Ltd) 81
Haven Nigeria Computer Co Ltd 121
Hunting Surveys (Nigeria) Ltd 125
International Computers (Nigeria) Ltd 132
Mesacom Electronics Instrumentations
  Ltd 168
Modelor Design Aids Ltd 174
Modulor Group 174
Narumal & Sons (Nigeria) Ltd 180
National Cash Register (WA) Ltd 181
NCR 181
Netarcomms Nigeria Ltd 186
Rimax Computer Services Ltd 262
Tara Consulting Nigeria Ltd 286

Construction plant

Ace Builders & Building Material
  Stockists (The) 5
Acrow Ltd 6
Afrotec Technical Services Nigeria Ltd 14
Agribuild Nigeria Ltd 14
Akinadod Akinloye Aboderin Ltd 16
Blackwood Hodge (Nigeria) Ltd 44
Bosag Builders 46
Briscoe, R T, (Nigeria) Ltd 49
Caaso Constructional Works Ltd 51
Camplant Engineering Sales & Service
  Ltd 52
Commind Nigeria Ltd 64
Compass Trading Co Ltd 65
Conveyancer (Nigeria) Ltd 67
Dragages Nigeria Ltd 81
Fanz Holdings Ltd 96
Hansen, Jos & Soehne (Nigeria) Ltd 120
Holman Brothers (Nigeria) Ltd 123
Kolinah Industries Nigeria Ltd 148
Marini Group 164
Matzen & Timm (Nigeria) Ltd 166
Morpol Industrial Corporation Ltd 176
Nigerian Technical Co Ltd 218
Odeco Ltd 228
Power & Communication Engineering
  Nigeria Ltd 251
Safni Ltd 266
Scoa Nigeria Ltd 270
Scoatrac (A Division of Scoa (Nigeria)
  Ltd) 270
Sehl International 272
Selwood Pumps 272
Servo Nigerian Enterprises Ltd 273
Siab Engineering Company Nigeria Ltd 274
Silverball Integrated Engineering Co
  Nigeria Ltd 274
Stephens, Henry, Engineering
  Company Ltd 281
Stronghold (Nigeria) Ltd 282
Structec 282
United Nigeria Motors Ltd 305
UTC Nigeria Ltd (Formerly Union
  Trading Company of Nigeria Ltd) 311
West African Engineering Company
  Nigeria Ltd (WAECO) 318
Whessoe Engineering Ltd 320
Wolff, Otto, (Nigeria) & Company Ltd 322

Consultants (business)

A G Leventis & Company (Nigeria) Ltd 3
Abbey Group of Insurance Brokers,
  Life & Pensions Consultants 4
Abebiyi Sonaike & Company 4
Aboderin & Glahé Nigeria Ltd 5
Adamu Management International 6
Ajanga International Agency 15
Amass Nigeria Ltd 23
Arewa Hotels (Developments) Ltd 27
Arthur Andersen & Company 29
Bana Consultants Nigeria Ltd 35
Berif International Company 41
Bode International Nig Agencies 45
Boma Associates (WA) Ltd 45
(BRMC) 51
Business Research Management
  Center 51
CEC & Co (Nigeria) Ltd 54
Central Investment Company Ltd 55
City Group Organization 62
Coopers & Lybrand Associates Ltd 68
Daniksi Ltd 74
Danlon Associates 74
Dar Al-Handasah Consultants &
  Partners 75
Delta Property Development Co Ltd 77
Dotun Okubanjo & Associates Ltd 81
Emos Dynamics Co (Nigeria) Ltd 91
Femce Marketing Company 98
Funcke, C, & Co (Nigeria) Ltd 105
Gaby and Company (Nigeria) 106
Gränges Nigeria Ltd 113
I I Commercial Services (IICS) 125
Idem Consultants 127
Investment Promotions Ltd 135
Irede Properties and Investment
  Company Ltd 135
Itiku & Co Ltd 136
J & H International Agency 137
Kosm (West Africa) Ltd 149
Lanlek (Nigeria) Associates 152
Linbolsen Multi-Lingual Services Ltd 156
Macgregor & Ojutalayo 159
Martins, Akin, (Nigeria) Ltd 165
Matef Ltd 166
Maurice Project Centre Ltd 166
Metra Nigeria 169
Metropol Management Consulting
  Services Ltd 170
MMCS Ltd 170
Modulor Group 174
Nabena, Benjamin, Nabenson
  Promotions 178
New Nigeria Development Company
  Ltd 189
Nichimen Company (Nigeria) Ltd 190
Niger Raw Materials Ltd 192
Nigerian Agricultural Promotions
  Company Ltd 199
Nigerian Diversified Investments Ltd 204
Nigerian Institute of Management 209
Nigerian Joint Agencies Ltd 209
Nordmann, Rassmann & Company
  (Nigeria) Ltd 222
Odeng Engineering Company Ltd 228
Omo Group Organisation 233
Ono & Partners 235
Oscarte (Nigeria) Ltd 236
Pan African Consultancy Services
  (Nigeria) Ltd 241
Peat Marwick Ani, Ogunde & Company 244
Price Waterhouse 253
Prideco - Projects & Industrial
  Equipment Co (Nigeria) Ltd 253
Project Management Ltd 254
Reliance Business Consultations 260
Safni Ltd 266
Scobi Associates 271
Secom Ltd 271
Segun International Group Ltd 272
Skoup & Co Ltd 275
Superform Africa Company Ltd 285
Tara Consulting Nigeria Ltd 286
Urbahn, Max O, International Ltd 310
Voss & Umlauft Nigeria Ltd 314
Walton Solomon & Associates 315
World Courier Nigeria Ltd 323
Yodesons (Nigeria) Ltd 323

Consultants (engineering)

Abayomi, Olufawo, & Partners	3
Adobi Organisation	8
Afro Elektro Konsult Ltd	13
Amana Consulting Engineers	22
Ameniger Construction Company Ltd	23
Americo Ltd	24
APC International Nigeria Ltd	25
ARC-Models Company	27
Arcus Consultant Ltd	27
Baertle, J, & Co (Nig) Ltd	34
Becker-Voigt, H	37
Berenshot Moret Bosboom	40
Berg Geotechnical Engineering (Nigeria) Ltd	40
Biobaku Faber & Partners	43
BRGM (Nigeria) Ltd	49
(BRMC)	51
Brown & Root Nigeria Ltd	50
Business & Industrial Consultants	50
Business Research Management Center	51
Caaso Constructional Works Ltd	51
Cansult Ltd	53
Cetaconsult (Nigeria) Ltd	55
City Group Organization	62
Communications Consultants Nigeria Ltd	65
Comprehensive Engineering Consultants	65
Construction & Support Services Nigeria Ltd	66
Construction Management Services	66
Coutinho, Caro & Co (Nigeria) Ltd	69
Design Group Nigeria	78
Deutsche Kaiser Gruppe (Interkontinental)	78
DHV Consultants Nigeria Ltd	79
Ebel Bau Nigeria Ltd	85
Edison Group & Parnters	86
Eksons (Nig) Ltd	87
Emirate Technical Services	91
Engineering Construction Co Ltd (ECC)	92
Formerly Mitsui & Co (Nigeria) Ltd	166
(Formerly Oscar Faber (Nigeria))	43
Foster Wheeler (Nigeria) Ltd	103
Foundation Construction Ltd	103
Foundation Engineering (Nigeria) Ltd	103
Gauff Consultants (Nigeria) Ltd	107
Geco Engineering Co (Nigeria) Ltd	107
Geocomsa & Co (Nigeria) Ltd	108
Geodetic Surveys Ltd	108
German-Nigerian Engineering Company Ltd (Gernig)	110
Grandi Lavori (Nigeria) Ltd	113
Gränges Nigeria Ltd	113
Haskoning Nigeria Ltd (Formerly Nedeco)	121
Hay, Barry, Odunsi & Associates	121
Herwa Ltd	122
Inco Consultants (Nigeria) Ltd	129
Insumma (Nigeria) Ltd	130
Integrated Consultants (Nigeria) Ltd	130
International Planning Associates	134
Joe Oyegoke Associates	139
Kaeler (West Africa) Ltd	142
Keppler Hausbau (Nigeria) Ltd	146
Kloeckner Ina Nigeria Ltd	148
Kosm (West Africa) Ltd	149
Kragha & Associates	149
Lavalin Nigeria Ltd	153
Lonogu Enterprises Ltd	157
Louis Berger Inc Nigeria	158
Maachi-Valle and Associates	158
Mandilas Ltd	162
Mapcotec (Nigeria) Ltd	163
Matzen & Timm (Nigeria) Ltd	166
Maurice Project Centre Ltd	166
MBK Nigeria Ltd	166
Mehr, Hans, (Nigeria) Ltd	167
Minister Technical Services	172
Modelor Design Aids Ltd	174
MRT Consulting Engineers (Nigeria) Ltd	177
Nabena, L R, & Sons Ltd	179
Netherlands Harbourworks (Nigeria) Ltd	187
Nidanconsult	191
Niger Consultants Ltd	192
Nigerian Engineering and Construction Company Ltd (NECCO)	205
Nigerian Mapping Company Ltd	210
Niger-Techno Ltd	221
Nuccon	226
Nukom Engineering Ltd	226
O'Bahor, J A, & Company Ltd	227
Odeng Engineering Company Ltd	228
Olatunde Laleye and Partners	232
Omenjor & Ramsauer Electrical Company	233
Osot Associates Consulting Engineers	237
Ove Arup & Partners Nigeria Ltd	238
Paktank Nigeria Ltd	240
Pan African Consultancy Services (Nigeria) Ltd	241
Pan African Surveys Ltd	241
Pencol International (Nigeria) Ltd	244
Petroleum Consultants (Nigeria) Ltd	245
Poloni & Company Ltd	251
Ponti & Company Ltd	251
PRC (Nigeria) Ltd	252
Prideco - Projects & Industrial Equipment Co (Nigeria) Ltd	253
Rajendram, R, and Associates	257
Rapid Electrical & Mechanical Company Nigeria Ltd (REMCO)	257
Reynolds Construction Company (Nigeria) Ltd	261
Rhine-Schelde-Verolme Engineers	261
Safni Ltd	266
Salzgitter (WA) Ltd	266
Sandwell, P R, & Co (Nigeria) Ltd	267
Seismograph Service (Nigeria) Ltd (SSL)	272
Sepi Estero Consultants (Nigeria) Ltd	273
Shawmont Nigeria Ltd	274
Siab Engineering Company Nigeria Ltd	274
Silverball Integrated Engineering Co Nigeria Ltd	274
SNC (Nigeria) Ltd	276
Structeng Associates	283
Superform Africa Company Ltd	285
Sverdrup & Parcel & Associates	285
Techint Engineering (Nigeria) Ltd	287
Techjob Associates	287
Tradon Nigeria Ltd	292
Voss & Umlauft Nigeria Ltd	314
Walton Solomon & Associates	315
Ward, Ashcroft & Parkman (Nigeria) Ltd	315
Widnell and Trollope Nigeria	321

Defence and armaments

Defence Industries Corporation of Nigeria	76
Ladejobi Products Nigeria Ltd	151
Nigerian Explosives & Plastics Co Ltd	205

Educational equipment and training services

All Purpose Nigeria Ltd	20
Arewa Advancement Enterprises Ltd	27
Aridi Industries (Nigeria) Ltd	28
Associated Laboratory Supplies Ltd	31
Bayajida Group of Companies	37
(BRMC)	51
Business Research Management Center	51
CEP	55
Chemdyes Nigeria Ltd	58
Chidiebere Transport Ltd	59
Ekerete, A, Ltd	87
Fanz Holdings Ltd	96
I I Commercial Services (IICS)	125
Joas Electrical Industries Ltd	139
Kucena-Damian (Nigeria) Ltd	149
Kufena Trading Co Ltd	150
Lanlek (Nigeria) Associates	152
Link Group International Ltd	156
Mareen Industries Ltd	163
Mesacom Electronics Instrumentations Ltd	168
Nabena, Benjamin, Nabenson Promotions	178

Nigerian Book Suppliers Ltd	200
Nigerian Institute of Management	209
NMB Modern Bookshops	222
Oshinmi Company Ltd	236
Pan African Consultancy Services (Nigeria) Ltd	241
PGL Group Ltd	245
Prime Feathers International Services Ltd	254
Promana Associates	255
Reliance Group of Companies	260
Scobi Associates	271
Superior Systems International Ltd	285
Thomade Enterprises (Nig) Ltd	289
Twilights Nigeria Ltd	297
United Educational Supplies Ltd	305
Universal Educational Supplies Ltd (Morison Arnold Ltd)	308
Urobo Agencies (Nigeria) Ltd	310
Vickins (Nigeria) Associates	313
Wiedemann & Walters (Nigeria) Ltd	321
Yinkus Book Centre Ltd	323

Electrical and electronic equipment

Abdul Azeez Electrical Centre	4
Adebowale Electrical Industries Ltd	6
Adejobi, Adeoye, Trading Stores Ltd	7
Adetona Awe (Nig) Enterprises	8
African Designs Development Centre Ltd	11
African Era and Company Ltd	11
Afro Commerce (WA) Ltd	13
Aircool Metal Industries (Nigeria) Ltd	15
Ajirotutu (Nigeria) Ltd	16
Akanji Commercial Enterprises Ltd	16
Akanji, D L, & Co (Nig) Ltd	16
Allied Electronics & Telecommunications Services Ltd	20
Asape (Nigeria) Company Ltd	29
Associated Electronic Products (Nigeria) Ltd	31
B & F Nigeria Ltd	34
Bayajida Group of Companies	37
Bayer (Nigeria) Ltd	37
Benora Instruments & Company	39
Binatone Electronics	43
Birma General Supplies Ltd	43
Black & Decker Nigeria Ltd	44
Bolingo Organisation	45
Briscoe, R T, (Nigeria) Ltd	49
Business & Industrial Consultants	50
CFAO (Nigeria) Ltd	56
Chemdyes Nigeria Ltd	58
Chrislow Associated Nigeria Ltd	59
Cneico (Nigeria) Ltd	63
Cutler-Hammer Nigeria Ltd	71
DAE International (Nigeria) Ltd	72
Daniksi Ltd	74
Diesel Generating Company Ltd	79
DPMS Ltd	81
Eddy's Electronics	85
Edrita & Company Ltd	86
Edun Commercial Agency	86
Ekisola Electrical Works Ltd	87
Electrical Material Supplies (EMS)	89
Electricare Ltd	89
Electro Technologies Nigeria Ltd (ELTEC)	89
Electronics Industrial Company (Nigeria) Ltd	90
Electronics Instrumentations Ltd	90
Eppellion International Ltd	92
Estate Electrical Industries (Nigeria) Ltd	93
Etco-Engineering & Technical Company (Nigeria) Ltd	93
(Formerly IBM Nig Ltd)	81
(Formerly Philips (Nig) Ltd)	31
Gaby and Company (Nigeria)	106
Gregson Trading Company Ltd	114
Group Elektro Power Nigeria Ltd	114
Hagemeyer (Nigeria) Ltd	119
Hammond, Michael, Engineering Ltd	119
Hilson Nigeria Ltd	122
Holt, John, Ltd	123
Hulls Services Ltd	125
International Agencies Ltd	131
International Contracts & Consultancy Services Ltd	132

INDEX: Business Activity Subdivided by Country

International Yettco (Nigeria) Ltd 134
Interworld Enterprises Nigeria Ltd 135
Itidal-Epid Enterprises of Nigeria 136
ITT Nigeria Ltd 136
J & H International Agency 137
Joas Electrical Industries Ltd 139
Jobba Trading Company 139
Johnson Foluso International
  Enterprises (JOFI) 139
Kabelmetal Nigeria Ltd 141
Kaycee (Nigeria) Ltd 145
Kolinton Technical Industries Ltd 148
Landmark Industrial Supplies Ltd 152
Latderma Enterprises 153
Littleways International Ltd 157
Lonogu Enterprises Ltd 157
Maclisle Complex Ltd 159
Maiden Electronics Works Ltd 159
Mandilas Ltd 162
Matuwo Electronics Co 166
Mesacom Electronics Instrumentations
  Ltd 168
Miccom Engineering Works Ltd 170
Mifi (Nigeria) Ltd 172
Mike Merchandise Co Ltd 172
Minnesota Nigeria Ltd 172
Mitton Refrigeration Service 173
Mofat Engineering Company Ltd 175
Moore Obioha, C, Sons & Company
  Ltd 176
Moukarim Industries Ltd 177
Nabena, Benjamin, Nabenson
  Promotions 178
Namco Nigeria Ltd 179
Netarcomms Nigeria Ltd 186
New Africa Development Company Ltd 188
Newmark Electric Co Ltd 190
Newmark Electric Company Ltd 190
Nigerchin Electrical Development
  Company Ltd 193
Nigeria Engineering Works Ltd 195
Nigerian Electric Fitting Ltd 204
Nigerian Electronics Company Ltd 204
Nimesco (Nigeria) Ltd 221
Nobgroup of Companies 222
Norman Industries Ltd 223
Normann, C, International Company 223
Northern Cable Processing and
  Manufacturing Company Ltd 224
Nucleus Electronics Ltd 226
Odeco Ltd 228
Oguine Brothers 230
Ohakwe & Associates (Nigeria) Ltd 230
Okenabirhie Enterprises Ltd 231
Olutone Electronics 233
Oluwakemi Motors & Finance
  Company Ltd 233
Olympic Group Ltd 233
Pan Electric Ltd 242
Petraco, De, Industries Ltd 245
Plessecomms Nigeria Ltd (Formerly
  Plessey (Nigeria) Ltd) 250
Polamp (Nigeria) Ltd 250
Princegate Trading & Contracting
  Company Ltd 254
Promana Associates 255
Radio Vision Centre (Nigeria) Ltd 257
Rex Radio Electronic Company Ltd 261
Roaag Company (Nigeria) Ltd 263
Runsewe Group of Companies 265
Sanyo (Nigeria) Ltd 267
Scan African Nigeria Ltd 269
Sebo Technical Industries Nigeria Ltd 271
Senn-Sound (West Africa) Ltd 272
Servo Nigerian Enterprises Ltd 273
Siej Agencies 274
Sodik-Asea (Nigeria) Ltd 277
Sporty Fancy & General Stores Ltd 279
Technae (Nigeria) Ltd 287
Technophon Electrical Enterprises
  Company Ltd 288
Teju Industries Ltd 288
Telerex Electronics Ltd 288
Thomade Enterprises (Nig) Ltd 289
Thompson Dickson Technical Co Ltd 289
Times Leisure Services Ltd 290
Tommy Building & Construction
  Company Ltd 291
UAC of Nigeria Ltd 297
Unigwe, Fred Balonwu, Group of
  Companies 302
Unije, B C, & Sons Ltd 302
Urobo Agencies (Nigeria) Ltd 310
VP (Nigeria) Ltd 315

VYB (Nigeria) Ltd 315
Weide & Co (Group of Companies) Ltd 316
West African Surveys Ltd 319
Wozabeth Trading Company 323
Yodesons (Nigeria) Ltd 323
Zabadne & Company Ltd 324
Zard, C, & Company Ltd 324

Electrical engineering

Allied Electronics &
  Telecommunications Services Ltd 20
Ameniger Construction Company Ltd 23
Analex Group Ltd 24
Asagba, M A, & Sons 29
Awosanmi & Sons Engineering Works 33
B B C Brown Boveri (Nigeria) Ltd 34
Bolori Brothers & Co Ltd (Bolbros) 45
Bosag Builders 46
Chidiebere Transport Ltd 59
City Group Organization 62
Citymark (West Africa) Ltd 62
Commonwealth Commodity Company
  International 64
Corpio Constructions (Nigeria) Ltd 69
Deutsche Kaiser Gruppe
  (Interkontinental) 78
Drake & Scull (Nigeria) Ltd 81
Electro Technologies Nigeria Ltd
  (ELTEC) 89
Elettro Engineering 90
Etco-Engineering & Technical
  Company (Nigeria) Ltd 93
Felicity Engineering Co Ltd 98
George Engineering Co Ltd 109
Green, A D, & Co Ltd 114
Group Elektro Power Nigeria Ltd 114
Hammond, Michael, Engineering Ltd 119
Heplac Nigeria Ltd 122
Igwe Brothers & Co Ltd 128
International Contracts & Consultancy
  Services Ltd 132
Kent Engineering Nigeria Ltd 146
Kilpatrick, James, (Nigeria) Ltd 146
Littleways International Ltd 157
Lonogu Enterprises Ltd 157
Marryat, Daniel, (Nigeria) Ltd 165
Mascot I Abali & Brothers Ltd 165
Mofat Engineering Company Ltd 175
Mouldex Ltd 177
New Africa Development Company Ltd 188
Newmark Electric Company Ltd 190
Niger Construction Ltd 191
Nigerian Company for Energy
  Engineering Ltd (NICOGEN) 202
Nkwonta, D O, & Sons Enterprises Ltd 222
Nobgroup of Companies 222
Northern Cable Processing and
  Manufacturing Company Ltd 224
Nwonye, I O M, & Sons Company Ltd 227
O'Bahor, J A, & Company Ltd 227
Oblozo & Partners Power Construction
  Company Ltd 227
Oguine Brothers 230
Ogunmefun Works Ltd 230
Ohakwe & Associates (Nigeria) Ltd 230
Omenjor & Ramsauer Electrical
  Company 233
Port & Marine Services Ltd 251
Power & Communication Engineering
  Nigeria Ltd 251
Rajendram, R, and Associates 257
Rapid Electrical & Mechanical
  Company Nigeria Ltd (REMCO) 257
Reynolds Construction Company
  (Nigeria) Ltd 261
Richas Engineering Works Company
  Ltd 261
Safni Ltd 266
Schroeder, H F, (WA) Ltd 270
Silverball Integrated Engineering Co
  Nigeria Ltd 274
Smeaton Ltd 275
Sodik-Asea (Nigeria) Ltd 277
Sointeco (Nigeria) Ltd 277
Songhai Group of Companies 278
Technical Constructions (Nigeria) Ltd 287
Transelek Nigeria Ltd 293
Trindel (Nigeria) Ltd 295

Wayne (West Africa) Ltd 316
Westend Engineering Ltd 320
Whessoe Engineering Ltd 320

Fertilizers

Adejumo Fam (Nigeria) Ltd 7
Agrotec Services Ltd 15
Basf (Nigeria) Ltd 37
Commind Nigeria Ltd 64
Compagnie Francaise de l'Afrique
  Internationale 65
Co-Operative Supply Association Ltd 68
Fisco-Chemicals (Nigeria) Ltd 100
Gobecco Trading Company Ltd 111
International Contracts & Consultancy
  Services Ltd 132
Olympic Group Ltd 233
Petro-Organico (Nigeria) Ltd 245
Ramson Mellamby & Company Ltd 257
Seepc (Nigeria) Ltd 271
Sehl International 272
United Development Trading Company
  Ltd 305
UTC Nigeria Ltd (Formerly Union
  Trading Company of Nigeria Ltd) 311

Fishing and fish processing

Asra Seafoods (Nigeria) Ltd 30
Bolingo Organisation 45
Commonwealth Commodity Company
  International 64
Globe Fishing Industries Ltd 111
Hamzer, G N A, & Co (Nigeria) Ltd 119
Ibru Sea Foods Ltd 126
Inter Continental Fishing (Nigeria) Ltd 131
Juli Importers & Exporters Enterprises 140
Niger Sea Foods Ltd 192
Nigeria National Fish Company Ltd 196
Nigerian National Fish Company Ltd 211
Nigerian National Shrimp Company
  Ltd 213
Obelawo Farcha Fishing Industries Ltd 227
Universal Fishing Company Ltd 308
West African Shrimps Ltd 319

Food and food processing

A G Leventis & Company (Nigeria) Ltd 3
Abukon Nigeria Ltd 5
Adarice Company Ltd 6
Addis Engineering Ltd 6
Agricultural Development Corporation
  (Anambra State) 14
Agro Industries & Development
  Schemes Co (Nig) Ltd 15
Alfa-Laval (Nigeria) Ltd 19
Allied Biscuit Company Ltd 20
Anambra Vegetable Oils Products
  Nigeria Ltd 25
(AVOP) 25
Bendel Chemical Industries Ltd 38
Benue Plateau Rice Company Ltd 40
Bibson Associates Ltd 42
Biscuit Manufacturing Company of
  Nigeria Ltd 43
Bolingo Organisation 45
Cadbury Nigeria Ltd 51
Calaro Oil Palm Estate Ltd 52
CFAO (Nigeria) Ltd 56
Champion Confectionery Co (Nigeria)
  Ltd 57
Charlie and Franco Ltd 57
Chattalas Brothers Ltd 57
Chellaram, K, & Sons (Nigeria) Ltd 57
Chrisray Nigeria Ltd 59
Christlieb, A C, (Nigeria) Ltd 59
Chukwurah Agriculture Industries Ltd 61
Clarke, W F, (Nigeria) Ltd 62
Cocoa Industries Ltd 63

Cocoa Producers Alliance	63
Co-Operative Supply Association Ltd	68
Daily Need Chemists Ltd	72
De Facto Bakeries & Catering Ltd	76
Desam Development Company Ltd	78
Eleiyele Cashew Factory	90
Ethiope Food Industries Ltd	94
Eurotrade (Nigeria) Ltd	94
Fan Milk Ltd	96
Fanz Holdings Ltd	96
Flour Mills of Nigeria Ltd	102
Food Specialities (Nigeria) Ltd	102
Foods Division of UAC of Nigeria Ltd	102
Foremost Dairies (Nigeria) Ltd	102
Formerly Benue Plateau Biscuits Co Ltd	180
Fredano Trading Co Ltd	103
Funtua Cottonseed Crushing Company Ltd	105
Global Stars (Nigeria) Ltd	111
Grace Bakeries	113
Guthrie (Nigeria) Ltd	115
Hamzer, G N A, & Co (Nigeria) Ltd	119
Ibru Organisation (Ibru Ltd)	126
Idehen, J I, & Sons (Nigeria) Ltd	127
Idehen Poultry Farm	127
International Biscuits Ltd	132
Kabba Co-Operative Credit & Marketing Union Ltd	141
Kano Confectionery Ltd	143
Kano Sugar Industry Nigeria Ltd	144
Kaura Biscuit and Macaroni Factory Ltd	145
Kedam Holdings (Nigeria) Ltd	145
Kwa Falls Oil Palm Estate Ltd	150
Ladejobi Products Nigeria Ltd	151
Ladgroup Ltd	151
Lafia Canning Factory	151
Las & Co Ltd	153
Life Flour Mill Ltd	155
Lipton of Nigeria Ltd	156
Lisabi Mills (Nigeria) Ltd	156
Makin Ltd	161
Management Enterprises Ltd	161
Marketing and Shipping Enterprises Ltd	165
Mogaji Osona Enterprises Ltd	175
Moon Confectionery Ltd	175
Mosheshe Group of Companies	176
Munro, Brian, Ltd	178
Nasco Biscuits (Nigeria) Ltd	180
Nasreddin Group International (Nigeria) Ltd	180
National Grains Production Company Ltd	181
National Root Crops Production Company Ltd	183
National Salt Company of Nigeria Ltd	183
New Nigeria Salt Company Ltd	189
NFS (Food and Cold Storage) Ltd	190
Nidoco Ltd	191
Nifeipiri Poultries Ltd	191
Niger Biscuits Company Ltd	191
Niger Sea Foods Ltd	192
Nigeria Cold Stores Ltd	194
Nigerian Cocoa Board	202
Nigerian Consolidated Food Producers Ltd	203
Nigerian Food Company Ltd	206
Nigerian Groundnut Board	207
Nigerian Oil Mills Ltd	213
Nigerian Processing Company Ltd	215
Nigerian Starch Mills Ltd	217
Nigerian Sugar Company Ltd	217
Nigerian Sweets and Confectionery Company Ltd	218
Nigerian Yeast & Alcohol Manufacturing Company Ltd	220
Northern Nigeria Flour Mills Ltd	224
Odus Bakeries	229
Okitipupa Oil Palm Co Ltd	231
Olaogun Enterprises Ltd	231
Olau Olu Modern Bakery Ltd	232
Onigbinde, M A, & Sons Ltd	235
Ono & Partners	235
Ovaltine (West Africa) Ltd	238
Pioneer Biscuit Factory Ltd	248
Pioneer Starch Industries (Nigeria) Ltd	248
Plateau Foods Processing Company Ltd	249
Port Express Services Ltd	251
Port Harcourt Flour Mills Ltd	251
Poultry & Animal Products (Nigeria) Ltd	251
Prime Feathers International Services Ltd	254
Rabiu, Isiyaku, & Sons Ltd	256
Raji Bakeries Ltd	257
Risonpalm Ltd	262
Rivers Vegetable Oil Company Ltd	263
Savannah Sugar Company Ltd	269
Sobat Ltd	276
Soccer Chewing Gum Enterprises Ltd	276
Star Sweets Co Ltd	280
Tate & Lyle (Nigeria) Ltd	286
Toyin Rising Bakery	292
Trebor (Nigeria) Ltd	294
UAC of Nigeria Ltd	297
UTC Nigeria Ltd (Formerly Union Trading Company of Nigeria Ltd)	311
Valley Foods Nigeria Ltd	311
Vegetable & Fruit Processing Ltd	312
Vegetable Oils (Nigeria) Ltd	312
West Africa Milk Company (Nigeria) Ltd	317
West African Cold Storage Co of Nigeria Ltd	318
West African Shrimps Ltd	319
Yassin Confectionery & Sweet Company Ltd	323

Freight forwarding and customs agents

Aeromaritime (Nigeria) Ltd	9
Akwiwu Motors Ltd	17
Alraine (Nigeria) Ltd	21
Amatemeso Shipping Agencies Ltd	23
Anopit Ltd	25
Ayo, Lawrence, & Sons Ltd	34
Balogun, A A, & Sons (Nigeria) Ltd	35
Ben Agency Service	38
Cepuz International Agencies	55
CFAO (Nigeria) Ltd	56
Charlie and Franco Ltd	57
Claretta Maritime Services Ltd	62
Coastal Services (Nigeria) Ltd	63
Combined Maritime Agencies (Nigeria) Ltd	64
Continental Lines (Africa) Ltd	66
Cross Lines Ltd	70
Dafinasi Enterprises Ltd	72
Danwawu Shipping Cargo Handling & Transport Co Ltd	74
DHL International Nigeria Ltd	78
Eastern (Overseas) Agencies Ltd	85
Equatorial Lines	92
Express International Maritime Ltd	95
Fallad Commercial Enterprises Ltd	96
Formerly Mitsui & Co (Nigeria) Ltd	166
Gaby and Company (Nigeria)	106
Goas Agencies Ltd	111
IAS Cargo Airlines	126
Ijomah International Co Ltd	128
Intercare Ltd	131
International Maritime Services	133
JOKI (Nigeria) Ltd	140
Kennedy Transport (Nigeria) Ltd	145
Kunza Heed (W.A.) Enterprises	150
Laas Ltd	150
Lagos & Niger Shipping Agencies Ltd	151
Maiden Maritime (Nigeria) Ltd	160
Majem Trading Company	160
MBK Nigeria Ltd	166
Middleton River Brothers (Nigeria) Ltd	171
Modearo (Nigeria) Ltd	173
Napak Services (Nigeria) Ltd	179
National Freight Company	181
Neptune Transport Services Ltd	186
New Nigeria Merchants Ltd	189
Nigerian Aviation Handling Company Ltd	200
Nigerian General Superintendence Co Ltd	207
Nigerian Maritime Services Ltd	210
Nigerian Removal & Storage Co Ltd (NIRSCO)	215
Ogheneovo Ventures Ltd	229
Ojuri Maritime Services	231
Palm Line Agencies (Nigeria)	240
Pan African Airlines (Nigeria) Ltd	241
Pan Atlantic Shipping & Transport Agencies Ltd	242
Panalpina World Transport (Nigeria) Ltd	242
Par Excellence (Nigeria) Ltd	243
Peezone Freight Service Agency	244
Poco Container Removals Ltd	250
Primus (Nigeria) Ltd	254
Sams Agencies & Maritime Service (Nig)	266
Sawyerr Enterprises (Nigeria) Ltd	269
Speed-Bird Clearing and Forwarding Agency Ltd	279
Stephens, Henry, Group of Companies	281
Tradewinds Express (Nigeria) Ltd	292
Trans Atlantic Shipping Agency Ltd	292
Trans Nigeria Road Haulage Ltd	293
Transcap Ltd	293
Transmarco Agencies (Nigeria) Ltd	293
Triana Ltd	294
TSTC Coastal Agency	295
Tuntaric Nigeria Ltd	295
Uche, A O, & Sons (Nigeria) Ltd	299
Umarco (Nigeria) Ltd	301

Furniture

Afprint Nigeria Ltd	9
All-African Woodworking Industry Ltd	20
Aridi Industries (Nigeria) Ltd	28
Bestform Industries Co Ltd	41
Bhojsons & Company (Nigeria) Ltd	42
Birma General Supplies Ltd	43
Bisrod Furniture Company Ltd	44
Blessed Furniture Enterprises	44
Bonomi, S G, Ltd	45
Borno Engineering & Steel Manufacturers Ltd	46
Business Equipment & Machinery Ltd (BEAM) (Division of UAC of Nigeria Ltd)	50
CFC Furniture Co (En) Ltd	56
CFC Furniture Co (WC) Ltd	56
City Group Organization	62
Complete Home Enterprises (Nig) Ltd	65
Concorde Furniture Manufacturing Co Ltd	65
Controlled Plastics Ltd	67
Costain (West Africa) Ltd	69
Daddo International (Nigeria) Ltd	72
Debs Modern Industries Ltd	76
Delta Furniture & Furnishing Ind Ltd	76
Dexso Furniture Factory Ltd	78
Dunon Furniture Industry Ltd	83
Duro International (Nigeria) Ltd	84
Eastern Wrought Iron Ltd	85
Epe Plywood Industries Ltd	92
Ernestco Ltd	93
Eterna Electrical Engineering Works Ltd	94
Eze, I O, & Sons Ltd	95
Ezeilo, C C	96
Fawaz Steelwood & Chemicals (Kano) Ltd	97
Fawehinmi Furniture Factory Ltd	98
Femo (West Africa) Ltd	99
(Formerly Polyplast Industrial Co Ltd)	67
Furniture House Ltd	105
Golden Furniture & Construction Co Ltd	112
Goodwill, Francis, Ltd	112
Guobadia Furniture & Construction Company (Nigeria) Ltd	115
Hamzer, G N A, & Co (Nigeria) Ltd	119
Harmony House Furniture Co Ltd	120
Hassan Furniture & Joinery Company Ltd	121
Ijagbemi, S A, & Sons (Nigeria) Ltd	128
International Contracts & Consultancy Services Ltd	132
Jac-Ogho (Nigeria) Enterprises	137
Jarmakani Industries (Nig) Ltd	137
Jire Engineering Ltd	138
Kojusola Foam Industries Ltd	148
Lecco Engineering Construction Co Ltd	154
Macpon Engineering and Construction Company Ltd	159
Mag Furniture and Interior Designs Ltd	159
Makira Kwarin Mabuga Metal Wood Manufacturing Company Ltd	161
Marbs Furniture Industry Ltd	163
Metal & Wood Furniture Construction Company Ltd	168

Metal Fabricator (Nigeria) Ltd	169
Metal Furniture (Nigeria) Ltd	169
Metriscope Nigeria Ltd	169
Mifi (Nigeria) Ltd	172
Modern Domus Ltd	174
Moukarim Industries Ltd	177
Moukarim Metalwood Factory Ltd	177
Ndah, G, & Sons Foundation	185
Nigeria Construction and Furniture Company Ltd (NCFC)	194
Nigeria Engineering Works Ltd	195
Nigeria Reliance Furniture Company	197
Nigerian Engineering and Construction Company Ltd (NECCO)	205
Nigerian Iron & Wood Factory Ltd	209
Nigerian Merchants & Produce Suppliers	210
Nigerian Office Stationery Supply Stores Ltd	213
Nigerian Romanian Wood Industries Ltd	215
Nigerian Sewing Machine Manufacturing Company Ltd	216
Nigerian Toys Manufacturing Company Ltd (NITOMAC)	219
Nigertal Industries Ltd	221
Northern Sawmill & Furniture Manufacturing Co Ltd	225
Norwo Trading Company Ltd	226
Omo Group Organisation	233
Ozo Brothers Cabinet Works Ltd	239
Pecco Ltd	244
Promana Associates	255
Raccaform Ltd	256
Raccah & Chaker Factory Ltd	256
Sabon Sara Nigeria Ltd	266
Santana Furniture Factory Ltd	267
Scano (Nigeria) Enterprises Ltd	269
Sokoto Furniture Factory Ltd	277
Standard Industrial Development Company Ltd	280
Superfine Furniture & Trading Company Ltd	284
Swenig Furniture Company Ltd	285
Thomas Furniture Company Ltd	289
Tommy Building & Construction Company Ltd	291
Toronto Organisation (Nigeria) Ltd	291
Ugbabe Furniture & Construction Company Ltd	299
Ugochukwu Chemical Industries Ltd	301
Uncle Fado and Sons Furniture Factory Ltd	301
Vono Products Ltd	314
West African Aluminium Products (Nigeria)	317
Wrought Iron (Nigeria) Ltd	323
Yusufu Modern Industries Co	324

Glass

African Glass Company Ltd (Formerly Central Glass (Nigeria) Ltd)	11
Arroways of Nigeria	28
Brossette (Nigeria) Ltd	50
Cogemat (Nigeria) Ltd	63
Delta Glass Company Ltd	76
Diborsons Business Enterprises	79
Edrita & Company Ltd	86
Feso Mirror and Glass Works Ltd	99
MBTG	168
Metal Box Toyo Glass Nigeria Ltd	168
Nigerian Glass Containers & Metal Manufacturers Ltd	207
Ojeniyi, Adelegan, Trading Company Nigeria	230
PGN Ltd	245
Reliance Group of Companies	260
Shalhoub Brothers Ltd	274
Triplex Safety Glass (Nigeria) Ltd	295
West African Glass Industry Ltd	318

Government bodies

Crown Agents For Overseas Governments and Administrations	71
Federal Ministry of Industries	98
National Electric Power Authority (NEPA)	181
New Agency of Nigeria	188
Nigeria National Supply Company Ltd	197
Nigerian Enterprises Promotion Board (NEPB)	205
Nigerian Ports Authority (NPA)	214
Nigerian Television Authority	218
Ondo State Investment Corporation	234
Tradev Ltd	292

Handicrafts, pottery and jewellery

Airegin Enterprises & Agencies Ltd	15
Aye Marble & Terrazzo Industrial Works	33
Benora Instruments & Company	39
Edun Commercial Agency	86
Faltas, A M, (West Africa) Ltd	96
Fimcon Ltd	100
Nigerian Watch-Making Industry Ltd	219
Oluwakemi Motors & Finance Company Ltd	233
Oluwakemi (Swiss) Nigeria Embroidery Industries Ltd	233
Premier Engineering Works Ltd	253
Zabadne & Company Ltd	324

Hardware

Arewa Tradewinds (Nig) Co Ltd	28
Bewac Ltd	41
Bhojsons & Company (Nigeria) Ltd	42
Charlton Trading Company (Nigeria) Ltd	57
Chellaram, K, & Sons (Nigeria) Ltd	57
Cneico (Nigeria) Ltd	63
Compass Trading Co Ltd	65
Co-Operative Supply Association Ltd	68
Cosmos Metal & Electrics Ltd	69
(CTC)	57
Deazula Trading Company (Nigeria) Ltd	76
Diborsons Business Enterprises	79
Duro International (Nigeria) Ltd	84
Eastern Enamelware Factory Ltd	84
Fimcon Ltd	100
Freedom Development Company Ltd	105
General Metalware Company Nigeria Ltd	108
Grand Industrial Company Ltd	113
Hagemeyer (Nigeria) Ltd	119
Iffna Co Ltd	127
International Enamelware Industry Ltd	132
Ises Ltd	135
Kaycee (Nigeria) Ltd	145
Landmark Industrial Supplies Ltd	152
Lecco Engineering Construction Co Ltd	154
Nabena, L R, & Sons Ltd	179
Nails & General Steel Manufacturing Industry Ltd	179
NCO Merchants Brothers Company	185
Nigeria Industrial Group Ltd	196
Nigerian Enamelware Company Ltd (NEWCO)	204
Nigerian Wire Industries Ltd	220
Northern Enamelware Company Ltd	224
Ojeniyi, Adelegan, Trading Company Nigeria	230
Omo-Bare & Sons (Nigeria) Ltd	233
Osborne, E, Nigeria Ltd	236
Ositadinma International Ltd	237
Parkes, Josiah, & Sons (Nigeria) Ltd	243
Pressed Metal Industry Ltd	253
Sporty Fancy & General Stores Ltd	279
Tilley Gyado Group of Companies	290
United Consolidated Industries Ltd	305
UTC Nigeria Ltd (Formerly Union Trading Company of Nigeria Ltd)	311
Ventures, Coopers Benly, & Company Ltd (The)	313
Zard, C, & Company Ltd	324

Hotels and catering

Airoe Construction & Civil Engineering Co Ltd	15
Akija Hotel Ltd	16
Akpenlamen Co Ltd	17
Alex L M Davou Fom & Sons Enterprise Ltd	18
Arewa Hotels (Developments) Ltd	27
Bendel Hotels Board	38
Bolingo Organisation	45
Bristol Hotel	49
Central Hotel	55
De Facto Bakeries & Catering Ltd	76
Delta Hotels Ltd	77
Eko Holiday Inn	87
Faltas, A M, (West Africa) Ltd	96
Fisayo Holdings Ltd	100
Grenigas Ltd	114
Jemine Enterprises Ltd	138
Kaduna Hotels Co Ltd	141
Kandara Palace Hotel Ltd	143
Kano Residential Hotel	144
Kano State Hotels Management Board	144
KLF Ltd	147
Kole-James & Co Ltd	148
Lagos Airport Hotel Ltd	151
Luncheon Vouchers Nigeria Ltd	158
Mainland Hotel	160
Manatec Company Ltd	161
Nigeria Hotels Ltd	195
(Nigeria Hotels Ltd)	55
Nigerian Caterers & Supermarkets Ltd	201
Nwandu, D A, & Sons Enterprises Ltd	226
Plateau Hotels & Tourism Company Ltd	249
Plateau Tourism, Development & Transport Co Ltd	250
Regent Hotel	259
Rendezvous Group Hotels (Nigeria) Ltd	261
Rivers State Tourist & Hotel Corporation	263
Runsewe Group of Companies	265
Safni Ltd	266
Tamaco Ltd	286
Tilley Gyado Group of Companies	290
Tourist Company of Nigeria Ltd	291
Uwai and Sons Enterprises	311
Ven Hotels Ltd	312

Household goods and appliances

Abdul Azeez Electrical Centre	4
Adejobi, Adeoye, Trading Stores Ltd	7
Afprint Nigeria Ltd	9
Agroline (Nigeria) Ltd	15
Allied Metal & Chemical Works Ltd	20
ALUMACO	21
Aluminium Manufacturing Company of Nigeria Ltd	21
Associated Electronic Products (Nigeria) Ltd	31
Associated Metal & Allied Works Ltd	31
Battery Manufacturing Co (Nig) Ltd	37
Beggmatic Automations Ltd	38
Benora Instruments & Company	39
Berec Nigeria Ltd	40
Bhojsons & Company (Nigeria) Ltd	42
Binatone Electronics	43
Bisiolu Enterprises Ltd	44
Borno Engineering & Steel Manufacturers Ltd	46
Brightstar Industries Ltd	49
Candles & Polish Works Ltd	53
Cogemat (Nigeria) Ltd	63
Daddo International (Nigeria) Ltd	72
Delta Glass Company Ltd	76
Dolmech Engineering (Nig) Ltd	80
Eddy's Electronics	85
Electrical Material Supplies (EMS)	89
Electricare Ltd	89
Eximport & Company Nigeria Ltd	95
Femo (West Africa) Ltd	99
(Formerly Philips (Nig) Ltd)	31
Freedom Development Company Ltd	105
Gazal Industrial Enterprises Ltd	107
Grenigas Ltd	114

Hapel Nigeria Ltd 120
International Enamelware Industry Ltd 132
Interworld Enterprises Nigeria Ltd 135
Ises Ltd 135
Joas Electrical Industries Ltd 139
Jobba Trading Company 139
Johnson Wax Nigeria Ltd 140
Kaycee (Nigeria) Ltd 145
Kolinah Industries Nigeria Ltd 148
Kolinton Technical Industries Ltd 148
Modern Industries Ltd 174
Morison, J L, Sons & Jones (Nigeria) Ltd 176
MULMACO 178
Multi Aluminium Manufacturing Company Ltd 178
Nasreddin Group International (Nigeria) Ltd 180
Nidogas Company Ltd 191
Niger Match Company Ltd 192
Nigeria Candle Stick Manufacturing Company Ltd 194
Nigerian Cutlery Ltd 203
Nigerian Electronics Company Ltd 204
Nigerian Match & Chemical Industries Ltd 210
Nigerian Metal Fabricating Ltd 210
Nigerian Sewing Machine Manufacturing Company Ltd 216
Nipol Ltd 221
Northern Enamelware Company Ltd 224
Northern Nigerian Technical Service Ltd 225
Okenabirhie Enterprises Ltd 231
Omo Group Organisation 233
Pan Electric Ltd 242
Petraco, De, Industries Ltd 245
Polamp (Nigeria) Ltd 250
Prestige Stores Nigeria Ltd 253
Prime Feathers International Services Ltd 254
Princegate Trading & Contracting Company Ltd 254
Ramson Mellamby & Company Ltd 257
Reckitt & Colman (Nigeria) Ltd 259
Safa Splints Ltd 266
Shalhoub Brothers Ltd 274
Sporty Fancy & General Stores Ltd 279
Star Match Company Ltd 280
Sungas Company Ltd 284
Teju Industries Ltd 288
Times Leisure Services Ltd 290
Tower Aluminium (Nigeria) Ltd 291
UAC of Nigeria Ltd 297
Union Carbide (Nigeria) Ltd 302
United Match Company of Nigeria Ltd 305
Universal Steels Ltd 308
Utilgas Nigerian and Overseas Gas Company Ltd 311
Ventures, Coopers Benly, & Company Ltd (The) 313
Vono Products Ltd 314
West Africa Household Utilities Manufacturing Company (Nigeria) Ltd 317
Wilmer Industries Nigeria Ltd 322
Zabadne & Company Ltd 324
Zenith Containers Company Ltd 324
Zerolas Batteries Company Ltd 324

Industrial equipment and heavy machinery

Acim 6
Acrow Ltd 6
Addis Engineering Ltd 6
Adejobi, Adeoye, Trading Stores Ltd 7
Agribuild Nigeria Ltd 14
Ajirotutu (Nigeria) Ltd 16
Alfa-Laval (Nigeria) Ltd 19
Allgemein Business Associates 20
Associated Exports (W.A.) Ltd 31
Avery Nigeria Ltd 33
B & F Nigeria Ltd 34
Beggmatic Automations Ltd 38
Bewac Ltd 41
Blackwood Hodge (Nigeria) Ltd 44
Boma Associates (WA) Ltd 45
Bosag Builders 46

Briscoe, R T, (Nigeria) Ltd 49
Cimeco Enterprises (Nigeria) Ltd 61
City Group Organization 62
Commind Nigeria Ltd 64
Compass Trading Co Ltd 65
Controlled Plastics Ltd 67
Conveyancer (Nigeria) Ltd 67
DAE International (Nigeria) Ltd 72
Desam Development Company Ltd 78
Diesel Generating Company Ltd 79
Diesel Sales and Service (Nigeria) Ltd 79
Disscol Ltd 79
Eurotrade (Nigeria) Ltd 94
(Formerly Polyplast Industrial Co Ltd) 67
Fusi Industrial Supplies Co Ltd 105
General Metalware Company Nigeria Ltd 108
Grenigas Ltd 114
Hansen, Jos & Soehne (Nigeria) Ltd 120
Holman Brothers (Nigeria) Ltd 123
Ibru Organisation (Ibru Ltd) 126
Incar Nigeria Ltd 129
Industrial & Safety Equipment (Nigeria) Ltd 129
Innocent Hope Overseas Company 130
ITT Nigeria Ltd 136
Kaeler (West Africa) Ltd 142
KLF Ltd 147
Kolinah Industries Nigeria Ltd 148
Leo's Group of Companies Ltd 154
Lonogu Enterprises Ltd 157
Maclisle Complex Ltd 159
Mascot I Abali & Brothers Ltd 165
Matzen & Timm (Nigeria) Ltd 166
Mehr, Hans, (Nigeria) Ltd 167
Metrocom International Ltd 170
Motorways Nigeria Ltd 177
Mouldex Ltd 177
Nabena, L R, & Sons Ltd 179
Nigeria General Motors Ltd 195
Nigeria Marine & Trading Company Ltd 196
Nigerian & Overseas Products Ltd 198
Nigerian Motors Industries Ltd 211
Nigerian Technical Co Ltd 218
Odeco Ltd 228
Oruche, Joe, Trading Company Ltd 236
Pan Nigerian Agency 242
Plastex Nigeria Ltd 249
Prideco - Projects & Industrial Equipment Co (Nigeria) Ltd 253
Roaag Company (Nigeria) Ltd 263
Rutam Ltd 265
Salzgitter (WA) Ltd 266
Scan African Nigeria Ltd 269
Scoa Nigeria Ltd 270
Scoatrac (A Division of Scoa (Nigeria) Ltd) 270
Sho's Engineering Company Ltd 274
Siab Engineering Company Nigeria Ltd 274
Silverball Integrated Engineering Co Nigeria Ltd 274
Siram Industrial Products Ltd 275
Sointeco (Nigeria) Ltd 277
Spicers (Nigeria) Ltd 279
Stag Engineering Nigeria Ltd 280
Stokvis (Nigeria) Ltd 282
Tarpaulin Industries (WA) Ltd 286
Teddy Continental Company 288
Topaz (Nigeria) Ltd 291
Tractor & Equipment 292
Tractors Under-Carriage Industry Nigeria Ltd 292
Tradon Nigeria Ltd 292
Wasco Ropes Ltd 315
Whessoe Engineering Ltd 320
Wiedemann & Walters (Nigeria) Ltd 321
Woermann, C, (Nigeria) Ltd 322
Wolff, Otto, (Nigeria) & Company Ltd 322

Insurance and re-insurance

Abbey Group of Insurance Brokers, Life & Pensions Consultants 4
African Alliance Insurance Co Ltd 9
African Insurance Company Ltd 11
African Ivory Insurance Company Ltd 11
African Prudential Insurance Company Ltd (The) 12

African Reinsurance Corporation 13
Akin-George, J, & Company 16
American International Insurance 24
Amicable Assurance Company Ltd 24
Ark Stewart Wrightson 28
Arrowhead Insurance Co (Nig) Ltd 29
Bendel Insurance Company Ltd 38
Braithwaite, T A, (Insurance Brokers) & Co 47
British India General Insurance Co (Nigeria) Ltd 49
British-American Insurance Company (Nigeria) Ltd 49
Century Insurance Co (Nigeria) Ltd 55
City Group Organization 62
Commerce Assurance Ltd 64
Crusader Insurance Co (Nigeria) Ltd 71
Equity & General Accident Insurance Company Ltd 92
Express Insurance Company Ltd 95
Fanz Holdings Ltd 96
(Formerly Nigerian Amicable Assurance Company Ltd) 24
Glanvill Enthoven & Company (Nigeria) 110
Great Nigeria Insurance Company Ltd 113
Guinea Insurance Company Ltd 114
H Clarkson Edu & Partners 117
Hamzer, G N A, & Co (Nigeria) Ltd 119
Harmony Insurance Co (Nigeria) Ltd 120
Herwa Insurance Ltd 122
Hogg Robinson Nigeria 123
Insurance Brokers of Nigeria 130
Intercare Ltd 131
International Maritime Services 133
Kapital Insurance Company Ltd 144
Kayson Company Ltd 145
Law Union and Rock Insurance Co of Nigeria Ltd 153
Leadway Assurance Company Ltd 153
Lion of Africa Insurance Co Ltd 156
Lombard Insurance Co Ltd 157
Manilla Insurance Company Ltd 162
Marine and General Assurance Company Ltd 164
Mercury Assurance Co Ltd 167
Motor and General Insurance Company 177
National Insurance Corporation of Nigeria 181
NEM Insurance Company (Nigeria) Ltd 185
New India Assurance Company (Nigeria) Ltd 188
New Insurance Company (Nigeria) Ltd 188
New Nigeria Insurance Company Ltd 189
New-Gate Insurance Co Ltd 190
NICON 181
Niger Insurance Company Ltd (The) 192
Nigeria Reinsurance Corporation 197
Nigerian General Insurance Company Ltd (The) 206
Nigerian Life & Pensions Consultants 210
Nigerian Safety Insurance Company Ltd 216
Nigerian Victory Assurance Company Ltd 219
Omo Group Organisation 233
Orumokpo & Sons (Nigeria) Ltd 236
Phoenix of Nigeria Assurance Company Ltd 247
Piccadilly Insurance Company Ltd 248
Progressive Insurance Company Ltd 254
Renaissance Assurance Company Ltd 260
Rivbank Insurance Company Ltd 262
Roomans Eneli Flynn & Company 264
Rotag Assurance Company Ltd 265
Royal Exchange Assurance (Nigeria) Ltd 265
Sentinel Assurance Company Ltd 272
Sun Insurance Office (Nigeria) Ltd 283
United Nigeria Insurance Company Ltd (The) 305
Unity Life and Fire Insurance Company Ltd 307
Universal Insurance Company Ltd 308
Valid Assurance Company Ltd 311
Veritas Insurance Company Ltd 313
West African Provincial Insurance Company Ltd 319

Irrigation services and equipment

Advance (Nig) Ltd ... 8
Agrotec Services Ltd ... 15
Balakhany (Nigeria) Ltd ... 35
Bewac Ltd ... 41
Disscol Ltd ... 79
Edok-Eter-Mandilas Ltd ... 86
Emanento Company Agency ... 90
Fanz Holdings Ltd ... 96
Guthrie (Nigeria) Ltd ... 115
Louis Berger Inc Nigeria ... 158
Monier Construction Company (Nig) Ltd ... 175
Nigercare International Company (Nigeria) Ltd ... 193
Nigerian Agricultural Promotions Company Ltd ... 199
Nigerian Foundries Ltd ... 206
Nirotec (A Division of Nigerian Ropes Ltd) ... 221
Obatraco Group of Companies ... 227
P W Nigeria Ltd ... 239
Pipes Below Ground Ltd ... 248
Roaag Company (Nigeria) Ltd ... 263
Safni Ltd ... 266
Siab Engineering Company Nigeria Ltd ... 274
Silverball Integrated Engineering Co Nigeria Ltd ... 274
Socea (Nigeria) Ltd ... 277
Structec ... 282
Uren Construction Engineering Company Ltd ... 310
UTC Nigeria Ltd (Formerly Union Trading Company of Nigeria Ltd) ... 311
Zartech Ltd ... 324

Leather and shoes

Ambrosini, L, Ltd ... 23
Bata Nigeria Ltd ... 37
Dauphin (Nigeria) Ltd ... 75
Eko Leatherware Factory ... 87
Fashion Shoe Company (Nigeria) Ltd ... 97
Federation Products (Nigeria) Ltd ... 98
Femo (West Africa) Ltd ... 99
Fimcon Ltd ... 100
Great Northern Tanning Co Ltd ... 113
Holt's Nigerian Tanneries Ltd ... 123
Iddo Plastics Ltd ... 127
Igbomina Investment Co Nigeria Ltd ... 128
International Tanners Ltd ... 134
Latderma Enterprises ... 153
Leather Tanning Industry Nigeria Ltd ... 154
Lennards Nigeria Ltd ... 154
Limson & Co Ltd ... 156
Metropolitan Industries (Nig) Ltd ... 170
Modern Shoe Industry Ltd ... 174
Neital Nigeria Ltd ... 185
Nigerian Commercial Factory Ltd ... 202
Nigerian Industrial Auxiliaries Ltd ... 208
Nigerian Leather Works Company Ltd ... 209
Nigerian Perfecta Shoes Ltd ... 214
Nigerian Shoe & Rubber Products Company Ltd ... 217
Oredola Okeya Trading Company Ltd ... 236
Pacific Printers Ltd ... 240
Passat Industries Ltd ... 243
Prestige Industries Ltd ... 253
Prestige Stores Nigeria Ltd ... 253
South Pacific Chemical & Plastics Engineering Company Ltd ... 279

Leisure goods

Abdul Azeez Electrical Centre ... 4
Adefusika Trading Company Ltd ... 7
African Era and Company Ltd ... 11
Amagra International Music House ... 21
Aye Marble & Terrazzo Industrial Works ... 33
Bhandari & Company (Nigeria) Ltd ... 42
Bidat Sportswear Company Ltd ... 42

Binatone Electronics ... 43
Decca (West Africa) Ltd ... 76
Dolphin Dive West Africa ... 80
Dubic International Ltd ... 83
Ekerete, A, Ltd ... 87
EMI (Nigeria) Ltd ... 91
Eximport & Company Nigeria Ltd ... 95
Fatsports Industries Ltd ... 97
Glendora Enterprises ... 111
Ibukun-Olu Enterprises ... 127
Igbomina Investment Co Nigeria Ltd ... 128
Latderma Enterprises ... 153
Moneme & Sons Bookshops ... 175
Morison, J L, Sons & Jones (Nigeria) Ltd ... 176
Nigerian Toys Manufacturing Company Ltd (NITOMAC) ... 219
Nigerpools Company Ltd ... 220
Oceanic & Coastal Marine Ltd ... 228
Oredola Okeya Trading Company Ltd ... 236
Phonogram Ltd ... 248
Principal Bookshop & Commercial Stores Ltd ... 254
Record Manufacturers of Nigeria Ltd ... 259
Record Market (Nigeria) Ltd ... 259
Take Your Choice Record Stores Ltd ... 286
Times Leisure Services Ltd ... 290
Ventures, Coopers Benly, & Company Ltd (The) ... 313

Livestock and animal feeds

Adesanya, A O, Nigeria Ltd ... 8
Agricultural Development Corporation (Anambra State) ... 14
Agrotec Services Ltd ... 15
Arroways of Nigeria ... 28
Calaro Oil Palm Estate Ltd ... 52
Chukwurah Agriculture Industries Ltd ... 61
Compagnie Francaise de l'Afrique Internationale ... 65
Ejinaka and Thornber Ltd ... 87
Eurotrade (Nigeria) Ltd ... 94
Funtua Cottonseed Crushing Company Ltd ... 105
Idehen, J I, & Sons (Nigeria) Ltd ... 127
Kolinah Industries Nigeria Ltd ... 148
Livestock Feeds Ltd ... 157
Management Enterprises Ltd ... 161
Mandrides, P S, & Co Ltd ... 162
Mereoleh Brothers Co (Nigeria) Ltd ... 168
National Grains Production Company Ltd ... 181
Nifeipiri Poultries Ltd ... 191
Nigerian Consolidated Food Producers Ltd ... 203
Nigerian Starch Mills Ltd ... 217
Odeco Ltd ... 228
Ofi Livestock Industries Ltd ... 229
Olaogun Enterprises Ltd ... 231
Olehson Brothers Company (Nigeria) Ltd ... 232
(Olehson's Agro Animal Kingdom) ... 232
Pfizer Products Ltd ... 245
Poultry & Animal Products (Nigeria) Ltd ... 251
Seepc (Nigeria) Ltd ... 271
Takko Engineering Ltd ... 286
Upjohn Nigeria Pty Ltd ... 310

Mechanical engineering

Adejobi, Adeoye, Trading Stores Ltd ... 7
Analex Group Ltd ... 24
Anglo-German Company (Intercontinental) Ltd ... 25
Audu Lukat Motors Ltd ... 33
Awosanmi & Sons Engineering Works ... 33
B & F Nigeria Ltd ... 34
Benora Instruments & Company ... 39
Berliet Nigeria Ltd ... 41
Bolori Brothers & Co Ltd (Bolbros) ... 45
Bozgomero of Nigeria Ltd ... 47
Camplant Engineering Sales & Service Ltd ... 52

Chidiebere Transport Ltd ... 59
City Group Organization ... 62
Citymark (West Africa) Ltd ... 62
Coutinho, Caro & Co (Nigeria) Ltd ... 69
Damen Shipyards Nigeria Ltd ... 74
Dolmech Engineering (Nig) Ltd ... 80
Dornier-Nigeria Aeronautical Engineering ... 81
Drake & Scull (Nigeria) Ltd ... 81
DSD Nigeria Ltd ... 82
Etco-Engineering & Technical Company (Nigeria) Ltd ... 93
Etuk Motors Technical Company Ltd ... 94
Fado Engineering Co Ltd ... 96
George Engineering Co Ltd ... 109
Group Elektro Power Nigeria Ltd ... 114
Heplac Nigeria Ltd ... 122
International Contracts & Consultancy Services Ltd ... 132
Kent Engineering Nigeria Ltd ... 146
Kilpatrick, James, (Nigeria) Ltd ... 146
Lonogu Enterprises Ltd ... 157
Marryat, Daniel, (Nigeria) Ltd ... 165
Mothercat Overseas (Nigeria) Ltd ... 177
Moukarim Metalwood Factory Ltd ... 177
Mouldex Ltd ... 177
Nabena, Benjamin, Nabenson Promotions ... 178
Niger Construction Ltd ... 191
Nigerian Company for Energy Engineering Ltd (NICOGEN) ... 202
Nirotec (A Division of Nigerian Ropes Ltd) ... 221
Nkwonta, D O, & Sons Enterprises Ltd ... 222
Nobgroup of Companies ... 222
O'Bahor, J A, & Company Ltd ... 227
Rajendram, R, and Associates ... 257
Rapid Electrical & Mechanical Company Nigeria Ltd (REMCO) ... 257
Richas Engineering Works Company Ltd ... 261
Safni Ltd ... 266
Scoa lard - a Division of Scoa Nigeria Ltd ... 270
Siab Engineering Company Nigeria Ltd ... 274
Silverball Integrated Engineering Co Nigeria Ltd ... 274
Smeaton Ltd ... 275
Sointeco (Nigeria) Ltd ... 277
Tradon Nigeria Ltd ... 292
Trindel (Nigeria) Ltd ... 295
VYB (Nigeria) Ltd ... 315
Whessoe Engineering Ltd ... 320
Wiedemann & Walters (Nigeria) Ltd ... 321

Metals, metal processing and fabrication

Abdullai Group of Companies Nigeria Ltd ... 4
ACE Metal Construction (Nigeria) Ltd ... 5
Adoks Engineering Ltd ... 8
Aisa Trading Company Ltd ... 15
Ajaokuta Steel Company Ltd ... 16
Alcan Aluminium of Nigeria Ltd ... 18
Alcan Aluminium Products Ltd ... 18
Allied Metal & Chemical Works Ltd ... 20
ALUMACO ... 21
Aluminium Manufacturing Company of Nigeria Ltd ... 21
Alusteel Construction Ltd ... 21
Architectural Metal Products Ltd ... 26
Arewa Metal Containers Ltd ... 27
Arewa Steel Works Company (Nig) Ltd ... 27
Aridi Industries (Nigeria) Ltd (ARMECO) ... 28 27
Asiatic Industries Ltd ... 30
Asiatic Industries Ltd ... 30
Associated Metal & Allied Works Ltd ... 31
Associated Ores Mining Company Ltd ... 31
Balin Builders & Aluminium Industries Ltd ... 35
Balmore Trading Company Ltd ... 35
Bendel Steel Structures Ltd ... 39
Bhandari & Company (Nigeria) Ltd ... 42
Borno Engineering & Steel Manufacturers Ltd ... 46
Bright Aluminium Products Co Ltd ... 49
Bright Steel Structures Co Ltd ... 49

Brown & Root Nigeria Ltd 50
Casting Nigeria Ltd 54
Chrisray Nigeria Ltd 59
Cogemat (Nigeria) Ltd 63
Coksee Engineering Works Ltd 63
Complete Home Enterprises (Nig) Ltd 65
Contex Nigeria Ltd 66
Continental Iron & Steel Co Ltd 66
Cosmos Metal & Electrics Ltd 69
Crittall-Hope Nigeria Ltd 70
Delta Steel Company Ltd 77
Dema Engineering Ltd 78
Dolmech Engineering (Nig) Ltd 80
Dorman Long & Amalgamated
  Engineering Ltd 80
Eldorado (Nigeria) Ltd 89
Electrode Nigeria Ltd 89
Fatmok Associates 97
Feso Mirror and Glass Works Ltd 99
Fuason Industries (Nigeria) Ltd 105
General Metal Products Ltd 108
George Cohen (Nigeria) Ltd 108
Gold & Base Metal Mines of Nigeria
  Ltd 112
Hoesch Pipe Mills (Nig) Ltd 123
Ijagbemi, S A, & Sons (Nigeria) Ltd 128
International Steel Industry Ltd 134
Iron Products Industries Ltd 135
Kaeler (West Africa) Ltd 142
Kano Welding & Steel Construction Co
  Ltd 144
Kedam Holdings (Nigeria) Ltd 145
Leman Industries (Kaduna) Ltd 154
Make Ltd 160
Makeri Smelting Company Ltd 161
Mandarin Industries Company Ltd 161
Memco Steel Co Ltd 167
Metal Box Nigeria Ltd 168
Metal Construction (WA) Ltd 169
Metalum Ltd 169
Midland Galvanizing Products Ltd 171
Mitsubishi Shoji Kaisha (Nigeria) Ltd 173
Modern Foundry Products Ltd 174
Moukarim Industries Ltd 177
Moukarim Metalwood Factory Ltd 177
MULMACO 178
Multi Aluminium Manufacturing
  Company Ltd 178
Naco Nigeria Ltd 179
Nails & General Steel Manufacturing
  Industry Ltd 179
NCIE Ltd 185
Neptune Constructions Ltd 186
Nigerchin Electrical Development
  Company Ltd 193
Nigeria Engineering Works Ltd 195
Nigeria General Motors Ltd 195
Nigeria Steel Products Ltd 197
Nigerian Aluminium Development Co
  Ltd (NADECO) 199
Nigerian Aluminium Engineering
  Company Ltd (NAECO) 199
Nigerian Aluminium Extrusions Ltd
  (NIGALEX) 199
Nigerian Commercial & Industrial
  Enterprises Ltd 202
Nigerian Enamelware Company Ltd
  (NEWCO) 204
Nigerian Foundries Ltd 206
Nigerian Hardware Industries Ltd 208
Nigerian Industrial Complex
  Amalgamation Ltd 208
Nigerian Metal Fabricating Ltd 210
Nigerian Smelting & Refining Company
  Ltd 217
Nigerian Steel Development Authority
  (NSDA) 217
Nigerian Thermoplastics Ltd 219
Nigerian Wire Industries Ltd 220
Nigersteel Company Ltd 220
Nigerwest Steel Company Ltd 221
Northern Steel Works Ltd 225
Northern Wire & Steelworks Ltd 226
Ogunnire Modern Furniture (Nigeria)
  Ltd 230
Pioneer Metal Products Company Ltd 248
Plastic and Engineering Works Ltd 249
Pressed Metal Industry Ltd 253
Pressed Metal Works Ltd 253
Primary Steel (Nigeria) Ltd 253
Raccaform Ltd 256
Romain, H W, & Son Ltd 264
Sabon Sara Nigeria Ltd 266
Salzgitter (WA) Ltd 266

Sanusi Brothers (Nigeria) Ltd 267
Sem Steels (Nigeria) Ltd 272
Sem-Edo Wire Industries Ltd 272
Seswa, Steel and Engineering Services
  (WA) Ltd 273
Steel Works Ltd 281
Stronghold (Nigeria) Ltd 282
Structural Steel Works Ltd 283
Tower Aluminium (Nigeria) Ltd 291
Toyo Menka Kaisha Ltd 292
Unisteel Works Ltd 303
Universal Steels Ltd 308
Universal Welding & Construction
  Company Ltd 309
Van Leer Containers (Nigeria) Ltd 312
Wasco Ropes Ltd 315
Waterglass Boatyard & Steel
  Construction Ltd 316
Wellyplates 317
West African Aluminium Products
  (Nigeria) 317
Western Steel Works 320
Whessoe Engineering Ltd 320
Wimpey-Brown & Root (Nigeria) Ltd 322
Wolff, Otto, (Nigeria) & Company Ltd 322
Wrought Iron (Nigeria) Ltd 323

Mining, mineral processing and
quarrying

Abdullai Group of Companies Nigeria
  Ltd 4
Abereoje (Nigeria) Ltd 4
Agbenor Mining Syndicate 14
Alheri Mining Co Ltd 19
Amalgamated Tin Mines of Nigeria Ltd 22
Amari Mines Ltd 22
Ashamu, E O, & Sons (Holdings) Ltd 29
Associated Ores Mining Company Ltd 31
Ayana Mining Syndicate 33
Barlow Mines Ltd 36
Birom Mines Ltd 43
Bisichi-Jantar (Nigeria) Ltd 44
Bolokor MK Ltd 45
BRGM (Nigeria) Ltd 49
Chuwang Gyang & Sons Ltd 61
CNMD Co 63
Czechoslovak Nigerian Minerals
  Development Co Ltd 63
Daniel, C C, Mining Industry 74
Eburutu Mining Syndicate 85
Egbon Mining Syndicate Ltd 87
Ejukorlem, D K, & Co Ltd 87
ENO Industries Ltd 92
Ex-Lands Nigeria Ltd 95
Fidelity Mining Syndicate 100
Gumo Mining Syndicate 115
Gyartagere Explosives & Chemicals Co
  Ltd 117
Harboni Ltd 120
Indo Mining Co (Nigeria) Ltd 129
Industrial Clays Nigeria Ltd 129
Jecima Mining Syndicate 138
Jos Alluvials Ltd 140
Kaduna Prospectors (Nigeria) Ltd 142
Kassa Mines Ltd 145
Kragha & Associates 149
Kufena Trading Co Ltd 150
Kuru Ltd 150
Lisabi Mining Association Ltd 156
Mansa Construction Co Ltd 162
Mbanejo Brothers Ltd 166
Metals & Minerals (Nigeria) Ltd 169
Mingi Mining Co Ltd 172
Nata'Ata, Alhaji, and Sons 180
Nigerian Alluvials Ltd 199
Nigerian Coal Corporation 202
Nigerian Embel Tin Smelting Company 204
Nigerian Metals Ltd 210
Nigerian Mineral Development
  Company Ltd 210
Nigerian Mining Corporation 211
Northern Tin Company Ltd 225
Oguejiofor, Alex, Company Ltd 230
Okpe Mining Syndicate 231
Okwuosa Mining Industry 231
Ron Mining and Development
  Company Ltd 264
Songhai Group of Companies 278

Tin & Associated Minerals Ltd 290
Warri Mining Syndicate 315
Zang, D B 324
Zarmaganda Tin Mines Ltd 324
Zawang Mining Company 324
Zelan Mining Company Ltd 324

Motor vehicles and components

Advance (Nig) Ltd 8
Allen, J, Co Ltd 20
Anambra Motor Manufacturing Co Ltd
  (ANAMMCO) 24
Aridi Industries (Nigeria) Ltd 28
Asemota Motors (Nigeria) Ltd 29
Associated Battery Manufacturers
  (Nigeria) Ltd 30
Audu Lukat Motors Ltd 33
Auto Components Ltd 33
Awaye Continental Motors Co Ltd 33
Awosanmi & Sons Engineering Works 33
B & C Autopanel Engineering Ltd 34
B & F Nigeria Ltd 34
Bakrin Enterprises Ltd 35
Banjoko Firesafety Ltd 35
Bao Nigeria Ltd 36
Bendel Chemical Industries Ltd 38
Berliet Nigeria Ltd 41
Bewac Automotive Products Ltd 41
Bewac Ltd 41
Bibson Associates Ltd 42
Briscoe, R T, (Nigeria) Ltd 49
Bronik Motors Ltd 50
CFAO (Nigeria) Ltd 56
Chidiebere Transport Ltd 59
City Group Organization 62
Compass Trading Co Ltd 65
Conveyancer (Nigeria) Ltd 67
Dada-Obe Industries (Nigeria) Ltd 72
Delta Pioneer Company Ltd 77
Duro International (Nigeria) Ltd 84
Edewor International Ltd 86
Ekisola Electrical Works Ltd 87
Emanento Company Agency 90
Etuk Motors Technical Company Ltd 94
Federated Motor Industries 98
Fisayo Holdings Ltd 100
Godbless Motors Nigeria Ltd 111
Gregson Trading Company Ltd 114
Holt, John, Ltd 123
Hulls Services Ltd 125
Ibru Organisation (Ibru Ltd) 126
Ikeja Retreads (Nigeria) Ltd 128
Incar (Nigeria) Ltd 129
Incontra Nigeria Ltd 129
Intra Motors (Nigeria) Ltd 135
Lanre Bhadmus Industries Ltd 152
Lecco Engineering Construction Co
  Ltd 154
Leman Industries (Kaduna) Ltd 154
Leyland Nigeria Ltd 155
Lister Motors (Nigeria) Ltd 156
London Africa & Overseas Ltd 157
Mais Tyres Service (City Retreading
  Service) 160
Mandilas Ltd 162
Memco Steel Co Ltd 167
Metal Construction (WA) Ltd 169
Mid-Motors Nigerian Company Ltd 171
Moore Obioha, C, Sons & Company
  Ltd 176
Morpol Industrial Corporation Ltd 176
Motor Parts Industry Ltd 177
Motorways Nigeria Ltd 177
National Motors (Nigeria) Ltd 183
National Trucks Manufacturers Ltd 185
Niger Motors Ltd 192
Nigeria Coach Construction Ltd 194
Nigeria Steel Products Ltd 197
Nigerian Motors Industries Ltd 211
Nigerian Technical Co Ltd 218
Nigerian Transmission Company Ltd 219
Nigerlink Industries Ltd 220
Nobgroup of Companies 222
Northern Nigerian Technical Service
  Ltd 225
Odeng Engineering Company Ltd 228
Oluwakemi Motors & Finance
  Company Ltd 233

Omole Motors Ltd 234
Orumokpo & Sons (Nigeria) Ltd 236
Oshue Brothers & Company (Nigeria) Ltd 237
Owoyemi Motors & Finance Company Ltd 239
Pecco Ltd 244
Peugeot Automobile Nigeria Ltd 245
Phoenix Motors Ltd 247
Radiators Nigeria Ltd 256
Ribway Tyre Retreading Co Ltd 261
Rida National Distributors Ltd 261
Runsewe Group of Companies 265
Rutam Ltd 265
Sams Agencies & Maritime Service (Nig) 266
Scoa Motors (Nigeria) Ltd 270
Scoa Nigeria Ltd 270
Siram Industrial Products Ltd 275
Stephens, Henry, Engineering Company Ltd 281
Steyr Nigeria Ltd 281
Structural Steel Works Ltd 283
Sunshine Batteries Manufacturing Company 284
Tabansi Motors Ltd 286
Taike & Brothers Ltd 286
Taiwo Ajai Communications 286
Tractor & Equipment 292
Tractors Under-Carriage Industry Nigeria Ltd 292
Tudor Batteries (Nigeria) Ltd 295
Turners Engineering Products (Nigeria) Ltd 297
UAC of Nigeria Ltd 297
Unico Stores 301
Unipetrol Nigeria Ltd 302
United Nigeria Motors Ltd 305
Universal Monolithic Bearing Structure Ltd 308
Universal Vulcanizing Company Nigeria Ltd 309
UTC Nigeria Ltd (Formerly Union Trading Company of Nigeria Ltd) 311
Ventures, Coopers Benly, & Company Ltd (The) 313
Volkswagen of Nigeria Ltd 314
Volvo Ltd 314
Waterglass Boatyard & Steel Construction Ltd 316
Wellyplates 317
West African Automobile & Engineering Company Ltd (WAATECO) 317
West African Batteries Ltd 317
West African Tyre Retreading Company Ltd 319

Motorcycles and bicycles

Boulos Enterprises Ltd 47
Boulos Enterprises Ltd 47
Chidiebere Transport Ltd 59
Gobecco Trading Company Ltd 111
Holt, John, Ltd 123
Honda Motors Nigeria Ltd 125
Moore Obioha, C, Sons & Company Ltd 176
Nobgroup of Companies 222
Odutola Nigerian Industries Ltd 229
Owoyemi Motors & Finance Company Ltd 239
Raleigh Industries (Nigeria) Ltd 257
Sams Agencies & Maritime Service (Nig) 266

Office equipment and supplies

Adamu Management International 6
Arewa Advancement Enterprises Ltd 27
Aridi Industries (Nigeria) Ltd 28
Atlas Nigeria Ltd 32
Atssco Abbey Office Machine Service Stationery (Nig) Ltd 32
Bisrod Furniture Company Ltd 44

Boma Associates (WA) Ltd 45
Business Equipment & Machinery Ltd (BEAM) (Division of UAC of Nigeria Ltd) 50
Chemdyes Nigeria Ltd 58
Concorde Furniture Manufacturing Co Ltd 65
ECWA Productions Ltd 85
Emanento Company Agency 90
Enomah Office Equipment Ltd 92
Envelope & File Co of Nigeria 92
Eze, I O, & Sons Ltd 95
Gem Fasteners Industry (Nigeria) Ltd 107
Gicen Technical Services Ltd 110
Glendora Enterprises 111
Good-Name Stationery Stores 112
Goodwill, Francis, Ltd 112
Green Light Industries Ltd 114
Hagemeyer (Nigeria) Ltd 119
Hilson Nigeria Ltd 122
International Contact Centre 132
Itidal-Epid Enterprises of Nigeria 136
J & H International Agency 137
Jobba Trading Company 139
Kolynson Co Ltd 149
Krabo Nigeria Ltd 149
Kucena-Damian (Nigeria) Ltd 149
Kufena Trading Co Ltd 150
Lanlek (Nigeria) Associates 152
Majand & Company 160
Mass Stationery Stores Co (Nigeria) 165
Mesacom Electronics Instrumentations Ltd 168
Modulor Group 174
Moneme & Sons Bookshops 175
Nabena, Benjamin, Nabenson Promotions 178
National Cash Register (WA) Ltd 181
NCR 181
Nigeria Engineering Works Ltd 195
Nigerian Ball-Point Ben Industries Ltd 200
Nigerian Office Stationery Supply Stores Ltd 213
Niyi Office Stationery Supply Stores Ltd 222
NMB Modern Bookshops 222
Norwo Trading Company Ltd 226
Ogunnire Modern Furniture (Nigeria) Ltd 230
Okwesa, John, Ltd 231
Onward Paper Mill Ltd 235
Onward Stationery Stores Ltd 235
Oshinmi Company Ltd 236
Ositadinma International Ltd 237
Ott-Attafua, A, & Company Ltd 237
Petraco, De, Industries Ltd 245
Polly Pen & Ink Company (Nigeria) Ltd 251
Prime Feathers International Services Ltd 254
Principal Bookshop & Commercial Stores Ltd 254
Professional and Manufacturing Services (Nigeria) Ltd 254
Promana Associates 255
Pyramid Paper Products Ltd 255
Raccah & Chaker Factory Ltd 256
Rank Xerox (Nigeria) Ltd 257
Santana Furniture Factory Ltd 267
Spicers (Nigeria) Ltd 279
Sunny Stationery Supply & Bookshop 284
Takko Engineering Ltd 286
Tasius Nigeria Ltd 286
Templar Afrique (Nigeria) Ltd 288
Tenimasunwon Agency 288
Thomade Enterprises (Nig) Ltd 289
Thompson Dickson Technical Co Ltd 289
Tommy Building & Construction Company Ltd 291
Topaz (Nigeria) Ltd 291
UAC of Nigeria Ltd 297
Unique Trading Co Ltd 303
United Educational Supplies Ltd 305
Universal Educational Supplies Ltd (Morison Arnold Ltd) 308
UTC Nigeria Ltd (Formerly Union Trading Company of Nigeria Ltd) 311
Wozabeth Trading Company 323
Wyatt, Thomas, Nigeria Ltd 323

Oil and gas exploration and production

Ashland Oil (Nigeria) Company 29
CGG Nigeria Ltd 56
Delta Oil Nigeria Ltd 77
ELF Nigeria Ltd 90
Forex Neptune of Nigeria Ltd 103
Geodetic Surveys Ltd 108
GOCON 115
Great Basins Petroleum Co (Nigeria) Ltd 113
Gulf Oil Company (Nigeria) Ltd 115
Hunting Surveys (Nigeria) Ltd 125
Mobil Producing Nigeria (MPN) 173
Nigergas Ltd 193
Nigerian Agip Oil Company Ltd 198
Nigerian National Petroleum Corporation (NNPC) 211
Nigus Petroleum Nigeria 221
Pan Ocean Oil Corporation (Nigeria) 242
Phillips Oil Company (Nigeria) Ltd 247
Shell Petroleum Development Company of Nigeria Ltd 274
Stephens, Henry, Group of Companies 281
Tenneco Oil Company of Nigeria 288
Texas Overseas (Nigeria) Petroleum Co (TOPCON) 289
United Geophysical (Nigeria) Ltd 305
West African Surveys Ltd 319

Oil and gas services, equipment and pipeline contracting

ACM of Nigeria Ltd 6
Aero Contractors Company of Nigeria Ltd 8
Ajosi Oilfields Supply Company Ltd 16
Akanji Transport 16
Allied Oilfield Services (Nigeria) Ltd (AOS) 20
Amdumac Group (Nigeria) Ltd 23
Arax Airlines Ltd 26
B B C Brown Boveri (Nigeria) Ltd 34
Baker Nigeria Ltd 34
Baroid of Nigeria Ltd 36
(BOGI) 45
Bonny Oil & Gas Industries (Nigeria) Ltd 45
Bristow Helicopters (Nigeria) Ltd 49
Brown & Root Nigeria Ltd 50
Caleb Brett & Son (Nigeria) Ltd 52
Camco Ltd 52
Cameron Iron Works (Nigeria) Ltd 52
CECA (Nigeria) Ltd 54
Chemex Nigeria Ltd 58
Chidiebere Transport Ltd 59
Chiyoda Chemical Engineering & Construction Co 59
Cornerstone Organisation Ltd 69
Cotsgas (Nigeria) Ltd 69
Della Group Ltd 76
Dixilyn (Nigeria) Ltd 79
Dowell Schlumberger (Nigeria) Ltd 81
(Dresser Magcobar Minerals Ltd) 82
Dresser Nigeria Ltd 82
Earth Sciences Ltd 84
Flopetrol Nigeria Ltd 102
Forex Neptune of Nigeria Ltd 103
Gaby and Company (Nigeria) 106
Gas & Welding (Nigeria) Ltd 106
Geodetic Surveys Ltd 108
Geoservices Nigeria Ltd 109
Gida Technical Enterprises Company 110
Halliburton Nigeria Ltd 119
Hassan Transport (Nigeria) Ltd 121
Hunting Surveys (Nigeria) Ltd 125
Industrial Gases Ltd 130
International Contracts & Consultancy Services Ltd 132
KCA Drilling (Nigeria) Ltd 145
Kenting Africa Resource Services Ltd 146
Keydril Nigeria Ltd 146
Kragha & Associates 149
McDermott (Nigeria) Ltd 158
Metals & Minerals (Nigeria) Ltd 169
Montubi 175

National Oil and Chemical Marketing
Company Ltd 183
Nidogas Company Ltd 191
Niger Construction 191
Niger Oil Resources Ltd (Norco) 192
Niger Petroleum Co Ltd 192
Nigeria Drilling Company Ltd 195
Nigeria Marine & Trading Company
Ltd 196
Nigerian Diving Service Ltd 204
Nigerian Dredging and Marine Ltd 204
Nigerian Gas Industries 206
Nigerian National Petroleum
Corporation (NNPC) 211
Nigerian Oil Services Shipping &
Equipment Co Ltd (NOSSEC) 213
Nigerian Petroleum Refining Company
Ltd (NPRC) 214
Nigerian Petroleum Terminals Ltd 214
Nigerian Pipelines Ltd 214
Nigerian Ropes Ltd 215
Nigerian Services & Supply Company
Ltd (NISSCO) 216
Nordive (West Africa) Ltd 222
Ocean Inchcape (Nigeria) Ltd 227
Oceannering (Nigeria) Ltd 228
OGT Group of Companies Ltd 229
Oil Supply Centre Ltd (OSC) 230
Oloro Properties Ltd 232
Otis of Nigeria Ltd 237
Paktank Nigeria Ltd 240
Pan Ocean Oil Corporation (Nigeria) 242
Pencol International (Nigeria) Ltd 244
Petroleum Consultants (Nigeria) Ltd 245
Pipes Below Ground Ltd 248
Pressed Metal Works Ltd 253
Santa Fe Nigeria Development
Company Ltd 267
Saybolt (Nigeria) Ltd 269
Schlumberger (Nigeria) Ltd 270
Sea Trucks (Nigeria) Ltd 271
Sedco Nigeria Ltd 271
Seismograph Service (Nigeria) Ltd
(SSL) 272
Service & Supply Company of West
Africa Ltd (SASCO) 273
Snamprogetti 276
Sointeco (Nigeria) Ltd 277
Solus Schall (Nigeria) Ltd 278
Southeastern Drilling Co (Nigeria) Ltd
(SEDCO) 279
Standard Industrial Development
Company Ltd 280
Storm (Nigeria) Ltd 282
Techint Engineering (Nigeria) Ltd 287
Tidex Nigeria Ltd 290
Total Nigeria Ltd 291
Trans-Africa Engineering Ltd 293
Transworld Drilling Company Ltd 294
TSMPE (Tsvetmetpromexport) 295
Unipetrol Nigeria Ltd 302
United Geophysical (Nigeria) Ltd 305
Utilgas Nigerian and Overseas Gas
Company Ltd 311
Wasco Ropes Ltd 315
Wayne (West Africa) Ltd 316
Weatherford (Nigeria) Ltd 316
West Africa Offshore Ltd 317
West African Surveys Ltd 319
Westminster Dredging (Nigeria) Ltd 320
Westminster Offshore (Nigeria) Ltd 320
Whipstock (Nigeria) Ltd 321
Williams International (Nig) Ltd 321
Wimpey-Brown & Root (Nigeria) Ltd 322
Yondav Petrocomplex Ltd 324

Oil refining

African Petroleum Ltd 12

Optical and photographic equipment

Alban Pharmacy Ltd 18
Alex L M Davou Fom & Sons
Enterprise Ltd 18

Atlas Nigeria Ltd 32
Benora Instruments & Company 39
Bhojsons & Company (Nigeria) Ltd 42
CEP 55
Copiers (Nigeria) Ltd 68
Dotun Okubanjo & Associates Ltd 81
Hagemeyer (Nigeria) Ltd 119
Kingsway Chemists Ltd 147
Onigbinde, M A, & Sons Ltd 235
Prime Feathers International Services
Ltd 254
Stag Engineering Nigeria Ltd 280
Steiner, F, & Company Ltd 281
United Development Trading Company
Ltd 305
UTC Nigeria Ltd (Formerly Union
Trading Company of Nigeria Ltd) 311
Village Gate & Company Ltd 313

Packaging

Afromedia Plastics & Engineering Ltd 14
Associated Exports (W.A.) Ltd 31
Avon Crowncaps and Containers
(Nigeria) Ltd 33
Blue Straps Ltd 44
Bordpak Premier Packaging 46
Central Packages of Nigeria Ltd 55
Colodense Nigeria Ltd 63
Containers (Nigeria) Ltd 66
Controlled Plastics Ltd 67
Crown Cork and Seal Company
(Nigeria) Ltd 71
Diamond Plastics Ltd 79
Dynamic Industries Ltd 84
Formerly Benue Plateau Packages Ltd 180
(Formerly Polyplast Industrial Co Ltd) 67
Gaby and Company (Nigeria) 106
Industrial Gases Ltd 130
International Packing Industries of
Nigeria Ltd 133
International Plastics (Nigeria) Ltd 134
Kaeler (West Africa) Ltd 142
Kano Suit and Packing Cases Factory
Ltd 144
Kesington Industries Ltd 146
Lafia Canning Factory 151
MBTG 168
Metal Box Nigeria Ltd 168
Metal Box Toyo Glass Nigeria Ltd 168
Nasco Pack Ltd 180
Nigeria Kraft Bags Ltd 196
Nigerian Bag Manufacturing Company
Ltd 200
Nigerian Carton & Packaging
Manufacturing Company Ltd 201
Nigerian Glass Containers & Metal
Manufacturers Ltd 207
Nigerian Match & Chemical Industries
Ltd 210
Nigerian Soft Drinks Co Ltd 217
Nigerpak Ltd 220
Nipol Ltd 221
Ogubule Industrial Printers Ltd 230
Onise Polyware Ltd 235
Ovaltine (West Africa) Ltd 238
Paper Conversion Corporation
(Nigeria) Ltd 242
Paper Sack (Nigeria) Ltd 243
Pegasus Industries (Nigeria) Ltd 244
Poly Products (Nigeria) Ltd 251
Sera Printing Ltd 273
Seven-up Bottling Company Ltd 273
Stephens, Henry, Group of Companies 281
Studio Press (Nigeria) Ltd 283
Triana Ltd 294
Triumph (Nigeria) Ltd 295
Universal Packaging (Nigeria) Ltd 308
Van Leer Containers (Nigeria) Ltd 312
VK Plastiks & Marble Co 314
VYB (Nigeria) Ltd 315

Paint

Adefusika Trading Company Ltd 7

African Paints (Nig) Ltd 11
Apex Paints Ltd 26
Askar of Nigeria Ltd 30
Benora Instruments & Company 39
Berger Paints (Nigeria) Ltd 41
Bisiolu Enterprises Ltd 44
Bosag Builders 46
Brossette (Nigeria) Ltd 50
Chemical & Allied Products Ltd 58
Denchukwu Group of Companies 78
Diborsons Business Enterprises 79
Ernestco Ltd 93
Freedom Development Company Ltd 105
Home Charm Paints (Nigeria) Ltd 125
International Paints (WA) Ltd 133
Kailash Industries (Nigeria) Ltd 143
Kesington Industries Ltd 146
Kunza Heed (W.A.) Enterprises 150
Nigeria Marine & Trading Company
Ltd 196
Nigerian Explosives & Plastics Co Ltd 205
Nigerian Hoechst Ltd 208
Nwonye, I O M, & Sons Company Ltd 227
Regency (Overseas) Company Ltd 259
Reliance Group of Companies 260
Sodangi Enterprises 277
Theo & Theo Paints Company (Nigeria)
Ltd 289

Paper and paper products

Alpha Industries (Nigeria) Ltd 21
Amalgamated Industries Ltd 22
Apex (Eastern Nigeria) Ltd 26
Arbor Services Nigeria Ltd 26
Bordpak Premier Packaging 46
Botam (Nigeria) Ltd 46
Brown & Root Nigeria Ltd 50
Colodense Nigeria Ltd 63
Continental Medical Complex Ltd 66
Copiers (Nigeria) Ltd 68
Doal Enterprises Ltd 80
Dubic Industries Ltd 83
ECWA Productions Ltd 85
Emidson Nigeria Ltd 91
Femina Hygienical Products (Nigeria)
Ltd 99
Glendora Enterprises 111
International Packing Industries of
Nigeria Ltd 133
Kagho Industrial Enterprises Ltd 143
Kucena-Damian (Nigeria) Ltd 149
Lanlek (Nigeria) Associates 152
Leo-Jimbus Mercantile Agencies
(Nigeria) 154
Luncheon Vouchers Nigeria Ltd 158
NCO Merchants Brothers Company 185
Niger Sanitary Industry Ltd 192
Nigeria Kraft Bags Ltd 196
Nigerian Cards Ltd 201
Nigerian Carton & Packaging
Manufacturing Company Ltd 201
Nigerian Cement Company Ltd
(Nigercem) 201
Nigerian Commercial & Industrial
Enterprises Ltd 202
Nigerian Commercial Press 202
Nigerian National Paper Manufacturing
Company Ltd 211
Nigerian Newsprint Manufacturing
Company Ltd 213
Nigerian Paper Converters Company 213
Nigerian Paper Mill Ltd 214
Ochumba Press Ltd 228
Okenabirhie Enterprises Ltd 231
Okwesa, John, Ltd 231
Onward Paper Mill Ltd 235
Oshunkeye Brothers (Nigeria) Ltd 237
Ott-Attafua, A, & Company Ltd 237
Paper Conversion Corporation
(Nigeria) Ltd 242
Paper Sack (Nigeria) Ltd 243
Polythene Enterprises (Nigeria) Ltd 251
Professional and Manufacturing
Services (Nigeria) Ltd 254
Pyramid Paper Products Ltd 255
Sandwell, P R, & Co (Nigeria) Ltd 267
Sera Printing Ltd 273
Spicers (Nigeria) Ltd 279

Thomade Enterprises (Nig) Ltd 289
Thoresen & Company (Nigeria) Ltd 290
Triumph (Nigeria) Ltd 295
Universal Distributors Ltd 307
Universal Educational Supplies Ltd
  (Morison Arnold Ltd) 308
Universal Packaging (Nigeria) Ltd 308
Vickins (Nigeria) Associates 313
Wiggins Teape West Africa Ltd 321
Yinkus Book Centre Ltd 323

Petrochemicals

African Petroleum Ltd 12
Agip (Nigeria) Ltd 14
Benora Instruments & Company 39
Brown & Root Nigeria Ltd 50
Cotsgas (Nigeria) Ltd 69
Mobil Oil Nigeria Ltd 173
National Oil and Chemical Marketing
  Company Ltd 183
Petro-Organico (Nigeria) Ltd 245
Phillips Oil Company (Nigeria) Ltd 247
Sungas Company Ltd 284
Texaco Nigeria Ltd 288
Unipetrol Nigeria Ltd 302

Pharmaceutical and medical
supplies and services

Abbott Laboratories Nigeria Ltd 4
Abdullai Group of Companies Nigeria
  Ltd 4
Adejumo Fam (Nigeria) Ltd 7
Adetona Awe (Nig) Enterprises 8
Afro Arab Techni-Chemicals Ltd 13
Alban Pharmacy Ltd 18
Alex L M Davou Fom & Sons
  Enterprise Ltd 18
Anamapharmaceutical Industries Ltd 24
Associated Drug Company (Nig) Ltd 30
Associated Laboratory Supplies Ltd 31
Associated Pharmaceutical Products
  Ltd 31
Bayer Pharmaceuticals (Nigeria) Ltd 37
Beecham Ltd 38
Bendel Pharmaceuticals Ltd 39
Bhandari & Company (Nigeria) Ltd 42
Biode Pharmaceutical Industries Ltd 43
Biomedical Services Company Ltd 43
Bolingo Organisation 45
Boots Company (Nigeria) Ltd (The) 46
Briscoe, R T, (Nigeria) Ltd 49
Bristol Myers Company 49
Chemical & Allied Products Ltd 58
Chesebrough Ponds Industries Ltd 59
Christela Chemical Works Ltd 59
Christlieb, A C, (Nigeria) Ltd 59
Chukwurah Agriculture Industries Ltd 61
Ciba-Geigy Ltd 61
Commercial Medicine Stores Ltd 64
Continental Medical Complex Ltd 66
Continental Pharmaceuticals Ltd 66
Daily Need Chemists Ltd 72
Delta Scientific & Technical Co Ltd 77
DLP Pharmaceuticals Ltd 80
Drug Houses Nigeria Ltd 82
Drug Specialities (Nigeria) Ltd 82
Dumex Pharmaceuticals Ltd 83
Edmund & Edmund (Nigeria) Ltd 86
Electro Technologies Nigeria Ltd
  (ELTEC) 89
Embechem Ltd (Formerly May & Baker
  (Nigeria) Ltd) 90
Evans Medical (Nigeria) Ltd 95
Everett Trading & Manufacturing Co
  Ltd 95
Faltas, A M, (West Africa) Ltd 96
Femope Marketing Company 99
Fisco-Chemicals (Nigeria) Ltd 100
Formerly Johnson & Johnson (Nigeria)
  Ltd 121
(Formerly Merck Sharp & Dohme
  (Nigeria) Ltd) 31
Galenika Nigeria Ltd 106

Gas Producers Ltd 106
Glaxo (Nigeria) Ltd 111
Global Pharmaceutical and Chemical
  Agencies Ltd 111
Gobecco Trading Company Ltd 111
Guthrie (Nigeria) Ltd 115
Health Care Products (Nigeria) Ltd 121
Holt, John, Ltd 123
Hospital Equipment and Orthopaedic
  Supplies Ltd 125
Idechemists Ltd 127
Ilonex Pharmaceutical Company 128
Incontra Nigeria Ltd 129
Industrial Gases Ltd 130
Jire Engineering Ltd 138
Jolliters Chemists Nigeria Ltd 140
Juli Pharmacy and Stores Ltd 140
Karopharm Laboratories Ltd 145
Kingsway Chemists Ltd 147
Labstock (Nigeria) Ltd 150
Ladejobi Products Nigeria Ltd 151
Link Group International Ltd 156
Major & Company (Nigeria) Ltd 160
Makin Ltd 161
Mareen Industries Ltd 163
Markdealers (Nigeria) Ltd 164
Medac (Nigeria) Ltd 167
Mentholatum (Nigeria) Ltd 167
Metriscope Nigeria Ltd 169
Micheljohnson Ltd 171
Minnesota Nigeria Ltd 172
Morison, J L, Sons & Jones (Nigeria)
  Ltd 176
Nagarta Drug Company Ltd 179
National Veterinary Research Institute 185
Nevlon Pharmaceutical (Revlon) Ltd 187
Nicholas Laboratories Nigeria Ltd 191
Niger Sanitary Industry Ltd 192
Nigerian Hoechst Ltd 208
Nigerian Medical Supplies Ltd 210
Nimesco (Nigeria) Ltd 221
Olehson Brothers Company (Nigeria)
  Ltd 232
(Olehson's Agro Animal Kingdom) 232
Omotoso Pharmaceuticals Ltd 234
Orthopaedic Supplies Ltd 236
Ositadinma International Ltd 237
Pabod Supplies Ltd 240
Parke-Davis & Company (Nigeria) Ltd 243
Paterson Zochonis Industries Ltd 243
Pfizer Products Ltd 245
Pharchem Industries Ltd 247
Pharco (Nigeria) Ltd (Pharmaceutical
  Company of West Africa) 247
Pharma Dyn Chemical Products 247
Prime Feathers International Services
  Ltd 254
Ramonu Alabi, S B, & Company 257
Rioco (Nigeria) Ltd 262
Robins, A H, International Company
  Ltd 264
Roche (Nigeria) Ltd 264
Roussel (Nigeria) Ltd 265
Sandoz (Nigeria) Ltd 267
Smith Kline & French Nigeria Ltd 276
Squibb (Nigeria) Ltd 279
Stag Engineering Nigeria Ltd 280
Starline Nigeria Ltd 280
Sterling Products (Nigeria) Ltd 281
Swiss Nigerian Chemical Company Ltd 285
UAC of Nigeria Ltd 297
Umerah Commercial Agency Ltd 301
United African Drug Co (Nig) Ltd 303
United Arewa Chemists Ltd 303
Upjohn Nigeria Pty Ltd 310
Urobo Agencies (Nigeria) Ltd 310
Vitalink Pharmaceutical Industries Ltd 314
Watson & Sons (Electro-Medical)
  Nigeria Ltd 316
Welfare Pharmaceuticals Ltd 316
Wellcome Nigeria Ltd 316
West African Drug Company Ltd 318
Wyeth Nigeria Ltd 323
Zabadne & Company Ltd 324

Plant hire

Bibson Associates Ltd 42
Camplant Engineering Sales & Service
  Ltd 52

Conveyancer (Nigeria) Ltd 67
Damen Shipyards Nigeria Ltd 74
Desam Development Company Ltd 78
George Cohen (Nigeria) Ltd 108
Greenham Plant Hire 114
Lagos Plant Hire Services (Nigeria) Ltd 151
Odeco Ltd 228
Safni Ltd 266
Scoa Nigeria Ltd 270
Scoatrac (A Division of Scoa (Nigeria)
  Ltd) 270
Siab Engineering Company Nigeria Ltd 274
UAC of Nigeria Ltd 297

Plastics and plastic products

Afromedia Plastics & Engineering Ltd 14
Ashamu, E O, & Sons (Holdings) Ltd 29
Associated Electronic Products
  (Nigeria) Ltd 31
Basf (Nigeria) Ltd 37
Bendel Plastic Industries Ltd 39
Bewac Ltd 41
Caprihans Industries Ltd 53
Cave Plastics Ltd 54
Central Packages of Nigeria Ltd 55
Chemical & Allied Products Ltd 58
Christlieb, A C, (Nigeria) Ltd 59
Colodense Nigeria Ltd 63
Commind Nigeria Ltd 64
Controlled Plastics Ltd 67
Delta Pioneer Company Ltd 77
Diamond Plastics Ltd 79
Diborsons Business Enterprises 79
Dr Pepper Bottling Company of
  Nigeria Ltd 81
Dubosh Plastics (Nigeria) Ltd 83
Dynamic Industries Ltd 84
Eslon Nigeria Ltd 93
Excel Plastic Industries Ltd 95
Feso Mirror and Glass Works Ltd 99
Fibreglass Reinforced Plastics Co Ltd 100
(Formerly Philips (Nig) Ltd) 31
(Formerly Polyplast Industrial Co Ltd) 67
General Metalware Company Nigeria
  Ltd 108
General Technology Nigeria Ltd 108
Ibru Organisation (Ibru Ltd) 126
Iddo Plastics Ltd 127
International Plastics (Nigeria) Ltd 134
Ivory Products Ltd 136
Kaeler (West Africa) Ltd 142
Krabo Nigeria Ltd 149
Light Industries (Nigeria) Ltd 155
Maasarant Industries Ltd 158
Metalloplastica (Nigeria) Ltd 169
Metropolitan Industries (Nig) Ltd 170
National Oil and Chemical Marketing
  Company Ltd 183
NCO Merchants Brothers Company 185
Nigerian Bag Manufacturing Company
  Ltd 200
Nigerian Ball-Point Ben Industries Ltd 200
Nigerian Commercial Factory Ltd 202
Nigerian Industrial Auxiliaries Ltd 208
Nigerlink Industries Ltd 220
Niyi Ibikunle (Nigeria) Ltd 221
Northern Metal Works Co Ltd 224
Obatraco Group of Companies 227
Pegasus Industries (Nigeria) Ltd 244
Petro-Organico (Nigeria) Ltd 245
Plasco Sheets (Nigeria) Ltd 249
Plastex Nigeria Ltd 249
Plastic and Engineering Works Ltd 249
Plastic Manufacturing Company Ltd
  (PMC) 249
Plasto-Crown (Nigeria) Ltd 249
Polly Pen & Ink Company (Nigeria) Ltd 251
Poly Products (Nigeria) Ltd 251
Polythene Enterprises (Nigeria) Ltd 251
Pukke, Horst, & Co (Nigeria) Ltd 255
Record Manufacturers of Nigeria Ltd 259
Record Market (Nigeria) Ltd 259
Rehau Plastiks (Nigeria) Ltd 260
Rida National Plastics Ltd 262
Rosaab Industrial Design Ltd 264
Runsewe Group of Companies 265
Scoa Nigeria Ltd 270
Segun International Group Ltd 272

South Pacific Chemical & Plastics
Engineering Company Ltd | 279
State Plastics Design Company | 281
Subetra Nigeria Industries Ltd | 283
Swiss Nigerian Chemical Company Ltd | 285
Syndivel Plastic Industry Nigeria Ltd | 285
Take Your Choice Record Stores Ltd | 286
Tate & Lyle (Nigeria) Ltd | 286
United Consolidated Industries Ltd | 305
United Development Trading Company
Ltd | 305
Universal Monolithic Bearing Structure
Ltd | 308
Vinben (Nigeria) Ltd | 313
VK Plastiks & Marble Co | 314
Warmac Products Ltd | 315
Wilmer Industries Nigeria Ltd | 322
Zenith Containers Company Ltd | 324

Power equipment

Adebowale Electrical Industries Ltd | 6
Advance (Nig) Ltd | 8
Aeronutronic Ford Overseas Systems | 9
Afro Elektro Konsult Ltd | 13
Afrotec Technical Services Nigeria Ltd | 14
B B C Brown Boveri (Nigeria) Ltd | 34
Benora Instruments & Company | 39
Black & Decker Nigeria Ltd | 44
Blackwood Hodge (Nigeria) Ltd | 44
Boulos Enterprises Ltd | 47
Camplant Engineering Sales & Service
Ltd | 52
Conveyancer (Nigeria) Ltd | 67
Daddo International (Nigeria) Ltd | 72
Electro Technologies Nigeria Ltd
(ELTEC) | 89
General Electric USA of Nigeria Ltd | 108
Gilco Nigeria Ltd | 110
Hilson Nigeria Ltd | 122
International Contracts & Consultancy
Services Ltd | 132
ITT Nigeria Ltd | 136
Kabelmetal Nigeria Ltd | 141
Landmark Industrial Supplies Ltd | 152
Lonogu Enterprises Ltd | 157
Maclisle Complex Ltd | 159
Matzen & Timm (Nigeria) Ltd | 166
Mesacom Electronics Instrumentations
Ltd | 168
Motorola | 177
Mouldex Ltd | 177
Namco Nigeria Ltd | 179
National Electric Power Authority
(NEPA) | 181
Newmark Electric Co Ltd | 190
Nigerchin Electrical Development
Company Ltd | 193
Nigeria General Motors Ltd | 195
Nigerian & Overseas Products Ltd | 198
Nigerlink Industries Ltd | 220
Nirotec (A Division of Nigerian Ropes
Ltd) | 221
Nordmann, Rassmann & Company
(Nigeria) Ltd | 222
Northern Cable Processing and
Manufacturing Company Ltd | 224
Obatraco Group of Companies | 227
Odeco Ltd | 228
Ohakwe & Associates (Nigeria) Ltd | 230
Omenjor & Ramsauer Electrical
Company | 233
Phoenix Motors Ltd | 247
Power & Communication Engineering
Nigeria Ltd | 251
Pump Services Nigeria Ltd | 255
Roaag Company (Nigeria) Ltd | 263
Safni Ltd | 266
Scoa Nigeria Ltd | 270
Scoatrac (A Division of Scoa (Nigeria)
Ltd) | 270
Sodik-Asea (Nigeria) Ltd | 277
Sointeco (Nigeria) Ltd | 277
Songhai Group of Companies | 278
Stag Engineering Nigeria Ltd | 280
Stephens, Henry, Engineering
Company Ltd | 281
Stokvis (Nigeria) Ltd | 282
Tarpaulin Industries (WA) Ltd | 286

Thoresen & Company (Nigeria) Ltd | 290
Tractor & Equipment | 292
Uren Construction Engineering
Company Ltd | 310
UTC Nigeria Ltd (Formerly Union
Trading Company of Nigeria Ltd) | 311
West African Automobile &
Engineering Company Ltd
(WAATECO) | 317
West African Engineering Company
Nigeria Ltd (WAECO) | 318
Wiedemann & Walters (Nigeria) Ltd | 321
Woermann, C, (Nigeria) Ltd | 322
Yodesons (Nigeria) Ltd | 323
Zartech Ltd | 324

Precision engineering

Damen Shipyards Nigeria Ltd | 74
Leman Industries (Kaduna) Ltd | 154
Lonogu Enterprises Ltd | 157
Motorways Nigeria Ltd | 177
Rosaab Industrial Design Ltd | 264
Stag Engineering Nigeria Ltd | 280
Steiner, F, & Company Ltd | 281

Printing

Afprint Nigeria Ltd | 9
Algadama (Holdings) Ltd | 19
Alpha Industries (Nigeria) Ltd | 21
Atoki, Fred, Publishing Company Ltd | 32
Baraka Press & Publishers Ltd | 36
Boladele Brothers & Co Ltd | 45
Caxton Press (West Africa) Ltd | 54
CEC & Co (Nigeria) Ltd | 54
Coates Brothers (WA) Ltd | 63
Colodense Nigeria Ltd | 63
Continuous Printing Industry (Nigeria)
Ltd | 66
Copiers (Nigeria) Ltd | 68
CPI-Moore (Nigeria) Ltd | 69
CSS Bookshops | 71
CSS Press (Nigeria) Ltd | 71
Doal Enterprises Ltd | 80
Fisayo Holdings Ltd | 100
Gaskiya Corporation Ltd | 106
Goodwill Press & Bookshop | 113
Hamzer, G N A, & Co (Nigeria) Ltd | 119
Imo Newspapers Ltd | 129
International Contact Centre | 132
Itidal-Epid Enterprises of Nigeria | 136
J & H International Agency | 137
Kaeler (West Africa) Ltd | 142
Kingston Ltd | 147
Krabo Nigeria Ltd | 149
Kucena-Damian (Nigeria) Ltd | 149
Light Industries (Nigeria) Ltd | 155
Mai-Nasara & Sons Ltd | 160
Modelor Design Aids Ltd | 174
Monotype Nigeria Ltd | 175
National Cash Register (WA) Ltd | 181
NCR | 181
New Nigerian Newspapers Ltd | 189
Nigerian Commercial Press | 202
Nigerian Match & Chemical Industries
Ltd | 210
Nigerian Paper Converters Company | 213
Nigerian Printing & Publishing
Company Ltd | 215
Nigerian Railway Press | 215
Nigerian Security Printing and Minting
Company Ltd | 216
Ochumba Press Ltd | 228
OGT Group of Companies Ltd | 229
Ogubule Industrial Printers Ltd | 230
Okwesa, John, Ltd | 231
Onibonoje Press & Book Industries
(Nig) Ltd | 234
Oshinmi Company Ltd | 236
Oshunkeye Brothers (Nigeria) Ltd | 237
Ott-Attafua, A, & Company Ltd | 237
Pacific Printers Ltd | 240
Plateau Publishing Company Ltd | 250
Principal Bookshop & Commercial
Stores Ltd | 254

Punch (Nigeria) Ltd | 255
Record Manufacturers of Nigeria Ltd | 259
Ribway Group of Companies | 261
Rimax Computer Services Ltd | 262
Rivers State Newspaper Corporation | 263
Savanna Press Ltd | 268
Sera Printing Ltd | 273
Sketch Publishing Company Ltd | 275
Studio Press (Nigeria) Ltd | 283
Thoresen & Company (Nigeria) Ltd | 290
Times Press Ltd | 290
Timmy Printing Press | 290
Topaz (Nigeria) Ltd | 291
Unique Trading Co Ltd | 303
VYB (Nigeria) Ltd | 315
West, John, Publications Ltd | 319
Wiggins Teape West Africa Ltd | 321

Property and real estate

A G Leventis & Company (Nigeria) Ltd | 3
Abbas Organisation Nigeria Ltd | 4
Abebiyi Sonaike & Company | 4
Agbara Estates Ltd | 14
Akarolo Technical Company Nigeria
Ltd | 16
Akhigbe, Odibo, & Co Ltd | 16
Akpenlamen Co Ltd | 17
Ashamu, E O, & Sons (Holdings) Ltd | 29
Bolingo Organisation | 45
Deazula Trading Company (Nigeria)
Ltd | 76
Delta Property Development Co Ltd | 77
Desam Development Company Ltd | 78
Doal Enterprises Ltd | 80
Dokunmu, M A, & Sons Ltd | 80
Dubic International Ltd | 83
Ebun Oluwa Group of Companies | 85
Ferdinand Enterprises (Nigeria) Ltd | 99
Formerly John Holt Investment
Company Ltd | 138
Hamzer, G N A, & Co (Nigeria) Ltd | 119
Ibadan City Motors (Nigeria) Ltd | 126
Ibile Properties Ltd | 126
Irede Properties and Investment
Company Ltd | 135
JHI Ltd | 138
Kedam Holdings (Nigeria) Ltd | 145
Knight, Frank & Rutley (Nigeria) Ltd | 148
Las & Co Ltd | 153
Macgregor & Ojutalayo | 159
Mosheshe Group of Companies | 176
Nabena, Benjamin, Nabenson
Promotions | 178
Nabena, L R, & Sons Ltd | 179
Nasco Estate Company (Nigeria) Ltd | 180
Ndah, G, & Sons Foundation | 185
Nigercare International Company
(Nigeria) Ltd | 193
Pedro Lee Associates (Nigeria) Ltd | 244
Pillars Nigeria Ltd | 248
REA Real Property Investments
(Nigeria) Ltd | 259
Stephens, Henry, Group of Companies | 281
Tilley Gyado Group of Companies | 290
UAC of Nigeria Ltd | 297
Uba, C, & Brothers Trading Company
(WA) Ltd | 297
Ugochukwu and Sons Ltd | 299
United Development Trading Company
Ltd | 305
Wemabod Estates Ltd | 317
Woclif (Nigeria) Ventures | 322

**Publishing, broadcasting, films
and advertising**

Academy Press Ltd | 5
Admark (Nigeria) Ltd | 8
African Designs Development Centre
Ltd | 11
African Newspapers of Nigeria Ltd | 11
African Universities Press | 13
Afroguard Publications | 14
Algadama (Holdings) Ltd | 19

Algadama Nigeria Film Distributors Ltd 19
Aromolaran Publishers Nigeria Ltd 28
Atoki, Fred, Publishing Company Ltd 32
Baraka Press & Publishers Ltd 36
Bendel Newspapers Corporation 39
CEC & Co (Nigeria) Ltd 54
Challenge Bookshops 56
Cross River State Newspaper
  Corporation 71
CSS Bookshops 71
Decca (West Africa) Ltd 76
ECWA Productions Ltd 85
Ethiope Publishing Corporation 94
Evans Brothers (Nigeria) Ltd 95
Fagbamigbe, Olaiya, Ltd 96
Federal Radio Corporation of Nigeria 98
  (FRCN) 98
Gaskiya Corporation Ltd 106
Grant Advertising International
  (Nigeria) Ltd 113
Hamzer, G N A, & Co (Nigeria) Ltd 119
Heinemann Educational Books
  (Nigeria) Ltd 121
I I Commercial Services (IICS) 125
Imo Newspapers Ltd 129
Intermark Associates Ltd 131
International Contact Centre 132
Lanlek (Nigeria) Associates 152
Longman Nigeria Ltd 157
Macmillan Nigeria Publishers Ltd 159
Nelson, Thomas (Nigeria) Ltd 185
New Agency of Nigeria 188
New Breed Organisation Ltd 188
New Nigeria Press 189
New Nigerian Newspapers Ltd 189
Nigeria Publishers Services Ltd 197
Nigerian Book Suppliers Ltd 200
Nigerian Institute of Management 209
Nigerian Mapping Company Ltd 210
Nigerian Paper Converters Company 213
Nigerian Printing & Publishing
  Company Ltd 215
Nigerian Television Authority 218
Northern Nigeria Publishing Company
  Ltd (NNPC) 225
OGT Group of Companies Ltd 229
Olu Holloway Nigeria Ltd 232
Onibonoje Press & Book Industries
  (Nig) Ltd 234
Pearl & Dean (Nigeria) Ltd 244
Pilgrim Books Ltd 248
  (Pilgrim Books Ltd) 13
Plateau Publishing Company Ltd 250
Principal Bookshop & Commercial
  Stores Ltd 254
Punch (Nigeria) Ltd 255
Rimax Computer Services Ltd 262
Rivers State Newspaper Corporation 263
Rod Publicity Ltd 264
Scobi Associates 271
Sketch Publishing Company Ltd 275
Universal Educational Supplies Ltd
  (Morison Arnold Ltd) 308
University of Ife Press Ltd 309
University Press Ltd 310
West, John, Publications Ltd 319

Rubber and rubber goods

Afro Nigerian Import & Export Co Ltd 14
Boladele Brothers & Co Ltd 45
Cross River Estate Ltd 70
Czechs (Nigeria) Ltd 72
Daddo International (Nigeria) Ltd 72
Dunlop Nigerian Industries Ltd 83
Edokpolo, John, & Co Ltd 86
Goodyear Midwest Rubber Processing
  Co (Nigeria) Ltd 113
Jafco Impex Ltd 137
Juli Importers & Exporters Enterprises 140
Lanre Bhadmus Industries Ltd 152
Lewis & Peat (NRI) Ltd 155
Mais Tyres Service (City Retreading
  Service) 160
Michelin (Nigeria) Ltd 171
Mouldex Ltd 177
New African Industries Ltd 188
New Independent Rubber Company
  Ltd 188

Nigeria Marine & Trading Company
  Ltd 196
Nigerian Explosives & Plastics Co Ltd 205
Nigerian Industrial Auxiliaries Ltd 208
Nigerian Rubber Board 216
Oban (Nigeria) Rubber Estates Ltd 227
Odutola Nigerian Industries Ltd 229
Oshinmi Company Ltd 236
Pamol (Nigeria) Ltd 240
Petro-Organico (Nigeria) Ltd 245
Phoebus Economides Rubber Industry
  Ltd 247
Pioneer Chemical Manufacturing
  Company (Nigeria) Ltd 248
Ribway Group of Companies 261
Ribway Tyre Retreading Co Ltd 261
Sakpoba Rubber Estate 266
Spiropoulos, F G, & Company Ltd 279
Thomas, J A, Rubber Estates Ltd 289
Universal Vulcanizing Company Nigeria
  Ltd 309
Utagba-Uno Rubber Estates Ltd 310
Vitafoam Nigeria Ltd 313
West African Tyre Retreading
  Company Ltd 319
Zard, C, & Company Ltd 324

Safety and security equipment

Allied Bendix Ltd 20
Amass Nigeria Ltd 23
Banjoko Firesafety Ltd 35
Delta Pioneer Company Ltd 77
Don International Ltd 80
Fire Protection Services Ltd 100
George Hunters & Company Ltd 109
Gobecco Trading Company Ltd 111
Goodwill, Francis, Ltd 112
Guthrie (Nigeria) Ltd 115
Hitech (Nigeria) Ltd 122
Industrial & Safety Equipment (Nigeria)
  Ltd 129
Krabo Nigeria Ltd 149
Matson & Company (Nigeria) Ltd 166
Minnesota Nigeria Ltd 172
Nigerguards Ltd 193
Nigerian Explosives & Plastics Co Ltd 205
Nigerian General Security & Safety
  Company Ltd 207
Nigerian Investigation and Safety
  Company Ltd 209
Omot Fire Protection Engineering Ltd 234
Oscarte (Nigeria) Ltd 236
Preussag Drilling Engineers Nigeria
  Ltd 253
Reliance International (Nigeria) Ltd 260
Roaag Company (Nigeria) Ltd 263
Runsewe Group of Companies 265
Scan African Nigeria Ltd 269
Sentrycom Alarms (Nigeria) Ltd 273
Shekoni Industries Nigeria Ltd 274
Stronghold (Nigeria) Ltd 282
Tasius Nigeria Ltd 286
Teddy Continental Company 288
Triplex Safety Glass (Nigeria) Ltd 295
Vanni Holdings Ltd 312
Waterglass Boatyard & Steel
  Construction Ltd 316

Scientific instruments

Associated Electronic Products
  (Nigeria) Ltd 31
Associated Laboratory Supplies Ltd 31
Atlas Nigeria Ltd 32
Bhandari & Company (Nigeria) Ltd 42
Biomedical Services Company Ltd 43
Bolingo Organisation 45
CEP 55
Chemdyes Nigeria Ltd 58
Christela Chemical Works Ltd 59
Drug Specialities (Nigeria) Ltd 82
Edmund & Edmund (Nigeria) Ltd 86
Electronics Instrumentations Ltd 90
Eximport & Company Nigeria Ltd 95

Fanz Holdings Ltd 96
Fisco-Chemicals (Nigeria) Ltd 100
(Formerly Philips (Nig) Ltd) 31
Global Pharmaceutical and Chemical
  Agencies Ltd 111
Hilson Nigeria Ltd 122
Joart United Construction &
  Engineering Ltd 138
Labstock (Nigeria) Ltd 150
Leo's Group of Companies Ltd 154
Link Group International Ltd 156
Major & Company (Nigeria) Ltd 160
Mareen Industries Ltd 163
Micheljohnson Ltd 171
Naafco (Scientific Supplies) Ltd 178
Nigerian Medical Supplies Ltd 210
Nucleus Electronics Ltd 226
Orthopaedic Supplies Ltd 236
Ositadinma International Ltd 237
Pabod Supplies Ltd 240
Prime Feathers International Services
  Ltd 254
Unigwe, Fred Balonwu, Group of
  Companies 302
Urobo Agencies (Nigeria) Ltd 310
UTC Nigeria Ltd (Formerly Union
  Trading Company of Nigeria Ltd) 311

Shipping, shipbuilding and shipping services

Aeromaritime (Nigeria) Ltd 9
Akwiwu Motors Ltd 17
Alhassan Dantata & Sons Ltd 19
Allen, J, Co Ltd 20
Alraine (Nigeria) Ltd 21
Amalighterage & Timber Exporting Co
  Ltd 22
Amatemeso Shipping Agencies Ltd 23
Anglo-Norman Shipping (Nigeria) Ltd 25
Anopit Ltd 25
ANSIL 25
Ashamu, E O, & Sons (Holdings) Ltd 29
Asian African Container (Nigeria) Ltd 30
Aurora Produce & Shipping Co Ltd 33
Ben Agency Service 38
Caleb Brett & Son (Nigeria) Ltd 52
Central Water Transportation
  Company Ltd 55
Cepuz International Agencies 55
Charlie and Franco Ltd 57
Coastal Services (Nigeria) Ltd 63
Combined Maritime Agencies (Nigeria)
  Ltd 64
Continental Lines (Africa) Ltd 66
Damen Shipyards Nigeria Ltd 74
Danwawu Shipping Cargo Handling &
  Transport Co Ltd 74
Delta Boatyard Ltd 76
Desam Development Company Ltd 78
Eastern (Overseas) Agencies Ltd 85
Elder Dempster Agencies (Nigeria) Ltd 89
Equatorial Lines 92
Express International Maritime Ltd 95
Falcon Nigeria Ltd 96
Farrell Lines International (Nigeria) Ltd 97
Formerly Mitsui & Co (Nigeria) Ltd 166
Gaby and Company (Nigeria) 106
Goas Agencies Ltd 111
Hamzer, G N A, & Co (Nigeria) Ltd 119
Harrison, Peter, Nigeria Ltd 120
Hoegh Line (Nigeria) Ltd 122
Holt, John, Ltd 123
Ijomah International Co Ltd 128
Inland Containers (Nigeria) Ltd 130
Intercare Ltd 131
JOKI (Nigeria) Ltd 140
Kennedy Transport (Nigeria) Ltd 145
Kusba Shipping Agencies Ltd 150
Laas Ltd 150
Lagos & Niger Shipping Agencies Ltd 151
Lewis & Peat (NRI) Ltd 155
Maiden Maritime (Nigeria) Ltd 160
MBK Nigeria Ltd 166
Modearo (Nigeria) Ltd 173
Mosheshe Group of Companies 176
Napak Services (Nigeria) Ltd 179
Nedlloyd Lines 185
Neptune Transport Services Ltd 186

New Nigeria Merchants Ltd 189
Niger Delta Shipping Agencies Ltd 192
Niger River Transport Ltd 192
Nigeria Green Lines Ltd 195
Nigerian Maritime Services Ltd 210
Nigerian National Shipping Line Ltd 211
Nigerian Ports Authority (NPA) 214
Nigerian Shipbuilders Ltd 216
Ocean Inchcape (Nigeria) Ltd 227
Oceanic & Coastal Marine Ltd 228
Oceannering (Nigeria) Ltd 228
Odus Globe & Company Ltd 229
Ogheneovo Ventures Ltd 229
OGT Group of Companies Ltd 229
Ojuri Maritime Services 231
Oldmac Shipping Lines Nigeria Ltd 232
Olumo Dunwo Commercial Enterprises
Ltd 232
OSA Marine Services (Nigeria) Ltd 236
Osena Shipping Company Ltd 236
Palm Line Agencies (Nigeria) 240
Pan Atlantic Shipping & Transport
Agencies Ltd 242
Panalpina World Transport (Nigeria)
Ltd 242
Par Excellence (Nigeria) Ltd 243
Paty Import Company of Nigeria 243
Port & Marine Services Ltd 251
Port Express Services Ltd 251
Roro Terminal Company (Nigeria) Ltd 264
Sea Dantainer Lines Ltd 271
Segun International Group Ltd 272
Sobat Ltd 276
Stephens, Henry, Group of Companies 281
Tidex Nigeria Ltd 290
Tradon Nigeria Ltd 292
Trans Atlantic Shipping Agency Ltd 292
Transcap Ltd 293
Transmarco Agencies (Nigeria) Ltd 293
Triana Ltd 294
Trianon Shipping & Chartering Ltd 294
Tuntaric Nigeria Ltd 295
Uche, A O, & Sons (Nigeria) Ltd 299
Umarco (Nigeria) Ltd 301
Waterglass Boatyard & Steel
Construction Ltd 316
West African Shipping Agency
(Nigeria) Ltd 319
Westminster Dredging (Nigeria) Ltd 320
Wimpey-Brown & Root (Nigeria) Ltd 322
Witt & Busch (Shipyard) Ltd 322
Zapata Marine Service (Nigeria) Ltd 324

Telecommunications

Aeronutronic Ford Overseas Systems 9
Afro Elektro Konsult Ltd 13
Allied Electronics &
Telecommunications Services Ltd 20
Allscope Communications (Nigeria) Ltd 21
Aronaout Communications Ltd 28
Associated Electronic Products
(Nigeria) Ltd 31
B B C Brown Boveri (Nigeria) Ltd 34
Briscoe, R T, (Nigeria) Ltd 49
City Group Organization 62
Communications Associates of Nigeria
Ltd 64
COMSAC 64
Dizengoff West Africa (Nigeria) Ltd 79
Electro Technologies Nigeria Ltd
(ELTEC) 89
Electronics Instrumentations Ltd 90
(Formerly Philips (Nig) Ltd) 31
GEC (Telecommunications) Nigeria Ltd 107
General Electric USA of Nigeria Ltd 108
Gilco Nigeria Ltd 110
GTE Nigeria Ltd 114
Hansen, Jos & Soehne (Nigeria) Ltd 120
Harris International
Telecommunications 120
ITT Nigeria Ltd 136
Kabelmetal Nigeria Ltd 141
Littleways International Ltd 157
Maiden Electronics Works Ltd 159
Mattem (Nigeria) Enterprises 166
Mesacom Electronics Instrumentations
Ltd 168
Motorola 177

Netarcomms Nigeria Ltd 186
Newmark Electric Co Ltd 190
Newmark Electric Company Ltd 190
Nigerian External Telecommunications
Ltd 205
Nigerian Far East Company Ltd
(NIFECO) 205
Northern Cable Processing and
Manufacturing Company Ltd 224
Nucleus Electronics Ltd 226
Plesscomms Nigeria Ltd (Formerly
Plessey (Nigeria) Ltd) 250
Power & Communication Engineering
Nigeria Ltd 251
Radio Communications (Nigeria) Ltd 256
Samsung (Nigeria) Ltd 267
Senn-Sound (West Africa) Ltd 272
Sunshine Batteries Manufacturing
Company 284
Westend Engineering Ltd 320
Yodesons (Nigeria) Ltd 323

Textiles and clothing; textile equipment

ABA Textiles Mills Ltd 3
Afprint Nigeria Ltd 9
Akande Trading Co Nigeria Ltd 16
Aladaire Export Ltd 18
Amarillo Umbrella Company (Nigeria)
Ltd 23
Arcee Textile Industries Ltd 26
Arewa Textiles Ltd 28
Associated Textile Manufacturers Co
Ltd 32
Aswani Textile Industries Ltd 32
Atlantic Textile Manufacturing Co Ltd 32
Bagauda Textile Mill Ltd 34
Bayajida Group of Companies 37
Bhojsons & Company (Nigeria) Ltd 42
Bhojsons Industries Ltd 42
Bidat Sportswear Company Ltd 42
Bolingo Organisation 45
CFAO (Nigeria) Ltd 56
CFC Furniture Co (WC) Ltd 56
Chellaram, K, & Sons (Nigeria) Ltd 57
Cinsere Sewing Machine Industrial
Company Ltd 61
Continental Medical Complex Ltd 66
Coutinho, Caro & Co (Nigeria) Ltd 69
Cunix Industrial & Commercial Co Ltd 71
Dalamal Textile Mills Ltd 73
Doyin Investments Nigeria Ltd 81
Edo Textile Mills Ltd 86
Edrita & Company Ltd 86
Edun Commercial Agency 86
Enpee Industries Ltd 92
Excelsior Garment Factory Ltd 95
Fedco Foam (Nigeria) Ltd 98
Five Star Industries Ltd 101
Furniture House Ltd 105
Gaby and Company (Nigeria) 106
GDM Textiles Manufacturing Ltd 107
Gold Star Industries Ltd 112
Haffar Industrial Co Ltd 117
Hamzer, G N A, & Co (Nigeria) Ltd 119
Ikorodu Trading Company Ltd 128
Indian Bazaar (Nigeria) Ltd 129
Jaybee Industries (Nigeria) Ltd 138
Kaduna Textiles Ltd 142
Kailash Weaving & Garment
Manufacturing Co (Nigeria) Ltd 143
Kano Citizens Trading Company Ltd 143
Kano Dyeing and Printing Co Ltd 143
Kanotex Ltd 144
Kay Industries Nigeria Ltd 145
Kaycee (Nigeria) Ltd 145
Latderma Enterprises 153
Madras Manufacturing Co Ltd 159
Midwest Textile Mills Ltd 172
Millet Nigeria Ltd 172
Narumal & Sons (Nigeria) Ltd 180
NCO Merchants Brothers Company
(Newspin) Ltd 217
Nichemtex Industries Ltd 190
Nigeria Fibre Industry Company Ltd
(NIFINCO) 195
Nigeria Teijin Textiles Ltd 197
Nigerian Cotton Board 203
Nigerian Fibre Industries Company Ltd 206

Nigerian Hoechst Ltd 208
Nigerian International Exchange Ltd 209
Nigerian Spinners & Dyers Ltd 217
Nigerian Spinning and Weaving Co Ltd 217
Nigerian Suiting Manufacturing
Company Ltd 218
Nigerian Textile Mills Ltd 218
Nigerian Weaving & Processing
Company Ltd 219
Nigerian Weaving, Spinning & Printing
Company Ltd (NEWSPIN Ltd) 219
Nitol Ltd 221
Nornit Ltd 223
Norspin Ltd 223
Nortex (Nigeria) Ltd 223
Northern Nigeria Fibre Products Ltd 224
Northern Nigeria Textile Mills Ltd 225
Northern Textile Manufacturers Ltd 225
Novelty Industrial Company Ltd
(NOVIC) 226
Nubi Textile Mills (Nigeria) Ltd 226
Oluwakemi Motors & Finance
Company Ltd 233
Oluwakemi (Swiss) Nigeria Embroidery
Industries Ltd 233
Onise Polyware Ltd 235
President Clothing Co Ltd 253
Prestige Industries Ltd 253
Princegate Trading & Contracting
Company Ltd 254
Project Textile Mill (Nigeria) Ltd 255
Ribway Group of Companies 261
Ronke Commercial Enterprises 264
Salleh, Alhaji Baba M, & Sons (Nigeria)
Ltd 266
Scoa Nigeria Ltd 270
Speco Mill Textiles Ltd 279
Sunflag Knitting Mills (Nigeria) Ltd 283
Tarpaulin Industries (WA) Ltd 286
Taylorbird Fabric & Design Ltd 287
Textile Commodities Ltd 289
Textile Utilities Manufacturing Ltd 289
Tropical Tarpaulin Industry (Nigeria)
Ltd 295
UAC of Nigeria Ltd 297
Umaru, Lawan & Sons Ltd 301
United Nigerian Textiles Ltd 305
Universal Textile Industries Ltd 309
Uoo Trading Company Ltd 310
UTC Nigeria Ltd (Formerly Union
Trading Company of Nigeria Ltd) 311
Varaman Industries (Nigeria) Ltd 312
West African Thread Company Ltd 319
Western Nigeria Tarpaulin Industries
Ltd 320
Western Textile Industries Company
Ltd 320
Western Textile Mills Ltd 320
Woollen & Synthetic Textile
Manufacturing Ltd 322
Woven Textiles Ltd 323
Zamfara Textile Industries Ltd 324

Timber industries and saw mills

(A Division of UAC of Nigeria Ltd) 13
Abereoje (Nigeria) Ltd 4
Adefusika Trading Company Ltd 7
Adeome Company Ltd 8
Adeyemi Commercial Syndicate
Sawmills Ltd 8
African Industrial Timber Co Ltd 11
African Timber & Plywood 13
Algadama (Holdings) Ltd 19
All-African Woodworking Industry Ltd 20
Amalighterage & Timber Exporting Co
Ltd 22
Asaboro, Joseph 29
Calabar Veneer & Plywood Ltd 52
Coast Timber Co Ltd 63
Gaby and Company (Nigeria) 106
Holex Timber (Nigeria) Ltd 123
Idehen, J I, & Sons (Nigeria) Ltd 127
Kedam Holdings (Nigeria) Ltd 145
Kolinah Industries Nigeria Ltd 148
Midwestern Timber Manufacturers
Syndicate 172
Nabena, L R, & Sons Ltd 179
Nigerian Hardwood Company Ltd 208

Nigerian Romanian Wood Industries
  Ltd   215
Nirotec (A Division of Nigerian Ropes
  Ltd)   221
Obaskeki, G I, & Sons Ltd   227
Oladapo & Company Ltd   231
Piedmont Plywoods Nigeria Ltd   248
Sandwell, P R, & Co (Nigeria) Ltd   267
Structor   283
Sutherland, B K, & Company Ltd   285
Swiss Nigerian Wood Industries Ltd   285
Thomas Furniture Company Ltd   289
Thomas, J A, Rubber Estates Ltd   289
Tradon Nigeria Ltd   292
UAC of Nigeria Ltd   297
Wata Timber Company Ltd   316
West African Trades Corporation Ltd   319

Tobacco

International Cigarette Company Ltd   176
Intra Tobacco Manufacturing Co Ltd   135
Juli Importers & Exporters Enterprises   140
London & Kano Trading Co Ltd   157
Manufacturers Agencies   162
Morris, Philip, Nigeria Ltd   176
Nigerian Tobacco Company Ltd   219

Toiletries and cosmetics

Advance (Nig) Ltd   8
Anambra Vegetable Oils Products
  Nigeria Ltd   25
Associated Pharmaceutical Products
  Ltd   31
(AVOP)   25
Beecham Ltd   38
Bendel Chemical Industries Ltd   38
Boots Company (Nigeria) Ltd (The)   46
Bush, W J, & Company (Nigeria) Ltd   50
Chami, A B, & Co Ltd   57
Chellaram, K, & Sons (Nigeria) Ltd   57
Chesebrough Ponds Industries Ltd   59
Christlieb, A C, (Nigeria) Ltd   59
Continental Medical Complex Ltd   66
Daily Need Chemists Ltd   72
Daily Soap Ltd   73
Femina Hygienical Products (Nigeria)
  Ltd   99
Formerly Johnson & Johnson (Nigeria)
  Ltd   121
(Formerly Merck Sharp & Dohme
  (Nigeria) Ltd)   31
General Cosmetics Company Ltd   108
Haco Ltd   117
Health Care Products (Nigeria) Ltd   121
Holt, John, Ltd   123
Johnson Products of Nigeria Ltd   140
Kailash Industries (Nigeria) Ltd   143
Lafa Soap & Cosmetic Industry   151
Lanre Bhadmus Industries Ltd   152
Lever Brothers Nigeria Ltd   154
Modern Industries Ltd   174
Morison, J L, Sons & Jones (Nigeria)
  Ltd   176
Nevlon Pharmaceutical (Revlon) Ltd   187
Nicholas Laboratories Nigeria Ltd   191
Niger Sanitary Industry Ltd   192
Nigerian Chemical Services Ltd (NCS)   202
Odus Industries (Nigeria) Ltd   229
Olehson Brothers Company (Nigeria)
  Ltd   232
(Olehson's Agro Animal Kingdom)   232
Olympic Group Ltd   233
Paterson Zochonis Industries Ltd   243
Ramonu Alabi, S B, & Company   257
Richard Riko (Nigeria) Ltd   261
Rioco (Nigeria) Ltd   262
Robins, A H, International Company
  Ltd   264
Rokana Industries Ltd   264
Ronke Commercial Enterprises   264
Seward, A J, (A Division of UAC of
  Nigeria Ltd)   273
Smith Kline & French Nigeria Ltd   276

Squibb (Nigeria) Ltd   279
Sterling Products (Nigeria) Ltd   281
Telota Cosmetics Company Nigeria
  Ltd   288
United Arewa Chemists Ltd   303
United Consolidated Industries Ltd   305
Unity Soap Manufacturers Ltd   307
UTC Nigeria Ltd (Formerly Union
  Trading Company of Nigeria Ltd)   311
Village Gate & Company Ltd   313
Vitalink Pharmaceutical Industries Ltd   314
West African Drug Company Ltd   318

Transport

Aero Contractors Company of Nigeria
  Ltd   8
Aeromaritime (Nigeria) Ltd   9
Akanji Transport   16
Akwiwu Motors Ltd   17
Alraine (Nigeria) Ltd   21
Amalighterage & Timber Exporting Co
  Ltd   22
Arax Airlines Ltd   26
Bakare, S B, & Brothers Ltd   34
Bakrin Enterprises Ltd   35
Bimbotech (Nigeria) Ltd   43
Blackwood Hodge (Nigeria) Ltd   44
Bristow Helicopters (Nigeria) Ltd   49
Central Water Transportation
  Company Ltd   55
Chidiebere Transport Ltd   59
Coastal Services (Nigeria) Ltd   63
Continental Lines (Africa) Ltd   66
Conveyancer (Nigeria) Ltd   67
Cornerstone Organisation Ltd   69
Cross Lines Ltd   70
Dafinasi Enterprises Ltd   72
Deribe, Alhaji Mai, & Sons Ltd   78
Dubic International Ltd   83
Edrita & Company Ltd   86
Egbema Enterprises Ltd (EEL)   86
El-Kalil, M, Transport Ltd   90
Fallad Commercial Enterprises Ltd   96
Fas Brothers Ltd   97
Folam International Trading Company   102
Gamboru, Alhaji Madu Mala Sheriff   106
Gindiri Concrete Products Ltd   110
Hapel Nigeria Ltd   120
Haruna, Alhaji Mustapha, & Sons   121
Hassan Transport (Nigeria) Ltd   121
Ibukun Transport Ltd   126
Ijomah International Co Ltd   128
IMNL   133
Inland Containers (Nigeria) Ltd   130
International Messengers (Nigeria) Ltd   133
Jemine Enterprises Ltd   138
Kennedy Transport (Nigeria) Ltd   145
Khalil & Dibbo Transport Ltd   146
Kpohraror & Sons Group of
  Companies   149
Kunza Heed (W.A.) Enterprises   150
Lagos State Transport Corporation   152
Mala, Alhaji Zanna K, & Sons
  Company   161
Manila Construction Co (Nigeria) Ltd   162
Marghi Enterprises Ltd   163
Mashall, Alhaji Sani, Estates   165
Middleton River Brothers (Nigeria) Ltd   171
Minarfol Transport Co Ltd   172
Modearo (Nigeria) Ltd   173
Moore Obioha, C, Sons & Company
  Ltd   176
Musa, Alhaji Sani, & Sons   178
National Freight Company   181
Nedlloyd Lines   185
New Nigeria Merchants Ltd   189
Nigeria Airways Ltd   193
Nigerian & Overseas Products Ltd   198
Nigerian Railway Corporation   215
Nigerian Removal & Storage Co Ltd
  (NIRSCO)   215
Nobgroup of Companies   222
North East Line Corporation   223
Northern Transporters and Merchants
  Syndicate Ltd   225
Nweke, J E, & Sons Ltd   226
Odus Globe & Company Ltd   229
Ogheneovo Ventures Ltd   229

Ohanenye & Sons Ltd   230
Ojuri Maritime Services   231
Omole, Lawrence, & Sons Ltd   233
Onuselogu, C N, Enterprises Ltd   235
Orumokpo & Sons (Nigeria) Ltd   236
Paas Industries (Nigeria) Company Ltd   240
Pan African Airlines (Nigeria) Ltd   241
Pan Atlantic Shipping & Transport
  Agencies Ltd   242
Panalpina World Transport (Nigeria)
  Ltd   242
Pem Ltd   244
Port & Marine Services Ltd   251
Primus (Nigeria) Ltd   254
Rapid Electrical & Mechanical
  Company Nigeria Ltd (REMCO)   257
Rivers State Transport Corporation   263
Salleh, Alhaji Baba M, & Sons (Nigeria)
  Ltd   266
SB Shipping & Trading Agencies Ltd   269
Segun International Group Ltd   272
Shour Industrial Enterprises Ltd   274
Songhai Group of Companies   278
Stephens, Henry, Group of Companies   281
Superform Africa Company Ltd   285
Tabansi Motors Ltd   286
Tenimasunwon Agency   288
Tetengi, Alhaji Usman, & Sons Ltd   288
Tidex Nigeria Ltd   290
Trans Nigeria Road Haulage Ltd   293
Transmarco Agencies (Nigeria) Ltd   293
Triana Ltd   294
Uba, C, & Brothers Trading Company
  (WA) Ltd   297
Umaru, Lawan & Sons Ltd   301
Uwai and Sons Enterprises   311
West Africa Offshore Ltd   317
Whyte, W W, & Co Ltd   321
World Courier Nigeria Ltd   323
Yerima Hamman Wabi, Alhaji, & Sons   323

Travel and tourism

Adamu Management International   6
Airegin Enterprises & Agencies Ltd   15
Alex Travel Agency Ltd   18
Bakrin Enterprises Ltd   35
Daboul Travel Office   72
Habis Travels Ltd   117
Hamzer, G N A, & Co (Nigeria) Ltd   119
I I Commercial Services (IICS)   125
J & H International Agency   137
Kennedy Transport (Nigeria) Ltd   145
Mandilas Ltd   162
Maurice Project Centre Ltd   166
Nigeria Airways Ltd   193
Nigerian Maritime Services Ltd   210
Plateau Tourism, Development &
  Transport Co Ltd   250
Rivers State Tourist & Hotel
  Corporation   263
Scantravel Ltd   269
Segun International Group Ltd   272
Stephens, Henry, Group of Companies   281
Times Leisure Services Ltd   290
Transcap Ltd   293
UAC of Nigeria Ltd   297
Vanni Holdings Ltd   312
West African Shipping Agency
  (Nigeria) Ltd   319

Utilities and public services

Balakhany (Nigeria) Ltd   35
Bendel Line   38
Carl-Ploetner (Nigeria) Ltd   54
Cross Lines Ltd   70
Della Group Ltd   76
Hansen, Jos & Soehne (Nigeria) Ltd   120
Ibru Organisation (Ibru Ltd)   126
Lagos State Transport Corporation   152
Nigerian Electricity Supply Corporation
  (Nigeria) Ltd   204
Nigerian Railway Corporation   215
North East Line Corporation   223

Plateau Tourism, Development &
   Transport Co Ltd   250
Rivers State Transport Corporation   263

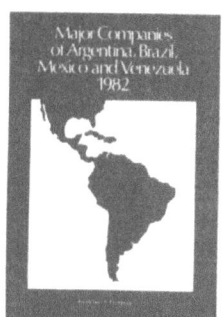 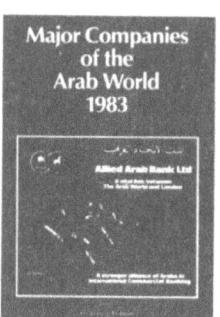 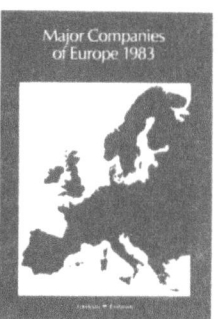 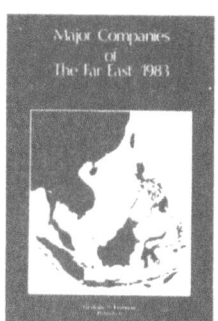 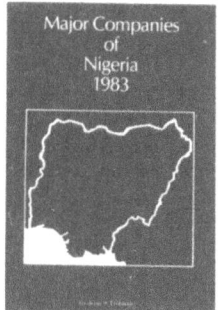

Advertisers' Index

The Ace Builders & Building Material
Stockists   5
Aeromaritime (Nigeria) Ltd   10
African Insurance Company Ltd   12
Akpenlamen Company Ltd   17
Alraine (Nigeria) Ltd   22
Amass Nigeria Ltd   23
BERG Engineering   40
Berif International Company   41
Boma Associates (WA) Ltd   45
Bordpak Premier Packaging   48
A C Christlieb (Nigeria) Ltd   60
Co-Operative & Commerce Bank
(Nigeria) Ltd   68
CPI-Moore (Nigeria) Ltd   70
Danlon Associates   75
DHL International Ltd   viii
Drug Specialities (Nigeria) Ltd   82
Edok-Eter Mandilas   88
Etco (Nigeria) Ltd   94
Flour Mills of Nigeria Ltd   104
GEC (Telecommunications) Nigeria Ltd   107
George Cohen (Nigeria) Ltd   109
GTE Nigeria Ltd   116
Guinea Insurance Co Ltd   118
Ijomah International Co Ltd   128
International Planning & Environment
Consultants (Nigeria) Ltd (INPLECON)   134
O.K. Isokariara & Sons (Nigeria) Ltd   136
Jeco Shipping   i
Kabelmetal Nigeria Ltd   141
Kaduna Co-Operative Bank Ltd   143
Leadway Assurance Co Ltd   153
Manilla Insurance Company Ltd   163
Marine & General Assurance Co Ltd   164
Metals & Minerals (Nigeria) Ltd   170
MISR (Nigeria) Ltd   173
Modearo Nigeria Ltd   174

Nasreddin Group International   182
National Bank of Nigeria Ltd   IFC
National Insurance Corporation   184
Neital Nigeria Ltd   186
Neptune Transport Services Ltd   187
Netarcomms Nigeria Ltd   187
Nigerguards Ltd   194
Nigeria Reinsurance Corporation   198
Nigerian Far East Company Ltd   ii
Nigerian Foundries Ltd   206
Nigerian Gas Industries   207
Overseas Technical Service   238
Panalpina World Transport Nigeria Ltd   vii
Pegasus Industries (Nigeria) Ltd   246
Port Express Services Ltd   252
R & A Services   258
Record Manufacturers of Nigeria Ltd   260
P R Sandwell & Company (Nigeria) Ltd   268
Siram Industrial Products Ltd   275
Sobat Ltd   276
Sun Insurance Office (Nigeria) Ltd   284
Transmarco Agencies (Nigeria) Ltd   294
Triana Ltd   296
Triplex Safety Glass   300
Turners Building Products (EMENE) Ltd   298
Union Bank of Nigeria Ltd   304
Unipetrol Nigeria Ltd   306
The United Nigeria Insurance Co Ltd   307
The Universal Insurance Co Ltd   309

Printed in Great Britain by
Page Bros (Norwich) Ltd

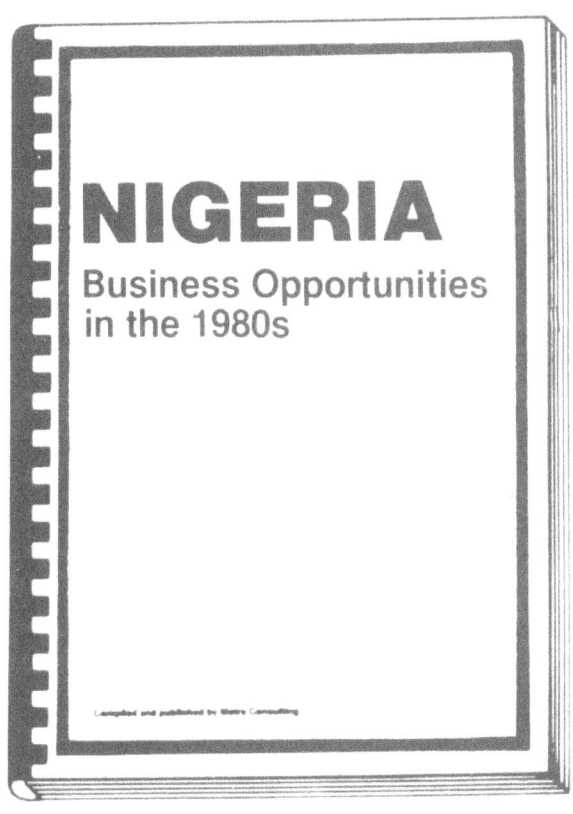